LITTLE AND FALACE'S

DENTAL MANAGEMENT *of the* Medically Compromised Patient

LITTLE AND FALACE'S

DENTAL MANAGEMENT *of the* Medically Compromised Patient

Eighth Edition

James W. Little, DMD, MS
Professor Emeritus
University of Minnesota
School of Dentistry
Minneapolis, Minnesota; Naples, Florida

Donald A. Falace, DMD, FDS RCSEd
Professor Emeritus
Oral Diagnosis and Oral Medicine
University of Kentucky College of Dentistry
Lexington, Kentucky

Craig S. Miller, DMD, MS
Professor of Oral Diagnosis and Oral Medicine
Provost Distinguished Service Professor
Department of Oral Health Practice
Department of Microbiology, Immunology and Genetics
The University of Kentucky College of Dentistry and College of Medicine
Lexington, Kentucky

Nelson L. Rhodus, DMD, MPH
Morse Distinguished Professor and Director
Division of Oral Medicine, Oral Diagnosis and Oral Radiology
University of Minnesota
School of Dentistry and College of Medicine
Minneapolis, Minnesota

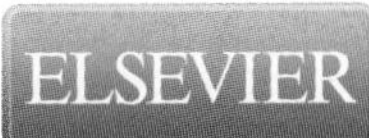

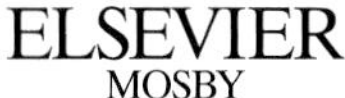

3251 Riverport Lane
St. Louis, Missouri 63043

Dental Management of the Medically Compromised Patient ISBN: 978-0-323-08028-6

Library of Congress Cataloging-in-Publication Data
Dental management of the medically compromised patient / James W. Little ... [et al.]. – 8th ed.
p. ; cm.
Includes bibliographical references and index.
ISBN 978-0-323-08028-6 (pbk. : alk. paper)
I. Little, James W., 1934-
[DNLM: 1. Dental Care. 2. Dental Care for Chronically Ill. 3. Oral Manifestations. WU 29]
617.6–dc23
2011052299

Vice President and Content Strategy Director: Linda Duncan
Executive Content Strategist: John Dolan
Senior Content Development Specialist: Courtney Sprehe
Publishing Services Manager: Catherine Jackson
Project Manager: Sara Alsup
Design Direction: Teresa McBryan
Cover Designer: Maggie Reid
Text Designer: Maggie Reid

Printed in China

Last digit is the print number: 9 8 7 6 5 4 3 2 1

We would like to dedicate this eighth edition to The American Academy of Oral Medicine that was founded by Dr. Samuel Charles Miller. The Academy's membership has dedicated their time and expertise to students, dentists, and patients in need. Working alongside dedicated professionals in our Academy to excel and improve the quality of life of our patients has motivated us with each new edition of our textbook. It has been our pleasure and privilege to observe and contribute to The American Academy of Oral Medicine's growth.

James W. Little
Donald A. Falace
Craig S. Miller
Nelson L. Rhodus

It is now 4 years since the seventh edition of *Dental Management of the Medically Compromised Patient* was published. The number of patients in this critically complex area of healthcare delivery continues to expand along with the scientific advances in etiology, pathophysiology, diagnosis, and treatment. The number of Americans over age 65, which now exceeds 15% of the population, is expected to increase by more than 20% within the next few decades. Thus the pool for such patients seeking and needing dental care grows. Furthermore, as longevity increases, so do the number of diseases and conditions that disable individuals, converting them to compromised patients.

With increasing longevity, and other factors such as obesity, poor diets, suboptimal exercise, new infections, as well as widespread use and abuse of drugs, the rising number of medically compromised patients will continue to grow. As a consequence, an ever increasing number of individuals with oral health problems will create demands and responsibilities on dental professionals with regards to services and standards of care. Education and readily available resource materials are essential to providing these services in an optimal and safe manner, and the thoroughly revised and updated eighth edition fills this role perfectly.

A multitude of diseases have an impact on oral healthcare services. Some examples follow. Cancer is an age-related disease that afflicts more than 1.5 million new patients each year in the United States. This in turn accounts for almost 25% of all deaths, and overall, is the second leading cause of death; in those under 85 years of age, cancer is the leading cause of death. Because of the number of new malignancies and the complications caused by aggressive therapy to increase survival rates, dental services and information—for example, oral complications of cancer treatments and rehabilitation—take on significant importance. Furthermore, this is a global problem with new cases of cancer exceeding 12 million each year.

Other examples of conditions that commonly affect dental-oral care are cardiovascular diseases, the number one killer of Americans, and diabetes. In Part 2, six chapters thoroughly cover all aspects of cardiovascular disease of interest for dental professionals. Diabetes (see Part 6, Chapter 14) is an exploding global problem with a profound effect on Americans, affecting more than 25 million with diagnosed diabetes, and an additional 12 million with undiagnosed diabetes. Diabetes has a large impact on dental health and care. It is the leading cause of end-stage renal disease and blindness among adults, and a major cause of heart disease and stroke. Diabetes is associated with obesity, poor diet, suboptimal physical activity, and aging. Projections estimate a possible doubling, or even tripling, in the coming decades if current trends continue. The list of medical diseases goes on, and underscores the need for current, reliable, and practical information to minimize or prevent potential problems related to general health, and ongoing oral-dental care. Knowledge of the pathophysiology of common medical diseases and conditions, along with the potential risks associated with some dental procedures and services, is essential.

Interrelationships between oral and general health involve most organ systems. Some examples of medical-dental interaction relate to hematologic, autoimmune, and infectious diseases that strike both the young and the elderly. These conditions include blood dyscrasias, vesiculobullous inflammatory diseases, and many bacterial, viral, and fungal infections. Thus a very common issue is the proper recognition and management of oral manifestations, control of blood-borne pathogens, and avoidance of complications when providing dental treatment. Again, to appropriately meet this challenge, updated information in a concise and understandable format is essential.

Because the majority of medically compromised patients need and/or seek oral healthcare, a working knowledge of the multitude of medically complex conditions is critical for dental professionals. This information will support and enable high standards for dental-oral healthcare delivery. This knowledge includes an understanding of medical conditions and compromised states and is necessary to help prevent, minimize, and alert clinicians to possible adverse side effects potentially associated with procedures and drugs used in dentistry. An understanding will assist in formulating treatment plans that are safe and compatible with a patient's medical status.

Care of the medically compromised patient often is complicated, and requires specialists. However, occurrence of compromised patients is so common that practitioners and students must know how to recognize and prevent problems associated with dental management, and to use consultations and referrals appropriately. This updated, revised, and expanded text recognizes and supplies this type of information with practical and organized overviews of diagnosis and management. This is accomplished in 30 well-organized and revised chapters by comprehensively covering diseases and conditions that lead to compromised states that affect a person's well-being. The 30 chapters, are presented in 9 logical parts that enhance user-friendly utility. The material is supported by summary tables for easy access to information, figures, and graphs to supplement text, and appendices that allow the reader to recognize disease states, be aware of potential complications, and select an approach to drug management. New Chapter 30 addresses the increasing problem of drug and alcohol abuse. An appendix on alternative and complementary medicine is helpful for background information regarding some of the more common agents.

Although the main focus is on the dental management of medically compromised patients, the text effectively includes a medical overview of each disease entity, including etiology, signs and symptoms, pathophysiology, diagnoses, treatment, and prognosis. Therefore, it also serves as a mini-text on common medical diseases and conditions. Because tobacco use is the most common cause of preventable deaths in the United States (more than 440,000 each year), Chapter 8 describes approaches that enable dental professionals to assess tobacco habits of patients and resources for cessation. Dental professionals have the opportunity to play a significant role in tobacco control. In its present format, this text serves as both a quick reference, and a somewhat in-depth resource for this critical interface of medicine and dentistry. It will help ensure high standards of care, and help reduce the occurrence of adverse reactions by improving knowledge and encouraging judgment in the management of at-risk patients.

In summary, treating the medically compromised patient is a complex part of dentistry, requiring competent practitioners with many attributes: sound technical skills, insight into medicine, familiarity with pharmacotherapeutics, and the capability of analyzing findings from patient histories and signs and symptoms. Therefore, the usefulness of this excellently updated, comprehensive text as a reference for students and practitioners is evident.

Sol Silverman, Jr., MA, DDS
Emeritus Professor of Oral Medicine
University of California, San Francisco

PREFACE

The need for an 8th edition of *Dental Management of the Medically Compromised Patient* became apparent because of the continued, ever-increasing flow of new knowledge and changing concepts in medicine and dentistry.

The purpose of the book remains to give the dental provider an up-to-date, concise, factual reference work describing the dental management of patients with selected medical problems. The more common medical disorders that may be encountered in a dental practice continue to be the focus. This book is not a comprehensive medical reference, but rather a book containing enough core information about each of the medical conditions covered to enable the reader to recognize the basis for various dental management recommendations. Medical problems are organized to provide a brief overview of the basic disease process, epidemiology, pathophysiology, signs and symptoms, laboratory findings, and currently accepted medical therapy of each disorder. This is followed by a detailed explanation and recommendations for specific dental management.

The accumulation of evidence-based research over the years has allowed us to make more specific dental management guidelines that should benefit those who read this text. This includes practicing dentists, practicing dental hygienists, dental graduate students in specialty or general practice programs, and dental and dental hygiene students. In particular, the text is intended to give the dental provider an understanding of how to ascertain the severity and stability of common medical disorders and make dental management decisions that afford the patient the utmost health and safety.

NEW TO THIS EDITION

A number of major changes have been made in this eighth edition. The assessment process has been standardized to include objective measures of disease severity and level of control (Chapter 1). One new chapter has been added, *Chapter 30: Alcohol and Substance Abuse*. This replaces material from *Chapter 11: Liver Disease* and *Chapter 29: Psychiatric Disorders* from the 7th edition. *Chapter 30: Dental Management of Older Adults* has been dropped from this edition. The use of bisphosphonates and its complications are discussed in *Chapter 23: Disorders of White Blood Cells* and *Chapter 26: Cancer and the Oral Care of the Patient* as the intravenous forms of these drugs are used to help manage multiple myeloma and bone metastases. Chapter 25 has been divided into two chapters, *Chapter 24: Acquired Bleeding and Hypercoagulable Disorders* and *Chapter 25: Congenital Bleeding and Hypercoagulable Disorders*. We also moved the material on Tuberculosis into *Chapter 7: Pulmonary Diseases*. Appendix A has been updated and reformatted to follow the P. A. B. C. D. sequence currently advocated for basic life support. Appendix B has been updated by including the most recent edition of the American Academy of Oral Medicine's Clinician's Guide to Treatment of Common Oral Conditions.

All chapters have been updated where necessary, and new dental considerations appear for steroid supplementation, antibiotic prophylaxis, and patients taking bisphosphonates. Many chapters have been provided with new figures, boxes, and tables. The Dental Management box has been redesigned from the other boxes and tables for more rapid identification. Here again, we reformatted these boxes, to follow the P. A. B. C. D. format, which emphasizes a standardized approach.

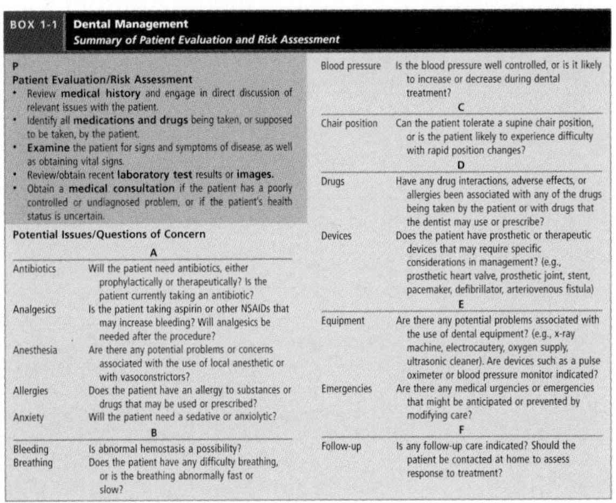

BOX 1-1 Dental Management
Summary of Patient Evaluation and Risk Assessment

P
Patient Evaluation/Risk Assessment
- Review **medical history** and engage in direct discussion of relevant issues with the patient.
- Identify all **medications and drugs** being taken, or supposed to be taken, by the patient.
- **Examine** the patient for signs and symptoms of disease, as well as obtaining vital signs.
- Review/obtain recent **laboratory test** results or **images.**
- Obtain a **medical consultation** if the patient has a poorly controlled or undiagnosed problem, or if the patient's health status is uncertain.

Potential Issues/Questions of Concern

A	
Antibiotics	Will the patient need antibiotics, either prophylactically or therapeutically? Is the patient currently taking an antibiotic?
Analgesics	Is the patient taking aspirin or other NSAIDs that may increase bleeding? Will analgesics be needed after the procedure?
Anesthesia	Are there any potential problems or concerns associated with the use of local anesthetic or with vasoconstrictors?
Allergies	Does the patient have an allergy to substances or drugs that may be used or prescribed?
Anxiety	Will the patient need a sedative or anxiolytic?
B	
Bleeding	Is abnormal hemostasis a possibility?
Breathing	Does the patient have any difficulty breathing, or is the breathing abnormally fast or slow?
Blood pressure	Is the blood pressure well controlled, or is it likely to increase or decrease during dental treatment?
C	
Chair position	Can the patient tolerate a supine chair position, or is the patient likely to experience difficulty with rapid position changes?
D	
Drugs	Have any drug interactions, adverse effects, or allergies been associated with any of the drugs being taken by the patient or with drugs that the dentist may use or prescribe?
Devices	Does the patient have prosthetic or therapeutic devices that may require specific considerations in management? (e.g., prosthetic heart valve, prosthetic joint, stent, pacemaker, defibrillator, arteriovenous fistula)
E	
Equipment	Are there any potential problems associated with the use of dental equipment? (e.g., x-ray machine, electrocautery, oxygen supply, ultrasonic cleaner). Are devices such as a pulse oximeter or blood pressure monitor indicated?
Emergencies	Are there any medical urgencies or emergencies that might be anticipated or prevented by modifying care?
F	
Follow-up	Is any follow-up care indicated? Should the patient be contacted at home to assess response to treatment?

Continued emphasis has been placed on the medications used to treat the medical conditions covered in this eighth edition. Dosages, side effects, and drug interactions with agents used in dentistry—including those used during pregnancy—are discussed in detail. Emphasis also has been placed on having contemporary equipment and diagnostic information to assess and monitor patients with moderate to severe medical disease.

Our sincere thanks and appreciation are extended to those many individuals who have contributed their time and expertise to the writing and revision of this text.

James W. Little
Donald A. Falace
Craig S. Miller
Nelson L. Rhodus

CONTENTS

Dental Management: A Summary

This table presents several important factors to be considered in the dental management of medically compromised patients. Each medical condition is outlined according to potential problems related to dental treatment, oral manifestations, prevention of these problems, and effects of complications on dental treatment planning.

This table has been designed for use by dentists, dental students, graduate students, dental hygienists, and dental assistants as a convenient reference work for the dental management of patients who have medical diseases discussed in this book.

Dental Management: A Summary

Potential Medical Problem Related to Dental Care	Oral Manifestations	Prevention of Problems	Treatment Planning Modification(s)
Infective Endocarditis (IE) ***Chapter 2***			

1. Dental procedures that involve the manipulation of gingival tissues or the periapical region of teeth or perforation of the oral mucosa can produce a bacteremia. Bacteremias can also be produced on a daily basis as the result of toothbrushing, flossing, chewing, or the use of toothpicks or irrigating devices. Although it is unlikely that a single dental procedure–induced bacteremia will result in infective endocarditis (IE), it is remotely possible that it can occur.
2. Patients with mechanical prosthetic heart valves may have excessive bleeding following invasive dental procedures as the result of anticoagulant therapy.
	• Oral petechiae may be found in patients with IE.	• Identify patients at greatest risk for adverse outcomes of IE, including patients with:
		  • Prosthetic cardiac valves
		  • A history of previous IE
		  • Certain types of congenital heart disease (i.e., unrepaired cyanotic congenital heart disease, including patients with palliative shunts and conduits, completely repaired congenital heart disease for the first 6 months after a procedure, or repaired congenital heart disease with residual defect)
		  • Cardiac transplantation recipients who develop cardiac valvulopathy
		• Prescribe antibiotic prophylaxis only for at-risk patients, as listed, who undergo dental procedures that involve manipulation of gingival tissue or the periapical region of teeth or perforation of the oral mucosa.
		• If prophylaxis is required for an adult, take a single dose 30 minutes to 1 hour before the procedure:
		  • Standard (oral amoxicillin 2 g)
		  • Allergic to penicillin (oral cephalexin 2 g, oral clindamycin* 600 mg, or azithromycin or clarithromycin 500 mg)
		    *NOTE: Cephalexin should not be used in patients with a history of anaphylaxis, angioedema, or urticaria with penicillins.
		  • Unable to take oral medications (intravenous [IV] or intramuscular [IM] ampicillin, cefazolin, or ceftriaxone)
		  • Allergic to penicillin and unable to take oral medications (IV or IM clindamycin phosphate, cefazolin, or ceftriaxone)
		• See Chapter 24 for management of potential bleeding problems associated with anticoagulant therapy.
			• Encourage the maintenance of optimal oral hygiene in all patients at increased risk for IE.
			• Provide antibiotic prophylaxis for only those patients with the highest risk for adverse outcomes of IE.
			• Provide antibiotic prophylaxis for all dental procedures, except:
			  • Routine anesthetic injections
			  • Taking of radiographs
			  • Placement of removable prosthodontic or orthodontic appliances
			  • Adjustment of orthodontic appliances
			  • Shedding of deciduous teeth or bleeding from trauma to the lips or oral mucosa
			• For patients selected for prophylaxis, perform as much dental treatment as possible during each coverage period.
			• A second antibiotic dose may be indicated if the appointment lasts longer than 6 hours, or if multiple appointments occur on the same day.
			• For multiple appointments, allow at least 10 days between treatment sessions so that penicillin-resistant organisms can clear from the oral flora. If treatment becomes necessary before 10 days have passed, select one of the alternative antibiotics for prophylaxis.
			• For patients with prosthetic heart valves who are taking anticoagulants, the dosage may have to be reduced on the basis of international normalized ratio (INR) level and the degree of invasiveness of the planned procedure (see Chapter 24).

Potential Medical Problem Related to Dental Care	Oral Manifestations	Prevention of Problems	Treatment Planning Modification(s)
Hypertension ***Chapter 3***			

1. Routine delivery of dental care to a patient with severe uncontrolled hypertension could result in a serious outcome such as angina, myocardial infarction, or stroke.
2. Stress and anxiety related to the dental visit may cause an increase in blood pressure, leading to angina, myocardial infarction, or stroke.
3. In patients taking nonselective beta blockers, excessive use of vasoconstrictors can potentially cause an acute elevation in blood pressure.
4. Some antihypertensive drugs can cause oral lesions or oral dryness and can predispose patients to orthostatic hypotension.
	• No oral complications are due to hypertension itself; however, adverse effects such as dry mouth, taste changes, and oral lesions may be drug-related.	• Detection of patients with hypertension and referral to a physician if poorly controlled or uncontrolled. Defer elective dental treatment if blood pressure (BP) is ≥180/110 mm Hg.
		• For patients who are being treated for hypertension, consider the following:
		  • Take measures to reduce stress and anxiety.
		  • Avoid the use of erythromycin or clarithromycin in patients taking a calcium channel blocker.
		  • Avoid the long-term use of nonsteroidal antiinflammatory drugs (NSAIDs).
		  • Provide oral sedative premedication and/or inhalation sedation.
		  • Provide local anesthesia of excellent quality.
		  • For patients who are taking a nonselective beta blocker, limit epinephrine to ≤2 cartridges of 1:100,000 epinephrine.
		  • Avoid epinephrine-containing gingival retraction cord.
		  • For patients with upper-level stage 2 hypertension, consider intraoperative monitoring of BP, and terminate appointment if BP reaches 180/110.
		  • Make slow changes in chair position to avoid orthostatic hypotension.
			• For patients with BP <180/110, and no evidence of target organ involvement, any treatment may be provided
			• For patients with BP ≥180/110, defer elective dental care
			• For patients with target organ involvement, refer to appropriate chapter for management recommendations

Continued

Dental Management: A Summary—cont'd

Potential Medical Problem Related to Dental Care	Oral Manifestations	Prevention of Problems	Treatment Planning Modification(s)

Angina Pectoris
Chapter 4
1. The stress and anxiety of a dental visit could precipitate an anginal attack, myocardial infarction, or sudden death.
2. For patients who are taking a nonselective beta blocker, the use of excessive amounts of epinephrine could precipitate a dangerous elevation in blood pressure.
3. Patients who are taking aspirin or other platelet aggregation inhibitor may experience excessive bleeding.
4. Questions may arise as to the necessity of antibiotic prophylaxis for patients with a history of coronary artery bypass graft, balloon angioplasty, or stent.
	• No oral complications are due to angina; however, adverse effects such as dry mouth, taste changes, and oral lesions may be drug related.
	• Excessive bleeding may occur as the result of the use of aspirin or other platelet aggregation inhibitors.
		Unstable Angina (major risk)
		• Elective dental care should be deferred; if care becomes necessary, it should be provided in consultation with the physician. Management may include establishment of an IV line; sedation; monitoring of electrocardiogram, pulse oximeter, and blood pressure; oxygen; cautious use of vasoconstrictors; and prophylactic nitroglycerin.
		Stable Angina—intermediate risk
		• Elective dental care may be provided, with the following management considerations:
		  • For stress/anxiety reduction: Provide oral sedative premedication and/or inhalation sedation if indicated, assess pretreatment vital signs and availability of nitroglycerin, and limit quantity of vasoconstrictor used.
		• For patients taking a nonselective beta blocker:
		  • Limit epinephrine to ≤2 cartridges of 1:100,000 epinephrine.
		  • Avoid use of epinephrine-impregnated gingival retraction cord.
		  • Avoid anticholinergics.
		  • Provide local anesthesia of excellent quality and adequate postoperative pain control.
		  • If patient is taking aspirin or another platelet aggregation inhibitor: Excess bleeding usually is manageable with local measures only; discontinuation of medication is not recommended.
		  • Antibiotic prophylaxis is *not* recommended for patients with a history of coronary artery bypass graft (CABG), angioplasty, or stent.
			Unstable Angina
			• Dental treatment should be limited to urgent care only such as treatment of acute infection, bleeding, or pain.
			Stable Angina
			• Any indicated dental treatment may be provided if appropriate management issues are considered.

Potential Medical Problem Related to Dental Care	Oral Manifestations	Prevention of Problems	Treatment Planning Modification(s)

Previous Myocardial Infarction *Chapter 4*
1. The stress and anxiety of a dental visit could precipitate an anginal attack, myocardial infarction, or sudden death in the office.
2. Patients may have some degree of heart failure.
3. If the patient has a pacemaker, some dental equipment may potentially cause electromagnetic interference.
4. In patients who are taking a nonselective beta blocker, excessive amounts of epinephrine may cause a dangerous elevation in blood pressure.
5. Patients who are taking aspirin or another platelet aggregation inhibitor or warfarin (Coumadin) may experience excessive postoperative bleeding.
6. Questions may arise about necessity of antibiotic prophylaxis for patients with a history of CABG, balloon angioplasty, or stent.
	• No oral complications are due to myocardial infarction; however, adverse effects such as dry mouth, taste changes, and oral lesions may be drug-related. Also, bleeding may be excessive because of use of aspirin, other platelet aggregation inhibitors, or warfarin (Coumadin).	*Recent Myocardial Infarction (<1 month)—major risk*
		• Elective dental care should be deferred; if care becomes necessary, it should be provided in consultation with the physician.
		• Management may include establishment of an IV line; sedation; monitoring of electrocardiogram, pulse oximeter, and blood pressure; oxygen; cautious use of vasoconstrictors; and prophylactic nitroglycerin.
		Past Myocardial Infarction (>1 month without symptoms)—intermediate risk
		• Elective dental care may be provided with the following management considerations:
		  • For stress/anxiety reduction: Provide oral sedative premedication and/or inhalation sedation if indicated, assess pretreatment vital signs and availability of nitroglycerin, and limit the quantity of vasoconstrictor used.
		  • For patients who are taking a nonselective beta blocker: Limit epinephrine to ≤2 cartridges of 1:100,000 epinephrine.
		  • Avoid use of epinephrine-impregnated gingival retraction cord.
		  • Avoid anticholinergics.
		  • Provide local anesthesia of excellent quality and adequate postoperative pain control.
		  • If the patient is taking aspirin or another platelet aggregation inhibitor, excessive bleeding is usually manageable by local measures only; discontinuation of medication is not recommended.
		  • If patient has a pacemaker or implanted defibrillator, avoid use of electrosurgery and ultrasonic scalers; antibiotic prophylaxis is not recommended for these patients.
		  • If patient is taking warfarin (Coumadin), the INR should be 3.5 or less before performance of invasive procedures.
		  • Antibiotic prophylaxis is not recommended for patients with a history of CABG, angioplasty, or stent.
			Recent Myocardial Infarction
			• Dental treatment should be limited to urgent care only, such as treatment of acute infection, bleeding, or pain.
			Past Myocardial Infarction
			• Any indicated dental treatment may be provided, taking into consideration appropriate management considerations.

Continued

Dental Management: A Summary—cont'd

Potential Medical Problem Related to Dental Care	Oral Manifestations	Prevention of Problems	Treatment Planning Modification(s)
Arrhythmias *Chapter 5* 1. The stress and anxiety of dental treatment or excessive amounts of epinephrine may induce life-threatening arrhythmias in susceptible patients. 2. Patients with preexisting arrhythmia are at increased risk for serious complications such as angina, myocardial infarction, stroke, heart failure, or cardiac arrest. 3. Patients with a pacemaker or a defibrillator may be at risk for possible malfunction caused by electromagnetic interference from some dental equipment; some question about the need for prophylactic antibiotics may arise. 4. In patients who are taking a nonselective beta blocker, excessive amounts of epinephrine may cause a dangerous elevation in blood pressure. 5. Patients with atrial fibrillation who are taking warfarin (Coumadin) are at risk for excessive postoperative bleeding. 6. Patients who are taking digoxin are at risk for arrhythmia if epinephrine is used; digoxin toxicity also is a potential problem.	• No oral complications are due to arrhythmia; however, adverse effects such as dry mouth, taste changes, and oral lesions may be drug-related. • Excessive bleeding or bruising may occur as the result of use of warfarin (Coumadin).	• Determine the nature, severity, and appropriate treatment of arrhythmia through history and clinical findings; if specific diagnosis is unclear, obtain medical consultation to confirm the following: • For high-risk arrhythmia (high-grade atrioventricular [AV] block, symptomatic ventricular arrhythmia, supraventricular arrhythmia with uncontrolled ventricular rate): 1. Elective dental care should be deferred; if care becomes necessary, it should be provided in consultation with the physician. 2. Management may include establishment of an IV line; sedation; monitoring of electrocardiogram, pulse oximeter, and blood pressure; oxygen; and cautious use of vasoconstrictors. • For intermediate- and low-risk arrhythmia (essentially all others): 1. Elective dental care may be provided with the following management considerations. Stress/anxiety reduction: provide oral sedative premedication and/or inhalation sedation if indicated; assess pretreatment vital signs; avoid excessive use of epinephrine (for patients who are taking a nonselective beta blocker, limit epinephrine to ≤2 cartridges of 1:100,000 epinephrine, avoid the use of epinephrine-impregnated gingival retraction cord, and provide local anesthesia of excellent quality and postoperative pain control). 2. For patients who are taking warfarin (Coumadin), the INR should be 3.5 or less before any invasive dental procedure; provide local measures for hemostasis. 3. For patients with a pacemaker or an implanted defibrillator, avoid the use of electrosurgery and ultrasonic scalers; antibiotic prophylaxis is *not* recommended for these patients. 4. For patients taking digoxin, avoid use of epinephrine because of increased risk of inducing arrhythmia; be observant for signs of digoxin toxicity (e.g., hypersalivation).	*High-Risk Arrhythmias* • Dental treatment should be limited to urgent care only, such as treatment of acute infection, bleeding, or pain. *All Other Arrhythmias* • Any indicated dental treatment may be provided as long as arrhythmia is controlled and appropriate management issues are considered.

Potential Medical Problem Related to Dental Care	Oral Manifestations	Prevention of Problems	Treatment Planning Modification(s)

Heart Failure
Chapter 6
1. Providing dental treatment to a patient with symptomatic or uncontrolled heart failure may result in worsening of symptoms, acute failure, arrhythmia, myocardial infarction, cardiac arrest, or stroke.
2. Patients with heart failure may have difficulty breathing and may not tolerate a supine chair position.
3. Heart failure is due to an underlying condition such as coronary artery disease or hypertension which may also require special management considerations.
4. In patients who are taking a nonselective beta blocker, excessive amounts of epinephrine may cause a dangerous elevation in blood pressure.
5. The use of epinephrine in patients who are taking digoxin may cause arrhythmia.
6. Digitalis may result in toxicity, so be on the alert.
	• No oral complications are caused by heart failure; however, adverse effects such as dry mouth, taste changes, and oral lesions may be drug-related.
	• Digoxin can cause an enhanced gag reflex.
		Symptomatic Heart Failure (NYHA class III or IV)
		• Elective dental care should be deferred and medical consultation obtained; if care becomes necessary, it should be provided in consultation with the physician.
		• Management may include establishment of an IV line; sedation; monitoring of electrocardiogram, pulse oximeter, and blood pressure; oxygen; cautious use of vasoconstrictors; and possibly, prophylactic nitroglycerin.
		Asymptomatic/Mild Heart Failure (NYHA class I and II and possibly III)
		• Elective dental care may be provided with the following management considerations:
		  • For stress/anxiety reduction: Provide oral sedative premedication and/or inhalation sedation if indicated, and assess pretreatment vital signs.
		  • For patients who are taking a nonselective beta blocker, limit epinephrine to ≤2 cartridges of 1:100,000 epinephrine, avoid the use of epinephrine-impregnated gingival retraction cord, and provide local anesthesia of excellent quality and postoperative pain control.
		  • Ensure a comfortable chair position; supine position may not be tolerated.
		  • If patient is taking digoxin, avoid the use of epinephrine.
		  • Avoid the use of nonsteroidal antiinflammatory drugs (NSAIDs).
			Symptomatic Heart Failure (NYHA class III or IV)
			• Dental treatment should be limited to urgent care only, such as treatment of acute infection, bleeding, or pain.
			Asymptomatic/Mild Heart Failure (NYHA class I and II)
			• Any necessary dental treatment may be provided.

Continued

Dental Management: A Summary—cont'd

Potential Medical Problem Related to Dental Care	Oral Manifestations	Prevention of Problems	Treatment Planning Modification(s)
Chronic Obstructive Pulmonary Disease *Chapter 7*			
1. Aggravation or worsening of compromised respiratory function	• Leukoplakia, erythroplakia, or squamous cell carcinoma may develop in chronic smokers of tobacco.	• Avoid treating if upper respiratory infection is present. • Use an upright chair position. • Use of local anesthesia is appropriate; minimize the use of bilateral mandibular or palatal blocks. • Do not use a rubber dam in patients with severe disease. • Use pulse oximetry to monitor oxygen saturation. • Use of low-flow oxygen is helpful. • Do not use nitrous oxide–oxygen sedation in patients with severe emphysema. • Low-dose oral diazepam is acceptable. • Avoid barbiturates, narcotics, antihistamines, and anticholinergics. • Usual daily steroid dose may be needed in patients who are taking systemic steroids for surgical procedures. • Avoid macrolide antibiotics (erythromycin, clarithromycin) and ciprofloxacin for patients who are taking theophylline. • Outpatient general anesthesia is contraindicated.	• None

Potential Medical Problem Related to Dental Care	Oral Manifestations	Prevention of Problems	Treatment Planning Modification(s)
Asthma *Chapter 7*			

1. Precipitation of an acute asthma attack	• Oral candidiasis is reported with the use of a corticosteroid inhaler inhaler without a "spacer," but it occurs rarely.
	• Maxillofacial growth can be altered when asthma is severe during childhood.
		• Identify asthmatic patient by history.
		• Determine character of asthma:
		  • Type (allergic or nonallergic)
		  • Precipitating factors
		  • Age at onset
		  • Level of control (frequency, severity of attacks [mild, moderate, severe])
		  • How usually managed
		  • Medications being taken
		  • Necessity for past emergency care
		  • Baseline forced expiratory volume at 1 second (FEV_1) stable (not decreasing)
		• Avoid known precipitating factors.
		• Consult with physician for severe persistent asthma.
		• Reduce the risk of an attack: Have the patient bring medication inhaler to each appointment, and recommend prophylaxis with an inhaler before each appointment for persons with moderate to severe persistent asthma.
		• Drugs to avoid:
		  • Aspirin-containing medications
		  • NSAIDs
		  • Narcotics and barbiturates
		  • Macrolide antibiotics (e.g., erythromycin), if the patient is taking theophylline
		  • Discontinue cimetidine 24 hours before IV sedation in patients who are taking theophylline.
		• Sulfite-containing local anesthetic solutions may need to be avoided.
		• Usual daily steroid dose may be needed for surgical procedures in patients who are taking systemic steroids.
		• Premedication (nitrous oxide or diazepam) may be needed for anxious patients.
		• Provide a stress-free environment.
		• Use a pulse oximeter.
		• Recognize signs and symptoms of a severe or worsening asthma attack (e.g., difficulty breathing, tachypnea).
			• None required.

Continued

Dental Management: A Summary—cont'd

Potential Medical Problem Related to Dental Care	Oral Manifestations	Prevention of Problems	Treatment Planning Modification(s)

Tuberculosis *Chapter 7*
1. Tuberculosis may be contracted by the dental health care worker from an actively infectious patient.
2. Patients and staff may be infected by a dentist who is actively infectious.
	• Oral ulceration (rare); tongue most common site; ulcer may occur on gingiva or palate
	• Tuberculosis involvement of cervical and submandibular lymph nodes (scrofula)
	• Calcified cervical lymph nodes may indicate previous infection/latent disease.
		• Caveat: Many patients with infectious disease cannot be identified by history or examination; therefore, all patients should be approached with the use of standard precautions (see Appendix B).
		• Patient with active sputum-positive tuberculosis:
		  • Consult with physician before treatment.
		  • Treatment is limited to emergency care (older than 6 years of age.)
		  • Treatment is provided in the hospital setting with proper isolation, sterilization, mask, gloves, gown, and ventilation.
		  • For patients younger than 6 years of age, treat as a normal (noninfectious) patient after consulting with the physician.
		  • For patients producing consistently negative sputum after undergoing at least 2 to 3 weeks of chemotherapy, treat as a normal patient.
		• Patients with a past history of tuberculosis:
		  • Patients should be approached with caution; obtain good history of disease and its treatment, and conduct appropriate review of systems.
		  • Obtain history of adequate treatment, periodic chest radiographs, and examination findings to rule out reactivation.
		  • Dental treatment should be postponed if:
		    1. Questionable history of adequate treatment
		    2. Lack of appropriate medical supervision since recovery
		    3. Signs or symptoms of relapse
		  • If present status is free of clinical disease, patient should be treated as for a normal patient.
			• None required.

Potential Medical Problem Related to Dental Care	Oral Manifestations	Prevention of Problems	Treatment Planning Modification(s)

		• Patients with recent conversion to a positive result on tuberculin skin testing (with purified protein derivative [PPD]):
		  • Should have been evaluated by the physician to rule out clinical disease
		  • May be receiving isoniazid (INH) prophylactically for 3 to 9 months
		  • Should be treated as a normal patient when the physician approves health status
		• Patients with signs or symptoms of tuberculosis:
		  • Should be referred to the physician and should have treatment postponed
		  • If treatment is necessary, provide treatment as for patient with active sputum-positive tuberculosis (above).	

Obstructive Sleep Apnea ***Chapter 9***			
1. Patients with untreated obstructive sleep apnea are at increased risk for hypertension, stroke, arrhythmia, myocardial infarction, and diabetes.	• Large tongue, long soft palate, long uvula, redundant parapharyngeal tissues, large tonsils, retrusive mandible	• Patients should be identified by history and clinical examination and referred to a sleep medicine specialist for diagnosis and treatment planning. • Signs and symptoms suggestive of obstructive sleep apnea include heavy snoring, witnessed apnea episodes during sleep, excessive daytime sleepiness, obesity, and large neck circumference. • Depending on the diagnosis and severity of the disease, treatment may include positive airway pressure, use of oral appliances, or various forms of upper airway surgery.	• Patients with obstructive sleep apnea may undergo any necessary dental treatment.

Continued

Dental Management: A Summary—cont'd

Potential Medical Problem Related to Dental Care	Oral Manifestations	Prevention of Problems	Treatment Planning Modification(s)
Viral Hepatitis Types B, C, D, and E *Chapter 10*			

1. Hepatitis may be contracted by the dentist from an infectious patient.
2. Patients or staff may be infected by the dentist who has active disease or is a carrier.
3. With chronic active hepatitis, the patient may have chronic liver dysfunction, which may be associated with a bleeding tendency or altered drug metabolism.
	• Bleeding
	• Lichenoid eruptions
	• Unpredictable drug metabolism
		• CAVEAT: Because most carriers are undetectable by history, all patients should be treated with the use of standard precautions (see Appendix B); risk may be decreased by the use of hepatitis B vaccine.
		• For patient with active hepatitis, use the following procedures:
		  • Consult with the physician (to determine status).
		  • Treat on an emergency basis only.
		• For patients with a history of hepatitis, use the following procedures:
		  • Consult with the physician (to determine status).
		  • Probable type determination:
		    1. Age at time of infection (type B uncommon at younger than 15 years of age)
		    2. Source of infection (if food or water, usually type A or E)
		    3. If blood transfusion–related, probably type C
		    4. If type is indeterminate, assay for hepatitis B surface antigen (HBsAg) may be considered.
		• With patients in high-risk categories, consider screening for HBsAg or anti–hepatitis C virus.
		• If patient is HBsAg- or hepatitis C virus–positive (carrier status):
		  • Consult with the physician to determine liver function status and/or recommendations for early treatment.
		  • Minimize the use of drugs metabolized by the liver.
		  • Monitor preoperative prothrombin time in chronic active hepatitis, if invasive/surgical procedures are planned.
		• Needlestick:
		  • Consult the physician.
		  • Consider hepatitis B immunoglobulin.
			• None required.

Potential Medical Problem Related to Dental Care	Oral Manifestations	Prevention of Problems	Treatment Planning Modification(s)
Alcoholic Liver Disease (Cirrhosis) *Chapter 10*			

1. Bleeding tendencies; unpredictable drug metabolism	• Neglect
	• Bleeding
	• Ecchymoses
	• Petechiae
	• Glossitis
	• Angular cheilosis
	• Impaired healing
	• Parotid enlargement
	• Candidiasis
	• Oral cancer
	• Alcohol breath odor
	• Bruxism
	• Dental attrition
	• Xerostomia
		• Identify alcoholic patients through the following methods:
		  • History
		  • Clinical examination
		  • Detection of odor on breath
		  • Information from friends or relatives
		• Consult with the physician to determine the status of liver dysfunction.
		• Perform clinical screening for alcohol abuse with the CAGE questionnaire, and attempt to guide patients during treatment.
		• Laboratory screening should include the following:
		  • Complete blood count with differential
		  • Aspartate aminotransferase, alanine aminotransferase
		  • Platelet count
		  • Thrombin time
		  • Prothrombin time
		• Minimize the use of drugs metabolized by the liver.
		• If screening tests are abnormal, consider antifibrinolytic agents, fresh frozen plasma, vitamin K, and platelets, for use during surgery.
		• Defer routine care if ascites (encephalopathy), is present.
			• Because oral neglect is commonly seen in persons who abuse alcohol, patients with this history should be required to demonstrate interest in and ability to care for dentition before any significant treatment is rendered.

Peptic Ulcer Disease *Chapter 11*			
1. Further injury to the intestinal mucosa caused by aspirin/other NSAIDs 2. Fungal overgrowth during or after systemic antibiotic use	• Rare—enamel dissolution associated with persistent regurgitation • Fungal overgrowth • Rare—vitamin B deficiency (glossopyrosis) with omeprazole use	• Avoid aspirin/other NSAIDs. • Avoid corticosteroids. • Examine oral cavity for signs of fungal overgrowth.	• Provide as stress-free an environment as possible.
Inflammatory Bowel Disease *Chapter 11*			
1. In patients who are being treated with steroids, stress may lead to serious medical problems.	• "Cobblestoning"—aphthous lesions • Pyostomatitis vegetans	• Additional steroids may be needed for surgical procedures. • Complete blood count is needed to monitor toxic hematologic effects of drugs. • If antibiotics are used, monitor for signs or symptoms (diarrhea, GI distress) of pseudomembranous colitis.	• Schedule appointments during remissions.

Continued

Dental Management: A Summary—cont'd

Potential Medical Problem Related to Dental Care	Oral Manifestations	Prevention of Problems	Treatment Planning Modification(s)
Pseudomembranous Colitis *Chapter 11* 1. Fungal overgrowth during or after course of antibiotics	• Rare—fungal overgrowth	• Select appropriate antibiotic, dosage, and duration. • Take precautions with prolonged antibiotic use in the elderly and those previously affected.	• Schedule appointments when the patient is free of disease symptoms.
End-Stage Renal Disease *Chapter 12* 1. Bleeding tendency 2. Hypertension 3. Anemia 4. Intolerance to nephrotoxic drugs metabolized by the kidney 5. Enhanced susceptibility to infection	• Mucosal pallor • Xerostomia • Metallic taste • Ammonia breath odor • Stomatitis • Loss of lamina dura • Bone radiolucencies • Bleeding tendency	• Consult with physician (to determine status). • Pretreatment screening (i.e., platelet count, prothrombin time, partial thromboplastin time, hematocrit, hemoglobin) for hematologic disorder done by dentist or patient's physician. • Closely monitor blood pressure before and during treatment. • Adjust dosage/avoid drugs excreted by the kidney and nephrotoxic drugs when glomerular filtration rate (GFR) <60 mL/min. • Meticulous attention should be paid to good surgical technique to minimize the risk of abnormal bleeding or infection. • Provide aggressive management of infection.	• Major emphasis on oral hygiene and optimal maintenance care to eliminate possible sources of infection. • No contraindications for routine dental care. • Extensive reconstructive crown and bridge procedures may not be indicated for patients with poor prognosis.
Hemodialysis *Chapter 12* 1. Bleeding tendency 2. Hypertension 3. Anemia 4. Intolerance to nephrotoxic drugs metabolized by the kidney 5. Bacterial endarteritis of arteriovenous fistula secondary to bacteremia 6. Hepatitis (active or carrier) 7. Bacterial endocarditis 8. Collapse of shunt	• Bleeding • Lichenoid eruptions	• Consultation with physician. • Delay dental treatment for at least 4 hours after dialysis to avoid heparin effects (potential for excessive bleeding); best to perform dental treatment on the day after dialysis. • Avoid drugs metabolized by kidney or nephrotoxic drugs. • American Heart Association does not recommend antibiotic prophylaxis for invasive dental procedures. • Monitor blood pressure closely—avoid placing blood pressure cuff on the arm containing the shunt used for dialysis. • Avoid intravenous medications in arm with shunt • Consider corticosteroid supplementation if indicated.	• None required.

Potential Medical Problem Related to Dental Care	Oral Manifestations	Prevention of Problems	Treatment Planning Modification(s)
Gonorrhea *Chapter 13*			

1. Remote possibility of transmission from oral or pharyngeal lesions of an infected patient	• Rare but varied expression, including generalized stomatitis, ulceration, and formation of pseudomembranous coating of oropharynx	CAVEAT: Many patients with sexually transmitted disease cannot be identified by history or examination; therefore, all patients must be approached with the use of standard precautions (see Appendix B).
		• For patients currently receiving treatment for gonorrhea, provide necessary care.
		• For patients with past history of gonorrhea, perform the following:
		  • Obtain a good history of disease and its treatment.
		  • Provide necessary care.
		• For patients with signs or symptoms suggestive of gonorrhea:
		  • Refer to physician for evaluation.
		  • Provide necessary care after disease treatment has been initiated.
			• None required.

Syphilis *Chapter 13*			

1. Syphilis may be contracted by the dentist from an actively infectious patient.
2. Patients or staff may be infected by the dentist who has syphilis.
	• Chancre
	• Mucous patch
	• Gumma
	• Interstitial glossitis
	• Congenital syphilis (associated with Hutchinson's incisors and mulberry molars)
		• For patients receiving treatment for syphilis:
		  • Consult with physician before treatment.
		  • Provide necessary care.
		  • Be aware that oral lesions of primary and secondary syphilis are infectious before initiation of antibiotic therapy.
		• For patients with a past history of syphilis:
		  • Approach with caution; obtain good history of disease, its treatment, and negative serologic tests for syphilis test after completion of therapy.
		  • Treat as normal patient if free of disease.
		• For patients showing signs or symptoms suggestive of syphilis:
		  • Refer to physician, and postpone treatment.
		  • The dentist may request/order serologic tests for syphilis before referral.
		  • Defer treatment until diagnosis established and medical treatment provided.
			• None required.

Continued

Dental Management: A Summary—cont'd

Potential Medical Problem Related to Dental Care	Oral Manifestations	Prevention of Problems	Treatment Planning Modification(s)
Genital Herpes *Chapter 13*			
1. Inoculation of oral cavity and potential transmission to dentist (fingers, eyes)	• Autoinoculation of type 2 herpes to oral cavity	CAVEAT: Many patients with sexually transmitted disease cannot be identified by history or examination; therefore, all patients must be approached with the use of standard precautions (see Appendix B). • Localized genital infection poses no problem; however, be aware of possibility of autoinoculation to dermal sites and the oral cavity by the patient. • For oral infection with HSV-1 or HSV-2 postpone elective dental care until lesion is healing (in scab phase or when it disappears).	• None usually required; patients prone to recurrence after dental treatment should be prescribed a systemic antiviral drug for prophylactic use for a few days.
Human Papillomavirus (HPV) Infection *Chapter 13*			
1. Inoculation of oral cavity and potential transmission to fingers	• Benign manifestations: papilloma, verruca vulgaris, condyloma acuminatum • Specific genotypes associated with risk for development of carcinoma	CAVEAT: Many patients with sexually transmitted disease cannot be identified by history or examination; therefore, all patients must be approached with the use of standard precautions (see Appendix B). • Localized genital infection poses no problem; however, be aware of the possibility of autoinoculation to the oral cavity by the patient. • Oral lesions should be excised and submitted for histologic examination. HPV typing should be considered.	• Discuss risks of transmission and the potential for development of carcinoma with high-risk types (HPV 16, 18, 31, 33, 35). Appropriate treatment and follow-up care should be provided.

Potential Medical Problem Related to Dental Care	Oral Manifestations	Prevention of Problems	Treatment Planning Modification(s)

Diabetes Mellitus
Chapter 14
1. In patients with uncontrolled diabetes:
a. Infection
b. Poor wound healing
c. Risk for systemic problems
2. Insulin reaction in patients treated with insulin
3. In diabetic patients, early onset of complications relating to cardiovascular system, eyes, kidneys, and nervous system (angina, myocardial infarction, cerebrovascular accident, renal failure, peripheral neuropathy blindness, hypertension, congestive heart failure)
	• Accelerated periodontal disease
	• Gingival proliferations
	• Periodontal abscesses
	• Xerostomia
	• Poor healing
	• Infection
	• Oral ulcerations
	• Candidiasis
	• Mucormycosis
	• Numbness, burning, or pain in oral tissues
		• Detection by the following methods:
		  • History
		  • Clinical findings
		  • Screening for blood glucose
		• Referral for diagnosis and treatment
		• Monitoring and control of hyperglycemia by assessment of blood glucose
		• Monitoring of hemoglobin A_{1c} (A1C) status
		• For patients receiving insulin (or sulfonylurea drugs), insulin reaction is prevented by the following methods:
		  • Eating normal meals before appointments
		  • Scheduling appointments in morning or mid-morning
		  • Informing the dentist of any symptoms of insulin reaction when they first occur
		  • Having sugar available in some form in cases of insulin reaction
		• Diabetic patients who develop oral infection may require increased insulin dosage and consultation with the physician, in addition to aggressive local and systemic management of infection (including antibiotic sensitivity testing).
		• Drug considerations include the following:
		  • Insulin reaction
		  • Insulin and drug interactions
		  • Hypoglycemic agents—on rare occasions can cause aplastic anemia, etc.
		  • Avoidance of general anesthesia in patients with severe diabetes
			• In patients with well-controlled diabetes, no alteration of treatment plan is indicated unless complications of diabetes are present, such as:
			  • Hypertension
			  • Congestive heart failure
			  • Myocardial infarction
			  • Angina
			  • Renal failure
			• Defer orthodontic and prosthodontic care until periodontal disease is well controlled.
			• Avoid periodontal or oral surgery if poor glycemic control.

Continued

Dental Management: A Summary—cont'd

Potential Medical Problem Related to Dental Care	Oral Manifestations	Prevention of Problems	Treatment Planning Modification(s)

Adrenal Insufficiency (AI)
Chapter 15
1. Inability to tolerate stress
2. Delayed healing
3. Susceptibility to infection
4. Hypertension (with prolonged steroid use)
	• Pigmentation of oral mucous membranes
	• Delayed healing
	• Possible oral infection
		• For routine dental procedures (excluding extractions):
		  • Patients currently taking corticosteroids—no additional supplementation generally required; be sure to obtain good local anesthesia and good postoperative pain control
		  • Patients with past history of regular corticosteroid usage; none generally required
		  • Patients using topical or inhalational steroids—generally no supplementation required
		• With secondary AI, provide usual daily steroid dose for surgical procedures.
		• With primary AI, for extractions or other surgery, extensive procedures, or extreme patient anxiety, with local anesthetic include the following:
		  • Discontinue drugs that decrease cortisol levels (e.g., ketoconazole) at least 24 hours before surgery with consent of the patient's physician.
		  • Give 25 mg/day hydrocortisone for minor oral and periodontal surgery, administered before procedure.
		  • Give 50-75 mg hydrocortisone at beginning of moderate oral surgery, and up to 1 day after. Return to preoperative glucocorticoid dose on postoperative day 2.
		  • Give 100-150 mg/day of hydrocortisone at beginning of major oral surgery or procedures involving general anesthesia; continue for 2-3 days.
		  • Monitor blood pressure throughout procedure and initial postoperative phase.
		  • Provide good pain control.
			• None required.

Potential Medical Problem Related to Dental Care	Oral Manifestations	Prevention of Problems	Treatment Planning Modification(s)
Hyperthyroidism (Thyrotoxicosis) ***Chapter 16***			

1. Thyrotoxic crisis (thyroid storm) may be precipitated in patients with untreated or incompletely treated thyrotoxicosis by:
a. Infection
b. Trauma
c. Surgical procedures
d. Stress
2. Patients with untreated or incompletely treated thyrotoxicosis may be very sensitive to actions of epinephrine and other pressor amines; thus, these agents must not be used; once the patient is well managed from a medical standpoint, these agents may be administered.
3. Thyrotoxicosis increases the risk for hypertension, angina, MI, congestive heart failure, and severe arrhythmias.
	• Osteoporosis may occur.
	• Periodontal disease may be more progressive.
	• Dental caries may be more extensive.
	• Premature loss of deciduous teeth and early eruption of permanent teeth may occur.
	• Early jaw development may be noted.
	• Tumors found at the midline of the posterior dorsum of the tongue must not be surgically removed until the possibility of functional thyroid tissue has been ruled out by ^{131}I uptake tests.
		• Detection of patients with thyrotoxicosis by history and examination findings
		• Referral for medical evaluation and treatment
		• Avoidance of any dental treatment for patient with thyrotoxicosis until good medical control is attained; however, any acute oral infection will have to be dealt with by antibiotic therapy and other conservative measures to prevent development of thyrotoxic crisis; suggest consultation with patient's physician during management of acute oral infection
		• Avoidance of epinephrine and other pressor amines in untreated or incompletely treated patient
		• Recognition of early stages of thyrotoxic crisis:
		  • Severe symptoms of thyrotoxicosis
		  • Fever
		  • Abdominal pain
		  • Delirious, obtunded, or psychotic
		• Initiation of immediate emergency treatment procedures:
		  • Seek immediate medical aid.
		  • Cool with cold towels, ice packs.
		  • Hydrocortisone (100-300 mg)
		  • Monitor vital signs.
		  • Start cardiopulmonary resuscitation (CPR) if needed.
			• Once under good medical management, the patient may receive any indicated dental treatment.
			• If acute infection occurs, the physician should be consulted regarding management.

4. Radioactive iodine complications	• Acute—salivary gland swelling, pain, loss of taste • Radioactive drug-induced: Chronic sialoadenitis—xerostomia, pain and dental caries	• Manage pain and xerostomia as described in Appendix C.	
5. Antithyroid agents: propylthiouracil, methimazole	• Sore throat, fever, mouth ulcers	• Possible agranulocytosis, refer to physician for evaluation and stopping the antithyroid medication.	

Continued

Dental Management: A Summary—cont'd

Potential Medical Problem Related to Dental Care	Oral Manifestations	Prevention of Problems	Treatment Planning Modification(s)
Hypothyroidism ***Chapter 16***			

1. Untreated patients with severe hypothyroidism exposed to stressful situations such as trauma, surgical procedures, or infection may develop hypothyroid (myxedema) coma.
2. Untreated hypothyroid patients may be highly sensitive to actions of narcotics, barbiturates, and tranquilizers.
	• Increase tongue size
	• Delayed eruption of teeth
	• Malocclusion
	• Gingival edema
		• Detection and referral of patients suspected of being hypothyroid for medical evaluation and treatment
		• Avoidance of narcotics, barbiturates, and tranquilizers in untreated hypothyroid patients
		• Recognition of initial stage of hypothyroid (myxedema) coma:
		  • Hypothermia
		  • Bradycardia
		  • Hypotension
		  • Epileptic seizures
		• Initiation of immediate treatment for myxedema coma:
		  • Seek immediate medical aid.
		  • Administer hydrocortisone (100-300 mg).
		  • Provide CPR as indicated.
			• In hypothyroid patients under good medical management, indicated dental treatment may be performed.
			• In patients with a congenital form of disease and severe mental retardation, assistance with hygienic procedures may be needed.

Thyroiditis ***Chapter 16***			
1. *Acute suppurative*—patient has acute infection, antibiotics are required.	• Usually none	• None	• Postpone elective dental care until infection has been treated.
2. *Subacute painful*—period of hyperthyroidism	• Pain may be referred to mandible.	• Include in differential diagnosis for jaw pain; see earlier under Hyperthyroidism.	• Avoid elective dental care if possible until symptoms of hyperthyroidism have cleared.
3. *Subacute painless*—up to 6-month period of hyperthyroidism	• None	• See earlier under Hyperthyroidism.	• Avoid elective dental care if possible until symptoms of hyperthyroidism have cleared.
4. *Hashimoto's*—leads to severe hypothyroidism	• Tongue may enlarge.	• See earlier under Hypothyroidism.	• In hypothyroid patients under good medical management, any indicated dental treatment can be performed. See above for uncontrolled disease.
5. *Chronic fibrosing (Riedel's)*—usually euthyroid	• None	• None	• None

Potential Medical Problem Related to Dental Care	Oral Manifestations	Prevention of Problems	Treatment Planning Modification(s)
Thyroid Cancer *Chapter 16*			

1. Usually none	• Usually none; metastasis to the oral cavity is rare.
	• Post-radiation induced chronic sialodenitis, xerostomia, risk for root caries.
		• Examine for signs and symptoms of thyroid cancer:
		  • Hard, painless lump in thyroid
		  • Dominant nodule in multinodular goiter
		  • Hoarseness, dysphagia, dyspnea
		  • Cervical lymphadenopathy
		  • Nodule that is affixed to underlying tissues
		  • Patient usually euthyroid
		• Patients found to have thyroid nodule(s) should be referred for fine needle aspiration biopsy.
			• For most patients, the dental treatment plan is not affected unless the cancer treatment includes external irradiation or chemotherapy. See summaries for Chapter 26. Patients with anaplastic carcinoma have a poor prognosis, and complex dental procedures usually are not indicated.

2. Levothyroxine suppression after surgery and radioiodine ablation is usual treatment for follicular carcinomas. Patient may have mild hyperthyroidism and may be sensitive to actions of pressor amines.	• Usually none	• Consult with patient's physician regarding permissible degree of hyperthyroidism in patients treated with thyroid hormone.	• Care with the use of epinephrine is indicated in patients treated with thyroid hormone.
3. Patients with multiple endocrine neoplasia-2 (MEN2) may have symptoms of hypertension and/or hypercalcemia.	• Patients with MEN2 can develop cystic lesions of the jaws related to hyperparathyroidism.		
4. Anaplastic carcinomas may be treated by external irradiation and/or chemotherapy. See problems listed in summaries for Chapter 26.	• See oral complications listed in summaries for Chapter 26.	• Manage complications of radiation therapy/chemotherapy as described in summaries for Chapter 26.	• Prognosis is poor with anaplastic carcinoma.

Continued

Dental Management: A Summary—cont'd

Potential Medical Problem Related to Dental Care	Oral Manifestations	Prevention of Problems	Treatment Planning Modification(s)
Pregnancy and Lactation ***Chapter 17*** 1. Dental procedures could harm the developing fetus through effects of: a. Radiation b. Drugs c. Stress 2. Supine hypotension in late pregnancy 3. Poor nutrition and diet can affect oral health. 4. Transmission of drugs to infant in breast milk 5. Lack of proper oral health care during pregnancy could harm the development of the fetus and affect time of delivery.	• Exaggeration of periodontal disease, "pregnancy gingivitis" • "Pregnancy tumor" • Tooth mobility	• Women of childbearing age: • Always use contemporary radiographic techniques, including lead apron and thyroid collar, when performing radiographic examination. • Do not prescribe drugs that are known to be harmful to the fetus, or whose effects are as yet unknown (see Table 17-3). • Encourage patients to maintain a balanced, nutritious diet. • For pregnant women: • Consider contacting the patient's physician to verify physical status and present management plan; ask for suggestions regarding patient's treatment, especially as it relates to drug administration. • Maintain optimal oral hygiene, including prophylaxis, throughout pregnancy. • Minimize oral microbial load (consider chlorhexidine and/or fluoride). • Avoid elective dental care during the first trimester. The second trimester and early third trimester are the best times for elective treatment. • Do not schedule radiographs during the first trimester; thereafter, take only those necessary for treatment, always with the use of a lead apron. • Avoid drugs known to be harmful to the fetus, or whose effects are unknown (see Table 17-3). • In advanced stages of pregnancy (late third trimester), do not place the patient in the supine position for prolonged periods; avoid aspirin/other NSAIDs. • For lactating mothers: • Most drugs are of little pharmacologic significance to lactation. • Do not prescribe drugs known to be harmful (see Table 17-3). • Administer drugs just after breast feeding.	• None, except that major reconstructive procedures, crown and bridge fabrication, and significant operations are best delayed until after delivery.

Potential Medical Problem Related to Dental Care	Oral Manifestations	Prevention of Problems	Treatment Planning Modification(s)
HIV Seropositive Asymptomatic ***Chapter 18***			
1. Transmission of infectious agents to dental personnel and patients, may include: a. Human immunodeficiency virus (HIV) b. Hepatitis B virus (HBV) c. Hepatitis C virus (HCV) d. Epstein-Barr virus (EBV) e. Cytomegalovirus (CMV) 2. To date, dental health care workers have not been infected with HIV through occupational exposure; six patients may have been infected by an HIV-infected dentist; thus, risk of HIV transmission in the dental setting is very low, but the potential exists. 3. Persons who are hepatitis carriers may transmit HBV or HCV to the unvaccinated or those lacking antibody.	• None in the early stage; however, increased incidence of certain oral lesions associated with AIDS is found when compared with noninfected persons (i.e., candidiasis).	• Identification of HIV-infected patient is difficult; interview questions should address promiscuous sexual behavior. • Infectious disease control procedures must be used for *all* patients. • Extreme care must be taken to avoid needlestick and instrument wounding. • All dental personnel should be vaccinated to be protected from HBV infection. • All asymptomatic antibody-positive (for HIV) patients may go on to develop AIDS; however, it may take as long as 15 years before a diagnosis of AIDS is made. • The HIV-infected patient's CD4+ cell count and viral titer must be monitored. • The patient's immune status, medications, and potential for opportunistic infections must be determined and monitored.	• None indicated.

Continued

Dental Management: A Summary—cont'd

Potential Medical Problem Related to Dental Care	Oral Manifestations	Prevention of Problems	Treatment Planning Modification(s)
HIV-Infected, Asymptomatic Patient (CD4+ lymphocyte count less than 500/µL but more than 200/µL) ***Chapter 18***			
1. Transmission of infectious agents to dental personnel and patients: a. HIV b. Hepatitis B virus c. Hepatitis C virus d. Epstein-Barr virus e. Cytomegalovirus Note: Transmission of HIV to patients who received care in dental offices has been reported. Transmission of HBV and HCV has been well documented on numerous occasions. 2. Patients with decreasing CD4+ lymphocytes may have significant immune suppression and be at increased risk for infection. 3. Patients with decreasing CD4+ lymphocytes may be thrombocytopenic and hence potential bleeders.	• Oral candidiasis • Hairy leukoplakia • Persistent lymphadenopathy • Salivary gland enlargement • With the exception of Kaposi sarcoma and non-Hodgkin lymphoma, other lesions listed under AIDS may be found with increased frequency.	• Use standard precautions in providing care for *all* patients. • Vaccinate dental personnel for protection from HBV infection. • Identify patients by presence of signs/symptoms associated with decreasing CD4+ cell counts; refer for medical evaluation, counseling, and management. • Establish platelet status and immune status of patients with low CD4+ cells (<500/µL) before performing invasive dental procedures (see AIDS, next entry). • Inform patients of various support groups available to help in terms of education and emotional, financial, legal, and other issues. • Identify potential drug-drug interactions.	• None indicated. • If patient is in "remission" with a CD4+ count >200/µL, routine and complex restorative procedures can be provided.

Potential Medical Problem Related to Dental Care	Oral Manifestations	Prevention of Problems	Treatment Planning Modification(s)
AIDS (CD4+ lymphocyte count less than 200 μL) *Chapter 18*			
1. Potential for transmission of infectious agents to dental personnel and patients: a. HIV b. Hepatitis B virus c. Hepatitis C virus d. Epstein-Barr virus e. Cytomegalovirus 2. Potential for transmission from dental health care workers to patients. 3. Patients with advanced disease have significant suppression of their immune system and may be at risk for infection resulting from invasive dental procedures. 4. Patients may be bleeders because of thrombocytopenia.	• Kaposi sarcoma • Non-Hodgkin's lymphoma • Oral candidiasis • Lymphadenopathy • Hairy leukoplakia • Xerostomia • Salivary gland enlargement • Venereal warts • Linear gingivitis erythema • Necrotizing ulcerative periodontitis • Necrotizing stomatitis • Herpes zoster • Primary or recurrent herpes simplex lesions • Major aphthous lesions • Herpetiform aphthous lesions • Petechiae, ecchymoses • Others (see Tables 18-5, 18-6)	• Use standard precautions in providing care for *all* patients. • Vaccinate dental personnel for protection from hepatitis B virus. • Through medical history and examination findings, identify undiagnosed cases and refer for medical evaluation, counseling, and management. • Give patients with significant immunosuppression antibiotic prophylaxis for surgical or invasive dental procedures, if neutrophil count is <500/μL. • Platelet count should be ordered before any surgical procedure is performed; if significant thrombocytopenia is present, platelet replacement may be needed. • The patient's immune status, medications (highly active antiretroviral therapy [HAART]), and potential for opportunistic infections must be determined and monitored. • Identify potential drug-drug interactions.	• Patients in advanced stages of disease should receive emergency and preventive dental care; elective dental treatment usually is not indicated at this stage.

Continued

Dental Management: A Summary—cont'd

Potential Medical Problem Related to Dental Care	Oral Manifestations	Prevention of Problems	Treatment Planning Modification(s)
Allergic Reaction (not severe) ***Chapter 19***			

1. Mild reaction occurring after patient exposure to known or likely allergenic agent, such as:
a. Drugs
b. Local anesthetic
c. Latex gloves or other rubber products (rubber dam, gutta percha)
	• Rash, itching	• Take careful history and identify patients who are allergic to agents used in dentistry, and who have a history of atopic reactions (e.g., asthma, hay fever, urticaria, angioneurotic edema).
		• Do not use agents to which the patient is allergic, as identified in the medical history.
		• For patients with a history of atopic reactions, use care when giving drugs and with use of materials associated with a high incidence of allergy such as penicillin; be prepared to deal with severe allergic reaction.
		• If patient develops allergic reaction to previously unsuspected drug or other material, consider the following:
		  • Nonemergency reaction, no further contact with agent—administer diphenhydramine 50 mg up to four times a day, orally or IM.
		  • Emergency reaction—with patient in supine position with patent airway and supplemental oxygen, inject 0.3 to 0.5 mL epinephrine 1:1000 IM; support respiration if necessary; check pulse; obtain medical assistance.
		  • When prescribing drugs, inform the patient regarding signs and symptoms of allergic reactions; advise the patient to call the dentist if such a reaction occurs, or to report to the nearest hospital emergency room.
			• Do not use agents to which the patient is allergic, as identified in the medical history.
			• Before administering local anesthetics, consider the following:
			  • Ask the patient about any allergic reactions to local anesthetic. (Most patients who say they are allergic will describe a fainting episode or a toxic reaction.) If an allergic reaction has occurred, identify the type of anesthetic used, and select one from various chemical groups.
			  1. Inject 1 drop (aspirate first) of alternate anesthetic, and wait 5 minutes; if no reaction occurs, proceed with injection of remaining anesthetic.
			  2. If anesthetic that patient has reacted to cannot be identified, consider the following procedures:
			    a. Refer to allergist for provocative dose testing, or
			    b. Use diphenhydramine (Benadryl) with epinephrine 1:100,000 as local anesthetic (1% solution, 1-4 mL).

Potential Medical Problem Related to Dental Care	Oral Manifestations	Prevention of Problems	Treatment Planning Modification(s)
Anaphylaxis ***Chapter 19*** 1. Severe reaction occurring after patient exposure to known or likely allergenic agent, such as: a. Drugs b. Local anesthetic c. Latex gloves or other rubber products (rubber dam, gutta percha)	• May develop itching of throat/palate, then skin rash and swelling of tissues in neck	• Take careful history and identify patients who are allergic to agents used in dentistry. • Avoid allergens (drugs/other agents). • If reaction is severe: • Identify anaphylactic reaction. • Call for medical help; activate EMS. • Place patient in the supine position. • Check for and maintain open airway. • Administer oxygen. • Check vital signs—respiration, blood pressure, pulse rate, and rhythm. • If vital signs depressed or absent, inject 0.3-0.5 mL of epinephrine 1:1000 IM into the tongue. • Provide CPR as indicated. • Repeat injection of epinephrine if no response is obtained.	• Do not use agents to which the patient is allergic, as identified in the medical history.
Urticaria (Angioedema) ***Chapter 19*** 1. Nonemergency; edematous swelling of lips, cheek, other tissue, after contact with allergen 2. Emergency; edematous swelling of tongue, pharynx, and larynx with obstruction of airway	• Soft tissue swelling	• Identify patients who have had allergic reactions through the history and what drug or materials caused the reaction. • Avoid the use of antigen in allergic persons. • If patient develops allergic reaction to previously unsuspected drug or other material, consider the following: • Nonemergency reaction, no further contact with agent—administer diphenhydramine 50 mg up to 4 times a day, orally or IM. • Emergency reaction—put patient in the supine position; with patent airway and oxygen, inject 0.3-0.5 mL epinephrine 1:1000 IM; support respiration if necessary; check pulse; obtain medical assistance. • For hereditary angioedema, consider use of danazol or C1 inhibitor concentrate as preventative measure. • For allergy to penicillin: • Administer erythromycin or another macrolide antibiotic. • In nonallergic person, administer by the oral route whenever possible—lowest incidence of sensitization. • Do not use in topical form.	• Do not use agents to which the patient is allergic, as identified in the medical history.

Continued

Dental Management: A Summary—cont'd

Potential Medical Problem Related to Dental Care	Oral Manifestations	Prevention of Problems	Treatment Planning Modification(s)
Rheumatoid Arthritis and Osteoarthritis *Chapter 20*			
1. Immunosuppression due to many antiinflammatory drugs—steroids, methotrexate, disease-modifying antirheumatic drugs (DMARDs), biologics 2. Potential for increased infections due to immunosuppresion (leukopenia) 3. Potential bleeding from long-term use of aspirin/other NSAIDs 4. Potential for adrenal suppression from long-term corticosteroid use	• Temporomandibular joint (TMJ) problems/disorders (TMDs) • Xerostomia • Bleeding • Infections	• Early risk assessment and intervention • Refer for medical care • Ensure patient receives regular medical care appointments	• Adjust chair position to keep patient more comfortable • TMD problems and limited jaw opening • Address and prevent xerostomia (increased caries rate) • Prevention of bleeding problems • Possible corticosteroid supplementation • Antibiotic prophylaxis (per previous)
Joint Replacements *Chapter 20*		Dentists have three options for managing dental patients with prosthetic joint replacements regarding antibiotic prophylaxis:	
1. Potential for late prosthetic joint infection		1. Informed consent. 2. Base clinical decisions on the 2003 ADA/AAOS consensus statement 3. Consultation with the patient's orthopedic surgeon to suggest following the 2003 guidelines until a new joint consensus statement is approved. If the orthopedist elects to recommend antibiotic prophylaxis for a patient who would not receive it on the basis of the 2003 guidelines, the orthopedist can write the prescription for the desired antibiotic.	• Defer dental care during immediate postoperative period • Use antibiotic prophylaxis for patients with prosthetic joint replacement for invasive dental procedures for the first two years following the placement of the joint replacement and in patients with "high risk" conditions: rheumatoid arthritis, type 1 diabetes, previous history of prosthetic joint infection, malnourishment, hemophilia, malignancy and severe immune suppression.
Giant Cell Arteritis *Chapter 20*			
1. Potential for jaw claudication, which may be mistaken for TMD symptoms	• TMD symptoms	• Include in differential diagnosis for pain in the temporal region. • Refer for medical care.	• Defer care during sympotomatic phase.

Potential Medical Problem Related to Dental Care	Oral Manifestations	Prevention of Problems	Treatment Planning Modification(s)
Systemic Lupus Erythematosus *Chapter 20*			
1. Potential for end-organ complications (e.g., heart, renal, skin, immune) 2. Immunosuppression due to many antiinflammatory drugs (e.g., steroids, methotrexate, DMARDs, biologics) 3. Potential for increased infections due to immunosuppression (leukopenia) 4. Potential bleeding from long-term use of aspirin/other NSAIDs 5. Potential for adrenal suppression from long-term corticosteroid use	• Infections • Oral ulcers (stomatitis) • Bleeding	• No specific recommendations for antibiotic prophylaxis, but antibiotics may be necessary if patient is immunosuppressed. • Differential diagnosis	• Prevention of bleeding problems • Possible corticosteroid supplementation
Lyme Disease *Chapter 20*			
1. Potential for facial palsy and paresthesia	• Facial palsy	• Differential diagnosis • Refer for medical care	• Defer care during symptomatic phase
Sjögren Syndrome *Chapter 20*			
1. Severe xerostomia, increased caries rate, candidiasis, glossitis/stomatitis 2. Salivary gland hypertrophy and potential transformation to lymphoma	• Xerostomia • Increased caries • Candidiasis • Glossitis/stomatitis	• Differential diagnosis • Multiple fluoride therapy (see Appendix C) • Sialagogues to stimulate salivary flow (see Appendix C) • Antifungal therapy • Increased oral hygiene	• Frequent prevention recalls and prophies • Rigid oral hygiene program • Close salivary gland monitoring (lymphoma) • Soothing ("Magic") mouthwash (see Appendix C)
Intravascular Access Devices (Uldall Catheter, Central IV Line, Broviac-Hickman Device) *Chapter 21*			
1. High rate of infection, but the role of transient dental bacteremias that cause these infections has not been established.	• None	• The Centers for Disease Control and Prevention (CDC) does not recommend antibiotic prophylaxis for invasive dental procedures.	• Modifications will depend on the reason for the intravascular device.

Continued

Dental Management: A Summary—cont'd

Potential Medical Problem Related to Dental Care	Oral Manifestations	Prevention of Problems	Treatment Planning Modification(s)
Solid Organ Transplantation ***Chapter 21***			
1. Infection from suppression of immune response by the following: a. Cyclosporine b. Azathioprine c. Prednisone d. Antithymocyte globulin e. Antilymphocyte globulin f. Orthoclone (monoclonal antibody), others 2. Acute rejection, reversible 3. Chronic rejection, nonreversible, includes the following: a. Graft failure—end-stage organ failure b. Bleeding—liver, kidney c. Drug overdosage—liver, kidney d. Death or need for transplantation of heart, liver e. Osteoporosis f. Drug-induced psychosis g. Anemia h. Leukopenia i. Thrombocytopenia j. Gingival hyperplasia k. Adrenocortical suppression l. Tumors (listed above) m. Poor healing n. Bleeding o. Infection	• Usually none • Diseases associated with excessive immunosuppression include: • Candidiasis • Herpes simplex • Herpes zoster • Hairy leukoplakia • Lymphoma • Kaposi sarcoma • Aphthous stomatitis • Squamous cell carcinoma of lip • Adverse effects of immunosuppressant drugs include: • Bleeding (spontaneous) • Infection • Ulceration • Petechiae • Ecchymoses • Gingival hyperplasia • Salivary gland dysfunction • Graft failure may manifest with: • Uremic stomatitis (kidney) • Bleeding (liver) • Petechiae (liver, kidney) • Ecchymoses (liver)	• Dental evaluation and treatment before transplantation includes the following: • Establish stable oral and dental status free of active dental disease. • Initiate aggressive oral hygiene program to maintain oral health. • Arrange medical consultation for patients with organ failure before performing needed dental treatment to establish the following: 1. Degree of failure 2. Current status of patient 3. Need for antibiotic prophylaxis 4. Need to modify drug selection or dosage 5. Need to take special precautions to avoid bleeding 6. If surgery is indicated, access to recent prothrombin time, partial thromboplastin time, and white cell count or differential may be needed. • Dental treatment after transplantation includes the following: • Immediate posttransplantation period (6 months): 1. Provide emergency dental care only. 2. Continue oral hygiene procedures. • Stable graft period: 1. Maintain oral hygiene. 2. Recall every 3 months. 3. Use universal precautions.	• Before transplantation, consider the following: • For patients with poor dental status, consider extractions and full dentures. • For patients with good dental status, perform the following: 1. Maintain dentition. 2. Establish aggressive oral hygiene program in the following areas: a. Toothbrushing, flossing b. Diet modification, if indicated c. Topical fluorides d. Plaque control, calculus removal e. Chlorhexidine or Listerine mouth rinse 3. Treat all active dental disease by: a. Extraction—nonrestorable teeth b. Endodontics—nonvital teeth c. Restoration of carious teeth d. Complex dental prostheses, other major work deferred until after transplantation

Potential Medical Problem Related to Dental Care	Oral Manifestations	Prevention of Problems	Treatment Planning Modification(s)
		5. Schedule medical consultation on the following topics: a. Need for antibiotic prophylaxis b. Need for precautions to avoid excessive bleeding c. Need for supplemental steroids d. Selection of drugs and dosage 6. Examine for clinical evidence of the following: a. Organ failure or rejection b. Overimmunosuppression (e.g., tumors, infection) 7. Monitor blood pressure at every appointment. 8. If evidence of drug adverse effects, graft rejection, or overimmunosuppression is found, refer patient to physician. • Chronic rejection period: 1. Perform immediate or emergency dental care only. 2. Follow guidelines for stable graft when treatment is performed.	• For patients with dental status between the defined extremes: 1. Decision to maintain natural dentition must be made on an individual patient basis. 2. Factors to be considered: a. Extent and severity of dental disease b. Importance of teeth to patient c. Cost of maintaining natural dentition d. Systemic status of patient and prognosis e. Physical ability to maintain good oral hygiene • After transplantation: • Immediate posttransplantation period—limit dental care to emergency needs. • Stable graft period—base treatment plan on needs and desires of the patient; recall every 3 to 6 months. • Chronic rejection period—limit dental care to immediate or emergency needs. • Maintain aggressive oral hygiene program throughout all periods. • Consult with physician to confirm patient's current status and the need for special precautions.

Continued

Dental Management: A Summary—cont'd

Potential Medical Problem Related to Dental Care	Oral Manifestations	Prevention of Problems	Treatment Planning Modification(s)
Heart Transplantation, Special Considerations *Chapter 21*			
In addition to risk of infection due to immune suppression: 1. Patient may be on long-term anticoagulation therapy; excessive bleeding may occur with surgical procedures. 2. Graft atherosclerosis may occur, increasing the risk for myocardial infarction. 3. No nerve supply exists to the transplanted heart; thus, pain will not be symptom of myocardial infarction. 4. Some patients require cardiac pacing; electrical equipment may interfere with the pacemaker. 5. Cardiac valvular disease may develop.	• Usually none • See Chapter 25	• Have physician modify anticoagulation regimen to achieve prothrombin time 2.5 times normal or less (INR, 3.5 or less), if surgical procedures are planned. • Consult with physician to establish status of coronary vessels of transplanted heart; if advanced graft atherosclerosis is present, manage as described in section on coronary atherosclerotic heart disease. • Be aware of signs and symptoms of myocardial infarction, other than pain; if these occur, obtain immediate medical assistance for patient. • Do not use ultrasonic scalers or electrosurgery unit in patients with a pacemaker.	• The American Heart Association (AHA) has stated that evidence regarding the need for antibiotic prophylaxis for prevention of endocarditis in patients with heart transplantation is inconclusive. • The AHA recommends that prophylaxis be considered for cardiac transplant patients who develop cardiac valvular disease. • If prophylaxis is planned, the standard amoxicillin regimen of the AHA would be appropriate.
Liver Transplantation, Special Considerations *Chapter 21*			
In addition to risk of infection due to immune suppression: 1. Drugs that may be toxic to the liver must not be prescribed. 2. Some patients may be on anticoagulation medication. 3. Excessive bleeding may occur with surgical procedures.	• See earlier under Solid Organ Transplantation.	• Avoid drugs that are toxic to the liver. • Have the physician modify the anticoagulation regimen to achieve an INR of 3.5 or less.	• The need for prophylactic antibiotics for invasive dental procedures in patients with stable liver transplants should be determined on an individual basis through medical consultation.
Kidney Transplantation, Special Considerations *Chapter 21*			
In addition to risk of infection due to immune suppression 1. Drugs that may be toxic to the kidney must not be prescribed.	• See earlier under Solid Organ Transplantation.	• Avoid drugs that are toxic to the kidney.	• The need for prophylactic antibiotics for invasive dental procedures in patients with stable kidney transplants should be determined on an individual basis through medical consultation.

Potential Medical Problem Related to Dental Care	Oral Manifestations	Prevention of Problems	Treatment Planning Modification(s)
Pancreas Transplantation *Chapter 21*			
1. No special considerations beyond those listed above for organ transplantation.	• See earlier under Solid Organ Transplantation.		• The need for prophylactic antibiotics for invasive dental procedures in patients with stable pancreas transplants should be determined on an individual basis through medical consultation.
Bone Marrow Transplantation *Chapter 21*			
1. Immune suppression and pancytopenia resulting from conditioning therapy, including: a. Total body irradiation b. Cyclophosphamide c. Busulfan 2. Problems during conditioning phase and critical phase (until transplanted marrow becomes functional) include: a. Infection b. Bleeding c. Poor healing 3. Immune suppression resulting from maintenance medications used to prevent graft-versus-host disease and: a. Cyclosporine b. Prednisone c. Methotrexate 4. Problems during maintenance phase include: a. Infection b. Others as listed earlier under Solid Organ Transplantation related to medication(s) being used 5. Graft-versus-host disease and chronic rejection: a. Infection b. Bleeding	• Mucositis • Gingivitis • Xerostomia • Candidiasis • Herpes simplex infections • Osteoradionecrosis • Gingival overgrowth (with cyclosporine)	• Avoid dental treatment during conditioning and critical phases of bone marrow transplantation. • Treat all active dental disease prior to bone marrow transplantation. • Observe requirements for antibiotic prophylaxis for invasive dental procedures: • Prophylaxis is indicated if procedures must be performed on an emergency basis during conditioning or critical phases of bone marrow transplantation. • Need should be determined through medical consultation. (See earlier under Solid Organ Transplantation for details of hygiene program and dental management.)	• If possible, treat active dental disease before transplantation. • Prognosis varies according to reason for transplantation, source of marrow to be transplanted, and techniques used to condition and maintain the patient; other factors that may affect prognosis include age and general health status; complex dental prostheses may not be indicated for many patients. • (See earlier under Solid Organ Transplantation for other suggested treatment planning considerations.) (For management of soft tissue complications, see Appendix C.)

Continued

Dental Management: A Summary—cont'd

Potential Medical Problem Related to Dental Care	Oral Manifestations	Prevention of Problems	Treatment Planning Modification(s)
Iron Deficiency Anemia *Chapter 22*			
1. Usually none 2. In rare cases, severe leukopenia and thrombocytopenia may result in problems with infection and excessive loss of blood.	• Paresthesias • Loss of papillae on dorsum of tongue • In rare cases, infection and bleeding complications • In patients with dysphagia, increased incidence of carcinoma of oral and pharyngeal areas (Plummer-Vinson syndrome)	• Detection and referral for diagnosis and treatment • Recognition that in women most cases are caused by physiologic process—menstruation or pregnancy • Recognition that in men most cases are the result of underlying disease—peptic ulcer, carcinoma of colon, other—requiring referral to the patient's physician	• Usually none indicated.
Glucose-6-Phosphate Dehydrogenase (G-6-PD) Deficiency *Chapter 22*			
1. Accelerated hemolysis of red blood cells	• Usually none	• Control infection. • Avoid drugs such as certain antibiotics, or that contain aspirin, or acetaminophen, which may increase risk for hemolytic anemia. • Be aware that these patients also often have increased sensitivity to sulfa drugs and chloramphenicol.	• Usually none unless anemia is severe; then, perform only procedures to meet urgent dental needs.
Pernicious Anemia *Chapter 22*			
1. Infection 2. Bleeding 3. Delayed healing	• Paresthesias of oral tissues (burning, tingling, numbness) • Delayed healing (severe cases), infection, bald red tongue, angular cheilosis • Petechial hemorrhages	• Detection and medical treatment (early detection and treatment can prevent permanent neurologic damage)	• None indicated, once the patient is under medical care.

Potential Medical Problem Related to Dental Care	Oral Manifestations	Prevention of Problems	Treatment Planning Modification(s)
Sickle Cell Anemia *Chapter 22*			

1. Sickle cell crisis	• Atypical trabecular pattern
	• Delayed eruption of teeth, growth abnormalities
	• Hypoplasia of teeth
	• Pallor of oral mucosa
	• Jaundice of oral mucosa
	• Bone pain
	• Osteoporosis
		• Consult with patient's physician to ensure that condition is stable.
		• Institute aggressive preventive dental care.
		• Avoid any procedure that may produce acidosis or hypoxia (avoid long, complicated procedures).
		• Drug modifications:
		  • Avoid excessive use of barbiturates and narcotics, because suppression of the respiratory center may occur, leading to acidosis, which can precipitate acute crisis. Use benzodiazepine instead.
		  • Avoid excessive use of salicylates, because "acidosis" may result, again leading to possible acute crisis; codeine and acetaminophen in moderate dosage can be used for pain control.
		  • Avoid the use of general anesthesia, because hypoxia can lead to precipitation of acute crisis.
		  • Nitrous oxide may be used, provided that 50% oxygen is supplied at all times; it is critical to avoid diffusion hypoxia at the termination of nitrous oxide administration. For nonsurgical procedures, use local without vasoconstrictor; for surgical procedures, use 1:100,000 epinephrine in anesthetic solution.
		  1. Aspirate before injecting.
		  2. Inject slowly.
		  3. Use no more than two cartridges.
		  4. It is necessary to prevent infection. Use prophylactic antibiotics for major surgical procedures.
		  5. If infection occurs, manage aggressively, with the use of:
		    a. Heat
		    b. Incision and drainage
		    c. Antibiotics
		    d. Corrective treatment (e.g., extraction, pulpectomy)
		  6. Avoid dehydration in patients with infection and in patients who are receiving surgical treatment.
			• Usually none, unless symptoms of severe anemia are present; then, only urgent dental needs should be met.

Continued

Dental Management: A Summary—cont'd

Potential Medical Problem Related to Dental Care	Oral Manifestations	Prevention of Problems	Treatment Planning Modification(s)
Aplastic Anemia *Chapter 22*			
1. Bleeding 2. Infection	• Gingival bleeding • Petechiae • Ecchymosis • Oral infection • Pallor of mucosa	• Referral for medical diagnosis and treatment • Medical consultation to determine current status of the patient under medical treatment • Some drugs (anticonvulsants, anthyroid drugs, select antidiabetic agents, diuretics and sulfonamides) are associated with higher incidence of aplastic anemia.	• During periods of low blood count (platelets, neutrophils, red blood cells), provide emergency care only. • Antimicrobial agents and supportive therapy are needed for oral infection (see Appendix C for specific treatment regimens).
Agranulocytosis *Chapter 23*			
1. Infection	• Oral ulcerations • Periodontitis • Necrotic tissue	• Referral for medical diagnosis and treatment • Drug considerations—some antibiotics (macrolides, penicillins, and cephalosporins) used for oral infections are associated with higher incidence of agranulocytosis. Avoid these antibiotics if possible.	• During periods of low blood count, provide emergency care only. Treatment should include the use of antimicrobial agents and supportive therapy for oral lesions (see Appendix C for specific treatment regimens).
Cyclic Neutropenia *Chapter 23*			
1. Infection	• Periodontal disease • Oral infection • Oral ulceration similar to that of aphthous stomatitis	• Antibiotics should be given to prevent infection. • Serial white blood cell (WBC) counts should be performed to identify the safest period for dental treatment (i.e., when the WBC count is closest to normal level).	• Modifications not required when the WBC count (neutrophils) is normal. • If the WBC count (neutrophils) is depressed severely, antibiotics should be provided to prevent postoperative infection.

Potential Medical Problem Related to Dental Care	Oral Manifestations	Prevention of Problems	Treatment Planning Modification(s)
Leukemia ***Chapter 23*** 1. Infection 2. Bleeding 3. Delayed healing 4. Mucositis	• Gingival swelling/ enlargement • Mucosal or gingival bleeding • Oral infection	• Referral for medical diagnosis, treatment, and consultation • Complete blood count to determine risk for anemia, bleeding, and infection • Antibiotics, antivirals, and antifungals provided during chemotherapy to prevent opportunistic oral infection • Chlorhexidine rinse/bland rinses to manage mucositis	• Inspect head, neck, and radiographs for undiagnosed or latent disease (e.g., retained root tips, impacted teeth) and infections that require managment before chemotherapy. • Eliminate infections before chemotherapy. • Extractions should be performed at least 10 days before initiation of chemotherapy. • Implement plaque control measures and chlorhexidine during chemotherapy. • Use prophylactic antibiotics if WBC count is less than 2000/μL, or neutrophil count is less than 500/μL (or 1000 at some institutions). • Platelet replacement may be required (if platelet count is <50,000/μL) when invasive dental procedures are performed.
Multiple Myeloma ***Chapter 23*** 1. Excessive bleeding after invasive dental procedures 2. Risk of infection because of decrease in normal immunoglobulins 3. Risks of infection and bleeding in patients who are being treated by irradiation or chemotherapy 4. Risk of osteonecrosis of the jaws in patients who are taking bisphosphonates (especially intravenously)	• Soft tissue tumors • Osteolytic lesions • Amyloid deposits in soft tissues • Unexplained mobility of teeth • Exposed bone	• Patients with oral soft tissue lesions and/or osseous lesions should have them biopsied by the dentist or should be referred for diagnosis and treatment as indicated. • Medical history should identify patients with diagnosed disease; medical consultation is needed to establish current status. (See sections on chemotherapy and radiation therapy on prevention and management of medical complications.) • Be aware of and take precautions for bisphosphonate-induced osteonecrosis of the jaws.	• For patients in terminal stage, provide supportive dental care only. • Long-term prognosis is poor, so complex dental procedures may not be indicated. • If thrombocytopenia or leukopenia is present, special precautions (platelet replacement, antibiotic therapy) are needed to prevent bleeding and infection when invasive dental procedures are performed. • Patients may be bleeders because of the presence of abnormal immunoglobulin M macroglobulins, which form complexes with clotting factors, thereby inactivating the clotting factors. (See sections on chemotherapy and radiation therapy for treatment plan modifications.)

Continued

Dental Management: A Summary—cont'd

Potential Medical Problem Related to Dental Care	Oral Manifestations	Prevention of Problems	Treatment Planning Modification(s)
Lymphomas: Hodgkin Disease, Non-Hodgkin Lymphoma, Burkitt's Lymphoma *Chapter 23*			
1. Increased risk for infection 2. Risks of infection and excessive bleeding in patients receiving chemotherapy 3. Minor risk of osteonecrosis in patients treated by radiation to the head and neck region (usually does not occur because radiation dosage seldom exceeds 50 Gy) 4. Xerostomia may occur in patients treated by irradiation to the head and neck region. 5. Non-Hodgkin lymphoma may be found in patients with AIDS; hence, transmission of infectious agents may be a problem.	• Extranodal oral tumors in Waldeyer's ring or osseous soft tissues • Xerostomia in patients treated by radiation; some of these patients prone to osteonecrosis • Burning mouth or tongue symptoms • Petechiae or ecchymoses if thrombocytopenia present because of tumor invasion of bone marrow • Cervical lymphadenopathy • Mucositis in patients treated by radiation therapy or chemotherapy	• Patients with generalized lymphadenopathy, extranodal tumors, and osseous lesions must be identified and referred for medical evaluation and treatment. • The dentist can biopsy extranodal or osseous lesions to establish a diagnosis; patients with lesions involving the lymph nodes should be referred for excisional biopsy. • Medical history should identify patients with diagnosed disease; medical consultation will be needed to establish current status. (See sections on chemotherapy and radiation therapy on management and prevention of medical complications.) • Before invasive procedures, a complete blood count should be obtained to determine risks for bleeding and infection. • Patients who have been treated by irradiation to the chest area may develop acute and chronic cardiovascular complications such as arrhythmias or valvular heart disease. Medical consultation is needed to confirm their current status.	• Patients in terminal phase should receive only supportive dental treatment. • Patients under "control" may receive any indicated treatment; however, complex restorative treatment may not be indicated in cases with a poor prognosis. • Platelet replacement may be needed for patients with thrombocytopenia. (See sections on radiation therapy and chemotherapy for treatment plan modifications.) • Consider prophylactic antibiotics if the WBC count is less than 2000/μL, or the neutrophil count is less than 500 (or 1000 at some institutions).
Bleeding Problem Suggested by Examination and History Findings But Lack of Clues to Underlying Cause *Chapter 24*			

1. Excessive blood loss after surgical procedures, scaling, other manipulations	• Excessive bleeding after dental procedures	• Screen patients with the following (if results of one or more tests are abnormal, refer for diagnosis and medical treatment):
		  • Prothrombin time
		  • Activated partial thromboplastin time
		  • Thrombin time
		  • Platelet count
		• Avoid use of aspirin and related drugs.
			• None, unless test result(s) abnormal; then, manage according to the nature of the underlying problem once diagnosis has been established by the physician.

Potential Medical Problem Related to Dental Care	Oral Manifestations	Prevention of Problems	Treatment Planning Modification(s)
Thrombocytopenia (Primary or Secondary) Caused by Chemicals, Radiation, or Leukemia *Chapter 24*			

1. Prolonged bleeding
2. Infection in patients with bone marrow replacement or destruction
3. A medical emergency can result from stress in patients being treated with steroids.
	• Spontaneous bleeding
	• Prolonged bleeding after certain dental procedures
	• Petechiae
	• Ecchymoses
	• Hematomas
		• Identification of patients to include the following:
		  • History
		  • Examination findings
		  • Screening tests— platelet count
		• Referral and consultation with hematologist
		• Correction of underlying problem or replacement therapy before surgery
		• Local measures to control blood loss (e.g., splint, Gelfoam, thrombin)
		• Prophylactic antibiotics may be considered in surgical cases to prevent postoperative infection if severe neutropenia is present.
		• Additional steroids should be used for patients being treated with steroids, if indicated (see section on adrenal insufficiency).
		• Aspirin/other NSAIDs, aspirin-containing compounds are not to be used; acetaminophen (Tylenol) with or without codeine may be used if analgesia is required.
			• In general, dental procedures can be performed if the platelet count is 30,000/μL or higher.
			• Extractions and minor surgery can be performed if the platelet count is 50,000/μL or higher.
			• Major oral surgery can be performed if the platelet count is 80,000/μL to 100,000/μL or higher.
			• Platelet transfusion will be needed for patients with platelet counts below the above values.
			• Patients with severe neutropenia (500/μL or less) may require antibiotics for certain surgical procedures (1000 at some institutions).
			• In children with primary thrombocytopenia, many will respond to steroids with increase in platelets to levels allowing dental procedures to be performed.

Vascular Wall Alterations (Scurvy, Infection, Chemical, Allergic, Autoimmune, Other Agents/Factors) *Chapter 24*			

1. Prolonged bleeding after surgical procedures or any insult to integrity of oral mucosa	• Excessive bleeding after scaling and surgical procedures
	• Petechiae
	• Ecchymoses
	• Hematomas
		• Identification of patients should include the following:
		  • History
		  • Clinical findings
		  • Screening tests—none reliable
		• Consultation with the hematologist should be obtained.
		• Local measures should be used to control blood loss: splints, Gelfoam, Oxycel, and surgical thrombin (see Table 24-6).
		• Prevention of allergy if causative, and if the antigen is identified.
			• Surgical procedures must be avoided in these patients unless the underlying problem has been corrected, or the patient has been prepared for surgery by the hematologist, and the dentist is prepared to control excessive loss of blood through local measures: splints, thrombin, microfibrillar collagen, Gelfoam, Oxycel, ε-aminocaproic acid (Amicar) (see Table 24-6).

Continued

Dental Management: A Summary—cont'd

Potential Medical Problem Related to Dental Care	Oral Manifestations	Prevention of Problems	Treatment Planning Modification(s)
Acquired Disorders of Coagulation (liver disease, broad-spectrum antibiotics, malabsorption syndrome, biliary tract obstruction, heparin, other agents/factors)			
Chapter 24			

1. Excessive bleeding after dental procedures that result in soft tissue or osseous injury	• Excessive bleeding
	• Spontaneous bleeding
	• Petechiae
	• Hematomas
		• Identification of patients with such disorders should include:
		  • History
		  • Examination findings
		  • Screening laboratory tests—prothrombin time (prolonged) in liver disease, platelet count (low if hypersplenism present)
		• Consultation and referral should be provided.
		• Preparation before the dental procedure may include vitamin K injection by the physician and platelet replacement if indicated.
		• Local measures are used to control blood loss (see Table 24-6).
		• For patients with liver disease, avoid or reduce dosage of drugs metabolized by the liver.
		• Do not use aspirin/other NSAIDs, aspirin-containing compounds.
			• No dental procedures should be performed unless the patient has been prepared on the basis of a consultation with the hematologist.

Anticoagulation with Coumarin Drugs (Warfarin)			
Chapter 24			

1. Excessive bleeding after dental procedures that result in soft tissue or osseous injury	• Excessive bleeding
	• Hematomas
	• Petechiae
	• In rare cases, spontaneous bleeding
		• Identify patients who are taking anticoagulants/coumarin in the following ways:
		  • History
		  • Screening laboratory test—international normalized ratio (INR), prothrombin time (PT)
		• Consultation should be obtained regarding level of anticoagulation:
		  • If INR is 3.5 or less, most surgical procedures can be performed.
		  • Dosage of anticoagulant should be reduced if INR is greater than 3.5 (it takes several days for INR to fall to desired level; confirmation should be obtained by new tests before surgery is completed).
		  • Patients undergoing major oral surgery should be managed on an individual basis; in most cases, INR should be below 3.0 at the time of surgery.
		  • Low-molecular-weight heparin bridging can be considered for major surgery.
		• ε-Aminocaproic acid (Amicar) rinses, just before surgery and every hour for 6-8 hours, will aid in control of bleeding. Local measures should be instituted to control blood loss after surgery (see Table 24-6).
			• No dental procedures should be performed unless medical consult has been obtained and level of anticoagulation is at an acceptable range; the procedure may have to be delayed by 2-3 days if the dosage of anticoagulant has to be reduced.
			• Avoid aspirin or aspirin-containing compounds. Use acetaminophen (Tylenol) for postoperative pain control.

Potential Medical Problem Related to Dental Care	Oral Manifestations	Prevention of Problems	Treatment Planning Modification(s)
Disseminated Intravascular Coagulation (DIC) ***Chapter 24***			

1. Excessive bleeding after invasive dental procedures; in chronic form of disease, widespread thrombosis may occur.	• Spontaneous gingival bleeding
	• Petechiae
	• Ecchymoses
	• Prolonged bleeding after invasive dental procedures
		• Identification of patients includes the following:
		  • History—excessive bleeding after minor trauma; spontaneous bleeding from nose, gingiva, gastrointestinal tract, urinary tract; recent infection, burns, shock and acidosis, or autoimmune disease; history of cancer most often associated with chronic form of disseminated intravascular coagulation (DIC), in which thrombosis rather than bleeding usually is the major clinical problem
		  • Examination findings include the following:
		    1. Petechiae
		    2. Ecchymoses
		    3. Spontaneous gingival bleeding; bleeding from nose, ears, and so on.
		  • Screening laboratory findings include the following:
		    1. Acute DIC—prothrombin time (prolonged), partial thromboplastin time (prolonged), thrombin time (prolonged), platelet count (decreased)
		    2. Chronic DIC—most tests may be normal, but fibrin-split products are present (positive result on D-dimer test).
		• Obtain referral and consultation with physician if invasive dental procedures must be performed, and include information on:
		  • Acute DIC—cryoprecipitate, fresh frozen plasma, and platelets
		  • Chronic DIC—anticoagulants such as heparin or vitamin K antagonists
		• Aspirin or aspirin-containing products are prohibited.
		• Local measures are used to control bleeding (see Table 24-6).
		• Antibiotic therapy may be considered to prevent postoperative infection.
			• Depending on the cause of DIC, the treatment plan should be altered as follows:
			  • With acute DIC—No routine dental care until medical evaluation and correction of cause
			  • With chronic DIC—No routine dental care until medical evaluation and correction of cause when possible; if prognosis is poor on the basis of underlying cause (advanced cancer), limited dental care is indicated.
			  • Avoid aspirin/other NSAIDs, aspirin-containing compounds.
			  • Do not use ε-aminocaproic acid (Amicar), tranexamic acid or desmopression, as these agents may complicate the disorder and result in increased bleeding.
			  • Acetaminophen with or without codeine can be used for postoperative pain.

Continued

Dental Management: A Summary—cont'd

Potential Medical Problem Related to Dental Care	Oral Manifestations	Prevention of Problems	Treatment Planning Modification(s)
Disorders of Platelet Release *Chapter 24*			

1. Excessive bleeding after invasive dental procedures	• Excessive bleeding may occur after surgery.
	• Petechiae, ecchymoses, and hematomas may be found when other platelet or coagulation disorders are present.
		• Identification of patient should include the following:
		  • History—recent use of aspirin, indomethacin, phenylbutazone, ibuprofen, or sulfinpyrazone; presence of other platelet or coagulation disorders
		  • Examination—often negative unless signs related to other platelet or coagulation disorders are present
		  • Screening laboratory tests— partial thromboplastin time (prolonged)
		• Most patients on drugs noted above without an additional platelet or coagulation problem will not bleed excessively after surgery.
		• Patients with prolonged partial thromboplastin time should be referred for evaluation before performance of any surgical procedures.
		• Elective surgery can be performed after withdrawal of drug for at least 3 days and management of other platelet or coagulation disorders by appropriate means.
			• Usually, no modifications are indicated for patients who have no other platelet or coagulation disorders.

Primary Fibrinogenolysis *Chapter 24*			

1. Excessive bleeding after invasive dental procedures	• Prolonged bleeding after invasive dental procedures
	• Jaundice of mucosa
	• Ecchymoses
		• Identification of patients should include the following:
		  • History—liver disease, cancer of lung, cancer of prostate, and heat stroke may cause this condition.
		  • Examination findings to consider:
		    1. Jaundice
		    2. Spider angiomas
		    3. Ecchymoses
		    4. Hematomas
		  • Screening laboratory tests:
		    1. Platelet count (often normal)
		    2. Prothrombin time (prolonged)
		    3. Partial thromboplastin time (prolonged)
		    4. Thrombin time (prolonged)
		  • Consultation and referral before any invasive dental procedure; ε-aminocaproic acid therapy will inhibit plasmin and plasmin activators.
			• Patients with advanced cancer should have treatment limited to emergency dental procedures and preventive measures; complex dental restorations in general are not indicated; in other patients, once preparation to avoid excessive bleeding has occurred (ε-aminocaproic acid), most dental treatment can be rendered.

Potential Medical Problem Related to Dental Care	Oral Manifestations	Prevention of Problems	Treatment Planning Modification(s)
Low-Molecular-Weight Heparin Therapy: Enoxaparin (Lovenox), Ardeparin (Normiflo), Dalteparin (Fragmin), Nadroparin (Fraxiparine), Reviparin (Clivarin), Tinzaparin (Innohep)			
Chapter 24			
1. Used in patients who have received prosthetic knee or hip replacement; patient takes medication for approximately 2 weeks after getting out of the hospital 2. Complications include the following: a. Excessive bleeding b. Anemia c. Fever d. Thrombocytopenia e. Peripheral edema	• Gingival bleeding • Petechiae • Ecchymoses • In rare cases, excessive bleeding after dental procedures	• Delay procedure until patient is off the medication. • Have physician stop medication and perform surgery the next day; once hemostasis is obtained, have the physician resume medication. • Perform surgery, and manage any excessive bleeding through local means (preferred if excessive bleeding is not anticipated).	• Usually none needed.
Antiplatelet Drug Therapy: Aspirin, Aspirin Plus Dipyridamole (Aggrenox), Ibuprofen (Advil, Motrin)			
Chapter 24			
1. Used for prevention of initial or recurrent myocardial infarction and stroke prevention 2. Complications include: a. Excessive bleeding b. Gastrointestinal bleeding c. Tinnitus d. Bronchospasm	• Gingival bleeding • Petechiae • Ecchymoses • In rare cases, excessive bleeding after dental procedures	• If no other complications occur, dental procedures and surgery can usually be performed.	• Usually none needed, unless there are other medical problems, such as recent MI or stroke.
Fibrinogen Receptor Therapy (Glycoprotein [GP] IIb/IIIa inhibitors—Abciximab, Tirofiban): ADP Inhibitors (clopidogrel [Plavix], ticlopidine [Ticlid])			
Chapter 24			
1. Used for prevention of recurrent myocardial infarction and stroke 2. Complications include: a. Excessive bleeding b. Gastrointestinal bleeding c. Neutropenia d. Thrombocytopenia	• Gingival bleeding • Petechiae • Ecchymoses • In rare cases, excessive bleeding after dental procedures • Adverse reactions increase risk for infection (neutropenia) and bleeding (thrombocytopenia).	• If no other complications occur, dental procedures and surgery may be performed.	• Usually none needed, unless there are other medical problems such as recent MI or stroke. • ADA and AHA issued a statement that dual-antiplatelet treatment (clopidogrel and aspirin) should not be discontinued for patients with stents when receiving invasive dental treatment.

Continued

Dental Management: A Summary—cont'd

Potential Medical Problem Related to Dental Care	Oral Manifestations	Prevention of Problems	Treatment Planning Modification(s)
Congenital Disorders of Coagulation (Hemophilia) ***Chapter 25***			

1. Excessive bleeding after dental procedures
2. HIV-, HBV-, and HCV-infected patients are potentially infectious (see Appendix B)
	• Spontaneous bleeding
	• Prolonged bleeding after dental procedures that injure soft tissue or bone
	• Hematomas
	• Oral lesions associated with HIV infection in patients who receive infected replacement products (most cases occurred before 1986)
		• Identification of patients includes the following:
		  • History—bleeding problems in relatives, excessive bleeding after trauma or surgery
		  • Examination findings:
		    1. Ecchymoses
		    2. Hemarthrosis
		    3. Dissecting hematomas
		  • Screening tests—prothrombin time (normal), activated partial thromboplastin time (prolonged), thrombin time (normal), platelet count (normal)
		• Consultation and referral should be provided for diagnosis and treatment and for preparation before dental procedures are performed.
		• Replacement options include the following:
		  • Cryoprecipitate (used rarely)
		  • Fresh frozen plasma (used rarely)
		  • Factor VIII concentrates, including:
		    1. Heat-treated concentrate
		    2. Purified factor VIII
		    3. Recombinant factor VIII
		    4. Porcine factor VIII
		  • For mild to moderate factor VIII deficiency, consider using:
		    1. 1-desamino-8-D-arginine vasopressin (desmopressin) (oral or nasal)
		    2. ε-Aminocaproic acid (Amicar) rinse or taken orally
		    3. Tranexamic acid (Cyklokapron); oral solution not available in the United States, injectable and tablets are
		    4. Factor VIII replacement for some cases
		    5. Often treated on an outpatient basis
			• No dental procedures should be performed unless the patient has been prepared on the basis of consultation with the hematologist.
			• Avoid aspirin/other NSAIDs, aspirin-containing compounds—use acetaminophen (Tylenol) with or without codeine.

Potential Medical Problem Related to Dental Care	Oral Manifestations	Prevention of Problems	Treatment Planning Modification(s)

		• For severe factor VIII deficiency, alleviate with such measures as:
		  • Agents used above for mild to moderate deficiency
		  • Higher dose(s) of factor VIII
		• Patients who are low responders (low antibody response to FVIII):
		  • Agents used for mild to moderate deficiency
		  • Very high dose(s) of factor VIII
		• Patients who are high responders (high antibody response to FVIII):
		  • No elective surgery
		  • Agents used for mild to moderate deficiency
		  • High doses of porcine factor VIII concentrate
		  • Nonactivated prothrombin/complex concentrate
		  • Activated prothrombin/complex concentrate
		  • Plasmapheresis
		  • Factor VIIa
		  • Steroids
		  • In rare cases, plasmapheresis
		• Treatment is provided on an outpatient basis in accordance with results of the consultation (mild to moderate deficiency, no inhibitors).
		• Local measures (e.g., splints, thrombin, microfibrillar collagen) are used for control of bleeding (see Table 25-6).
		• Aspirin/other NSAIDs, aspirin-containing compounds should be avoided.	

Continued

Dental Management: A Summary—cont'd

Potential Medical Problem Related to Dental Care	Oral Manifestations	Prevention of Problems	Treatment Planning Modification(s)
von Willebrand Disease ***Chapter 25***			

1. Excessive bleeding after invasive dental procedures	• Spontaneous bleeding
	• Prolonged bleeding after dental procedures that injure soft tissue or bone
	• Petechiae
	• Hematomas
		• Identification of patients should include:
		  • History of bleeding problems in relatives and of excessive bleeding after surgery or trauma, etc.
		  • Examination findings to include:
		    1. Petechiae
		    2. Hematomas
		  • Screening laboratory tests— possible prolonged partial thromboplastin time, platelet count may be low.
		• Consultation and referral should be provided for diagnosis and treatment and preparation before dental procedures.
		• Type I and many type II cases require the following:
		  • 1-desamino-8-D-arginine vasopressin (desmopression and Amicar)
		  • Local measures (see Table 25-6)
		  • May be treated on an outpatient basis
		• Type III and some type II patients require the following:
		  • Fresh frozen plasma
		  • Cryoprecipitate
		  • Special factor VIII concentrates (retain vWF)
		    1. Humate-P
		    2. Koate HS
		  • Local measures (see Table 25-6)
		• Outpatient treatment is possible on the basis of results of consultation.
		• Avoid aspirin/other NSAIDs, aspirin-containing compounds.
			• No invasive dental procedures should be performed unless the patient has been prepared on the basis of consultation with the hematologist.
			• Most dental procedures including complex restorations can be offered to these patients.
			• Emphasis is on maintaining good oral hygiene, topical fluorides, and diet.
			• Acetaminophen with or without codeine may be used for postoperative pain control.

Potential Medical Problem Related to Dental Care	Oral Manifestations	Prevention of Problems	Treatment Planning Modification(s)
Radiation-Treated Patients (Radiation to Head and Neck)			
Chapter 26 1. Patients treated by irradiation tend to develop the following problems during and just after completion of therapy: a. Mucositis b. Xerostomia c. Loss of taste d. Constricture of muscles (trismus) e. Secondary infections—viral, bacterial, fungal (candidiasis) f. Tooth sensitivity 2. Chronic problems caused by radiation therapy include the following: a. Xerostomia b. Cervical caries c. Osteonecrosis d. Muscle trismus e. Tooth sensitivity f. Loss of taste	• Mucositis • Candidiasis • Xerostomia • Loss of taste • Trismus • Sensitivity of teeth • Cervical caries, cuspal and rampant caries • Osteonecrosis	• Before radiation therapy is started, the dentist should be involved; after a complete examination, the following procedures should be done: • Extract teeth that cannot be repaired. • Extract teeth with advanced periodontal disease. • Perform preprosthetic surgery. • Restore large carious lesions. • Perform surgeries with adequate time for healing, or consider hyperbaric oxygen therapy. • Establish good oral hygiene. • Start daily prescription strength fluoride application with the use of a flexible tray. • Treat endodontically, or extract nonvital teeth. • Treat chronic tooth and jaw infections. • During radiation treatment, the dentist can be involved with the following: • Symptomatic treatment of mucositis (see Appendix C) • Management of xerostomia (see Appendix C) • Prevention of trismus by using mouth opening exercises or physical therapy • Chlorhexidine rinses for plaque control and an antifungal if candidiasis develops (see Appendix C) • Diagnosis and treatment of secondary infection—candidiasis, others (see Appendix C) • Continue daily fluoride treatment. • After radiation treatment, the dentist should ensure the following: • Have patient back for frequent recall appointments (every 3 to 4 months). • Continue emphasis on good oral hygiene. • Treat carious lesions when first detected. • Make every effort to avoid oral infection. • Manage xerostomia (see Appendix C). • Manage chronic loss of taste (see Appendix C).	• Once radiation treatment has been completed and more than 6000 cGy used, every effort should be made to avoid osteonecrosis: • Teeth should not be extracted. • Diseased teeth should be endodontically treated, if indicated. • Aggressive preventive measures are needed to prevent periodontal disease and cervical caries. • Most dental procedures other than extractions and surgical procedures can be done if performed atraumatically and without vascular compromise.

Continued

Dental Management: A Summary—cont'd

Potential Medical Problem Related to Dental Care	Oral Manifestations	Prevention of Problems	Treatment Planning Modification(s)
Patients Receiving Chemotherapy for Cancer *Chapter 26*			

1. Excessive bleeding secondary to bone marrow suppression (thrombocytopenia)
2. Prone to infection as a result of bone marrow suppression (leukopenia)
3. Severe anemia from bone marrow suppression
4. Thrombocytopenia, leukopenia, and anemia are possible complications of underlying cancer.
	• Mucositis
	• Excessive bleeding after minor trauma
	• Spontaneous gingival bleeding
	• Xerostomia
	• Infection
	• Poor healing
		• Before starting chemotherapy, the dentist should:
		• Eliminate gross infection in the following areas:
		  • Periapical
		  • Periodontal
		  • Soft tissue
		• Treat advanced carious lesions.
		• Tooth edges are smooth and not sharp.
		• Remove appliances.
		• Provide oral hygiene instructions.
		• Ensure that in children and young adults, the following issues are addressed:
		  • Mobile primary teeth are removed.
		  • Gingival operculum is removed.
		  • Adequate time is allowed for healing before induction.
		• During chemotherapy, the dentist should:
		  • Consult with oncologist before any invasive dental procedures.
		  • Perform the following if invasive procedures are required:
		    1. Consider antibiotic prophylaxis if WBC is less than 1000/μL or absolute neutrophil count (ANC) is less than 500/μL.
		    2. Consider platelet replacement if platelet count is less than 50,000/μL.
		  • Perform culture and antibiotic sensitivity testing of exudate from areas of infection.
		  • Control spontaneous bleeding with gauze, periodontal packing, and soft mouth guard.
			• Perform only emergency dental treatment during chemotherapy.
			• On the basis of the prognosis of underlying disease, consider limiting dental treatment to only immediate care needs for patients who are being treated in a palliative mode; however, children and adults who are being treated for leukemia may have a very good prognosis, and any indicated dental treatment may be performed; also, many patients with lymphoma may have a good prognosis.

Potential Medical Problem Related to Dental Care	Oral Manifestations	Prevention of Problems	Treatment Planning Modification(s)
		• Use topical fluoride for caries control. • Apply chlorhexidine rinses for plaque and candidiasis control (see Appendix C). • Provide symptomatic relief of mucositis and xerostomia (see Appendix C). • Be aware of and take precautions for bisphosphonate-induced osteonecrosis. • If severe anemia is present, avoid general anesthesia. • Consider modifying home care instructions on the basis of oral status, reduce or stop flossing and brushing if excessive bleeding or tissue irritation results; damp gauze can be used to wipe the gingiva and teeth; solution of water and baking soda can be used to rinse the mouth to clean ulcerated tissues. • Minimize food aversion during chemotherapy—fast before treatment (4 hours), eat novel nonimportant food just before treatment, and avoid nutritionally important foods during posttreatment nausea. • After completion of chemotherapy: • Monitor patient until all adverse effects of therapy have cleared. • Place patient on dental recall program. • Antibiotic prophylaxis is not indicated for these patients on the basis of available evidence; however, need should be decided on an individual patient basis following medical consultation. • Be aware of and take precautions for bisphosphonate-induced osteonecrosis.	

Continued

Dental Management: A Summary—cont'd

Potential Medical Problem Related to Dental Care	Oral Manifestations	Prevention of Problems	Treatment Planning Modification(s)

Seizure Disorder (Epilepsy)
Chapter 27
1. Occurrence of generalized tonic-clonic seizure in dental office
2. Drug-induced leukopenia and thrombocytopenia (phenytoin, carbamazepine, valproic acid)
3. Drug-induced gingival overgrowth that affects periodontal health
	• Gingival overgrowth caused by phenytoin (Dilantin)
	• Traumatic oral injuries
	• Drug-induced erythema multiforme
		• Identify epileptic patient by history, including:
		  • Type of seizure
		  • Age at onset
		  • Cause of seizures
		  • Medications
		  • Regularity of physician visits
		  • Degree of control
		  • Frequency of seizures, last seizure
		  • Precipitating factors
		  • History of seizure-related injuries
		• Well-controlled—normal care can be provided.
		• Poorly controlled—consultation with physician; medication change may be required.
		• Be awarene of adverse effects of anticonvulsants.
		• Patients taking valproic acid should avoid aspirin/other NSAIDs.
		• Avoid propoxyphene and erythromycin in patients taking carbamazepine.
		• Use a ligated mouth prop at beginning of the appointment.
			• Maintenance of optimal oral hygiene
			• Surgical reduction of gingival overgrowth, if indicated
			• Replacement of missing teeth with fixed prosthesis as opposed to removable
			• Metal prosthodontic devices used instead of porcelain when possible
			• Protect patient during a seizure, manage airway, and discontinue treatment afterward.

Stroke
Chapter 27
1. Dental treatment could precipitate or coincide with a stroke.
2. Bleeding is caused by drug therapy used to prevent clots.
3. Patient may be unable to understand, verbalize, or transfer easily to the dental chair.
	• An evolving stroke may be associated with unilateral loss of function or sensation.
	• After a stroke, may have unilateral atrophy and one-sided neglect.
		• Identify stroke-prone patient from history (e.g., hypertension, congestive heart failure, diabetes, transient ischemic attacks, age >75 years).
		• Reduce patient's risk factors for stroke (smoking, elevated cholesterol, hypertension).
		• For past history of stroke:
		  • For current transient ischemic attacks—No elective care
		  • Delay elective care for 6 months.
		  • Drug considerations include the following:
		    1. Aspirin and dipyridamole—be aware of potential bleeding problems if another bleeding problem is present.
		    2. Warfarin (Coumadin)—order INR; should be 3.5 or less before invasive procedures are performed.
			• Consider periodic panoramic films to assess carotid patency.
			• Plan is dependent on physical impairment.
			• All restorations should be made easily cleansable—porcelain occlusals should be prevented.
			• Modified oral hygiene aids may be needed.

Potential Medical Problem Related to Dental Care	Oral Manifestations	Prevention of Problems	Treatment Planning Modification(s)
		• Schedule short, morning appointments. • Monitor blood pressure. • Use minimal amount of vasoconstrictor in local anesthetic. • Avoid epinephrine-containing retraction cord. • Provide frequent dental recall and specialized toothbrushes (e.g., Collis curve toothbrush, mechanical brushes) to maintain adequate oral hygiene.	
Parkinson's Disease ***Chapter 27*** 1. Patient may be unable to perform oral hygiene procedures. 2. Patient may have a tremor or may be unable to cooperate during dental treatment.	• Excess salivation and drooling • Muscle rigidity and repetitive muscle movements contribute to poor oral hygiene • Antiparkisonian drugs may cause xerostomia, nausea, and tardive dyskinesia	• Provide frequent dental recall and specialized toothbrushes (e.g., Collis curve toothbrush, mechanical brushes) to maintain adequate oral hygiene. • Salivary substitutes and topical fluoride are beneficial. • Personal care providers should be educated about their role in assisting and maintaining the oral hygiene of these patients (also applies to stroke victims).	• Sedation may be required to overcome muscle rigidity.

Anxiety
Chapter 28
1. Extreme apprehension
2. Avoidance of dental care
3. Elevation of blood pressure
4. Precipitation of arrhythmia
5. Adverse effects and drug interactions with agents used in dentistry
	• Usually none
	• Oral lesions associated with adverse effects of medications
		• Behavioral aspects—the dentist should do the following:
		  • Provide effective communication (be open and honest).
		  • Explain what is going to happen.
		  • Make procedures as "pain-free" as possible.
		  • Encourage patient to ask questions at any time.
		  • Use relaxation techniques such as hypnosis, music, others.
		• Pharmacologic aspects—the dentist should provide the following as indicated:
		  • Oral sedation—alprazolam, diazepam, triazolam
		  • Inhalation sedation—nitrous oxide
		  • Intramuscular sedation—midazolam, meperidine
		  • Intravenous sedation—diazepam, midazolam, fentanyl
		  • Analgesics for pain control—salicylates/ NSAIDs, acetaminophen, codeine, oxycodone, fentanyl
		  • Adjunctive medications—antidepressants, muscle relaxants, steroids, anticonvulsants, antibiotics
			• Postpone complex dental procedures until patient is more comfortable in the dental environment.
			• It is important to develop trust and establish communication with patients with posttraumatic stress disorder.
			• May need to refer for diagnosis and treatment patients with panic attack or phobic symptoms related to dentistry.

Continued

Dental Management: A Summary—cont'd

Potential Medical Problem Related to Dental Care	Oral Manifestations	Prevention of Problems	Treatment Planning Modification(s)
Eating Disorder: Anorexia Nervosa and Bulimia Nervosa ***Chapter 28***			

1. Patients with anorexia are in a state of self-starvation (severe weight loss) and may be subject to hypotension, bradycardia, severe arrhythmia, and death.
2. Bulimic patients are at risk for serum electrolyte disturbances, esophageal or gastric rupture, cardiac arrhythmia, and death.
3. Patients with bulimia may induce vomiting through the use of physical means (finger in throat) or the use of ipecac (may cause myopathy or cardiomyopathy); laxatives and diuretics also are used by bulimics to purge.
4. Some patients may show signs and symptoms of both anorexia and bulimia.
	• With bulimia, the following may be noted:
	  • Dental erosion of the lingual surfaces of teeth (usually maxillary teeth)
	  • Patients with poor oral hygiene may be at increased risk for caries and periodontal disease.
	  • Extensive dental caries (associated with diet—lots of carbohydrates)
	  • Tooth sensitivity to thermal changes
	• With anorexia, the following may be noted:
	  • Intaroral findings are infrequent without concurrent bulimia.
	  • Sialodenosis
	  • If oral hygiene is poor, there is increased risk for caries and periodontal disease.
		• Patients with severe weight loss and no history of cancer or other illnesses, and who are hypotensive should be referred for medical evaluation and management.
		• Attempts should be made to ascertain the cause of dental erosion involving the lingual surfaces of teeth. Consider referral for medical and psychosocial evaluation.
		• Educate the patient as to the serious nature of the complications of anorexia (hypotension, severe arrhythmia, and death) and of bulimia (gastric and esophageal tears, cardiac arrhythmia, and death).
			• Avoid elective dental procedures until the patient is stable from a cardiac standpoint.
			• In general, for both anorexic and bulimic patients, the emphasis should be on oral hygiene maintenance and noncomplex repair, until significant improvement in medical health status has been obtained.
			• Complex restorative procedures should be avoided in bulimic patients until the purging has been controlled. However, crowns may have to be placed to stabilize a tooth or to protect it from thermal symptoms in patients who are still actively purging.

Potential Medical Problem Related to Dental Care	Oral Manifestations	Prevention of Problems	Treatment Planning Modification(s)
Anxiolytic Drugs (for Anxiety Control): Benzodiazepines—Chlordiazepoxide (Librium), Diazepam (Valium), Lorazepam (Ativan), Oxazepam (Serax), Alprazolam (Xanax) *Chapter 28*			

1. Drug adverse effects include the following:
a. Daytime sedation
b. Aggressive behavior
c. Amnesia (older adults)
2. Drug interactions (central nervous system [CNS] depression):
a. Antipsychotic agents
b. Antidepressants
c. Narcotics
d. Sedative agents
e. Antihistamines
f. Histamine H_2 receptor blockers
	• Usually no significant oral findings	• Advise patient not to drive when using these medications.
		• Use reduced dosage in older adults.
		• Limit reduce dosage for patients on other CNS depressant drugs.
		• Use in reduced dosage in patients taking:
		  • Cimetidine
		  • Ranitidine
		  • Erythromycin
		• Do not dispense to patients with narrow angle glaucoma.
			• When using sedative agents, narcotics or antihistamines, reduce dosage or do not use these agents.
			• All dental procedures can be provided to patients on these medications.
			• Use anxiolytic drugs in dentistry for short durations to avoid tolerance and dependency.

Depression and Bipolar Disorders *Chapter 29*			

1. Little or no interest in oral health
2. Factors increasing risk of suicide:
a. Age—adolescent and elderly at greatest risk
b. Chronic illness, alcoholism, drug abuse, and depression
c. Recent diagnosis of serious condition such as AIDS and cancer
d. Previous suicide attempts
e. Recent psychiatric hospitalization
f. Loss of a loved one
g. Living alone or little social contact
3. Taking medications that have significant adverse effects and that may interact with agents used by the dentist
	• Depression—poor oral hygiene and xerostomia associated with agents used to treat depression increase risks for caries and periodontal disease; facial pain syndromes and glossodynia
	• Manic disorder—injury to soft tissue and abrasion of teeth from overflossing and overbrushing
	• Oral lesions associated with the adverse effects of medications used to treat depression and mania
		• If patient appears very depressed:
		  • Ask about thoughts of suicide:
		    1. Does patient have a plan?
		    2. Does patient have the means to carry out the plan?
		  • Immediately refer patient who is suicidal for medical intervention.
		  • If possible, involve family member or relative.
		• Obtain good history, including medications (prescription, herbal, over-the-counter), and avoid using agents that may have significant interactions (see Table 29-7).
		• If history and examination findings suggest presence of significant drug adverse effects, refer patients to their physician.
			• Patients often have little interest in dental health or home care procedures, and poor dental repair is common.
			• Emphasis should be on maintaining the best possible oral health during depressive episodes.
			• Dental treatment should be directed toward immediate needs with elective and complex procedures put off until effective medical management of depression and mania is obtained.

Continued

Dental Management: A Summary—cont'd

Potential Medical Problem Related to Dental Care	Oral Manifestations	Prevention of Problems	Treatment Planning Modification(s)
Schizophrenia ***Chapter 29*** 1. Patient may be difficult to communicate with and uncooperative during dental care. 2. Significant drug adverse effects are common, and agents used by the dentist may interact with medications the patient is taking (see later section on antipsychotic [neuroleptic] drugs).	• Usually none • Oral lesions may be self-inflicted or may develop as adverse effects of medications used to treat the patient (see later section on antipsychotic drugs).	• Have family member or attendant accompany the patient. • Schedule morning appointments. • Avoid confrontational and authoritative attitudes. • Perform elective dental care only if patient is under good medical management. • Consider sedation with diazepam or oxazepam.	• Emphasis is on maintaining oral health and comfort by preventing and controlling dental disease. • Family member or attendant may have to assist patient with home care procedures. • Complex dental procedures usually are not indicated.

Antidepressant Drugs
Chapter 29
1. Drug adverse effects include the following:
a. Xerostomia
b. Hypotension
c. Orthostatic hypotension
d. Arrhythmia
e. Nausea and vomiting
f. Leukopenia, anemia, thrombocytopenia, agranulocytosis
g. Mania, seizures
h. Hypertension (venlafaxine)
i. Loss of libido
	• Usually, no significant oral findings associated with medications, unless the following drug adverse effects are present:
	  • Xerostomia—increases risk for caries, periodontal disease, and mucositis
	  • Leukopenia—infection
	  • Thrombocytopenia—bleeding
		• Identify by medical and drug history patients who are taking any of these medications.
		• Identify patients with significant drug adverse effects:
		  • History
		  • Examination—blood pressure, pulse rate, bleeding, soft tissue lesions, infection
		• Refer patients with significant drug adverse effects.
		• Consult with patient's physician to confirm current status and medications.
		• Minimize effects of orthostatic hypotension:
		  • Change chair position slowly.
		  • Support patients as they get out of the dental chair.
		• Avoid atropine in patients with glaucoma.
		• Use epinephrine with caution and only in small concentrations.
		• Look up specific medication the patient is taking to explore significant adverse effects associated with the drug and possible drug interactions with agents used in dentistry.
			• Avoid elective dental procedures until depression has been managed by medication or behavioral means.
			• Local anesthetic:
			  • Use without vasoconstrictor for most dental procedures.
			  • For surgical or complex restorative procedures:
			    1. Epinephrine is the vasoconstrictor of choice.
			    2. Use 1 : 100,000 concentration of epinephrine.
			    3. Aspirate before injecting.
			    4. In general, do not use more than 2 cartridges.
			• Do not use topical epinephrine to control bleeding or in retraction cord.
			• Provide treatment to deal with xerostomia (see Appendix C).

Potential Medical Problem Related to Dental Care	Oral Manifestations	Prevention of Problems	Treatment Planning Modification(s)
2. Drug interactions include the following: a. Epinephrine • Hypertensive crisis • Myocardial infarction b. Sedative, hypnotics, narcotics, and barbiturates may cause respiratory depression. c. Atropine: Increase intraocular pressure. d. Warfarin metabolism may be inhibited, thus causing bleeding. 3. Patients taking monoamine oxidase inhibitors (MOIs) must avoid foods that contain tyramine (may cause severe hypertension).		• Do not mix the different classes of antidepressant drugs	

Continued

Dental Management: A Summary—cont'd

Potential Medical Problem Related to Dental Care	Oral Manifestations	Prevention of Problems	Treatment Planning Modification(s)
Antimanic (Mood-Stabilizing) Drugs *Chapter 29*			
1. Lithium a. Adverse effects include the following: • Nausea, vomiting, diarrhea • Metallic taste • Xerostomia • Hypothyroidism • Diabetes insipidus • Arrhythmia • Sedation • Seizures b. Drug interactions (toxicity) include the following: • NSAIDs • Diuretics • Erythromycin 2. Valproic acid, carbamazepine, and lamotrigine a. Adverse effects include the following: • Nausea, ataxia, blurred vision • Tremor • Xerostomia • Agranulocytosis (infection) • Platelet dysfunction (bleeding) • Seizures, if abruptly stopped • Stevens-Johnson syndrome • Rare suicide ideation b. Drug interactions (toxicity) include the following: • Erythromycin • Isoniazid • Cimetidine	• Lithium (metallic taste) • Valproic acid and carbamazepine • Oral ulcerations • Bleeding • Infection • Tremor of the tongue	• Identify by medical and drug histories that patients are taking these medications. • Refer to physician when significant drug adverse effects occur. • Avoid the use of NSAIDs and erythromycin, or use at reduced dosage in patients on lithium. • Avoid the use of erythromycin, or use in reduced dosage in patients who are taking valproic acid or carbamazepine. • Patients taking lamotrigine who complain of tingling and itching of the skin should be referred to their physician for possible change in medication, as such symptoms may be the first indication that Stevens-Johnson syndrome may be developing.	• No special modifications are needed in the treatment plan of patients whose condition is well controlled with lithium or anticonvulsant drugs. • Patients with signs or symptoms of lithium toxicity should be referred to their physician for evaluation. • NSAIDs should be avoided or used at reduced dosage for pain control in patients who are taking lithium, to prevent lithium toxicity. • It also should be avoided in patients who are taking valproic acid or carbamazepine. • Patients on the anticonvulsant drugs (valproic acid or carbamazepine) who develop oral ulcerations, infection, or bleeding should be referred for medical evaluation.

Potential Medical Problem Related to Dental Care	Oral Manifestations	Prevention of Problems	Treatment Planning Modification(s)
Antipsychotic (Neuroleptic) Drugs *Chapter 29*			
1. Drug adverse effects include the following: a. Hypotension b. Acute dystonia, akathisia c. Parkinsonism d. Tardive dyskinesia e. Xerostomia, dry eyes f. Dizziness, postural hypotension g. Sexual dysfunction h. Seizures i. Neuroleptic malignant syndrome j. Agranulocytosis 2. Drug interactions include the following: a. Prolong or intensify the actions of the following: • Alcohol • Sedatives, hypnotics, opioids, antihistamines • Anesthetics (general) b. Antiarrhythmics—increase risk of arrhythmia c. Anticonvulsants—reduce effects of neuroleptic drugs d. Antihypertensives—increase risk of hypotension e. Erythromycin—increase serum level of neuroleptic drugs f. Sympathomimetics (epinephrine)—risk for hypotension	• No significant oral findings are associated with these medications, unless the following drug adverse effects are present: • Agranulocytosis—ulceration, infection • Xerostomia—mucositis, caries, periodontal disease • Leukopenia—infection • Thrombocytopenia—bleeding • Tardive dyskinesia—uncontrolled movement of the lips and tongue	• Identification of patients: • Obtain history of mental disorder (patient may be taking antipsychotic medication). • Ask patients to list all drugs that they are taking. • Identify patients with recent onset of adverse effects. • Refer patients with significant adverse effects. • Obtain consultation with patient's physician to confirm current status and medications. • Reduce dosage or avoid: • Epinephrine • Sedatives, hypnotics, opioids, antihistamines • Erythromycin	• Local anesthetic guidelines include the following: • Use without vasoconstrictor for most dental procedures, if possible. • For surgical or complex restorative procedures, epinephrine is the vasoconstrictor of choice: 1. Use 1:100,000 concentration. 2. Aspirate before injecting. 3. In general, limit to two or fewer cartridges. • Do not use topical epinephrine to control bleeding or in the retraction cord. • On the basis of patient needs and wants, any dental procedure can be provided. • Provide treatment to deal with xerostomia, if present (see Appendix C). • Patients with tardive dyskinesia may be difficult to manage; if this adverse effect has just started, refer patients to their physician for evaluation and possible change in medication.

Continued

Dental Management: A Summary—cont'd

Potential Medical Problem Related to Dental Care	Oral Manifestations	Prevention of Problems	Treatment Planning Modification(s)
Somatoform Disorders—Conversion Disorder, Pain Disorder, Factitious Disorder, Others *Chapter 29*			
1. Somatoform disorders: a. Isolated symptoms with no physical cause that do not conform to known anatomic pathways b. Psychological factors involved in the origin c. May serve as a defense to reduce anxiety (primary gain) d. Secondary gain reason for not working, attention from family e. When these patients are followed over time, in 10% to 50%, a physical disease process will become apparent. 2. Factitious disorders: a. Intentional production of physical or psychological signs b. Voluntary production of symptoms without external incentive c. More often seen in men and health care workers	• Examples of oral symptoms that can be related to somatoform disorders: • Burning tongue • Painful tongue • Numbness of soft tissues • Tingling sensations in oral tissues • Pain in the facial region • Oral examples of factitious injuries: • Self-extraction of teeth • Picking gingiva with fingernails • Nail file gingival injury • Chemical burning of the lips and oral mucosa • Thermal burning of lips and oral mucosa	• Refer patients found to have psychological disorders for diagnosis and management, but stay involved from a dental standpoint. • Discuss with patient the possible causes of symptoms, and rule out underlying systemic conditions that could account for the symptoms. • Continue to examine for signs and symptoms that may be related to an underlying systemic or local condition.	• Do not perform dental treatment on the basis of the patient's symptoms, unless a dental cause can be established. • A diagnosis of an oral somatoform disorder should not be made until after a thorough search over time has failed to uncover pathologic findings that could explain the symptoms. • Maintain good oral hygiene and dental repair for the patient, but avoid complex dental procedures until somatoform symptoms have been managed. • Patients may insist that the dentist "do something" to relieve the symptom, such as extraction or endodontic therapy; the dentist must avoid such nonindicated interventions. • Antidepressants and pain medication may be used to comfort the patient.

Potential Medical Problem Related to Dental Care	Oral Manifestations	Prevention of Problems	Treatment Planning Modification(s)
Drug and Alcohol Abuse ***Chapter 30***			
1. Drug abusers may try to obtain controlled substances from the dentist by fraudulent claims or behavior. 2. Patients may be undiagnosed alcohol or drug abusers. 3. Methamphetamine and cocaine abusers are at risk for acute hypertension if epinephrine is administered. 4. Patients with alcohol abuse may have excessive bleeding and unpredictable drug metabolism due to liver disease. 5. Dilated pupils, elevated blood pressure, or cardiac arrhythmias may indicate recent drug use and increases risk for stroke, arrhythmias, and myocardial infarction.	• Drug and/or alcohol abusers may have excessive caries and periodontal disease from oral neglect; amphetamine abuse often leads to extensive caries ("meth mouth"). • Alcohol abuse and associated altered drug metabolism by liver can alter anesthesia effectiveness. • Alcohol abuse is a risk factor for oral cancer, especially when coupled with tobacco use. • Drug and alcohol abuse may lead to xerostomia. • Alcohol abuse may lead to petechiae, ecchymosis, and parotid enlargement.	1. Be alert for signs or symptoms suggestive of substance abuse 2. Discuss concerns with the patient and refer to physician for further evaluation 3. If significant alcohol abuse is present, consider ordering liver function tests prior to surgical procedures 4. For suspected substance abusers, avoid prescribing controlled medications or if needed, prescribe only a limited amount with no refills 5. For recovering substance abusers, avoid prescribing controlled medications, if possible 6. For suspected methamphetamine or cocaine users, avoid the use of epinephrine	• If patient has a history or clinical findings consistent with active drug or alcohol abuse, elective dental care should be deferred and the person should be encouraged to seek medical care. • If oral neglect is evident, patient should be required to demonstrate interest in and ability to care for dentition before any significant dental treatment is undertaken.

PART I

Patient Evaluation and Risk Assessment

CHAPTER

1

Patient Evaluation and Risk Assessment

The practice of dentistry today is far different from that typical of only a decade or two ago, not only in techniques and procedures but also in the kinds of patients encountered. As a result of advances in medical science, people are living longer and are receiving medical treatment for disorders that were fatal only a few years ago. For example, damaged heart valves are surgically replaced, occluded coronary arteries are surgically bypassed or opened by balloons and stents, organs are transplanted, severe hypertension is medically controlled, and many types of malignancies and immune deficiencies are managed or controlled.

Because of the increasing numbers of dental patients, especially among the elderly, who have chronic medical problems, the dentist must remain knowledgeable about a wide range of medical conditions. Many chronic disorders or their treatments necessitate alterations in the provision of dental treatment. Failure to make appropriate treatment modifications may have serious clinical consequences.

The key to successful dental management of a medically compromised patient is a thorough evaluation of the patient followed by a thoughtful assessment of risk to determine whether a planned procedure can be safely tolerated. The fundamental question that must be addressed is whether the benefit of dental treatment outweighs the risk of a medical complication occurring either during treatment or as a result of treatment. This evaluation begins with a thorough review of the medical history, expanded as necessary by discussion of any relevant issues with the patient, and proceeds to identification of drugs or medications that the patient is taking (or is supposed to be taking), examining the patient for symptoms and signs of disease as well as obtaining vital signs, reviewing or obtaining current laboratory test results, and obtaining a medical consultation if needed. All of this information can then be applied to assess the risk for problems related to specific factors identified in the evaluation. This process is summarized in Box 1-1, using an "ABC"-type format.

MEDICAL HISTORY

A medical history must be taken for every patient who is to receive dental treatment. Two basic techniques are used to obtain a medical history. The first technique consists of an interview of the patient (medical model), in which the interviewer questions the patient and then records a narrative of the patient's verbal responses on a blank sheet. The second technique is the use of a printed questionnaire that the patient fills out. The latter approach is most commonly used in dental practice and is very convenient and efficient. It is important, however, that the medical information acquired in this manner be reviewed by the dentist and discussed or clarified with the patient as appropriate, to determine the significance of the findings and any necessary modifications in dental treatment.

Many questionnaires are commercially available today, in both electronic and hard copy versions. Dentists also may develop or modify questionnaires to meet the specific needs of their individual practices. Although medical history questionnaires may differ in organization and detail, most attempt to elicit information about the same basic medical problems. This section presents an overview of such medical conditions, organized by body systems, as well as other conditions and factors of relevance, that specifies the rationale for why certain questions are asked and highlights the significance of positive responses on the questionnaire or in the interview. Detailed information concerning most of these medical problems is found in the specific subsequent chapters.

Cardiovascular Disease

Patients with various forms of cardiovascular disease are especially vulnerable to physical or emotional challenges that may be encountered during dental treatment.

Heart Failure. Heart failure is not a disease per se but rather a clinical syndrome complex that results from an underlying cardiovascular problem such as coronary

BOX 1-1 Dental Management
Summary of Patient Evaluation and Risk Assessment

P

Patient Evaluation/Risk Assessment

- Review **medical history** and engage in direct discussion of relevant issues with the patient.
- Identify all **medications and drugs** being taken, or supposed to be taken, by the patient.
- **Examine** the patient for signs and symptoms of disease, as well as obtaining vital signs.
- Review/obtain recent **laboratory test** results or **images.**
- Obtain a **medical consultation** if the patient has a poorly controlled or undiagnosed problem, or if the patient's health status is uncertain.

Potential Issues/Questions of Concern

A	
Antibiotics	Will the patient need antibiotics, either prophylactically or therapeutically? Is the patient currently taking an antibiotic?
Analgesics	Is the patient taking aspirin or other NSAIDs that may increase bleeding? Will analgesics be needed after the procedure?
Anesthesia	Are there any potential problems or concerns associated with the use of local anesthetic or with vasoconstrictors?
Allergies	Does the patient have an allergy to substances or drugs that may be used or prescribed?
Anxiety	Will the patient need a sedative or anxiolytic?
B	
Bleeding	Is abnormal hemostasis a possibility?
Breathing	Does the patient have any difficulty breathing, or is the breathing abnormally fast or slow?
Blood pressure	Is the blood pressure well controlled, or is it likely to increase or decrease during dental treatment?
C	
Chair position	Can the patient tolerate a supine chair position, or is the patient likely to experience difficulty with rapid position changes?
D	
Drugs	Have any drug interactions, adverse effects, or allergies been associated with any of the drugs being taken by the patient or with drugs that the dentist may use or prescribe?
Devices	Does the patient have prosthetic or therapeutic devices that may require specific considerations in management? (e.g., prosthetic heart valve, prosthetic joint, stent, pacemaker, defibrillator, arteriovenous fistula)
E	
Equipment	Are there any potential problems associated with the use of dental equipment? (e.g., x-ray machine, electrocautery, oxygen supply, ultrasonic cleaner). Are devices such as a pulse oximeter or blood pressure monitor indicated?
Emergencies	Are there any medical urgencies or emergencies that might be anticipated or prevented by modifying care?
F	
Follow-up	Is any follow-up care indicated? Should the patient be contacted at home to assess response to treatment?

heart disease or hypertension. The underlying cause of the heart failure should be identified and its potential significance assessed. Patients with untreated or symptomatic heart failure are at increased risk for myocardial infarction (MI), arrhythmias, acute heart failure, or sudden death, and generally are not candidates for elective dental treatment. Chair position may influence ability to breathe, with some patients unable to tolerate a supine position. Vasoconstrictors should be avoided, if possible, in patients taking digitalis glycosides (digoxin) because the combination can precipitate arrhythmias (see Chapter 6). Stress reduction measures also may be advisable (Box 1-2).

Heart Attack. A history of a heart attack (myocardial infatction; MI) within the very recent past may preclude elective dental care, because during the immediate postinfarction period, patients are at increased risk for reinfarctions, arrhythmias, and heart failure. Patients may be taking medications such as antianginals, anticoagulants, adrenergic blocking agents, calcium channel blockers, antiarrhythmic agents, or digitalis. Some of these drugs may alter the dental management of patients because of potential interactions with vasoconstrictors in the local anesthetic, adverse side effects, or other considerations (see Chapter 4). Stress and anxiety reduction measures may be advisable (see Box 1-2).

BOX 1-2 General Stress Reduction Protocol

- Open communication about fears or concerns
- Short appointments (preferably morning)
- Preoperative sedation: short-acting benzodiazepine (e.g., triazolam 0.125-0.25 mg) 1 hour before the appointment and possibly the night before the day of the appointment
- Intraoperative sedation (N_2O-O_2)
- Profound local anesthesia: use topical before injection
- Adequate postoperative pain control
- Patient contacted on evening of the procedure

Angina Pectoris. Brief substernal pain resulting from myocardial ischemia, commonly provoked by physical activity or emotional stress, is a common and significant symptom of coronary heart disease. Patients with angina, especially unstable or severe angina, are at increased risk for arrhythmias, MI, and sudden death. A variety of vasoactive medications, such as nitroglycerin, β-adrenergic blocking agents, and calcium channel blockers, are used to treat angina. Caution is advised with the use of vasoconstrictors. Stress and anxiety reduction measures may be appropriate (see Box 1-2). Patients with unstable or progressive angina are not candidates for elective dental care (see Chapter 4).

High Blood Pressure. Patients with hypertension (blood pressure greater than 140/90 mm Hg) should be identified by history and the diagnosis confirmed by blood pressure measurement. Patients with a history of hypertension should be asked if they are taking or are supposed to be taking antihypertensive medication. Failure to take medication often is the cause of elevated blood pressure in a patient who reports being under treatment for hypertension. Current blood pressure readings and any clinical signs and symptoms that may be associated with severe, uncontrolled hypertension, such as visual changes, dizziness, spontaneous nosebleeds, and headaches, should be noted. Some antihypertensive medications, such as the nonselective β-adrenergic blocking agents, may require caution in the use of vasoconstrictors (see Chapter 3). The coadministration of calcium channel blockers with macrolide antibiotics (e.g., erythromycin, clarithromycin) can result in excessive hypotension. Stress and anxiety reduction measures also may be appropriate (see Box 1-2). Elective dental care should be deferred for patients with severe, uncontrolled hypertension (blood pressure of 180/110 mm Hg or higher) until the condition can be brought under control.

Heart Murmur. A heart murmur is caused by turbulence of blood flow that produces vibratory sounds during the beating of the heart. Turbulence may result from physiologic (normal) factors or pathologic abnormalities of the heart valves, vessels, or both. The presence of a heart murmur may be of significance in the dental patient in that it may be an indication of underlying heart disease. The primary goal is to determine the nature of the heart murmur; consultation with the patient's physician often is necessary to make this determination. Previously, the American Heart Association (AHA) recommended antibiotic prophylaxis for many patients with heart murmurs caused by valvular disease (e.g., mitral valve prolapse, rheumatic heart disease) in an effort to prevent infective endocarditis; however, current guidelines omit this recommendation on the basis of accumulated scientific evidence. If a murmur is due to certain specific cardiac conditions (e.g., previous endocarditis, prosthetic heart valve, complex congenital cyanotic heart disease), the AHA continues to recommend antibiotic prophylaxis for most dental procedures (see Chapter 2).

Mitral Valve Prolapse. In mitral valve prolapse (MVP), the leaflets of the mitral valve "prolapse" or balloon back into the left atrium during systole. As a result, tight closure of the leaflets may not occur, which can result in leakage or backflow of blood (regurgitation) from the ventricle into the atrium. Not all patients with MVP have regurgitation, however. In previously published guidelines, the AHA recommended that patients with MVP with regurgitation receive antibiotic prophylaxis for invasive dental procedures to prevent infective endocarditis. On the basis of accumulated scientific evidence, however, current guidelines do not include this recommendation (see Chapter 2).

Rheumatic Fever. Rheumatic fever is an autoimmune condition that can follow an upper respiratory β-hemolytic streptococcal infection and may lead to damage of the heart valves (rheumatic heart disease). The AHA currently does not recommend antibiotic prophylaxis for patients with a history of this condition (see Chapter 2).

Congenital Heart Disease. Patients with some forms of severe congenital heart disease are at increased risk for infective endocarditis, with significant morbidity and mortality. These are primarily patients with complex cyanotic heart disease (e.g., tetralogy of Fallot), and those who have had an incomplete surgical repair of a congenital defect, with a residual leak. These patients should receive antibiotic prophylaxis for most dental procedures. For patients with most other types of congenital heart disease the AHA currently does not recommend antibiotic prophylaxis (see Chapter 2).

Artificial Heart Valve. A diseased valve may be replaced with artificial or prosthetic valves. Such replacement valves are associated with a high risk for development of infective endocarditis, with significant morbidity and mortality. Accordingly, the AHA recommends that all patients with a prosthetic heart valve be given prophylactic antibiotics before most dental procedures (see Chapter 2). Patients with an artificial heart valve also may be on anticoagulant medication to prevent blood clots associated with the valve. In such patients, excessive bleeding may be encountered with surgical procedures; it is therefore necessary to determine the level of anticoagulation before any invasive procedure.

Arrhythmias. Arrhythmias frequently are related to heart failure or ischemic heart disease. Stress, anxiety, physical activity, drugs, and hypoxia are some elements that can precipitate arrhythmias. Vasoconstrictors in local anesthetics should be used cautiously in patients prone to arrhythmias, because they may be precipitated by excessive quantities or inadvertent intravascular injections. Stress reduction measures may be appropriate (see Box 1-2). Some of these patients take antiarrhythmic drugs, which may cause oral changes or other side effects. Patients with atrial fibrillation also may be on anticoagulant or antiplatelet medication, which is associated with increased risk for excessive bleeding with surgical procedures. Patients with certain arrhythmias may require a pacemaker or a defibrillator to regulate or pace heart rhythm by artificial means. Patients with such devices do not require antibiotic prophylaxis. Caution is advised with the use of certain types of electrical equipment (e.g., electrocautery, ultrasonic scaler) in patients with pacemakers or defibrillators because of the possibility of intermittent electromagnetic interference with the function of these devices (see Chapter 5). Elective dental care is not recommended for patients with severe, symptomatic arrhythmias.

Coronary Artery Bypass Graft/Angioplasty/Stent. These procedures are performed in patients with coronary heart disease to restore patency to blocked coronary arteries. One of the most common forms of cardiac surgery performed today is coronary artery bypass grafting (CABG). The grafted artery bypasses the occluded portion of the artery. These patients do not require antibiotic prophylaxis. Another method of restoring patency is by means of a balloon catheter, which is inserted into the partially blocked artery; the balloon is then inflated, which compresses the atheromatous plaque against the vessel wall. A metallic mesh stent then may be placed to aid in the maintenance of patency. After stent placement, patients often are prescribed one or more antiplatelet drugs to decrease the risk of blood clots associated with the stents and may therefore be at increased risk for excessive bleeding with surgical procedures. Patients who have had balloon angioplasty with or without placement of a stent do not require antibiotic prophylaxis (see Chapter 4).

Hematologic Disorders

Hemophilia or Inherited Bleeding Disorder. Patients with an inherited bleeding disorder such as hemophilia A or B, or von Willebrand's disease, are at risk for severe bleeding after any type of dental treatment that causes bleeding, including scaling and root planing. These patients must be identified and managed in cooperation with their physician or hematologist. Patients with severe factor deficiency may require factor replacement before invasive treatment, as well as aggressive postoperative measures to maintain hemostasis (see Chapter 25).

Blood Transfusion. Patients with a history of blood transfusions are of concern from at least two aspects. The underlying problem that necessitated a blood transfusion, such as an inherited or acquired bleeding disorder, must be identified, and alterations in the delivery of dental treatment may have to be made. These patients also may be carriers of hepatitis B or C or may have become infected with the human immunodeficiency virus (HIV) and must be identified. Laboratory screening or medical consultation may be appropriate to determine the status of liver function, and, as always, standard infection control procedures are mandatory (see Chapters 10, 18, and 24).

Anemia. A significant reduction in the oxygen-carrying capacity of the red blood cells may result from an underlying pathologic process such as acute or chronic blood loss, decreased production of red blood cells, or hemolysis. Some anemias, such as glucose-6-phosphate dehydrogenase (G6PD) deficiency and sickle cell disease, require dental management modifications. Oral lesions, infections, delayed wound healing, and adverse responses to hypoxia all are potential matters of concern (see Chapter 22).

Leukemia/Lymphoma. Depending on the type of leukemia or lymphoma, status of the disease, and type of treatment, some patients may have bleeding problems or delayed healing, or may be prone to infection. Gingival enlargement can be a sign of leukemia. Some adverse effects can result from the use of chemotherapeutic agents and may require dental management modifications (see Chapter 23).

Taking a "Blood Thinner"/Tendency to Bleed Longer Than Normal. A potentially significant problem is that of a patient with a history of abnormal bleeding, or one who is taking an anticoagulant or an antiplatelet drug. This is of obvious concern, especially if surgical treatment is planned. Information about an episode of unexplained bleeding should be obtained and evaluated. Many reports of abnormal bleeding are more apparent than real; additional questioning or screening laboratory tests may allow the dentist to make this distinction. Patients taking anticoagulant or antiplatelet medication will need to be evaluated to determine the risk for postoperative bleeding. Many patients can be treated without alteration of their medication regimens; however, laboratory testing may help to make this determination (see Chapters 24 and 25).

Neurologic Disorders

Stroke. Disorders that predispose to stroke such as hypertension and diabetes must be identified so that appropriate management alterations can be made. Elective dental care should be avoided in the immediate poststroke period because of an increased risk for subsequent strokes. Vasoconstrictors should be used cautiously. Anticoagulant medications and antiplatelet medications can cause excessive bleeding. Stress and anxiety reduction measures may be necessary (see Box 1-2). Some stroke victims may have residual paralysis, speech impairment, or other physical handicaps. Occasionally, calcified atheromatous plaques may be seen in the carotid arteries on panoramic films; presence of such lesions may be a risk factor for stroke (see Chapter 27).

Epilepsy, Seizures, and Convulsions. A history of epilepsy or grand mal seizures should be identified, and the degree of seizure control should be determined. Specific triggers of seizures (e.g., odors, bright lights) should be identified and avoided. Some medications used to control seizures may affect dental treatment because of drug actions or adverse side effects. For example, gingival overgrowth is a well-recognized adverse effect of diphenylhydantoin (Dilantin). Patients may discontinue the use of anticonvulsant medication without their doctor's knowledge and thus may be susceptible to seizures during dental treatment. Therefore, verification of patients' adherence to their medication schedule is important (see Chapter 27).

Behavioral Disorders/Psychiatric Treatment. Patients with a history of a behavioral disorder or psychiatric illness as well as the nature of the problem need to be identified. This information may help explain patients' unusual, unexpected, or bizzare behavior or complaints such as unexplainable or unusual conditions. Additionally, some psychiatric drugs have the potential to interact adversely with vasoconstrictors in local anesthetics. They also may produce adverse oral effects such as hyposalivation or xerostomia. Other adverse drug effects such as dystonia, akathisia, or tardive dyskinesia may complicate dental treatment. Some patients may be excessively anxious or apprehensive about dental treatment, requiring stress reduction measures (see Box 1-2, and Chapters 28 and 29).

Gastrointestinal Diseases

Stomach or Intestinal Ulcers, Gastritis, and Colitis. Patients with gastric or intestinal disease should not be given drugs that are directly irritating to the gastrointestinal tract, such as aspirin or nonsteroidal antiinflammatory drugs. Patients with colitis or a history of colitis may not be able to take certain antibiotics. Many antibiotics can cause a particularly severe form of colitis (i.e., pseudomembranous colitis), and elderly persons are more susceptible to this condition. Some drugs used to treat gastric or duodenal ulcers may cause dry mouth (see Chapter 11).

Hepatitis, Liver Disease, Jaundice, and Cirrhosis. Patients who have a history of viral hepatitis are of concern in dentistry because they may be asymptomatic carriers of the disease and can transmit it unknowingly to dental personnel or other patients. Of the several types of viral hepatitis, only hepatitis B, C, and D have carrier stages. Fortunately, laboratory tests are available to identify affected patients. Standard infection control measures are mandatory. Patients also may have chronic hepatitis (B or C) or cirrhosis, with associated impairment of liver function. This deficit may result in prolonged bleeding and less efficient metabolism of certain drugs, including local anesthetics and analgesics (see Chapter 10).

Respiratory Tract Disease

Allergies or Hives. Patients may be allergic to some drugs or materials used in dentistry. Common drug allergens include antibiotics and analgesics. Latex allergy also is common, and in patients so affected, alternative materials such as vinyl or powderless gloves and vinyl dam material can be used to prevent an adverse reaction. True allergy to amide local anesthetics is uncommon. Dentists should procure a history regarding allergy by specifically asking patients how they react to a particular substance. This information will help to distinguish a true allergy from intolerance or an adverse side effect that may have been incorrectly identified as an allergy. Symptoms and signs consistent with allergy include itching, urticaria (hives), rash, swelling, wheezing, angioedema, runny nose, and tearing eyes. Isolated signs and symptoms such as nausea, vomiting, heart palpitations, and fainting generally are not of an allergic origin but rather are manifestations of drug intolerance, adverse side effects, or psychogenic reactions (see Chapter 19).

Asthma. The type of asthma should be identified, as should the drugs taken and any precipitating factors or triggers. Stress may be a precipitating factor and should be minimized when possible (see Box 1-2). It often is helpful to ask whether the patient has visited the emergency room for acute treatment of asthma, because this historical detail would indicate more severe disease. A patient who uses an albuterol inhaler for treatment of acute attacks should be instructed to bring it to the dental appointment (see Chapter 7).

Emphysema/Chronic Bronchitis. Patients with chronic pulmonary diseases such as emphysema and chronic bronchitis must be identified. The use of medications or procedures that might further depress respiratory function or dry or irritate the airway should be avoided. Chair position may be a factor; some patients may not be able to tolerate a supine position. Use of a rubber dam may not be tolerated because of a choking or smothering feeling experienced by the patient. The use of high-flow oxygen should be avoided in patients with severe disease because it can decrease the respiratory drive (see Chapter 7). Since cigarette smoking is the cause of most cases of emphysema and chronic bronchitis, the dentist may be able to provide assistance to the patient who is interested in smoking cessation (see Chapter 8).

Tuberculosis. Patients with a history of tuberculosis (TB) must be identified, and information about the treatment received must be sought. A positive result on skin testing means specifically that the person has at some time been infected with TB, not necessarily that active disease is present. Most patients who become positive skin testers do not develop active disease. A diagnosis of active TB is made by chest x-ray imaging, sputum culture, and clinical examination. Some positive skin testers, who are at increased risk for the development of active disease, may be placed on chemophylaxis (e.g., isoniazid) as a preventive measure. Medical treatment for active disease includes the use of multiple medications taken for several months. A history of follow-up medical evaluation is important to detect reactivation of the disease or inadequate treatment. Patients with acquired immunodeficiency syndrome (AIDS) have a high incidence of tuberculosis, so the potential coexistence of these two conditions should be explored (see Chapter 7).

Sleep Apnea/Snoring. Patients with obstructive sleep apnea (OSA) are at increased risk for hypertension, MI, stroke, diabetes, and car crashes and should receive treatment for the disorder. Symptoms and signs include loud snoring, excessive daytime sleepiness, and witnessed breathing cessation during sleep. Patients who present with these symptoms should be referred to a sleep physician specialist for evaluation. Obesity and large neck circumference are common risk factors for the disease. The gold standard for treatment is positive airway pressure; however, many patients cannot tolerate this modality. Other treatment options include use of oral appliances and various forms of upper airway surgery (see Chapter 9).

Musculoskeletal Disease

Arthritis. Many types of arthritis have been identified; the most common of these are osteoarthritis and rheumatoid arthritis. Patients with arthritis may be taking a variety of medications that could influence dental care. Nonsteroidal antiinflammatory drugs, aspirin, corticosteroids, and cytotoxic and immunosuppressive drugs are examples. Tendencies for bleeding and infection should be considered. Chair position may be a factor for physical comfort. Patients with Sjögren syndrome, which may occur with rheumatoid arthritis or independently of that, have a dry mouth that can be very problematic. Patients with Sjögren also are at increased risk for lymphoma. Patients with arthritis may have problems with manual dexterity and oral hygiene. In addition, patients with arthritis may have involvement of the temporomandibular joints (see Chapter 20).

Prosthetic Joints. Some patients with artificial joints are thought to be at increased risk for infection of the prosthesis subsequent to dental treatment, and it is currently recommended that they should receive prophylactic antibiotics before any dental treatment that is likely to produce bacteremia. Included in this category are patients with rheumatoid arthritis, type 1 diabetes, recent joint replacement, and hemophilia, as well as those who are immunosuppressed. Patients with joint prostheses who do not fall into these risk categories are not recommended for antibiotic prophylaxis (see Chapter 20). This is a very controversial issue and the need for prophylactic antibiotics is currently under review by several professional organizations.

Endocrine Disease

Diabetes. Patients with diabetes mellitus must be identified to determine the type of diabetes, how it is being treated, and how well controlled it is. Patients with type 1 diabetes require insulin, whereas type 2 diabetes usually is controlled through diet and/or oral hypoglycemic agents; however, some patients with type 2 diabetes eventually also require insulin. Those with type 1 diabetes have a greater number of complications and are of greater concern regarding management than are those with type 2 diabetes. Symptoms and signs suggestive of diabetes include excessive thirst and hunger, frequent urination, weight loss, and frequent infections. Long-term complications include blindness, hypertension, and kidney failure, each of which also may affect dental management. Patients with diabetes typically do not handle infection very well and also may have exaggerated periodontal disease. Patients who take insulin are at risk for episodes of hypoglycemia in the dental office if meals are skipped or if infection is present (see Chapter 14).

Thyroid Disease. Patients with uncontrolled hyperthyroidism are potentially hypersensitive to stress and α_1-adrenergic effects of sympathomimetics, so the use of vasoconstrictors generally is contraindicated. In rare cases, infection or surgery can initiate a thyroid crisis—a serious medical emergency. These patients also may be easily upset emotionally and intolerant of heat, and they may exhibit tremors. Exophthalmos may be present. Patients with known hypothyroidism usually are taking a thyroid supplement; this medication regimen generally warrants no concern so long as the thyroid hormone level does not become too high. Thyroid cancer is a common form of head and neck cancer that often is curable if detected and treated early. Thus, palpation of the thyroid gland during the head and neck examination is important to detect swelling or nodules (see Chapter 16).

Genitourinary Tract Disease

Kidney Failure. Patients with chronic kidney disease or a kidney transplant must be identified. The potential for abnormal drug metabolism, immunosuppressive drug therapy, bleeding problems, hepatitis, infection, high blood pressure, and heart failure must be considered in management (see Chapter 12). Certain drugs that are nephrotoxic should be avoided. Patients on hemodialysis do not require antibiotic prophylaxis.

Sexually Transmitted Diseases. A variety of sexually transmitted diseases such as syphilis, gonorrhea, human immunodeficiency virus (HIV) infection, as well as AIDS, can have manifestations in the oral cavity because of oral-genital contact or secondary to hematogenous dissemination in the blood or immune suppression. The dentist may be the first to identify these conditions. In addition, some sexually transmitted diseases, including HIV infection, hepatitis B and C, and syphilis, can be transmitted to the dentist through direct contact with oral lesions or infectious blood (see Chapters 10, 13, and 18).

Other Conditions and Factors

Tobacco and Alcohol Use. The use of tobacco products is a risk factor that is associated with cancer, cardiovascular disease, pulmonary disease, and periodontal disease. Patients who use tobacco products should be asked whether they would like to quit and should be encouraged to do so (see Chapter 8). The dentist may be able to provide assistance for patients who are interested in smoking cessation. Excessive use of alcohol is a risk factor for malignancy and heart disease, and may lead to liver disease. The combination of excessive alcohol and tobacco use is a significant risk factor for oral cancer.

Drug Addiction and Substance Abuse. Patients who have a history of intravenous drug use are at increased risk for infectious diseases such as hepatitis B or C, AIDS, and infective endocarditis. Narcotic and sedative medications should be prescribed with caution, if at all, for these patients, because of the risk of triggering a relapse. This caveat also applies to patients who are recovering alcoholics. Vasoconstrictors should be avoided in patients who are cocaine or methamphetamine users because the combination may precipitate arrhythmias or severe hypertension. Patients who abuse prescription narcotics or other controlled substances may engage in "doctor shopping" and drug-seeking activity (see Chapter 30).

Tumors and Cancer. Patients who have had cancer are at risk for recurrence, so they should be closely monitored. Also, cancer treatment regimens including chemotherapeutic agents or radiation therapy may result in infection, gingival bleeding, oral ulcerations, dry mouth, mucositis, and impaired healing after invasive dental treatment, all of which represent significant management considerations. Patients with a history of intravenous bisphosphonate therapy for metastatic bone disease are at risk for osteonecrosis of the jaw, and surgical treatment should be managed cautiously (see Chapter 26).

Radiation Therapy and Chemotherapy. Patients with previous radiation treatment to the head, neck, or jaw must be carefully evaluated, because radiation can permanently destroy the blood supply to the jaws, leading to osteoradionecrosis after extraction or trauma. Irradiation of the head and neck can destroy the salivary glands, resulting in decreased saliva, increased dental caries, and mucositis. Fibrosis of masticatory muscles resulting in limited mouth opening also may occur. Chemotherapy can produce many undesirable adverse effects, most commonly a severe mucositis; however, such changes resolve with cessation of the chemotherapeutic agents (see Chapter 26).

Steroids. Cortisone and prednisone are examples of corticosteroids that are used in the treatment of many diseases. These drugs are important because their use can result in adrenal insufficiency and potentially render the patient unable to mount an adequate response to the stress of an infection or invasive dental procedure such as extractions or periodontal surgery. Generally, however, most routine dental procedures do not require administration of supplemental steroids (see Chapter 15).

Operations or Hospitalizations. A history of hospitalizations can provide a record of past serious illnesses that may have current significance. For example, a patient may have been hospitalized for cardiac catheterization for ischemic heart disease. Another example is that of a patient who is hospitalized for hepatitis C. In both instances, the patient may not have received medical follow-up care for the initial problem, so this aspect of the evaluation may be an indirect but effective way of identifying a current condition. Information about hospitalizations should include diagnosis, treatment, and complications. If a patient has undergone any operation, the reason for the procedure and any associated untoward events such as an anesthetic emergency, unusual postoperative bleeding, infection, or drug allergy should be ascertained.

Pregnancy. Women who are or may be pregnant may need special consideration in dental management. Caution typically is warranted in the taking of radiographs, administration of drugs, and timing of dental treatment. Good dental hygiene is important to maintain during pregnancy, for reasons discussed in Chapter 17.

Current Physician

As part of the medical history, information should be sought regarding the identity of the patient's physician, why the patient is under medical care, diagnoses, and treatment received. If the reason for seeing a physician was the need for a routine physical examination, the patient should be asked whether any problems were discovered and the date of the examination. The name, address, and phone number of the patient's physician should be recorded for future reference. A patient who does not have a physician may require a more cautious approach than a patient who sees a doctor regularly. This is especially true for the patient who has not seen a physician in several years, because of the possibility of the presence of undiagnosed problems. The response to this question also may provide insight into the priorities that the person assigns to health care.

Drugs, Medicines, or Pills

All drugs, medicines, supplements, or pills that a patient is taking, or is supposed to be taking, should be identified and investigated for actions, adverse side effects, and potential drug interactions. The interviewer should specifically mention "drugs, medicines, or pills of any kind," because frequently patients do not list over-the-counter drugs (e.g., aspirin) or herbal medicines. The dentist should have a reliable, up-to-date, comprehensive source for drug information, which may be available in print format or through an on-line database.

The patient's list of medications ("drug history") may provide the only clues to presence of an unreported medical disorder. The patient may have believed that a particular problem was not important enough to mention or may just have omitted the information inadvertently.

The patient may nevertheless report taking medication typically prescribed for a disease. For example, a patient with hypertension may fail to report a history of that problem yet may list medications used to treat hypertension. A patient with previously medically managed condition may have discontinued taking a prescribed medication owing to cost or other reasons, and questioning should uncover this possibility.

Functional Capacity

In addition to asking patients about specific diagnoses, it also is important to ask some screening questions regarding the ability of the patient to engage in normal physical activity (functional capacity). Ability to perform common daily tasks can be expressed in metabolic equivalents of tasks (METs), which quantify the body's use of oxygen. Thus, the patient's ability to meet MET levels as determined for specific activities reflects general physical status. An MET is a unit of oxygen consumption; 1 MET equals 3.5 mL of oxygen per kg of body weight per minute at rest.[1] It has been shown that the risk for occurrence of a serious perioperative cardiovascular event (e.g., MI, heart failure) is increased in patients who are unable to meet a 4-MET demand during normal daily activity.[2] Daily activities requiring 4 METs include level walking at 4 miles/hour or climbing a flight of stairs. Activities requiring greater than 10 METs include swimming and singles tennis. An exercise capacity of 10 to 13 METs indicates excellent physical conditioning. Thus, a patient who reports an inability to walk up a flight of stairs without shortness of breath, fatigue, or chest pain may be at increased risk for medical complications during dental treatment, especially when such limitation is combined with other risk factors.

PHYSICAL EXAMINATION

In addition to a medical history, the dental patient should be afforded the benefits of a simple, abbreviated physical examination to detect signs or symptoms of disease or adverse treatment outcomes. This evaluation should include assessment of general appearance, measurement of vital signs, and an examination of the head and neck.

General Appearance

Much can be learned about the patient's state of health from a purposeful but tactful visual inspection. Careful observation can lead to awareness and recognition of abnormal or unusual features or medical conditions that may exist and may influence the provision of dental care. This survey consists of an assessment of the general appearance of the patient and inspection of exposed body areas, including skin, nails, face, eyes, nose, ears, and neck. Each visually accessible area may demonstrate peculiarities that can signal underlying systemic disease or abnormalities.

The patient's outward appearance and movement also can give an indication of general state of health and well-being. Examples of possible trouble are a wasted, cachectic appearance; a lethargic demeanor; ill-kempt, dirty clothing and hair; body odors; a staggering or halting gait; extreme thinness or obesity; bent posture; and difficulty breathing. The dentist should remain sensitive to breath odors which may be associated with disease such as acetone associated with diabetes, ammonia associated with renal failure, putrefaction of pulmonary infections, and alcohol, possibly associated with alcohol abuse or subsequent liver disease.

Skin and Nails. The skin is the largest organ of the body; usually, large areas of skin are exposed and accessible for inspection. Changes in the skin and nails frequently are associated with systemic disease. For example, cyanosis can indicate cardiac or pulmonary insufficiency, yellowing (jaundice) may be caused by liver disease, pigmentation may be associated with hormonal abnormalities, and petechiae or ecchymoses can be a sign of a blood dyscrasia or a bleeding disorder (Figure 1-1). Alterations in the fingernails, such as clubbing (seen in cardiopulmonary insufficiency) (Figure 1-2), white discoloration (seen in cirrhosis), yellowing (from malignancy), and splinter hemorrhages (from infective endocarditis), usually are caused by chronic disorders. The dorsal surfaces of the hands are common sites for actinic keratosis and basal cell carcinomas, as are the bridge of the nose, infraorbital regions, and the ears (Figure 1-3). A raised, darkly pigmented lesion with irregular borders may be a melanoma.

Face. The shape and symmetry of the face are abnormal in a variety of syndromes and conditions. Well-recognized examples are the coarse and enlarged features of acromegaly (Figure 1-4), moon facies in Cushing syndrome

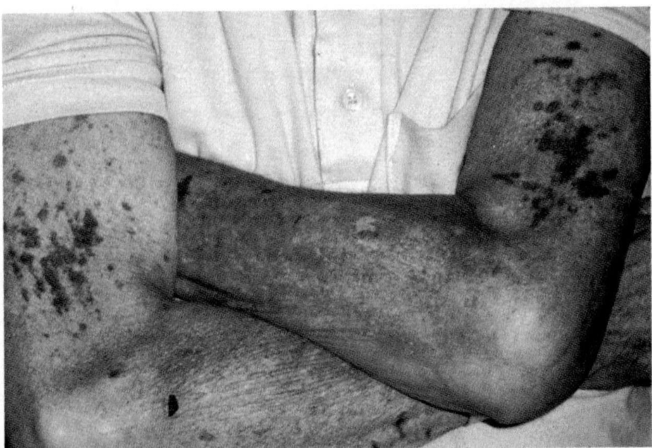

FIGURE 1-1 Petechiae and ecchymosis in a patient that may signal a bleeding disorder. *(Courtesy Robert Henry, DMD, Lexington, Kentucky.)*

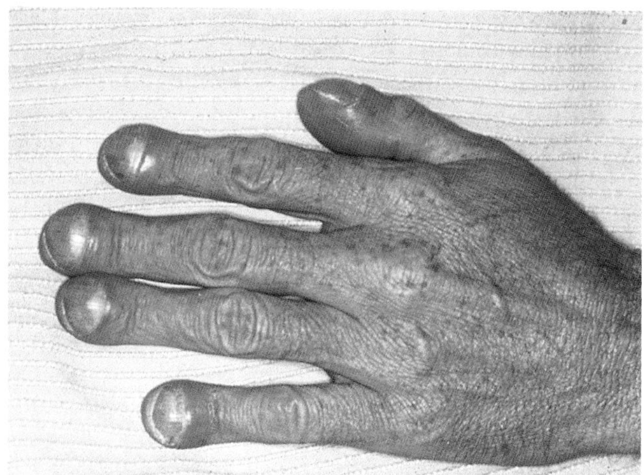

FIGURE 1-2 Clubbing of digits and nails may be associated with cardiopulmonary insufficiency.

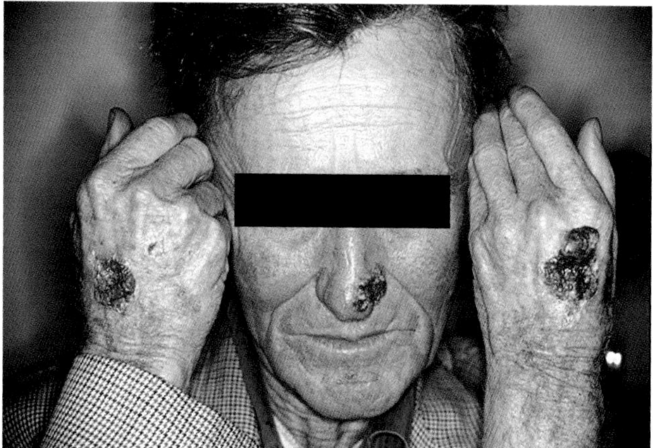

FIGURE 1-3 Basal cell carcinomas of the dorsum of the hands and the ala of the nose.

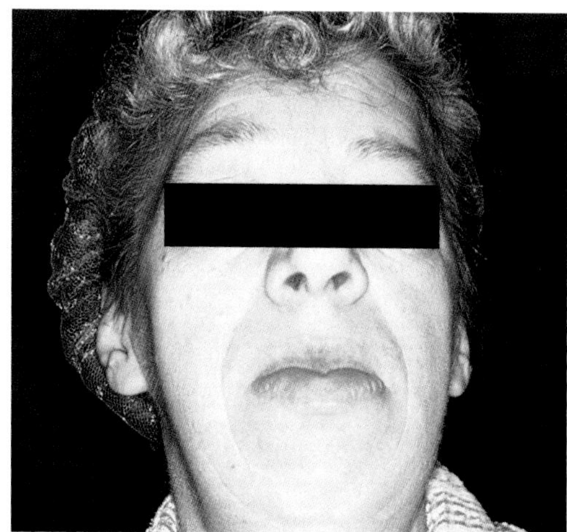

FIGURE 1-4 Patient with acromegaly.

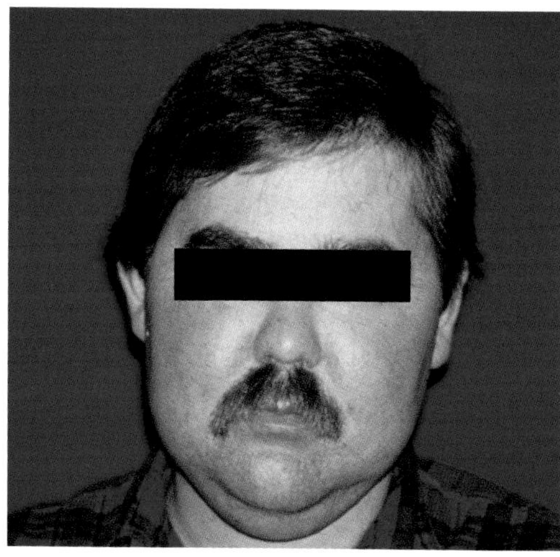

FIGURE 1-5 Patient who acquired cushingoid facies after several weeks of prednisone administration. *(From Bricker SL, Langlais RP, Miller CS:* Oral diagnosis, oral medicine, and treatment planning, *ed 2, Hamilton, Ontario, 2002, BC Decker.)*

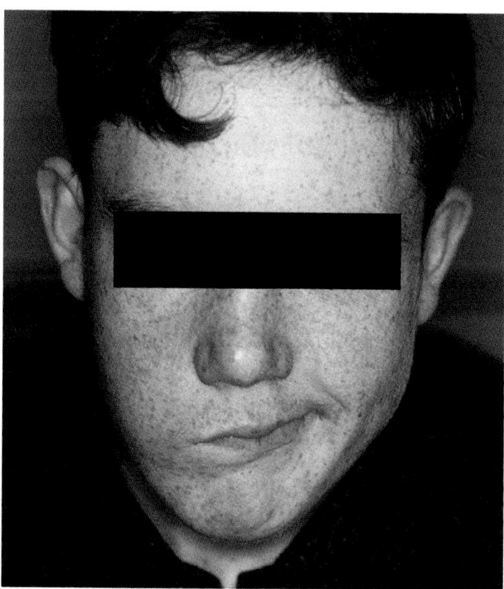

FIGURE 1-6 Unilateral facial paralysis in a patient with Bell's palsy.

(Figure 1-5), and the unilateral paralysis of Bell's palsy (Figure 1-6).

Eyes. The eyes can be sensitive indicators of systemic disease and should therefore be closely inspected. Patients who wear glasses should be requested to remove them during examination of the head and neck, to allow examination of the skin beneath them. Hyperthyroidism may produce a characteristic lid retraction, resulting in a wide-eyed stare (Figure 1-7). Xanthomas of the eyelids frequently are associated with hypercholesterolemia (Figure 1-8), as is arcus senilis in an older person. Scleral yellowing may be caused by liver disease. Reddening of the conjunctiva can result from the sicca syndrome or allergy.

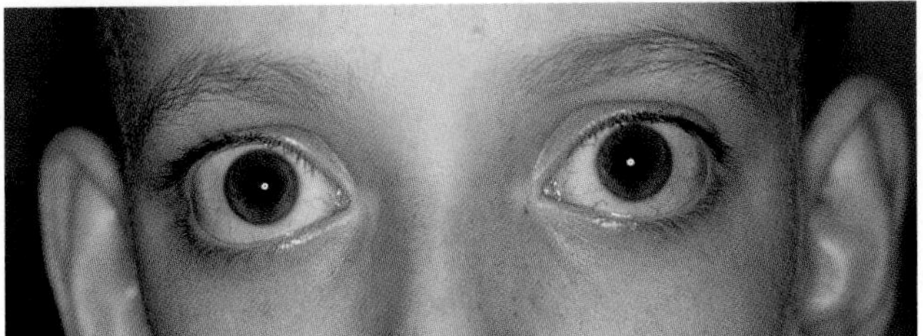

FIGURE 1-7 Lid retraction from hyperthyroidism.

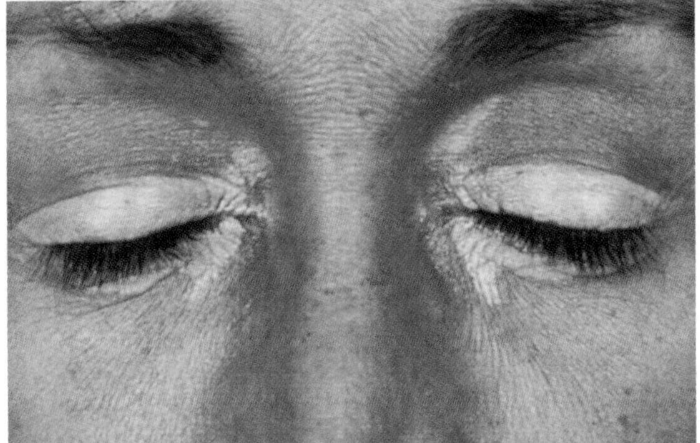

FIGURE 1-8 Xanthomas of the eyelids may signal hypercholesterolemia.

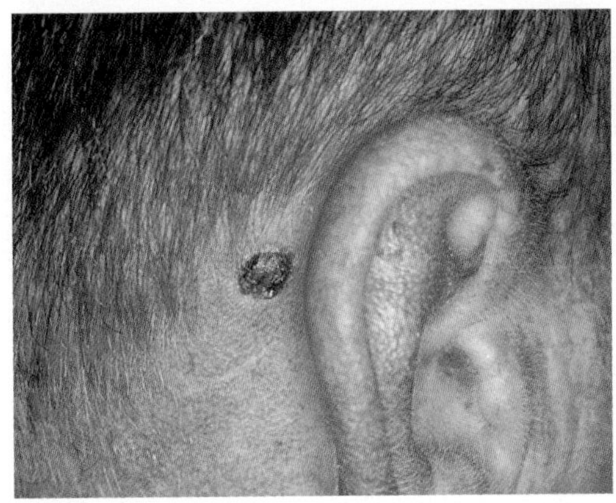

FIGURE 1-9 Malignant melanoma posterior to the ear.

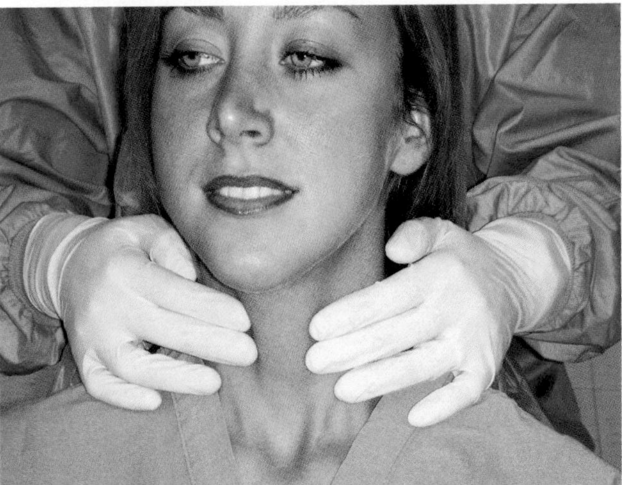

FIGURE 1-10 Bimanual palpation of the anterior neck.

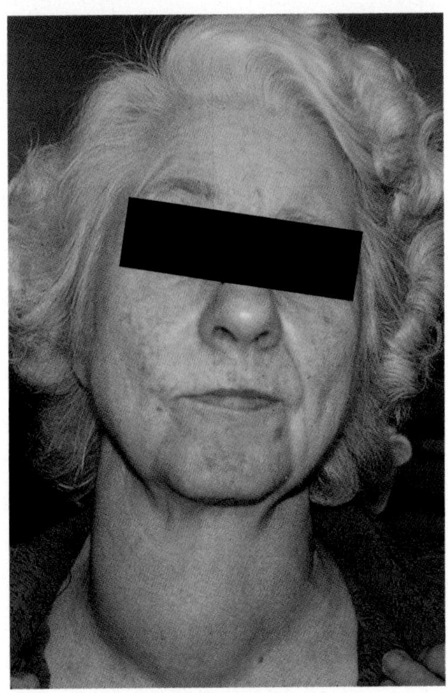

FIGURE 1-11 Midline neck enlargement from a goiter.

Ears. The ears should be inspected for gouty tophi in the helix or antihelix. An earlobe crease may be an indicator of coronary artery disease. Malignant or premalignant lesions (e.g., skin cancer) may be found on and around the ears (Figure 1-9).

Neck. The neck should be inspected for enlargement and asymmetry. Bilateral palpation of the thyroid gland should be performed (Figure 1-10). Depending on location and consistency, enlargement may be caused by goiter (Figure 1-11), infection, cysts (Figure 1-12), enlarged lymph nodes (Figure 1-13), malignancy, or vascular deformities.

Vital Signs

Vital signs consist of blood pressure, pulse, respiratory rate, temperature, height, and weight. In the dental setting, usually only blood pressure and pulse are measured directly. Respiratory rate is determined by observation. Temperature usually is measured when infection or systemic involvement is suspected. Height and weight can be determined by questioning the patient. Abnormal readings may require further investigation or referral.

The benefits of vital sign measurement during an initial examination are twofold. First, the establishment of baseline normal values ensures a standard of

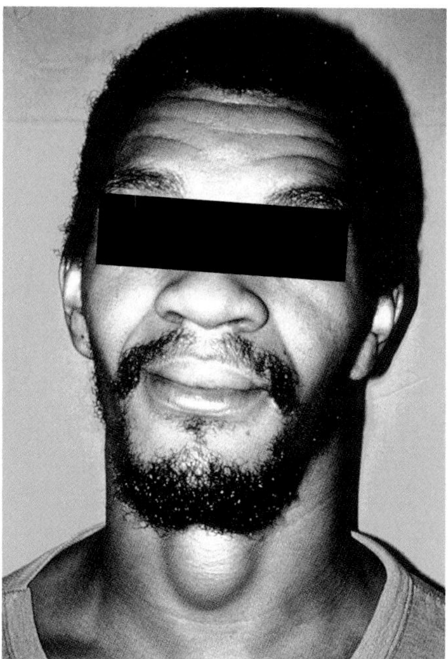

FIGURE 1-12 Midline neck enlargement caused by a thyroglossal duct cyst.

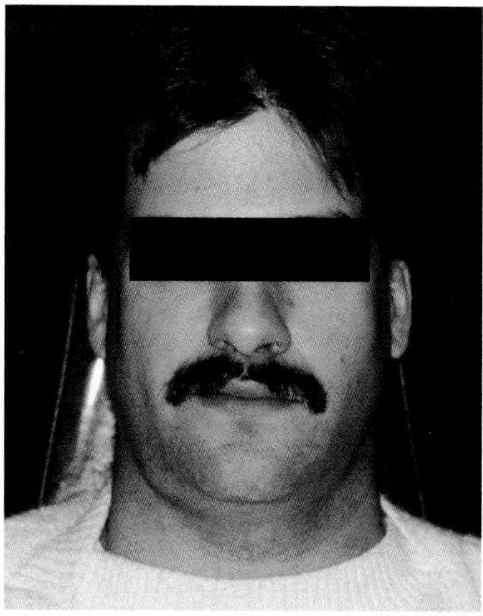

FIGURE 1-13 Enlarged lymph node beneath the right body of the mandible, resulting from a salivary gland infection.

comparison in the event of a medical emergency during treatment. If an emergency occurs, knowledge of the patient's normal values is helpful in determination of the severity of the problem. For example, if the unexpected event is a loss of consciousness accompanied by a drop in blood pressure to 90/50 mm Hg, the level of concern will be entirely different for a patient whose blood pressure normally is 110/65 mm Hg from that for a patient with hypertension whose blood pressure normally is 180/110 mm Hg. In the second instance, the patient may well be in a state of shock.

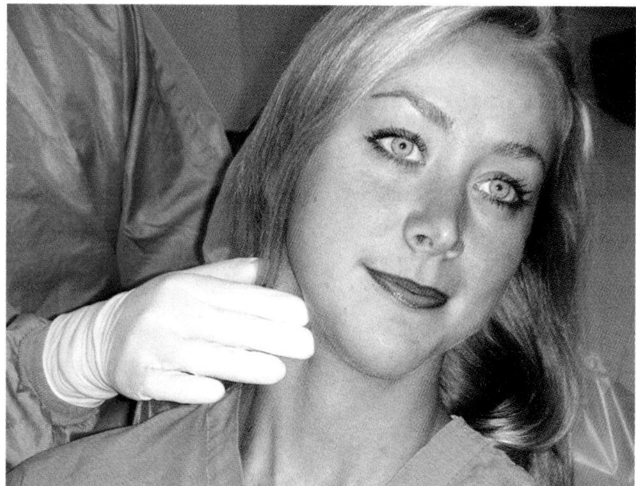

FIGURE 1-14 Palpation of the carotid pulse.

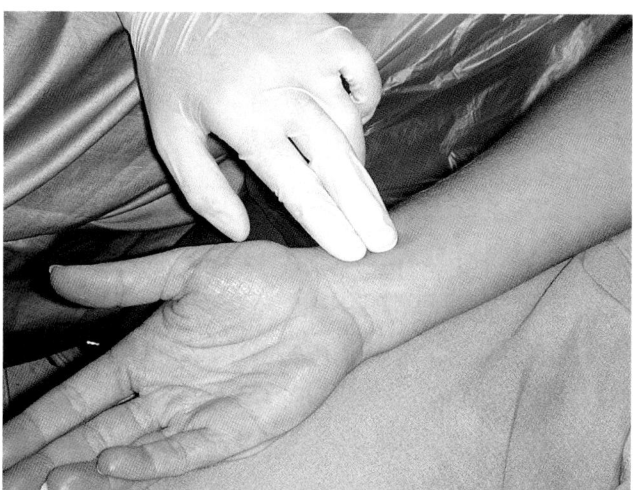

FIGURE 1-15 Palpation of the radial pulse.

A second benefit of vital sign measurement during an examination is in screening for abnormalities, either diagnosed or undiagnosed. For example, if a person with severe, uncontrolled hypertension that was not identified received dental treatment with no management alteration, the potential consequences could be serious. The purpose of this examination is merely detection of an abnormality—not diagnosis, which is the responsibility of the physician. If an abnormal finding is significant, the patient should be referred to a physician for further evaluation.

Pulse. The standard procedure for assessing the pulse rate is to palpate the carotid artery at the side of the trachea (Figure 1-14) or the radial artery on the thumb side of the wrist (Figure 1-15). The pulse should be palpated for 1 minute so that rhythm abnormalities are more likely to be detected. Alternatively, the pulse may be palpated for 30 seconds and the count multiplied by 2. Use of the carotid artery for pulse determination has some advantages. First, the carotid pulse is familiar in clinical practice because of cardiopulmonary resuscitation (CPR) training. Second, it is reliable because it is a large, central artery that supplies the brain; therefore, in emergency situations, it may remain palpable when peripheral arteries in the extremities are not. Finally, the carotid is easily located and palpated because of its size.

The carotid pulse can be palpated along the anterior border of the sternocleidomastoid muscle at approximately the level of the thyroid cartilage. Displacement of the sternocleidomastoid muscle slightly posteriorly allows palpation of the pulse with the examiner's first and middle fingers.

Rate. The average pulse rate in normal adults is 60 to 100 beats/minute. A pulse rate greater than 100 beats per minute is called *tachycardia,* whereas a slow pulse rate of less than 60 beats/minute is called *bradycardia.* An abnormal pulse rate may be a sign of a cardiovascular disorder, but the pulse also may be influenced by anemia, exercise, conditioning, anxiety, drugs, or fever.

Rhythm. The normal pulse is a series of rhythmic beats that occur at regular intervals. When the beats occur at irregular intervals, the pulse is called *irregular, dysrhythmic,* or *arrhythmic.* To detect an arrhythmia, palpation of the pulse for 1 full minute is suggested for accuracy.

Blood Pressure. Blood pressure is determined by indirect measurement in the upper extremities with a blood pressure cuff and stethoscope (Figure 1-16). The cuff should be of the correct width to give an accurate recording. The bladder within the cuff ideally should encompass 80% of the circumference of the arm, with the center of the bladder positioned over the brachial artery. The standard cuff width for an average adult arm is 12 to 14 cm. A cuff that is too small yields falsely elevated values, whereas a cuff that is too large yields falsely low values. Narrower cuffs are available for use with children, and wider cuffs or thigh cuffs are available for use with obese or larger patients. As an alternative for an obese patient, a standard-size cuff can be placed on the forearm below the antecubital fossa, and the radial artery may be palpated so that only the approximate systolic pressure can be determined.[3] The blood pressure cuff should not be placed on the arm with an arteriovenous shunt for hemodialysis. Instruments that measure blood pressure at the wrist or on a finger have become popular; however, their use is not recommended because of potential inaccuracies.[3] The stethoscope should be of good standard quality. The bell end (cup) is preferred for auscultation of the brachial artery; however, use of the diaphragm (flat surface) is common in practice and is acceptable.

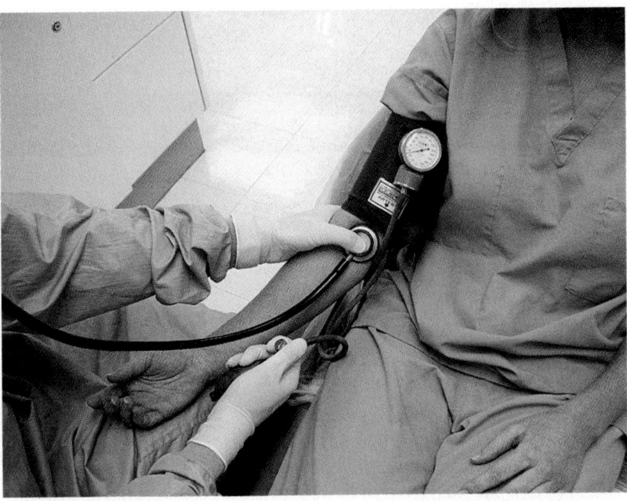

FIGURE 1-16 Blood pressure cuff and stethoscope in place.

The auscultation method of blood pressure measurement has gained universal acceptance. This technique, advocated by the AHA, is as follows[3]: The patient should be comfortably seated without the legs crossed. Before placement of the cuff, the brachial artery is located. The cuff is then placed snugly on the bared upper arm, with the lower border appearing approximately an inch above the antecubital fossa. The standard cuff typically has a mark or arrow that designates the midpoint of the bladder, which is centered above the previously palpated brachial artery (at the medial aspect of the tendon of the biceps). Then, while the radial pulse is palpated, the cuff is inflated until the radial pulse disappears (approximate systolic pressure); it is then inflated an additional 20 to 30 mm Hg. The stethoscope is placed over the previously palpated brachial artery at the bend of the elbow in the antecubital fossa (not touching the cuff), and no sounds should be heard. The pressure release valve is then slowly turned, allowing the needle to fall at a rate of 2 to 3 mm Hg per second. As the needle falls, a point is noted at which beating sounds (Korotkoff sounds) first become audible. The pressure at this point is recorded as the systolic pressure.

As the needle continues to fall, the sound of the beats becomes louder and then gradually diminishes until a point is reached at which a sudden, marked diminution in intensity occurs. The weakened beats are heard for a few moments longer and then disappear altogether (Figure 1-17). The most reliable index of diastolic pressure is the point at which sound completely disappears. Occasionally, muffled sounds can be heard continuously at pressures far below the true diastolic pressure. When this occurs, the initial point of muffling is used as the diastolic pressure measurement. Pulse pressure is defined as the difference between the systolic and diastolic pressures. In older patients with a wide pulse pressure, Korotkoff sounds may become inaudible between systolic and diastolic pressures and then may reappear as cuff deflation is continued. This phenomenon is known as the *auscultatory gap.*[4]

In the average healthy adult, normal systolic pressure ranges between 90 and 120 mm Hg and generally

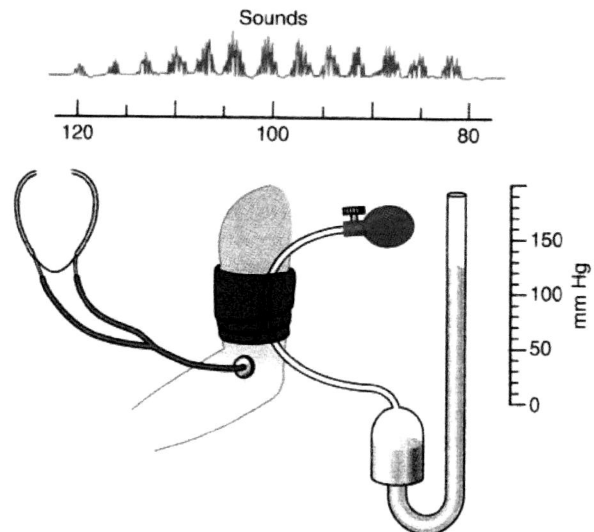

FIGURE 1-17 The typical sound pattern obtained when blood pressure in a normotensive adult is recorded. *(From Guyton AC, Hall JE:* Textbook of medical physiology, *ed 11, Philadelphia, 2006, Saunders.)*

increases with age. Normal diastolic pressure ranges between 60 and 80 mm Hg. Hypertension in adults is defined as blood pressure of 140/90 mm Hg or greater[4] (Table 1-1). It is recommended that blood pressure be measured twice during the appointment, separated by several minutes, and the average taken as the final measurement.

Respiration. The rate and depth of respiration should be noted through careful observation of movement of the chest and abdomen in the quietly breathing patient. The respiratory rate in a normal resting adult is approximately 12 to 16 breaths/minute. The respiratory rate in small children is higher than that in adults. Notice should be made of patients with labored breathing, rapid breathing, or irregular breathing patterns because all may be signs of systemic problems, especially cardiopulmonary disease. A common finding in apprehensive patients is hyperventilation (rapid, prolonged, deep breathing or sighing), which may result in lowered carbon dioxide levels and may cause disturbing symptoms and signs, including perioral numbness, tingling in the fingers and toes, nausea, a "sick" feeling, and carpopedal spasms.

Temperature. Temperature is not usually recorded during a routine dental examination but rather is determined when a patient has febrile signs or symptoms such as might be found with an abscessed tooth or a mucosal or gingival infection. Normal oral temperature is 98.6° F (37° C) but may vary by as much as plus or minus 1° F over 24 hours and usually is highest in the afternoon. Normal rectal temperature is about 1° F higher than oral, and normal axillary temperature is about 1° F lower than oral.

Weight. Patients should be questioned about any recent unintentional gain or loss of weight. A rapid loss of weight may be a sign of malignancy, diabetes, tuberculosis, or other wasting disease, whereas a rapid weight gain can be a sign of heart failure, edema, hypothyroidism, or neoplasm. Obesity is a risk factor for many health problems including heart disease and diabetes.

Head and Neck Examination

Examination of the head and neck may vary in its comprehensiveness but should include inspection and palpation of the soft tissues of the oral cavity, maxillofacial region, and neck, as well as evaluation of cranial nerve function. (See standard texts on physical diagnosis for additional descriptions.)

CLINICAL LABORATORY TESTS

Laboratory evaluation can be an important part of the evaluation of a patient's health status. Whether ordering tests personally or referring the patient to a physician for such testing, the dentist should be familiar with indications for clinical laboratory testing, what tests measure, and what abnormal results mean. When laboratory test

TABLE 1-1 Classification of Blood Pressure (BP) in Adults and Recommendations for Follow-up

BP Classification	Systolic BP (mm Hg)		Diastolic BP (mm Hg)	Recommended Follow-up
Normal	<120	*and*	<80	Recheck in 2 years
Prehypertension	120-139	*or*	80-89	Recheck in 1 year
Stage 1 hypertension	140-159	*or*	90-99	Confirm within 2 months
Stage 2 hypertension	≥160	*or*	≥100	Evaluate or refer to source of care within 1 month For patients with higher pressures (e.g., >180/110 mm Hg), evaluation and treatment referral are needed immediately or within 1 week, depending on the clinical situation and complications

Adapted from the National Heart, Lung, and Blood Institute: The seventh report of the Joint National Committee on Prevention, Detection, Evaluation, and Treatment of High Blood Pressure: the JNC 7 report, *Bethesda, Maryland, US Department of Health and Human Services, Public Health Service, National Institutes of Health, National Heart, Lung, and Blood Institute, August 2004.*

results are reported, they are accompanied by normal values for that particular laboratory. Some indications for clinical laboratory testing in dentistry are

- Aiding in the detection of suspected disease (e.g., diabetes, infection, bleeding disorders, malignancy)
- Screening high-risk patients for undetected disease (e.g., diabetes, AIDS, chronic kidney disease)
- Establishing normal baseline values before treatment (e.g., anticoagulant status, white blood cells, platelets)
- Addressing medicolegal considerations (e.g., possible bleeding disorders, hepatitis B infection)

A comprehensive discussion of laboratory tests is beyond the scope of this chapter; however, Table 1-2 lists several common laboratory tests and ranges of normal values.

PHYSICIAN REFERRAL AND CONSULTATION

On the basis of medical history, physical examination, and laboratory screening, contact with the patient's physician for consultation or referral purposes may be warranted. Requests for information should be made in writing by letter or fax if possible; however, a phone call may be more expedient or convenient. The principal advantages of a phone call are the opportunity to obtain immediate information and the chance to ask follow-up questions. Unfortunately, the physician often is not available to take the call, and a nurse or receptionist must relay the response of the physician. It is imperative that the conversation be recorded in the progress notes to ensure inclusion in the permanent record. In addition, a follow-up fax or letter should be sent to the physician summarizing the conversation and asking that any treatment modifications be faxed to the office. These communications should be entered into the patient's chart. The advantage of a letter or fax is that it provides a written statement of the physician's reply that can simply be added to the patient record.

Potential Issues/Questions of Concern

Based on the information collected during the patient evaluation, several fundamental issues or possible concerns may arise that may have impact on the ultimate dental management plan. These issues should be identified and addressed in systematic fashion in order to determine the need for treatment modifications. The checklist for this purpose presented in Box 1-1 is in "ABC"-type format for ease of use.

TABLE 1-2 Clinical Laboratory Tests and Normal Values

Test	Range of Normal Values
Complete Blood Count	
White blood cells	4500-10,000/mL
Red blood cells: male	4.5-5.9 × 106 10^6/μL
Red blood cells: female	4.5-5.1 × 10^6/μL
Platelets	150,000-450,000/μL
Hematocrit: male	41.5-50.4%
Hematocrit: female	35.9-44.6%
Hemoglobin: male	13.5-17.5 g/dL
Hemoglobin: female	12.3-15.3 g/dL
Mean corpuscular volume (MCV)	80-96 μm^3
Mean corpuscular hemoglobin (MCH)	27.5-33.2 pg
Mean corpuscular hemoglobin concentration (MCHC)	33.4-35.5%
Differential White Blood Cell Count	**Mean %**
Segmented neutrophils	56
Bands	3
Eosinophils	2.7
Basophils	0.3
Lymphocytes	34
Monocytes	4
Hemostasis	
Prothrombin time (PT)	10-13 seconds
Activated partial thromboplastin time (aPTT)	25-35 seconds
Thrombin time (TT)	9-13 seconds

Test	Range of Normal Values
Serum Chemistry	
Glucose, fasting	70-110 mg/dL
Blood urea nitrogen (BUN)	8-23 mg/dL
Creatinine	0.6-1.2 mg/dL
Bilirubin, indirect—unconjugated	0.1-1.0 mg/dL
Bilirubin, direct—conjugated	<0.3 mg/dL
Calcium, total	9.2-11 mg/dL
Magnesium	1.8-3.0 mg/dL
Phosphorus, inorganic	2.3-4.7 mg/dL
Serum Electrolytes	
Sodium	136-142 mEq/L
Potassium	3.8-5.0 mEq/L
Chloride	95-103 mEq/L
Bicarbonate	21-28 mmol/L
Serum Enzymes	
Alkaline phosphatase	20-130 IU/L
Alanine aminotransferase	4-36 μ/L
Aspartate aminotransferase	8-33 μ/L
Amylase	16-120 Somogyi units/dL
Creatine kinase: male	55-170 U/L
Creatine kinase: female	30-135 U/L

Data from McPherson RA, Pincus MR, editors: Henry's clinical diagnosis and management by laboratory methods, *ed 21, Philadelphia, Saunders, 2007, pp 1404-1418.*

RISK ASSESSMENT

Once the patient evaluation (medical history, identification of drugs and medications, clinical examination, review of laboratory test results, consultations) is complete, and the items in the ABC checklist have been considered, the collected data must be thoughtfully assessed to determine whether the patient can safely undergo the planned dental treatment (risk-benefit profile). One widely used method of expressing medical risk is the American Society of Anesthesiologists (ASA) Physical Classification System. This system originally was developed to classify patients according to perioperative risk with general anesthesia; however, it has been adapted for outpatient medical and dental use and for all types of surgical and nonsurgical procedures, regardless of the type of anesthesia used.

Briefly, the classification is as follows:

ASA I Normal healthy patient

ASA II Patient with mild systemic disease (e.g., mild asthma, well-controlled hypertension). No significant impact on daily activity; unlikely to have an impact on anesthesia and surgery.

ASA III Patient with significant or severe systemic disease that limits daily activity (e.g., hemodialysis, class 2 heart failure). Significant impact on daily activity; probable impact on anesthesia and surgery.

ASA IV Patient with severe systemic disease that is a constant threat to life or that requires intensive therapy (e.g., acute MI, respiratory failure requiring mechanical ventilation). Serious limitation of daily activity; likely major impact on anesthesia and surgery.

(ASA V is the category for a moribund patient not expected to survive the next 24 hours.)

The implication is that as the classification level increases (ASA II through IV), so does the risk. Although it generally is helpful to classify patients using the ASA system, the usefulness of this system is limited.

Risk assessment more practically involves the evaluation of four components:

- The *nature, severity, control, and stability of the patient's medical condition* as determined by the initial evaluation
- The *functional capacity or ability* of the patient to respond to a physical or an emotional demand
- The *emotional status* of the patient
- The *type and magnitude of the planned procedure* (invasive or noninvasive)

All factors must be carefully weighed for each patient, to determine an accurate risk profile (Figure 1-18).

Risk assessment cannot be approached as a cookbook exercise. Each situation requires thoughtful consideration to determine whether the benefits of having dental treatment outweigh the potential risks to the patient. For example, a patient may have symptomatic heart failure,

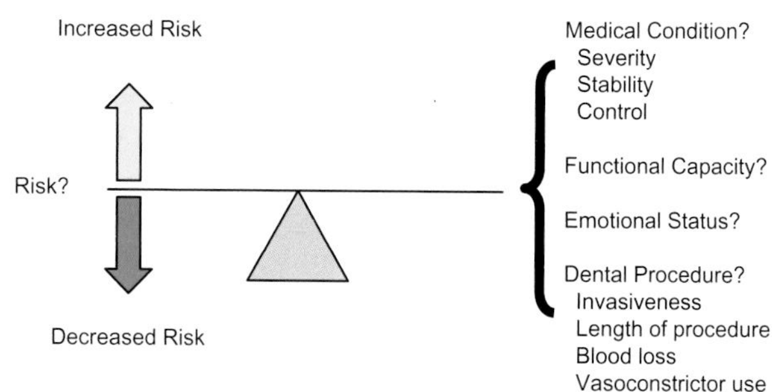

FIGURE 1-18 Risk assessment by weighing of key determining factors.

but the risk is minimal if the planned dental procedure is limited to taking radiographs (noninvasive) and the patient is not anxious or fearful. Conversely, in the same patient, the risk may be significant if the planned procedure is a full mouth extraction (invasive) and the patient is very anxious. Therefore, the dentist must carefully weigh the physical and emotional state of the patient against the invasiveness and trauma of the planned procedure. In general, nonsurgical dental procedures carry lower risk, whereas surgical procedures are associated with higher risk. In addition, the longer the procedure and the greater the blood loss, the greater the risk. Also, more risk is associated with the use of general anesthesia than with local anesthesia. Again, the question that must be answered is whether the expected benefit of the planned dental treatment outweighs the risk of a medical complication, either occurring during treatment or arising as a result of treatment. Fortunately, in most cases, the benefit of needed dental treatment far outweighs any risk; in some instances, however, the risk is great enough to mandate deferral of dental treatment.

TREATMENT MODIFICATIONS

Once it is decided to provide dental treatment (on the ground that its expected benefit outweighs the associated risk of a medical complication), modifications may need to be made in the delivery of such treatment. Fortunately, most treatment modifications are simple to make, as is evident in the following examples:

- Giving prophylactic antibiotics before to an AHA-specified dental procedure in a patient at risk for infective endocarditis
- Determining the international normalized ratio (INR) before surgery in a patient taking warfarin (Coumadin)
- Ensuring food intake before dental treatment in a diabetic patient on insulin

- Prescribing an anxiolytic drug for an anxious patient with stable angina
- Limiting the amount of vasoconstrictor in a patient who takes a nonselective beta blocker
- Administering nitrous oxide–oxygen to an anxious patient with poorly controlled hypertension
- Using an upright chair position for a patient with heart failure
- Avoiding the use of electrosurgery in a patient with a pacemaker
- Avoiding elective radiographs in a pregnant patient
- Using additional local measures for hemostasis in a patient taking sodium warfarin (Coumadin)
- Prescribing antibiotics for periodontal disease after extractions in a patient with poorly controlled diabetes

Thus, through systematic assessment of risk and identification of potential problems, simple modifications in the delivery of dental treatment can be made in an effort to reduce risk to the patient. It should be recognized, however, that risk is always increased when a medically compromised patient is treated; the goal is to reduce that risk as much as possible. The dentist should always try to anticipate possible urgencies or emergencies and be prepared to manage them if they arise.

STRESS AND ANXIETY REDUCTION

In all patients, especially those with medical problems, stress and anxiety control is important and helps to reduce risk (see Box 1-2). Establishment of good rapport and trust is of paramount importance. Allowing the patient to ask questions and encouraging frank and open discussions are equally important. Explaining what is to be done before treatment is initiated often helps put the patient at ease. Short morning appointments may be better tolerated than appointments later in the day. In patients with pronounced anxiety or fear about a planned dental procedure, oral premedication with an anxiolytic or sedative drug 1 hour before an appointment is recommended. In addition, an anxiolytic or sedative can be prescribed the night before the appointment to ensure a good night's rest. One of the most commonly used drugs for this purpose is triazolam, a short-acting benzodiazepine. Other drugs such as diazepam, oxazepam, lorazepam, or hydroxyzine also may be used. If an anxiolytic or a sedative is prescribed, patients should be cautioned not to drive or operate machinery while under the influence of the drug. Intraoperative monitoring by pulse oximetry is recommended for those who are sedated with oral medication. In addition to oral premedication, intraoperative inhalation sedation with nitrous oxide–oxygen may be considered for additional anxiolysis and sedation. This may be especially beneficial for patients with cardiovascular disease because oxygen is continuously administered during the procedure.

Injection of local anesthetic is the procedure that most patients fear; therefore, every effort should be made to avoid pain during administration. Keeping the needle and syringe out of the patient's sight until it is ready to use is important. Topical anesthetic should be applied, followed by slow advancement of the needle and slow injection of the solution after aspiration. Adequate time should then be allowed after injection to ensure adequate anesthesia before the start of work. It is imperative to ensure profound local anesthesia to prevent intraoperative pain.

At the completion of the appointment, it should be determined whether postoperative pain is likely; if so, consideration may be given to administering a long-acting local anesthetic (e.g., bupivicaine) before the patient is dismissed. Appropriate analgesia also should be prescribed. Analgesics also can be started preemptively, before the procedure, and may provide enhanced effectiveness. Instructions should be provided to the patient, along with a phone number to call if the patient needs to contact the dentist. An especially helpful tactic is to call the patient on the evening of the appointment day to see how he or she is doing.

OLDER PATIENTS

Older patients constitute a growing segment of the population. It is estimated that by 2020, one in six Americans will be 65 years of age or older. Compared with younger patients, older patients tend to have more medical problems and therefore take more medications. Half of people older than 65 have two or more chronic illnesses, and one third of all prescription medications are taken by the elderly. Of persons aged 65 or older, only 39% report that their health is either good or excellent. Older patients are unique in that they often suffer from multiple comorbid conditions of variable degree, with an increased frequency of nonspecific signs or symptoms, drug interactions or side effects, frailty, cognitive impairment, and physical disability. It is therefore important to be mindful of these realities and to approach dental care in the older patient with extra consideration and caution.

REFERENCES

1. Fletcher GF, et al: Exercise standards. A statement for healthcare professionals from the American Heart Association Writing Group, *Circulation* 91:580-615, 1995.
2. Fleisher LA, et al: ACC/AHA 2007 guidelines on perioperative cardiovascular evaluation and care for noncardiac surgery: executive summary: a report of the American College of Cardiology/American Heart Association Task Force on Practice Guidelines (Writing Committee to Revise the 2002 Guidelines on Perioperative Cardiovascular Evaluation for Noncardiac Surgery), *Circulation* 116:1971-1996, 2007.
3. Pickering TG, et al: Recommendations for blood pressure measurement in humans and experimental animals: Part 1: blood

pressure measurement in humans: a statement for professionals from the Subcommittee of Professional and Public Education of the American Heart Association Council on High Blood Pressure Research, *Circulation* 111:697-716, 2005.

4. National Heart, Lung, and Blood Institute: *The seventh report of the Joint National Committee on Prevention, Detection, Evaluation, and Treatment of High Blood Pressure: the JNC 7 report,* Bethesda, Maryland, US Department of Health and Human Services, Public Health Service, National Institutes of Health, National Heart, Lung, and Blood Institute, August 2004.

PART II

Cardiovascular Disease

2

Infective Endocarditis

Infective endocarditis (IE) is a microbial infection of the endothelial surface of the heart or heart valves that most often occurs in proximity to congenital or acquired cardiac defects.[1] A clinically and pathologically similar infection that may occur in the endothelial lining of an artery, usually adjacent to a vascular defect (e.g., coarctation of the aorta) or a prosthetic device (e.g., arteriovenous [AV] shunt), is called *infective endarteritis*. Although bacteria most often cause these diseases, fungi and other microorganisms also may cause such infection; thus, the designation *infective* is used in keeping with this multimicrobial origin. The term *bacterial endocarditis* (BE) is in common use, reflecting the fact that most cases of IE are due to bacteria; however, *IE* has become the preferred nomenclature and is therefore used in this chapter.

Previously, IE was classified as acute or subacute, to reflect the rapidity of onset and duration of symptoms before diagnosis; however, this classification was found to be somewhat arbitrary. It has now largely been replaced by a classification that is based on the causative microorganism (e.g., streptococcal endocarditis, staphylococcal endocarditis, candidal endocarditis) and the type of valve that is infected (e.g., native valve endocarditis [NVE], prosthetic valve endocarditis [PVE]). IE also is classified according to the source of infection—that is, whether it is community-acquired or hospital-acquired—or whether the patient is an intravenous drug user (IVDU).

IE is a disease of significant morbidity and mortality that is difficult to treat; therefore, emphasis has long been directed toward prevention. Historically, various dental procedures have been reported to be a significant cause of IE, because bacterial species found in the mouth frequently have been found to be the causative agent. Furthermore, whenever a patient is given a diagnosis of IE caused by oral flora, dental procedures performed at any point within the previous several months typically have been blamed for the infection. As a result, antibiotics have been administered before certain invasive dental procedures in an attempt to prevent infection. Of note, however, the effectiveness of such prophylaxis in humans has never been substantiated, and accumulating evidence more and more questions the validity of this practice.

EPIDEMIOLOGY

IE is a serious, life-threatening disease that affects more than 15,000 patients each year in the United States; the overall mortality rate approaches 40%.[2] IE is a relatively rare disease that occurs most frequently in middle-aged and elderly persons and is more common in men than in women. The incidence rate varies with the population studied. In the general population, the incidence has remained relatively stable over the past 3 decades, ranging between 0.16 and 5.4 cases per 100,000 person-years.[3] A somewhat higher incidence has been reported, however, in more recent studies. A community study in Minnesota reported an incidence of 5 to 7 cases per 100,000 person-years, and a study in the metropolitan Philadelphia area reported an overall incidence of 11.6 per 100,000 person-years.[4,5] In the Philadelphia study, the rate of community-acquired IE was found to be 4.45 per 100,000 person-years, which is comparable to that reported in previous studies; however, the higher overall incidence was attributed to a high prevalence of intravenous drug users (IVDUs) in the population studied.

When populations at enhanced risk are considered, the incidence rate is increased. One study reported the lifetime risk of acquiring IE with various conditions.[6] In that study, the risk ranged from 5 per 100,000 person-years in the general population to 2160 per 100,000 person-years in patients who underwent surgical replacement of an infected prosthetic valve (Table 2-1). Previously, the most common underlying condition predisposing to endocarditis was rheumatic heart disease (RHD) (Figure 2-1); however, in developed countries, the frequency of RHD has markedly declined over the past several decades, and this disorder has become a much less significant factor. Mitral valve prolapse (MVP) (Figure 2-2), which accounts for 25% to 30% of adult cases of NVE, is now the most common underlying condition among patients who acquire IE.[5] Aortic valve disease (either stenosis or regurgitation or both) (Figure 2-3) appears to account for about 30% of cases.[7] Congenital heart disease (e.g., patent ductus arteriosus, ventricular septal defect, bicuspid aortic valve) (Figure 2-4) is the substrate for IE in 10% to 20% of younger adults

TABLE 2-1 Lifetime Risk of Acquiring Infective Endocarditis

Predisposing Condition/Factor	No. of Patients/100,000 Patient-Years
General population	5
Mitral valve prolapse without audible cardiac murmur	4.6
Mitral valve prolapse with audible murmur of mitral regurgitation	52
Rheumatic heart disease	380-440
Mechanical or bioprosthetic valve	308-383
Cardiac valve replacement surgery for native valve	630
Previous endocarditis	740
Prosthetic valve replacement in patients with PVE	2160

PVE, Prosthetic valve endocarditis.
Data from Steckelberg JM, Wilson WR: Risk factors for infective endocarditis, Infect Dis Clin North Am *7:9-19, 1993.*

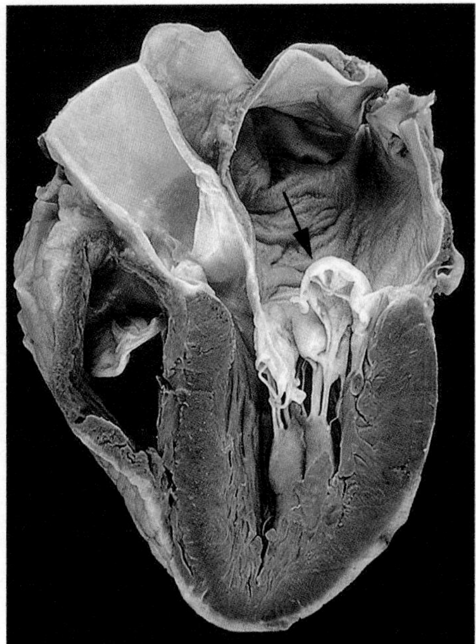

FIGURE 2-2 Prolapse of the posterior mitral valve leaflet into the left atrium. *(Courtesy William D. Edwards, MD, Mayo Clinic, Rochester, Minnesota. From Schoen FJ, Mitchell RN: The heart. In Kumar V, et al, editors:* Robbins and Cotran pathologic basis of disease, *ed 8, Philadelphia, 2010, Saunders.)*

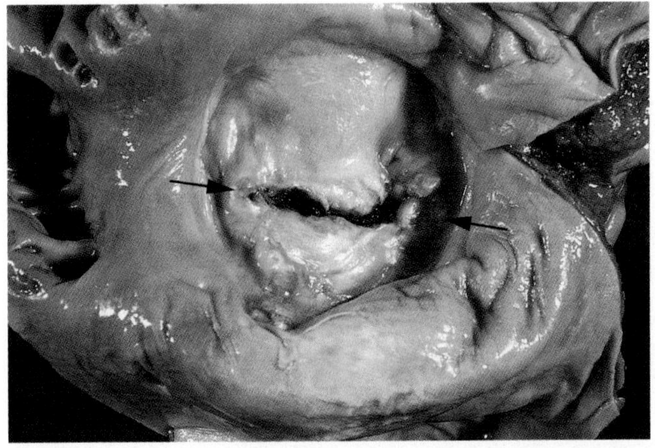

FIGURE 2-1 Mitral stenosis with diffuse fibrous thickening and distortion of the valve leaflets in chronic rheumatic heart disease. *(From Schoen FJ, Mitchell RN: The heart. In Kumar V, et al, editors:* Robbins and Cotran pathologic basis of disease, *ed 8, Philadelphia, 2010, Saunders.)*

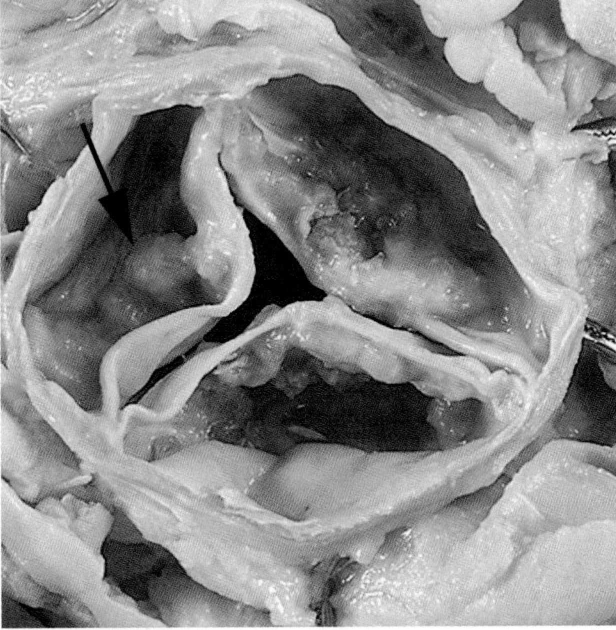

FIGURE 2-3 Calcific aortic stenosis of a previously normal valve. Nodular masses of calcium are heaped up within the sinuses of Valsalva. *(From Schoen FJ, Mitchell RN: The heart. In Kumar V, et al, editors:* Robbins and Cotran pathologic basis of disease, *ed 8, Philadelphia, 2010, Saunders.)*

and in 8% of older adults.[1] Tetralogy of Fallot, the most common type of congenital cyanotic heart disease, generally requiring extensive reconstructive surgery for survival (Figure 2-5), accounts for less than 2% of cases. The incidence of PVE (Figure 2-6) is increasing, and this entity accounts for about one third of all cases of IE. Of note, in many patients with IE, a predisposing cardiac condition cannot be identified (Table 2-2).

The incidence of IE among IVDUs ranges from 150 to 2000 per 100,000 person-years.[8] Conversely, among patients with IE, the concomitant rate of intravenous drug abuse ranges from 5% to 20%.[9] Several unique features characterize the IE in IVDUs. In most cases, the

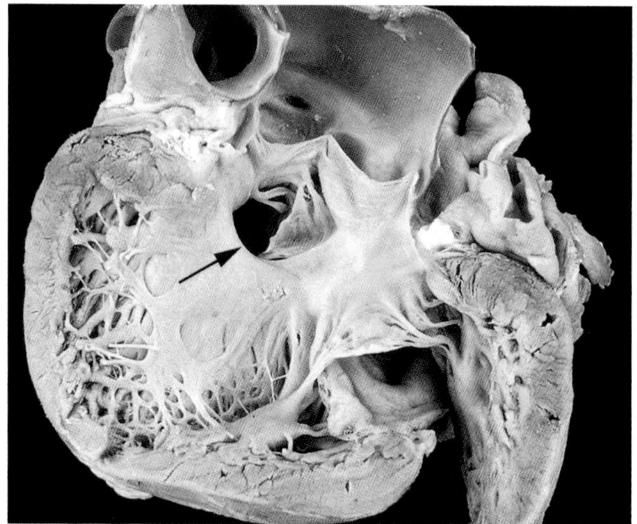

FIGURE 2-4 Gross photograph of a ventricular septal defect (defect denoted by *arrow*). *(Courtesy William D. Edwards, MD, Mayo Clinic, Rochester, Minnesota. From Schoen FJ, Mitchell RN: The heart. In Kumar V, et al, editors:* Robbins and Cotran pathologic basis of disease, *ed 8, Philadelphia, 2010, Saunders.)*

cardiac valves are normal before infection. Such infection usually affects the valves of the right side of the heart (tricuspid), and *Staphylococcus aureus* is the most common pathogen.[10] Thus, because of these unique characteristics, IE in IVDUs historically has not been linked to dental treatment.

ETIOLOGY

About 90% of community-acquired cases of native valve IE are due to streptococci, staphylococci, or enterococci, with streptococci being the most common causative

TABLE 2-2 Predisposing Conditions Associated with Infective Endocarditis (IE)

Underlying Condition	Frequency of IE
Mitral valve prolapse	25-30%
Aortic valve disease	12-30%
Congenital heart disease	10-20%
Prosthetic valve	10-30%
Intravenous drug abuse	5-20%
No identifiable condition	25-47%

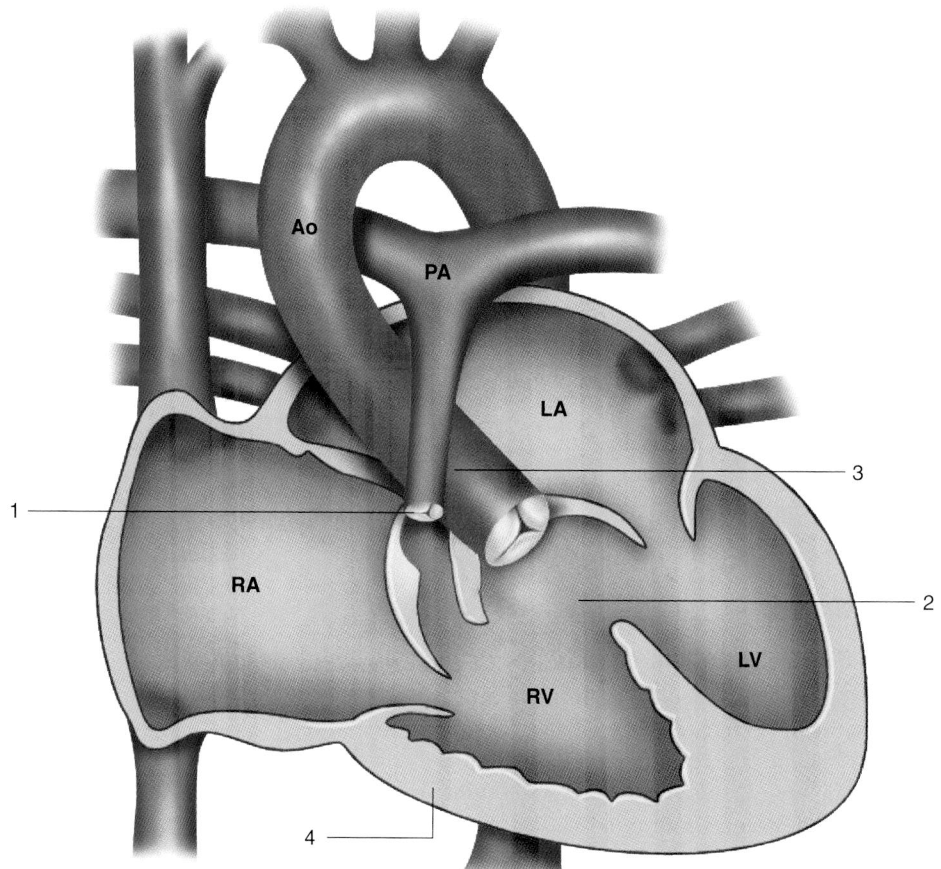

FIGURE 2-5 Tetralogy of Fallot. **1,** Pulmonary stenosis. **2,** Ventricular septal defect. **3,** Overriding aorta. **4,** Right ventricular hypertrophy. *Ao,* Aorta; *LA,* left atrium; *LV,* left ventricle; *PA,* pulmonary artery; *RA,* right atrium; *RV,* right ventricle. *(Redrawn from Mullins CE, Mayer DC:* Congenital heart disease: a diagrammatic atlas, *New York, 1988, Wiley-Liss.)*

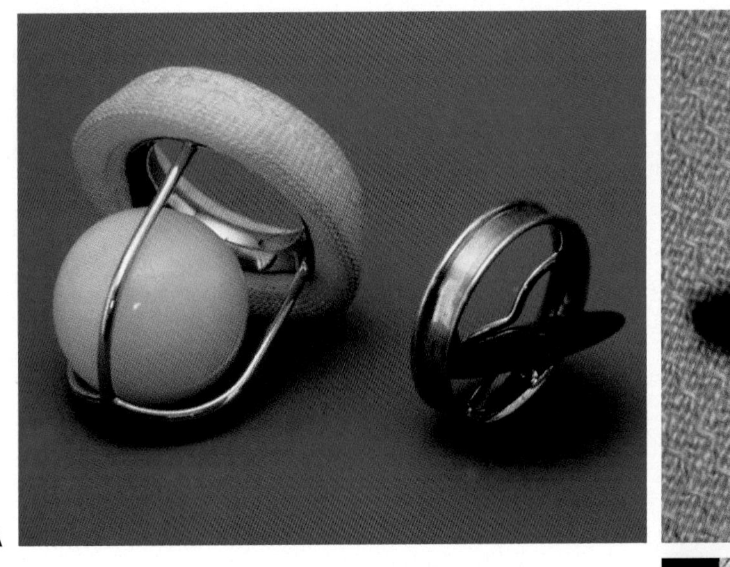

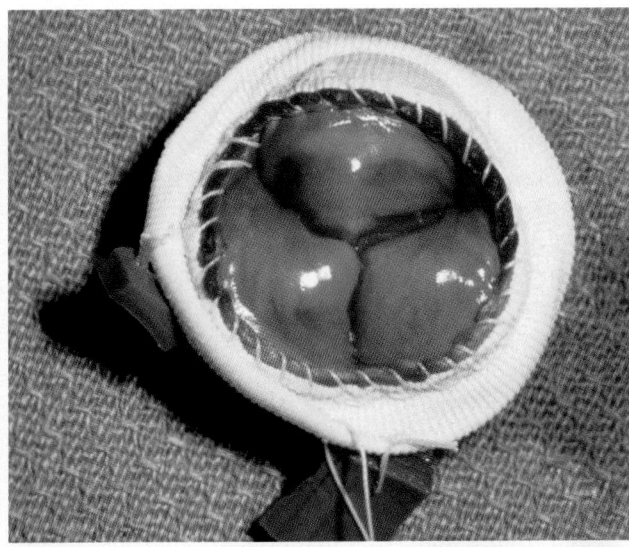

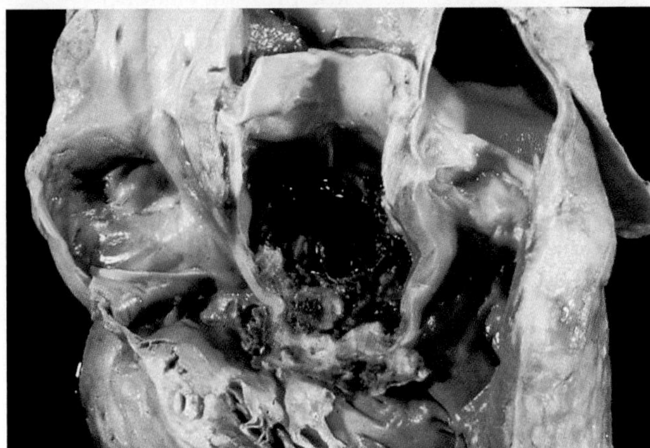

FIGURE 2-6 **Prosthetic cardiac valves. A,** Starr-Edwards caged ball mechanical valve. **B,** Hancock porcine bioprosthetic valve. **C,** Prosthetic valve endocarditis.

organisms.[3] In IE associated with intravenous drug abuse or secondary to health care contact, staphylococci are the most common pathogen identified. Overall, streptococci continue to be the most common cause of IE, but staphylococci have been gaining increasing importance. Viridans streptococci (α-hemolytic streptococci), constituents of the normal oral flora and gastrointestinal (GI) tract, remain the most common cause of community-acquired NVE, without regard for intravenous drug abuse, and they cause 30% to 65% of cases of IE.[1] The species that most commonly cause endocarditis are *Streptococcus sanguis, Streptococcus oralis (mitis), Streptococcus salivarius, Streptococcus mutans,* and *Gemella morbillorum* (formerly called *Streptococcus morbillorum*). Group D streptococci, which include *Streptococcus bovis* and the enterococci *(Enterococcus faecalis),* are normal inhabitants of the GI tract and account for 5% to 18% of cases of IE. *Streptococcus pneumoniae* has decreased in prevalence and now accounts for only 1% to 3% of cases of IE.[11] Group A β-hemolytic streptococci rarely cause IE.[1]

Staphylococci are the cause of at least 30% to 40% of cases of IE; of these, 80% to 90% are due to coagulase-positive *S. aureus.*[2] *S. aureus,* the cause of most cases of acute IE, is the most common pathogen in IE associated with intravenous drug abuse. It also is the most common pathogen in nonvalvular cardiovascular device infections.[12] Of note, *S. aureus* is not a normal constituent of the oral flora. In PVE, staphylococci are the most common pathogens in early and intermediate infections; however, streptococci predominate in late PVE. The proportion of cases of *S. aureus*–related IE appears to be increasing at community-based and university hospitals. This increase appears to be due in large part to increasing health care contact, such as through surgical procedures or the use of indwelling catheters.

Other microbial agents that less commonly cause IE include the HACEK group *(Haemophilus, Actinobacillus, Cardiobacterium, Eikenella, Kingella), Pseudomonas aeruginosa, Corynebacterium pseudodiphtheriticum, Listeria monocytogenes, Bacteroides fragilis,* and fungi.

PATHOPHYSIOLOGY AND COMPLICATIONS

Although the precise mechanism whereby IE occurs has not been fully elucidated, it is thought to be the result of a series of complex interactions of several factors involving endothelium, bacteria, and the host immune response. The sequence of events leading to infection usually begins with injury or damage to an endothelial surface, most often of a cardiac valve leaflet. Although IE can occur on normal endothelium, most cases begin with a damaged surface, usually in proximity to an anatomic defect or prosthesis. Endothelial damage can result from any of a variety of events, including the following[1]:

- Directed flow from a high-velocity jet onto the endothelium
- Flow from a high- to a low-pressure chamber
- Flow across a narrowed orifice at high velocity

Fibrin and platelets then adhere to the roughened endothelial surface, where they form small clusters or masses, resulting in a condition called *nonbacterial thrombotic endocarditis* (NBTE) (Figure 2-7). A similar and frequently indistinguishable condition is found in some patients with systemic lupus erythematosus and is called *Libman-Sacks verrucous endocarditis*. Initially, these masses are sterile and do not contain microorganisms. With the occurrence of a transient bacteremia, however, bacteria can be seeded into and adhere to the mass. Additional platelets and fibrin are then deposited onto the surface of the mass, which serves to sequester and protect the bacteria, which undergo rapid multiplication within the protection of the vegetative mass (Figure 2-8). Once the vegetative process is established, the metabolic activity and cellular division of the bacteria are diminished, which decreases the effectiveness of antibiotics. Bacteria are slowly and continually released from the vegetations and shed into the bloodstream, resulting in a continuous bacteremia; fragments of the friable vegetations break off and embolize. A variety of host immune responses to bacteria may occur. This sequence of events results in the clinical manifestations of IE.

The clinical outcome of IE depends on several factors, including[1]

- Local destructive effects of intracardiac (valvular) lesions
- Embolization of vegetative fragments to distant sites, resulting in infarction or infection
- Hematogenous seeding of remote sites during continuous bacteremia
- Antibody response to the infecting organism, with subsequent tissue injury caused by deposition of preformed immune complexes or antibody-complement interaction with antigens deposited in tissues

Although combination antibiotic and surgical treatment is effective for many patients, complications are common and serious. The most common complication of IE, and the leading cause of death, is heart failure, which results from severe valvular dysfunction. This pathologic process most commonly begins as a problem with aortic valve involvement, followed by mitral and then tricuspid valve infection. Embolization of vegetation fragments often leads to further complications such as stroke. Myocardial infarction can occur as the result of embolism of the coronary arteries, and distal emboli can produce peripheral metastatic abscesses. Pulmonary emboli, usually septic in nature, occur in 66% to 75% of IVDUs who have tricuspid valve endocarditis.[10] Emboli also may involve other systemic organs, including the liver, spleen, and kidney, as well as abdominal mesenteric vessels. The incidence of embolic events is markedly reduced by the initiation of antibiotic therapy.[1] Renal dysfunction also is common and may be due to immune complex glomerulonephritis or infarction.[13]

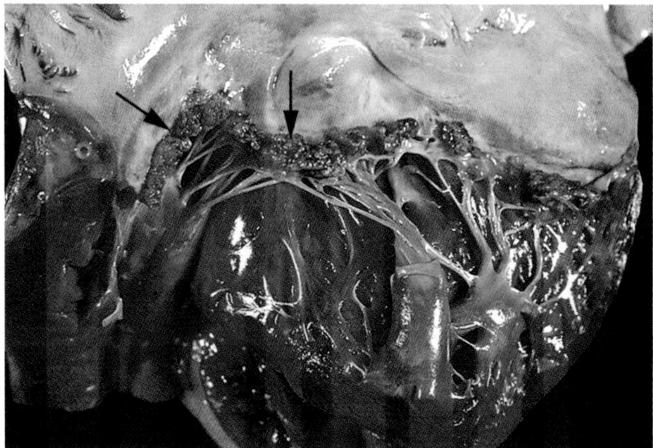

FIGURE 2-7 Nonbacterial thrombotic endocarditis (NBTE). *(From Schoen FJ, Mitchell RN: The heart. In Kumar V, et al, editors:* Robbins and Cotran pathologic basis of disease, *ed 8, Philadelphia, 2010, Saunders.)*

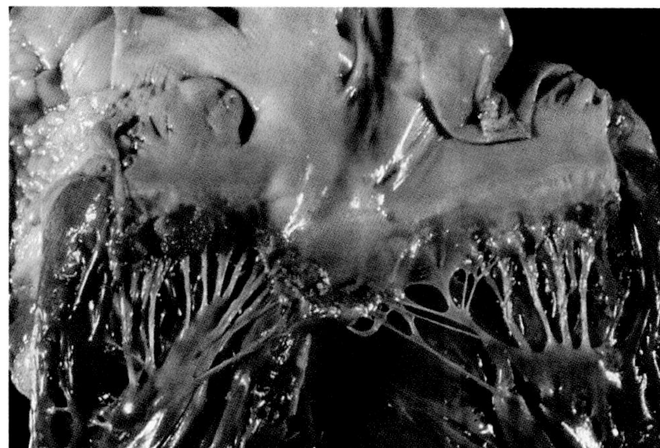

FIGURE 2-8 Viridans streptococcal endocarditis of mitral valve. *(Courtesy W. O'Conner, MD, Lexington, Kentucky.)*

SIGNS AND SYMPTOMS

The classic findings in IE include fever, heart murmur, and positive blood culture, although the clinical presentation may vary. Of particular significance is that the interval between the presumed initiating bacteremia and the onset of symptoms of IE is estimated to be less than 2 weeks in more than 80% of patients with IE.[1,14] In many cases of IE that have been purported to be due to dentally induced bacteremia, the interval between the dental appointment and the diagnosis of IE has been much longer than 2 weeks (sometimes months), so it is very unlikely that the initiating bacteremia was associated with dental treatment.

Fever, the most common sign of IE, occurs in up to 80% to 95% of patients.[3] It may be absent, however, in the elderly or in patients with heart failure or renal failure. New or changing heart murmurs, systolic or diastolic, are found in 80% to 85% of patients.[1] Heart murmurs often are not heard initially in patients who are IVDUs but appear later in the course of the disease. This sequence is characteristic of tricuspid valve IE caused by *S. aureus*. Peripheral manifestations of IE due to emboli and/or immunologic responses are less frequently seen since the advent of antibiotics. These include petechiae of the palpebral conjunctiva, the buccal and palatal mucosa, and extremities (Figure 2-9), Osler's nodes (small, tender, subcutaneous nodules that develop in the pulp of the digits) (Figure 2-10), Janeway lesions (small, erythematous or hemorrhagic, macular nontender lesions on the palms and soles), splinter hemorrhages in the nail beds (Figure 2-11), and Roth spots (oval retinal hemorrhages with pale centers) (Figure 2-12). Other signs include splenomegaly and clubbing of the digits (Figure 2-13). Sustained bacteremia is typical of IE, and blood cultures are positive in most cases. Although up to 30%

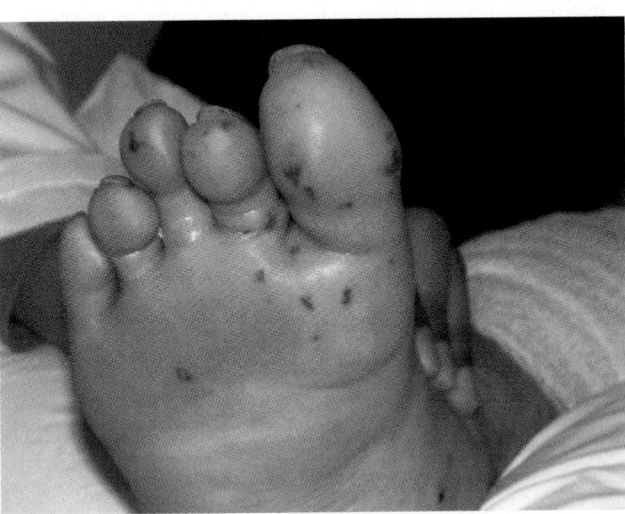

FIGURE 2-9 Petechiae in infective endocarditis. *(From Fowler VG Jr, Bayer AS: Infective endocarditis. In Goldman L, Ausiello D, editors:* Cecil medicine, *ed 23, Philadelphia, 2008, Saunders.)*

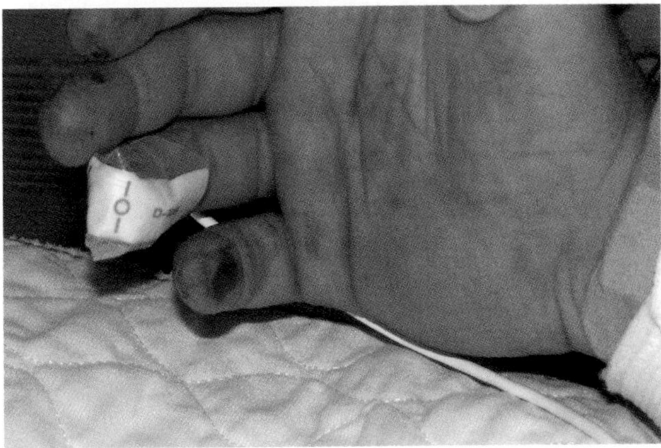

FIGURE 2-10 Osler's node in infective endocarditis. *(From Fowler VG Jr, Bayer AS: Infective endocarditis. In Goldman L, Ausiello D, editors:* Cecil medicine, *ed 23, Philadelphia, 2008, Saunders.)*

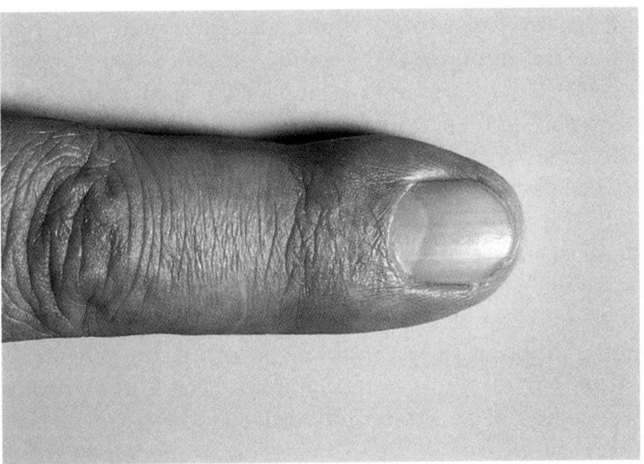

FIGURE 2-11 Splinter hemorrhages of the nail beds in infective endocarditis. *(From Porter SR, et al:* Medicine and surgery for dentistry, *ed 2, London, 1999, Churchill Livingstone.)*

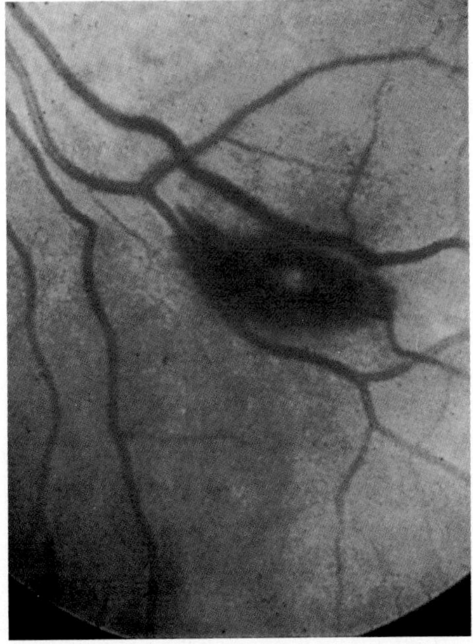

FIGURE 2-12 A Roth spot in the retina in infective endocarditis. *(From Forbes CD, Jackson WF:* Color atlas and text of clinical medicine, *ed 3, Edinburgh, 2003, Mosby.)*

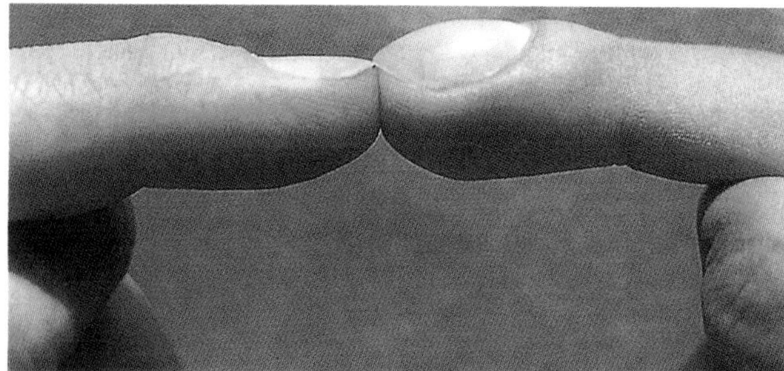

FIGURE 2-13 Nail clubbing may appear within a few weeks of development of IE. *(From Zipes DP, et al, editors:* Braunwald's heart disease: a textbook of cardiovascular medicine, *ed 7, Philadelphia, 2005, Saunders.)*

of cases of IE initially are found to be "culture-negative," when strict diagnostic criteria are used, only 5% of cases are culture-negative.[15] Many patients with negative blood cultures have taken antibiotics before the diagnosis of IE. Three separate sets of blood cultures obtained over a 24-hour period are recommended in the evaluation of a patient for suspected IE.[16]

The diagnosis of IE should be considered for a patient with fever along with one or more of the following *cardinal elements* of IE: a predisposing cardiac lesion or behavior pattern, bacteremia, embolic phenomena, and evidence of an active endocardial process.[1] The clinical presentation in IE is variable, and other conditions can cause similar signs and symptoms. The Duke criteria were developed and later modified to facilitate the definitive diagnosis of IE.[16,17] Application of this set of diagnostic criteria involves ascertaining the presence or absence of major and minor criteria.

Major criteria are two of the aforementioned cardinal elements:

- Positive blood cultures
- Evidence of endocardial involvement (e.g., positive findings on echocardiography, presence of new valvular regurgitation)

Minor criteria include the following factors:

- Predisposing heart condition or IV drug use
- Fever
- Vascular phenomena including embolic events
- Immunologic phenomena
- Microbiologic evidence other than positive blood culture

Definitive diagnosis of IE requires the presence of two major criteria, one major and three minor criteria, or five minor criteria.

LABORATORY FINDINGS

Other than blood culturing, laboratory tests used for the diagnosis and treatment of IE are basic and nonspecific and may include a complete blood count with differential, electrolyte panel, renal function tests, urinalysis, plain chest radiograph, and electrocardiogram (ECG).[1,3] Patients with IE frequently are found to have a normocytic, normochromic anemia that tends to worsen as the disease progresses. The white blood cell count may or may not be elevated. Urinalysis often reveals microscopic hematuria and proteinuria. Appearance on the chest film may be abnormal with evidence of heart failure. ECG may show evidence of conduction block with myocardial involvement or infarction. Other abnormal findings may include an elevated erythrocyte sedimentation rate, increased immune globulins, circulating immune complexes, and positive rheumatoid factor.

Echocardiography, transthoracic or transesophageal, is used to confirm the presence of vegetation in patients suspected of having IE; it has become a cornerstone in the diagnostic process. Echocardiographic evidence of vegetation is one of the major findings included in the Duke criteria.

MEDICAL MANAGEMENT

Before the advent of antibiotics, IE almost always was fatal. This poor outcome has changed dramatically with early diagnosis and the institution of antibiotic therapy or surgical treatment, or both. Although the survival rate has greatly improved, the overall mortality rate still hovers around 40%.[2] However, the mortality rate varies significantly among groups of patients with IE of differing causes. For example, for viridans group streptococcal PVE, the reported mortality rate is approximately 20%, but that for viridans group streptococcal NVE is 5% or less.[11] For *S. aureus* endocarditis in non-IVDU patients, the mortality rate ranges between 25% and 40%, and for fungal endocarditis, the mortality rate exceeds 80%. For IE of the tricuspid valve in IVDUs, the mortality rate is between 2% and 4%.[10] The management of patients with IE requires effective antibiotic therapy and, in cases involving significant structural damage, surgical intervention.

Recently, guidelines for the diagnosis, antimicrobial therapy, and management of infective endocarditis have been revised as an American Heart Association (AHA) Scientific Statement.[11] Most strains of viridans streptococci, "other" streptococci (including *Streptococcus pyogenes*), and nonenterococcal group D streptococci (primarily *S. bovis*) are exquisitely sensitive to penicillins, with a minimal inhibitory concentration (MIC) of less than 0.2 μg/mL. Bacteriologic cure rates of 98% or higher may be anticipated in patients who complete 4 weeks of therapy with parenteral penicillin or ceftriaxone for NVE caused by highly penicillin-susceptible viridans group streptococci or *S. bovis*. The addition of gentamicin sulfate to penicillin exerts a synergistic killing effect on viridans group streptococci and *S. bovis*. A 2-week regimen of penicillin or ceftriaxone combined with single-daily-dose gentamicin is appropriate for uncomplicated cases of endocarditis caused by highly penicillin-susceptible viridans group streptococci or *S. bovis* in patients at low risk for adverse events caused by gentamicin therapy. For patients who are unable to tolerate penicillin or ceftriaxone, vancomycin is the most effective alternative.

Patients with endocarditis arising as a complication after surgery to place prosthetic valves or other prosthetic material that is caused by a highly penicillin-susceptible strain (MIC of 0.12 μg/mL or less) should receive 6 weeks of therapy with penicillin or ceftriaxone, with or without gentamicin for the first 2 weeks. Those with endocarditis caused by a strain that is relatively or highly resistant to penicillin (MIC greater than 0.12 μg/mL) should receive 6 weeks of therapy with penicillin or ceftriaxone combined with gentamicin. Vancomycin therapy is recommended only for patients who are unable to tolerate penicillin or ceftriaxone.

Regardless of whether IE is community- or hospital-acquired, most *S. aureus* organisms produce β-lactamase; therefore, the condition is highly resistant to penicillin G. The drug of choice for treatment of IE caused by methicillin-susceptible *S. aureus* (MSSA) is one of the semisynthetic, penicillinase-resistant penicillins such as nafcillin or oxacillin sodium. For patients with native valve *S. aureus* endocarditis, a 6-week course of oxacillin or nafcillin with the optional addition of gentamicin for 3 to 5 days is recommended. Staphylococcal PVE is treated as for NVE, except that treatment is given for a longer period. For strains resistant to oxacillin, vancomycin is combined with rifampin and gentamicin.

Surgical intervention may be necessary to facilitate a cure for IE or to repair damage caused by the infection. Indications for surgery include moderate to severe heart failure caused by valvular dysfunction, unstable or obstructed prosthesis, infection uncontrollable by antibiotics alone, fungal endocarditis, and intracardiac complications with PVE.

DENTAL MANAGEMENT

Antibiotic Prophylaxis

Dental treatment has long been implicated as a significant cause of IE. Conventional wisdom has taught that in a patient with a predisposing cardiovascular disorder, IE most often was due to a bacteremia that resulted from a dental procedure, and that through the administration of antibiotics before those procedures, IE could be prevented. On the basis of these assumptions, over the past half-century, the AHA has published 10 sets of recommendations for antibiotic prophylaxis for dental patients at risk for acquiring IE[18-26] (Table 2–3). These recommendations, first published in 1955 and revised every few years, varied in terms of identification of risk conditions,

TABLE 2-3 Selected Previous Iterations of American Heart Association–Recommended Antibiotic Regimens (1955-1997) for Dental/Respiratory Tract Procedures in Adults

Year	Primary Regimen for Dental Procedures
1955	600,000 U of aqueous penicillin and 600,000 U of procaine penicillin in oil containing 2% aluminum monostearate administered IM 30 minutes before the operative procedure.
1957	For 2 days before surgery, 200,000 to 250,000 U of penicillin by mouth 4 times a day. On day of surgery, 200,000 to 250,000 U by mouth 4 times a day and 600,000 U aqueous penicillin with 600,000 units procaine penicillin IM 30 minutes before surgery. For 2 days after, 200,000 to 250,000 U by mouth 4 times a day.
1960	*Step 1:* Prophylaxis 2 days before surgery with 600,000 U of procaine penicillin IM on each day. *Step 2:* Day of surgery: 600,000 U procaine penicillin IM, supplemented by 600,000 U of crystalline penicillin IM 1 hour before surgical procedure. *Step 3:* For 2 days after surgery: 600,000 U procaine penicillin IM each day.
1965	Day of procedure: Procaine penicillin 600,000 U, supplemented by 600,000 U of crystalline penicillin IM 1 to 2 hours before the procedure. For 2 days after procedure: Procaine penicillin 600,000 U IM each day
1972	600,000 U of procaine penicillin G with 200,000 U of crystalline penicillin G IM 1 hour before procedure and once daily for 2 days after the procedure.
1977	Aqueous crystalline penicillin G (1,000,000 U IM) mixed with procaine penicillin G (600,000 U IM). Give 30 minutes to 1 hour before procedure, and then give penicillin V 500 mg orally every 6 hours for 2 doses.
1984	Penicillin V 2 g orally 1 hour before procedure; then give 1 g 6 hours after initial dose.
1990	Amoxicillin 3 g orally 1 hour before procedure; then give1.5 g 6 hours after initial dose.
1997	Amoxicillin 2 g orally 1 hour before procedure.

From Wilson W, et al: American Heart Association Rheumatic Fever, Endocarditis, and Kawasaki Disease Committee; American Heart Association Council on Cardiovascular Disease in the Young; American Heart Association Council on Clinical Cardiology; American Heart Association Council on Interdisciplinary Working Group: Prevention of infective endocarditis: guidelines from the American Heart Association: a guideline from the American Heart Association Rheumatic Fever, Young, and the Council on Clinical Cardiology, Council on Cardiovascular Surgery and Anesthesia, and the Quality Care of Outcomes Research interdisciplinary Working Group. Circulation *116(15):1736-54, 2007 Oct 9.*

selection of antibiotics, timing of antibiotic administration, and route of administration of antibiotics. It is important to recognize that although these recommendations were a rational and prudent attempt to prevent life-threatening infection, they were largely based on circumstantial evidence, expert opinion, clinical experience, and descriptive studies in which surrogate measures of risk were used.[14] Furthermore, the effectiveness of these recommendations has never been proved in humans. Recently, accumulating evidence suggests that many of the widely held assumptions on which these previous recommendations were made may not be accurate.

Source and Frequency of Bacteremia

The primary assumption that has driven the previous recommendations was that dental procedures were the source of most of the bacteremias that led to IE; therefore, antibiotics given just prior to dental procedures would prevent IE. Although it is undisputed that many dental procedures can cause bacteremia,[27-31] it also is clear that bacteremia can result from many normal daily activities such as toothbrushing, flossing, manipulation of toothpicks, use of oral water irrigation devices, and chewing[27,30,32-41] (Table 2-4). Because the average person living in the United States makes fewer than two dental visits per year, it follows that the frequency of and exposure to bacteremia are far greater through routine daily activities.[14] It is thus likely that the frequency and cumulative duration of exposure to bacteremia from routine daily events over 1 year are much higher than those resulting from a single dental procedure.[42,43] Accordingly, it is inconsistent to recommend antibiotic prophylaxis for patients undergoing dental procedures (which can be done) but not for these same patients engaging in routine daily activities (which would be impractical and/or impossible).[14]

TABLE 2-4 Reported Frequency of Bacteremia Associated with Various Dental Procedures and Oral Manipulation

Dental Procedure/Oral Manipulation	Reported Frequency of Bacteremia
Tooth extraction	10-100%
Periodontal surgery	36-88%
Scaling and root planing	8-80%
Teeth cleaning	≤40%
Rubber dam matrix/wedge placement	9-32%
Endodontic procedures	≤20%
Toothbrushing and flossing	20-68%
Use of wooden toothpicks	20-40%
Use of water irrigation devices	7-50%
Chewing food	7-51%

Data from Wilson W, et al: American Heart Association Rheumatic Fever, Endocarditis, and Kawasaki Disease Committee; American Heart Association Council on Cardiovascular Disease in the Young; American Heart Association Council on Clinical Cardiology; American Heart Association Council on Interdisciplinary Working Group: Prevention of infective endocarditis: guidelines from the American Heart Association: a guideline from the American Heart Association Rheumatic Fever, Young, and the Council on Clinical Cardiology, Council on Cardiovascular Surgery and Anesthesia, and the Quality Care of Outcomes Research interdisciplinary Working Group. Circulation *116(15):1736-54, 2007 Oct 9.*

Magnitude of Bacteremia

Another assumption often made is that the magnitude of bacteremias resulting from dental procedures is more likely to cause IE than that seen with bacteremias resulting from normal daily activities. No published data support this contention. Furthermore, the magnitude of bacteremia resulting from dental procedures is relatively low (with bacterial counts of fewer than 10^4 colony-forming units/mL), is similar to that of bacteremia resulting from normal daily activities, and is far less than that (10^6 to 10^8 colony-forming units/mL) needed to cause experimental BE in animals.[30,44,45] It also has been shown that in patients with poor oral hygiene, the frequency of positive blood cultures just before dental extraction was similar to that after extraction.[46,47] Thus, although the infective dose required to cause IE in humans is unknown, the number of microorganisms in blood after a dental procedure or associated with daily activities is similarly low, and cases of IE caused by oral bacteria probably result from frequent exposure to low inocula of bacteria in the bloodstream, resulting from routine daily activities and not from a dental procedure.[14] Also noteworthy is that most patients with viridians streptococci IE have not undergone a dental procedure within the 2 weeks before the onset of symptoms.[48-50] These findings imply that emphasis on maintaining good oral hygiene and eradicating dental or oral disease is key to decreasing the frequency of bacteremia produced by normal daily activities. The importance of oral hygiene was demonstrated in recent studies by Lockhart[46] and Brennan[51] and their co-workers, which found that the incidence of bacteremia after toothbrushing was significantly related to poor oral hygiene and gingival bleeding after toothbrushing.

BLEEDING AND BACTEREMIA

Previous AHA recommendations have suggested that on the basis of the likelihood that significant bleeding will be encountered during the procedure, prophylaxis should be provided for some dental procedures but not for others. This specific recommendation often has been confusing for the practitioner and has resulted in conflicting and arbitrary decisions, because it is impossible to predict, with any accuracy, the likelihood that significant bleeding will be encountered during a given dental procedure. To add to the confusion, it has been shown that visible bleeding during a dental procedure is not a reliable predictor of bacteremia.[43] Collective published data suggest that the vast majority of dental office visits result in some degree of bacteremia, and that it is not clear which dental procedures are more or less likely to cause transient bacteremia or to result in a greater magnitude of bacteremia than that caused by bacteremia produced by routine daily activities such as chewing food, toothbrushing, or flossing.[14]

Efficacy of Antibiotic Prophylaxis

The assumption that antibiotics given to at-risk patients before a dental procedure will prevent or reduce a bacteremia that can lead to IE is controversial. Some studies have reported that antibiotics administered before a dental procedure reduced the frequency, nature, or duration of bacteremia,[47,53-56] although others did not.[28,57-61] More recent studies suggest that amoxicillin therapy has a statistically significant impact on reducing the incidence, nature, and duration of bacteria associated with dental procedures, but it does not eliminate bacteremia.[52-54,60] However, no data show that such a reduction caused by antibiotic therapy reduces the risk of or prevents IE. No prospective, randomized, placebo-controlled trials have been conducted to examine the efficacy of antibiotic prophylaxis for preventing IE in patients who undergo a dental procedure; and it is highly unlikely that any such studies will ever be done because of the complex logistical, ethical, and medicolegal issues that would be involved. Some retrospective studies, however, have suggested that prophylaxis is beneficial, but these studies are small in size and report insufficient clinical data.[14] Also, in many of the cases cited in retrospective studies, the time interval between purported occurrence of bacteremia and onset of symptoms was much longer than 2 weeks.

A study from the Netherlands by van der Meer and colleagues[61] investigated the efficacy of antibiotic prophylaxis for preventing IE in dental patients with native or prosthetic cardiac valves. Investigators concluded that dental or other procedures probably caused only a small fraction of cases of IE, and that prophylaxis would prevent only a small number of cases, even if it were 100% effective. In a case control study undertaken by the same authors,[62] among patients for whom prophylaxis was provided, 5 of 20 cases of IE occurred despite administration of antibiotics (for a 75% efficacy rate at best), leading to the conclusion that prophylaxis was not effective. A more recent large, multicenter, case control study was undertaken in the Philadelphia area by Strom and colleagues[50] to evaluate the relationship between antibiotic prophylaxis and cardiac risk factors. These investigators concluded that dental treatment was not a risk factor for IE even in patients with valvular heart disease, and that few cases of IE could be prevented with prophylaxis even if it were 100% effective. Finally, a recent French study[63] estimated that only about 2.6% of cases of IE occurred annually in patients undergoing unprotected dental procedures, and that a "huge number of prophylaxis doses would be necessary to prevent a very low number of IE cases."

Risk of Bacterial Endocarditis Due to Dental Procedures

Although the absolute risk for IE caused by a dental procedure is impossible to measure precisely, the best available estimates are as follows[14]: If dental treatment causes 1% of all cases of IE due to viridans group streptococci annually in the United States, the overall risk in the general population is estimated to be as low as 1 case of IE per 14 million dental procedures. The estimated absolute risk rates for IE caused by a dental procedure in patients with underlying cardiac conditions are as follows: mitral valve prolapse, 1 per 1.1 million procedures; congenital heart disease, 1 per 475,000; rheumatic heart disease, 1 per 142,000; presence of a prosthetic cardiac valve, 1 per 114,000; and previous IE, 1 per 95,000 dental procedures.

Thus, although it has long been assumed that dental procedures may cause IE in patients with underlying cardiac risk factors, and that antibiotic prophylaxis is effective, scientific proof to support these assumptions is lacking. The AHA[14] has concluded that "of the total number of cases of IE that occur annually, it is likely that an exceedingly small number of these cases are caused by bacteremia-producing dental procedures. Accordingly, only an extremely small number of cases of IE might be prevented by antibiotic prophylaxis, even if it were 100% effective. The vast majority of cases of IE caused by oral microflora most likely result from random bacteremias caused by routine daily activities." Thus, on the basis of accumulated available evidence, the AHA in 2007 revised the previous (1997) recommendations.

CURRENT AMERICAN HEART ASSOCIATION RECOMMENDATIONS (2007)[14]

In summarizing the foregoing data, the AHA guidelines cite the following reasons for revision of the previous recommendations:

- IE is much more likely to result from frequent exposure to random bacteremia associated with daily activities than from bacteremia caused by a dental procedure.
- Prophylaxis may prevent an exceedingly small number of cases of IE, if any, in patients who undergo a dental procedure.
- The risk of antibiotic-associated adverse events exceeds the benefit, if any, from prophylactic antibiotic therapy.
- Maintenance of optimal oral health and hygiene may reduce the incidence of bacteremia from daily

activities and is more important than prophylactic antibiotics for reducing the risk of IE resulting from a dental procedure.

Patients Recommended to Receive Antibiotic Prophylaxis[14]

Because no published data demonstrate convincingly that the administration of prophylactic antibiotics prevents bacteremia from an invasive procedure, it would seem logical that antibiotic prophylaxis should no longer be recommended before dental procedures for any patient. Indeed, a recent Cochrane review[64] concluded that there is a lack of evidence to support the use of prophylactic penicillin to prevent endocarditis related to dental procedures. However, the AHA notes:

> We cannot exclude the possibility that there may be an exceedingly small number of cases of IE that could be prevented by prophylactic antibiotics in patients who undergo an invasive procedure. However, if prophylaxis is effective, such therapy should be restricted to those patients with the highest risk of adverse outcome from IE who would derive the greatest benefit from prevention of IE. In patients with underlying cardiac conditions associated with the highest risk for adverse outcome from IE, IE prophylaxis for dental procedures may be reasonable, even though we acknowledge that the effectiveness is unknown.

A similar approach is advocated in recently revised Guidelines for the Prevention of Endocarditis by the Working Party of the British Society for Antimicrobial Chemotherapy,[65] as well as in a recent update of the 1992 French guidelines.[66] The British document states that in view of the lack of evidence of benefit, the most logical step is to withhold antibiotic prophylaxis for dental procedures. However, it was acknowledged that many clinicians would be reluctant to accept these "radical, but logical" changes, so a compromise was accepted in which prophylaxis would be indicated only for those high-risk patients with the potentially most serious outcomes from IE. Of note, however, the National Institute for Health and Clinical Excellence (NICE), which provides guidance for clinical care to the National Health Service in the United Kingdom, does not recommend antibiotic prophylaxis for any at-risk patient undergoing dental treatment.[67]

Previous AHA recommendations used the lifetime risk for acquiring IE related to underlying cardiac disorders in the selection of patients to receive antibiotic prophylaxis when undergoing dental procedures (see Table 2-1). Current guidelines, however, recommend antibiotic prophylaxis on the basis of risk of adverse outcomes (significantly increased morbidity and mortality) from IE. Consequently, prophylaxis is recommended only for those patients with the potentially most serious outcomes from IE. For example, with viridans group streptococcal or enterococcal IE, outcomes of disease can vary widely, ranging between a relatively benign infection and death, with a mortality rate of less than 5% reported for streptococcal NVE.[11] However, patients with those underlying conditions listed in Box 2-1 virtually always experience an adverse outcome, so they are recommended to receive prophylaxis.

BOX 2-1 Cardiac Conditions Associated with the Highest Risk of Adverse Outcomes from Endocarditis for Which Prophylaxis with Dental Procedures Is Recommended

- Prosthetic cardiac valve
- Previous infective endocarditis
- Congenital heart disease (CHD)*
  - Unrepaired cyanotic CHD, including those with palliative shunts and conduits
  - Completely repaired CHD with prosthetic material or device by surgery or catheter intervention during the first 6 months after the procedure†
  - Repaired CHD with residual defects at the site or adjacent to the site of a prosthetic patch or prosthetic device, which inhibits endothelialization
- Cardiac transplant recipients who develop cardiac valvulopathy

*Except for the conditions listed in this box, antibiotic prophylaxis is no longer recommended for any other form of CHD.

†Prophylaxis is recommended, because endothelialization of prosthetic material occurs within 6 months after the procedure.

From Wilson W, et al: American Heart Association Rheumatic Fever, Endocarditis, and Kawasaki Disease Committee; American Heart Association Council on Cardiovascular Disease in the Young; American Heart Association Council on Clinical Cardiology; American Heart Association Council on Interdisciplinary Working Group: Prevention of infective endocarditis: guidelines from the American Heart Association: a guideline from the American Heart Association Rheumatic Fever, Young, and the Council on Clinical Cardiology, Council on Cardiovascular Surgery and Anesthesia, and the Quality Care of Outcomes Research interdisciplinary Working Group. Circulation *116(15):1736-54, 2007 Oct 9.*

Dental Procedures for Which Antibiotic Prophylaxis Is Recommended[34]

Previous AHA recommendations listed specific dental procedures for which antibiotic prophylaxis was recommended on the basis of the likelihood that significant bleeding would be encountered. However, a review of the published data suggests that transient viridans group streptococcal bacteremia may result from *any* dental procedure that involves manipulation of the gingival or periapical region of the teeth or perforation of the oral mucosa, even in the absence of visible bleeding. Therefore, antibiotic prophylaxis is recommended only for patients with conditions listed in Box 2-1 who undergo any dental procedure that involves the manipulation of gingival tissues or the periapical region of a tooth, and for those procedures that perforate the oral mucosa (Box 2-2). This recommendation does not include routine local anesthetic injections through noninfected tissue,

BOX 2-2 Dental Procedures in Patients with Cardiac Conditions* for Which Endocarditis Prophylaxis Is Recommended

- All dental procedures that involve manipulation of gingival tissue or the periapical region of teeth or perforation of the oral mucosa
- This includes all dental procedures except the following procedures and events:
  - Routine anesthetic injections through noninfected tissue
  - Taking of dental radiographs
  - Placement of removable prosthodontic or orthodontic appliances
  - Adjustment of orthodontic appliances
  - Shedding of deciduous teeth and bleeding from trauma to the lips or oral mucosa

*See Box 1-1.

From Wilson W, et al: American Heart Association Rheumatic Fever, Endocarditis, and Kawasaki Disease Committee; American Heart Association Council on Cardiovascular Disease in the Young; American Heart Association Council on Clinical Cardiology; American Heart Association Council on Interdisciplinary Working Group: Prevention of infective endocarditis: guidelines from the American Heart Association: a guideline from the American Heart Association Rheumatic Fever, Young, and the Council on Clinical Cardiology, Council on Cardiovascular Surgery and Anesthesia, and the Quality Care of Outcomes Research interdisciplinary Working Group. Circulation *116(15):1736-54, 2007 Oct 9.*

taking of dental radiographs, placement of removable prosthodontic or orthodontic appliances, adjustment of orthodontic appliances, or the shedding of deciduous teeth and bleeding from trauma to the lips or oral mucosa.

Antibiotic Prophylaxis Regimens[14]

In the limited patient population for which antibiotic prophylaxis is recommended, prophylaxis should be directed against viridans group streptococci. Unfortunately, over the past 2 decades, a significant increase has been noted in the proportion of strains of viridans group streptococci that are resistant to the antibiotics recommended in previous AHA recommendations. In many studies, typical resistance rates of viridans group streptococci for penicillin range from 17% to 50%, for ceftriaxone from 22% to 42%, for macrolides from 22% to 58%, and for clindamycin from 13% to 27%.[14] Although these data are indeed alarming, the effect on selection of prophylactic antibiotics is unclear. The AHA states:

> The impact of viridans group streptococcal resistance on antibiotic prevention of IE is unknown. If resistance in vitro is predictive of lack of clinical efficacy, the high resistance rates of viridans group streptococci provide additional support for the assertion that prophylactic therapy for a dental procedure is of little, if any, value. It is impractical to recommend prophylaxis with only those antibiotics, such as vancomycin or a fluoroquinolone, that are highly active in vitro against viridans group streptococci. There is no evidence that such therapy is effective for prophylaxis of IE, and their use might result in the development of resistance of viridans group streptococci and other microorganisms to these and other antibiotics.

Antibiotic prophylaxis should be administered in a single dose 30 to 60 minutes before the procedure. If the antibiotic is *inadvertently* not administered before the procedure, the dosage may be administered up to 2 hours after the procedure. Table 2-5 lists the recommended antibiotic regimens for use for dental procedures in patients from Box 2-1. Because of the possibility of cross-allergenicity, the use of cephalosporins is *not* recommended for patients who have a history of anaphylaxis, angioedema, or urticaria (immediate-onset IgE-mediated hypersensitivity) caused by the administration of penicillin. An important point in this context is that the use of antibiotics is not without risk, with the potential for allergic reactions, adverse side effects, and the promotion of antibiotic resistance.

Study results are contradictory regarding the efficacy of oral antimicrobial mouth rinses (e.g., chlorhexidine, povidone-iodine) to reduce the frequency of bacteremia associated with dental procedures; however, the preponderance of evidence suggests that no clear benefit is associated with their use. Of note, however, the British Society for Antimicrobial Therapy guidelines do recommend the preoperative use of chlorhexidine (0.2%) mouthwash, while the NICE guidelines state that chlorhexidene mouthrinses should not be used.[65]

It is important that the dentist continue to identify from the medical history those patients with cardiac conditions that increase risk for IE, such as mitral valve prolapse, rheumatic heart disease, or systemic lupus erythematosus. Patients with these conditions should be under the care of a physician for monitoring the status of their valvular heart disease and potential complications. The establishment and maintenance of optimal oral hygiene are of critical importance in these patients. Also, when treating a patient with a cardiac condition associated with an increased risk for IE, the dentist should remain alert to the presence of signs or symptoms of IE (e.g., fever) and make the appropriate physician referral as indicated. This precaution applies whether or not the patient has received prophylactic antibiotics for dental procedures.

Special Situations[14]

Patients Already Taking Antibiotics. In patients who are already taking penicillin or amoxicillin for eradication of an infection (e.g., sinus infection) or for long-term secondary prevention of rheumatic fever, presence of viridans group streptococci that are relatively resistant to penicillin or amoxicillin is likely. Therefore, clindamycin,

TABLE 2-5 Antibiotic Regimens for Dental Procedures

Situation	Agent	Regimen: Single Dose 30-60 Minutes Before Procedure	
		Adults	**Children**
Oral	Amoxicillin	2 g	50 mg/kg
Unable to take oral medication	Ampicillin *or*	2 g IM or IV	50 mg/kg IM or IV
	Cefazolin *or* Ceftriaxone	1 g IM or IV	50 mg/kg IM or IV
Allergic to penicillins or ampicillin (oral)	Cephalexin*† *or*	2 g	50 mg/kg
	Clindamycin	600 mg	20 mg/kg
	Azithromycin *or* Clarithromycin	500 mg	15 mg/kg
Allergic to penicillins or ampicillin and unable to take oral medication	Cefazolin *or* Ceftriaxone†	1 g IM or IV	50 mg/kg
	Clindamycin phosphate	600 mg IM or IV	20 mg/kg IM or IV

IM, Intramuscularly; *IV*, Intravenously.
*Or other first- or second-generation oral cephalosporin in equivalent adult or pediatric dosage.
†Cephalosporins should not be used in a person with a history of anaphylaxis, angioedema, or urticaria after receiving penicillins or ampicillin.
From Wilson W, et al: American Heart Association Rheumatic Fever, Endocarditis, and Kawasaki Disease Committee; American Heart Association Council on Cardiovascular Disease in the Young; American Heart Association Council on Clinical Cardiology; American Heart Association Council on Interdisciplinary Working Group: Prevention of infective endocarditis: guidelines from the American Heart Association: a guideline from the American Heart Association Rheumatic Fever, Young, and the Council on Clinical Cardiology, Council on Cardiovascular Surgery and Anesthesia, and the Quality Care of Outcomes Research interdisciplinary Working Group. Circulation *116(15):1736-54, 2007 Oct 9.*

azithromycin, or clarithromycin should be selected for prophylaxis if treatment is immediately necessary. Because of cross-resistance with cephalosporins, this class of antibiotics should be avoided. An alternative approach is to wait for at least 10 days after completion of antibiotic therapy before administration of prophylactic antibiotics. In this instance, the usual regimen can be used.

Patients Undergoing Cardiac Surgery. It is recommended that a preoperative dental evaluation be performed and necessary dental treatment be provided whenever possible before initiation of cardiac valve surgery or replacement or repair of congenital heart disease, in an effort to decrease the incidence of late PVE caused by viridans group streptococci.

Prolonged Dental Appointment. The duration of a dental appointment in relation to the effective plasma concentration of an administered antibiotic is not addressed in these recommendations; however, for a lengthy appointment, this may be a matter of concern. With amoxicillin, which has a half-life of approximately 80 minutes, the average peak plasma concentration of 4 μg/mL is reached about 2 hours after oral administration of a 250-mg dose.[68] Most of the penicillin-sensitive viridans group streptococci have an MIC requirement of 0.2 μg/mL.[11] Thus, a 2-g dose of amoxicillin should produce an acceptable MIC for at least 6 hours. If a procedure lasts longer than 6 hours, it may be prudent to administer an additional 2-g dose.

Other Considerations[14]

No evidence suggests that coronary artery bypass graft surgery is associated with long-term risk for infection; thus, antibiotic prophylaxis is not recommended for patients undergoing this procedure. Patients who have had a heart transplant are at increased risk for acquired valvular dysfunction, especially during episodes of rejection. Endocarditis that occurs in this instance is associated with a high risk of adverse outcome; therefore, IE prophylaxis may be reasonable in these patients, although its usefulness has not been established. Patients with mechanical or tissue prosthetic valves often will be taking long-term anticoagulant medication (e.g., warfarin) to prevent valve-associated thrombosis. These patients are at risk for excessive bleeding during and after surgical procedures (see Chapter 24).

Implementation of the Recommendations

In view of the significant changes that have been made since previous AHA recommendations for antibiotic prophylaxis were published, it can be anticipated that patients may have questions and may be concerned about the implementation of the current recommendations. Patients with various valvular disorders (e.g., mitral valve prolapse, rheumatic heart disease) who have been told for many years that they needed antibiotics because of the risk for IE caused by dental treatment are now informed that they no longer require antibiotics when they go to the dentist. Additionally, patients who were previously told that they required antibiotic prophylaxis only for invasive dental procedures (i.e., only those patients with conditions listed in Box 2-1) are now told that antibiotic prophylaxis is recommended for essentially all dental treatment. The AHA recommends discussing the reasons for the revision with the patient in an effort to alleviate concern. The *Journal of the American Dental Association* in its July 2007 issue includes a letter explaining the rationale for the changes, which can be copied for use as a patient handout.

A reasonable approach is to share the new recommendations with the patient and explain the rationale for changes, emphasizing that they are based on an extensive review of current scientific evidence. In addition, the dentist should consult with the patient's physician to ensure that he or she is aware of the current AHA recommendations, and to discuss their implementation in treatment of the patient. These conversations should be documented in the patient's progress notes.

Nonvalvular Cardiovascular Devices

In a 2003 AHA scientific statement,[69] guidelines are provided regarding antibiotic prophylaxis for patients with various types of nonvalvular cardiovascular devices (e.g., coronary artery stents, hemodialysis grafts) who are undergoing dental procedures. Table 2-6 provides a list of various devices, along with reported incidence of infection. After performing an extensive review of available data, the AHA reporting committee concluded that no convincing evidence suggests that microorganisms associated with dental procedures cause infection of nonvalvular vascular devices at any time after implantation. Indeed, infections of these devices most often are due to staphylococci, gram-negative bacteria, or other microorganisms associated with implantation of the device or

TABLE 2-6 Nonvalvular Cardiovascular Device–Related Infections

Type of Device	Incidence of Infection (%)
Intracardiac	
Pacemakers (temporary and permanent)	0.13-19.9
Defibrillators	0.00-3.2
Left ventricular assist devices	25-70
Total artificial hearts	To be determined
Ventriculoatrial shunts	2.4-9.4
Pledgets	Rare
Patent ductus arteriosus occlusion devices	Rare
Atrial septal defect and ventriculoseptal defect occlusion devices	Rare
Conduits	Rare
Patches	Rare
Arterial	
Peripheral vascular stents	Rare
Vascular grafts, including for hemodialysis	1.0-6
Intraaortic balloon pumps	≤5-26
Angioplasty/angiography	<1
Coronary artery stents	Rare
Patches	1.8
Venous	
Vena cava filters	Rare

From Baddour LM, et al: Nonvalvular cardiovascular device–related infections, Circulation *108:2015-2031, 2003.*

TABLE 2-7 Catheters Used for Venous and Arterial Access

Catheter Type	Entry Site	Comments
Peripheral venous catheters (short)	Usually inserted into veins of forearm or hand	Phlebitis with prolonged use; rarely associated with bloodstream infection
Peripheral arterial catheters	Usually inserted into radial artery; can be placed in femoral, axillary, brachial, posterior tibial arteries	Low infection risk; rarely associated with bloodstream infection
Midline catheters	Inserted through antecubital fossa into proximal basilica or cephalic veins; does not enter central veins, peripheral catheters	Anaphylactoid reactions have been reported with catheters made of elastomeric hydrogel; lower rates of phlebitis than with short peripheral catheters
Nontunneled central venous catheters	Percutaneously inserted into central veins (subclavian, internal jugular, or femoral)	Account for most catheter-related bloodstream infections
Pulmonary artery catheters	Inserted through a Teflon introducer into a central vein (subclavian, internal jugular, or femoral)	Usually heparin bonded; similar rates of bloodstream infection as central venous catheters
Peripherally inserted central venous catheters (PICCs)	Inserted into basilica, cephalic, or brachial veins and advanced to superior vena cava	Lower rate of infection than nontunneled central venous catheters
Tunneled central venous catheters	Implanted into subclavian, internal jugular, or femoral veins	Cuff inhibits migration of organisms into catheter tract; lower rate of infection than with nontunneled central venous catheters
Totally implantable	Tunneled beneath skin with subcutaneous port access with a needle; implanted in subclavian or internal jugular vein	Lowest risk for catheter-related bloodstream infections; improved patient self-image; no need for local catheter site care; surgery required for catheter removal
Umbilical catheters	Inserted into umbilical vein or umbilical artery	Risk for catheter-related bloodstream infection similar with use of umbilical vein and with use of artery

Adapted from O'Grady NP, et al: Guidelines for the prevention of intravascular catheter–related infections. Centers for Disease Control and Prevention, MMWR Recomm Rep *51:1-29, 2002.*

resulting from wound or other active infections. Accordingly, the AHA does not recommend routine antibiotic prophylaxis for patients with any of these devices who undergo dental procedures. Prophylaxis is recommended, however, for selected patients with these devices:

- Those undergoing incision and drainage of infected tissue (abscesses)
- Those patients with residual valve leak after device placement for attempted closure of leaks associated with patent ductus arteriosus, atrial septal defect, or ventricular septal defect

Intravascular Catheters

Concerns often arise regarding the need for antibiotic prophylaxis to prevent infection in patients with various types of intravenous or intraarterial catheters. Examples are peripheral venous catheters, peripheral arterial catheters, midline catheters, nontunneled central venous catheters, pulmonary artery catheters, peripherally inserted central venous catheters (PICCs), tunneled central venous catheters, totally implantable catheters, and umbilical catheters (Table 2-7). The causative microorganisms in these infections include coagulase-negative staphylococci, *S aureus,* enterococci, gram-negative rods, *Escherichia coli, Enterobacter* and *Candida* spp., *P aeruginosa,* and *Klebsiella pneumoniae.* None of these, with the exception of *Candida,* are normal inhabitants of the oral cavity; thus, they do not introduce risk for infection with oral procedures. The Centers for Disease Control and Prevention (CDC), in its published Guidelines for the Prevention of Intravascular Catheter-Related Infections,[70] does not include any recommendation for antibiotic prophylaxis for patients with any of these devices who are undergoing dental procedures. Likewise, a recent review found no evidence to support the administration of prophylactic antibiotics to prevent catheter-related infections associated with an invasive dental procedure in patients with chronic indwelling central venous catheters.[71]

The practice of providing antibiotics for dental patients with various types of medical problems (other than for endocarditis prophylaxis) to prevent metastatic infection from oral flora is controversial. In almost every instance, no evidence of need or efficacy has been documented.[72,73] Box 2-3 lists several of those conditions for which antibiotics have been advocated.

BOX 2-3 Other Conditions, Unrelated to Endocarditis Prophylaxis, for Which Antibiotic Prophylaxis Has Been Advocated, but Without Evidence for Need or Efficacy[72,73]

Organ transplants
Prosthetic joints
Cerebrospinal fluid shunts
Immunosuppressive drugs (e.g., steroids, DMARDs, chemotherapy)
Autoimmune disease (e.g., systemic lupus erythematosus)
Insulin-dependent diabetes
HIV infection/AIDS
Splenectomy
Severe neutropenia
Sickle cell anemia
Breast implants
Penile implants

AIDS, Acquired immunodeficiency syndrome; *DMARDs,* Disease-modifying antirheumatic drugs; *HIV,* Human immunodeficiency virus.

REFERENCES

1. Karchmer AW: Infective endocarditis. In Libby P, et al, editors: *Braunwald's heart disease. a textbook of cardiovascular medicine*, ed 8, Philadelphiax, 2008, Saunders, pp 1713-1738.
2. Bashore TM, Cabell C, Fowler V Jr: Update on infective endocarditis, *Curr Probl Cardiol* 31:274-352, 2006.
3. Fowler VG Jr, Bayer A: Infective endocarditis. In Goldman L, Ausiello D, editors: *Cecil medicine*, ed 23, Philadelphia, 2008, Saunders, pp 537-548.
4. Berlin JA, et al: Incidence of infective endocarditis in the Delaware Valley, 1988-1990, *Am J Cardiol* 76:933-936, 1995.
5. Tleyjeh IM, et al: Temporal trends in infective endocarditis: a population-based study in Olmsted County, Minnesota, *JAMA* 293:3022-3028, 2005.
6. Steckelberg JM, Wilson WR: Risk factors for infective endocarditis, *Infect Dis Clin North Am* 7:9-19, 1993.
7. de Sa DD, et al: Epidemiological trends of infective endocarditis: a population-based study in Olmsted County, Minnesota, *Mayo Clin Proc* 85:422-426, 2010.
8. Mylonakis E, Calderwood SB: Infective endocarditis in adults, *N Engl J Med* 345:1318-1330, 2001.
9. Miro JM, del Rio A, Mestres CA: Infective endocarditis in intravenous drug abusers and HIV-1 infected patients, *Infect Dis Clin North Am* 16:273-295, 2002.
10. Mathew J, et al: Clinical features, site of involvement, bacteriologic findings, and outcome of infective endocarditis in intravenous drug users, *Arch Intern Med* 155:1641-1648, 1995.
11. Baddour LM, et al: Infective endocarditis: diagnosis, antimicrobial therapy, and management of complications: a statement for healthcare professionals from the Committee on Rheumatic Fever, Endocarditis, and Kawasaki Disease, Council on Cardiovascular Disease in the Young, and the Councils on Clinical Cardiology, Stroke, and Cardiovascular Surgery and Anesthesia, *American Heart Association—Circulation* 11123:e394-434, 2005.
12. Baddour LM, et al: Nonvalvular cardiovascular device-related infections, *Clin Infect Dis* 38:1128-1130, 2004.
13. Majumdar A, et al: Renal pathological findings in infective endocarditis, *Nephrol Dial Transplant* 15:1782-1787, 2000.
14. Wilson W, et al: Prevention of infective endocarditis: guidelines from the American Heart Association: a guideline from the American Heart Association Rheumatic Fever, Young, and the Council on Clinical Cardiology, Council on Cardiovascular Surgery and Anesthesia, and the Quality Care of Outcomes Research interdisciplinary Working Group, *Circulation* 116(15):1736-1754, 2007 Oct 9.
15. Hoen B, et al: Infective endocarditis in patients with negative blood cultures: analysis of 88 cases from a one-year

nationwide survey in France, *Clin Infect Dis* 20:501-506, 1995.
16. Li JS, et al: Proposed modifications to the Duke criteria for the diagnosis of infective endocarditis, *Clin Infect Dis* 30:633-638, 2000.
17. Durack DT, Lukes AS, Bright DK: New criteria for diagnosis of infective endocarditis: utilization of specific echocardiographic findings. Duke Endocarditis Service, *Am J Med* 96:200-209, 1994.
18. Jones T, et al: Prevention of rheumatic fever and bacterial endocarditis through control of streptococcal infections, *Circulation* 11:317-320, 1955.
19. Prevention of rheumatic fever and bacterial endocarditis through control of streptococcal infections, *Pediatrics* 155:642-646,1955.
20. Rammelkamp, CH, et al (Committee on Prevention of Rheumatic Fever and Bacterial Endocarditis, American Heart Association): Treatment of streptococcal infections in the general population, *Circulation* 15:154-158 [Abstract], 1957.
21. Hussar AE: Prevention of bacterial endocarditis, *Circulation* 31:953-954, 1965.
22. Prevention of bacterial endocarditis, American Heart Association, *J Am Dent Assn* 85:1377-1379, 1972.
23. Kaplan EL: Prevention of bacterial endocarditis, *Circulation* 56:139A-143A, 1977.
24. Shulman ST, et al: Prevention of bacterial endocarditis: a statement for health professionals by the Committee on Rheumatic Fever and Infective Endocarditis of the Council on Cardiovascular Disease in the Young, *Circulation* 70:1123A-1127A, 1984.
25. Dajani AS, et al: Prevention of bacterial endocarditis. Recommendations by the American Heart Association, *JAMA* 264:2919-2922, 1990.
26. Dajani AS, et al: Prevention of bacterial endocarditis: recommendations by the American Heart Association, *J Am Dent Assoc* 128:1142-1151, 1997.
27. Lockhart PB: The risk for endocarditis in dental practice, *Periodontol* 23:127-135, 2000.
28. Lockhart PB, Durack DT: Oral microflora as a cause of endocarditis and other distant site infections, *Infect Dis Clin North Am* 13:833-850, vi, 1999.
29. Pallasch TJ, Slots J: Antibiotic prophylaxis and the medically compromised patient. *Periodontol* 10:107-138, 1996.
30. Roberts GJ, et al: Duration, prevalence and intensity of bacteraemia after dental extractions in children, *Heart* 92:1274-1277, 2006.
31. Takai S, et al: Incidence and bacteriology of bacteremia associated with various oral and maxillofacial surgical procedures, *Oral Surg Oral Med Oral Pathol Oral Radiol Endod* 99:292-298, 2005.
32. Cobe HM: Transitory bacteremia, *Oral Surg Oral Med Oral Pathol* 7:609-615, 1954.
33. Sconyers JR, Crawford JJ, Moriarty JD: Relationship of bacteremia to toothbrushing in patients with periodontitis, *J Am Dent Assoc* 87:616-622, 1973.
34. Faden HS: Dental procedures and bacteremia (letter), *Ann Intern Med* 81:274, 1974.
35. Felix JE, Rosen S, App GR: Detection of bacteremia after the use of an oral irrigation device in subjects with periodontitis, *J Periodontol* 42:785-787, 1971.
36. O'Leary TJ, et al: Possible penetration of crevicular tissue from oral hygiene procedures. II. Use of the toothbrush, *J Periodontol* 41:163-164, 1970.
37. O'Leary TJ, et al: Possible penetration of crevicular tissue from oral hygiene procedures. I. Use of oral irrigating devices, *J Periodontol* 41:158-162, 1970.
38. Rise E, Smith JF, Bell J: Reduction of bacteremia after oral manipulations, *Arch Otolaryngol* 90:198-201, 1969.
39. Round H, Kirkpatrick HJR, Hails CG: Further investigations on bacteriological infections of the mouth, *Proc R Soc Med* 29:1552-1556, 1936.
40. Schlein RA, et al: Toothbrushing and transient bacteremia in patients undergoing orthodontic treatment, *Am J Orthod Dentofacial Orthop* 99:466-472, 1991.
41. Crasta K, et al: Bacteraemia due to dental flossing, *J Clin Periodontol* 36:323-332, 2009.
42. Guntheroth WG: How important are dental procedures as a cause of infective endocarditis? *Am J Cardiol* 54:797-801, 1984.
43. Roberts GJ: Dentists are innocent! "Everyday" bacteremia is the real culprit: a review and assessment of the evidence that dental surgical procedures are a principal cause of bacterial endocarditis in children, *Pediatr Cardiol* 20:317-325, 1999.
44. Durack DT, Beeson PB: Experimental bacterial endocarditis. II. Survival of a bacteria [*sic*] in endocardial vegetations, *Br J Exp Pathol* 53:50-53, 1972.
45. Lucas VS, et al: Comparison of lysis filtration and an automated blood culture system (BACTEC) for detection, quantification, and identification of odontogenic bacteremia in children, *J Clin Microbiol* 40:3416-3420, 2002.
46. Lockhart PB, et al: Poor oral hygiene as a risk factor for infective endocarditis-related bacteremia, *J Am Dent Assoc* 140:1238-1244, 2009.
47. Asi KS, Gill AS, Mahajan S: Postoperative bacteremia in periodontal flap surgery, with and without prophylactic antibiotic administration: a comparative study, *J Indian Soc Periodontol* 14:18-22, 2010.
48. Durack DT: Prevention of infective endocarditis, *N Engl J Med* 332:38-44, 1995.
49. Durack DT: Antibiotics for prevention of endocarditis during dentistry: time to scale back? *Ann Intern Med* 129:829-831, 1998.
50. Strom BL, et al: Dental and cardiac risk factors for infective endocarditis. A population-based, case-control study, *Ann Intern Med* 129:761-769, 1998.
51. Brennan MT, et al: The impact of oral disease and nonsurgical treatment on bacteremia in children, *J Am Dent Assoc* 138:80-85, 2007.
52. Lockhart PB, et al: Impact of amoxicillin prophylaxis on the incidence, nature, and duration of bacteremia in children after intubation and dental procedures, *Circulation* 109:2878-2884, 2004.
53. Roberts GJ, Radford P, Holt R: Prophylaxis of dental bacteraemia with oral amoxycillin in children, *Br Dent J* 162:179-182, 1987.
54. Shanson DC, et al: Erythromycin stearate, 1.5 g, for the oral prophylaxis of streptococcal bacteraemia in patients undergoing dental extraction: efficacy and tolerance, *J Antimicrob Chemother* 15:83-90, 1985.
55. Pineiro A, et al: Bacteraemia following dental implants' placement, *Clin Oral Implants Res* 21:913-918, 2010.
56. Morozumi T, et al: Effects of irrigation with an antiseptic and oral administration of azithromycin on bacteremia caused by scaling and root planing, *J Periodontol* 81:1555-1563, 2010.
57. Hall G, Heimdahl A, Nord CE: Bacteremia after oral surgery and antibiotic prophylaxis for endocarditis, *Clin Infect Dis* 29:1-8, 1999.
58. Hall G, Heimdahl A, Nord CE: Effects of prophylactic administration of cefaclor on transient bacteremia after dental extraction, *Eur J Clin Microbiol Infect Dis* 15:646-649, 1996.
59. Hall G, et al: Prophylactic administration of penicillins for endocarditis does not reduce the incidence of postextraction bacteremia, *Clin Infect Dis* 17:188-194, 1993.

60. Lockhart PB: An analysis of bacteremias during dental extractions. A double-blind, placebo-controlled study of chlorhexidine, *Arch Intern Med* 156:513-520, 1996.
61. van der Meer JT, et al: Epidemiology of bacterial endocarditis in The Netherlands. II. Antecedent procedures and use of prophylaxis, *Arch Intern Med* 152:1869-1873, 1992.
62. Van der Meer JT, et al: Efficacy of antibiotic prophylaxis for prevention of native-valve endocarditis, *Lancet* 339:135-139, 1992.
63. Duval X, et al: Estimated risk of endocarditis in adults with predisposing cardiac conditions undergoing dental procedures with or without antibiotic prophylaxis, *Clin Infect Dis* 42:e102-e107, 2006.
64. Oliver R, et al: Antibiotics for the prophylaxis of bacterial endocarditis in dentistry, *Cochrane Database Syst Rev* (4):CD003813, 2008.
65. Gould FK, et al: Guidelines for the prevention of endocarditis: report of the Working Party of the British Society for Antimicrobial Chemotherapy, *J Antimicrob Chemother* 57:1035-1042, 2006.
66. Danchin N, Duval X, Leport C: Prophylaxis of infective endocarditis: French recommendations 2002, *Heart* 91:715-718, 2005.
67. Richey R, Wray D, Stokes T: Prophylaxis against infective endocarditis: summary of NICE guidance, *BMJ* 336:770-771, 2008.
68. Petri WA: Penicillins, cephalosporins, and other β-lactam antibiotics. In Brunton LL, Lazo JS, Parker KL, editors: *Goodman and Gilman's The Pharmacological Basis of Therapeutics*, ed 11, New York, 2006, McGraw-Hill, pp 1127-1154.
69. Baddour LM, et al: Nonvalvular cardiovascular device-related infections, *Circulation* 108:2015-2031, 2003.
70. O'Grady NP, et al: Guidelines for the prevention of intravascular catheter-related infections. Centers for Disease Control and Prevention, *MMWR Recomm Rep* 51:1-29, 2002.
71. Hong CH, et al: Antibiotic prophylaxis for dental procedures to prevent indwelling venous catheter-related infections, *Am J Med* 123:1128-1133, 2010.
72. Lockhart PB, et al: The evidence base for the efficacy of antibiotic prophylaxis in dental practice, *J Am Dent Assoc* 138:458-474, 2007.
73. Little JW, et al: Antibiotic prophylaxis in dentistry: an update, *Gen Dent* 56:20-28, 2008.

3

Hypertension

Hypertension is an abnormal elevation in arterial pressure that can be fatal if sustained and untreated. People with hypertension may not display clinical signs or symptoms for many years but eventually can experience symptomatic damage to several target organs, including kidneys, heart, brain, and eyes. In adults, a sustained systolic blood pressure of 140 mm Hg or greater and/or a sustained diastolic blood pressure of 90 mm Hg or greater is defined as hypertension. The Seventh Report of the Joint National Committee on Prevention, Detection, Evaluation, and Treatment of High Blood Pressure (JNC 7) provided several revisions to the previous 1997 report[1] (Table 3-1). These guidelines include an updated classification that redefines "normal" blood pressure as 120/80 mm Hg and introduces a new category of "prehypertension" (systolic blood pressures ranging from 120 to 139 and diastolic pressures ranging from 80 to 89 mm Hg), which encompasses the previously designated categories of "normal" and "borderline" hypertension. This revision reflects the findings that health risks are increased with blood pressures higher than 115/75 mm Hg and that lowering blood pressure in patients with what was formerly considered "normal" or "borderline" blood pressure can result in decreased frequency of adverse vascular events such as stroke and myocardial infarction (MI). In addition, the previously designated stages 2 and 3 of hypertension were combined into a single stage 2 category, because treatment for both groups is essentially the same. Table 3-1 also includes recommendations for follow-up care based on initial blood pressure measurements. A separate publication provides similar information on the classification, detection, diagnosis, and management of hypertension in children and adolescents, while updating 1996 guidelines.[2] In children and adolescents, hypertension is defined as elevated blood pressure that persists on repeated measurement at the 95th percentile or greater for age, height, and gender (Tables 3-2 and 3-3). For example, according to Table 3-3, a 6-year-old girl who is at the 50th percentile in height would be considered to have hypertension if her blood pressure was persistently 111/74 mm Hg or greater.

The dental health professional can play a significant role in the detection and control of hypertension and may well be the first to detect a patient with an elevation in blood pressure or with symptoms of hypertensive disease. Along with detection, monitoring is an equally valuable service, because patients who are receiving treatment for hypertension may nevertheless fail to achieve adequate control because of poor compliance or inappropriate drug selection or dosing. The JNC 7 specifically encourages the active participation of all health care professionals in the detection of hypertension and the surveillance of treatment compliance.[1] Only a physician can make the diagnosis of hypertension and decide on its treatment. The dentist, however, should detect abnormal blood pressure measurements, which then become the basis for referral to or consultation with a physician.

Management of the dental patient with hypertension poses several potentially significant considerations. These include identification of disease, monitoring, stress and anxiety reduction, prevention of drug interactions, and awareness and management of adverse drug side effects.

Of note, new guidelines (JNC 8) are currently under review and scheduled to be published in 2012.

GENERAL DESCRIPTION

Prevalence

With 35 million office visits annually, hypertension is the most common primary diagnosis in America.[1] Before 1990, the prevalence of hypertension was steadily declining; however, recent evidence indicates that the trend has reversed, and hypertension is once again on the rise.[3] According to National Health and Nutrition Examination Survey (NHANES) data for the period 1999 to 2000, at least 65 million adults in the United States have high blood pressure (HBP) or are taking antihypertensive medication.[4] This estimate equals about one fourth of the population and represents a 30% increase from 1988 to 1994.[5] In a typical practice population of 2000 patients, therefore, around 500 will have hypertension. This marked increase is attributed to aging of the population and to the epidemic increase in obesity. The National High Blood Pressure Education Program was begun in 1972, and in a little more than 3 decades, it has had

TABLE 3-1 Classification of Blood Pressure (BP) in Adults and Recommendations for Follow-up

BP Classification	Systolic BP (mm Hg)		Diastolic BP (mm Hg)	Recommended Follow-up
Normal	<120	*and*	<80	Recheck in 2 years
Prehypertension	120-139	*or*	80-89	Recheck in 1 year
Stage 1 hypertension	140-159	*or*	90-99	Confirm within 2 months
Stage 2 hypertension	≥160	*or*	≥100	Evaluate or refer to source of care within 1 month. For those with higher pressures (e.g., >180/110 mm Hg), evaluate and treat immediately or within 1 week, depending on the clinical situation and complications

Adapted from the National Heart, Lung, and Blood Institute: The seventh report of the Joint National Committee on Prevention, Detection, Evaluation, and Treatment of High Blood Pressure: the JNC 7 report, *Bethesda, Maryland, US Department of Health and Human Services, Public Health Service, National Institutes of Health, National Heart, Lung, and Blood Institute, August 2004.*

TABLE 3-2 Classification of Blood Pressure in Children and Adolescents

Classification	SBP or DBP Percentile*
Normal	<90th
Prehypertension	90th to <95th, or pressure exceeds 120/80 even with <90th percentile up to <95th percentile
Stage 1 hypertension	95th to 99th percentile plus 5 mm Hg
Stage 2 hypertension	>99th percentile plus 5 mm Hg

*For gender, age, and height, as measured on at least three separate occasions.

DBP, Diastolic blood pressure; *SBP,* Systolic blood pressure.

Data from the National Heart, Lung, and Blood Institute: The Fourth Report on the Diagnosis, Evaluation, and Treatment of High Blood Pressure in Children and Adolescents, *Bethesda, Maryland, US Department of Health and Human Services, Public Health Service, National Institutes of Health, National Heart, Lung, and Blood Institute, May 2005.*

TABLE 3-3 95th Percentile of Blood Pressure by Selected Ages, by 50th and 75th Height Percentiles, and by Gender in Children and Adolescents

	Girls' SBP/DBP		Boys' SBP/DBP	
Age (yr)	50th Percentile for Height	75th Percentile for Height	50th Percentile for Height	75th Percentile for Height
1	104/58	105/59	103/56	104/57
6	111/74	113/74	114/74	115/75
12	123/80	124/81	123/81	125/82
17	129/84	130/85	136/87	138/87

DBP, Diastolic blood pressure; *SBP,* Systolic blood pressure.

Data from the National Heart, Lung, and Blood Institute: The Fourth Report on the Diagnosis, Evaluation, and Treatment of High Blood Pressure in Children and Adolescents, *Bethesda, Maryland, US Department of Health and Human Services, Public Health Service, National Institutes of Health, National Heart, Lung, and Blood Institute, May 2005.*

significant success.[1] The number of people with HBP who are aware of their condition has increased from 51% to 70%, and the percentage of those receiving treatment for HBP has increased from 31% to 59%. The proportion of patients taking medication whose blood pressure is controlled to 140/90 increased from 10% to 34% during the same period. Concomitant with increased awareness and treatment has been a significant decline in number of deaths from coronary heart disease (50%) and from stroke (57%), although this decline has slowed in recent years.[1] Although these trends are encouraging, 30% of patients with HBP remain unaware of their disease, 40% of patients with HBP are not being treated, and more than 60% of hypertensive patients are taking medications but have not achieved adequate control of the condition.

Diagnosis and treatment of hypertension were once based largely on diastolic blood pressure; with growing recognition of the importance of systolic blood pressure, however, this is no longer the case. Isolated systolic hypertension gradually increases with age such that among patients older than 50 years of age, it is the most prevalent form of hypertension.

The prevalence of high blood pressure increases with aging, such that more than half of all Americans aged 65 and older have hypertension.[6] If people live long enough, more than 90% will develop hypertension.[7] Systolic blood pressure continues to rise throughout life, but diastolic blood pressure rises until around age 50 and then levels off or falls; as a result, after the age of 50, isolated systolic hypertension becomes the more prevalent pattern. In one study, isolated systolic hypertension was identified in 87% of inadequately controlled patients older than 60 years of age.[8] Isolated diastolic hypertension most commonly is seen before age 50. Diastolic blood pressure is a more potent cardiovascular risk factor than is systolic blood pressure until age 50; thereafter, systolic blood pressure is more important.[9]

Prevalence varies with race as well and is highest among African Americans. In general, it is lower among Hispanics than among whites; however, variation has been noted among racial subgroups. For example, the prevalence of hypertension among Mexican Americans is lower than among non-Hispanic whites, although among Puerto Rican Americans, it is higher.[10] Prevalence generally is higher in Asian Americans, Native Americans, and Native Alaskans than in whites; however, again, variation is seen among subgroups.[11]

Etiology

About 90% of patients have no readily identifiable cause for their disease, which is referred to as *primary* (essential) hypertension. In the remaining 10% of patients, an underlying cause or condition may be identified; for these patients, the term *secondary* hypertension is applied. Box 3-1 is a listing of the most common identifiable causes of secondary hypertension. Lifestyle can play an important role in the severity and progression of hypertension; obesity, excessive alcohol intake, excessive dietary sodium, and physical inactivity are significant contributing factors.

Pathophysiology and Complications

In primary hypertension, the basic underlying defect is a failure in the regulation of vascular resistance. The pulsating force is modified by the degree of elasticity of the walls of larger arteries and the resistance of the arteriolar bed. Control of vascular resistance is multifactorial, and abnormalities may exist in one or more areas. Mechanisms of control include neural reflexes and ongoing maintenance of sympathetic vasomotor tone and other effects mediated by neurotransmitters such as norepinephrine, extracellular fluid, and sodium stores; the renin-angiotensin-aldosterone pressor system; and locally active hormones and substances such as prostaglandins, kinins, adenosine, and hydrogen ions (H^+). In isolated systolic hypertension, which commonly is seen in elderly persons, the underlying problem is one of central arterial stiffness and loss of elasticity.[7]

Many physiologic factors may have an effect on blood pressure. Increased viscosity of the blood (e.g., polycythemia) may cause an elevation in blood pressure resulting from an increase in resistance to flow. A decrease in blood volume or tissue fluid volume (e.g., anemia, hemorrhage) reduces blood pressure. Conversely, an increase in blood volume or tissue fluid volume (e.g., sodium/fluid retention) increases blood pressure. Increases in cardiac output associated with exercise, fever, or thyrotoxicosis also may increase blood pressure.

A linear relationship exists between blood pressures at any level above normal and an increase in morbidity and mortality rates from stroke and coronary heart disease. Blood pressures above 115 mm Hg systolic and 75 mm Hg diastolic are associated with increased risk of cardiovascular disease.[12] It is estimated that about 15% of all blood pressure–related deaths from coronary heart disease occur in persons with blood pressure in the prehypertensive range.[13] However, the higher the blood pressure, the greater the chances of heart attack, heart failure, stroke, and kidney disease. For every increase in blood pressure of 20 mm Hg systolic and 10 mm Hg diastolic, a doubling of mortality related to ischemic heart disease and stroke occurs.[1] Hypertension precedes the onset of vascular changes in the kidney, heart, brain, and retina that lead to such clinical complications as renal failure, stroke, coronary insufficiency, MI, congestive heart failure, dementia, encephalopathy, and blindness. If the condition goes untreated, about 50% of hypertensive patients die of coronary heart disease or congestive heart failure, about 33% of stroke, and 10% to 15% of renal failure.[14]

BOX 3-1 Identifiable Causes of Hypertension

- Sleep apnea
- Drug-induced or drug-related
- Chronic kidney disease
- Primary aldosteronism
- Renovascular disease
- Chronic steroid therapy and Cushing syndrome
- Pheochromocytoma
- Coarctation of the aorta
- Thyroid or parathyroid disease

Data from the National Heart, Lung, and Blood Institute: The seventh report of the Joint National Committee on Prevention, Detection, Evaluation, and Treatment of High Blood Pressure: the JNC 7 report, *Bethesda, Maryland, US Department of Health and Human Services, Public Health Service, National Institutes of Health, National Heart, Lung, and Blood Institute, August 2004.*

CLINICAL PRESENTATION

Signs and Symptoms

Hypertension may remain an asymptomatic disease for many years, with the only sign being an elevated blood pressure. Blood pressure is measured with the use of a sphygmomanometer (Figure 3-1). Pressure at the peak of ventricular contraction is the *systolic pressure. Diastolic pressure* represents the total resting resistance in the arterial system after passage of the pulsating force produced by contraction of the left ventricle. The difference between diastolic and systolic pressures is called *pulse pressure. Mean arterial pressure* is roughly defined as the sum of the diastolic pressure plus one-third the pulse pressure. Patients commonly are found to have significant variability in blood pressures. *Labile* hypertension is the term that was previously used to describe the status of a subgroup of patients with wide variability in blood pressure readings; however, this term has fallen into disuse because it is now recognized that variability in blood pressure is the norm rather than the exception. About 15% to 20% of patients with untreated stage 1 hypertension have what is called *white coat hypertension,* which is defined as persistently elevated blood

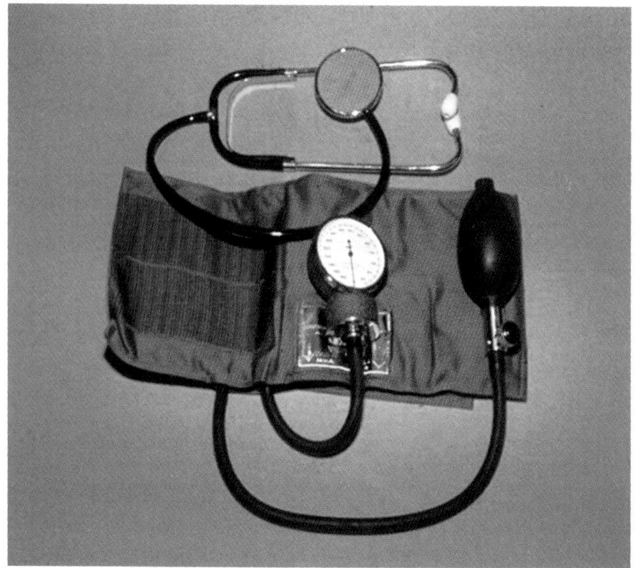

FIGURE 3-1 Standard blood pressure cuff (sphygmomanometer) and stethoscope.

BOX 3-2 Signs and Symptoms of Hypertensive Disease

Early
- Elevated blood pressure readings
- Narrowing and sclerosis of retinal arterioles
- Headache
- Dizziness
- Tinnitus

Advanced
- Rupture and hemorrhage of retinal arterioles
- Papilledema
- Left ventricular hypertrophy
- Proteinuria
- Congestive heart failure
- Angina pectoris
- Renal failure
- Dementia
- Encephalopathy

pressure only in the presence of a health care worker but not elsewhere.[6] In these patients, accurate blood pressure readings may require self-measurement at home or 24-hour ambulatory monitoring. Persons with blood pressure elevation in this setting are at lower risk for hypertensive complications than are those with sustained hypertension.

Before the age of 50, hypertension typically is characterized by an elevation in both diastolic and systolic pressures. *Isolated diastolic hypertension,* defined as a systolic pressure of 140 or less and a diastolic pressure of 90 or greater, is uncommon and most often is found in younger adults. Although the prognostic significance of this condition remains unclear and controversial, it appears that it may be relatively benign.[15] *Isolated systolic hypertension* is defined as a systolic pressure of 140 or higher and a diastolic blood pressure of 90 or less; it generally is found in older patients and constitutes an important risk factor for cardiovascular disease. Occasionally, isolated systolic blood pressure elevation is found in older children and young adults, often male. In these age groups, this form of hypertension is due to the combination of rapid growth in height and very elastic arteries, which accentuate the normal amplification of the pressure wave between the aorta and the brachial artery, resulting in high systolic pressure in the brachial artery but normal systolic pressure in the aorta.[6]

The earliest sign of hypertension is an elevated blood pressure reading; however, funduscopic examination of the retina may show early changes of hypertension consisting of narrowed arterioles with sclerosis. As indicated earlier, hypertension may remain an asymptomatic disease for many years, but when symptoms do occur, they include headache, tinnitus, and dizziness. These symptoms are not specific for hypertension, however, and may be experienced just as commonly by normotensive persons.[14]

Late signs and symptoms are related to involvement of various target organs, including kidney, brain, heart, or eye (Box 3-2). In advanced cases, retinal vessel hemorrhage, exudate, and papilledema may occur and are indicative of accelerated malignant hypertension, which is a medical emergency and requires immediate intervention. Hypertensive encephalopathy is characterized by headache, irritability, alterations in consciousness, and other signs of central nervous system (CNS) dysfunction. Other findings in advanced cases may include enlargement of the left ventricle with impairment of cardiac function, leading to congestive heart failure. Renal involvement can result in hematuria, proteinuria, and renal failure. Persons with hypertension may report fatigue and coldness in the legs, resulting from the peripheral arterial changes that may occur in advanced hypertension. Patients with hypertension often demonstrate an accelerated cognitive decline with aging.[16] Although these changes may be seen in patients with both primary and secondary hypertension, additional signs or symptoms may be present in secondary hypertension associated with underlying disease.

Laboratory Findings

The JNC 7[1] recommends that patients who have sustained hypertension be screened through routine laboratory tests, including 12-lead electrocardiogram, urinalysis, blood glucose, hematocrit, and a serum potassium, creatinine, calcium, and lipid profile. Results of these tests serve as baseline laboratory values that the physician should obtain before initiating therapy. Additional tests should be ordered if clinical and laboratory findings suggest the presence of an underlying cause for hypertension.

MEDICAL MANAGEMENT

Evaluation of a patient with hypertension includes a thorough medical history, a complete physical examination, and routine laboratory tests as described earlier. Additional diagnostic tests or procedures may be performed to detect secondary causes of hypertension or to make a definitive diagnosis. Patients found to have an identifiable cause for their hypertension should be treated for that disorder. Those without an identifiable cause are diagnosed with primary hypertension.

Classification and diagnosis of blood pressure (see Table 3-1) are based on an average of two or more properly measured blood pressure readings obtained in the seated patient on each of two or more office visits.[1] Measurement of blood pressure most commonly is achieved using the auscultatory method with a mercury, aneroid, or hybrid sphygmomanometer (see Figure 3-1). Mercury sphygmomanometers have long been considered the most accurate of such devices and the "gold standard;" however, because of increasing environmental concerns about mercury and the risk of breakage and spill, their use has become limited. Aneroid digital devices are the type most commonly used in dental offices. They are easy to use and provide reasonably accurate readings; however, they require regular calibration, and at least two readings should be taken.[17]

Patients with a diagnosis of prehypertension are not usually candidates for drug therapy but rather are encouraged to adopt lifestyle modifications to decrease their risk of developing the disease. Prehypertension is not a disease but rather a designation that reflects the fact that these patients are at increased risk for the development of hypertension. Lifestyle modifications include losing weight; adopting a diet rich in vegetables, fruits, and low-fat dairy products; reducing intake of foods high in cholesterol and saturated fats; decreasing sodium intake; limiting alcohol intake; and engaging in daily aerobic physical activity (Box 3-3). It is considered essential that patients with prehypertension, as well as those with diagnosed hypertension, follow these recommendations, because lifestyle modifications have been shown to effectively reduce blood pressure, prevent or delay the incidence of hypertension, enhance antihypertensive drug therapy, and decrease cardiovascular risk.[1] If lifestyle modifications are found to be inadequate for achieving desired blood pressure reduction, drug therapy is initiated.

The JNC 7[1] suggests that all people with hypertension—stages 1 and 2—should be treated. The treatment goal for most patients with hypertension is to reduce blood pressure to less than 140/90 mm Hg. For hypertensive patients with diabetes or kidney disease, however, the goal is less than 130/80 mm Hg. Evidence demonstrates

BOX 3-3 Lifestyle Modifications for Prevention and Reduction of High Blood Pressure

- Weight loss
- DASH (Dietary Approaches to Stop Hypertension) diet
  - Fruits
  - Vegetables
  - Low-fat dairy products
- Reduced intake of cholesterol-rich foods
- Reduced intake of saturated and total fats
- Reduced sodium intake to less than 2.4 g/day
- Regular aerobic physical activity on most days (30 minutes of brisk walking)
- Limited alcohol intake to no more than 1 oz/day (2 drinks for men and 1 drink for women)

Data from the National Heart, Lung, and Blood Institute: The seventh report of the Joint National Committee on Prevention, Detection, Evaluation, and Treatment of High Blood Pressure: the JNC 7 report, *Bethesda, Maryland, US Department of Health and Human Services, Public Health Service, National Institutes of Health, National Heart, Lung, and Blood Institute, August 2004.*

the clear benefits of aggressive treatment of hypertension. In clinical trials, antihypertensive therapy resulted in an average reduction in stroke incidence of 35% to 40%; MI, 20% to 25%; and heart failure, greater than 50%.[18]

Many drugs are currently available to treat hypertension (Table 3-4). Those most commonly used include thiazide diuretics, angiotensin-converting enzyme inhibitors (ACEIs), angiotensin receptor blockers (ARBs), beta blockers (BBs), and calcium channel blockers (CCBs). Other drugs that are less frequently used include α_1-adrenergic blockers and central α_2 agonists, as well as other centrally acting drugs, and direct vasodilators. Figure 3-2 depicts the algorithm suggested by the JNC 7 for the treatment of hypertension. If lifestyle modification is ineffective at lowering blood pressure adequately, then thiazide diuretics are most often the first drugs of choice, given either alone or in combination with ACEIs, ARBs, BBs, or CCBs, depending on the degree of elevation of blood pressure. For early stage 1 hypertension, single-drug therapy may be effective; however, for later stage 1 and for stage 2 hypertension, two or more drug combinations are necessary. The presence of certain comorbid conditions or factors such as heart failure, previous MI, diabetes, or kidney disease may be a compelling reason to select specific drugs or classes of drugs that have been found to be beneficial in clinical trials.

Patients with severe, uncontrolled hypertension, defined as blood pressure of 180/110 or higher, may require urgent or immediate treatment, including hospitalization.[1] Hypertensive emergencies are characterized by a severe elevation in blood pressure *with* evidence of impending or progressive target organ dysfunction such as hypertensive encephalopathy, intracerebral hemorrhage, acute MI, left ventricular failure with pulmonary edema, or unstable angina pectoris. These patients require immediate blood pressure reduction

TABLE 3-4 Drugs Used in the Management of Hypertension

Drug	Vasoconstrictor Interactions	Oral Manifestations	Other Considerations
Diuretics			
Thiazide Diuretics			
Chlorothiazide (Diuril) Chlorthalidone [generic] Hydrochlorothiazide (HCTZ) (HydroDIURIL, Microzide) Polythiazide (Renese) Indapamide (Lozol) Metolazone (Mykrox) Metolazone (Zaroxolyn)	None	Dry mouth, lichenoid reactions	Orthostatic hypotension; avoid prolonged use of NSAIDs—may reduce antihypertensive effects
Loop Diuretics			
Bumetanide (Bumex) Furosemide (Lasix) Torsemide (Demadex)			
Potassium-Sparing Diuretics			
Amiloride (Midamor) Triamterene (Dyrenium)			
Aldosterone Receptor Blockers			
Eplerenone (Inspra) Spironolactone (Aldactone)			
Combination			
Aldactazide, Dyazide			
Beta Blockers (BBs)			
Nonselective			
Propranolol (Inderal) Timolol (Blocadren) Nadolol (Corgard) Pindolol (Visken) Penbutolol (Levatol) Carteolol (Cartrol)	*Nonselective*—potential increase in blood pressure (use maximum of 0.036 mg epinephrine); avoid levonordefrin	Taste changes, lichenoid reactions	Avoid prolonged use of NSAIDs—may reduce antihypertensive effects
Cardioselective			
Metoprolol (Lopressor) Acebutolol (Sectral) Atenolol (Tenormin) Betaxolol (Kerlone) Bisoprolol (Zebeta)	*Cardioselective:* Normal use		
Combined Alpha and Beta Blockers			
Carvedilol (Coreg) Labetalol (Normodyne, Trandate)	Because both β_1- and β_2-adrenergic receptor sites are blocked, the potential for an adverse interaction is present; however, it is unlikely to occur because of compensatory α-adrenergic receptor blockade	Taste changes	Orthostatic hypotension; avoid prolonged use of NSAIDs—may reduce antihypertensive effects
Angiotensin-Converting Enzyme (ACE) Inhibitors			
Benazepril (Lotensin) Captopril (Capoten) Enalapril (Vasotec) Fosinopril (Monopril) Lisinopril (Prinivil; Zestril) Moexipril (Univasc) Perindopril (Aceon) Quinapril (Accupril) Ramipril (Altace)	None	Angioedema of lips, face, tongue; taste changes; oral burning	Orthostatic hypotension; avoid prolonged use of NSAIDs—may reduce antihypertensive effects

Drug	Vasoconstrictor Interactions	Oral Manifestations	Other Considerations
Angiotensin Receptor Blockers (ARBs)			
Candesartan (Atacand) Eprosartan (Teveten) Irbesartan (Cozaar) Olmesartan (Benicar) Telmisartan (Micardis) Valsartan (Diovan)	None	Angioedema of the lips, face, tongue	Orthostatic hypotension
Calcium Channel Blockers (CCBs)			
Diltiazem (Cardizem) Verapamil (Calan) Amlodipine (Norvasc) Felodipine (Plendil) Isradipine (DynaCirc) Nicardipine (Cardene) Nifedipine (Procardia) Nisoldipine (Sular)	None	Gingival hyperplasia	
α_1-Adrenergic Blockers			
Doxazosin (Catapres) Prazosin (Minipress) Terazosin (Hytrin)	None	Dry mouth, taste changes	Orthostatic hypotension, avoid prolonged use of NSAIDs—may reduce antihypertensive effects
Central α_2-Adrenergic Agonists and Other Centrally Acting Drugs			
Clonidine (Catapres) Methyldopa (Aldomet) Reserpine (generic) Guanfacine (Tenex)	None	Dry mouth, taste changes	Orthostatic hypotension
Direct Vasodilators			
Hydralazine (Apresoline) Minoxidil (Loniten)	None	Lupus-like oral and skin lesions, lymphadenopathy	Orthostatic hypotension; avoid prolonged use of NSAIDs—may reduce antihypertensive effects

NSAIDs, Nonsteroidal antiinflammatory drugs.

(within 1 hour) and should be admitted to an intensive care unit (ICU).[14]

Patients with severe hypertension but with less ominous clinical signs and symptoms such as headache, shortness of breath, nosebleeds, or severe anxiety require urgent treatment, but this level of hypertension does not constitute an emergency. The underlying problem in these patients most often is found to be noncompliance or an inadequate medication regimen. They should receive timely treatment to reduce blood pressure but without the immediacy of concern associated with evidence of progressive target organ damage. Treatment may include the administration of a short-acting oral antihypertensive agent followed by several hours of observation and subsequent adjustments in the medication regimen. Patients typically do not require admission to the ICU. Of note, severe, uncontrolled hypertension may occur with complete absence of symptoms. Patients diagnosed with this condition should receive timely medical treatment, but it is not considered an emergent or urgent situation.

DENTAL MANAGEMENT

Medical Considerations

The first task of the dentist is to identify patients with hypertension, both diagnosed and undiagnosed. A medical history, including the diagnosis of hypertension, how it is being treated, identification of antihypertensive drugs, compliance status, presence of hypertension-associated symptoms and signs, and level of stability of the disease, should be obtained. On occasion, patients may fail to report that they have been diagnosed with hypertension yet may report taking medications, including herbal medications, typically advocated to treat high blood pressure. This may be the only way for the clinician to uncover information revealing that the patient

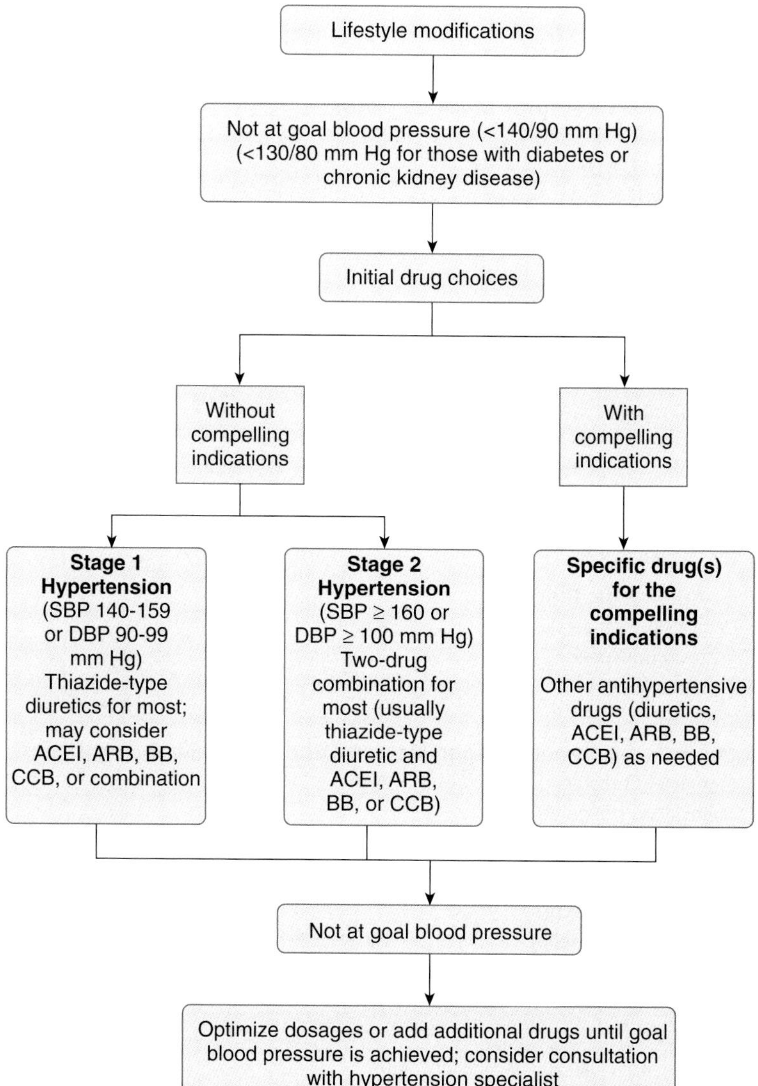

FIGURE 3-2 The treatment of hypertension. *(Redrawn from the National Heart, Lung, and Blood Institute:* The seventh report of the Joint National Committee on Prevention, Detection, Evaluation, and Treatment of High Blood Pressure: the JNC 7 report, *Bethesda, Maryland, US Department of Health and Human Services, Public Health Service, National Institutes of Health, National Heart, Lung, and Blood Institute, August 2004.)*

has hypertension. Patients also may be receiving treatment for complications of hypertensive disease, such as congestive heart failure, cerebrovascular disease, MI, renal disease, peripheral vascular disease, or diabetes mellitus. These conditions should be identified as well, because they may necessitate modification of the dental management plan.

In addition to a medical history, all patients should undergo blood pressure measurement (see Chapter 1). Blood pressure measurements should be routinely performed for all new patients and at recall appointments. More frequent blood pressure measurements are indicated for patients who are not compliant with treatment, whose hypertension is poorly controlled, or who have comorbid conditions such as heart failure or previous MI or stroke. In patients who are being treated for hypertension but have blood pressures above normal, the most common reason for the persistence of HBP is noncompliance or inadequate treatment; they should be encouraged to return to their physician for follow-up care. The patient who has not been diagnosed with hypertension but who has an abnormally elevated blood pressure should also be encouraged to see his or her physician. When a patient with upper-level stage 2 blood pressure is receiving dental treatment, consideration should be given to leaving the blood pressure cuff on the patient's arm and periodically checking the pressure during the appointment. The dentist should not make a diagnosis of hypertension but rather should inform the patient that the blood pressure reading is elevated, and that a physician should evaluate the condition.

The primary concern in dental management of a patient with hypertension is that during the course of treatment, a sudden, acute elevation in blood pressure might occur, potentially leading to a serious outcome such as stroke or MI. Such acute elevations in blood pressure may result from the release of endogenous catecholamines in response to stress and anxiety, from injection of exogenous catecholamines in the form of vasoconstrictors in the local anesthetic, or from absorption of a vasoconstrictor from the gingival retraction cord. Other concerns include potential drug interactions between the patient's antihypertensive medications and the drugs used in dental practice, and oral adverse effects that may be caused by antihypertensive medications.

Two important questions should be answered before dental treatment is provided for a patient with hypertension:

- What are the associated risks of treatment in this patient?
- At what level of blood pressure is treatment unsafe for the patient?

The American College of Cardiology and the American Heart Association have jointly published practice guidelines for the perioperative evaluation of patients with cardiovascular disease for whom noncardiac surgery of various types is planned.[19] These guidelines provide a framework to estimate the risk for occurrence of a stroke, MI, acute heart failure, or sudden death as a result of the surgery. Oral and maxillofacial surgery and periodontal surgery both are forms of noncardiac surgery; thus, these guidelines are directly applicable. In addition, the guidelines may be extrapolated and applied to nonsurgical dental treatment, as well. In the practice guidelines,[19] the determination of risk includes the evaluation of three factors: (1) the risk imposed by the patient's cardiovascular disease, (2) the risk imposed by the surgery or procedure, and (3) the risk imposed by the functional reserve or capacity of the patient.

The risk imposed by the presence of a *specific cardiovascular condition or disease* is stratified into major, intermediate, and minor risk categories (Box 3-4). Uncontrolled blood pressure, defined as 180/110 mm Hg or greater, is classified as a *minor* risk condition; however, the practice guidelines include a statement that blood pressure should be brought under control before any surgery is performed. Of note, the JNC 7 classification recommends timely or immediate referral for patients with blood pressure of 180/110 or higher, depending on the presence or absence of symptoms (see Table 3-1). Risk imposed by the *type of surgery* (or procedure) also is stratified into high (>5% risk), intermediate (<5% risk), and low (<1% risk) risk categories. In general, risk is greatest with vascular or emergency surgery, prolonged procedures, and procedures associated with excessive blood loss and general anesthesia (Box 3-5). Head and neck surgery, which may include major oral and maxillofacial procedures and extensive periodontal procedures, is classified as *intermediate* risk. Superficial surgical procedures, which include minor oral and periodontal surgery and nonsurgical dental procedures, are classified as *low* risk. Thus, it would appear that the risk associated with most general, outpatient dental procedures is very low.

BOX 3-4 Clinical Predictors of Increased Perioperative Cardiovascular Risk*

Major Risk Factors
- Unstable coronary syndromes
  - Acute or recent myocardial infarction[†] with evidence of important ischemic risk in clinical signs and symptoms or noninvasive study
  - Unstable or severe angina (Canadian class III or IV)[†‡§]
- Decompensated heart failure
- Significant arrhythmias
- Severe valvular disease

Intermediate Risk Factors
- History of ischemic heart disease
- History of compensated or previous heart failure
- History of cerebrovascular disease
- Diabetes mellitus
- Renal insufficiency

Minor Risk Factors
- Advanced age (>70 years)
- Abnormal ECG (left ventricular hypertrophy, left bundle branch block, ST-T abnormalities)
- Rhythm other than sinus rhythm
- Uncontrolled systemic hypertension (blood pressure ≥180/110 mm Hg)

ECG, Electrocardiogram.
*Cardiac events of myocardial infarction, heart failure, or death.
[†]The American College of Cardiology National Database Library defines *recent MI* as occurring more than 7 days but within 1 month (at or before 30 days) before the procedure and *acute MI* as occurring within 7 days.
[‡]May include "stable" angina in patients who are unusually sedentary.
[§]*Data from Campeau L: Grading of angina pectoris,* Circulation *54:522-523, 1976. The Canadian classification is a system of grading angina severity (grades I to IV), with grade I angina occurring only with strenuous exertion and grade IV angina occurring with any physical activity or at rest.*
Data from Fleisher LA, et al: ACC/AHA 2007 guidelines on perioperative cardiovascular evaluation and care for noncardiac surgery: a report of the American College of Cardiology/American Heart Association Task Force on Practice Guidelines *(Writing Committee to Revise the 2002 Guidelines on Perioperative Cardiovascular Evaluation for Noncardiac Surgery).* Circulation *116:e418-e499, 2007.*

The third factor involved in risk assessment is determination of the ability of the patient to perform certain physical activities *(functional capacity)* and is defined in metabolic equivalents (METs) (see Chapter 1). Perioperative cardiac risk is increased in patients who are unable to meet a 4-MET demand during most normal daily activities, which is equivalent to climbing a flight of stairs. Thus, a patient who reports inability to climb a flight of stairs without chest pain, shortness of breath, or fatigue would be at increased risk during a procedure.

Table 3-5 provides dental management recommendations for patients with various levels of blood pressure. In summary, patients with blood pressures less than 80/110 mm Hg can undergo any necessary dental treatment, both surgical and nonsurgical, with very little risk of an adverse outcome. For patients found to have

TABLE 3-5 Dental Management and Follow-up Recommendations Based on Blood Pressure

Blood Pressure (mm Hg)	Dental Treatment Recommendation	Follow-up Recommendation
≤120/80	Any required	No physician referral necessary
≥120/80 *but* <140/90	Any required	Encourage patient to see physician
≥140/90 *but* <160/100	Any required	Encourage patient to see physician
≥160/100 *but* <180/110	Any required; consider intraoperative monitoring of blood pressure for upper-level stage 2 hypertension	Refer patient to physician promptly (within 1 month)
≥180/110	Defer elective treatment	Refer to physician as soon as possible; if patient is symptomatic, refer immediately

BOX 3-5 Cardiac Risk* Stratification for Noncardiac Surgical Procedures

High (Reported Cardiac Risk Often Greater Than 5%)
- Aortic and other major vascular surgery
- Peripheral vascular surgery

Intermediate (Reported Cardiac Risk Generally Less Than 5%)
- Intraperitoneal and intrathoracic surgery
- Carotid endarterectomy
- Head and neck surgery
- Orthopedic surgery
- Prostate surgery

Low (Reported Cardiac Risk Generally Less Than 1%)
- Endoscopic procedures
- Superficial procedures
- Cataract surgery
- Breast surgery
- Ambulatory surgery

*Combined incidence of cardiac death and nonfatal myocardial infarction.
Adapted from Fleisher LA, et al: ACC/AHA 2007 guidelines on perioperative cardiovascular evaluation and care for noncardiac surgery: executive summary: a report of the American College of Cardiology/American Heart Association Task Force on Practice Guidelines *(Writing Committee to Revise the 2002 Guidelines on Perioperative Cardiovascular Evaluation for Noncardiac Surgery).* Circulation *116:1971-1996, 2007.*

asymptomatic blood pressure of 180/110 mm Hg or greater (uncontrolled hypertension), elective dental care should be deferred, and a physician referral for evaluation and treatment within 1 week is indicated. Patients with uncontrolled blood pressure associated with symptoms such as headache, shortness of breath, or chest pain should be referred to a physician for immediate evaluation. In patients with uncontrolled hypertension, certain problems such as pain, infection, or bleeding may necessitate urgent dental treatment. In such instances, the patient should be managed in consultation with the physician, and measures such as intraoperative blood pressure monitoring, electrocardiogram monitoring, establishment of an intravenous line, and sedation may be used. The decision must always be made as to whether the benefit of proposed treatment outweighs the potential risks.

Once it has been determined that the hypertensive patient can be safely treated, a management plan should be developed (Box 3-6). For all patients, the dentist should make every effort to reduce as much as possible the stress and anxiety associated with dental treatment. This consideration is of particular importance in patients with hypertension. A critical factor in providing an anxiety-free situation is the relationship established among the dentist, office staff, and the patient. Patients should be encouraged to express and discuss their fears, concerns, and questions about dental treatment.

Stress management is important for patients with hypertension to lessen the chances of endogenous release of catecholamines during the dental visit (see Chapter 1). Long or stressful appointments are best avoided. Short morning appointments seem best tolerated. If the patient becomes anxious or apprehensive during the visit, the appointment may be terminated and rescheduled for another day. Anxiety can be reduced for many patients by oral premedication with a short-acting benzodiazepine such as triazolam (Halcion; Pharmacia & Upjohn, Kalamazoo, Michigan), taken 1 hour before the start of the dental appointment. Dose is dictated by the age and size of the patient and is determined in accordance with prescribing guidelines for the agent selected. Nitrous oxide plus oxygen for inhalation sedation is an excellent intraoperative anxiolytic for use in patients with hypertension. Care is indicated to ensure adequate oxygenation at all times, avoiding postdiffusion hypoxia at the termination of administration. Hypoxia is to be avoided because of the resultant rebound elevation in blood pressure that may occur. During treatment of a patient with upper-level stage 2 hypertension, it may be advisable to leave the blood pressure cuff on the patient's arm, and to periodically check the pressure. If the blood pressure rises above 179/109 mm Hg, the procedure should be terminated, the patient referred to his or her physician, and the appointment rescheduled.

Because many of the antihypertensive agents tend to produce orthostatic hypotension as a side effect, rapid changes in chair position during dental treatment should be avoided. When treatment has concluded for that

BOX 3-6 Dental Management
Recommendations for Patients with Hypertension

P

Patient Evaluation/Risk Assessment (see Box 1-1)

- Evaluate and determine if hypertension exists.
- Refer patient to physician if blood pressure is poorly controlled or if the condition is untreated.

Potential Issues/Factors of Concern

A	
Antibiotics	Avoid the use of erythromycin and clarithromycin (not azithromycin) with calcium channel blockers, because the combination can enhance hypotension.
Analgesics	Avoid long-term (>2 weeks) use of NSAIDs, because these agents may interfere with effectiveness of some antihypertensive medications.
Anesthesia	Modest doses of local anesthetic with 1:100,000 or 1:200,000 epinephrine (e.g., 1 or 2 carpules) at a given time are of little clinical consequence in patients with blood pressure <180/110 mm Hg. Greater quantities may be tolerated reasonably well, but with increased risk. Levonordefrin should be avoided. In patients with uncontrolled hypertension (blood pressure >180/110 mm Hg), the use of epinephrine may be tolerated but should be discussed with the physician.
Allergies	No issues
Anxiety	Patients with hypertension who are anxious or fearful are especially good candidates for preoperative oral and/or intraoperative inhalation sedation. Apply good stress management protocols.
B	
Bleeding	Excessive bleeding due to hypertension is possible but unlikely.
Breathing	No issues
Blood pressure	Patients with a blood presure <180/110 mm Hg may receive any necessary dental treatment. For patients with a pressure reading >180/110 mm Hg, dental treatment should be deferred until blood pressure is brought under control. If urgent or emergency dental treatment is required, it should be done in as limited and conservative a manner as possible.
C	
Chair position	Avoid rapid position changes owing to possibility of antihypertensive drug-associated orthostatic hypotension.
D	
Drugs	Several of the antihypertensive drugs have reported oral manifestations. The nonselective β-adrenergic blockers can potentially interact with epinephrine, but such interaction is dose-dependent and very unlikely to occur at the usual doses.
Devices	For patients with stage II hypertension (blood pressure >160/100 mm Hg), periodic monitoring of pressure during treatment may be advisable.
E	
Equipment	No issues
Emergencies	Patients with hypertension are at increased risk for cardiovascular disease; thus, although unlikely, angina, stroke, arrhythmia, and MI should all be anticipated as possible occurrences.
F	
Follow-up	Schedule follow-up appointment if patient is referred to physician.

appointment, the dental chair should be returned slowly to an upright position. After sufficient time to permit adjustment to the change in posture, the patient should be physically supported while slowly getting out of the chair, to ensure that good balance and stability have been regained. A patient who experiences dizziness or lightheadedness should be directed to sit back down to allow safe recovery of equilibrium.

Ambulatory (outpatient) general anesthesia in the dental office generally is recommended only for patients whose status on the American Society of Anesthesiologists (ASA) classification is ASA I (status of a healthy, normal patient) or ASA II (presence of mild to moderate systemic disease). Some patients with severe hypertension may be excluded.

Use of Vasoconstrictors. Profound local anesthesia is critical for pain and anxiety control and is especially important for patients with hypertension or other cardiovascular disease, to decrease endogenous catecholamine release. The effectiveness of local anesthesia is enhanced by the inclusion of a vasoconstrictor in the local anesthetic solution, which delays systemic absorption, increases the duration of anesthesia, and provides local hemostasis. These properties allow for enhanced quality and duration of pain control and markedly facilitate performance of the technical procedures. Thus, the advantages of including a vasoconstrictor in the local anesthetic are obvious. Concerns have emerged, however, that the use of local anesthetic with a vasoconstrictor in a patient with hypertension could result in a potentially serious spike in blood pressure.

The cardiovascular response to conventional doses of injected epinephrine, both in patients who are healthy and in those with hypertension, usually is of little clinical importance. A metaanalysis of several clinical studies determined that the mean resting venous plasma epinephrine concentration is 39 pg/mL; this is approximately doubled by the intraoral injection of a single

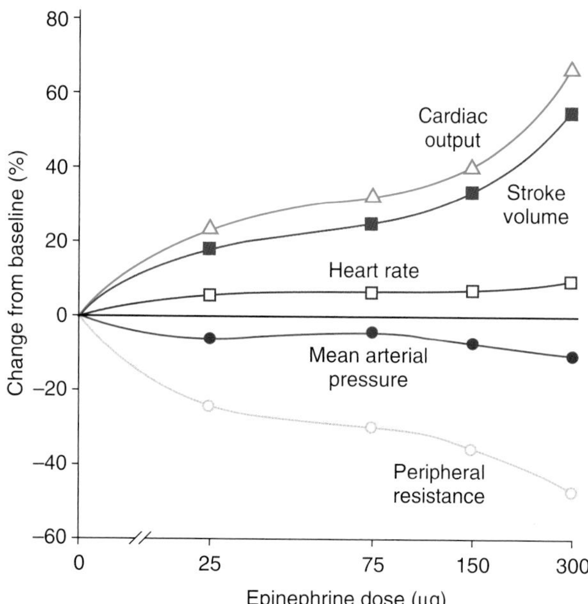

FIGURE 3-3 Cardiovascular effects of epinephrine when used in regional anesthesia. *(Redrawn from Jastak JT, Yagiela JA, Donaldson D:* Local anesthesia of the oral cavity, *Philadelphia, 1995, Saunders.)*

cartridge of 2% lidocaine with 1 : 100,000 epinephrine.[20] This resulting elevation in plasma epinephrine is linear and dose-dependent. Although large doses of epinephrine may cause a significant rise in blood pressure and heart rate, small doses such as those contained in one or two cartridges of lidocaine with 1 : 100,000 epinephrine cause minimal physiologic changes (Figure 3-3). This fact is due to a preponderance of action among β_2 receptors and a decrease in diastolic pressure; thus, mean arterial pressure is essentially unchanged, with only a minimal increase in heart rate.

Several clinical investigations have evaluated changes in plasma epinephrine concentration and hemodynamic parameters in healthy patients after dental injections of 2% lidocaine with 1 : 100,000 epinephrine. After injection of 1.8 mL (one cartridge), plasma levels increased two- to three-fold, but no significant changes were observed in heart rate or blood pressure.[21-23] With 5.4 mL of solution (three cartridges), however, plasma levels increased five- to six-fold; these changes were accompanied by significant increases in heart rate and systolic blood pressure, but with no adverse symptoms or sequelae.[24,25] The critical question, then, is how a particular patient with hypertension or other cardiovascular disease will react to these dose challenges of epinephrine.

A systematic review of the literature on the cardiovascular effects of epinephrine in hypertensive dental patients[26] concluded that although the quantity and quality of pertinent articles were problematic, the increased risk of adverse events among patients with uncontrolled hypertension was low, and the reported occurrence of adverse events associated with the use of epinephrine in local anesthetic agents was minimal. This review was cited by the JNC 7[1] report and supported its conclusions. Another recent review of the subject noted an absence of adverse case reports involving epinephrine in local anesthetics and cited the numerous studies that demonstrated the safety and efficacy of these preparations.[27]

Thus, the existing evidence indicates that use of modest doses (one or two cartridges of 2% lidocaine with 1 : 100,000 epinephrine) carries little clinical risk in patients with hypertension, the benefits of its use far outweighing any potential problems. Use of more than this amount at one time may be tolerated, but with increasing risk for adverse hemodynamic changes. Levonordefrin should be avoided in patients with hypertension, however, because of its comparative excessive α_1 stimulation. The use of epinephrine generally is not advised in patients with uncontrolled hypertension, in whom elective dental care should be deferred. If urgent treatment becomes necessary, however, a decision must be made regarding the use of epinephrine, which will be dictated by the situation. A reasonable conclusion from all of the available evidence is that the benefits of use of epinephrine outweigh the increased risks, so long as modest doses (e.g., one or two carpules) are used at one time, and care is taken to avoid inadvertent intravascular injection. Consultation with the patient's physician is advisable before a definitive decision is made.

An additional concern when patients with hypertension are treated is the potential for adverse drug interactions between vasoconstrictors and antihypertensive drugs—specifically, the nonselective β-adrenergic blocking agents. The basis for concern with use of nonselective β-adrenergic blocking agents (e.g., propranolol) is that the normal compensatory vasodilatation of skeletal muscle vasculature mediated by β_2 receptors is inhibited by these drugs, and injection of epinephrine, levonordefrin, or any other pressor agent may result in uncompensated peripheral vasoconstriction because of unopposed stimulation of α_1 receptors. This vasoconstrictive effect could potentially cause a significant elevation in blood pressure and a compensatory bradycardia.[28,29] Several cases of this interaction have been reported in the literature, but it appears to be dose-dependent.[30-32] Adverse interactions are even less likely to occur in patients who take cardioselective beta blockers.[25] Although the *potential* exists for adverse interactions between vasoconstrictors and the nonselective β-adrenergic-blocking agents, available evidence and clinical experience suggest that epinephrine in small doses of one to two cartridges containing 1 : 100,000 epinephrine can be used safely.[33] Indeed, Brown and Rhodus[27] concluded in their review that adverse drug interactions between beta blockers and epinephrine were extremely unlikely; however, they noted that levonordefrin should be avoided. Topical vasoconstrictors generally should not be used for local hemostasis in patients with hypertension. When performing crown and bridge procedures for patients with hypertension, the dentist should avoid using gingival retraction cord that contains epinephrine, because this material contains highly concentrated epinephrine, which can be quickly absorbed through abraided gingival sulcus tissues, resulting in tachycardia and elevated blood pressure. As an alternative, one study reported that tetrahydrozoline (Visine; Pfizer Inc, New York, New York), oxymetazoline (Afrin; Schering-Plough, Summit, New Jersey), and phenylephrine (Neo-Synephrine; Bayer, Morristown, New Jersey) may be used to soak the cord, providing hemostatic effects similar to those obtained with epinephrine but with minimal cardiovascular effects.[34]

Several other effects are of concern with antihypertensive agents and dental management. Some antihypertensive agents, especially alpha blockers, alpha-beta blockers, and diuretics, may predispose patients to development of orthostatic hypotension and potentiate the actions of anxiolytic and sedative drugs. Also, erythromycin and clarithromycin can exacerbate the hypotensive effect of calcium channel blockers. Anxiolytics and sedatives may be used for patients who take these antihypertensive medications; however, the usual dosage may need to be reduced. The efficacy of antihypertensive drugs may be decreased by the prolonged use of nonsteroidal antiinflammatory drugs—an interaction that should be considered if these drugs are used for analgesia, although the use of nonsteroidal antiinflammatory drugs for a few days is of little clinical importance.[35]

Treatment Planning Modifications

Patients with blood pressures less than 180/110 mm Hg can receive any indicated dental treatment; however, those with elevated blood pressures (140/90 and above) should be encouraged to see their physician for further investigation. Elective dental procedures should be deferred for the patient who has uncontrolled hypertension (blood pressure of 180/110 or higher) (see Table 3-5).

Oral Manifestations. Oral complications have not been associated with hypertension itself. The development of facial palsy has been described in the occasional patient with malignant hypertension.[36] Excessive bleeding after surgical procedures or trauma has been reported in patients with severe hypertension; such bleeding in this patient population is not common, however, and its association with hypertension is controversial. Patients who take antihypertensive drugs, especially diuretics, may report dry mouth. Mercurial diuretics may cause oral lesions with an allergic or toxic basis. Lichenoid reactions have been reported with thiazides, methyldopa, propranolol, and labetalol. ACEIs may cause neutropenia, resulting in delayed healing or gingival bleeding. Angioedema and a persistent cough may be caused by ACEIs.[37] Oral burning also has been reported to be caused by ACEIs.[38] Calcium channel blockers can cause gingival overgrowth (Figure 3-4; see also Table 3-4).

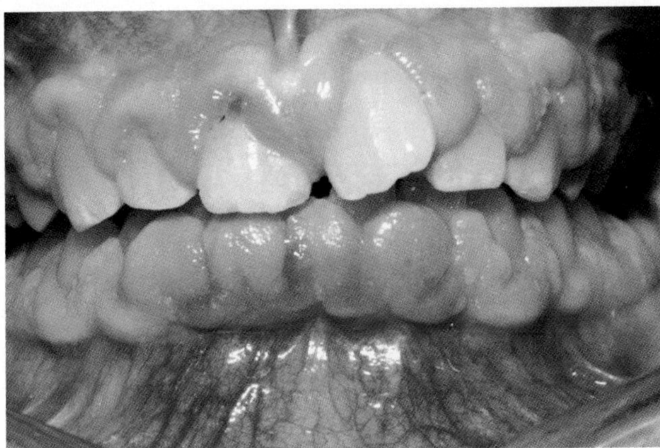

FIGURE 3-4 Gingival hyperplasia in a patient taking a calcium channel blocker. *(Courtesy Dr. Terry Wright.)*

REFERENCES

1. National Heart, Lung, and Blood Institute: The seventh report of the Joint National Committee on Prevention, Detection, Evaluation, and Treatment of High Blood Pressure: the JNC 7 report, Bethesda, Maryland, US Department of Health and Human Services, Public Health Service, National Institutes of Health, National Heart, Lung, and Blood Institute, August 2004.
2. National Heart, Lung, and Blood Institute: The Fourth Report on the Diagnosis, Evaluation, and Treatment of High Blood Pressure in Children and Adolescents, Bethesda, Maryland, US Department of Health and Human Services, Public Health Service, National Institutes of Health, National Heart, Lung, and Blood Institute, May 2005.
3. Hajjar I, Kotchen JM, Kotchen TA: Hypertension: trends in prevalence, incidence, and control. *Annu Rev Public Health* 27:465-490, 2006.
4. Fields LE, et al: The burden of adult hypertension in the United States 1999 to 2000: a rising tide, *Hypertension* 44:398-404, 2004.
5. Burt VL, et al: Prevalence of hypertension in the US adult population. Results from the Third National Health and Nutrition Examination Survey, 1988-1991, *Hypertension* 25:305-313, 1995.
6. Pickering TG, et al: Recommendations for blood pressure measurement in humans and experimental animals: Part 1: blood pressure measurement in humans: a statement for professionals from the Subcommittee of Professional and Public Education of the American Heart Association Council on High Blood Pressure Research, *Circulation* 111:697-716, 2005.
7. Victor RG: Arterial hypertension. In Goldman L, Ausiello D, editors: *Cecil medicine*, ed 23, Philadelphia, 2008, Saunders, pp 430-450.
8. Franklin SS, et al: Predominance of isolated systolic hypertension among middle-aged and elderly U.S. hypertensives: analysis based on National Health and Nutrition Examination Survey (NHANES) III, *Hypertension* 37:869-874, 2001.
9. Franklin SS: Hypertension in older people: part 1, *J Clin Hypertens (Greenwich)* 8:444-449, 2006.
10. Hypertension-related mortality among Hispanic subpopulations—United States, 1995-2002, *MMWR Morb Mortal Wkly Rep* 55:177-180, 2006.

11. Smith SC Jr, et al: Discovering the full spectrum of cardiovascular disease: Minority Health Summit 2003: report of the Obesity, Metabolic Syndrome, and Hypertension Writing Group, *Circulation* 111:e134-e139, 2005.
12. Lewington S, et al: Age-specific relevance of usual blood pressure to vascular mortality: a meta-analysis of individual data for one million adults in 61 prospective studies, *Lancet* 360:1903-1913, 2002.
13. Miura K, et al: Relationship of blood pressure to 25-year mortality due to coronary heart disease, cardiovascular diseases, and all causes in young adult men: the Chicago Heart Association Detection Project in Industry, *Arch Intern Med* 161:1501-1508, 2001.
14. Victor RG, Kaplan AL: Systemic hypertension: mechanisms and diagnosis. In Libby P, et al, editors: *Braunwald's heart disease: a textbook of cardiovascular medicine*, ed 8, Philadelphia, 2008, Saunders, pp 1027-1048.
15. Pickering TG: Isolated diastolic hypertension, *J Clin Hypertens (Greenwich)* 5:411-413, 2003.
16. Reinprecht F, et al: Hypertension and changes of cognitive function in 81-year-old men: a 13-year follow-up of the population study "Men born in 1914," Sweden, *J Hypertens* 21:57-66, 2003.
17. Wan Y, et al: Determining which automatic digital blood pressure device performs adequately: a systematic review, *J Hum Hypertens* 24:431-438, 2010.
18. Neal B, MacMahon S, Chapman N: Effects of ACE inhibitors, calcium antagonists, and other blood-pressure-lowering drugs: results of prospectively designed overviews of randomised trials. Blood Pressure Lowering Treatment Trialists' Collaboration, *Lancet* 356:1955-1964, 2000.
19. Fleisher LA, et al: ACC/AHA 2007 guidelines on perioperative cardiovascular evaluation and care for noncardiac surgery: executive summary: a report of the American College of Cardiology/American Heart Association Task Force on Practice Guidelines (Writing Committee to Revise the 2002 Guidelines on Perioperative Cardiovascular Evaluation for Noncardiac Surgery), *Circulation* 116:1971-1996, 2007.
20. Yagiela J: Local anesthetics. In Dionne R, Phero J, editors: *Management of pain and anxiety in dental practice*, New York, 1991, Elsevier Science Publishing.
21. Cioffi GA, et al: The hemodynamic and plasma catecholamine responses to routine restorative dental care, *J Am Dent Assoc* 111:67-70, 1985.
22. McInnes GT: Integrated approaches to management of hypertension: promoting treatment acceptance, *Am Heart J* 138(3 Pt 2):252-255, 1999.
23. Tolas AG, Pflug AE, Halter JB: Arterial plasma epinephrine concentrations and hemodynamic responses after dental injection of local anesthetic with epinephrine, *J Am Dent Assoc* 104:41-43, 1982.
24. Beilin LJ, Puddey IB, Burke V: Lifestyle and hypertension, *Am J Hypertens* 12(9 Pt 1):934-945, 1999.
25. Jastak J, Yagiela J, Donaldson D: *Local anesthesia of the oral cavity*, Philadelphia, 1995, WB Saunders.
26. Bader JD, Bonito AJ, Shugars DA: A systematic review of cardiovascular effects of epinephrine on hypertensive dental patients, *Oral Surg Oral Med Oral Pathol Oral Radiol Endod* 93:647-653, 2002.
27. Brown RS, Rhodus NL: Epinephrine and local anesthesia revisited, *Oral Surg Oral Med Oral Pathol Oral Radiol Endod* 100:401-408, 2005.
28. Houben H, Thien T, van't Laar A: Effect of low-dose epinephrine infusion on hemodynamics after selective and nonselective beta-blockade in hypertension, *Clin Pharmacol Ther* 31:685-690, 1982.
29. Reeves RA, et al: Nonselective beta-blockade enhances pressor responsiveness to epinephrine, norepinephrine, and angiotensin II in normal man, *Clin Pharmacol Ther* 35:461-466, 1984.
30. Foster CA, Aston SJ: Propranolol-epinephrine interaction: a potential disaster, *Plast Reconstr Surg* 72:74-78, 1983.
31. Kram J, et al: Propranolol (letter), *Ann Intern Med* 80:282, 1974.
32. Mito RS, Yagiela JA: Hypertensive response to levonordefrin in a patient receiving propranolol: report of case, *J Am Dent Assoc* 116:55-57, 1988.
33. Hersh EV, Giannakopoulos H: Beta-adrenergic blocking agents and dental vasoconstrictors, *Dent Clin North Am* 54:687-696, 2010.
34. Bowles WH, Tardy SJ, Vahadi A: Evaluation of new gingival retraction agents, *J Dent Res* 70:1447-1449, 1991.
35. Oates JA, et al: Clinical implications of prostaglandin and thromboxane A_2 formation (1), *N Engl J Med* 319:689-698, 1988.
36. Scully C, Cawson R: *Medical problems in dentistry*, ed 5, Edinburgh, 2005, Churchill Livingstone.
37. Tai S, Mascaro M, Goldstein NA: Angioedema: a review of 367 episodes presenting to three tertiary care hospitals, *Ann Otol Rhinol Laryngol* 119:836-841, 2010.
38. Brown RS, et al: A retrospective evaluation of 56 patients with oral burning and limited clinical findings, *Gen Dent* 54:267-271, 2006.

4

Ischemic Heart Disease

Coronary atherosclerotic heart disease is a major health problem in the United States and in other industrialized nations. Atherosclerosis is the thickening of the intimal layer of the arterial wall caused by the accumulation of lipid plaques. The atherosclerotic process results in a narrowed arterial lumen with diminished blood flow and oxygen supply. Atherosclerosis is the most common underlying cause of not only coronary heart disease (angina and myocardial infarction [MI]) but also cerebrovascular disease (stroke) and peripheral arterial disease (intermittent claudication).

Symptomatic coronary atherosclerotic heart disease often is referred to as *ischemic heart disease*. Ischemic symptoms are the result of oxygen deprivation secondary to reduced blood flow to a portion of the myocardium. Other conditions such as embolism, coronary ostial stenosis, coronary artery spasm, and congenital abnormalities also may cause ischemic heart disease.

GENERAL DESCRIPTION

Incidence and Prevalence

More than 70 million Americans (about 25% of the population) are estimated to have some form of cardiovascular disease, with about 13 million having coronary heart disease.[1] The annual mortality rate for cardiovascular diseases as a group has been declining since 1940. From 1970 to 2000, mortality from coronary heart disease decreased by 50% and from stroke by 60%.[2] Despite this decline, cardiovascular diseases continue to pose the most serious threat to health in America, accounting for about 33% of all deaths.[1] Coronary heart disease is the leading cause of death in the United States after age 65, and it is responsible for 1.2 million new or recurrent heart attacks annually, of which 40% are fatal.[1] Autopsy studies in the United States have shown that cardiovascular disease begins at an early age, and that one in six American teenagers already has pathologic intimal thickening of the coronary arteries.[3] Autopsy studies of soldiers killed during the Korean and Vietnam conflicts and of trauma victims have shown that atherosclerosis begins early in life, although its symptoms and complications typically manifest later, in midlife.[4,5] The average dental practice with 2000 patients can be expected to include at least 100 patients with ischemic heart disease.

Etiology

The cause of coronary atherosclerosis is not known; however, research indicates that the disease is related to a variety of risk factors. These risk factors include male gender, older age, a family history of cardiovascular disease, hyperlipidemia, hypertension, cigarette smoking, physical inactivity, obesity, insulin resistance and diabetes mellitus, mental stress, and depression. In addition to these conventional risk factors, markers of inflammation such as C-reactive protein, homocysteine, fibrinogen, and lipoprotein(a) have been found to be associated with atherosclerosis.[1]

Before the age of 75, the risk of coronary atherosclerosis is greater for men than for women.[1] MI and sudden death are rare in premenopausal women; however, after menopause, a rapid reduction occurs in this gender difference. The fact that men are more prone to the clinical manifestations of coronary atherosclerosis is accentuated in nonwhite populations (e.g., African Americans, Native Americans, Hispanics). Studies have confirmed that people with parents or siblings affected by coronary atherosclerotic heart disease are at risk for development of the disease at a younger age than that typical for those without such a history.

Elevation in serum lipid levels is a major risk factor for atherosclerosis. Increased levels of low-density lipoprotein (LDL) cholesterol pose the greatest risk for coronary atherosclerosis, whereas increased levels of high-density lipoprotein (HDL) cholesterol have been shown to reduce the risk.[6] Persons with elevated triglyceride or β-lipoprotein levels have an increased risk for the disease. A diet rich in total calories, saturated fats, cholesterol, sugars, and salts also enhances the risk.

Increased blood pressure appears to be one of the most significant risk factors for coronary atherosclerotic heart disease.[1] In general, systolic blood pressure (SBP) is more strongly related to the incidence of cardiovascular disease than is diastolic blood pressure, especially in the elderly.[6] SBP rises throughout life, and diastolic blood pressure (DBP) tends to level off or decrease after the age of 50. Most epidemiologic studies, however, recognize the importance of both DBP and SBP in the assessment of cardiovascular risk. It has been shown that morbidity and mortality increase linearly with blood pressures greater than 115/75 mm Hg.[2] In the Framingham Study, even prehypertension (defined as SBP of 130 to 139 and DBP of 85 to 89) was associated with a risk of cardiovascular disease double that for lower pressures.[7]

Cigarette smoking is the single most important modifiable risk factor for coronary heart disease (see Chapter 8). Multiple prospective studies have clearly documented that, compared with nonsmokers, persons who smoke 20 or more cigarettes daily have a two- to four-fold increase in coronary heart disease.[8] This increased risk appears to be proportionate to the number of cigarettes smoked per day. In a 5-year study of 4165 smokers with coronary atherosclerotic heart disease, the death rate was reduced for people who stopped smoking.[9] The death rate was 22% for 2675 persons who continued smoking and 15% for 1490 who stopped. In the Framingham Study, participants who discontinued smoking lowered their risk of MI within 2 years.[10] Pipe and cigar smoking apparently convey little risk for development of heart disease.

Patients with diabetes mellitus have a greater incidence of coronary atherosclerotic heart disease and more extensive lesions. They develop the condition at an earlier age than that typical for persons who do not have diabetes. Almost 41 million Americans have some degree of abnormal glucose tolerance (prediabetes)—a condition along with obesity that markedly increases the risk for type 2 diabetes and premature atherosclerosis.[11] Patients with diabetes have two- to eight-fold higher rates of future cardiovascular events as compared with age-matched and ethnically matched nondiabetic patients.[12] Three fourths of all deaths among diabetic patients result from coronary heart disease.[13] Compared with unaffected persons, diabetic patients have a greater degree of atherosclerosis in the major arteries and in the microvascular circulation. Although hyperglycemia is associated with microvascular disease, insulin resistance itself promotes atherosclerosis even before it produces frank diabetes, and available data corroborate the role of insulin resistance as an independent risk factor for atherothrombosis.[14] *Metabolic syndrome* is the term used to describe a cluster of pathologic findings consisting of obesity, insulin resistance, low HDL cholesterol, elevated triglycerides, and hypertension, all of which are risk factors for atherosclerosis. The recognized importance of this clinical syndrome as a setting for the development of atherosclerosis reflects a synergistic effect of the multiple risk factors. The prevalence of metabolic syndrome among adults in the United States is estimated to be 34% to 38%, increasing with age.[15]

Other risk factors for the development of atherosclerosis have emerged and include elevated levels of C-reactive protein (inflammatory marker), fibrinogen (procoagulant), plasminogen activator inhibitor (thrombolytic), and homocysteine.[6]

Numerous studies have reported an association between periodontal disease and cardiovascular disease, raising the question of whether periodontal disease is a risk factor for cardiovascular disease.[16] Although the mechanism to explain this relationship is unclear, it is hypothesized that the chronic inflammatory burden of periodontal disease may lead to impaired functioning of the vascular endothelium.[17] This is merely an association, however, and causation has not been proved.[18] Additional interventional studies will be required to further elucidate this relationship.

No single risk factor is responsible for the development of coronary atherosclerosis, but many factors act synergistically. Evidence suggests that modification of those risk factors that can be controlled, such as cigarette smoking, hypertension, hyperlipidemia, and diabetes, may reduce or modify the clinical effects of the disease.

Pathophysiology and Complications

Understanding of the pathophysiology of atherosclerosis has evolved significantly over the past 2 or 3 decades. In essence, the basic model has gone from the concept of a cholesterol storage disease with a buildup of plaque on the surface of an artery, analogous to rust buildup in a pipe, to one of an inflammatory disorder of the cellular lining of the arteries, with inflammation playing a fundamental role at all stages of the disease.[4,19] Furthermore, it is now clear that narrowing of the arteries does not necessarily presage MI, and that simply treating narrowed blood vessels does not prolong life. In fact, vascular events rarely result from plaque growth but more often follow the rupture of a less prominent plaque, resulting in clot formation or thrombus.

Libby and Theroux[19] have elegantly described the formation of atheromatous plaques. The first steps in the formation of an atheromatous plaque remain largely conjectural; however, they involve an inflammatory repair response of the injured arterial intima. Chronic minimal injury to the arterial endothelium is common and results from both physiologic and pathologic processes. Physiologic injury often occurs as the result of disturbed blood flow at bending points or bifurcations (branch points) in the artery. Endothelial injury or dysfunction also may be caused by hypercholesterolemia, glycation end products in diabetes, irritants in tobacco smoke, circulating vasoactive amines, immune complexes, and infection.

Atheroma formation is initiated by adherence of monocytes to an area of injured or altered endothelium. Usually, monocytes do not adhere to intact endothelium; however, triggers of atherosclerosis such as a high saturated fat diet, smoking, hypertension, hyperglycemia, obesity, and insulin resistance initiate the expression of adhesion molecules by the endothelial cells, thus promoting attachment. The attached monocytes then migrate into the intima of the vessel and become macrophages. Lipids derived from plasma LDLs also enter through the injured or dysfunctional endothelium, forming extracellular deposits or small pools. Macrophages then engulf lipid molecules to become *foam cells,* which are characteristic features of the *fatty streak.* Foam cells are joined by T lymphocytes, and together they produce a variety of inflammatory cytokines, which promote the migration and proliferation of smooth muscle cells and collagen to surround the foam cells, thereby forming a fibrous covering or cap. The arrival of the smooth muscle cells triggers a coalescence of the foam cells and small extracellular pools of lipid into a larger pool or lipid core. The T lymphocytes secrete cytokines that inhibit the further production of collagen, possibly leading to weakening and thinning of the fibrous cap and rendering it susceptible to rupture. With rupture or disruption of the plaque surface, tissue factor comes into contact with blood, and a thrombus is subsequently formed (Figure 4-1).

Plaques may grow and proliferate outwardly, away from the lumen of the artery, or inwardly, into the lumen. With inward proliferation, the size of the lumen is progressively reduced (stenosis). Thus, blood flow may be chronically decreased, and when the demand for oxygen exceeds supply, the outcome is ischemic pain. Ischemic symptoms may be produced when occlusion reaches 75% of the cross-sectional area of the artery[20] (Figure 4-2). Of interest, however, in most instances of an acute coronary event, the vessels typically are less than 50% occluded by plaque growth.[21]

Most acute coronary syndromes (e.g., unstable angina, myocardial infarction) are caused by physical disruption or fracture of the atheromatous plaque, most commonly of a plaque that did not cause extreme stenosis. In plaque rupture, the fibrous cap tears, allowing arterial blood to enter the lipid core, where contact with tissue factor and collagen induces platelet adhesion and aggregation and activation of the coagulation cascade. This series of events results in thrombus formation and sudden expansion of the lesion. Blood flow through the affected artery may become compromised or completely blocked.

Atherosclerosis usually is a focal disease that commonly occurs in certain areas or regions of arteries while sparing others. Those affected include the brain, heart, aorta, and peripheral arteries (Figure 4-3). For example, the proximal left anterior descending coronary artery is a common area of atherosclerotic involvement; however, the internal mammary artery is rarely affected. The lumen of an affected artery may be circumferentially narrowed evenly or eccentrically, depending on the location and extent of the plaque.

The outcome of the atherosclerotic process is extremely variable. Some lesions never progress past the fatty streak phase; however, in most Western societies, the presence of frank plaques is the norm. Even so, most

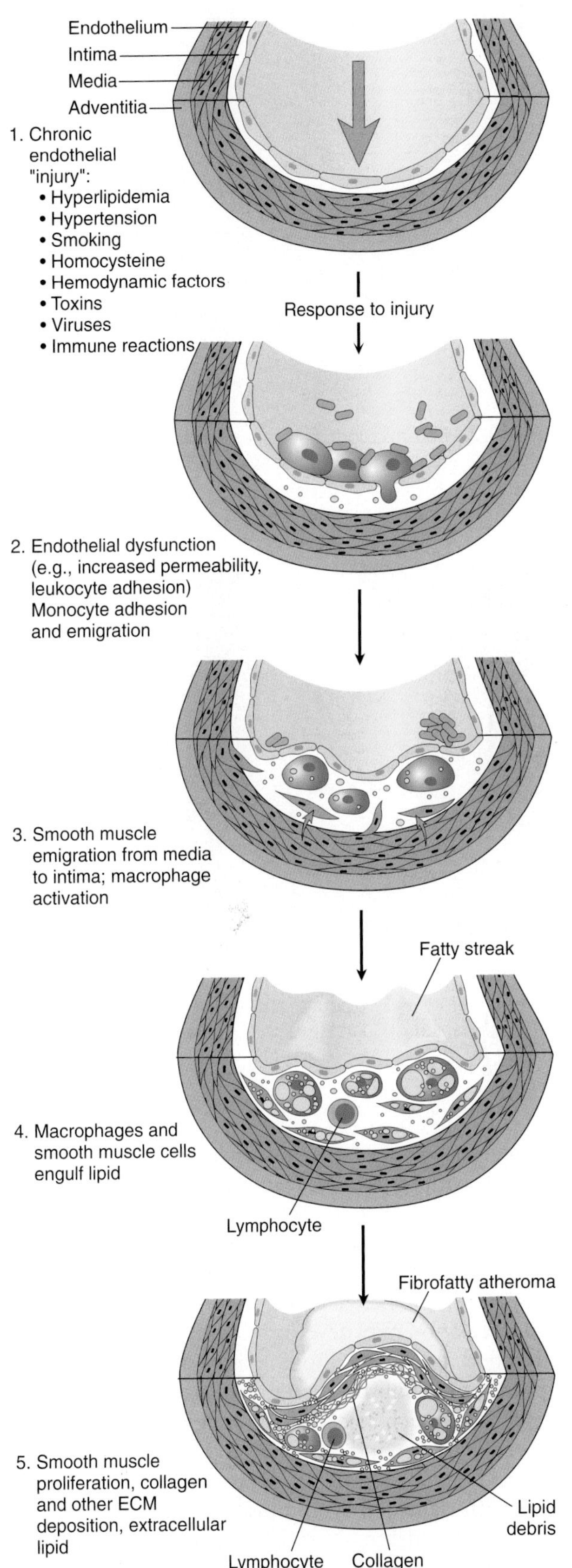

FIGURE 4-1 Evolution of arterial wall changes in the response to injury hypothesis. *ECM,* Extracellular matrix. *(From Schoen FJ: Blood vessels. In Kumar V, et al editors:* Robbins and Cotran pathologic basis of disease, *ed 8, Philadelphia, 2010, Saunders.)*

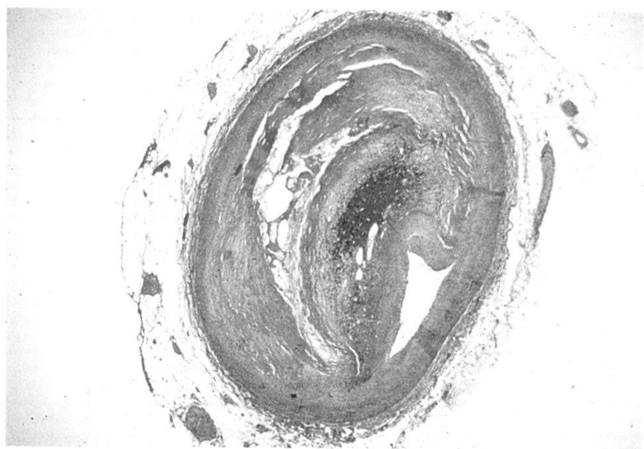

FIGURE 4-2 Photomicrograph of a cross section of a coronary artery with severe stenosis and narrowing. *(Courtesy W. O'Conner, MD, Lexington, Kentucky.)*

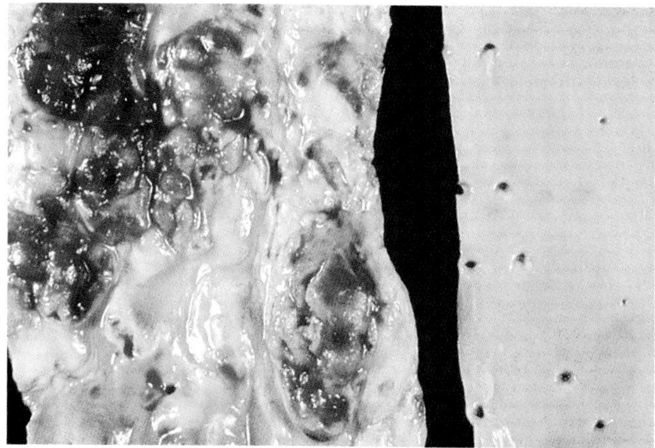

FIGURE 4-3 The segment of aorta on the *left* demonstrates advanced atheromatous plaques, and the specimen on the *right* side is unaffected. *(Courtesy W. O'Conner, MD, Lexington, Kentucky.)*

atheromatous plaques are not associated with clinical signs and symptoms and may never produce clinical manifestations.[19] Several factors may be responsible, including arterial remodeling, in which the plaque grows outward away from the lumen with a compensatory increase in the diameter of the vessel. In addition, collateral circulation may develop to compensate for diminished blood flow. For those lesions that do produce symptoms, flow-limiting intact plaques typically precipitate symptoms such as chest pain (angina) when oxygen need exceeds demand, as during exercise. However, plaque rupture produces an acute or unstable clinical picture with signs and symptoms such as angina at rest, MI, or sudden death. Not all plaques have the same propensity to rupture, and risk depends on the physical and biochemical characteristics of the plaque.

Intraarterial complications of coronary atherosclerosis consist of luminal narrowing, intramural hemorrhage, thrombosis, embolism, and aneurysm. Intramural hemorrhage, which results from weakening of the intimal tissues, may lead to thrombosis. The localized blood also may serve as an irritant to precipitate a reflex reaction, resulting in spasm of the collateral vessels. Once formed, a thrombus may become encapsulated and may undergo fibrous organization and recanalization.

If the degree of ischemia that results from coronary atherosclerosis is significant and the oxygen deficit is prolonged, the area of myocardium supplied by that vessel may undergo necrosis. Reduced blood flow may result from thrombosis of the affected artery, a hypotensive episode, an increased demand for blood, or emotional stress. The infarct, or area of necrosis, may be subendocardial or transmural, the latter involving the entire thickness of the myocardium (Figure 4-4). The extent of involvement is reflected in the electrocardiogram (ECG), in which the ST segment is not elevated in cases with only partial obstruction to blood flow and limited myocardial necrosis, but elevation of the ST segment is seen in cases with more profound ischemia and a larger area of necrosis. Complications of MI include weakened heart muscle, resulting in acute congestive heart failure, postinfarction angina, infarct extension, cardiogenic shock, pericarditis, and arrhythmias. Causes of death in patients who have had an acute MI include ventricular fibrillation, cardiac standstill, congestive heart failure, embolism, and rupture of the heart wall or septum.[22]

CLINICAL PRESENTATION

Symptoms

Chest pain is the most important symptom of coronary atherosclerotic heart disease. The pain may be brief, as in angina pectoris resulting from temporary ischemia of the myocardium, or it may be prolonged, as in unstable angina or acute MI. Ischemic myocardial pain results from an imbalance between the oxygen supply and the oxygen demand of the muscle. Atherosclerotic narrowing of the coronary arteries is an important cause of this imbalance. The exact mechanism or agents involved in producing the cardiac pain are not known.

Angina pectoris usually is described as a sensation of aching, heavy, squeezing pressure or tightness in the midchest region. The area of discomfort often is reported to be approximately the size of a fist and may radiate into the left or right arm to the neck or lower jaw. In rare cases, it may be present in only one of these distant sites, and the patient is free of central chest pain. The pain is of brief duration, lasting 5 to 15 minutes if the provoking stimulus is stopped or for a shorter time if nitroglycerin is used. Angina is defined in terms of its pattern of symptom stability. *Stable angina* is pain that is predictably reproducible, unchanging, and consistent over time. Pain typically is precipitated by physical effort such as walking or climbing stairs but also may occur

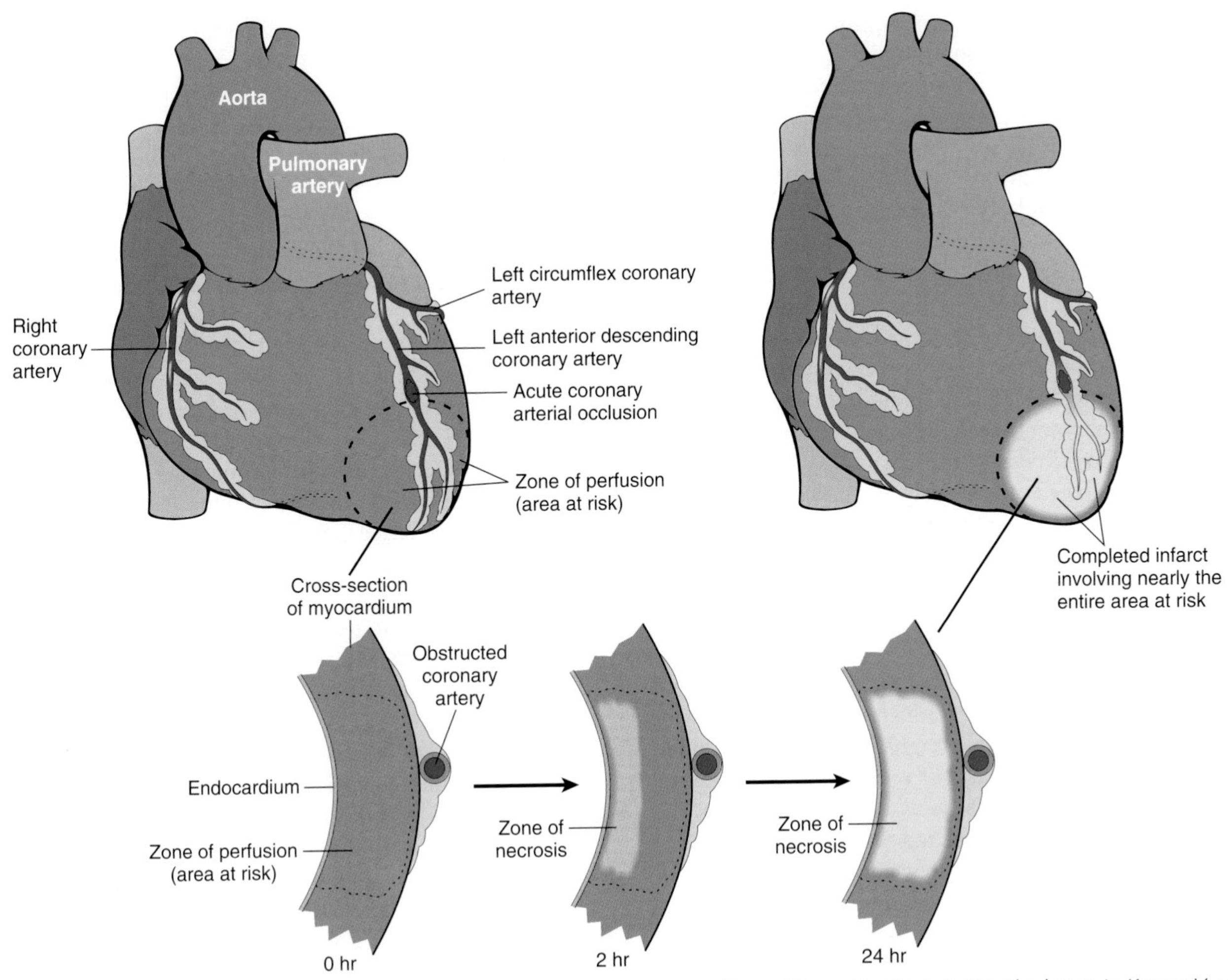

FIGURE 4-4 Progression of myocardial necrosis after coronary artery occlusion. *(From Schoen FJ, Mitchell, RN: The heart. In Kumar V, et al, editors:* Robbins and Cotran pathologic basis of disease, *ed 8, Philadelphia, 2010, Saunders.)*

with eating or stress. Pain is relieved by cessation of the precipitating activity, by rest, or with the use of nitroglycerin. *Unstable angina* is defined as new-onset pain, pain that is increasing in frequency, pain that is increasing in intensity, pain that is precipitated by less effort than before, or pain that occurs at rest. This pain is not readily relieved by nitroglycerin. The key feature is the changing character (increasing intensity) or pattern of the pain. Patients with stable angina have a relatively good prognosis. Patients with unstable angina have a poorer prognosis and often experience an acute MI within a short time. The term *acute coronary syndrome* describes a continuum of myocardial ischemia that ranges from unstable angina at one end to non–ST segment MI at the other.[21] Differentiation requires diagnostic and laboratory testing. A relatively uncommon form of angina, *Prinzmetal's variant angina,* occurs at rest and is caused by focal spasm of a coronary artery, usually with varied amounts of atherosclerosis.[20] Angina also may occur in persons with normal coronary vessels.

Patients with coronary atherosclerosis who experience prolonged pain as a result of myocardial ischemia usually have unstable angina or are having an acute MI. This pain usually is more severe and lasts longer than 15 minutes but has the same general character as that described for stable angina. Its location is the same as for the brief pain that results from temporary myocardial ischemia, and it may radiate in the same pattern. Use of vasodilators or cessation of activity does not relieve the pain caused by infarction. Neither brief nor prolonged pain resulting from myocardial ischemia is aggravated by deep breathing. Of interest, women and men report different symptoms of MI, with fewer women experiencing chest pain but more often experiencing fatigue and dyspnea.[23]

Sudden cardiac death accounts for 300,000 deaths annually in the United States and is often, but not always, due to cardiac arrhythmia.[24] Most cardiac arrest survivors have structural heart disease; nearly 75% have coronary artery disease. Predominant symptoms and signs that most often precede sudden death include chest pain, cough, shortness of breath, fainting, dizziness, palpitations, and fatigue. The most common cause of sudden death is ventricular fibrillation, a form of abnormal electrical activity resulting from interruption of the heart's electrical conduction system.

Palpitations of the heart (disagreeable awareness of the heartbeat) may be present in patients with coronary atherosclerotic heart disease with normal or abnormal rhythm. The complaint is not directly related to the seriousness of the underlying cardiac problem. Syncope, a transient loss of consciousness resulting from inadequate cerebral blood flow, also may occur in patients with coronary atherosclerotic heart disease.

Symptoms and signs of congestive heart failure developing as a complication of coronary atherosclerotic heart disease and its sequelae include dyspnea, orthopnea, paroxysmal nocturnal dyspnea, edema, hemoptysis, fatigue, weakness, and cyanosis. Fatigue and weakness may be manifest early in the course of heart disease, before the onset of congestive failure (see Chapter 6).

Signs

Clinical signs of coronary atherosclerotic heart disease are few, and the patient's clinical appearance may be entirely normal. Most clinical signs relate to other underlying cardiovascular disease or conditions such as congestive failure. Conditions such as corneal arcus and xanthoma of the skin are related to hyperlipidemia and hypercholesterolemia. Blood pressure may become elevated, and abnormalities in the rate and/or rhythm of the pulse may occur. Diminished peripheral pulses in the lower extremities may be noted, along with bruits in the carotid arteries. Panoramic radiographs of the jaws may occasionally demonstrate carotid calcifications in the areas of C_3 and C_4, consistent with atherosclerotic plaques in the carotid arteries (see Chapter 27). Retinal changes are common in hypertensive disease and diabetes mellitus. Signs associated with advanced coronary atherosclerotic heart disease usually reflect the presence of congestive heart failure. Distention of neck veins, peripheral edema, cyanosis, ascites, and enlarged liver may be noted.

Laboratory Findings

Blood tests are used in the evaluation of patients with symptoms of angina pectoris to screen for abnormalities that may contribute to or worsen coronary heart disease. These tests include complete blood count to rule out anemia, thyroid function tests to exclude hyperthyroidism, renal function tests to exclude renal insufficiency, lipid screening for hypercholesterolemia, glucose screening for diabetes, homocysteine level determination, and C-reactive protein assay. Other diagnostic modalities that are specific for coronary heart disease include resting ECG, chest x-ray studies, exercise stress testing, ambulatory (Holter) electrocardiography, stress thallium-201 perfusion scintigraphy, exercise echocardiography, ambulatory ventricular function monitoring, and cardiac catheterization and angiography.[25]

Along with physical examination and diagnostic testing, serum enzyme determinations are necessary to establish the diagnosis of acute MI and to determine the extent of infarction. Serum markers of acute MI most commonly used in clinical practice include troponin I, troponin T, and creatine kinase isoenzyme (CK-MB). These enzymes are released only when cell death (infarction) or injury to the myocyte occurs. Troponins are proteins that are derived from the breakdown of myocardial sarcomeres. For investigation of acute MI, troponin assays have largely replaced creatine kinase (CK) and CK-MB determinations because these markers are more specific in differentiating cardiac muscle damage from trauma to skeletal muscle or other organs. Very little difference has been noted between the two troponins. Plasma troponins are virtually absent in normal persons and are found only after cardiac injury. Troponins are first detectable 2 to 4 hours after the onset of an acute MI, are maximally sensitive at 8 to 12 hours, peak at 10 to 24 hours and persist for 5 to 14 days.[22]

CK-MB is another enzymatic marker of cardiac cell injury with characteristics similar to those of the troponins; however, in addition to its presence in damaged heart, CK-MB is found after injury to skeletal muscle and other tissues. Despite this relative lack of specificity, elevated levels of CK-MB usually are considered to be the result of an MI. CK-MB is detectable within 3 to 4 hours after infarction; it reaches peak values at 12 to 24 hours and persists for 2 to 4 days.[22] In many cardiac centers, troponin assay has replaced CK-MB determination as the diagnostic test of choice for MI because of its sensitivity and specificity, and as a result of cost issues. In any case, definitive diagnosis of MI requires serial testing over several days, rather than reliance on single test results. Testing for levels of B-natriuretic peptide, which is produced largely by the left ventricle, also aids in determining the extent of ventricular damage and the prognosis of heart failure.

MEDICAL MANAGEMENT

Angina Pectoris

Medical management of a patient with chronic stable angina consists of a varied array of interventions:

- Identification and treatment of associated diseases that can precipitate or worsen angina
- Reduction in risk factors for cardiovascular disease
- Behavioral modifications and lifestyle interventions
- Pharmacologic management
- Revascularization by percutaneous catheter–based techniques or by coronary artery bypass surgery (Box 4-1)

BOX 4-1 Medical Management of Patients with Stable Angina Pectoris

- Identification and treatment of associated diseases that can precipitate or worsen angina (anemia, obesity, hyperthyroidism, sleep apnea)
- Reduction in risk factors for cardiovascular disease (hypertension, smoking, hyperlipidemia)
- Behavioral modification and lifestyle intervention (weight loss, exercise)
- Pharmacologic management
  - Nitrates
  - Beta blockers
  - Calcium channel blockers
  - Antiplatelet agents
- Revascularization
  - Percutaneous transluminal coronary angioplasty with stenting
  - Coronary artery bypass grafting

Management may include general lifestyle measures such as an exercise program; weight control; restriction of salt, cholesterol, and saturated fatty acids; cessation of smoking; and control of exacerbating conditions such as anemia, hypertension, and hyperthyroidism. Patients who have significant angina are encouraged to avoid long hours of work, take rest periods during the working day, obtain adequate rest at night, use mild sedatives, take frequent vacations, and, in some cases, change their occupation or retire. Patients should avoid known precipitating factors that may bring on cardiac pain, such as cold weather, hot and humid weather, big meals, emotional upset, cigarette smoking, and drugs (e.g., amphetamines, caffeine, ephedrine, cyclamates, alcohol).

Drug therapy consists of nitrates (nitroglycerin or long-acting nitrates), antiplatelet agents, statins, β-adrenergic blockers, calcium channel blockers, and ACE inhibitors (Table 4-1). Nitrates are vasodilators, predominantly venodilators, and are a cornerstone of the pharmacologic management of angina. Their mechanism of action is unknown; however, researchers believe their effect may be caused by a decrease in cardiac load, resulting in decreased oxygen demand. Nitrates also may alleviate coronary artery spasm. Nitroglycerin may be used acutely for the relief of anginal pain and prophylactically to prevent angina. It comes in a variety of forms, including tablet, lingual spray, ointment, and transdermal patch. Nitroglycerin tablets are placed under the tongue to dissolve; the spray can be administered beneath the tongue or onto the oral mucosa. Nitrates are taken orally to prevent anginal symptoms and are supplied in tablet form, as an ointment for topical application, or as long-acting transdermal nitrate patches that are applied to the skin. Nitrates are used to reduce symptoms of angina, but they do not slow, alter, or reverse the progression of coronary artery disease.

Beta blockers, which are effective in the treatment of many patients with angina, compete with catecholamines for β-adrenergic receptor sites, resulting in decreased heart rate and myocardial contractility and reducing myocardial oxygen demand. *Nonselective* beta blockers block the β_1 and β_2 receptors, whereas *cardioselective* beta blockers preferentially block the β_1 receptors at normal therapeutic doses. Nonselective beta blockers may cause unwanted effects, such as increasing the tone of vascular smooth muscle and causing both vasoconstriction of peripheral vessels and contraction of bronchial smooth muscle. Thus, nonselective beta blockers are not prescribed for patients with a history of asthma. Injections of sympathomimetic drugs such as epinephrine or levonordefrin may result in elevation of blood pressure in patients taking nonselective beta blockers; therefore, caution is indicated in use of these agents.

Calcium channel blockers are effective in the treatment of chronic stable angina when given alone or in combination with beta blockers and nitrates. These drugs decrease intracellular calcium, resulting in vasodilatation of coronary, peripheral, and pulmonary vasculature, along with decreased myocardial contractility and heart rate.

The statins inhibit 3-hydroxy-3-methylglutaryl–coenzyme A reductase (HMG-CoA) in the liver, thereby leading to enhanced expression of the LDL receptors that capture blood cholesterol. They are therefore used to lower LDL cholesterol and increase HDL cholesterol and have been shown to decrease the risk for a major coronary event and the risk of death.[20] Statins also are antiinflammatory.

Angiotensin-converting enzyme (ACE) inhibitors are indicated for use in patients with coronary heart disease who also have diabetes, left ventricular dysfunction, or hypertension.[20] The benefit of these agents appears to be primarily due to their antihypertensive effects.

Antiplatelet therapy with aspirin is another cornerstone of treatment in patients with angina.[20] Regular use of aspirin in patients with stable angina is associated with a significant reduction in fatal events, and in patients with unstable angina, aspirin decreases the chances of fatal and nonfatal MI. Aspirin, in daily doses of 75 to 325 mg, is recommended for all patients with acute and chronic ischemic heart disease, regardless of the presence or absence of symptoms.[20] Clopidogrel, another antiplatelet agent, has been shown to have effects equivalent to those of aspirin; it is used in place of or in combination with aspirin. Ticlopidine and dipyridamole have not been shown to have any beneficial effects and are not recommended for use.

Revascularization is an option for patients with stable or unstable angina. Available procedures for revascularization include percutaneous transluminal coronary angioplasty, stents, and coronary artery bypass grafting. Percutaneous transluminal coronary angioplasty, also known as *balloon angioplasty,* involves the use of a

TABLE 4-1 Drugs Used in the Management of Angina

Drug	Vasoconstrictor Interactions	Oral Side/ Adverse Effects	Other Considerations
Nitrates			
Nitroglycerin Nitrogard Nitrolingual Nitro-Bid Nitrek Nitrostat Nitro-Time Nitrol Nitro-Tab Nitrogard Nitro-Dur Minitran Isosorbide dinitrate Dilatrate-SR Isordil Isosorbide 5-mononitrate Monoket Imdur Ismo	None	Dry mouth	Orthostatic hypotension, headache
Beta Blockers			
Nonselective: Blockade of β_1 and β_2 Receptors			
Propranolol/LA (Inderal) Nadolol (Corgard) Carteolol (Cartrol) Timolol (Blocadren) Penbutolol (Levatol) Pindolol (Visken) Sotalol (Betapace)	Increase in blood pressure possible with sympathomimetics, cautious use recommended (maximum 0.036 mg epinephrine; 0.20 mg levonordefrin)	Taste changes, lichenoid reactions	Orthostatic hypotension
Cardioselective: Blockade of β_1 Receptors Only			
Metoprolol/XL (Lopressor) Atenolol (Tenormin) Acebutolol (Sectral) Labetalol (Normodyne, Trandate)	Minimal effect with sympathomimetics; normal use		
Calcium Channel Blockers			
Bepridil (Vascor) Diltiazem/CD (Cardizem, Cartia, Dilacor, Diltia, Taztia, Tiazac) Felodipine (Plendil) Isradipine (DynaCirc) Nifedipine/PA/XL (Adalat, Nifedical, Procardia) Verapamil/SR (Calan, Isoptin, Verelan, Covera) Amlodipine (Norvasc) Nicardipine/SR (Cardene) Nisoldipine (Sular) Nitrendipine	None	Gingival hyperplasia, dry mouth, lichenoid eruptions (rare)	None
Platelet Aggregation Inhibitors			
Aspirin	None	None	Increased bleeding, but not clinically significant with daily doses ≤325 mg
Clopidogrel (Plavix)	None	None	Increased bleeding time

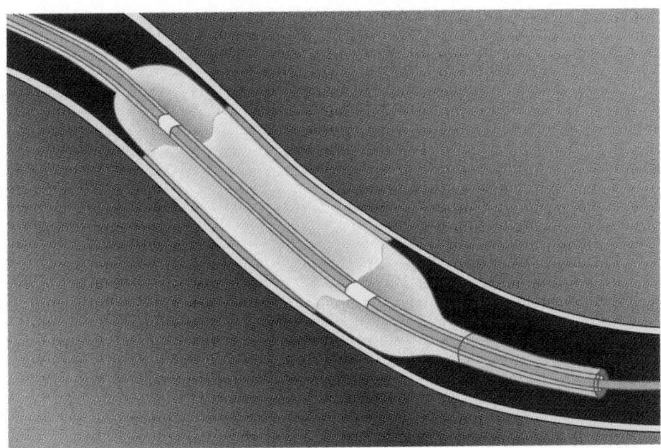

FIGURE 4-5 Balloon angioplasty catheter. *(From Teirstein PS: Percutaneous coronary interventions. In Goldman L, Ausiello D, editors:* Cecil textbook of medicine, *ed 23, Philadelphia, 2008, Saunders.)*

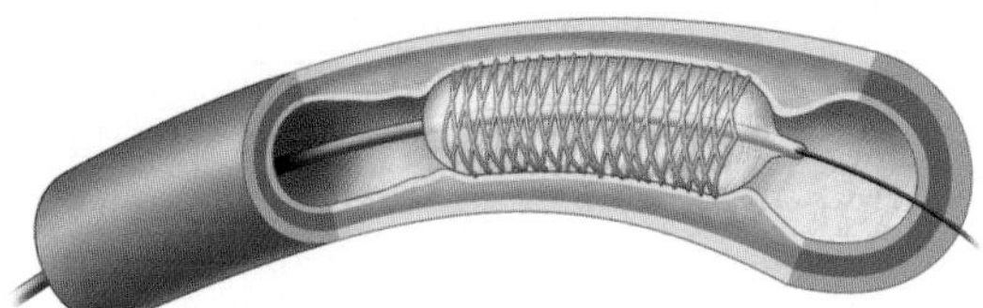

FIGURE 4-6 Expandable metallic stent. The stent is left in place after deflation and withdrawal of the balloon catheter.

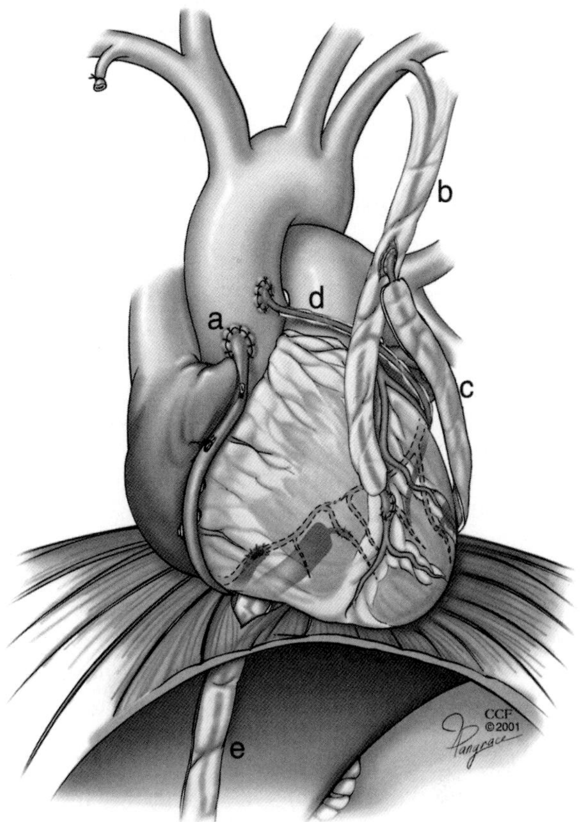

FIGURE 4-7 **Types of bypass grafts.** Bypass grafts include reversed saphenous vein graft from aorta to right coronary artery (*a*), in situ left internal mammary artery graft to anterior descending coronary artery (*b*), Y graft of right internal mammary artery from left internal mammary artery to circumflex coronary artery (*c*), radial artery graft from aorta to circumflex coronary artery (*d*), and in situ gastroepiploic graft to posterior descending branch of the right coronary artery (*e*). *(From Lytle BW: Surgical treatment of coronary artery disease. In Goldman L, Ausiello D, editors:* Cecil textbook of medicine, *ed 23, Philadelphia, 2008, Saunders.)*

small, inflatable balloon catheter over a thin guidewire that is threaded through the occluded segment of the artery. Once in place, the balloon is inflated, and compresses the plaque and thrombus against the arterial wall, with consequent enlargement of the lumen of the vessel (Figure 4-5). Widening of the lumen results in an immediate increase in blood flow, and provides symptomatic relief for ischemia. However, stenosis recurs within 6 months in 10% to 50% of patients, along with a return of symptoms.[26]

One method of decreasing the occurrence of restenosis with percutaneous transluminal coronary angioplasty involves the use of a thin, expandable, metallic mesh stent positioned by the balloon and expanded against the plaque and vessel wall, then left in place. The stent functions as a permanent scaffold to help maintain vessel patency (Figure 4-6). The use of stents has decreased the incidence of restenosis to about 20% to 30%; however, it has not prevented restenosis from occurring.[26] Currently, two types of stents are used: bare metal and drug-eluting. The bare metal stents maintain mechanical patency; however, they do not prevent endothelial proliferation that results in restenosis. Drug-eluting stents, however, are coated with antiproliferative agents that are very effective in controlling restenosis. Drug-eluting stents carry an increased risk for thrombosis for up to 1 year, however, so patients with such stents require long-term use of aspirin and/or clopidogrel.

Other non–balloon angioplasty methods are rotational atherectomy and the use of lasers. With percutaneous intervention, a successful outcome is achieved in more than 95% of patients, with very few complications.[26]

Coronary artery bypass graft (CABG) surgery is an effective means of controlling symptoms in the management of unstable angina; it can improve the long-term survival rate in certain subsets of patients. It also is effective in controlling symptoms in patients whose pain persists despite medical control. With coronary artery bypass grafting, a segment of artery or vein is harvested or released from a donor site; it is then grafted to the affected segment of coronary artery, thus bypassing the area of occlusion (Figure 4-7). Two primary graft donor sites are used: the saphenous vein from the leg and the internal mammary artery from the chest. Of the two, the internal mammary artery graft is sturdier and much less susceptible to graft atherosclerosis and occlusion than are vein grafts. Within 10 years postoperatively, 30% of saphenous vein grafts become occluded, while internal mammary artery grafts are much more resistant to occlusion. The arterial grafts are preferred for first bypass procedures when possible. Reoperation is difficult because of surgical site scarring and the limited supply of graft donor material. The perioperative morality rate for primary elective CABG procedures is less than 1%.[27]

Myocardial Infarction

Patients who have experienced an acute MI should be hospitalized or should receive emergency treatment as soon as possible (Box 4-2). The basic management goal is to minimize the size of the infarction and prevent death from lethal arrhythmias. The size and extent of the infarct are critical in the determination of outcome. Early administration of aspirin is recommended, with 160 to 325 mg being chewed and swallowed to decrease platelet aggregation and limit thrombus formation. The definitive treatment for patients with acute MI depends on the extent of ischemia as reflected on the ECG, which shows the presence or absence of ST segment elevation (Figure 4-8). An MI *without* ST segment elevation (non-STEMI) is due to partial blockage of coronary blood flow. An MI *with* ST segment elevation is due to complete blockage of coronary blood flow and more profound ischemia involving a relatively large area of myocardium. This distinction is clinically important because early fibrinolytic therapy improves outcomes in STEMI but not in non–STEMI.[21]

BOX 4-2 Medical Management of Patients with Acute Myocardial Infarction

- Rapid hospitalization and determination of ST segment changes
- Aspirin administration
- Early thrombolytic therapy (for patients with ST segment elevation only)
    - Streptokinase
    - Alteplase
    - Reteplase
    - Tenectaplase
- Early revascularization
    - Thrombolysis (for patients with ST segment elevation only)
    - Percutaneous transluminal coronary angioplasty with stenting
    - Coronary artery bypass grafting
- Pharmacologic therapy
    - Antiplatelet drugs (glycoprotein IIa/IIIb inhibitor, aspirin, clopidogrel)
    - Nitrates
    - β-Adrenergic blockers
    - Calcium channel blockers
    - Angiotensin-converting enzyme (ACE) inhibitors
    - Lipid-lowering drugs
    - Anticoagulants (unfractionated heparin, low-molecular-weight heparin)
    - Morphine
    - Sedative-hypnotics
- Oxygen

The management of acute MI has undergone significant change over the past several years with the recognition that early recanalization with thrombolytic therapy and/or percutaneous coronary intervention can result in significant reduction in morbidity and mortality associated with STEMI. The greatest benefit is realized when patients receive thrombolytic drugs within the first 3 hours after infarction. The early use of thrombolytic drugs may decrease the extent of necrosis and myocardial damage and dramatically improve outcome and prognosis. Thrombolytic (or fibrinolytic) drugs used in the treatment of acute MI include streptokinase (SK), alteplase (t-PA), and reteplase (r-PA), and tenecteplase (t-PA). For most patients with STEMI, the preferred method for revascularization is percutaneous coronary angioplasty. In patients with STEMI, non–STEMI, or unstable angina (acute coronary syndrome), anticoagulation often is effected with unfractionated heparin or low-molecular-weight heparin; in addition, glycoprotein IIa/IIIb inhibitors (abciximab, eptifibatide, tirofiban) are administered intravenously for their antiplatelet effects. General pharmacologic measures for patients with acute MI include the use of nitrates, beta blockers, calcium channel blockers, ACE inhibitors, and lipid-lowering agents. Antiplatelet drugs achieve significant decreases in morbidity and mortality rates, and aspirin is the drug of choice. Daily doses of 81 to 325 mg are recommended. Clopidogrel (Plavix; Bristol-Myers Squibb/Sanofi Pharmaceuticals, New York, New York) and ticlopidine (Ticlid; Roche Laboratories, Inc., Nutley, New Jersey) are other antiplatelet drugs that may be used, although ticlopidine has been supplanted by clopidogrel because of superior outcomes reported with the latter. For pain relief, morphine sulfate is the drug of choice. Sedatives and anxiolytic medications also may be used. Oxygen may be administered by nasal cannula during the acute period to enhance oxygen saturation of the blood and keep the heart workload at a minimum level. The development of an arrhythmia in a patient who has had an AMI constitutes an emergency that must be treated aggressively with antiarrhythmic drugs. During the first several weeks after an infarction, the conduction system of the heart may be unstable, and patients are prone to serious arrhythmias and reinfarction. A pacemaker may be used with severe myocardial damage and resultant heart failure.

DENTAL MANAGEMENT

Medical Considerations

Risk assessment for the dental management of patients with ischemic heart disease involves three determinants:

1. *Severity* of the disease
2. *Type and magnitude* of the dental procedure
3. *Stability and cardiopulmonary reserve* of the patient

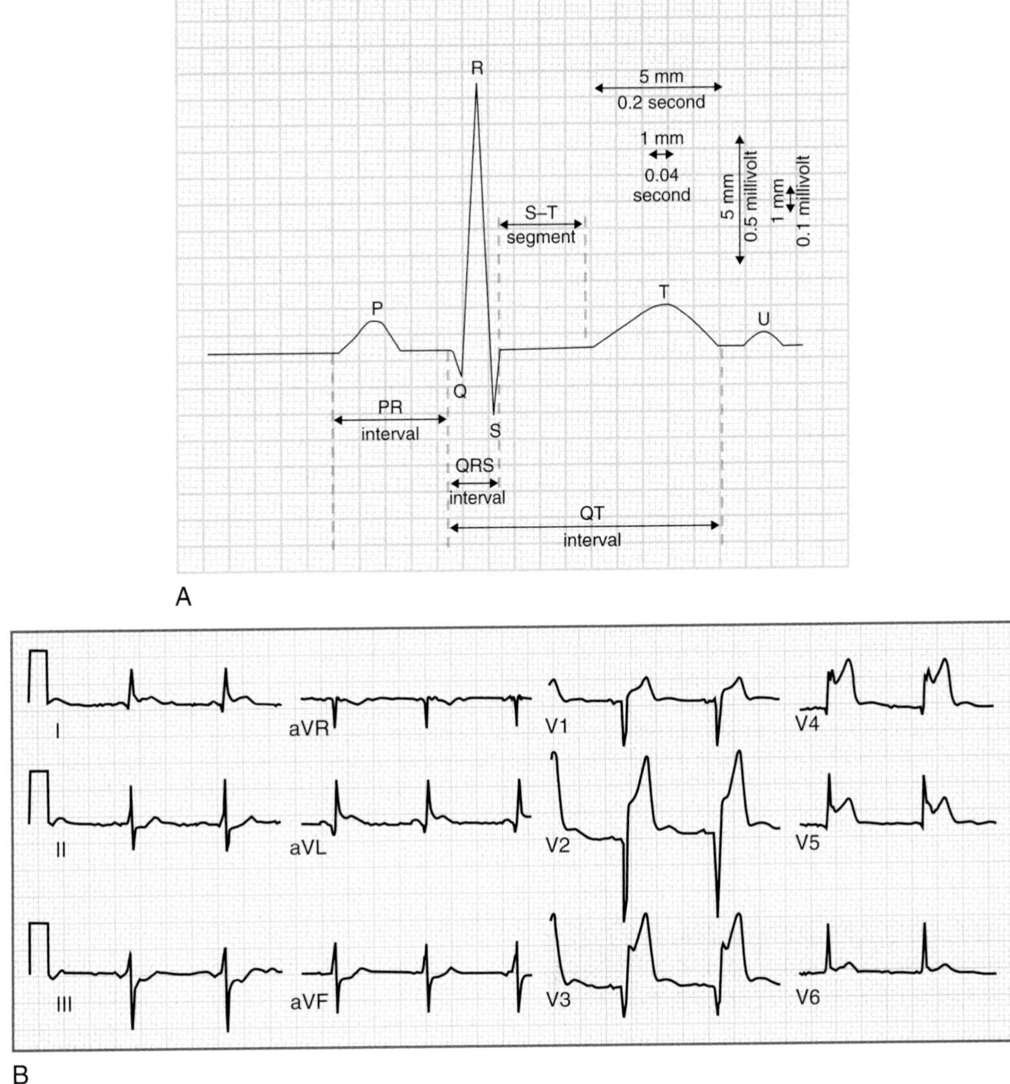

FIGURE 4-8 A, Waves and intervals on a normal electrocardiogram (ECG). The ST segment characteristically lies only very slightly above the baseline tracing. **B,** Electrocardiographic tracing shows an acute anterior/lateral MI. ST segment elevation is evident in leads I, aV_L, and V_{1-6}. *(**A,** From Ganz L, Curtiss E: Electrocardiography. In Goldman L, Ausiello D, editors:* Cecil textbook of medicine, *ed 23, Philadelphia, 2008, Saunders. **B,** Courtesy Dr. Thomas Evans. From Anderson JL: ST-elevation acute myocardial infarction and complications of myocardial infarction. In Goldman L, Ausiello D, editors:* Cecil textbook of medicine, *ed 23, Philadelphia, 2008, Saunders.)*

All must be factored into a dental management plan so that a rational and safe decision can be made—specifically, to determine whether a patient can safely tolerate a planned procedure. The American College of Cardiology and the American Heart Association[28] have published risk stratification guidelines for patients with various types of heart disease who are undergoing noncardiac surgical procedures. These guidelines can provide a framework for determination of associated risk for surgical as well as for nonsurgical dental procedures (Boxes 4-3 and 4-4). For example, recent MI (within the past 7 to 30 days) and unstable angina are classified as clinical predictors of major risk for perioperative complications. By contrast, a past history of ischemic heart disease (i.e., stable (mild) angina and past history of MI) is considered one of the intermediate risk factors for perioperative complications. Accordingly, a past history of ischemic heart disease with no other clinical risk factors, as shown in Box 4-3, is unlikely to be associated with significant risk for an adverse event during dental procedures.

The type and magnitude of the planned procedure also must be considered. On the basis of these guidelines, extensive oral and maxillofacial surgical procedures, and perhaps some of the more extensive periodontal surgical procedures, would fall into the intermediate cardiac risk category under "head and neck procedures," with a 1% to 5% risk. Minor oral surgery and periodontal surgery, would fall within the low-risk, "superficial surgery" or "ambulatory surgery" category, with less than 1% risk. Although not included in the list, nonsurgical dental

BOX 4-3 Clinical Predictors of Increased Perioperative Cardiovascular Risk—Myocardial Infarction, Heart Failure, or Death

Major Clinical Risk Factors
- Unstable coronary syndromes
  - Acute or recent myocardial infarction (*) associated with important ischemic risk as indicated by clinical signs and symptoms or by noninvasive study
  - Unstable or severe angina (Canadian class III or IV)[†‡]
- Decompensated heart failure (NYHA class 4: worsening or new-onset heart failure)
- Significant arrhythmias
  - High-grade atrioventricular block
  - Mobitz type 2 atrioventricular block
  - Third-degree atrioventricular block
  - Symptomatic ventricular arrhythmias in the presence of underlying heart disease
  - Supraventricular arrhythmias with uncontrolled ventricular rate
  - Symptomatic bradycardia
  - Newly recognized ventricular tachycardia
- Severe valvular disease
  - Severe aortic stenosis
  - Symptomatic mitral stenosis

Intermediate Clinical Risk Factors
- History of ischemic heart disease
- History of compensated or previous heart failure
- History of cerebrovascular disease
- Diabetes mellitus
- Renal insufficiency

Minor Clinical Risk Factors
- Advanced age (>70 years)
- Abnormal ECG electrocardiogram (left ventricular hypertrophy, left bundle branch block, ST-T wave abnormalities)
- Rhythm other than sinus (e.g., atrial fibrillation)
- Uncontrolled systemic hypertension (≥180/110 mm Hg)

*The American College of Cardiology National Database Library defines *recent MI* as occurring after than 7 days but within1 month (at or before 30 days) before the procedure and *acute MI* as occurring within 7 days.
[†]May include "stable" angina in patients who are unusually sedentary.
[‡]*Data from Campeau L: Grading of angina pectoris,* Circulation *54:522-523, 1976. The Canadian classification is a system of grading angina severity (grades I to IV), with grade I angina occurring only with strenuous exertion and grade IV angina occurring with any physical activity or at rest.*
Data from Fleisher LA, et al: ACC/AHA 2007 guidelines on perioperative cardiovascular evaluation and care for noncardiac surgery: executive summary: a report of the American College of Cardiology/American Heart Association Task Force on Practice Guidelines *(Writing Committee to Revise the 2002 Guidelines on Perioperative Cardiovascular Evaluation for Noncardiac Surgery).* Circulation *116:1971-1996, 2007.*

BOX 4-4 Cardiac Risk* Stratification for Noncardiac Surgical Procedures

High (Reported Cardiac Risk Often Greater Than 5%)
- Aortic and other major vascular surgery

Intermediate (Reported Cardiac Risk Generally Less Than 5%)
- Intraperitoneal and intrathoracic surgery
- Carotid endarterectomy
- Head and neck surgery
- Orthopaedic surgery
- Prostate surgery

Low (Reported Cardiac Risk Generally Less Than 1%)
- Endoscopic procedures
- Superficial procedures
- Cataract surgery
- Breast surgery
- Ambulatory surgery

*Combined incidence of cardiac death and nonfatal myocardial infarction.
Adapted from Fleisher LA, et al: ACC/AHA 2007 guidelines on perioperative cardiovascular evaluation and care for noncardiac surgery: executive summary: a report of the American College of Cardiology/American Heart Association Task Force on Practice Guidelines *(Writing Committee to Revise the 2002 Guidelines on Perioperative Cardiovascular Evaluation for Noncardiac Surgery).* Circulation *116:1971-1996, 2007.*

procedures are likely to carry even less of a risk, considering that local anesthesia is used, minimal blood loss is anticipated, and procedures typically are of short duration. Procedures that are performed with the patient under general anesthesia and have the potential for significant blood and fluid loss with resultant adverse hemodynamic effects pose the highest risk.

The final element included in the AHA/ACC Guidelines is the ability of the patient to perform basic physical tasks. The energy expended in performing these tasks is measured in metabolic equivalents of tasks (METs), which is a measure of oxygen consumption. Studies have shown that a person who cannot perform at a minimum of a 4 MET level is at increased risk for a cardiovascular event. Climbing a flight of stairs requires a 4-MET effort; thus, a person who cannot climb a flight of stairs without chest pain or shortness of breath is at increased risk.

These risk stratification guidelines may be applied to various dental management scenarios. For example, a patient with unstable angina or recent MI is assigned to the major cardiac risk category. It also is likely that this person would have difficulty climbing a flight of stairs. By contrast, if the planned dental procedure is limited to routine clinical examination with x-rays (extremely low risk category), and the patient is stable and not anxious, the risk for an adverse occurrence is minimal; thus, alterations in the dental management approach would be unnecessary. If, however, a patient with stable angina or a past history of MI (intermediate risk category), with minimal cardiac reserve, is scheduled for multiple extractions and implant placement (low to intermediate risk category), the risk for an adverse perioperative event is more significant, and a more complex dental management plan may be required.

Angina Pectoris/Past History of Myocardial Infarction. A determination should be made regarding the presence, severity, and stability of ischemic symptoms. A patient with stable angina characteristically describes the occurrence of chest pain in a consistent, recurring, and predictable pattern. Pain is precipitated by typical physical activity such as exercising, mowing the lawn, or climbing stairs and subsides within 5 to 15 minutes with rest or the use of nitroglycerin. Pain occurs in a chronic, unchanging pattern over time. These patients pose an intermediate cardiac risk.

A patient with unstable angina conversely may describe the recent onset of chest pain, or progressively worsening chest pain that occurs with physical exertion or at rest. A pattern of increasing severity, frequency, or duration of pain is typical. Pain occurring at rest or during sleep is particularly ominous. Patients with unstable angina should be considered to be at major cardiac risk and are not candidates for elective dental care.

Patients who have had an MI in the past may or may not have ischemic symptoms. For an asymptomatic patient with no other risk factors, risk for an adverse event is minimal. If, however, symptoms such as chest pain, shortness of breath, dizziness, or fatigue are present, the patient falls in the major risk category, and elective dental care should be deferred and medical consultation obtained. Likewise, a patient who has a history of MI in association with other clinical risk factors is at increased risk for an adverse event, and medical consultation should be obtained before elective dental care.

Based on the assessment of medical risk, the type of planned dental procedure, and the stability and anxiety level of the patient, general management strategies for patients with stable angina or a past history of MI without ischemic symptoms (intermediate risk category) and no other risk factors may include the following: short appointments in the morning, comfortable chair position, pretreatment vital signs, availability of nitroglycerin, oral sedation, nitrous oxide–oxygen sedation, profound local anesthesia, limited amount of vasoconstrictor, avoidance of epinephrine-impregnated retraction cord, and effective postoperative pain control. For patients who have had balloon angioplasty with placement of a coronary artery stent, or for those who have undergone a CABG procedure, antibiotic prophylaxis is not recommended[29] (Box 4-5). In addition, NSAIDs should be avoided in patients with established

BOX 4-5 Dental Management

Considerations for Patients with Stable (Mild) Angina or Past History of Myocardial Infarction (MI), Without Ischemic Symptoms

P
Patient Evaluation/Risk Assessment
Potential Issues/Concerns

A	
Antibiotics	No issues
Analgesics	Ensure adequate postoperative pain control.
Anesthesia	Avoid use of excessive amounts of epinephrine; limit to two carpules of 1:100,000 epinephrine at a time (within 30-45 minutes); greater quantities may be tolerated well clinically but with increasing risk.
Allergy	No issues
Anxiety	Use stress reduction protocol (see Chapter 1). Consider the use of preoperative oral sedation (short-acting benzodiazepine) 1 hour before procedure, as well as using N_2O-O_2 inhalational sedation intraoperatively.
B	
Bleeding	If patient is taking aspirin or other antiplatelet medication, anticipate some excessive bleeding, but modification of drug regimen is not required.
Breathing	No issues
Blood pressure	No issues
C	
Chair position	Ensure a comfortable chair position and avoid rapid position changes.
D	
Drugs	The use of excessive amounts of epinephrine with nonselective beta blockers can potentially cause a spike in blood pressure, but this is unlikely and appears to be dose-dependent; avoid the use of epinephrine-impregnated retraction cord.
Devices	Patients who have coronary artery stents do not require antibiotic prophylaxis; however, they are likely to be taking aspirin and/or clopidogrel (or other antiplatelet medication) to decrease the chance of stent-related thrombus. Anticipate excessive bleeding, but it generally is unnecessary to discontinue these medications.
E	
Equipment	Consider taking preoperative vital signs and the use of a pulse oximeter if oral sedation is used, or if the patient becomes symptomatic.
Emergencies	Precipitation of an angina attack, MI, arrhythmia, or cardiac arrest is possible. Have nitroglycerin readily available as well as oxygen. Be prepared to perform CPR and activate EMS.
F	
Follow-up	Ensure that patient is maintaining regular follow-up visits with physician.

CPR, Cardiopulmonary resuscitation; *EMS,* Emergency medical services.

cardiovascular disease, especially those whose cardiac history includes an MI. In a recent study, the use of NSAIDs in patients with previous MI was shown to increase the risk for a subsequent myocardial infarction, even after only 7 days of NSAID administration.[30] In this study, only naproxen did not increase the risk. Whether shorter duration of use decreases the risk is not clear, but this correlation seems likely; thus, we recommend that NSAIDs be used with caution, if at all, in patients who have had a previous MI, and that if an NSAID is used, naproxen be the drug of choice, administered for less than 7 days.

For patients with symptoms of unstable angina or those who have had an MI within the past 30 days (major risk category), elective care should be postponed (Box 4-6). If treatment becomes necessary, it should be performed as conservatively as possible and directed primarily toward pain relief, infection control, or the control of bleeding, as appropriate. Consultation with the physician is advised. Additional management recommendations may include establishing and maintaining an intravenous line, continuously monitoring the ECG and vital signs, using a pulse oximeter, and administering nitroglycerin prophylactically just before the initiation of treatment.[25] These measures may require that the patient be treated in a special patient care facility or hospital dental clinic.

Vasoconstrictors. The use of vasoconstrictors in local anesthetics poses potential problems for patients with ischemic heart disease because of the possibility of precipitating cardiac tachycardias, arrhythmias, and increases in blood pressure. Local anesthetics without vasoconstrictors may be used as needed. If a vasoconstrictor is necessary, patients with intermediate clinical risk factors and those taking nonselective beta blockers can safely be given up to 0.036 mg epinephrine (two cartridges containing 1:100,000 epinephrine) at one appointment; intravascular injections are to be avoided.

BOX 4-6 Dental Management

Considerations for Patients with Unstable Angina or History of Recent Myocardial Infarction (MI) (within Past 30 Days)

P

Patient Evaluation/Risk Assessment

- Avoid elective dental care.
- If care becomes necessary, consult with physician to develop treatment plan.
- Patient is best treated in a hospital dental clinic or special care facility.

Potential Issues/Factors of Concern

A	
Antibiotics	No issues
Analgesics	Ensure adequate postoperative pain control.
Anesthesia	Avoid use of vasoconstrictor if possible. If vasoconstrictor is needed, avoid excessive amounts of epinephrine; limit to two carpules of 1:100,000 epinephrine at a time (within 30-45 minutes); greater quantities may be tolerated well clinically but with increasing risk. May need to discuss use with physician.
Allergy	No issues
Anxiety	Use stress reduction protocol (see Chapter 1). Consider the use of preoperative oral sedation (short-acting benzodiazepine) 1 hour before procedure, as well as using N_2O-O_2 inhalational sedation intraoperatively.
B	
Bleeding	If patient is taking aspirin or other antiplatelet medication, anticipate some excessive bleeding, but modification of drug regimen is not required.
Breathing	No issues
Blood pressure	Continuous monitoring of blood pressure and pulse is recommended.
C	
Chair position	Ensure a comfortable chair position and avoid rapid position changes.
D	
Drugs	Consider administering prophylactic nitroglycerin just before procedure. Provide continuous oxygen by nasal cannula or nasal mask. The use of excessive amounts of epinephrine with nonselective beta blockers can potentially cause a spike in blood pressure, but this is unlikely and appears to be dose-dependent; avoid the use of epinephrine-impregnated retraction cord.
Devices	Patients who have coronary artery stents do not require antibiotic prophylaxis; however, they are likely to be taking aspirin and/or clopidogrel (or other antiplatelet medication) to decrease the chance of stent-related thrombus. Anticipate excessive bleeding, but it generally is unnecessary to discontinue these medications.
E	
Equipment	Recommended management includes placement of intravenous line, continuous ECG monitoring, ongoing monitoring of vital signs, and use of a pulse oximeter.
Emergencies	Precipitation of an angina attack, MI, arrhythmia, or cardiac arrest is possible. Have nitroglycerin readily available as well as oxygen. Be prepared to perform CPR and activate EMS.
F	
Follow-up	Ensure that patient is maintaining regular follow-up visits with physician.

CPR, Cardiopulmonary resuscitation; *ECG*, Electrocardiogram; *EMS*, Emergency medical services.

Greater quantities of vasoconstrictor may well be tolerated, but increasing quantities increase the risk of adverse cardiovascular effects. For patients at higher risk, the use of vasoconstrictors should be discussed with the physician. Studies have shown, however, that modest quantities of vasoconstrictors may be used safely even in high-risk patients when accompanied by oxygen, sedation, nitroglycerin, and excellent pain control measures.[31-33]

For patients at all levels of cardiac risk, the use of gingival retraction cord impregnated with epinephrine should be avoided because of the rapid absorption of a high concentration of epinephrine and the potential for adverse cardiovascular effects. As an alternative, plain cord saturated with tetrahydrozoline HCl 0.05% (Visine; Pfizer Inc, New York, New York) or oxymetazoline HCl 0.05% (Afrin; Schering-Plough, Summit, New Jersey) provides gingival effects equivalent to those of epinephrine without adverse cardiovascular effects.[34]

Bleeding. Patients who take daily aspirin and/or other antiplatelet agents (e.g., clopidogrel) can expect some increase in surgical and postoperative bleeding, but this is generally not clinically significant and can be controlled with local measures only. Discontinuation of these agents before dental treatment generally is unnecessary. Patients who are taking warfarin for anticoagulation can safely undergo dental or surgical procedures, provided that the INR is 3.5 or less (see Chapter 24). Discontinuation of antiplatelet agents and anticoagulants (e.g., warfarin) before dental treatment and routine extractions generally is unnecessary.

Oral Manifestations

No lesions or oral complications are the direct result of coronary atherosclerotic heart disease. Drugs used in the treatment of this disease and its complications, however, may produce oral changes such as dry mouth, taste aberrations, and stomatitis. In rare cases, patients with angina occurring as a manifestation of coronary atherosclerotic heart disease may experience pain referred to the neck, lower jaw, or teeth. The pattern of onset of pain with physical activity and its disappearance with rest usually serves as a clue to its cardiac origin.

REFERENCES

1. Roger VL, et al: Heart disease and stroke statistics—2011 update: a report from the American Heart Association, *Circulation* 123:e18-e209, 2011.
2. National Heart, Lung, and Blood Institute: *The seventh report of the Joint National Committee on Prevention, Detection, Evaluation, and Treatment of High Blood Pressure: the JNC 7 report*, Bethesda, Maryland, US Department of Health and Human Services, Public Health Service, National Institutes of Health, National Heart, Lung, and Blood Institute, August 2004.
3. Tuzcu EM, et al: High prevalence of coronary atherosclerosis in asymptomatic teenagers and young adults: evidence from intravascular ultrasound, *Circulation* 103:2705-2710, 2001.
4. Libby P: Inflammation and cardiovascular disease mechanisms, *Am J Clin Nutr* 83:456S-460S, 2006.
5. Virmani R, et al: Coronary artery atherosclerosis revisited in Korean war combat casualties, *Arch Pathol Lab Med* 111:972-976, 1987.
6. Criqui MH: Epidemiology of cardiovascular disease. In Goldman L, Ausiello D, editors: *Cecil textbook of medicine*, ed 23, Philadelphia, 2008, Saunders, pp 301-305.
7. Vasan RS, et al: Impact of high-normal blood pressure on the risk of cardiovascular disease, *N Engl J Med* 345:1291-1297, 2001.
8. Garrett BE, et al: Cigarette smoking—United States, 1965-2008, *MMWR Surveill Summ* 60(suppl):109-113, 2011.
9. Vlietstra RE, et al: Effect of cigarette smoking on survival of patients with angiographically documented coronary artery disease. Report from the CASS registry, *JAMA* 255:1023-1027, 1986.
10. Kannel WB: Hypertension, blood lipids, and cigarette smoking as co-risk factors for coronary heart disease, *Ann N Y Acad Sci* 304:128-139, 1978.
11. Inzucchi SE, Sherwin RS: Type 2 diabetes mellitus. In Goldman AL, Ausiello D, editors: *Cecil textbook of medicine*, ed 23, Philadelphia, 2008, Saunders, pp 1748-1760.
12. Howard BV, et al: Prevention Conference VI: Diabetes and cardiovascular disease: Writing Group I: epidemiology, *Circulation* 105:e132-137, 2002.
13. Gu K, Cowie CC, Harris MI: Mortality in adults with and without diabetes in a national cohort of the U.S. population, 1971-1993, *Diabetes Care* 21:1138-1145, 1998.
14. Summary of revisions for the 2007 Clinical Practice Recommendations, *Diabetes Care* 30(Suppl 1):S3, 2007.
15. Ford ES, Li C, Zhao G: Prevalence and correlates of metabolic syndrome based on a harmonious definition among adults in the US, *J Diabetes* 2:180-193, 2010.
16. Beck JD, et al: Periodontal disease and coronary heart disease: a reappraisal of the exposure, *Circulation* 112:19-24, 2005.
17. Elter JR, et al: The effects of periodontal therapy on vascular endothelial function: a pilot trial, *Am Heart J* 151:47, 2006.
18. Lam OL, et al: A systematic review of the effectiveness of oral health promotion activities among patients with cardiovascular disease, *Int J Cardiol* 2010 Dec 20 [Epub ahead of print].
19. Libby P, Theroux P: Pathophysiology of coronary artery disease, *Circulation* 111:3481-3488, 2005.
20. Theroux P: Angina pectoris. In Goldman AL, Ausiello D, editors: *Cecil textbook of medicine*, ed 23, Philadelphia, 2008, Saunders, pp 477-491.
21. Waters DD: Acute coronary syndrome: unstable angina and non-ST segment elevation myocardial infarction. In Goldman AL, Ausiello D, editors: *Cecil textbook of medicine*, ed 23, Philadelphia, 2008, Saunders, pp 491-500.
22. Anderson JL: ST segment elevation acute myocardial infarction and complications of myocardial infarction. In Goldman AL, Ausiello D, editors: *Cecil textbook of medicine*, ed 23, Philadelphia, 2008, Saunders, pp 500-518.
23. Canto JG, et al: Symptom presentation of women with acute coronary syndromes: myth vs reality, *Arch Intern Med* 167:2405-2413, 2007.
24. Lerman BB: Ventricular arrhythmias. In Goldman AL, Ausiello D, editors: *Cecil textbook of medicine*, ed 23, Philadelphia, 2008, Saunders, pp 414-425.
25. Niwa H, et al: Safety of dental treatment in patients with previously diagnosed acute myocardial infarction or unstable angina pectoris, *Oral Surg Oral Med Oral Pathol Oral Radiol Endod* 89:35-41, 2000.

26. Teirstein PS: Percutaneous coronary interventions. In Goldman AL, Ausiello D, editors: *Cecil textbook of medicine*, ed 23, Philadelphia, 2008, Saunders, pp 518-522.
27. Lytle BW: Surgical treatment of coronary artery disease. In Goldman AL, Ausiello D, editors: *Cecil textbook of medicine*, ed 23, Philadelphia, 2008, Saunders, pp 522-524.
28. Fleisher LA, et al: *ACC/AHA 2007 guidelines on perioperative cardiovascular evaluation and care for noncardiac surgery: executive summary: a report of the American College of Cardiology/American Heart Association Task Force on Practice Guidelines* (Writing Committee to Revise the 2002 Guidelines on Perioperative Cardiovascular Evaluation for Noncardiac Surgery), *Circulation* 116:1971-1996, 2007.
29. Baddour LM, et al: Nonvalvular cardiovascular device-related infections, *Circulation* 108:2015-2031, 2003.
30. Schjerning Olsen AM, et al: Duration of treatment with nonsteroidal anti-inflammatory drugs and impact on risk of death and recurrent myocardial infarction in patients with prior myocardial infarction: a nationwide cohort study, *Circulation* 123:2226-2235, 2011.
31. Cintron G, et al: Cardiovascular effects and safety of dental anesthesia and dental interventions in patients with recent uncomplicated myocardial infarction, *Arch Intern Med* 146:2203-2204, 1986.
32. Findler M, et al: Dental treatment in very high risk patients with active ischemic heart disease, *Oral Surg Oral Med Oral Pathol* 76:298-300, 1993.
33. Niwa H, Sato Y, Matsuura H: Safety of dental treatment in patients with previously diagnosed acute myocardial infarction or unstable angina pectoris, *Oral Surg Oral Med Oral Pathol Oral Radiol Endod* 89:35-41, 2000.
34. Bowles WH, Tardy SJ, Vahadi A: Evaluation of new gingival retraction agents, *J Dent Res* 70:1447-1449, 1991.

5

Cardiac Arrhythmias

Cardiac arrhythmia, which refers to any variation in the normal heartbeat, includes disturbances in rhythm, rate, or the conduction pattern of the heart. Cardiac arrhythmias are present in a significant percentage of the population, many of whom will seek dental treatment. Most arrhythmias are of little clinical concern, for either the patient or the dentist; however, some can produce symptoms, and a few may be life-threatening. Potentially fatal arrhythmias can be precipitated by strong emotion such as anxiety or anger,[1,2] and by various drugs,[3] both of which are factors likely to be encountered in the dental setting. Therefore, patients with significant arrhythmias must be identified before undergoing dental treatment.

GENERAL DESCRIPTION

Incidence and Prevalence

Cardiac arrhythmias are relatively common in the general population; and their prevalence increases with age. They occur more frequently in elderly persons, people with a long history of smoking, patients with underlying ischemic heart disease, and patients taking certain drugs or have various systemic diseases.[4] In the United States, arrhythmias are present in 12.6% of people older than 65 years of age,[5] with a rate of 13.6 per 100,000 reported for the general population.[6] Arrhythmias directly account for more than 36,000 deaths annually and constitute the underlying or contributing cause in almost 460,000 cases.[7] The most common type of persistent arrhythmia is atrial fibrillation (AF), which affects approximately 2.6 million people.[7]

Little and associates[8,9] found the prevalence of cardiac arrhythmias in a large population of more than 10,000 general dentistry patients to be 17.2%, and more than 4% of those were serious, potentially life-threatening cardiac arrhythmias. In two similar studies performed in health care settings, a prevalence of 15% for arrhythmias, with 1.7% to 4% considered as potentially serious, has been reported.[10,11] To manage their arrhythmias, more than 500,000 people in North America have implanted pacemakers.[12]

Etiology

Cardiac contractions are controlled by a complex system of specialized excitatory and conductive neuronal circuitry (Figure 5-1). The normal pattern of sequential depolarization involves the structures of the heart in the following order: (1) sinoatrial (SA) node, (2) atrioventricular (AV) node, (3) bundle of His, (4) right and left bundle branches, and finally (5) subendocardial Purkinje network.[13] The electrocardiogram (ECG) is a recording of this electrical activity. The primary anatomic pacemaker for the heart is the SA node, a crescent-shaped structure 9 to 15 mm long that is located at the junction of the superior vena cava and the right atrium. The SA node regulates the functions of the atria and is responsible for production of the P wave (atrial depolarization) on the ECG (Figure 5-2). The ends of the sinus nodal fibers connect with atrial muscle fibers. The generated action potential travels along the muscle fibers (internodal pathways) and eventually arrives at and excites the AV node, which serves as a gate that regulates the entry of atrial impulses into the ventricles. It also slows the conduction rate of impulses generated within the SA node. From the AV node, impulses travel along the AV bundle (His bundle) within the ventricular septum, which divides into right and left bundle branches. The bundle branches then terminate in the small Purkinje fibers, which course throughout the ventricles and become continuous with cardiac muscle fibers. Simultaneous depolarization of the ventricles produces the QRS complex on ECG. The T wave is formed by repolarization of the ventricles. Repolarization of the atria occurs at about the same time as depolarization of the ventricles and thus is usually obscured by the QRS wave.[13]

Normal cardiac function depends on cellular automaticity (impulse formation), conductivity, excitability, and contractility. Disorders in automaticity and conductivity constitute the underlying cause of the vast majority of cardiac arrhythmias. Under normal conditions, the SA node is responsible for impulse formation, resulting in a sinus rhythm with a normal rate of 60 to 100 beats per minute.[14] However, other cells or groups of cells also are capable of generating impulses (ectopic pacemakers), and under certain conditions, these may emerge outside of the normal conduction system. After a normal impulse is generated (depolarization), cells of the SA node need time for recovery and repolarization and are said to be *refractory;* during this time, they cannot conduct an impulse. Disturbances causing complete refractoriness result in a block, and those inducing partial refractoriness result in delay of conductivity.

Disorders of conductivity (block or delay) paradoxically may lead to rapid cardiac rhythm through the mechanisms of reentry. Reentry arrhythmias occur when accessory or ectopic pacemakers reexcite previously depolarized fibers before they would become depolarized in the normal sequential impulse pathway, typically producing tachyarrhythmias. The type of arrhythmia may suggest the nature of its cause. For example, paroxysmal atrial tachycardia with block suggests digitalis toxicity.[14]

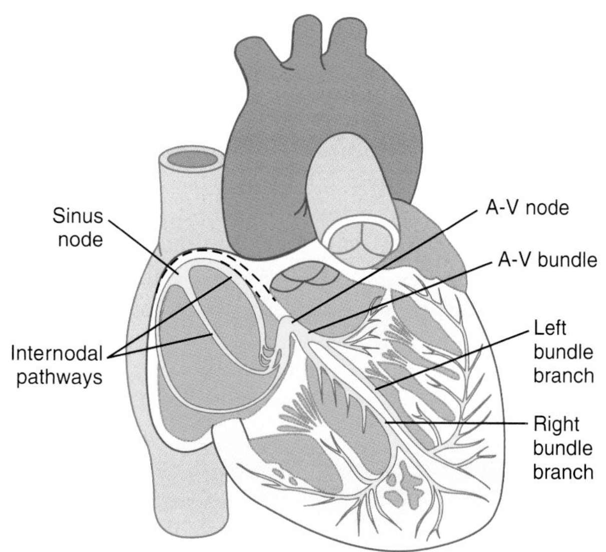

FIGURE 5-1 The electrical conduction system of the heart. *(From Hall JE:* Guyton and Hall textbook of medical physiology, *ed 12, Philadelphia, 2011, Saunders.)*

However, many cardiac arrhythmias are not specific for a given cause. In such cases, a careful search is undertaken to identify the cause of the arrhythmia. The most common causes include primary cardiovascular disorders, pulmonary disorders (e.g., embolism, hypoxia), autonomic disorders, systemic disorders (e.g., thyroid disease), drug-related adverse effects, and electrolyte imbalances.[3,15] Cardiac arrhythmias also are associated with many systemic diseases (Table 5-1) and various drugs or other substances including foods[3,14,16,17] (Table 5-2).

Pathophysiology and Complications

The outcome of an arrhythmia often depends on the nature of the arrhythmia and the physical condition of the patient. For example, a young healthy person with paroxysmal atrial tachycardia may have minimal symptoms, whereas an elderly patient who has heart disease with the same arrhythmia is at risk for developing shock, congestive heart failure, or myocardial ischemia. Furthermore, evidence suggests that patients with certain types of cardiac arrhythmias (e.g., AF) are susceptible to ischemic events within the dental office.[18]

Arrhythmias are classified by site of origin (Box 5-1). Any arrhythmia that arises above the bifurcation of the His bundle into right and left bundle branches is classified as supraventricular.[19] Supraventricular cardiac arrhythmias may be broadly categorized into tachyarrhythmias and bradyarrhythmias. Brief descriptions of some of the more common arrhythmias likely to be encountered in dental patients are provided.

Supraventricular Arrhythmias

Sinus Nodal Disturbances

- **Sinus arrhythmia.** Sinus arrhythmia is characterized by phasic variation in sinus cycle length.[14] In the *respiratory* type, heart rate increases with inhalation and decreases with exhalation. It is seen predominantly in the young and reflects variations in parasympathetic and sympathetic signals to the heart and is considered a normal event. *Nonrespiratory* sinus

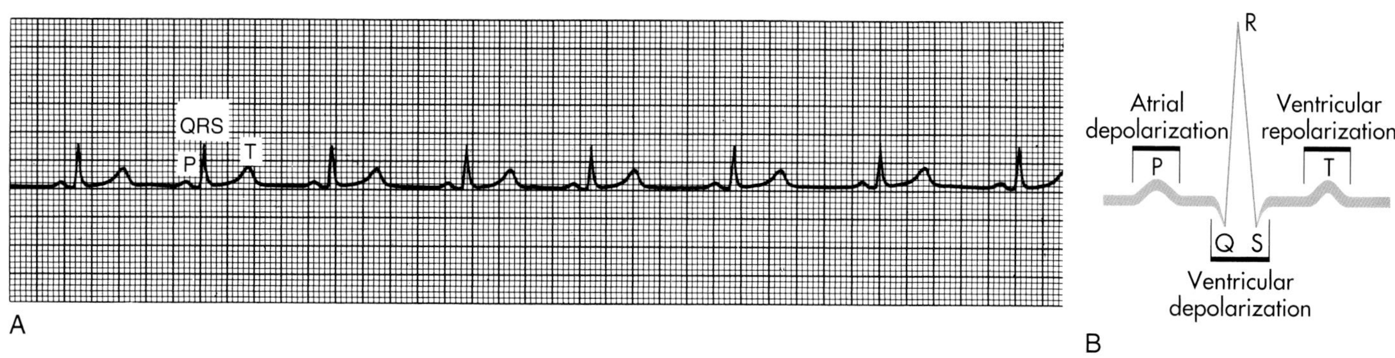

FIGURE 5-2 **A,** Electrocardiographic tracing of the cardiac cycle. **B,** Normal electrocardiographic deflections. The normal electrocardiogram consists of a P wave, representing atrial depolarization; a QRS complex, representing ventricular depolarization; and a T wave, representing rapid repolarization of the ventricles. *(**A,** From Goldberger AL, Goldberger E:* Clinical electrocardiography: a simplified approach, *ed 4, St. Louis, 1990, Mosby. **B,** From Pagana KD, Pagana TJ:* Mosby's manual of diagnostic and laboratory tests, *ed 4, St. Louis, 2010, Mosby.)*

TABLE 5-1 Cardiac Arrhythmias Associated with Various Systemic Diseases

Arrhythmia	Associated Systemic Conditions
Sinus bradycardia	Infectious diseases, hypothermia, myxedema, obstructive jaundice, increased intracranial pressure, myocardial infarction
Atrial extrasystoles	Congestive heart failure, coronary insufficiency, myocardial infarction
Sinoatrial block	Rheumatic heart disease, myocardial infarction, acute infection
Sinus tachycardia	Febrile illness, infection, anemia, hyperthyroidism
Atrial tachycardia	Obstructive lung disease, pneumonia, myocardial infarction
Atrial flutter	Ischemic heart disease, mitral stenosis, myocardial infarction, open heart surgery
Atrial fibrillation	Myocardial infarction, mitral stenosis, ischemic heart disease, thyrotoxicosis, hypertension
Atrioventricular block	Rheumatic heart disease, ischemic heart disease, myocardial infarction, hyperthyroidism, Hodgkin disease, myeloma, open heart surgery
Ventricular extrasystole	Ischemic heart disease, congestive heart failure, mitral valve prolapse
Ventricular tachycardia	Mitral valve prolapse, myocardial infarction, coronary atherosclerotic heart disease
Ventricular fibrillation	Blunt cardiac trauma, mitral valve prolapse, anaphylaxis, cardiac surgery, rheumatic heart disease, cardiomyopathy, coronary atherosclerotic heart disease

arrhythmia is unrelated to respiratory effort and is seen in digitalis intoxication.

- **Sinus tachycardia.** *Tachycardia* in an adult is defined as a heart rate greater than 100 beats per minute, with otherwise normal findings on the ECG.[14] The rate usually is between 100 and 180 beats per minute. This condition most often is a physiologic response to exercise, anxiety, stress, or emotion. Pathophysiologic causes include fever, hypotension, hypoxia, infection, anemia, hyperthyroidism, and heart failure. Drugs that may cause sinus tachycardia include atropine, epinephrine, alcohol, nicotine, and caffeine.
- **Sinus bradycardia.** *Bradycardia* is defined as a heart rate less than 60 beats per minute, with an otherwise normal ECG tracing.[14] It often coexists with a sinus arrhythmia. It is relatively common among well-conditioned athletes and healthy young adults and decreases in prevalence with advancing age. Pathophysiologic causes of bradycardia include intracranial tumor, increased intracranial pressure, myxedema, hypothermia, and gram-negative sepsis. Bradycardia

TABLE 5-2 Drugs/Foods that Can Induce Cardiac Arrhythmias

Cardiac Arrhythmia	Precipitating Drugs/ Food Substance
Bradycardia	Digitalis Morphine Beta blockers Calcium channel blockers
Tachycardia	Atropine Epinephrine Nicotine Ephedrine Caffeine
Premature atrial beats	Alcohol Nicotine Tricyclic antidepressants Caffeine
Ventricular extrasystoles	Digitalis Alcohol Epinephrine Amphetamines
Ventricular tachycardia	Digitalis Quinidine Procainamide Potassium Sympathetic amines

BOX 5-1 Classification of Common Cardiac Arrhythmias

Supraventricular Arrhythmias

- Sinus nodal disturbances
  - Sinus arrhythmia
  - Sinus tachycardia
  - Sinus bradycardia
- Disturbances of atrial rhythm
  - Premature atrial complexes
  - Atrial flutter
  - Atrial fibrillation
  - Atrial tachycardias
- Tachycardias involving the atrioventricular (AV) junction
  - Preexcitation syndrome (Wolff-Parkinson-White)
- Heart block
  - AV block/complete AV block

Ventricular Arrhythmias

- Premature ventricular complexes
- Ventricular tachycardia
- Ventricular fibrillation

Disorders of Repolarization

- Long QT syndrome

may occur during vomiting and vasovagal syncope and as the result of carotid sinus stimulation. Drugs that may cause bradycardia include lithium, amiodarone, beta blockers, clonidine, and calcium channel blockers.

Disturbances of Atrial Rhythm

- **Premature atrial complexes.** Impulses arising from ectopic foci anywhere in the atrium may result in premature atrial beats. Premature atrial complexes, or contractions, occur frequently in otherwise healthy people but often occur during infection, inflammation, or myocardial ischemia.[14] They may be provoked by smoking, lack of sleep, excessive caffeine, or alcohol.[13] They are common in conditions associated with dysfunction of the atria such as congestive heart failure.
- **Atrial flutter.** Atrial flutter is characterized by a rapid, regular atrial rate of 250 to 350 beats per minute. It is rare in healthy persons and most often occurs in association with septal defects, pulmonary emboli, mitral or tricuspid valve stenosis or regurgitation, or chronic ventricular failure.[14] It ialso may be noted in patients with hyperthyroidism, alcoholism, or pericarditis.
- **Atrial fibrillation.** AF is the most common sustained arrhythmia in adults.[19] It is characterized by rapid, disorganized, and ineffective atrial contractions that occur at a rate of 350 to 600 beats per minute. The ventricular response is highly irregular. The atria do not contract effectively, thereby promoting the formation of intraarterial clots, along with consequent embolism and stroke. Thus, patients with AF who are at risk for stroke (e.g., history of previous stroke, systemic emboli, valvular heart disease, hypertension, diabetes, coronary heart disease, heart failure) should be placed on a regimen of warfarin for antithrombotic therapy, with a target international normalized ratio (INR)[20] of 2.0 to 3.0.[14,21] Patients who cannot take warfarin, as well as those who do not have risk factors for stroke, may be managed with dabigatran or aspirin therapy. AF is associated with a history of congestive heart failure, valvular heart disease and stroke, left atrial enlargement, abnormal mitral or aortic valve function, or treated systemic hypertension, as well as with advanced age.[12,22] It may occur intermittently or may be chronic. Symptoms are variable and depend on underlying cardiac status, ventricular rate, and loss of atrial contraction. Treatment consists of medication or cardioversion.
- **Atrial tachycardias.** Any tachycardia arising above the AV junction for which the ECG shows a P wave configuration different from that for sinus rhythm is called *atrial tachycardia.*[19] Atrial tachycardia is characterized by an atrial rate between 150 and 200 beats per minute[14] and may result from enhanced normal automaticity, abnormal automaticity, triggered activity, or reentry. It commonly is seen in patients with coronary artery disease, myocardial infarction (MI), cor pulmonale (right ventricular hypertrophy and pulmonary hypertension), or digitalis intoxication.

Tachycardias Involving the AV Junction

- **Preexcitation syndrome (e.g., Wolff-Parkinson-White syndrome).** The atria and ventricles are electrically insulated from each other by fibrous tissue that forms the anatomic AV junction. Normally, impulses are transmitted from atria to ventricles across this electrical bridge; however, in some persons, additional electrical bridges connect the atria and ventricles, bypassing the normal pathways and forming the basis for preexcitation syndromes such as Wolff-Parkinson-White syndrome.[19] The basic defect in this disorder involves premature activation (preexcitation) of the ventricles by way of an accessory AV pathway that allows the normal SA-AV pathway to be bypassed. This accessory pathway allows rapid conduction and short refractoriness, with impulses passed rapidly between atria and ventricles, and it provides a route for reentrant (backflow) tachyarrhythmias. Resultant paroxysmal tachycardia is characterized by a normal QRS complex, a regular rhythm, and ventricular rates of 150 to 250 beats per minute, along with sudden onset and termination.[14] Wolff-Parkinson-White syndrome is found in all age groups but is more prevalent among men and decreases with age. For most patients with recurrent tachycardia, the prognosis is good, but sudden death occurs rarely, at a frequency of 0.1%.[14]

Heart Block

- **AV block.** Heart block is a disturbance of impulse conduction that may be permanent or transient, depending on the underlying anatomic or functional impairment. Conduction impairment in heart block is classified by severity, with the various forms divided into three categories.[14] During *first-degree* heart block, conduction time is prolonged, but all impulses are conducted. *Second-degree* heart block occurs in two forms: Mobitz type I (Wenckebach) and type II. Type I heart block is characterized by progressive lengthening of conduction time until an impulse is not conducted. Type II heart block denotes occasional or repetitive sudden block of conduction of an impulse without previous lengthening of conduction time. When no impulses are conducted, complete or *third-degree* block is present. AV block occurs when the atrial impulse is conducted with delay or is not conducted at all to the ventricles at a time when the AV junction is not physiologically refractory.[14] Conduction delay may occur at the AV node, within the His-Purkinje system (bundle branches), or at both sites. AV block may be first-degree or second-degree block, or it may be complete. AV block may be caused by a multitude of conditions such as surgery, electrolyte disturbance, myoendocarditis, tumor, myxedema, rheumatoid nodules, Chagas' disease,* calcific aortic stenosis, polymyositis, and amyloidosis. In children, the most common cause is congenital. Drugs (e.g., digitalis, propranolol, potassium, quinidine) also may cause AV heart block. Symptoms increase in severity with increasing degree of block.

Ventricular Arrhythmias

- **Premature ventricular complexes.** Premature ventricular complexes (PVCs) (or contractions) are very common arrhythmias that are characterized by the premature occurrence of an abnormally shaped QRS complex (ventricular contraction), followed by a pause. PVCs may occur alone, as bigeminy (every other beat is a PVC), as trigeminy (every third beat is a PVC), or with higher periodicity. The combination of two consecutive PVCs is called a couplet; three or more in a row at a rate of 100 beats per minute are referred to as ventricular tachycardia.[23] PVCs may be provoked by a variety of medications, by electrolyte imbalance, by tension states, and by excessive use of tobacco, caffeine, and alcohol. In patients without structural heart disease, PVCs have no prognostic significance and no impact on longevity or limitation of activity.[18] The prevalence of PVCs increases with age; they are associated with male gender and are related to low serum potassium concentration. Among patients with previous MI or valvular heart disease, however, frequent PVCs are associated with an increased risk of death.[12]
- **Ventricular tachycardia.** The occurrence of three or more ectopic ventricular beats (PVCs) at a rate of 100 or more per minute is defined as *ventricular tachycardia* (VT). VT may be sustained or episodic. Sustained VT that persists for 30 seconds or longer may require termination because of hemodynamic instability. VT can quickly degenerate into ventricular fibrillation. A variant of VT called *torsades de pointes* is characterized by QRS complexes of changing amplitude that appear to twist around the isoelectrical line; this rhythm occurs at rates of 200 to 250 beats per minute.[24] VT almost always occurs in patients with heart disease, most commonly ischemic heart disease and cardiomyopathy.[14] Certain drugs such as digitalis, sympathetic amines (epinephrine), potassium, quinidine, and procainamide may induce VT.[25]
- **Ventricular flutter and fibrillation.** Ventricular flutter and ventricular fibrillation (VF) are lethal arrhythmias characterized by chaotic, disorganized electrical activity that results in failure of sequential cardiac contraction and inability to maintain cardiac output.[23] The distinction between flutter and fibrillation can be difficult and is of academic interest only; therefore, the two can be discussed together. If these disorders are not rapidly treated within 3 to 5 minutes, death will ensue. VF occurs most commonly as a sequela of ischemic heart disease.

Disorders of Repolarization

- **Long QT syndrome.** Long QT syndrome is a disorder of the conduction system in which the recharging of the heart during repolarization (i.e., the QT interval) is delayed. It is caused by a genetic mutation in myocardial ion channels and by certain drugs, or may be the result of a stroke. The condition can lead to fast, chaotic heartbeats, which can trigger unexplained syncope, a seizure, or sudden death.[24,26]

CLINICAL PRESENTATION

Signs and Symptoms

Arrhythmias may be symptomatic or asymptomatic; however, symptoms alone cannot be relied on to determine the seriousness of an arrhythmia. Some arrhythmias such as PVCs may be highly symptomatic, yet are not associated with an adverse outcome, whereas some patients with atrial fibrillation have no symptoms at all but may be at significant risk for stroke.[27] The symptoms most commonly associated with cardiac arrhythmias include palpitations, lightheadedness, feeling faint, syncope, and those related to congestive heart failure (e.g., shortness of breath, orthopnea). The only clinical sign of an arrhythmia is a pulse that is too fast, too slow, or irregular (Box 5-2).

Laboratory Findings

The ECG is the primary tool used in the identification and diagnosis of cardiac arrhythmias. Additional tests that may be used include exercise or stress testing,

BOX 5-2 Signs and Symptoms of Cardiac Arrhythmias

Signs
- Slow heart rate (<60 beats/min)
- Fast heart rate (>100 beats/min)
- Irregular rhythm

Symptoms
- Palpitations, fatigue
- Dizziness, syncope, angina
- Congestive heart failure:
  - Shortness of breath
  - Orthopnea
  - Peripheral edema

---

*Chagas' disease, also known as American trypanosomiasis, is a tropical acute and chronic parasitic disease of the Americas caused by the flagellate protozoan *Trypanosoma cruzi* usually transmitted by an insect bite.

long-term or ambulatory ECG (Holter) recording, baroreceptor reflex sensitivity testing, body surface mapping, and upright tilt-table testing. Electrode catheter techniques allow for intracavitary recordings of the specialized conducting systems, which aid greatly in the diagnosis of arrhythmias.[27]

MEDICAL MANAGEMENT

Management of cardiac arrhythmias involves medications, cardioversion, pacemakers, implanted cardioverter-defibrillators (ICDs), radiofrequency catheter ablation, and surgery. Patients with asymptomatic arrhythmias usually require no therapy; those with symptomatic arrhythmias typically are treated first with medications. Patients who do not respond to medications may be treated by cardioversion, ablation, or implanted pacemaker or ICD. Surgery may be necessary for the treatment of patients with certain arrhythmias. Emergency cardioversion is indicated for any tachyarrhythmias that compromise hemodynamics or are life-threatening (e.g., cardiac arrest).

Antiarrhythmic Drugs

Generally, molecular targets for optimal action of antiarrhythmic drugs involve channels within the cellular membranes through which ions are diffused rapidly. Antiarrhythmic drugs are therefore classified on the basis of their effect on sodium, potassium, or calcium channels and whether they block beta receptors[28,29] (Table 5-3). *Class I* drugs have "local anesthetic" properties or membrane-stabilizing effects and work by primarily blocking the fast sodium channels. *Class II* drugs are β-adrenergic-blocking agents. *Class III* drugs prolong the duration of the cardiac action potential and enhance refractoriness through their effects on potassium channels. *Class IV* drugs are calcium channel blockers. Although this classification implies a single action for each class, the reality is that they typically have multiple sites of action across different classification categories. For example, procainamide blocks both sodium and potassium channels, and amiodarone blocks sodium, potassium, and calcium channels.[30]

Many of the antiarrhythmic drugs have very narrow therapeutic ranges, so optimum blood levels that are not too high or too low may be difficult to achieve. Thus, undermedicated patients may be at increased risk for an adverse event during dental treatment; conversely, in those who are overmedicated, drug toxicity also is a possibility. Patients with AF often are prescribed warfarin sodium (Coumadin; Bristol-Myers Squibb, Princeton, New Jersey) to prevent atrial thrombosis and embolism; the target INR (therapeutic range) is between 2.0 and 3.0. A newer antithrombin drug, dabigatran (Pradaxa, Boehringer Ingelheim, Ridgefield, Connecticut), also has been approved by the U.S. Food and Drug Administration (FDA) for the prevention of stroke in patients with nonvalvular AF.

Implanted Permanent Pacemakers

A permanent, implanted pacemaker consists of a lithium battery–powered generator implanted subcutaneously in the left infraclavicular area that produces an electrical impulse that is transmitted by a lead inserted into the heart through the subclavian vein to an electrode in contact with endocardial or myocardial tissue (Figure 5-3). The leads may be either unipolar (stimulating only one chamber) or, more commonly, bipolar (stimulating two chambers). With a bipolar pacemaker, one lead usually is inserted into the right atrium, and the second lead is positioned within the right ventricle.[31]

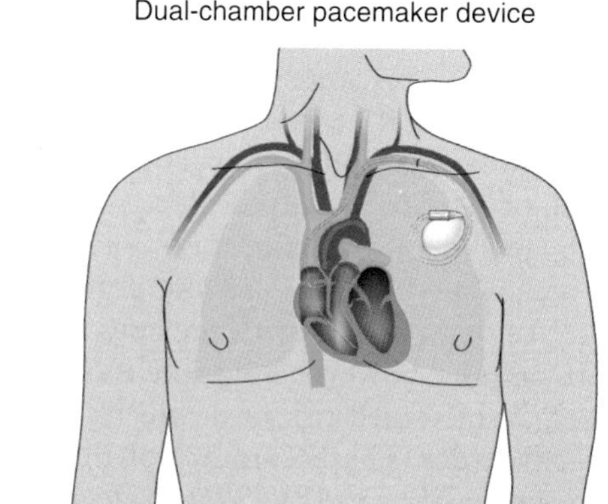

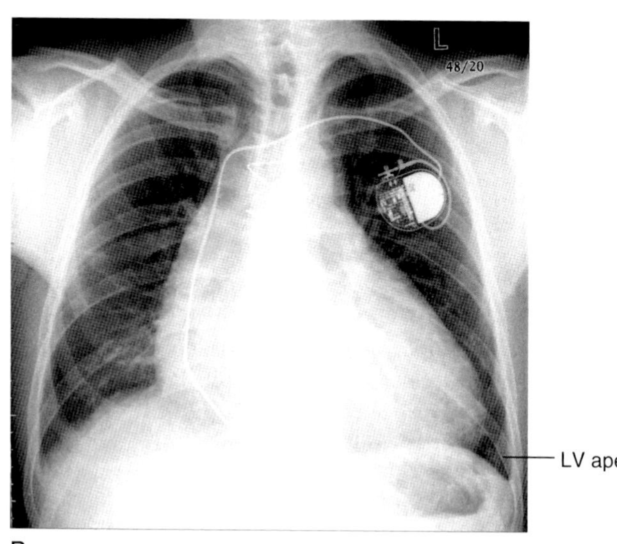

FIGURE 5-3 A, The site of implantation of a permanent pacemaker (note: can be inserted in the left or right intraclavicular chest wall). **B,** A chest x-ray showing a pacemaker in a patient. *(**A,** Courtesy Matt Hazzard, University of Kentucky. **B,** From Bonow RO, et al, editors:* Braunwald's heart disease: a textbook of cardiovascular medicine, *ed 9, Philadelphia, 2012, Saunders.)*

TABLE 5-3 Drugs Used to Treat Arrhythmias

Drug	Vasoconstrictor Interactions	Oral Side/ Adverse Effects	Other Considerations
Class I: Sodium Channel Blockers			
Quinidine	None	Bitter taste, dry mouth, petechiae, gingival bleeding	Syncope, hypotension, nausea, vomiting, thrombocytopenia
Procainamide	None	Bitter taste, oral ulcerations	Worsening of arrhythmias, lupus-like syndrome, rash, myalgia, fever, agranulocytosis
Disopyramide (Norpace)	None	Dry mouth	Urinary hesitancy, constipation
Mexiletine (Mexitil)	None	Dry mouth	Tremor, dizziness, diplopia, nausea, vomiting
Propafenone (Rythmol)	None	Taste aberration, dry mouth	Worsening of arrhythmias, dizziness, nausea, vomiting
Flecainide (Tambocor)	None	Metallic taste	Worsening of arrhythmias, confusion, irritability
Class II: Beta Blockers			
Propranolol (Inderal)—nonselective beta blocker	Possible increase in blood pressure is possible with nonselective beta blockers; cautious use of vasoconstrictors is recommended (maximum, 0.036 mg epinephrine, 0.20 mg levonordefrin)	Taste changes; lichenoid reactions	Hypotension, bradycardia, fatigue; avoid long-term use of NSAIDs
Also: acebutolol, esmolol, metoprolol, atenolol, timolol	With cardioselective beta blockers, use vasoconstrictors normally		
Class III: Agents for Prolonged Action Potential and Refractoriness			
Amiodarone (Cordarone)	None	Taste aberration	Interstitial pneumonitis, hyper- or hypothyroidism, elevated liver enzymes, bluish skin discoloration
Sotalol (Betapace)—nonselective beta blocker	Increase in blood pressure is possible with nonselective beta blockers; cautious use of vasoconstrictors is recommended (maximum, 0.036 mg epinephrine, 0.20 mg levonordefrin)	Taste changes; lichenoid reactions	Hypotension, bradycardia, torsades de pointes, fatigue; avoid long-term use of NSAIDs
Class IV: Calcium Channel Blockers			
Verapamil (Calan) *Also:* Diltiazem	None	Gingival overgrowth	Hypotension, bradycardia
Miscellaneous			
Digoxin (Lanoxin)	Increased risk for arrhythmias; avoid if possible	Hypersalivation (toxicity)	Precipitation of arrhythmias, toxicity (headache, nausea, vomiting, altered color perception, malaise)

NSAIDs, Nonsteroidal antiinflammatory drugs.

Pacemakers are capable of very specific individualized pacing programs or modes, depending upon the individual's needs. A classification code is used to describe the various pacing modes of a pacemaker unit, which include the chamber that is paced, the chamber that is sensed, inhibitory or tracking function capability, rate modulation capability, and capability for antitachycardia pacing and/or the delivery of a shock.[31] Most pacemakers are of the demand variety, which can detect the patient's natural heartbeat and prevent competitive pacemaker firing; they are rate adaptive. Newer units contain pacing circuits that allow for programming, memory, and telemetry. In general, pacemakers are indicated to treat bradycardias in patients with acquired AV block, congenital AV block, chronic bifascicular and trifascicular block, AV block associated with acute MI, sinus node dysfunction, hypersensitive carotid sinus and neurocardiogenic syncope, and certain forms of cardiomyopathy. They also are indicated for the prevention and termination of certain tachyarrhythmias.[32]

Complications are infrequent but have been reported as a result of pacemaker placement. These include pneumothorax, perforation of the atrium or ventricle, subsequent dislodgment of the leads, infection, and erosion of the pacemaker pocket.[31] Infective endocarditis rarely may occur; however, antibiotic prophylaxis for dental treatment is not recommended.[33-35]

Implantable Cardioverter-Defibrillators

An ICD is a device that is similar to a pacemaker and is implanted in the same way as for a pacemaker. ICDs are capable not only of delivering a shock but of providing antitachycardia pacing (ATP) and ventricular bradycardia pacing. Most ICDs have a single lead that is inserted into the right ventricle and function by continuously monitoring a patient's cardiac rate and delivering ATP or a shock when the rate exceeds a predetermined cutoff point, such as in VT or VF.[36] ATP has the advantage of terminating a rhythm disturbance without delivering a shock. ICDs generally are larger than pacemakers, and their batteries do not last as long as those of a pacemaker, the life span of the latter being 5 to 10 years. Antibiotic prophylaxis for dental treatment in patients with these devices is not recommended.[35]

Electromagnetic Interference. Electromagnetic interference (EMI)[37] from nonintrinsic electrical activity can temporarily interfere with the function of a pacemaker or ICD. The pacemaker or ICD senses these extraneous signals and misinterprets them, which may cause rate alterations, sensing abnormalities, asynchronous pacing, noise reversion, or reprogramming.[38] Numerous sources of EMI are present in daily life, industry, and medical and dental settings (Box 5-3). Examples of EMI sources in daily life are cell phones, metal detectors, high-voltage power lines, and some home appliances (e.g., electric razor). EMI sources in the workplace include welding equipment and induction furnaces. In the medical setting, magnetic resonance imaging scanners, electrosurgery, neurostimulators, defibrillators, TENS (transcutaneous electrical nerve stimulation) units, and instrumentation from radiofrequency catheter ablation, therapeutic diathermy, therapeutic ionizing radiotherapy, and ultrasonic lithotripsy all are documented sources of potentially harmful EMI.[39] The effects of EMI on pacemakers and ICDs vary with the intensity of the electromagnetic field, the frequency of the spectrum of the signal, the distance and positioning of the device relative to the source, the electrode configuration, nonprogrammable device characteristics, programmed settings, and patient characteristics.[38] Electrical and magnetic fields are reduced inversely with the square of the distance from the source. It also has been demonstrated that devices from different manufacturers differ in their susceptibility to various sources of EMI.[38]

Several studies suggest that dental devices may cause EMI with pacemakers and ICDs. In studies performed in vitro, electrosurgery units, ultrasonic bath cleaners, ultrasonic scaling devices, and battery-operated curing lights have produced EMI with pacemakers and ICDs.[40-43] Amalgamators, electrical pulp testers and apex locators, handpieces, electric toothbrushes, microwave ovens, and x-ray units did not cause any significant EMI with the pacemakers and ICDs tested.[40,41,44,45] Internal shielding has been increased on newer generators to minimize the adverse effects of such interference.

BOX 5-3 Sources of Electromagnetic Interference for Pacemakers/ICDs

Daily Living
- Cell phones, metal detectors
- High-voltage power lines
- Household appliances (e.g., electric razors)

Industrial
- Arc welders, induction furnaces

Medical
- Magnetic resonance imaging scanners
- Electrosurgery, therapeutic diathermy
- Neurostimulators, defibrillators
- Transcutaneous electrical nerve stimulation (TENS) units
- Radiofrequency catheter ablation
- Therapeutic ionizing radiotherapy
- Lithotripsy

Dental
- Electrosurgery, ultrasonic bath cleaners
- Ultrasonic scalers, battery-operated curing light

Radiofrequency Catheter Ablation

Radiofrequency catheter ablation is a technique whereby a catheter (electrode) is introduced percutaneously into a vein and is threaded into the heart. The catheter is positioned in contact with the area determined by electrophysiologic testing to be the anatomic source of an arrhythmia. Radiofrequency energy is then delivered through the electrode catheter whose tip is in contact with the target tissue, which results in resistive heating of the tissue, producing irreversible tissue destruction of an area 5 to 6 mm in diameter and 2 to 3 mm deep, destroying the ectopic pacemaker. This technique can eliminate a variety of supraventricular and ventricular tachycardias that previously required long-term pharmacologic treatment for suppression or surgery for cure.[31]

Surgery

Surgery is another therapeutic approach that is used to treat patients with tachycardia. Direct surgical approaches designed to interrupt accessory pathways consist of resection of tissue and ablation. In addition to direct surgical approaches, indirect approaches such as aneurysmectomy, coronary artery bypass grafting, or relief of valvular regurgitation or stenosis may be useful in selected patients.[28]

Cardioversion and Defibrillation

Transthoracic delivery of an electric shock can be performed electively (cardioversion), to terminate persistent or refractory arrhythmias, or on an emergency basis (defibrillation), to terminate a lethal arrhythmia. Direct current defibrillators deliver an electrical charge by way of two paddles (electrodes) placed on the chest wall. One electrode is placed on the left chest over the region of the apex, and the other on the right side of the chest just to the right of the sternum and below the clavicle (Figure 5-4). The shock terminates arrhythmias caused by reentry by simultaneously depolarizing large portions of the atria and ventricles, thereby causing reentry circuits to disappear momentarily.[31] Defibrillation usually is instantaneous, and cardiac pumping resumes within a few seconds. It may have to be repeated if defibrillation is unsuccessful (i.e., if a regular heartbeat is not occurring). The most common arrhythmias treated by cardioversion/defibrillation are VF, VT, AF, and atrial flutter. Treatment of patients with VF is always emergent; treatment of patients with VT may be elective or emergent, depending on the patient's hemodynamic status. Treatment of those with atrial flutter and AF usually is elective.

Several types of automated external defibrillators (AEDs) are available for use in the dental office for emergency defibrillation. An AED should be considered for inclusion in the dentist's emergency medical kit. The use of AEDs is now taught as part of basic and advanced cardiopulmonary resuscitation courses, and familiarity with these devices and their application among laypersons is encouraged by public health agencies. These devices, now commonly found in public areas, are simple and easy to use, and emergency defibrillation is a critical part of successful resuscitation for a victim of cardiac arrest.

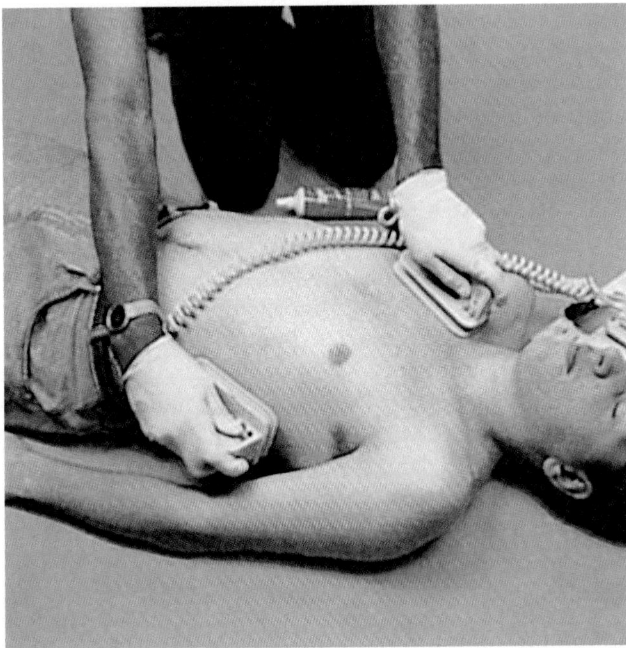

FIGURE 5-4 Cardioversion/defibrillation paddles in place on a patient. *(From Sanders MJ:* Mosby's paramedic textbook, *ed 3, St. Louis, 2005, Mosby.)*

DENTAL MANAGEMENT

Medical Considerations

Stress associated with dental treatment or use of excessive amounts of injected epinephrine may lead to life-threatening cardiac arrhythmias in susceptible dental patients. Patients with an existing arrhythmia, diagnosed or undiagnosed, are at increased risk for adverse events in the dental environment. In addition, patients at risk for developing an arrhythmia may be in danger in the dental office if they are not identified and measures are not taken to minimize situations that can precipitate an arrhythmia. Other patients may have their arrhythmias under control with the use of drugs or a pacemaker but require special consideration when receiving dental treatment. The keys to successful dental management of patients prone to developing a cardiac arrhythmia and those with an existing arrhythmia are identification and prevention. Even under the best of circumstances, however, a patient may develop a cardiac arrhythmia that requires immediate emergency measures.

Identification of patients with a history of an arrhythmia, those with an undiagnosed arrhythmia, and those prone to developing a cardiac rhythm disturbance is the first step in risk assessment and in avoiding an untoward event (Box 5-4). This process is accomplished by obtaining a thorough medical history, including a pertinent review of systems, and taking and evaluating vital signs (pulse rate and rhythm, blood pressure, respiratory rate). In a review of systems, patients should be asked about the presence of signs or symptoms related to the cardiovascular and pulmonary systems. Patients who report palpitations, dizziness, chest pain, shortness of breath, or syncope may have a cardiac arrhythmia or other cardiovascular disease and should be evaluated by a physician. Patients with an irregular cardiac rhythm (even without symptoms) also may require consultation with the physician to determine its significance.

Patients with a known history of arrhythmia should be interviewed carefully to ascertain the type of arrhythmia (if known), how it is being treated, medications being taken, presence of a pacemaker or defibrillator, effects on their activity, and stability of their disease. Because the classification and diagnosis of arrhythmia often are complex, patients often do not know the specific diagnosis that has been assigned to their disorder; thus, the physician must be relied on to provide this

BOX 5-4 Identifying Patients with Cardiac Arrhythmias

Patients with cardiac arrhythmias may be identified by:

- Assessing the medical history*:
  - Type of arrhythmia
  - Frequency of occurrence and severity
  - How treated
  - Presence of pacemaker or defibrillator
  - Level of control/stability
- Understanding risk for arrhythmia is increased in the presence of other cardiovascular or pulmonary disease.
- Identifying the patient who does not report an arrhythmia but may be taking one or more of the antiarrhythmic drugs.
- Pertinent review of systems—asking about the presence of symptoms that could be caused by arrhythmias (palpitations, dizziness, chest pain, shortness of breath, syncope).
- Obtaining vital signs suggestive of arrhythmia (rapid pulse rate, slow pulse rate, irregular pulse).
- Refering patient to physician if signs or symptoms are present that are suggestive of a cardiac arrhythmia or other cardiovascular disease.

*Consultation with the patient's physician may be required to obtain or verify this information.

BOX 5-5 Perioperative Risk and Dental Treatment for Patients with Cardiac Arrhythmias

Arrhythmias Associated with Major Perioperative Risk

- High-grade atrioventricular (AV) block
- Symptomatic ventricular arrhythmias in the presence of underlying heart disease
- Supraventricular arrhythmias with uncontrolled ventricular rate
  Dental management: Avoid elective dental care.

Arrhythmias Associated with Intermediate Perioperative Risk

- Abnormal Q waves on electrocardiogram (ECG) (marker of previous myocardial infarction)
  Dental management: Elective dental care is appropriate.

Arrhythmias Associated with Minor Perioperative Risk

- ECG abnormalities consistent with:
  - Left ventricular hypertrophy
  - Left bundle branch block
  - ST-T wave abnormalities
  - Any rhythm other than sinus (e.g., atrial fibrillation)
  Dental management: Elective dental care is appropriate.

Data from Fleisher LA, et al: ACC/AHA 2007 guidelines on perioperative cardiovascular evaluation and care for noncardiac surgery: a report of the American College of Cardiology/American Heart Association Task Force on Practice Guidelines (Writing Committee to Revise the 2002 Guidelines on Perioperative Cardiovascular Evaluation for Noncardiac Surgery). Circulation. *2007;116:e418-e499.*

information. It is important to identify any known triggers, such as stress, anxiety, or medications. The presence of other heart, thyroid, kidney, or chronic pulmonary disease also should be determined, because such disorders may be a cause of or contributor to the arrhythmia and may necessitate additional changes in dental management. If any questions or uncertainties arise, a medical consultation should be sought regarding the patient's diagnosis and current status, and to aid the dentist in assessing risk for aggravating or precipitating a cardiac arrhythmia, stroke, or MI during or in relation to dental treatment.

The dentist must make a determination of the risk involved in providing dental treatment to a patient with a history of arrhythmia and must decide whether the benefits of treatment outweigh any risk. This often requires consultation with the physician. The American College of Cardiology (ACC) and the American Heart Association (AHA) have published guidelines that can help make this determination.[46] These guidelines are intended for use by physicians who are evaluating patients with cardiovascular disease to determine whether they can safely undergo surgical procedures. They also may be applied to the provision of dental care and may be of significant value to the dentist in making a determination of risk.

Box 5-5 is based on these ACC/AHA guidelines and provides an estimate of the risk that a serious event (acute MI, unstable angina, or sudden death) may occur during noncardiac surgery in patients with various arrhythmias. Patients with a significant arrhythmia (i.e., high-grade AV block, symptomatic ventricular arrhythmias in the presence of cardiovascular disease, and supraventricular arrhythmias with an uncontrolled ventricular rate) are at major risk for complications and are not candidates for elective dental care. Dental care should be deferred until a consultation with the physician has occurred. The presence of other types of arrhythmias carries significantly less risk. The presence of pathologic Q waves (marker of a previous MI) is a clinical predictor of intermediate risk for perioperative complications; other ECG abnormalities, including left ventricular hypertrophy, left bundle branch block, and ST-T wave abnormalities, as well as any rhythm other than sinus rhythm, are associated with minor perioperative risk. Patients with these types of arrhythmias can undergo elective dental treatment with only minimally increased risk for an adverse event.

The type and magnitude of the planned dental procedure also must be considered in determination of perioperative risk. Box 5-6 provides an estimate of cardiac risk for specific surgical procedures in patients with cardiovascular disease. Although dental procedures are not specifically listed, they would certainly be included in the low risk category, associated with less than a 1% chance

BOX 5-6 Cardiac Risk* Stratification for Noncardiac Surgical Procedures

High (Reported Cardiac Risk Often Greater Than 5%)
- Emergent major operations, particularly in the elderly
- Aortic and other major vascular surgery
- Peripheral vascular surgery
- Anticipated prolonged surgical procedures associated with large fluid shifts and/or blood loss

Intermediate (Reported Cardiac Risk Generally Less Than 5%)
- Carotid endarterectomy
- Head and neck surgery
- Intraperitoneal and intrathoracic surgery
- Orthopedic surgery
- Prostate surgery

Low (Reported Cardiac Risk Generally Less Than 1%)
- Endoscopic procedures
- Superficial procedures
- Cataract surgery
- Breast surgery

*Combined incidence of cardiac death and nonfatal myocardial infarction.
Adapted from Fleisher LA, et al: ACC/AHA 2007 guidelines on perioperative cardiovascular evaluation and care for noncardiac surgery: a report of the American College of Cardiology/American Heart Association Task Force on Practice Guidelines (Writing Committee to Revise the 2002 Guidelines on Perioperative Cardiovascular Evaluation for Noncardiac Surgery). Circulation. *2007;116:e418-e499.*

of an adverse perioperative event. Nonsurgical dental procedures are likely to pose even less risk than that for surgical procedures. More extensive oral and maxillofacial surgical procedures, and perhaps some of the more extensive periodontal surgical procedures, probably would be included in the intermediate cardiac risk category under "head and neck procedures," with a risk of less than 5%. Procedures associated with the highest risk (greater than 5%) include emergency major surgery in elderly persons, aortic or vascular surgery, and peripheral vascular surgery. These procedures are performed with the patient under general anesthesia and carry the potential for significant blood and fluid loss with resultant adverse hemodynamic effects. Therefore, it seems clear that the vast majority of dental procedures, whether surgical or nonsurgical, are associated with low to very low risk for an adverse event in patients with arrhythmias and other cardiovascular diseases.

Stress and Anxiety Reduction. Based on the assessment of medical risk, the type of planned dental procedure, and the stability and anxiety level of the patient, stress reduction strategies for patients with arrhythmias of low to intermediate risk may include the following: establishing good rapport, scheduling short appointments in the morning, ensuring comfortable chair position, pretreatment assessment of vital signs, preoperative oral sedation, intraoperative use of nitrous oxide–oxygen sedation, ensuring excellent local anesthesia, and providing effective postoperative pain control (see Chapter 1). On occasion, it may be necessary to provide urgent dental care to a patient with a significant arrhythmia. If treatment becomes necessary, it should be performed as conservatively as possible and should be directed primarily toward pain relief, infection control, or control of bleeding. Consultation with the patient's physician is advised. Additional management recommendations may include establishing and maintaining an intravenous line, continuously monitoring the ECG and vital signs, and using a pulse oximeter. These measures may require that the patient be treated in a special patient care facility or hospital dental clinic (Box 5-7).

Use of Vasoconstrictors. The use of vasoconstrictors in local anesthetics poses potential problems for patients with arrhythmias because of the possibility of precipitating cardiac tachycardia or another arrhythmia. A local anesthetic without vasoconstrictor may be used as needed. If a vasoconstrictor is deemed necessary, patients in the low to intermediate risk category and those taking nonselective beta blockers can safely be given up to 0.036 mg epinephrine (two cartridges containing 1:100,000 epinephrine); intravascular injections are to be avoided.[47] Greater quantities of vasoconstrictor may well be tolerated, but increasing quantities are associated with increased risk for adverse cardiovascular effects. Vasoconstrictors should be avoided in patients taking digoxin because of the potential for inducing arrhythmias.[48,49] For patients at major risk for arrhythmias, the use of vasoconstrictors should be avoided, but if their use is considered essential, it should be discussed with the physician (see Box 5-7). Studies have shown that modest amounts of vasoconstrictor can be used safely in high-risk cardiac patients when accompanied by oxygen, sedation, nitroglycerin, and excellent pain control measures.[50-52]

For patients at all levels of cardiac risk, the use of gingival retraction cord impregnated with epinephrine should be avoided because of the associated rapid absorption of a high concentration of epinephrine and the potential for adverse cardiovascular effects. As an alternative, plain cord saturated with tetrahydrozoline HCl 0.05% (Visine; Pfizer, New York, New York), or with oxymetazoline HCl 0.05% (Afrin; Schering-Plough, Summit, New Jersey), provides gingival effects equivalent to those of epinephrine without the adverse cardiovascular effects.[53]

Warfarin (Coumadin). Patients with atrial fibrillation often are given anticoagulant therapy (warfarin) to prevent thrombus formation, embolism, and stroke; thus, they are at risk for increased bleeding. The target range for anticoagulation in patients with atrial fibrillation usually is an INR between 2 and 3 times the normal value.[54] Studies have shown that minor oral surgery, such as simple extractions, can be performed without altering or stopping the warfarin regimen, provided that the INR

BOX 5-7 Dental Management
Considerations in Patients with Cardiac Arrhythmias

P

Patient Evaluation/Risk Assessment (see Box 1-1)

- Evaluate and determine whether an arrhythmia exists.
- Obtain medical consultation if the patient's heart condition is poorly controlled or if the condition is undiagnosed, or if the cause or nature of the arrhythmia is uncertain.

Potential Issues/Factors of Concerns

A	
Analgesics	Provide good postoperative analgesia to minimize pain and associated stress.
Antibiotics	For patients with pacemakers or ICDs, antibiotic prophylaxis to prevent bacterial endocarditis is not recommended. Some antibiotics (e.g., metronidazole, extended-spectrum penicillins) are known to increase the INR in patients on warfarin (Coumadin); caution in their use is advised.
Anesthesia	Ensure profound local anesthesia. Epinephrine-containing local anesthetic can be used with minimal risk if the dose is limited to 0.036 mg epinephrine (two capsules containing 1:100,000 concentration). Higher doses may be tolerated, but the risk of complications increases with dose. Avoid the use of epinephrine in retraction cord.
Anxiety	Establish good rapport, and schedule short morning appointments. Use anxiety reduction techniques: • Provide preoperative sedation (short-acting benzodiazepine the night before and/or 1 hour before the appointment). • Administer intraoperative sedation (nitrous oxide–oxygen).
Allergy	No Issues
B	
Bleeding	In patients taking warfarin: • Review current INR lab results (within 24 hours of surgical procedure). • If INR is within the therapeutic range (2.0-3.5), dental treatment, including minor oral surgery, can be performed without stopping or altering the warfarin regimen. In patients taking dabigatran when major oral surgery is planned: • Review current thrombin clotting time, activated partial thromboplastin time or ecarin clotting time lab results. • Ensure patient has normal renal function. In patients taking warfarin, dabigatran or other anticoagulant/antiplatelet: • Use local hemostatic measures and products including gelatin sponge, oxidized cellulose or chitosan products in sockets, suturing, gauze pressure packs, and preoperative stents. Tranexamic acid or ε-aminocaproic acid can be used as mouth rinse and/or to soak gauze for placement at bleeding site.
Blood pressure	Obtain pretreatment vital signs and monitor pulse and blood pressure throughout stressful and invasive procedures.
C	
Chair position	Ensure comfortable chair position. Raise chair slowly, and in case of slow heart rate or hypotension, stabilize patient in upright position before dismissing.
D	
Devices	Pacemakers and ICDs may experience electromagnetic interference with dental equipment such as ultrasonic scalers, ultrasonic bath cleaners, electrosurgery devices, or battery-operated curing lights.
Drugs	In patients taking digoxin, watch for signs or symptoms of toxicity (e.g., hypersalivation, visual changes); avoid epinephrine or levonordefrin.
E	
Equipment	Have emergency medical kit readily available.
Emergencies and urgent care	For high-risk patient who requires urgent care, consider treating in special care clinic or hospital where a defibrillator can be used if needed. After consulting with physician, provide limited care only for pain control, treatment of acute infection, or control of bleeding, as appropriate. The following measures may be used as needed: • Placement of intravenous line • Sedation • Electrocardiogram (ECG) monitoring • Pulse oximetry • Blood pressure monitoring • Avoiding or limiting epinephrine
F	
Follow-up	Patients who have had surgery should be contacted to ensure that the postoperative course proceeds without complications.

ICD, implantable cardioverter-defibrillator; *INR*, International normalized ratio.

is within the therapeutic range. (Depending upon the reason for the anticoagulant, the therapeutic range of the INR is between 2.0 and 3.5.)[55-58] Management recommendations also include the use of local measures such as placing of gelatin sponges, oxidized cellulose or chitosan hemostatic products in the sockets, suturing, gauze sponges for pressure pack, or stents during the surgery; and the topical use of tranexamic acid or ε-aminocaproic acid as a mouthrinse and/or to soak sponges postoperatively (see Box 5-7). For more significant surgery, consultation with the physician should be obtained.

Dabigatran (Pradaxa). Patients who have atrial fibrillation may be taking the newer anticoagulant dabigatran to prevent thrombus formation, embolism, and stroke. Dabigatran is an oral antithrombin medication that is reported to cause less major bleeding than warfarin, when used at recommended doses.[59] Thus, it is not predicted to cause concern for major bleeding during and after invasive dental procedures. However, few studies to date have evaluated this drug in a dental setting, and patients who receive higher doses, as in the elderly and those who have kidney function impairment, are at increased risk for major bleeding.[60] Accordingly, dentists are advised to use good local hemostatic procedures for patients taking this drug.

Pacemakers/ICDs and Antibiotic Prophylaxis. Patients with pacemakers or ICDs are not at risk for bacterial endocarditis related to dental procedures; thus, antibiotic prophylaxis is not indicated.[33,34,46]

Pacemakers/ICDs and Electromagnetic Interference. The risk of encountering significant EMI with a pacemaker in the dental office is low. Box 5-3 lists known sources of EMI. In the dental setting, only electrosurgery, ultrasonic bath cleaners, curing lights, and ultrasonic scalers have been shown to produce potential interference.[40,41] Therefore, these devices should not be used on or around a patient with a pacemaker (see Box 5-7).

Digoxin Toxicity. Because the therapeutic range for digoxin is very narrow, toxicity can easily occur (see Box 5-7). This is a special concern in elderly persons and in those with hypothyroidism, renal insufficiency, dehydration, hypokalemia, hypomagnesemia, or hypocalcemia. Patients with electrolyte disturbances generally are more susceptible to digoxin toxicity. Signs of toxicity include hypersalivation, nausea and vomiting, headache, drowsiness, and visual distortions, with objects appearing yellow or green.[61] Thus, the dentist should be alert to these changes and should refer the patient reporting such changes to the physician.

Treatment Planning Considerations

A patient who is susceptible to cardiac arrhythmias can receive virtually any indicated dental procedure once the arrhythmia has been identified and the aforementioned steps are taken. Complex dental procedures should be scheduled over several appointments to avoid overstressing the patient (see Box 5-7).

Oral Manifestations

The only significant oral complications found in patients with arrhythmias are those that occur as a result of adverse effects of medications used to control arrhythmia. Table 5-3 lists the oral manifestations potentially associated with use of antiarrhythmic drugs.

REFERENCES

1. Lampert R, et al: Emotional and physical precipitants of ventricular arrhythmia, *Circulation* 106:1800-1805, 2002.
2. Culic V, et al: Triggering of ventricular tachycardia by meteorologic and emotional stress: protective effect of beta-blockers and anxiolytics in men and elderly, *Am J Epidemiol* 160:1047-1058, 2004.
3. Mirvis DM, Goldberger AL: Electrocardiography. In Zipes D, et al, editors: *Braunwald's heart disease: a textbook of cardiovascular medicine*, ed 7, Philadelphia, 2005, Saunders.
4. Guize L, et al: [Cardiac arrhythmias in the elderly, *Bull Acad Natl Med* 190:827-841, 2006.
5. Lok NS, Lau CP: Prevalence of palpitations, cardiac arrhythmias and their associated risk factors in ambulant elderly, *Int J Cardiol* 54:231-236, 1996.
6. Gaziano JM: Global burden of cardiovascular disease. In Zipes D, et al, editors: *Braunwald's heart disease: a textbook of cardiovascular medicine*, ed 7, Philadelphia, 2005, Saunders.
7. Lloyd-Jones D, et al: Executive summary: heart disease and stroke statistics—2010 update: a report from the American Heart Association, *Circulation* 121:948-954, 2010.
8. Little JW, et al: Dental patient reaction to electrocardiogram screening, *Oral Surg Oral Med Oral Pathol* 70:433-439, 1990.
9. Little JW, et al: Evaluation of an EKG system for the dental office, *Gen Dent* 38:278-281, 1990.
10. Simmons MS, et al: Screening dentists for risk factors associated with cardiovascular disease, *Gen Dent* 42:440-445, 1994.
11. Rhodus NL, Little JW: The prevalence of cardiac arrhythmias in dental and dental hygiene students, *Calif Inst Cont Educ Dent* 5:23-26, 1998.
12. Stephenson LW: History of cardiac surgery. In Cohn LH, editor: *Cardiac surgery in the adult*, ed 3, New York, 2008, McGraw-Hill, pp 3-28.
13. Guyton AC, Hall JE: *Textbook of medical physiology*, ed 11, Philadelphia, 2006, Saunders.
14. Olgin JE, Zipes D: Specific arrhythmias: diagnosis and treatment. In Zipes D, et al, editors: *Braunwald's heart disease: a textbook of cardiovascular medicine*, ed 7, Philadelphia, 2005, Saunders.
15. Novo S, et al: Increased prevalence of cardiac arrhythmias and transient episodes of myocardial ischemia in hypertensives with left ventricular hypertrophy but without clinical history of coronary heart disease, *Am J Hypertens* 10:843-851, 1997.
16. Calkins H: Principles of electrophysiology. In Goldman L, Ausiello D, editors: *Cecil textbook of medicine*, ed 22, Philadelphia, 2004, Saunders.
17. Barnes BJ, Hollands JM: Drug-induced arrhythmias, *Crit Care Med* 38(6 Suppl):S188-S197, 2010.
18. Matsuura H: The systemic management of cardiovascular risk patients in dentistry, *Anesth Pain Control Dent* 2:49-61, 1993.
19. Akhtar M: Cardiac arrhythmias with supraventricular origin, In Goldman L, Ausiello D, editors: *Cecil textbook of medicine*, ed 23, Philadelphia, 2008, Saunders.
20. Shariff G, et al: Relationship between oral bacteria and hemodialysis access infection, *Oral Surg Oral Med Oral Pathol Oral Radiol Endod* 98:418-422, 2004.
21. Pineo G, Hull RD: Coumarin therapy in thrombosis, *Hematol Oncol Clin North Am* 17:201-216, viii, 2003.
22. Hirsh J, et al: Antithrombotic and thrombolytic therapy: American College of Chest Physicians Evidence-Based Clinical Practice Guidelines (8th Edition), *Chest* 133(6 Suppl):110S-112S, 2008.
23. Lerman BB: Ventricular arrhythmias and sudden death. In Goldman L, Ausiello D, editors: *Cecil textbook of medicine*, ed 23, Philadelphia, 2008, Saunders.

24. Goldenberg I, Moss AJ. Long QT syndrome, *J Am Coll Cardiol* 51:2291-2300, 2008.
25. Taira CA, et al: Cardiovascular drugs inducing QT prolongation: facts and evidence, *Curr Drug Saf* 5:65-72, 2010.
26. Rochford C, Seldin RD: Review and management of the dental patient with Long QT syndrome (LQTS), *Anesth Prog* 56:42-48, 2009.
27. Miller JM, Zipes D: Diagnosis of cardiac arrhythmias. In Zipes D, et al, editors: *Braunwald's heart disease: a textbook of cardiovascular medicine*, ed 7, Philadelphia, 2005, Saunders.
28. Miller JM, Zipes D: Therapy for cardiac arrhythmias. In Zipes D, et al, editors: *Braunwald's heart disease: a textbook of cardiovascular medicine*, ed 7, Philadelphia, 2005, Saunders.
29. Mazzini MJ, Monahan KM: Pharmacotherapy for atrial arrhythmias: present and future, *Heart Rhythm* 5(6 Suppl):S26-S31, 2008.
30. Woolsey RL: Antiarrhythmic drugs. In Goldman L, Ausiello D, editors: *Cecil textbook of medicine*, ed 22, Philadelphia, 2004, Saunders.
31. Morady F: Electrophysiologic interventional procedures and surgery. In Goldman L, Ausiello D, editors: *Cecil textbook of medicine*, ed 22, Philadelphia, 2004, Saunders.
32. Gregoratos G, et al: ACC/AHA/NASPE 2002 guideline update for implantation of cardiac pacemakers and antiarrhythmia devices: summary article. A report of the American College of Cardiology/American Heart Association Task Force on Practice Guidelines (ACC/AHA/NASPE Committee to Update the 1998 Pacemaker Guidelines), *J Cardiovasc Electrophysiol* 13:1183-1199, 2002.
33. Baddour LM, et al. Nonvalvular cardiovascular device-related infections, *Circulation* 108:2015-2031, 2003.
34. Dajani AS, et al: Prevention of bacterial endocarditis: recommendations by the American Heart Association, *J Am Dent Assoc* 128:1142-1151, 1997.
35. Baddour LM, et al: Update on cardiovascular implantable electronic device infections and their management: a scientific statement from the American Heart Association, *Circulation* 121:458-477, 2010.
36. Hayes DL, Zipes D: Cardiac pacemakers and cardioverter-defibrillators. In Zipes D, et al, editors: *Braunwald's heart disease: a textbook of cardiovascular medicine*, ed 7, Philadelphia, 2005, Saunders.
37. Femiano F, et al: Pyostomatitis vegetans: a review of the literature, *Med Oral Patol Oral Cir Bucal* 14:E114-E117, 2009.
38. Pinski SL, Trohman RG: Interference in implanted cardiac devices, part I, *Pacing Clin Electrophysiol* 25:1367-1381, 2002.
39. Pinski SL, Trohman RG: Interference in implanted cardiac devices, part II, *Pacing Clin Electrophysiol* 25:1496-1509, 2002.
40. Miller CS, Leonelli FM, Latham E: Selective interference with pacemaker activity by electrical dental devices, *Oral Surg Oral Med Oral Pathol Oral Radiol Endod* 85:33-36, 1998.
41. Roedig JJ, et al: Interference of cardiac pacemaker and implantable cardioverter-defibrillator activity during electronic dental device use, *J Am Dent Assoc* 141:521-526, 2010.
42. Brand HS, et al: Interference of electrical dental equipment with implantable cardioverter-defibrillators, *Br Dent J* 203:577-579, 2007.
43. Brand HS, et al: [Electromagnetic interference of electrical dental equipment with cardiac pacemakers.], *Ned Tijdschr Tandheelkd* 114:373-376, 2007.
44. Wilson BL, et al: Safety of electronic apex locators and pulp testers in patients with implanted cardiac pacemakers or cardioverter/defibrillators, *J Endod* 32:847-852, 2006.
45. Garofalo RR, et al: Effect of electronic apex locators on cardiac pacemaker function, *J Endod* 28:831-833, 2002.
46. Fleisher LA, et al. ACC/AHA 2007 guidelines on perioperative cardiovascular evaluation and care for noncardiac surgery: a report of the American College of Cardiology/American Heart Association Task Force on Practice Guidelines (Writing Committee to Revise the 2002 Guidelines on Perioperative Cardiovascular Evaluation for Noncardiac Surgery). *Circulation* 116:e418-e499, 2007.
47. Hersh EV, Giannakopoulos H: Beta-adrenergic blocking agents and dental vasoconstrictors, *Dent Clin North Am* 54:687-696, 2010.
48. Blinder D, Shemesh J, Taicher S: Electrocardiographic changes in cardiac patients undergoing dental extractions under local anesthesia, *J Oral Maxillofac Surg* 54:162-165, 1996.
49. Blinder D, et al: Electrocardiographic changes in cardiac patients having dental extractions under a local anesthetic containing a vasopressor, *J Oral Maxillofac Surg* 56:1399-1402, 1998.
50. Cintron G, et al: Cardiovascular effects and safety of dental anesthesia and dental interventions in patients with recent uncomplicated myocardial infarction, *Arch Intern Med* 146:2203-2204, 1986.
51. Findler M, et al: Dental treatment in very high risk patients with active ischemic heart disease, *Oral Surg Oral Med Oral Pathol* 76:298-300, 1993.
52. Niwa H, Sato Y, Matsuura H: Safety of dental treatment in patients with previously diagnosed acute myocardial infarction or unstable angina pectoris, *Oral Surg Oral Med Oral Pathol Oral Radiol Endod* 89:35-41, 2000.
53. Bowles WH, Tardy SJ, Vahadi A: Evaluation of new gingival retraction agents, *J Dent Res* 70:1447-1449, 1991.
54. Fuster V, et al: ACC/AHA/ESC 2006 Guidelines for the Management of Patients with Atrial Fibrillation: a report of the American College of Cardiology/American Heart Association Task Force on Practice Guidelines and the European Society of Cardiology Committee for Practice Guidelines (Writing Committee to Revise the 2001 Guidelines for the Management of Patients With Atrial Fibrillation): developed in collaboration with the European Heart Rhythm Association and the Heart Rhythm Society, *Circulation* 114:e257-e354, 2006.
55. Jafri SM: Periprocedural thromboprophylaxis in patients receiving chronic anticoagulation therapy, *Am Heart J* 147:3-15, 2004.
56. Jeske AH, Suchko GD: Lack of a scientific basis for routine discontinuation of oral anticoagulation therapy before dental treatment, *J Am Dent Assoc* 134:1492-1497, 2003.
57. Wahl MJ: Myths of dental surgery in patients receiving anticoagulant therapy, *J Am Dent Assoc* 131:77-81, 2000.
58. Aframian DJ, Lalla RV, Peterson DE: Management of dental patients taking common hemostasis-altering medications, *Oral Surg Oral Med Oral Pathol Oral Radiol Endod* 103(S45):e1-e11, 2007.
59. Cairns JA, et al: Canadian cardiovascular society atrial fibrillation guidelines 2010: prevention of stroke and systemic thromboembolism in atrial fibrillation and flutter, *Can J Cardiol* 27:74-90, 2011.
60. Legrand M, et al. The use of dabigatran in elderly patients, *Arch Int Med* 171:1285-1286, 2011.
61. Dowd FJ: Cardiac glycosides and other drugs used in heart failure. In Yagiela JA, Dowd FJ, Neidle EA, editors: *Pharmacology and therapeutics for dentistry*, ed 5, St. Louis, 2004, Mosby.

6

Heart Failure (or Congestive Heart Failure)

Heart failure (HF) is primarily a condition of the elderly and as such it is a major and growing public health problem in the United States.[1] Approximately 5 million patients in this country have HF, and more than 550,000 patients are diagnosed with HF for the first time each year.[1] The incidence of HF approaches 10 per 1000 population after age 65, and approximately 80% of patients hospitalized with HF are older than 65 years of age.[1] The disorder is the primary reason for 12 to 15 million office visits and 6.5 million hospital days each year.[1] From 1990 to 1999, the annual number of hospitalizations increased from approximately 810,000 to more than 1 million for HF as a primary diagnosis and from 2.4 million to 3.6 million for HF as a primary or secondary diagnosis. In 2001, nearly 53,000 patients died of HF as a primary cause. The number of HF deaths has increased steadily despite advances in treatment, in part because of increasing numbers of patients living with HF as a consequence of better treatment and "salvage" after acute myocardial infarction (MI) experienced earlier in life.[1]

HF, often called *congestive heart failure* (CHF), is not an actual diagnosis; rather, it manifests as a symptom complex that can be the result of any of a number of specific diseases (Box 6-1). HF represents the end stage of many of the cardiovascular diseases. HF is essentially the inability of the heart to supply enough blood circulation to meet the body's needs.[2] The American College of Cardiology/American Heart Association (ACC/AHA) 2010 Guideline Update for the Diagnosis and Management of Chronic Heart Failure in the Adult defines HF as a complex clinical syndrome that can result from any structural or functional cardiac disorder that impairs the ability of the ventricle to fill with or eject blood.[1]

Patients with untreated or poorly managed HF are at high risk during dental treatment for complications such as cardiac arrest, stroke (cerebrovascular accident), and MI. On encountering such a patient, the dentist must be able to recognize the problem from the history and clinical findings; then the patient can be referred for medical diagnosis and management, and the patient's physician consulted to develop a safe and effective dental management plan.[3-6]

GENERAL DESCRIPTION

Incidence and Prevalence

The prevalence of HF is significantly increasing, primarily as a result of advances in medical technology in preserving and maintaining life after cardiovascular events. Approximately 6 million people in the United States have HF, with more than 550,000 new patients diagnosed each year.[7] The annual incidence of new cases of HF increases with age, from less than 1 per 1000 patient-years among those younger than 45 years of age, to 10 per 1000 patient-years for those older than 65 years, to 30 per 1000 patient-years (3%) for those older than 85. Prevalence figures follow a similar pattern of progression, increasing from 0.1% before the age of 50 to 55 years to almost 10% after age 80 years.[6-8]

HF is the most common Medicare diagnosis-related group (i.e., hospital discharge diagnosis), and more Medicare dollars are spent for the diagnosis and treatment of HF than for any other clinical entity.[9] Similar data for these epidemiologic categories are reported worldwide. A study from the Mayo Clinic noted a 40% increase in the incidence of heart failure over the 20-year period ending in 2005.[10] Because it is the chronic outcome of several cardiovascular diseases over time, HF is primarily a condition of the elderly, as noted. A typical dental practice serving 2000 patients would expect to treat approximately 14 persons with HF.

The HF syndrome is characterized by signs and symptoms of intravascular and interstitial volume overload and/or manifestations of inadequate tissue perfusion (Figure 6-1). Because HF often goes undiagnosed, patients may not know that they have the condition, so the dentist must be particularly aware of its signs and symptoms. HF may occur as a result of (1) impaired myocardial contractility (systolic dysfunction, commonly characterized as reduced left ventricular ejection fraction [LVEF][11]); (2) increased ventricular stiffness or impaired myocardial relaxation (diastolic dysfunction, which commonly is associated with a relatively normal LVEF); (3) a variety of other cardiac abnormalities, including obstructive or regurgitant valvular disease, intracardiac shunting, or disorders of heart rate or rhythm; or (4) states in which the heart is unable to compensate for increased peripheral blood flow or metabolic requirements[11,12] (Figure 6-2).

Conditions that cause myocardial necrosis damage and/or produce chronic pressure or volume overload on the heart can induce myocardial dysfunction and HF.[11,12]

Box 6-1 lists the potential causes of HF, with the most common causes identified. The most common underlying cause of HF in the United States is coronary heart disease, or coronary artery disease (secondary to atherosclerosis), accounting for 60% to 75% of cases, with cardiomyopathy, hypertension, and valvular heart disease also well-recognized contributory conditions.[11,12] The second most common cause of HF, accounting for about one fourth of all cases, is dilated cardiomyopathy (DCM). DCM is a syndrome characterized by cardiac enlargement with impaired systolic function of one or both ventricles, often accompanied by signs and symptoms of HF. About half of all cases of DCM have no identifiable cause and are therefore considered idiopathic. Known causes of cardiomyopathy include alcohol abuse, hereditary cardiomyopathies, and viral infections.[11,12] Although hypertension often is not a primary cause of HF, it is a major contributor to HF, with more than 75% of HF patients having a long-standing history of hypertension. Valvular heart disease used to be a more significant cause of HF; today, however, with declining rates of rheumatic heart disease and congenital heart disease in the United States, the frequency of HF resulting from valvular disease has decreased as well.[11,12] Type 2 diabetes mellitus also may be a risk factor for development of HF.[12,13]

Although the mortality rates for MI and stroke are declining, HF continues to be a major contributor to morbidity and mortality. In the past 20 years, the number

BOX 6-1 Most Common Causes of Heart Failure

- Coronary heart disease
- Cardiomyopathy
- Hypertension
- Valvular heart disease
- Myocarditis
- Infective endocarditis
- Congenital heart disease
- Pulmonary hypertension
- Pulmonary embolism
- Endocrine disease

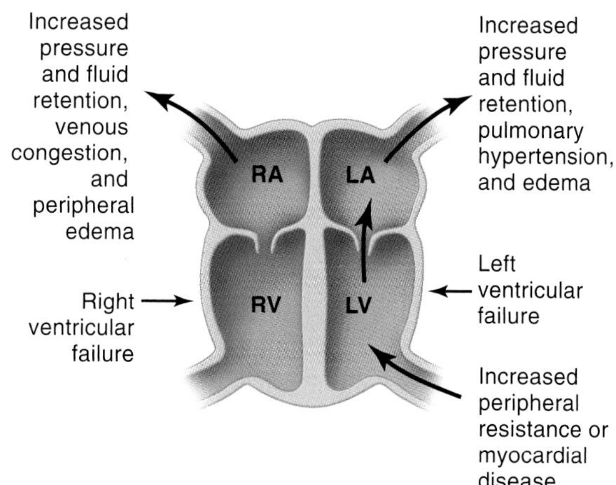

FIGURE 6-1 Effects of right- and left-sided heart failure.

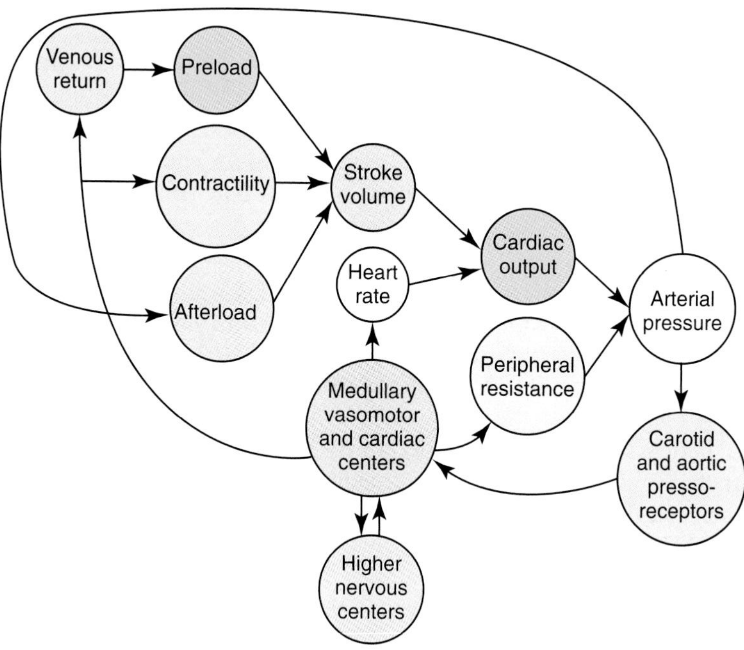

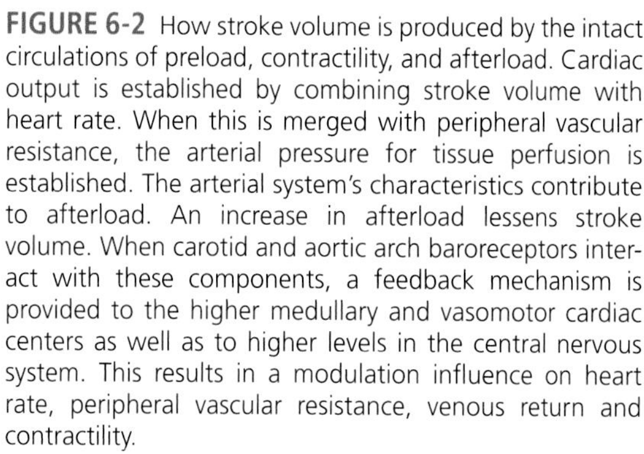

FIGURE 6-2 How stroke volume is produced by the intact circulations of preload, contractility, and afterload. Cardiac output is established by combining stroke volume with heart rate. When this is merged with peripheral vascular resistance, the arterial pressure for tissue perfusion is established. The arterial system's characteristics contribute to afterload. An increase in afterload lessens stroke volume. When carotid and aortic arch baroreceptors interact with these components, a feedback mechanism is provided to the higher medullary and vasomotor cardiac centers as well as to higher levels in the central nervous system. This results in a modulation influence on heart rate, peripheral vascular resistance, venous return and contractility.

of HF hospitalizations increased more than 165%.[14] In the United States, approximately 56,000 deaths each year are primarily caused by HF, and it is listed as a contributing cause in 262,000 deaths. The prognosis for patients with HF is poor. Of patients who survive an acute onset of HF, only 35% of men and 50% of women are alive after 5 years.[7,15]

Pathophysiology and Complications

Heart failure is caused by the inability of the heart to function efficiently as a pump, which results in either an inadequate emptying of the ventricles during systole or an incomplete filling of the ventricles during diastole. This in turn results in a decrease in cardiac output, with consequent delivery of an inadequate volume of blood to the tissues, or in a backup of blood, causing systemic congestion. HF may involve one or both ventricles. Most of the acquired disorders that lead to HF result in initial failure of the left ventricle. Left ventricular heart failure (LVHF) often is followed by failure of the right ventricle. In adults, left ventricular involvement is almost always present even if the clinical manifestations are primarily those of right ventricular dysfunction (fluid retention without dyspnea or rales). HF may result from an acute insult to cardiac function, such as with a large MI, or, more commonly, from a chronic process.[2,16] By the time most patients are seen for medical treatment, the pathoanatomic changes of HF usually are present on both sides of the heart. The cardinal manifestations of HF are dyspnea and fatigue.[11,12]

HF can result from an acute injury to the heart such as with MI or, more commonly, from a chronic process such as that associated with hypertension or cardiomyopathy. Failure of the heart most often begins with LVHF brought on by an increased workload or disease of the heart muscle.[11,12] The determination of left ventricular failure often is based on a finding of an abnormal *ejection fraction,* which is the percentage of blood ejected from the left ventricle during systole. Normal values for ejection fraction determined with the patient at rest range between 55% and 70%.[11,12] Although arbitrary, an LVEF of 45% to 50% often is used as a threshold value to diagnose left ventricular failure. The outstanding symptom of left ventricular failure is dyspnea, which results from the accumulation or congestion of blood in the pulmonary vessels—hence the designation *congestive.* Acute pulmonary edema often is the result of left ventricular failure. Left-sided heart failure leads to pulmonary hypertension, which increases the work of the right ventricle pumping against increased pressure, often culminating in right-sided heart failure.[11,12]

The most common cause of right-sided heart failure is preceding failure of the left ventricle.[16] The outcomes of right ventricular failure are systemic venous congestion and peripheral edema (see Figures 6-1 and 6-2). Failure of the right side of the heart alone is uncommon. The most common cause of pure right-sided heart failure is emphysema.

Ventricular failure leads to dilation and hypertrophy of the ventricle as it attempts to compensate for its inability to keep up with the workload. Venous pressure and myocardial tone increase along with the increase in blood volume. The net effect is diastolic dilation, which serves to increase the force and volume of the subsequent systolic contraction. These changes lead to dyspnea, orthopnea, and pulmonary edema. When right-sided ventricular enlargement occurs as a result of a lung disorder (e.g., emphysema) that produces pulmonary hypertension, the condition is called *cor pulmonale.*[11,12]

Signs and symptoms of HF appear when the heart no longer functions properly as a pump. As the cardiac output falls, an increasing disproportion is observed between the required hemodynamic load and the capacity of the heart to handle the load. With decreasing cardiac output, stimulation of the renin-angiotensin system and the sympathetic nervous system (i.e., neurohumoral responses) occurs in an attempt to compensate for the loss of function.[11,12,16] The effects of these responses include increased heart rate and myocardial contractility, increased peripheral resistance, sodium and water retention, redistribution of blood flow to the heart and brain, and an increased efficiency of oxygen utilization by the tissues. If these responses result in improved cardiac output with an elimination of symptoms, the condition is termed *compensated* HF. Symptomatic HF is termed *decompensated* HF.[11,12,14]

The American Heart Association/American College of Cardiology (AHA/ACC) classification of HF consists of four stages, reflecting the fact that HF is a progressive disease for which the outcome can be modified by early identification and treatment.[1] Stages A and B denote the status of patients with risk factors that predispose to the development of HF, such as coronary artery disease, hypertension, and diabetes, but who do not have any symptoms of HF[8,17,18] (see Box 6-5).

The difference between stage A and stage B is that in *stage A,* patients do not demonstrate left ventricular hypertrophy (LVH) or dysfunction, whereas in *stage B,* LVH and/or dysfunction (structural heart disease) is present. *Stage C* is the disease designation for patients with past or present symptoms of HF associated with underlying structural heart disease (the bulk of patients), and *stage D,* for patients with refractory HF who might be eligible for specialized, advanced treatment or for end-of-life care. This classification system complements the New York Heart Association (NYHA) classification system, which is discussed in the next section ("Signs and Symptoms").[1]

HF is a progressive disease, and symptoms will worsen over time owing to the ongoing deterioration of cardiac structure and function. The prognosis is better if the underlying cause can be treated. At 1 year after the diagnosis of HF, 20% of patients will succumb to the disease. In people diagnosed with HF, sudden death occurs at a rate six to nine times that for the general population.[11,12]

CLINICAL PRESENTATION

Signs and Symptoms

The symptoms and signs of HF (Boxes 6-2 and 6-3) reflect respective ventricular dysfunction. Left ventricular failure produces pulmonary vascular congestion with resulting pulmonary edema and dyspnea. Dyspnea is the most common symptom of HF and usually is present only with exertion or physical activity. Dyspnea experienced by the patient at rest is an indication of severe HF.[11,12]

BOX 6-2 Symptoms of Heart Failure

Dyspnea (perceived shortness of breath)
Fatigue and weakness
Orthopnea (dyspnea experienced with patient in recumbent position)
Paroxysmal nocturnal dyspnea (dyspnea awakening patient from sleep)
Acute pulmonary edema (cough or progressive dyspnea)
Exercise intolerance (inablility to climb a flight of stairs)
Fatigue (especially muscular)
Dependent edema (swelling of feet and ankles after standing or walking)
Report of weight gain or increased abdominal girth (fluid accumulation; ascites)
Right upper quadrant pain (liver congestion)
Anorexia, nausea, vomiting, constipation (bowel edema)
Hyperventilation followed by apnea during sleep (Cheyne-Stokes respiration)

BOX 6-3 Signs of Heart Failure

Rapid, shallow breathing
Cheyne-Stokes respiration (hyperventilation alternating with apnea)
Inspiratory rales (crackles)
Heart murmur
Gallop rhythm
Increased venous pressure
Enlargement of cardiac silhouette on chest radiograph
Pulsus alternans
Distended neck veins
Large, tender liver
Jaundice
Peripheral edema
Ascites
Cyanosis
Weight gain
Clubbing of fingers

Orthopnea is positional dyspnea that is precipitated or worsened by the patient's assuming a recumbent or semirecumbent position. Most patients with mild to moderate HF do not exhibit orthopnea when the condition is treated adequately. Paroxysmal nocturnal dyspnea (PND) is an attack of sudden, severe shortness of breath awakening the patient from sleep, usually within 1 to 3 hours after the patient goes to bed, and resolving within 10 to 30 minutes after the patient awakens, often gasping for air. The occurrence of PND is uncommon. Both orthopnea and PND are relatively specific indicators of HF and are due to increased venous return encouraged by the recumbent position with resulting increase in pulmonary venous pressure and alveolar edema. Central regulation of respiration also may be impaired in patients with advanced HF, resulting in alternating cycles of rapid, deep breathing (hyperventilation) with periods of central apnea—a pattern called *Cheyne-Stokes respiration.* PND is a common clinical feature associated with Cheyne-Stokes respiration in patients with HF.

Exercise intolerance (e.g., inability to climb a flight of stairs) is one of the hallmark symptoms of HF and is due to a combination of dyspnea and reduced blood and oxygen supply to the skeletal muscles. Fatigue (especially muscle fatigue) is a common, nonspecific symptom of HF. The findings on pulmonary examination in patients with HF usually are unremarkable. However, rales (or crackles), representing alveolar fluid, are a classic feature of HF when present. The chest radiograph may reveal enlargement and displacement of the cardiac silhouette or abnormalities of the pulmonary vasculature. Evidence of interstitial fluid or pleural effusion also may be seen[1,19-25] (Figure 6-3). Right ventricular failure results in systemic venous congestion and peripheral edema. Evidence of systemic venous congestion may include the presence of distended neck veins (Figure 6-4), a large tender liver, peripheral edema (Figure 6-5), and ascites (Figure 6-6). The retention of fluid results in weight gain and may increase body girth as a consequence of accumulation of fluid in the peritoneal cavity. On occasion, patients with chronic HF may exhibit clubbing of the fingers[1,19-22] (Figure 6-7).

Cardiac examination usually reveals evidence of the underlying cardiac abnormality, as well as compensatory or degenerative changes in cardiac structure. Auscultation often reveals a laterally displaced apical impulse caused by left ventricular hypertrophy. A murmur of mitral regurgitation may be heard, as well as an S_3 or S_4 gallop. Pulsus alternans, a regular rhythm with alternating strong and weak ventricular contractions, is pathognomonic for left ventricular failure but is not present in most patients with heart failure. Central venous pressure is increased.[1,19-22]

The NYHA has developed a widely used classification system of HF (Box 6-4) that is based on the severity of symptoms and the amount of effort needed to elicit symptoms. It is complementary to the AHA/ACC staging

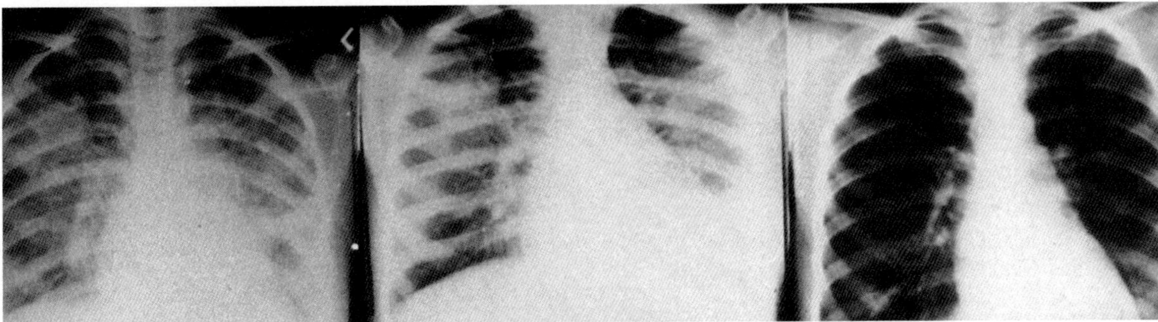

FIGURE 6-3 Serial chest radiographs demonstrating the resolution of pulmonary edema (*left* to *right*). Note the enlargement of the cardiac silhouette. *(Courtesy J. Noonan, MD, Lexington, Kentucky.)*

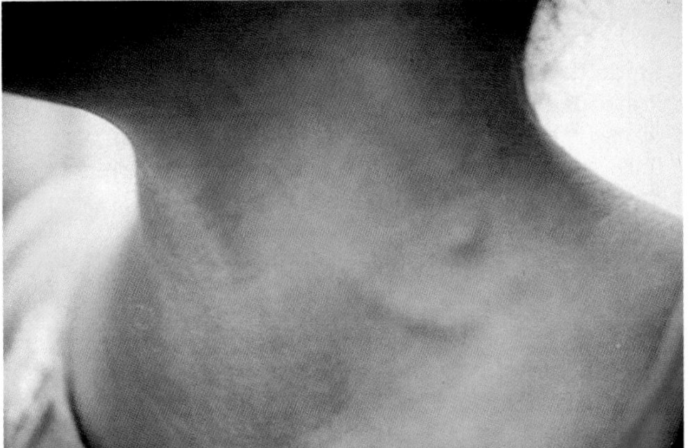

FIGURE 6-4 Distended jugular vein in patient with heart failure.

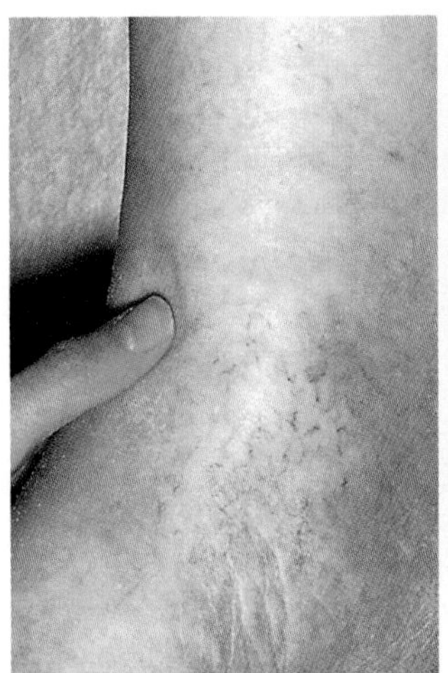

A

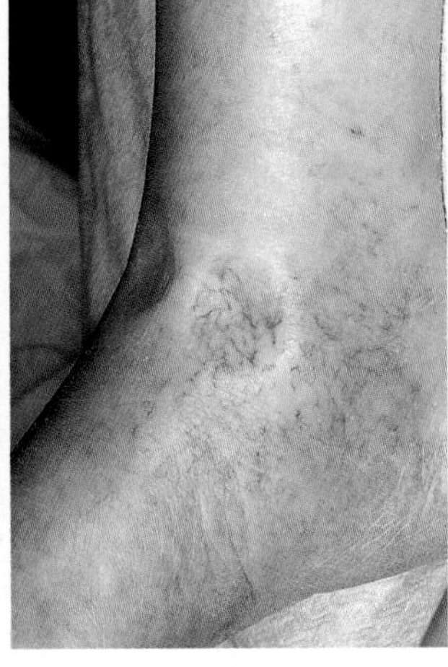

B

FIGURE 6-5 Pitting edema in a patient with heart failure. A depression ("pit") remains in the edematous tissue for some minutes after firm fingertip pressure is applied. *(From Forbes CD, Jackson WF:* Color atlas and text of clinical medicine, *Edinburgh, 2004, Mosby.)*

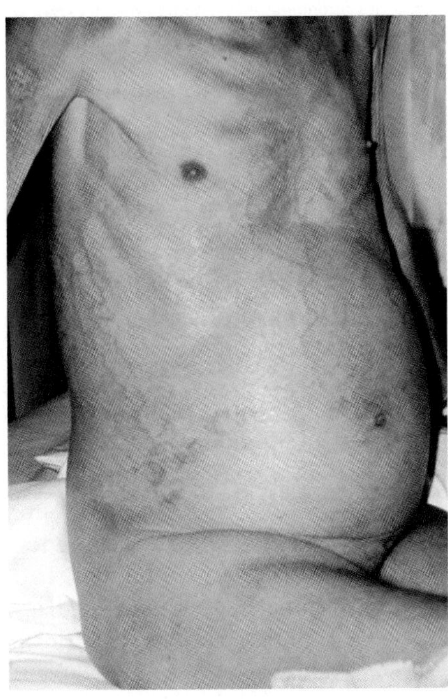

FIGURE 6-6 Ascites. *(Courtesy P. Akers, MD, Evanston, Illinois.)*

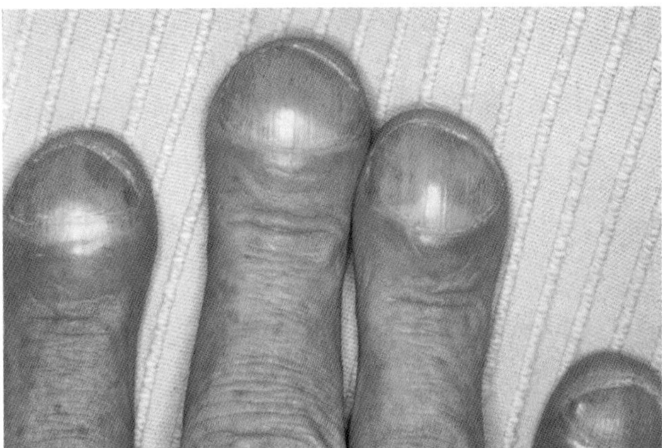

FIGURE 6-7 Clubbing of the fingers in a patient with congestive heart failure.

BOX 6-4 NYHA Classification of Heart Failure

- *Class I:* No limitation of physical activity. No dyspnea, fatigue, or palpitations with ordinary physical activity.
- *Class II:* Slight limitation of physical activity. Patients experience fatigue, palpitations, and dyspnea with ordinary physical activity but are comfortable at rest.
- *Class III:* Marked limitation of activity. Less than ordinary physical activity results in symptoms, but patients are comfortable at rest.
- *Class IV:* Symptoms are present with the patient at rest, and any physical exertion exacerbates the symptoms.

NYHA, New York Heart Association.

system described earlier and essentially is a subclassification of stage C.[1,19-22,26] The features of NYHA classes I to IV range in severity from absence of clinical symptoms with ordinary physical activity to presence of symptoms with the patient at rest, worsened with any level of exertion.

Laboratory Findings

A variety of specialized tests are used to diagnose HF and monitor affected patents, depending on the etiology. Among these are plain radiography of the chest, electrocardiogram, echocardiography, radionuclide angiography or ventriculography, exercise stress test, ambulatory electrocardiogram (Holter) monitoring, and cardiac catheterization. Determination of the ejection fraction, which was previously described, will be valuable in assessing the level of severity of HF. Measurements of plasma levels of norepinephrine, atrial natriuretic peptide, and renin have possible prognostic value and may be helpful clinically. Routine investigations may include complete blood count, renal function testing and electrolyte panel, liver function testing, blood glucose assay, lipid profile, and thyroid function testing.[19-22]

MEDICAL MANAGEMENT

Despite advances in the care of patients with heart failure, outcomes are not significantly improving.[27] The medical management of HF is complex and generally is applied in a graduated approach, depending on the AHA/ACC stage of the disease (Box 6-5). For stages A and B, management begins with risk reduction and includes the identification and treatment of underlying medical problems including hypertension, atherosclerotic disease, diabetes, obesity, and metabolic syndrome (consisting of abdominal obesity, elevated blood glucose, dyslipidemia, and hypertension). In addition, behavioral modification is promoted and includes smoking cessation, weight loss as appropriate, reduction of risk factors for cardiovascular disease, mild aerobic exercise, adequate rest, and avoidance of alcohol and illicit drugs.

BOX 6-5 Medical Management of Patients with Heart Failure (HF) by AHA/ACC Stage

Stage A: Patients at High Risk for HF, but without Structural Heart Disease or Symptoms of HF

Treatment of hypertension, encourage smoking cessation, treatment of lipid disorders, encouragement of regular exercise, discourage alcohol intake, illicit drug use, and control of metabolic syndrome

ACE inhibitors or ARBs as appropriate for treatment of vascular disease or diabetes

Stage B: Patients with Structural Heart Disease, but without Signs or Symptoms of HF

All measures for stage A, *plus*

ACE inhibitors (or ARBs) as appropriate

Beta blockers as appropriate

Stage C: Patients with Structural Heart Disease with Previous or Current Symptoms of HF

All measures for stages A and B, dietary salt restriction, *plus*

Drugs for routine use: diuretics, ACE inhibitors, beta blockers

Drugs in selected patients: aldosterone antagonists, ARBs, digitalis, hydralazine-nitrates

Devices in selected patients: biventricular pacing device, implantable defibrillator

Stage D: Patients with Refractory HF Requiring Special Interventions

Appropriate measures from stages A, B, and C

Heart transplant recipients: chronic inotropes, permanent mechanical support, experimental drugs or surgery

Compassionate end-of-life care/hospice care

ACE, Angiotensin-converting enzyme; *AHA/ACC,* American Heart Association/American College of Cardiology; *ARBs,* Angiotensin receptor blockers.
(Data from Hunt SA, et al: ACC/AHA 2005 guideline update for the diagnosis and management of chronic heart failure in the adult: a report of the American College of Cardiology/American Heart Association Task Force on Practice Guidelines *[Writing Committee to Update the 2001 Guidelines for the Evaluation and Management of Heart Failure].)*

Unfortunately, compliance with treatment recommendations is notoriously poor.[27] Drug therapy may be indicated for the treatment of vascular disease or diabetes in stage A, as well as for ventricular dysfunction in stage B* (see Box 6-5).

For management of stage C HF, all measures from stage A and B apply, with the addition of salt restriction and drug therapy (Table 6-1). Drug therapy begins with diuretics to control fluid retention. Several types of diuretics are used including loop diuretics, thiazide diuretics, and potassium-sparing diuretics. Diuretics are used for three purposes: They are the only drugs that can adequately control fluid retention, they produce more rapid symptomatic relief than that achievable with other drugs, and they modulate other drugs used to treat HF. Although diuretics are effective in decreasing the signs

*References 2, 6, 12, 17, 19-22, 28-30.

TABLE 6-1 Drugs Used for the Treatment of Heart Failure

Drug	Vasoconstrictor Interactions	Oral Side/Adverse Effect(s)	Other Consideration(s)
Diuretics			
Loop Diuretics Bumetanide (Bumex) Furosamide (Lasix) Torsemide (Demadex)	None	Dry mouth	Orthostatic hypotension
Thiazide Diuretics Chlorothiazide (Diuril) Chlorthalidone (Thalitone) Hydrochlorothiazide (HCTZ) Indapamide (Lozol) Metolazone (Mykrox)	None	Dry mouth	Orthostatic hypotension
Potassium-Sparing Diuretics Amiloride (Midamor) Spironolactone (Aldactone) Triamterene (Dyrenium)	None	Dry mouth	Orthostatic hypotension
ACE Inhibitors Benazepril (Lotensin) Captopril (Capoten) Enalapril (Vasotec) Fosinopril (Monopril) Lisinopril (Prinivil) Moexapril (Univasc) Perindopril (Coversyl) Quinapril (Accupril) Ramipril (Altace) Trandolapril (Mavik)	None	Angioedema of lip, face, or tongue; taste changes; burning mouth; lichenoid reactions	Orthostatic hypotension; avoid prolonged use of NSAIDs
Angiotensin Receptor Blockers Candesarten (Atacand) Eprosartan (Teveten) Irbesartan (Avapro) Losartan (Cozaar) Olmesartan (Benicar) Telmisartan (Micardis) Valsartan (Diovan)	None		Orthostatic hypotension
Aldosterone Inhibitors Eplerenone (Inspra) Spironolactone (Aldactone)	None		Orthostatic hypotension
Beta Blockers *Cardioselective* Acebutolol (Sectral) Atenolol (Tenormin) Betaxolol (Kerlone) Bisoprolol (Zebeta) Labetolol (Normodyne) Metoprolol (Lopressor) *Nonselective* Carteolol (Cartrol) Carvedilol (Coreg) (alpha/beta blocker) Nadolol (Corgard) Penbutolol (Levatol) Pindolol (Visken) Propranolol (Inderal) Timolol (Blocadren)	*Cardioselective:* use vasoconstrictors normally *Nonselective:* possible increase in BP is possible; cautious use of vasoconstrictors is recommended (maximum 0.036 mg epinephrine; 0.20 mg levonordefrin)	Lichenoid reactions	Orthostatic hypotension; avoid long-term use of NSAIDs
Digitalis Digoxin (Lanoxin)	Increased risk for arrhythmias; avoid if possible	Increased gag reflex; hypersalivation (sign of toxicity)	Erythromycin and clarithromycin can increase toxic effects of digoxin—*avoid*
Vasodilators Hydralazine (Apresoline) Isosorbide dinitrate (Isordil)	None	Lupus-like oral lesions, lymphadenopathy, dry mouth	Orthostatic hypotension

NSAIDs, Nonsteroidal antiinflammatory drugs.

and symptoms of fluid retention, they cannot maintain the clinical stability of patients with HF when used alone. Spironolactone, a potassium-sparing diuretic, also blocks the action of aldosterone (aldosterone antagonist) and, when used in patients with class IV symptoms, has been shown to reduce the risk of death by 25% to 30%. Other than spironolactone, the diuretics do not influence the natural history of chronic HF[31,32] (see Box 6-5).

In addition to diuretics, drugs that modulate or decrease neurohormonal activity have become the foundation of treatment of HF. These drugs decrease the morbidity and mortality associated with HF by inhibiting the cardiotoxic effects of the neurohormonal system, thereby retarding the progression of HF. Several types of neurohormonal antagonists are used to treat HF, including angiotensin-converting enzyme (ACE) inhibitors, β-adrenergic blockers, and angiotensin receptor blockers (ARBs). The ACE inhibitors are first-line drugs for treatment of HF and have been shown to reduce the risk of death and the need for hospitalization by 20% to 30%. These agents, which typically are prescribed along with or after diuretic therapy, decrease the need for large doses of diuretics, as well as limiting some of the adverse metabolic effects of the diuretics (see Box 6-5). In addition to ACE inhibitors, β-adrenergic blockers are advocated; when used in combination with the ACE inhibitors, beta blockers appear to reduce both the risk of death and the need for hospitalization for heart failure by 30% to 40%.[19-22] A treatment algorithm for medical management of heart failure is presented in Figure 6-8.

The digitalis glycosides have been used in the treatment for HF for many years, with digoxin being the most commonly prescribed. With the advent of the ACE inhibitors, however, their use has declined. Digoxin has not been shown to decrease either the risk of death or need for hospitalization, as opposed to the ACE inhibitors and beta blockers, both of which do provide these benefits. Digoxin is, however, effective in alleviating symptoms, so it is principally used to treat residual symptoms not controlled by other drugs. In addition, digoxin is the preferred agent in patients with HF who have atrial fibrillation and a rapid ventricular response. A significant problem with digitalis glycosides is their narrow therapeutic range and the resulting toxicity that can easily occur (Box 6-6). Other drugs used to treat HF unresponsive to ACE inhibitors include ARBs and direct-acting

BOX 6-6 Clinical Manifestations of Digitalis Toxicity

Headache, nausea, vomiting
Hypersalivation
Altered vision and color perception
Fatigue, malaise, drowsiness
Arrhythmias (tachycardias or bradycardias)

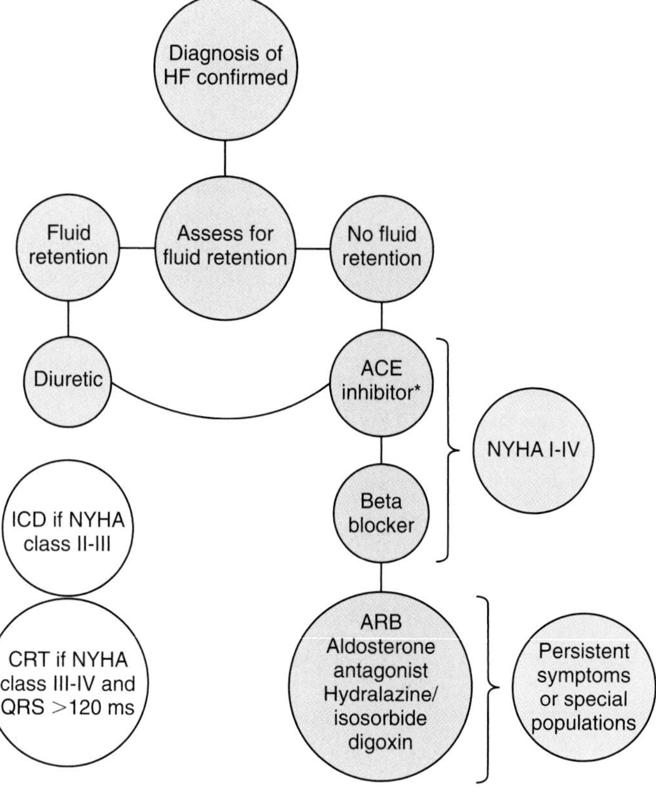

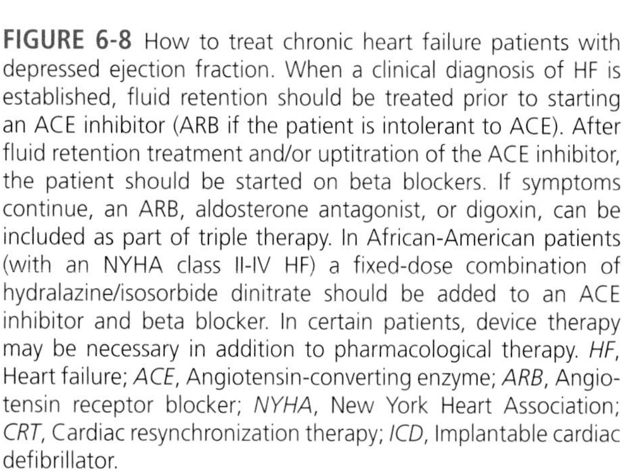

FIGURE 6-8 How to treat chronic heart failure patients with depressed ejection fraction. When a clinical diagnosis of HF is established, fluid retention should be treated prior to starting an ACE inhibitor (ARB if the patient is intolerant to ACE). After fluid retention treatment and/or uptitration of the ACE inhibitor, the patient should be started on beta blockers. If symptoms continue, an ARB, aldosterone antagonist, or digoxin, can be included as part of triple therapy. In African-American patients (with an NYHA class II-IV HF) a fixed-dose combination of hydralazine/isosorbide dinitrate should be added to an ACE inhibitor and beta blocker. In certain patients, device therapy may be necessary in addition to pharmacological therapy. *HF*, Heart failure; *ACE*, Angiotensin-converting enzyme; *ARB*, Angiotensin receptor blocker; *NYHA*, New York Heart Association; *CRT*, Cardiac resynchronization therapy; *ICD*, Implantable cardiac defibrillator.

vasodilators (hydralazine, isosorbide dinitrate). For all patients with HF, drugs that are known to worsen the clinical status should be avoided. These include nonsteroidal antiinflammatory drugs (NSAIDs), most antiarrhythmic agents, and calcium channel blockers. In selected patients, other nonpharmacologic measures may be indicated, such as biventricular pacing or the use of an implantable defibrillator.[19-22] Owing to the deterioration of renal function in patients with HF, therapy aimed at counterregulatory responses mediated by adenosine is promising. Randomized clinical trials have been conducted with rolofyllin, an adenosine A_1 receptor agonist. Thus far, however, these latter agents have not been effective for treating HF.[33] As with many conditions, the success of medical therapy depends in large degree on patient compliance with treatment recommendations. Because the medical management regimen in many of these patients includes a plethora of drugs, it is important to monitor and encourage compliance. A recent study, however, demonstrated that even after telemonitoring and multiple verbal reminders, the overall impact on improving outcomes in HF was not significant.[27]

If drug therapy is found to be inadequate to control the severe, refractory HF (stage D), mechanical and surgical intervention may be provided. Available procedures and techniques include intraaortic balloon counterpulsation, placement of a left ventricular assist device, and heart transplantation. Recently, use of an implantable cardioverter-defibrillator (ICD) has demonstrated benefit in treating patients with HF of NYHA class II or III.[34,35] When cardiac resynchronization therapy is added to ICD placement, the mortality and morbidity rates in patients with HF are decreased.[35] The final measure is end-of-life care with hospice.[19-22] Recent reports on use of continuous-flow left ventricular assist devices have demonstrated significant improvements in survival of patients with HF as well as quality of life and functional capacity.[30,36]

DENTAL MANAGEMENT

Medical Considerations

A major risk in providing dental treatment for a patient with symptomatic HF is that the symptoms could abruptly worsen with resultant acute failure, a fatal arrhythmia, stroke, or MI. Identification of patients with a history of HF, those with undiagnosed HF, or those prone to developing HF is the first step in risk assessment and in avoiding an untoward event. As noted earlier, HF is a symptom complex that is the end result of an underlying disease such as coronary heart disease, hypertension, or cardiomyopathy; therefore, the cause of HF must be identified and steps taken for appropriate dental management. Identification is accomplished by obtaining a thorough medical history, including a pertinent review of systems, and taking and evaluating the vital signs (pulse rate and rhythm, blood pressure, respiratory rate). All of the patient's medications, prescription and otherwise, should be identified as well. In a review of systems, the patient is asked about the presence of signs or symptoms related to the cardiovascular and pulmonary systems. Shortness of breath, orthopnea, PND, fatigue, or exercise intolerance may indicate HF or other cardiovascular disease. Inability to climb a flight of stairs without shortness of breath or fatigue may reflect poor functional capacity or diminished cardiopulmonary reserve, with an increased risk for adverse outcome. Patients with a previous history of HF or who are asymptomatic have *compensated* HF (NYHA class I). Those who are symptomatic have *decompensated* HF (NYHA classes II, III, and IV) (see Box 6-4).[19-22,26,30]

The dentist must make a determination of the risk involved in providing dental treatment to a patient with HF and then decide if the benefits of treatment outweigh the risk. This determination often will require consultation with the patient's physician. The ACC and the AHA[1] have published guidelines that can help to make this determination. These guidelines are intended for use by physicians who are evaluating patients with cardiovascular disease to determine if they can safely undergo surgical procedures. They also can be applied to the provision of dental care and be of significant value to the dentist in making a determination of risk.[3]

The guidelines suggest that decompensated HF constitutes a major risk for the occurrence of a serious event (acute MI, unstable angina, or sudden death) during treatment.[1] Thus, patients with symptoms of HF (i.e., with decompensated HF—NYHA class II, III, or IV) generally are not candidates for elective dental care, and treatment is deferred until medical consultation can be obtained (Box 6-7). Patients who have a history of HF but who are asymptomatic (i.e., those with compensated HF, designated NYHA class I) are at intermediate risk for occurrence of a serious event. With good functional capacity and reserve (as demonstrated by the ability to climb a flight of stairs) (see Chapter 1), however, they generally can safely undergo any required treatment with little likelihood of problems. Thus, patients with NYHA class I status can receive routine outpatient dental care. Even in these patients, however, the disease should not be considered "mild," because decompensation could indeed occur during dental treatment.[26] Many patients with NYHA class II HF and some with class III disease also may undergo routine treatment in an outpatient setting after approval by their physician. It is very important, however, to recognize the potential for decompensation of even previously well-compensated HF during a dental procedure. The most common reason for such decompensation is the patient's failure to take presccribed medications properly. Therefore, the dentist must maintain awareness of the patient's clinical status, including medication compliance, with use of close monitoring as appropriate, and be prepared for an emergency.[3]

BOX 6-7 Dental Management
Considerations in Patients with Heart Failure (HF)

P

Patient Evaluation/Risk Assessment (see Box 1-1)

- Careful evaluation is needed to determine the nature, severity, control, and stability of the heart disease.

Potential Issues/Factors of Concern

A	
Analgesics	No issues.
Antibiotics	Patients with HF may be more susceptible to infection (leukopenia), but usually this is not a problem. There is no need for antibiotic prophylaxis unless the patient has a prosthetic heart valve or another cardiac condition (refer to AHA guidelines).
Anesthesia	It is very important to achieve and maintain excellent anesthesia in order to reduce stress and prevent cardiac crisis. Use of epinephrine (1:100,000) at a dose of no more than 2 carpules in local anesthetics generally causes no problems, but patients should be monitored closely. Clinicians should provide good postoperative pain control. General anesthesia should be avoided.
Anxiety	Patients with untreated or poorly controlled HF may appear very anxious and stressed and are at risk for cardiac crisis. Use of special anxiety/stress reduction techniques (see Chapter 1) may be indicated.
Allergy	No issues.
B	
Bleeding	Excessive bleeding may occur in the patient with untreated or poorly controlled HF, because the medical treatment regimen typically includes anticoagulants (e.g., warfarin, clopidogrel), which are associated with greater risk for postsurgical bleeding and development of hypotension.
Blood pressure	Monitor blood pressure (BP) throughout procedure because it may significantly increase or decrease in patients with poorly controlled disease. Also monitor blood loss. IF BP drops below 100/60 mm Hg and patient is unresponsive to fluid replacement and vasopressive measures, seek immediate medical attention.
C	
Chair position	Positioning usually is not a problem if the patient is under good medical management; however, a patient who is becoming hypotensive and syncopal from cardiac stress and pulmonary congestion may not tolerate the supine position.
Consultation	Once the patient is under good medical management, the dental treatment plan can be implemented without changes. Initially, however, consultation with the patient's physician to establish the level of control (as reflected in ejection fraction or other functional measures) is recommended as part of the management program.
D	
Devices	Dental patients with a diagnosis of HF may have pacemakers, implanted defibrillators, or prosthetic valves, in which case published guidelines should be followed.
Drugs	Patients with HF typically are on many medications. The dentist should be aware of potential side effects and interactions. The use of epinephrine or other pressor amines (either in gingival retraction cord or as agents to control bleeding) must be avoided. Digitalis toxicity may present a problem, so caution should be exercised in treating those patients.
E	
Equipment	No issues.
Emergencies	A cardiac crisis, once precipitated, may progress to cardiac arrest. This condition therefore constitutes a medical emergency, and it may be necessary to call 911; the patient who is ambulatory and stable should be advised to seek urgent medical care. Ongoing vital signs must be monitored, and cardiopulmonary resuscitation initiated; if necessary, arrange for transport of patient to emergency medical facilities.
F	
Follow-up	Careful follow-up interview of the patient is indicated to determine disease severity and level of control.

AHA, American Heart Association.

The remaining patients with NYHA class III HF and all those with class IV disease are best treated in a special care facility such as a hospital dental clinic with continuous monitoring.

In most cases of HF, the dentist will need to obtain a medical consultation with the patient's cardiologist to determine the patient's physical status, laboratory test results, level of control, compliance with medications and recommendations, and overall stability.[3]

Recommendations for management include short, stress-free appointments (see Box 6-7). Patients with HF may not tolerate a supine chair position because of pulmonary edema and will need a semisupine or upright chair position. For patients taking a digitalis glycoside (digoxin), epinephrine should be avoided, if possible, because the combination can potentially precipitate arrhythmias.[32,37] Generally, epinephrine in moderate doses is well tolerated, even in patients with advanced

HF.[38] If use of epinephrine is considered essential, caution in all aspects of administration is advised. A maximum of 0.036 mg epinephrine (i.e., two cartridges of 2% lidocaine with 1:100,000 epinephrine) is recommended, with care taken to avoid inadvertent intravascular injection. Use of epinephrine-impregnated gingival retraction cord should be avoided.[38] Patients should be observed for signs of digitalis toxicity such as hypersalivation. If toxicity is suspected, prompt referral for medical evaluation is indicated. For patients with NYHA class III or IV HF, vasoconstrictors should be avoided, but if use of such agents is considered essential, a physician consultation should be scheduled beforehand. NSAIDs also should be avoided, because they can exacerbate symptoms of HF. Nitrous oxide plus oxygen sedation can be used if adequate O_2 flow (at least 30%) is maintained. Supplemental low-flow oxygen alone also may be used.[3]

Treatment Planning Modifications

In general, patients with HF who are under good medical management can receive any indicated dental treatment so long as the dental management plan deals effectively with the problems presented by the condition, the underlying cause, and the effects of prescribed medications. By contrast, patients with symptomatic HF require further evaluation and physician consultation to determine necessary changes in dental management.

Oral Manifestations

There are no oral manifestations related to HF per se; however, many of the drugs used to manage HF can cause dry mouth and oral lesions (see Table 6-1). In addition, digitalis may exaggerate the gag reflex, an important consideration in dental treatment.[39,40]

REFERENCES

1. Hunt SA, et al: 2009 focused update incorporated into the ACC/AHA guidelines for the diagnosis and management of heart failure, *Circulation* 121:391-479, 2010.
2. Jessup A: Cardiovascular medicine, II: heart failure. In Federman DD, Nabel EG, editors: *ACP medicine*, New York, 2010, BC Decker, pp 870-912.
3. Herman WW, Ferguson HW: Dental care for patients with heart failure: an update, *J Am Dent Assoc* 141:845-853, 2010.
4. Wang G, et al: Costs of heart failure-related hospitalizations in patients aged 18 to 64 years, *Am J Manag Care* 16:769-776, 2010.
5. Vaartjes I, et al: Age- and gender-specific risk of death after first hospitalization for heart failure, *BMC Public Health* 10:637, 2010.
6. Metra M, et al: Cardiovascular and noncardiovascular comorbidities in patients with chronic heart failure, *J Cardiovasc Med (Hagerstown)* 12:76-84, 2011.
7. Kalogeropoulos A, et al: Epidemiology of incident heart failure, *Arch Intern Med* 169:708-714, 2009.
8. Francis GS, et al: ACCF/AHA/ACP/HFSA/ISHLT 2010 clinical competence statement on management of patients with advanced heart failure and cardiac transplant: a report of the ACCF/AHA/ACP Task Force on Clinical Competence and Training, *Circulation* 122:644-672, 2010.
9. Writing Group Members, Lloyd-Jones D, et al: Heart disease and stroke statistics, *Circulation* 119:480-486, 2009.
10. Owen TE, et al: Trends in prevalence and outcome of heart failure with preserved ejection fraction, *N Engl J Med* 355:251-262, 2006.
11. Abraham WT, et al: Rationale and design of the treatment of hyponatremia based on lixivaptan in NYHA class III/IV cardiac patient evaluation (THE BALANCE) study, *Clin Transl Sci* 3:249-253, 2010.
12. Khalaf KI, Taegtmeyer H: Insulin sensitizers and heart failure: an engine flooded with fuel, *Curr Hypertens Rep* 12:399-401, 2010.
13. Leung AA, et al: Risk of heart failure in patients with recent-onset type 2 diabetes: population-based cohort study, *J Card Fail* 15:152-157, 2009.
14. Alattar FT, et al: Fractional excretion of sodium predicts worsening renal function in acute decompensated heart failure, *Exp Clin Cardiol* 15:e65-e69, 2010.
15. Mann DL: Heart failure and cor pulmonale. In Fauci AS, et al, editors: *Harrison's principles of internal medicine*, ed 17, New York, 2008, McGraw-Hill, pp 1442-1499.
16. Phan TT, Frenneaux M: The pathophysiology of diastolic heart failure, *F1000 Biol Rep* 2:16, 2010.
17. Timoteo AT, et al: Impact of obesity on results after primary angioplasty in patients with ST segment elevation acute myocardial infarction, *Rev Port Cardiol* 29:999-1008, 2010.
18. Stevenson LW, et al: Chronic ambulatory intracardiac pressures and future heart failure events, *Circ Heart Fail* 3:580-587, 2010.
19. Jessup M, et al: 2009 focused update: ACCF/AHA Guidelines for the Diagnosis and Management of Heart Failure in Adults: a report of the American College of Cardiology Foundation/American Heart Association Task Force on Practice Guidelines: developed in collaboration with the International Society for Heart and Lung Transplantation, *Circulation* 119:1977-2016, 2009.
20. Massie BM: Heart failure: pathophysiology and diagnosis. In Goldman L, Ausiello D, editors: *Cecil textbook of medicine*, ed 22, Philadelphia, 2007, Saunders.
21. Massie BM, et al: Irbesartan in patients with heart failure and preserved ejection fraction, *N Engl J Med* 359:2456-2467, 2008.
22. Ghany M, Hoofnagle JH: Approach to the patient with liver disease. In Fauci AS, et al, editors: *Harrison's principles of internal medicine*, ed 17, New York, 2010, McGraw-Hill.
23. Barkman A: Heart failure. In Porth CM, Matfin G, editors: *Pathophysiology: concepts of altered health states*, ed 8, Philadelphia, 2009, Lippincott Williams & Wilkins, pp 606-620.
24. Anter E, Jessup M, Callans DJ: Atrial fibrillation and heart failure, *Circulation* 119:2516-2525, 2009.
25. Bashore TM, et al: Heart disease. In McPhee SJ, Papadakis MA, Tierney LM, editors: *Current medical diagnosis and treatment 2009*, ed 48, New York, 2009, McGraw-Hill Medical, pp 287-375.
26. Witte KK, Clark AL: NYHA class I heart failure is not 'mild,' *Int J Cardiol* 146:128-129, 2011.
27. Chaundry S, et al: Telemonitoring in patients with heart failure, *N Engl J Med* 363:2301-2311, 2010.
28. Waterworth S, Gott M: Decision making among older people with advanced heart failure as they transition to dependency and death, *Curr Opin Support Palliat Care* 4:238-242, 2010.
29. Padilla H, Michael Gaziano JM, Djoussé L: Alcohol consumption and risk of heart failure: a meta-analysis, *Phys Sportsmed* 38:84-89, 2010.

30. Jessup M: Defining success in heart failure: the end-point mess, *Circulation* 121:1977-1980, 2010.
31. Agha SA, et al: Echocardiography and risk prediction in advanced heart failure: incremental value over clinical markers, *J Card Fail* 15:586-592, 2009.
32. Conrado VC, et al: Cardiovascular effects of local anesthesia with vasoconstrictor during dental extraction in coronary patients, *Arq Bras Cardiol* 88:507-513, 2007.
33. Massie BM, et al: Rolofyllin, an adenosine A_1-receptor agonist in acute heart failure, *N Engl J Med* 363:1419-1425, 2010.
34. Cleland JG, et al: The effect of cardiac resynchronization on morbidity and mortality in heart failure, *N Engl J Med* 352:1539-1549, 2005.
35. Tang A, et al: Cardiac resynchronization therapy for mild-to-moderate heart failure, *N Engl J Med* 363:2385-2392, 2010.
36. Jaarsma T, et al: Quality of life and symptoms of depression in advanced heart failure patients and their partners, *Curr Opin Support Palliat Care* 4:233-237, 2010.
37. Friedlander AH, et al: Atrial fibrillation: pathogenesis, medical-surgical management and dental implications, *J Am Dent Assoc* 140:167-177, 2009.
38. Neves RS, et al: Effects of epinephrine in local dental anesthesia in patients with coronary artery disease, *Arq Bras Cardiol* 88:545-5551, 2007.
39. House AA: Pharmacological therapy of cardiorenal syndromes and heart failure, *Contrib Nephrol* 164:164-172, 2010.
40. Klapholz M: Beta-blocker use for the stages of heart failure, *Mayo Clin Proc* 84:718-729, 2009.

PART III

Pulmonary Disease

CHAPTER

7

Pulmonary Disease

Chronic obstructive pulmonary disease (bronchitis and emphysema) and asthma are common pulmonary diseases that cause obstruction in airflow. They are discussed in this chapter along with tuberculosis (TB), the most prevalent contagious disease in the world.

CHRONIC OBSTRUCTIVE PULMONARY DISEASE

Chronic obstructive pulmonary disease (COPD) is a general term for pulmonary disorders characterized by chronic airflow limitation from the lungs that is not fully reversible. COPD encompasses two main diseases: chronic bronchitis and emphysema. *Chronic bronchitis* is defined as a condition associated with excessive tracheobronchial mucus production (at the bronchial level) sufficient to cause a chronic cough with sputum production for at least 3 months in at least 2 consecutive years in a patient in whom other causes of productive chronic cough have been excluded. *Emphysema* is defined as the presence of permanent enlargement of the air spaces distal to the terminal bronchioles accompanied by destruction of alveolar walls or septa (at the acinar level) without obvious fibrosis.[1] These conditions are related, often represent the progression of disease, and may have overlapping symptoms, making differentiation difficult. Accordingly, experts have recommended use of the designation COPD over the traditional terms chronic bronchitis and emphysema. COPD currently is diagnosed on the basis of the presence of cough, sputum production, and dyspnea, together with an abnormal measurement of lung function.[2]

EPIDEMIOLOGY

COPD is the third leading cause of death in the United States and is estimated to affect more than 24 million people. COPD affects approximately 8% of adults and 14% of older adults in the United States.[1,3] The disease is more common in men, and the death rate for men is 83 per 100,000; the rate in women is 57 per 100,000.[3] COPD is disabling, second only to arthritis as the leading cause of long-term disability and functional impairment. Prevalence, incidence, and hospitalization rates increase with age and are now similar for men and women.[4] The disease is underdiagnosed in most populations. On the basis of current figures, the average dental practice of 2000 patients is estimated to have about 130 patients who experience features of COPD.

Etiology

Worldwide, the most important cause of COPD is tobacco smoking. Approximately 12.5% of current smokers and 9% of former smokers have COPD.[4] Smoking also accounts for 85% to 90% of COPD-related deaths in both men and women. The risk for development of COPD is dose-related and increases with the number of cigarettes smoked per day and duration of smoking.[5,6] The risk of death from COPD is 13 times higher in female smokers and 12 times higher in male smokers than in nonsmokers of the same gender.[5] Despite the increased risk, only about one in five chronic smokers develop COPD. This observation suggests that genetic susceptibility to the production of inflammatory mediators (i.e., cytokines) in response to smoke exposure plays an important role. In addition to cigarette smoking, long-term exposure to occupational and environmental pollutants and the absence or deficiency of α_1-antitrypsin are other factors that contribute to COPD. α_1-antitrypsin is made in the liver and neutralizes neutrophil elastase.

Pathophysiology and Complications

Chronic exposure to cigarette smoke induces pathophysiologic responses of the airways and lung tissue. Chronic bronchitis involves the large and small airways. In the large airways, tobacco smoke and irritants induce thickened bronchial walls with inflammatory cell infiltrate, increased size of the mucous glands, and goblet cell hyperplasia. Obstruction is exacerbated in the small airways by narrowing, scarring, increased sputum production, mucous plugging, and collapse of peripheral airways resulting from the loss of surfactant[7] (Figure 7-1). Obstruction is present on both inspiration and expiration.

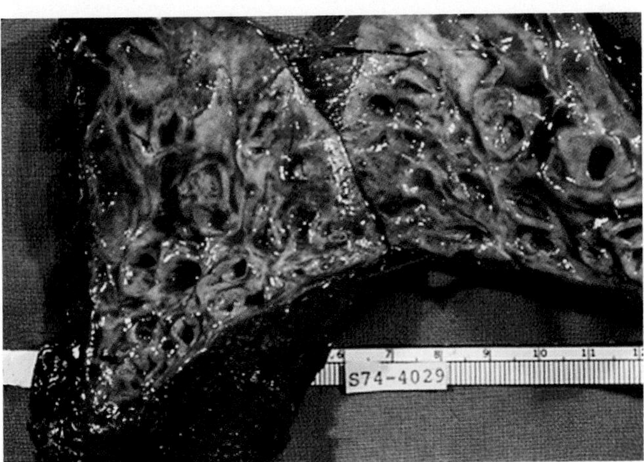

FIGURE 7-1 Gross pathologic specimen shows lung changes (thickened bronchial walls, narrowing of small airways) due to chronic bronchitis. *(Courtesy McLay RN, et al:* Tulane gross pathology tutorial, Tulane University School of Medicine, *New Orleans, Louisiana, 1997.)*

Emphysematous changes occur as chronic smoke inhalation injures lung parenchyma. The alveolar epithelium is damaged, causing a release of inflammatory mediators that attract activated macrophages and neutrophils. These inflammatory cells release enzymes (elastase) that destroy the alveolar walls, resulting in enlarged air spaces distal to the terminal bronchioles and loss of elastic recoil of the lungs (Figure 7-2). Obstruction is caused by the collapse of these unsupported and enlarged air spaces and is evident on expiration—not inspiration.[7]

COPD usually is progressive, and the course is one of deterioration and periodic exacerbations, unless intervention is provided early in its onset.[6] The types of complications that develop vary depending on the site of damage. With continued exposure to primary etiologic factors (cigarette smoking, environmental pollutants), COPD usually results in progressive dyspnea and hypercapnia to the point of severe debilitation (clinically

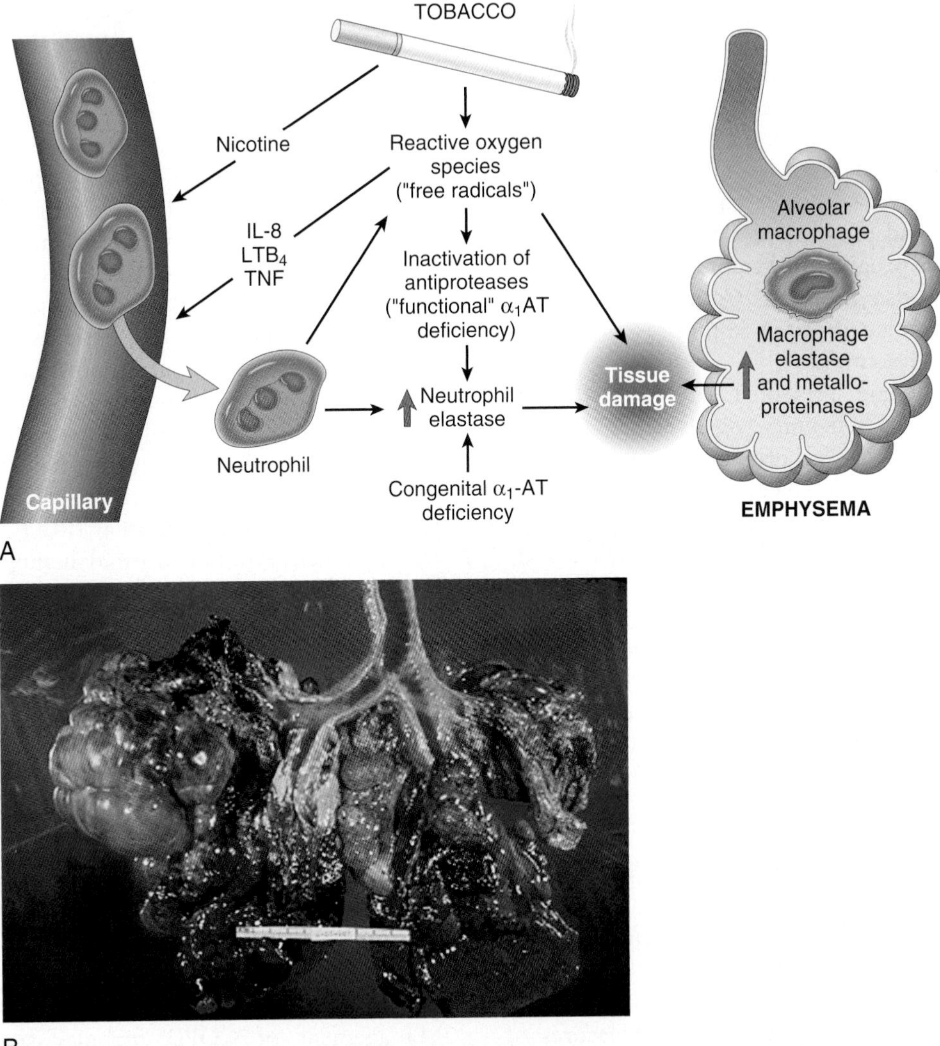

FIGURE 7-2 **A,** Pathogenesis of emphysema involving imbalance in proteases-antiproteases that results in tissue damage and collapse of alveoli. **B,** Gross pathologic specimen of an emphysemic lung. *(**A,** From Kumar V, Abbas A, Fausto N, editors:* Robbins & Cotran pathologic basis of disease, *ed 8, Philadelphia, 2010, Saunders.* ***B,*** *Courtesy McLay RN, et al:* Tulane gross pathology tutorial, Tulane University School of Medicine, *New Orleans, Louisiana, 1997.)*

significant disability will develop in 15% to 20% of the patients).[8] Recurrent pulmonary infections with *Haemophilus influenzae, Moraxella catarrhalis,* and *Streptococcus pneumoniae* are especially common with bronchitis. These acute exacerbations are managed with antibiotics. Pulmonary hypertension can develop and, in the absence of supplemental oxygen therapy, lead to cor pulmonale (right-sided heart failure). Patients with emphysema more frequently are found to have enlarged air spaces, with a higher incidence of thoracic bullae and pneumothorax. Poor quality of sleep secondary to nocturnal hypoxemia is common with COPD. Although COPD is an irreversible process for which no cure exists, avoidance of pulmonary irritants can be of significant benefit in decreasing the morbidity and mortality rates for both diseases.

BOX 7-1 Predominant Findings in Patients with Chronic Obstructive Pulmonary Disease

History: Exposure to risk factors
Clinical: Cough, sputum production, exertional dyspnea
Laboratory: Spirometry revealing airflow limitation, blood gas abnormalities
Imaging: Chest radiograph/computed tomography scan revealing prominent bronchovascular markings and/or evidence of hyperinflation

- Features of *chronic bronchitis:* onset at the age of approximately 50 years, overweight, chronic productive cough, copious mucopurulent sputum, mild dyspnea, frequent respiratory infections, elevated PCO_2, decreased PO_2 (hypoxia), cor pulmonale, chest radiograph showing prominent blood vessels and large heart
- Features of *emphysema:* onset at the age of approximately 60 years, thin physique, barrel-chested, seldom coughing, scanty sputum, severe dyspnea, few respiratory infections, normal PCO_2, decreased PO_2, chest radiograph showing hyperinflation and small heart

CLINICAL PRESENTATION

Signs and Symptoms

The onset phase of COPD takes many years in most patients and usually begins after age 40. Symptoms develop slowly, and many patients are unaware of the emerging condition. Key indicators are a chronic cough with sputum production that may be intermittent, unproductive or productive, scanty or copious, and dyspnea that is persistent and progressive or worsens with exercise. As the disease progresses, weight loss and decreased exercise capacity also are seen. Comorbid conditions include cardiovascular disease, respiratory infections, osteoporosis, and fractures.[9]

Traditional teaching presented patients who had chronic bronchitis as sedentary, overweight, cyanotic, edematous, and breathless; accordingly, they were known as "blue bloaters." Patients diagnosed with emphysema were traditionally known as "pink puffers" because they demonstrated enlarged chest walls for a "barrel-chested" appearance, weight loss with disease progression, severe exertional dyspnea with a mild nonproductive cough, lack of cyanosis, and pursing of the lips with efforts to forcibly exhale air from the lungs. Currently, it is recognized that most patients with COPD may exhibit features of both diseases (Box 7-1).

Laboratory Findings

Diagnosing COPD in its early stages can be difficult, but the possibility of this clinical entity should be considered in any patient who experiences dyspnea with previously tolerated activities and demonstrates chronic cough with or without sputum production, as well as exposure to risk factors, especially cigarette smoking. Measures of expiratory airflow are the key diagnostic procedures performed. Forced vital capacity (FVC) and forced expiratory volume in 1 second (FEV_1) are determined by spirometry—a simple objective test that measures the amount of air a person can breathe out (Figure 7-3). A diagnosis of COPD is assigned when patients have pulmonary symptoms and FEV_1 less than 70% of predicted volume (FVC) in the absence of any other pulmonary disease. The four stages of COPD are shown in Box 7-2.[2]

Arterial blood gas measurement and chest radiographs aid in the diagnosis. Patients with chronic bronchitis have an elevated partial pressure of carbon dioxide (PCO_2) and decreased partial pressure of oxygen (PO_2) (as measured by arterial blood gases), leading to secondary erythrocytosis, an elevated hematocrit value, and compensated respiratory acidosis. Patients with emphysema have a relatively normal (PCO_2) and a decreased (PO_2), which maintain normal hemoglobin saturation, thus avoiding erythrocytosis. Total lung capacity and residual volume are markedly increased. The ventilatory drive of hypoxia also is reduced in both types of COPD.

Chest radiographs and computed tomography scans assist in classifying COPD and identifying comorbid conditions. In chronic bronchitis, typical radiographic abnormalities consist of increased bronchovascular markings at the base of the lungs (Figure 7-4). In emphysema, films demonstrate persistent and marked overdistention of the lungs, flattening of the diaphragm, and emphysematous bullae.

MEDICAL MANAGEMENT

Management of COPD includes smoking cessation, influenza and pneumococcal vaccinations, and use of short- and long-acting bronchodilators. Other recommended measures include regular exercise, good nutrition, and adequate hydration. Use of bronchodilator

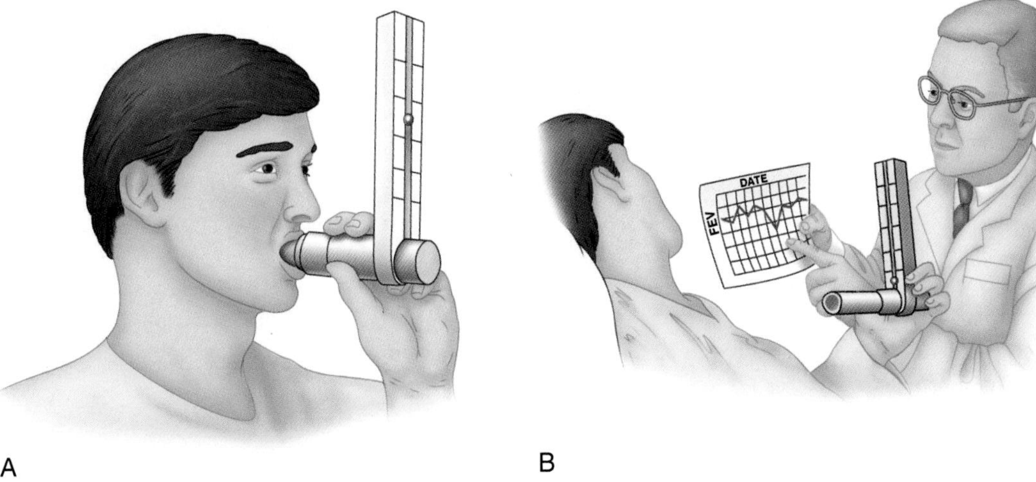

FIGURE 7-3 **A,** Measure of forced expiratory volume by spirometry. **B,** Discussion of daily spirometry results with physician.

BOX 7-2 Stages of Chronic Obstructive Pulmonary Disease

Stage I—mild COPD: defined by an FEV_1/FVC ratio of less than 70% and an FEV_1 of 80% or more of that predicted
Stage II—moderate COPD: worsening airflow limitation and FEV_1/FVC less than 70% and FEV_1 of 50% to less than 80% predicted
Stage III—severe COPD: FEV_1/FVC less than 70% and FEV_1 of 30% to less than 50% predicted, with further worsening of airflow limitation
Stage IV—very severe COPD: FEV_1/FVC less than 70%; FEV_1 less than 30% predicted, with chronic respiratory failure and exacerbations that may be life-threatening

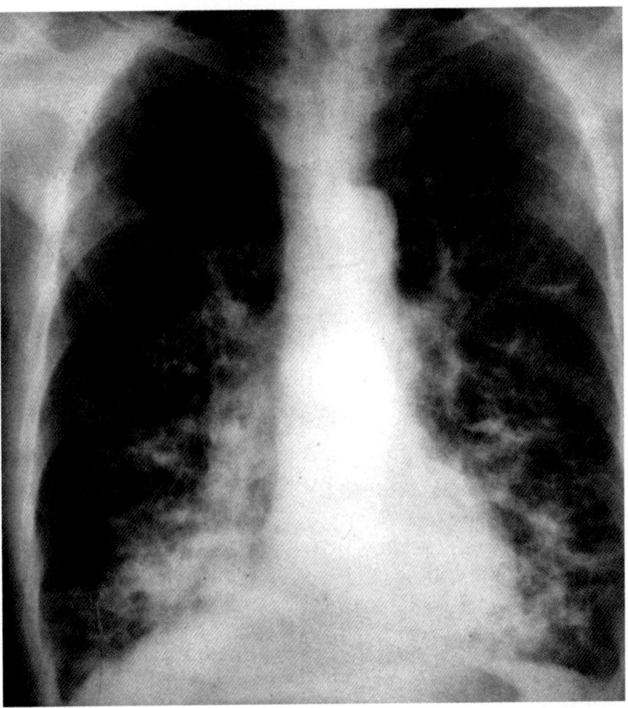

FIGURE 7-4 Chest radiograph of a patient with chronic obstructive pulmonary disease showing prominent vascular markings (consistent with chronic bronchitis).

drugs are recommended in a stepwise manner, as shown in Figure 7-5.[2,10] Other drugs used in the management of COPD are listed in Table 7-1.

Bronchodilators serve as the cornerstone of management, with inhaled and regular therapy preferred. The primary inhaled agents are short- and long-acting anticholinergics (e.g., ipratropium, tiotropium) that reduce glandular mucus and relax smooth muscle by blocking acetylcholine at the muscarinic receptors; and short- and long-acting β_2-adrenergic bronchodilators that relax smooth muscle by increasing cyclic adenosine monophate levels. Combining bronchodilators can lead to pronounced benefits, because they work by different mechanisms. Inhaled corticosteroids are added to the regimen for symptomatic patients at stage III or above who have repeated exacerbations.[2] Phosphodiesterase inhibitors are alternative agents used. Theophylline, a methylxanthine nonselective phosphodiesterase inhibitor, relaxes bronchial smooth muscle cells, but has a limited role in COPD management because of its narrow therapeutic range and likelihood of adverse effects (especially in the elderly).[11] When used, theophylline is administered as a slow-release formulation. More recently, phosphodiesterase-4–selective inhibitors (e.g., roflumilast, cilomilast) have been developed as agents for reducing exacerbations in patients with more advanced COPD.

Antibiotics are used for pulmonary infections, and low-flow supplemental O_2 (2 L/minute) is recommended when the patient's PO_2 is 88% or less.[2,12] Other important treatment options include pulmonary rehabilitation,

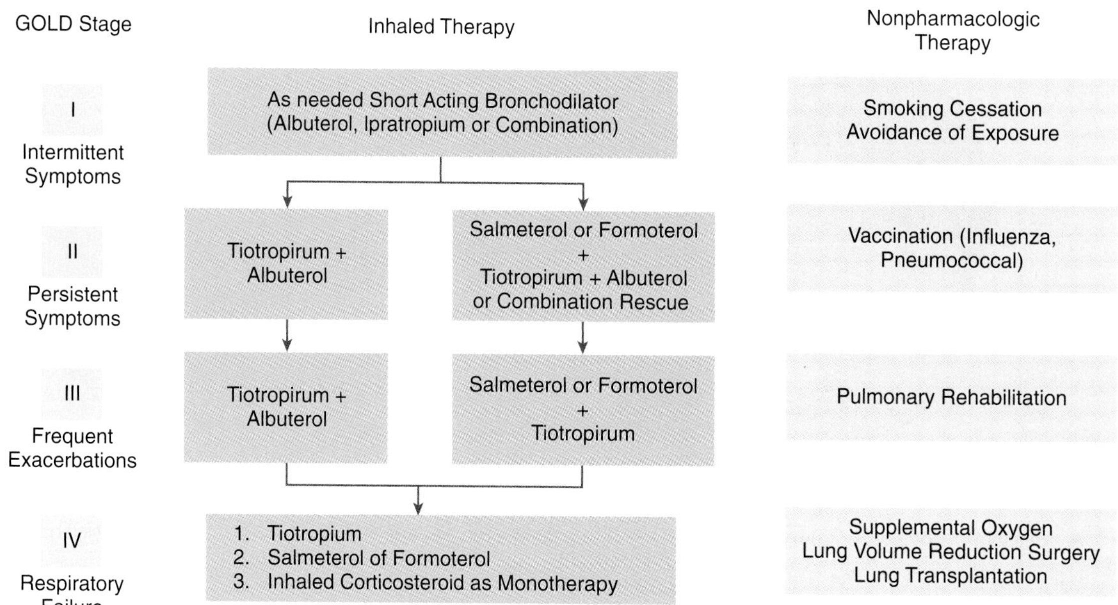

FIGURE 7-5 Clinical algorithm for treatment based on Global Initiative for Chronic Obstructive Lung Disease (GOLD) stages. *(Redrawn from Cooper CB, Tashkin DP: Recent developments in inhaled therapy in stable chronic obstructive pulmonary disease,* BMJ *330:640-644, 2005.)*

screening for comorbid conditions, and continual monitoring for disease progression.

DENTAL MANAGEMENT

Prevention of Potential Problems

Most patients with COPD have a history of smoking tobacco. Dental health care providers can make an important contribution to the management of patients with COPD by encouraging those who smoke to quit. By providing information on the diseases associated with smoking, dental health providers may help patients to start thinking seriously about giving up the habit. Many interventional approaches (e.g., nicotine replacement, bupropion therapy) are available, and providers should help the patient implement the method with which they feel most comfortable (see Chapter 8).[13,14]

Before initiating dental care, clinicians should assess the severity of the patient's respiratory disease and the degree to which it has been controlled. A patient coming to the office for routine dental care who displays shortness of breath at rest, a productive cough, upper respiratory infection, or an oxygen saturation level less than 91% (as determined by pulse oximetry) is unstable. Accordingly, the appointment should be rescheduled and an appropriate referral for medical attention should be made. If the patient is stable and the breathing is adequate, efforts should be directed toward the avoidance of anything that could further depress respiration (Box 7-3). Patients should be placed in a semisupine or upright chair position for treatment, rather than in the supine position, to prevent orthopnea and a feeling of respiratory discomfort. Pulse oximetry monitoring is advised. Humidified low-flow O_2—generally at a rate of 2 to 3 L/minute—may be provided and should be considered for use when the oxygen saturation level is less than 95%.

No contraindication to the use of local anesthetic has been identified. However, the use of bilateral mandibular blocks or bilateral palatal blocks can cause an unpleasant airway constriction sensation in some patients. This concern may be more important in the management of a patient with severe COPD with a rubber dam, or when medications are administered that dry mucous secretions. Humidified low-flow O_2 can be provided to alleviate the unpleasant airway feeling produced by nerve blocks, use of a rubber dam, and/or medications.

If sedative medication is required, low-dose oral diazepam (Valium) may be used. Nitrous oxide–oxygen inhalation sedation should be used with caution in patients with mild to moderate chronic bronchitis. It should not be used in patients with severe COPD and emphysema, because the gas may accumulate in air spaces of the diseased lung. If this sedation modality is used in the patient with chronic bronchitis, flow rates should be reduced to no greater than 3 L/minute, and the clinician should anticipate induction and recovery times with nitrous oxide approximately twice as long as those in healthy patients.[15] Narcotics and barbiturates should not be used, because of their respiratory depressant properties. Anticholinergics and antihistamines generally should be used with caution in patients with COPD, on account of their drying properties and the resultant increase in mucus tenacity; because patients with chronic bronchitis may already be taking these types of

TABLE 7-1 Drugs Used in Outpatient Management of Chronic Obstructive Pulmonary Disease (COPD) and Asthma

Drug	Trade Name	Dental Treatment Considerations
Antiinflammatory Drugs		
Corticosteroids—Inhaled		
Beclomethasone dipropionate	Vanceril, Beclovent	Not intended for acute asthma attack; may contribute to the development of oral candidiasis if used improperly or excessively
Budesonide	Pulmicort	
Dexamethasone	Decadron	
Flunisolide	AeroBid	
Fluticasone propionate	Flonase	
Triamcinolone acetonide	Azmacort	
Corticosteroids—Systemic		
Prednisone	Deltasone or generic	Not intended for acute asthma attack; possible adrenal suppression, cushingoid features with long-term use
Prednisolone	Delta-Cortef	
Methylprednisolone	Solu-Medrol	
Antileukotrienes		
5-Lipoxygenase Inhibitor		Not intended for acute asthma attack
Zileuton	Zyflo	
Leukotriene D_4 Receptor Antagonists		
Zafirlukast (Accolate)		
Montelukast	Singulair	
Nonsteroidal—Chromones		
Cromolyn sodium	Intal inhaler	Not intended for acute asthma attack
Nedocromil	Tilade inhaler	
β-Adrenergic Bronchodilators		
Fast-Acting Nonselective β-Agonist Inhalers		
Epinephrine*	Primatene Mist, Bronkaid (available in parenteral form also)	For use during acute asthma attack
Ephedrine†	Eted II	
Intermediate-Acting Nonselective β-Agonist Inhalers (3 to 6 hours)		
Isoproterenol‡	Isuprel	Not best choice for use during acute asthma attack
Isoetharine	Bronkosol	
Metaproterenol§	Alupent, Metaprel, others	
β_2-Selective Agonist Inhalers		
Albuterol‡	Proventil, Ventolin	For use during acute asthma attack
Bitolterol mesylate	Tornalate	
Fenoterol	Berotec	
Levalbuterol	Xopenex	
Pirbuterol	Maxair, Maxair Autohaler	
Terbutaline‡	Brethaire, Bricanyl	
Long-Acting β_2-Selective Agonist Inhalers (>12 hours)		
Salmeterol (slow onset, long duration)	Serevent	Not intended for acute asthma attack
Formoterol (rapid onset, long duration)	Foradil	
Anticholinergic Bronchodilators (Quaternary Ammonium Derivatives of Atropine)		
Ipratropium bromide	Atrovent	Not intended for acute asthma attack; generally used in combination with other antiasthma drugs
Tiotropium (long-acting)	Spiriva	
Phosphodiesterase (PD) Inhibitors		
Theophylline (nonselective)	Theo-Dur	Adverse drug interaction with erythromycin and azithromycin; serum drug levels should be monitored for toxicity
Roflumilast (selective PD-4)	Daxas, Daliresp	Adverse effects of headache, coughing may affect diagnostic workup and treatment
Cilomilast (selective PD-4)	Ariflo	

*Inhalation and parenteral.
†Oral and parenteral.
‡Inhalation, oral, and parenteral.
§Inhalation and oral. Some combination drugs are formoterol + budesonide propionate (Symbicort) and salmeterol + fluticasone propionate (Advair).
Injectable α_1-proteinase inhibitor formulations (Aralast, Prolastin, Zemaira) are available for treatment of emphysema due to inherited α_1-antitrypsin deficiency.

BOX 7-3 Dental Management
Considerations in Patients with Chronic Obstructive Pulmonary Disease (COPD)

P

Patient Evaluation/Risk Assessment (see Box 1-1)

- Evaluate and determine whether COPD is present.
- Obtain medical consultation if the condition is poorly controlled (as manifested by dyspnea, coughing, or frequent upper respiratory infections) or undiagnosed, or if the diagnosis is uncertain. Review history and clinical findings for concurrent heart disease.
- Encourage current smokers to stop smoking.

Potential Issues/Factors of Concern

A	
Analgesics	No issues.
Antibiotics	Avoid erythromycin, macrolide antibiotics, and ciprofloxacin in patients taking theophylline. In patient who has received courses of antibiotics for upper respiratory infections, oral and lung flora may include antibiotic-resistant bacteria.
Anesthesia	Local anesthesia can be used without change in technique. Avoid outpatient general anesthesia.
Anxiety	Avoid nitrous oxide–oxygen inhalation sedation in patients with severe (stage 3 or worse) COPD. Consider low-dose oral diazepam or another benzodiazepine, although these agents may cause oral dryness.
Allergy	No issues.
B	
Bleeding	No issues.
Blood pressure	Patients with COPD can have cardiovascular comorbidity. Assess blood pressure.
C	
Chair position	Semisupine or upright chair position may be better for treatment in these patients.
D	
Devices	Avoid use of rubber dam in patients with severe disease. Use pulse oximetry to monitor oxygen saturation. Spirometry readings are helpful in determining level of control.
Drugs	Avoid use of barbiturates and narcotics, which can depress respiration. Avoid use of antihistamines and anticholinergic drugs because they can further dry mucosal secretions. Supplemental steroids are unlikely to be needed to perform routine dental care; the usual morning corticosteroid dose should be taken on the day of surgical procedures.
E	
Equipment	Monitor oxygen saturation with pulse oximeter during sedation and invasive procedures. Use low-flow (2 to 3 L/minute) supplemental O_2 when oxygen saturation drops below 95%; it may become necessary when oxygen saturation drops below 91%.
Emergencies	No issues.
F	
Follow-up	At each follow-up appointment, encourage patient to quit smoking, and examine oral cavity for lesions that may be related to smoking. Avoid treatment if upper respiratory infection is present.

medications, concurrent administration could result in additive effects.

Patients with COPD often have comorbid conditions such as hypertension and coronary heart disease that require dental management considerations (see Chapters 3 and 4). Patients taking systemic corticosteroids may require supplementation for major surgical procedures because of adrenal suppression (see Chapter 15). Macrolide antibiotics (e.g., erythromycin, azithromycin) and ciprofloxacin hydrochloride should be avoided in patients taking theophylline because these antibiotics can retard the metabolism of theophylline, resulting in theophylline toxicity.[16] The dentist should be aware of the manifestations of theophylline toxicity. Signs and symptoms include anorexia, nausea, nervousness, insomnia, agitation, thirst, vomiting, headache, cardiac arrhythmias, and convulsions. Outpatient general anesthesia is contraindicated for most patients with COPD.

Treatment Planning Modifications

No technical treatment planning modifications are required in patients with COPD.

Oral Complications and Manifestations

Patients with COPD who are chronic smokers have an increased likelihood of developing halitosis, extrinsic tooth stains, nicotine stomatitis, periodontal disease, premalignant mucosal lesions, and oral cancer. Anticholinergics are associated with dry mouth. In rare instances, theophylline has been associated with the development of Stevens-Johnson syndrome.

ASTHMA

DEFINITION

Asthma is a chronic inflammatory disease of the airways characterized by reversible episodes of increased airway hyperresponsiveness resulting in recurrent episodes of dyspnea, coughing, and wheezing.[17] The bronchiolar lung tissue of patients with asthma is particularly sensitive to a variety of stimuli. Overt attacks may be provoked by allergens, upper respiratory tract infection, exercise, cold air, certain medications (salicylates, nonsteroidal antiinflammatory drugs, cholinergic drugs, and β-adrenergic blocking drugs), chemicals, smoke, and highly emotional states such as anxiety, stress, and nervousness.

EPIDEMIOLOGY

Incidence and Prevalence

Asthma affects 300 million persons worldwide and accounts for 1 of every 250 deaths worldwide. In the United States, its prevalence has more than doubled since the 1960s, from about 2% to 7% or greater (affecting 23 million people).[18] Asthma is a disease primarily of children, with 10% of children (6 million) affected.[17] Females have higher rates of asthma than males, although the prevalence is higher during childhood in boys. Higher body mass index (BMI) increases the risk for asthma in women.[19] The disease affects 6% of older adults.[20] It occurs in all races, with a slightly higher prevalence among African Americans and a lower prevalence among Hispanics than among other races or ethnic groups.[21] Patients with asthma in the United States make over 1.8 million visits to emergency departments annually, and more than 4000 asthma-related deaths occur annually. On the basis of current figures, the average dental practice is estimated to include at least 100 patients who have asthma.

Etiology

Asthma is a multifactorial and heterogeneous disease whose exact cause is not completely understood. Its development requires interaction between the environment and genetic susceptibility, with clinical manifestations resulting from dysfunction of the airway epithelium, smooth muscle, immune cells, and neuronal elements. Many triggers of asthma are recognized; these factors traditionally have been grouped into one of four categories based on pathophysiology: extrinsic (allergic or atopic), intrinsic (idiosyncratic, nonallergic, or nonatopic), drug-induced, and exercise-induced. Today, from a management perspective, the type of trigger is more important than the category.

Allergic or *extrinsic asthma* is the most common form and accounts for approximately 35% of all adult cases. It is an exaggerated inflammatory response that is triggered by inhaled seasonal allergens such as pollens, dust, house mites, and animal danders. Allergic asthma usually is seen in children and young adults.[22] In these patients, a dose-response relationship exists between allergen exposure and immunoglobulin E (IgE)–mediated sensitization, positive skin testing to various allergens, and associated family history of allergic disease. Inflammatory responses are mediated primarily by type 2 helper T (T_H2) cells, which secrete interleukins and stimulate B cells to produce IgE (Figure 7-6). During an attack, allergens interact with IgE antibodies affixed to mast cells, basophils, and eosinophils along the tracheobronchial tree. The complex of antigen with antibody causes leukocytes to degranulate and secrete vasoactive autocoids and cytokines such as bradykinins, histamine, leukotrienes, and prostaglandins.[23] Histamine and leukotrienes cause smooth muscle contraction (bronchoconstriction) and increased vascular permeability, and they attract eosinophils into the airway.[24] The release of platelet-activating factor sustains bronchial hyperresponsiveness. Release of E-selectin and endothelial cell adhesion molecules, neutrophil chemotactic factor, and eosinophilic chemotactic factor of anaphylaxis is responsible for recruitment of leukocytes (neutrophils and eosinophils) to the airway wall, which increases tissue edema and mucus secretion. T lymphocytes prolong the inflammatory response (late-phase response), and imbalances in matrix metalloproteinases and tissue inhibitor metalloproteinases may contribute to fibrotic changes.

Intrinsic asthma accounts for about 30% of asthma cases and seldom is associated with a family history of allergy or with a known cause. Patients usually are nonresponsive to skin testing and demonstrate normal IgE levels. This form of asthma generally is seen in middle-aged adults, and its onset is associated with endogenous factors such as emotional stress (implicated in at least 50% of affected persons), gastroesophageal acid reflux, or vagally mediated responses.[24]

Ingestion of drugs (e.g., aspirin, nonsteroidal antiinflammatory drugs, beta blockers, angiotensin-converting [ACE] enzyme inhibitors) and some food substances (e.g., nuts, shellfish, strawberries, milk, tartrazine food dye yellow color no. 5) can trigger asthma.[25] Aspirin causes bronchoconstriction in about 10% of patients with asthma, and sensitivity to aspirin occurs in 30% to 40% of people with asthma who have pansinusitis and nasal polyps (the so-called "triad asthmaticus").[25] The ability of aspirin to block the cyclooxygenase pathway appears causative. The buildup of arachidonic acid and leukotrienes mediated by the lipoxygenase pathway results in bronchial spasm.[25,26]

Metabisulfite preservatives of foods and drugs (specifically in local anesthetics containing epinephrine) may cause wheezing when metabolic levels of the enzyme sulfite oxidase are low.[27] Sulfur dioxide is produced in the absence of sulfite oxidase. The buildup of sulfur dioxide in the bronchial tree precipitates an acute asthma attack.[25]

Exercise-induced asthma is stimulated by exertional activity. Although the pathogenesis of this form of asthma is unknown, thermal changes during inhalation of cold air provoke mucosal irritation and airway hyperactivity. Children and young adults are more severely affected because of their high level of physical activity.

Infectious asthma is a term previously used to describe persons who developed asthma because of the inflammatory response to bronchial infection. Now it is

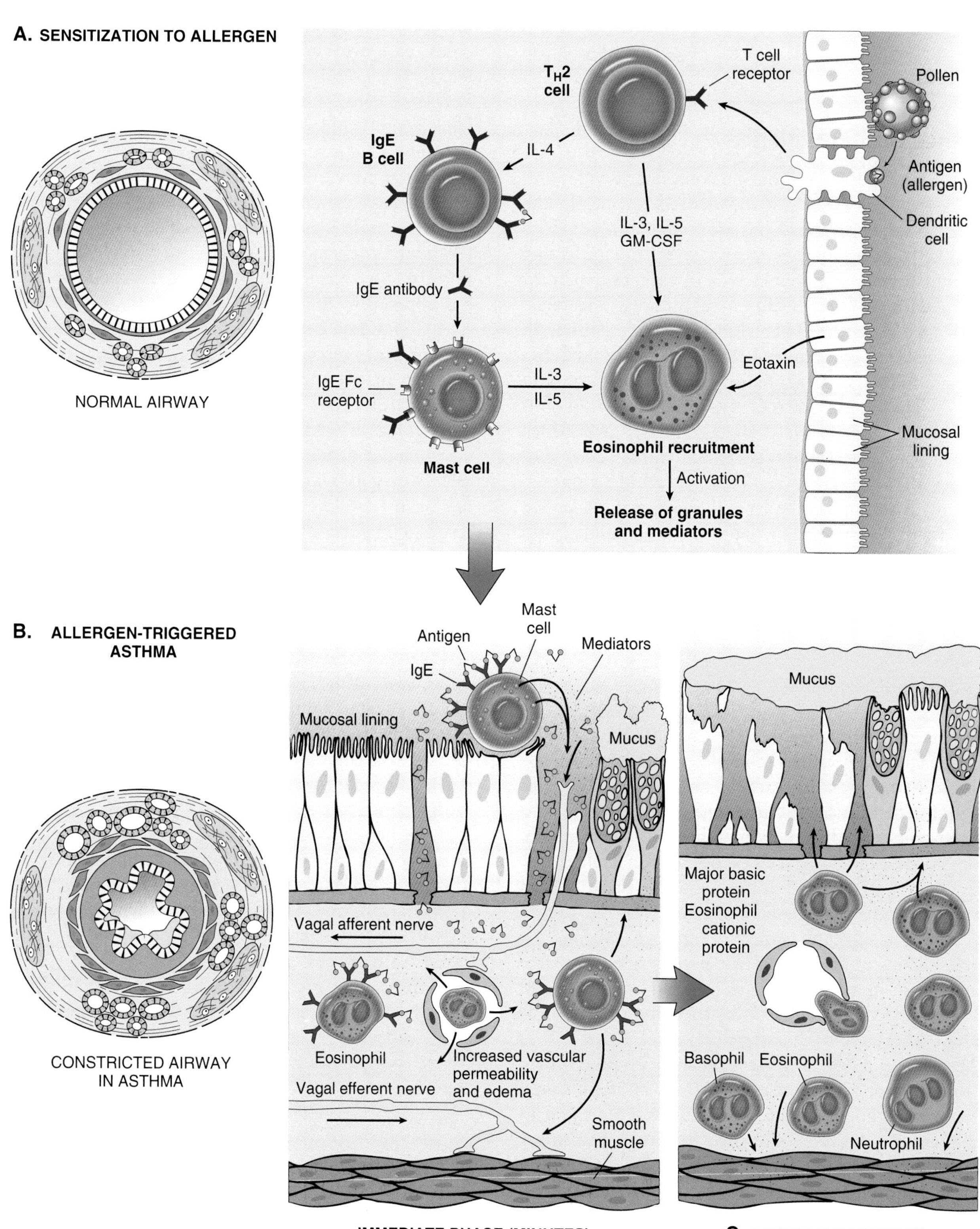

FIGURE 7-6 Processes involved in allergic (extrinsic) asthma. *(From Kumar V, Abbas A, Fausto N, editors:* Robbins & Cotran pathologic basis of disease, *ed 8, Philadelphia, 2010, Saunders.)*

recognized that several respiratory viral infections during infancy and childhood can result in the development of asthma. Also, causative agents of respiratory infections (bacteria, dermatologic fungi I *Trichophyton*), and *Mycoplasma* organisms) can exacerbate asthma. Treatment of the respiratory infection generally improves control of bronchospasm and constriction.

PATHOPHYSIOLOGY AND COMPLICATIONS

In asthma, obstruction of airflow occurs as the result of bronchial smooth muscle spasm, inflammation of bronchial mucosa, mucus hypersecretion, and sputum plugging. The most striking macroscopic finding in the asthmatic lung is occlusion of the bronchi and bronchioles by thick, tenacious mucous plugs (Figure 7-7). Histologic findings are those of inflammation and airway remodeling, including (1) thickening of the basement membrane (from collagen deposition) of the bronchial epithelium, (2) edema, (3) mucous gland hypertrophy and goblet cell hyperplasia, (4) hypertrophy of the bronchial wall muscle, (5) accumulation of mast cell and inflammatory cell infiltrate, (6) epithelial cell damage and detachment, and (7) blood vessel proliferation and dilation.[28] These changes contribute to decreased diameter of the airway, increased airway resistance, and difficulty in expiration.

Asthma is relatively benign in terms of morbidity. Most patients can expect a reasonably good prognosis, especially those in whom the disease develops during childhood. In many young children, the condition resolves spontaneously after puberty. In one reported series, however, two thirds of asthmatic children still had symptoms at age 21 years.[29] In a small percentage of patients, both young and old, the condition can progress to COPD and respiratory failure, or status asthmaticus, the most serious manifestation of asthma, may occur. Status asthmaticus is a particularly severe and prolonged asthmatic attack (one lasting longer than 24 hours) that is refractory to usual therapy. Signs include increased and progressive dyspnea, jugular venous pulsation, cyanosis, and pulsus paradoxus (a fall in systolic pressure with inspiration). Status asthmaticus often is associated with a respiratory infection and can lead to exhaustion, severe dehydration, peripheral vascular collapse, and death. Although death directly attributable to asthma is relatively uncommon, the disease causes more than 4000 deaths per year in the United States. Asthma deaths occur more often in persons older than 45 years of age, are largely preventable, and often are related to delays in delivery of appropriate medical care.[29]

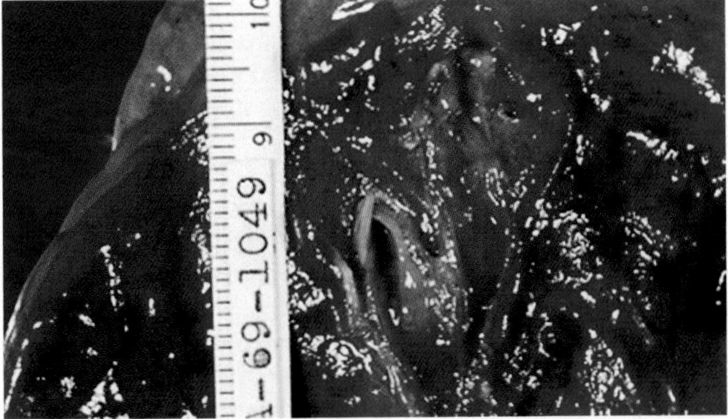

FIGURE 7-7 Section of a lung with the bronchioles occluded by mucous plugs. *(Courtesy McLay RN, et al:* Tulane gross pathology tutorial, Tulane University School of Medicine, *New Orleans, Louisiana, 1997.)*

CLINICAL PRESENTATION

Signs and Symptoms

Asthma is a disease of episodic attacks of airway hyperresponsiveness. For reasons that are unclear, attacks often occur at night but also may follow or accompany exposure to an allergen, exercise, respiratory infection, or emotional upset and excitement. Typical symptoms and signs of asthma consist of reversible episodes of breathlessness (dyspnea), wheezing, cough that is worse at night, chest tightness, and flushing. Onset usually is sudden, with peak symptoms occurring within 10 to 15 minutes. Inadequate treatment results in emergency department visits for about 25% of patients.[29] Respirations become difficult and are accompanied by expiratory wheezing. Tachypnea and prolonged expiration are characteristic. Termination of an attack commonly is accompanied by a productive cough with thick, stringy mucus. Episodes usually are self-limiting, although severe attacks may necessitate medical assistance.[30]

Laboratory Findings

Diagnostic testing by a physician is important in the differentiation of asthma from other airway diseases. Experienced clinical judgment and recognition of the signs and symptoms are essential, because laboratory tests for asthma are relatively nonspecific and no single test is diagnostic. Commonly ordered tests include 6-minute walk test, spirometry before and after administration of a short-acting bronchodilator, chest radiographs (to detect hyperinflation), skin testing (for specific allergens), bronchial provocation (by histamine or methacholine chloride challenge) testing, sputum smear examination and cell counts (to detect neutrophilia or eosinophilia), arterial blood gas determination, and antibody-based enzyme-linked immunosorbent assay (ELISA) for measurement of environmental allergen exposure.[31] Spirometry is widely applied in diagnosing asthma because by definition, the associated airflow obstruction must be episodic and at least partially reversible. Reversibility is demonstrated by an increase in pulmonary function (i.e., FEV_1) of 12% or greater from baseline after therapy or an increase of 10% or more in predicted FEV_1 after inhalation of a short-acting bronchodilator. Also, a recent drop in FEV_1 can be interpreted as a predictive of an asthma attack (see Figure 7-3), and a drop of more than 10% during exercise fulfills the diagnosis of exercise-induced asthma. Fractional exhaled nitric oxide determination is an additional noninvasive test used to aid in the diagnosis and management of asthma.[32]

Classification

Patients with chronic asthma are clinically classified as having intermittent or persistent disease (mild, moderate, or severe asthma). Severity is based on frequency of symptoms, impairment of lung function and risk of attacks (Box 7-4). Persons with mild persistent asthma have symptoms once per week but less than once daily and an FEV_1 greater than 80%. Symptoms generally last less than an hour. Patients with moderate asthma have FEV_1 greater than 60% but less than 80% and daily symptoms that affect sleep and activity level and, on occasion, require occasional emergency care. Asthma is severe when patients have less than 60% FEV_1, which results in ongoing symptoms that limit normal activity. Attacks are frequent or continuous, occur at night, and result in emergency hospitalization.

MEDICAL MANAGEMENT

The goals of asthma therapy are to limit exposure to triggering agents, allow normal activities, restore and maintain normal pulmonary function, minimize frequency and severity of attacks, control chronic and nocturnal symptoms, and avoid adverse effects of medications.[33] Experts agree that these goals are best accomplished by educating patients and involving them in the prevention or elimination of precipitating factors (e.g., smoking cessation) and comorbid conditions (rhinosinusitis, obesity) that confound management, establishment of a plan for regular self-monitoring, and provision of regular follow-up care.[33] Specifically, it is recommended that a written education and action plan be given to each patient, with appropriate support and instructions for its use. Inexpensive peak expiratory flowmeters should be used regularly at home and levels recorded daily in diaries. For patients with known allergies, the importance of avoidance of allergens to prevent attacks should be underscored. This can be conveyed by monitoring of allergen levels (tobacco smoke and pollutants) in the patient's home, provision of desensitization intradermal injections, and monitoring of the pulmonary function zone on the basis of daily peak flow meter results (spirometry). Unfortunately, poor control of asthma often is related to low socioeconomic status (e.g., the patient cannot afford medication), increased anxiety, poor compliance, and unfavorable home environment.

BOX 7-4 Classification of Asthma and Recommended Drug Management

Classification	Recommended Drug Management
Intermittent Symptoms less than once per week, brief exacerbations, asymptomatic between exacerbations, nocturnal symptoms less than twice a month, FEV_1 80% of predicted or more, less than 20% variability	No daily medication or short-acting β_2 agonist as needed
Mild Persistent Symptoms less than once per week but more than once a day exacerbations that affect activity and sleep, nocturnal symptoms more than twice a month (limited exercise tolerance; rare ED visit), FEV_1 80% of predicted or more, less than 20-30% variability	Low-dose inhaled corticosteroids or other antiinflammatory, as needed; short-acting β_2 agonist
Moderate Persistent Daily symptoms, daily use of inhaled short-acting beta agonist, exacerbations that may affect activity and sleep, nocturnal symptoms more than once a week (occasional ED visit), FEV_1 60-80% of predicted, greater than 30% variability	Low- or medium-dose inhaled corticosteroids + long-acting bronchodilator, as needed; short-acting β_2 agonist
Severe Persistent Daily symptoms, frequent (more than 4 times a month) exacerbations and nocturnal asthma symptoms, exercise intolerance, FEV_1 60% or less, greater than 30% variability (often resulting in hospitalization)	High-dose inhaled corticosteroids + long-acting bronchodilator + oral corticosteroid, as needed; short-acting β_2 agonist

ED, Emergency department; *FEV_1,* Forced expiratory volume in 1 second.
Adapted from Bateman ED, et al: Global strategy for asthma management and prevention: GINA executive summary, Eur Respir J *31:143-178, 2008.*

Antiasthmatic drug selection is based on the type and severity of asthma and whether the drug is to be used for long-term control or quick relief. Current guidelines recommend a "stepped-care" approach with the use of inhaled antiinflammatory agents as first-line drugs (the preferred inhalational agent is a corticosteroid preparation, with a leukotriene inhibitor as an alternative) for the long-term management and prophylaxis of persistent asthma (Figure 7-8). β-adrenergic agonists are recommended for intermittent asthma and are secondary agents that should be added (i.e., not to be used alone) for persistent asthma when antiinflammatory drugs are inadequate alone. Alternative drugs include mast cell stabilizers (cromolyn and nedocromil), immunomodulators, and theophylline. Combination therapy with these medications often is used to improve lung function.[33]

Inhaled corticosteroids are the most effective antiinflammatory medications currently available for the treatment of persistent asthma.[34,35] They act by reducing the inflammatory response and preventing the formation of cytokines, adhesion molecules, and inflammatory enzymes. Aerosol dosage is two (for mild to moderate disease) to four times daily (severe asthma). Onset of action usually is after 2 hours, and peak effects occur 6 hours later. Long-term use of steroid inhalers rarely is associated with systemic adverse effects, provided the maximum recommended dose of 1.5 mg per day of inhaled beclomethasone dipropionate (Vanceril) or equivalent is not exceeded. Use of systemic steroids is reserved for asthma unresponsive to inhaled corticosteroids and bronchodilators, and for use during the recovery phase of a severe acute attack. Inhaled steroids often are used in combination with long-acting β_2-adrenergic bronchodilators (salmeterol or formoterol). Newer agents such as omalizumab (Xolair) that block IgE (monoclonal antibody against human IgE) are used for additive therapy in patients with severe persistent asthma who have allergy triggers; however, cost and the injectable-only formulation are major considerations with this drug.[36]

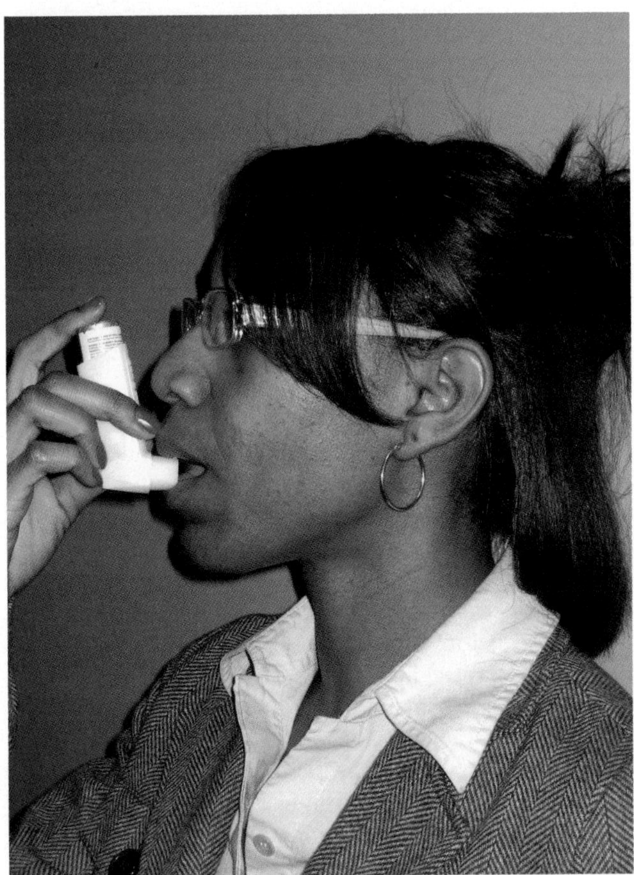

FIGURE 7-8 Use of an inhaler by a patient.

For relief of acute asthma attacks, inhaled short-acting β_2-adrenergic agonists are the drugs of choice because of their fast and notable bronchodilatory and smooth muscle relaxation properties (see Table 7-1). Short-acting β_2-adrenergic agonists produce bronchodilation by activating β_2 receptors on airway smooth muscle cells, generally in 5 minutes or less.[23] Inhalation corticosteroids, inhaled cromolyn sodium, and oral anticholinergics are not used for this purpose because of their slow onset of action.

β_2-adrenergic agonists (administered by a metered-dose inhaler) and cromolyn sodium (Intal) and nedocromil may be used in preventing exercise-induced bronchospasm. They are taken about 30 minutes before initiation of physical activity. Cromolyn and nedocromil decrease airway hyperresponsiveness by stabilizing the membrane of mast cells and interfering with chloride channel function, so that mediators are not released when challenged by exercise or cold air. Theophylline is a mild to moderate bronchodilator to be used as an alternative. Monitoring of its serum concentration is essential.

DENTAL MANAGEMENT

Prevention of Potential Problems

The underlying primary goal in dental management of patients with asthma is to prevent an acute asthma attack (Box 7-5). The first step in achieving this goal is to identify patients with asthma by history, followed by assessment to elucidate the surrounding details of the problem, along with prevention of precipitating factors.

Through a good history, the dentist should be able to determine the severity and stability of disease. Questions should be asked that ascertain the type of asthma (e.g., allergic versus nonallergic), the precipitating substances, the frequency and severity of attacks, the times of day when attacks occur, whether this is a current or past problem, how attacks usually are managed, and whether the patient has received emergency treatment for an acute attack. The clinician must be cognizant of the indications of severe disease: frequent exacerbations, exercise intolerance, FEV_1 less than 60%, use of several medications, and a history of visits to an emergency facility for treatment of acute attacks (see Box 7-4).

BOX 7-5 Dental Management
Considerations in Patients with Asthma

P

Patient Evaluation/Risk Assessment (see Box 1-1)

- Evaluate and identify asthma as a medically confirmed or likely diagnosis along with its severity and type if present.
- Obtain medical consultation if asthma is poorly controlled (as indicated by wheezing or coughing, or a recent hospitalization) or is undiagnosed, or if the diagnosis is uncertain. Ecourage current smokers to stop smoking.

Potential Issues/Factors of Concern

A	
Analgesics	No issues.
Antibiotics	Avoid erythromycin, macrolide antibiotics, and ciprofloxacin in patients taking theophylline.
Anesthesia	The clinicians may elect to avoid solutions containing epinephrine or levonordefrin because of sulfite preservative.
Anxiety	Provide stress-free environment through establishment of rapport and openness to reduce risk of anxiety-induced asthma attack. If sedation is required, use of nitrous oxide–oxygen inhalation sedation and/or small doses of oral diazepam is recommended.
Allergy	Asthmatics with nasal polyps are increased risk for allergy to aspirin. Avoid aspirin use.
B	
Bleeding	No issues.
Blood pressure	Monitor blood pressure during asthma attack to observe for the development of status asthmaticus.
C	
Chair position	Semisupine or upright chair position for treatment may be better tolerated.
D	
Devices	Instruct patient to bring current medication inhaler to every appointment; use prophylactically in moderate to severe disease. Obtain spirometry reading to determine level of control. Use pulse oximetry to monitor oxygen saturation during dental procedure.
Drugs	Avoid precipitating odorants and drugs (aspirin). Avoid use of barbiturates and narcotics, which can depress respiration and release histamine, respectively. Supplemental steroids are unlikely to be needed in routine dental care; provide usual morning corticosteroid dose the morning of surgical procedures.
E	
Equipment	Use low-flow (2 to 3 L/minute) supplemental O_2 when oxygen saturation drops below 95%; it also may become necessary when oxygen saturation drops below 91%.
Emergencies	Recognize signs and symptoms of a severe or worsening asthma attack: inability to finish sentences with one breath, ineffectiveness of bronchodilators to relieve dyspnea, recent drop in FEV_1 as determined by spirometry, tachypnea with respiratory rate of 25 breaths/minute or more, tachycardia with heart rate of 110 beats/minute or greater, diaphoresis, accessory muscle usage, paradoxical pulse. Administer fast-acting bronchodilator (NOTE: ccorticosteroids have delayed onset of action), oxygen, and, if needed, subcutaneous epinephrine (1:1000) in a dose of 0.3 to 0.5 mL. Activate emergency medical system (EMS); repeat administration of fast-acting bronchodilator every 20 minutes until EMS personnel arrive.
F	
Follow-up	Ensure that patient is receiving adequate medical follow-up care on a routine basis.

The stability of the disease can be assessed during the interview component of the history and by clinical examination and the results of laboratory measures. Features such as shortness of breath, wheezing, increased respiratory rate (more than 50% above normal), FEV_1 that has fallen more than 10% or to below 80% of peak FEV_1, an eosinophil count that is elevated to above 50/mm^3, poor drug use compliance, and emergency department visits within the previous 3 months suggest inadequate treatment and poor stability. Also, the use of more than 1.5 canisters of a beta agonist inhaler per month (more than 200 inhalations per month) or doubling of monthly use indicates high risk for a severe asthma attack.[37] For severe and unstable asthma, consultation with the patient's physician is advised. Routine dental treatment should be postponed until better control is achieved.

Modifications during the preoperative and operative phases of dental management of a patient with asthma can minimize the likelihood of an attack. Patients who have nocturnal asthma should be scheduled for late-morning appointments, when attacks are less likely. Use of operatory odorants (e.g., methyl methacrylate) should be reduced before the patient is treated. Patients should be instructed to regularly use their medications, to bring their inhalers (bronchodilators) to each appointment, and to inform the dentist at the earliest sign or symptom of an asthma attack. Prophylactic inhalation of a patient's bronchodilator at the beginning of the appointment is a valuable method of preventing an asthma attack. Alternatively, patients may be advised to bring their spirometer and daily expiratory record to the office. The dentist may request that the patient exhale into the spirometer and record the expired volume. A significant drop in lung function (to below 80% of peak FEV_1 or a greater than 10% drop from previously recorded values) indicates that prophylactic use of the inhaler or referral to a physician is needed.[38] The use of a pulse oximeter also is valuable for determining the patient's oxygen saturation level. In healthy patients, this value remains between 97% and 100%, whereas a drop to 91% or below indicates poor oxygen exchange and the need for intervention.

Because stress is implicated as a precipitating factor in asthma attacks and dental treatment may result in decreased lung function,[39] all dental staff members should make every effort to identify patients who are anxious and provide a stress-free environment through establishment of rapport and openness. Preoperative and intraoperative sedation may be desirable. If sedation is required, nitrous oxide–oxygen inhalation is best. Nitrous oxide is not a respiratory depressant, nor is it an irritant to the tracheobronchial tree. Oral premedication may be accomplished with small doses of a short-acting benzodiazepine. Reasonable alternatives with children are hydroxyzine (Vistaril), for its antihistamine and sedative properties, and ketamine, which causes bronchodilation. Barbiturates and narcotics, particularly meperidine, are histamine-releasing drugs that can provoke an attack. Outpatient general anesthesia generally is contraindicated for patients with asthma.

Selection of local anesthetic may require adjustment. In 1987, the U.S. Food and Drug Administration[27] (FDA) warned that drugs that contained sulfites were a cause of allergic-type reactions in susceptible individuals. Sulfite preservatives are found in local anesthetic solutions that contain epinephrine or levonordefrin, although the amount of sulfite in a local anesthetic cartridge is less than the amount commonly found in an average serving of certain foods. Although rare, at least one case of an acute asthma attack precipitated by exposure to sulfites has been reported.[40] Thus, the use of local anesthetic without epinephrine or levonordefrin may be advisable for patients with moderate to severe disease. Because relevant data remain limited, the dentist should discuss with the patient any past responses to local anesthetics and allergy to sulfites and should consult with the physician on this issue. As an alternative, local anesthetics without a vasoconstrictor may be used in at-risk patients.

Patients with asthma who are medicated over the long term with systemic corticosteroids may require supplementation for major surgical procedures if their health is poor (see Chapter 15). However, long-term use of inhaled corticosteroids rarely causes adrenal suppression unless the daily dosage exceeds 1.5 mg of beclomethasone dipropionate or its equivalent.

Administration of aspirin-containing medication or other nonsteroidal antiinflammatory drugs to patients with asthma is not advisable, because aspirin ingestion is associated with the precipitation of asthma attacks in a small percentage of patients. Likewise, barbiturates and narcotics are best not used, because they also may precipitate an asthma attack. Antihistamines have beneficial properties but should be used cautiously because of their drying effects. Patients who are taking theophylline preparations should not be given macrolide antibiotics (i.e., erythromycin and azithromycin) or ciprofloxacin hydrochloride, because these agents interact with theophylline to produce a potentially toxic blood level of theophylline. To prevent serious toxicity, the dentist should ask the patient who takes theophylline whether the dosage is being monitored on the basis of serum theophylline levels (recommended to be less than 10 µg/mL). Approximately 3% of patients who take zileuton exhibit elevated alanine transaminase levels, reflecting liver dysfunction that may affect the metabolism of dentally administered drugs.[41]

Management of Potential Problems: Asthma Attack

An acute asthma attack requires immediate therapy. The signs and symptoms (see Box 7-5) should be recognized quickly and an inhaler provided rapidly. A short-acting β_2-adrenergic agonist inhaler (Ventolin, Proventil) is the most effective and fastest-acting bronchodilator. It should be administered at the first sign of an attack. Long-lasting β_2 agonist drugs like salmeterol (Serevent) and corticosteroids do not act quickly and are not given for an immediate response, but they may provide a delayed response. With a severe asthma attack, use of subcutaneous injections of epinephrine (0.3 to 0.5 mL, 1:1000) or inhalation of epinephrine (Primatene Mist) is the most potent and fastest-acting method for relieving the bronchial constriction. Supportive treatment includes providing positive-flow oxygenation, repeating bronchodilator doses as necessary every 20 minutes, monitoring vital signs (including oxygen saturation, if possible, which should reach 90% or higher), and activating the emergency medical system, if needed.[42]

Treatment Planning Modifications

No specific treatment planning modifications are required for the patient with asthma.

Oral Complications and Manifestations

Nasal symptoms, allergic rhinitis, and mouth breathing are common with extrinsic asthma. Patients with asthma who are mouth breathers may have altered nasorespiratory function, which may be associated with increased upper anterior and total anterior facial height, higher palatal vault, greater overjet, and a higher prevalence of crossbite.[43]

The medications taken by patients who have asthma may contribute to oral disease. For example, β_2-agonist inhalers reduce salivary flow by 20% to 35%, decrease plaque pH,[44] and are associated with increased prevalence of gingivitis and caries in patients with moderate to severe asthma.[45,46] Gastroesophageal acid reflux is common in patients with asthma and is exacerbated by the use of β-agonists and theophylline. This reflux can contribute to erosion of enamel. Oral candidiasis (acute pseudomembranous type) occurs in approximately 5% of patients who use inhalation steroids for long periods at high dose or frequency.[47] However, development of this condition is rare if a "spacer" or aerosol-holding chamber is attached to the metered-dose inhaler and the mouth is rinsed with water after each use.[48] The condition readily responds to local antifungal therapy (i.e., nystatin, clotrimazole, or fluconazole). Patients should receive instructions on the proper use of their inhaler and the need for oral rinsing. Headache is a frequent adverse effect of antileukotrienes and theophylline. The clinician should be aware of this adverse effect when diagnosing disease in patients with orofacial pain complaints.

TUBERCULOSIS

DEFINITION

Tuberculosis[8] (TB) is an important human disease caused by an infectious and communicable organism, *Mycobacterium tuberculosis*. TB represents a major global health problem that is responsible for illness and deaths in large segments of the world's population. The disease is spread by inhalation of infected droplets and usually demonstrates a prolonged quiescent period. *M. tuberculosis* replication leads to an inflammatory and granulomatous response in the host, with consequent development of classic pulmonary and systemic symptoms. Although *M. tuberculosis* is by far the most common causative agent in this human infection, other species of mycobacteria occasionally are encountered, such as *M. avium* complex, *M. kansasii, M. abscessus, M. xenopi, M. bovis, M. africanum, M. microti*, and *M. canetti*. These mycobacterial species may cause systemic diseases (manifesting as pulmonary lymphadenitis, cutaneous or disseminated) that are referred to as *mycobacterioses*.[47]

EPIDEMIOLOGY

Incidence and Prevalence

TB has a worldwide incidence of 9 to 10 million; the World Health Organization (WHO) estimates that one third of the world population—representing 2 billion people—is infected. This disease kills more adults worldwide each year than does any other single pathogen.[49-51] In contrast, the occurrence of TB in the United States steadily decreased during the past century and has dropped at a rate of 5% per year over the past 50 years. Peak prevalence in Western countries occurred around the beginning of the 19th century. By the turn of the 20th century, approximately 500 new cases of active TB per 100,000 population were identified annually in the United States. By the mid-1980s, reports to the Centers for Disease Control and Prevention (CDC) indicated that the rate had decreased to 9.3 per 100,000 population. A resurgence in TB occurred between 1985 and 1992, when rates rose to 10.6 per 100,000, or 26,000 cases, primarily because of adverse social and economic factors, the acquired immunodeficiency syndrome (AIDS) epidemic, and immigration of foreign-born persons who had TB.[52] Since then, the rate has steadily declined. In 2009, 11,540 cases of TB were reported—representing a rate of 3.8 per 100,000.[53] This was the lowest rate reported during the past century. Although the figures are encouraging, the disease continues to occur in almost every state of the United States and affects 5% to 10% of the population (approximately 15 to 30 million people). Moreover, 54% of new U.S. cases occur in foreign-born persons who migrate or travel to the U.S.—a rate that has continually increased since 1993.[53]

Although the present rate for the United States as a whole is low, racial and ethnic minorities, residents of inner city ghettos, the elderly, the urban poor, people living in congregate facilities (community dwellings, prisons, and shelters), and patients who have AIDS have occurrence rates that are several times the national average (Box 7-6). Higher risk for the disease (an 8% chance of developing TB per year) also has been noted in human immunodeficiency virus (HIV)-positive persons and in those who are immunosuppressed from use of medications.[8-12] TB is diagnosed most often in men (with

BOX 7-6 Groups at High Risk for Tuberculosis (TB)

- Close contacts of persons who have TB
- Skin test converters (within past 2 years)
- Residents and employees of high-risk congregate settings (correctional facilities, nursing homes, mental institutions, homeless shelters, health care facilities)
- Recent immigrants/foreign-born persons (and migrant workers) from countries that have a high TB incidence or prevalence
- Persons who visit areas with a high prevalence of active TB, especially if visits are frequent or prolonged
- Populations defined as having increased incidence of latent *M. tuberculosis* infection: medically underserved persons, those with low income, persons who abuse drugs or alcohol
- Infants, children, and adolescents exposed to persons who are at increased risk for latent *M. tuberculosis* infection or active TB, or have a positive result on tuberculin skin testing

HIV, Human immunodeficiency virus.
(Adapted From Mazurek GH, et al: Updated guidelines for using Interferon Gamma Release Assays to detect Mycobacterium tuberculosis *infection—United States, 2010,* MMWR Recomm Rep *59(RR-5):1-25, 2010.)*

a male-to-female ratio of 1.6:1); in Hispanics, African Americans, and Asian Americans (at rates 7.3, 8.3, and 23 times higher than that for whites, respectively); and in persons between 25 and 64 years of age.[53]

Factors important in reducing the spread of TB in the United States during the past century have included improved sanitation and hygiene measures and the use of effective antituberculosis drugs. Unfortunately, failure to complete a course of therapy (a recognized problem in more than 20% of patients) and improper drug selection have contributed to the persistence of this disease and to the rise in the development of multidrug-resistant TB (MDR-TB), which has accounted for 1% of cases in the United States since 1997 but constitutes 5.4% of cases worldwide.[53,54] MDR-TB disproportionately affects foreign-born persons in the United States, with countries such as China, India, and the Russian Federation accounting for more than 50% of all cases reported globally.

Etiology

In most cases of human TB, the causative agent is *M. tuberculosis*, an acid-fast, nonmotile, intracellular rod that is an obligate aerobe. As an aerobe, this organism exists best in an atmosphere of high oxygen tension; therefore, it most commonly infects the lung.

M. tuberculosis typically is transmitted by way of infected airborne droplets of mucus or saliva that are forcefully expelled from the lungs, most commonly through coughing but also by sneezing and during talking. The quantity and size of expelled droplets influence transmission. Smaller droplets evaporate readily, leaving bacteria and other solid material as floating particles that are easily inhaled. Larger droplets quickly settle to the ground. Transmission by way of fomites rarely occurs.[47,55] Transmission by ingestion (e.g., of contaminated milk) occurs but is rare because of the use of pasteurized milk. A secondary mode of transmission—by ingestion—is possible when a patient coughs up infected sputum, thereby inoculating oral tissues. Oral lesions of TB may be initiated through this mechanism.

The interval from infection to development of active TB is widely variable, ranging from a few weeks to decades. Most cases of TB result from reactivation of a dormant tubercle; only 5% to 10% of cases arise de novo at the time of the initial infection. The number of organisms inhaled and the level of immunocompetency largely determine whether exposed person will contract the disease.

Pathophysiology and Complications

TB can involve virtually any organ of the body, although the lung is the most common site of infection. The typical infection of primary pulmonary TB begins with inhalation of infected droplets. These droplets are carried into the alveoli, where bacteria are engulfed by macrophages. Replication occurs within alveolar macrophages, and spread of infection occurs locally to regional (hilar) lymph nodes. The combination of a primary granulomatous lung lesion and an infected hilar lymph node is known as a Ghon complex. If the infection is not controlled locally, distant dissemination through the bloodstream may occur. However, the vast majority of disseminated bacteria are destroyed by natural host defenses. At approximately 2 to 8 weeks after onset, delayed hypersensitivity to the bacteria develops that is mediated by T ($CD4^+$) helper lymphocytes. This condition manifests as conversion of the tuberculin skin testing (using purified protein derivative [PPD], as described later on) from negative to positive. Subsequently, a chronic granulomatous inflammatory reaction develops that involves activated epithelioid macrophages and formation of granulomas. These natural host defenses usually control and contain the primary pulmonary TB infection, resulting in latent tuberculosis infection (LTBI). If not contained, the nidus of infection (granuloma) may become a productive tubercle with central necrosis and caseation. Cavitation may occur (Figure 7-9), resulting in the dumping of organisms into the airway for further dissemination into other lung tissue or the exhaled air.

Limitation and local containment of infection may be influenced by a variety of factors, including host resistance, host immune capabilities, and virulence of the mycobacterium. Once the infection has been successfully interrupted, the lesion heals spontaneously and then

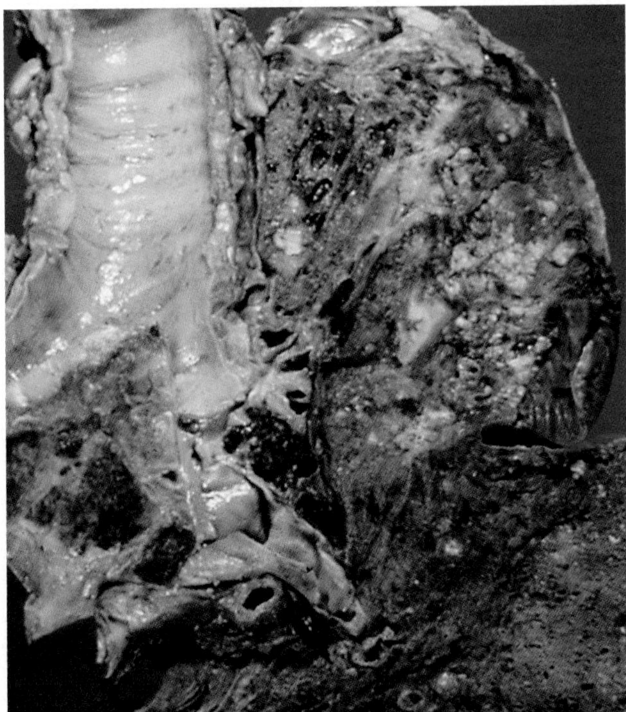

FIGURE 7-9 Gross specimen of a tuberculous lung, demonstrating caseating granulomas and cavitation. *(Courtesy R. Powell, Lexington, Kentucky.)*

undergoes inspissation, hardening, encapsulation, and calcification. Although the lesion "heals," some bacteria may remain dormant. If infection is not interrupted, dissemination of bacilli may occur through the lung parenchyma, resulting in extensive pulmonary lesions and lymphohematogenous spread. Widespread infection with multiple organ involvement is called *miliary tuberculosis*.

Primary pulmonary TB is seen most often in infants and children; however, cavitation is rare in these age groups, and children generally do not actively produce or expectorate sputum; they instead usually swallow any pulmonary secretions. Expression of the disease differs somewhat in teenagers and adults in that lymph node involvement and lymphohematogenous spread are not prominent features. However, cavitation commonly occurs. The usual form of disease found in adults is called *secondary* or *reinfection TB*, which occurs with delayed reactivation of persistent dormant viable bacilli and probably represents relapse of a previous infection. This form of the disease usually is confined to the lungs, and cavitation is common. Reasons for relapse include inadequate treatment of the primary infection and the influences of illness, immunosuppressive agents, immunodeficiency disease (as in AIDS), and age.

Some of the more common sequelae of TB include progressive primary TB, cavitary disease, pleurisy and pleural effusion, meningitis, and disseminated or miliary TB. Isolated organ involvement other than that of the lung may occur, with the pericardium, peritoneum, kidneys, adrenal glands, and bone (known as Pott's disease when occurring in the spine) commonly affected.[56] The tongue and other tissues of the oral cavity also are involved, albeit infrequently. Factors that increase the risk of a poor clinical outcome are listed in Box 7-7.

Approximately 5% to 10% of persons who develop TB die of the disease. However, the rate of deaths attributable to TB is much higher (54%) in young persons who have AIDS.[57] The advent of effective chemotherapy undoubtedly has been the most significant reason for today's lower mortality rate among nonimmunosuppressed, TB-infected persons.

BOX 7-7 Persons at Increased Risk for Progression of Infection to Active Tuberculosis

- Persons with human immunodeficiency virus infection
- Infants and children younger than 5 years of age
- Persons who are receiving immunosuppressive therapy such as with tumor necrosis factor-α (TNF-α) antagonists, or systemic corticosteroids equivalent to 15 mg or more of prednisone per day, or immunosuppressive drug therapy after organ transplantation
- Persons who were recently infected with *M. tuberculosis* (within the past 2 years)
- Persons with a history of untreated or inadequately treated active tuberculosis, including persons with fibrotic changes on chest radiograph consistent with previous active tuberculosis
- Persons with silicosis, diabetes mellitus, chronic renal failure, leukemia, lymphoma, solid organ transplant, or cancer of the head, neck, or lung
- Persons who have had a gastrectomy or jejunoileal bypass
- Persons who are underweight (weigh less than 90% of their ideal body weight) or malnourished
- Cigarette smokers and persons who abuse drugs or alcohol
- Populations defined locally as having an increased incidence of active tuberculosis, possibly including medically underserved or low-income populations

From Mazurek GH, et al: Updated guidelines for using Interferon Gamma Release Assays to detect Mycobacterium tuberculosis *infection—United States, 2010,* MMWR Recomm Rep *59(RR-5):1-25, 2010.*

CLINICAL PRESENTATION

Signs and Symptoms

Primary infection with *M. tuberculosis* in about 90% of patients results in few manifestations other than a positive result on tuberculin skin testing and characteristic radiographic changes. Progression of clinical disease usually is associated with underlying conditions (young and old ages) and diseases that depress the immune response. Once symptoms become apparent, they typically are nonspecific and could be associated with any infectious disease. They include cough, lassitude and malaise, anorexia, unexplained weight loss, night sweats, and fever. Temperature elevation commonly occurs in the evening or during the night and is accompanied by profuse sweating.

Specific local symptoms of the disease are dependent on the organ involved. Persistent cough is the symptom most commonly associated with pulmonary TB, although it may appear late in the course of the disease. Cough is common with cavitary disease. The sputum produced is characteristically scanty and mucoid, but it becomes purulent with progressive disease. Hemoptysis (blood in sputum) is infrequent, occurring in about 20% of cases. Dyspnea is a feature of advanced disease.

Manifestations of extrapulmonary disease occur in about 10% to 20% of cases, more often in HIV-infected persons, and may include localized lymphadenopathy with the development of sinus tracts, back pain over the affected spine, gastrointestinal disturbances (in intestinal TB), dysuria and hematuria (in renal involvement), heart failure, and neurologic deficits.[58] In contrast, findings in some patients on physical examination may be inconclusive.

Laboratory Findings

Laboratory tests are directed toward determining whether the patient has active infection or LTBI. Active infection is considered when there is a positive acid-fast bacillus sputum smear, a history of cough and weight loss, and characteristic chest radiographic findings. The definitive diagnosis of TB is based on culture or direct molecular tests (e.g., nucleic acid amplification) that identify *M. tuberculosis* or other mycobacterial species from body fluids and tissues, usually sputum. Three consecutive morning sputum specimens are obtained for culturing to ensure positive results.[47] With traditional culture techniques, several weeks are required to grow mycobacteria on solid medium; however, the use of selective broth (BACTEC-460, Becton-Dickson, Sparks, Md) or similar systems reduces the time to about 1 week.[58-60] Cultures should be accompanied by antimicrobial susceptibility testing for all isolates of *M. tuberculosis* because of the rising incidence of multiple drug resistance and extensively drug-resistant TB. Antibiotic sensitivity testing takes about 7 to 10 days. Molecular tests (nucleic acid amplification and probe kits) are advantageous because they provide results within 24 hours. Some tests (skin testing, sputum smears, cultures, and chest films) are less reliable when the patient has HIV infection.

Radiographic findings in TB include patchy or lobular infiltrates in the apical posterior segments of the upper lobes or in the middle or lower lobes, with cavitation and hilar adenopathy in active "progressive primary" TB. Healed primary lesions leave a calcified peripheral nodule associated with a calcified hilar lymph node (Ghon complex).

Two tests are used for the diagnosis of LTBI: the tuberculin (Mantoux) skin test[61] (TST) and the interferon-gamma release assay (IGRA).[51,62] The TST is 95% sensitive and 95% specific for determining whether the patient has been infected with *M. tuberculosis*. This test is of limited utility in immunocompromised persons and during the first 6 to 8 weeks, when the bacillus is incubating, because false-negative results are likely. Also, for various reasons, 10% to 25% of people with active TB have false-negative skin test results.[62] A positive test result presumptively means that the person has been infected. It does not mean that the person has clinically active TB. Some positive skin reactions indicate infection with other mycobacterial species. Physical examination and tests that identify *M. tuberculosis* are required for diagnosis.

The TST is administered by intradermal injection of 0.1 mL of PPD, which contains 5 units of tuberculin (culture extract from *M. tuberculosis*), on the volar or dorsal surface of the forearm. The test measures the delayed hypersensitivity response by evidence of induration noted 48 to 72 hours later. The size of the induration determines whether the results are read as negative (induration size less than 5 mm) or positive (with 10 and 15 mm used as cut points), interpreted in light of the presence of risk factors or abnormalities on the chest radiograph (Table 7-2). Induration of 15 mm or greater is considered positive evidence of TB in all persons tested.[51] A positive result on PPD testing necessitates a physical examination, a radiographic evaluation, and, if necessary, sputum culture to rule out active disease. Without treatment, approximately 5% of skin test converters develop TB within 2 years; another 5% develop it later.[63] Thus, all persons who are at risk for development of TB—including dentists—should undergo tuberculin skin testing annually.

IGRAs performed on fresh whole blood are diagnostic tests that may be used in place of the TST (except in children younger than 5 years of age). IGRAs measure the person's immune reactivity to white blood cells infected with *M. tuberculosis,* which release interferon-γ when mixed with antigens from the mycobacteria. These assays are advantageous because they can detect recent infections, results are available within 24 hours, and

TABLE 7-2 Significance for Various Patient Groups of Positive Results on Purified Protein Derivative (PPD) Testing

Groups at Risk for Progression to Active TB Disease, Stratified by Induration Size		
Induration ≥5 mm	***Induration ≥10 mm***	***Induration ≥15 mm***
HIV-seropositive patients Patients with recent contact with a person with active TB disease Persons whose chest radiograph shows changes consistent with previous untreated TB Organ transplant recipients or patients on immunosuppression regimens (taking the equivalent of >15 mg/day of prednisone for 1 month or longer; taking TNF-α antagonists)	Children <5 years of age Infants, children, and adolescents exposed to adults at high risk for developing active TB Recent immigrants Injection drug users Persons with clinical conditions associated with high risk for TB* Mycobacteriology laboratory personnel Residents and employees of congregate facilities	All persons in this category are considered to have TB (despite absence of risk factors for TB)

HIV, Human immunodeficiency virus; *TB,* Tuberculosis; *TNF-α,* Tumor necrosis factor-α.
*Silicosis, diabetes mellitus, chronic renal failure, leukemia, lymphoma, and head, neck, or lung cancer; weight loss of more than 10% of ideal body weight; gastrectomy, jejunoileal bypass.

previous bacille Calmette-Guérin (BCG) vaccination does not cause a false-positive result. Like the TST, however, they cannot discriminate active from latent infection.[64]

MEDICAL MANAGEMENT

The International Standards for Tuberculosis Care (ISTC) recommendations[65] include the following: The diagnosis should be established promptly and accurately; standardized treatment regimens should be used; treatment should be supervised; the response to treatment should be monitored; and appropriate public health measures should be carried out. Of particular concern are patient compliance and completion of therapy, as well as exposure of personal contacts, who may be at risk for the disease.[66]

Effective chemotherapy for TB is dependent on (1) patient education and compliance, (2) appropriate selection of drugs, (3) multiple drug use, and (4) drug administration continued for a sufficient period of time. The ISTC and the CDC currently recommend that all patients receive at least a four-drug regimen isoniazid, rifampin, ethambutol, and pyrazinamide.[66] The four-drug regimen is given for 8 weeks, and a sputum specimen is collected to determine response to therapy. If the specimen is negative for *M. tuberculosis,* isoniazid and rifampin are given daily or twice-weekly for the next 4 months, for a total of 6 months of therapy. If, however, at 2 months the sputum is positive, cavitational disease is present on the initial chest film, or the patient is HIV-seropositive, then isoniazid and rifampin are continued for an additional 7 months. A larger combination of drugs (standard four drugs plus three additional agents) is used when drug resistance is established by drug susceptibility testing (Box 7-8).

BOX 7-8 Common Drug Regimens for the Treatment of Tuberculosis (TB)[49,65]

Non–Drug-Resistant TB

- Four-drug regimen (isoniazid + rifampin + ethambutol + pyrazinamide) for 2 months
- Then two-drug therapy (isoniazid and rifampin) for 4 months; continued for 7 months if patient is seropositive for HIV or if chest radiograph revealed cavitation on initial examination

Confirmed Multidrug-Resistant TB*

- Ethambutol + pyrazinamide + fluoroquinolone, ethionamide, or an injectable drug—streptomycin, amikacin, kanamycin, or capreomycin—to which the organism is susceptible, continued for at least 12 months. Treatment regimens are individualized in accordance with several factors including resistance pattern, extent of disease, and presence of comorbid conditions.

*Multidrug-resistant TB is defined as TB resistant to therapy with isoniazid and rifampin.

After the initiation of chemotherapy, reversal of infectiousness is dependent on proper drug selection and patient compliance. Within 3 to 6 months, approximately 90% of patients become noninfectious, and their sputum cultures convert to negative.[67] Patients are allowed to return to normal public contact on the basis of reversal of infectiousness and continued chemotherapy. In 2005, only 83% of patients completed indicated therapy.[53]

Because of its contagiousness and the problem of less than ideal compliance with treatment regimens, protection measures have been introduced to control the spread of disease.[23] Public health measures include screening close contacts for the disease, hospitalizing patients with potentially infectious TB, and treating infected patients in isolation rooms with negative air pressure.[68,69] In addition, "directly observed therapy" is used to ensure that patients who have TB take the appropriate medicine at the appropriate time for the duration of therapy.

MDR-TB is the most threatening feature of the disease and occurs in approximately 1% of cases in the United States and more than 10% of cases in parts of the former Soviet Union (Russian Federation) and China.[49,53] Ninety percent of drug resistance cases (defined by the WHO as resistant to the two strongest antituberculosis drugs, isoniazid and rifampin) occur in HIV-infected persons and in many countries where TB is endemic.[60] Transmission of drug-resistant TB has occurred between patients, between patients and health care workers, and between patients and family members. In 2008, 500,000 persons worldwide were estimated to have MDR-TB. Mortality rates range from 70% to 90%, and survival has been reported to be 4 to 16 weeks from the time of diagnosis. To limit the spread of MDR-TB, sputum cultures should be tested for drug-resistant bacteria if drug resistance is likely or sputum specimens remain positive. Current guidelines recommend that at least four antituberculosis medications be prescribed in a stepwise manner, and treatment be provided in a hospital using directly observed therapy.

Asymptomatic patients in whom skin testing (or IGRA) yielded a negative result that when repeated converted to positive are considered to be latently infected with *M. tuberculosis.* Once physical examination, radiographs, and sputum culturing have established that the disease is not active, patients who have LTBI are candidates for treatment if they are at high risk for disease progression (see Box 7-7). Most commonly, isoniazid (INH), 300 mg daily for 9 months (10 mg/kg for 9 months in children), is recommended.[66] Rifampicin (rifampin) alone for 4 months or with INH for 3 months can be used as an alternative. Although these regimens usually prevent the occurrence of active disease, the person retains hypersensitivity to PPD, so skin tests will continue to give a positive result. Major efforts toward development of a TB vaccine are under way.[70]

DENTAL MANAGEMENT

Medical Considerations

Many patients with infectious disease, including TB, cannot be clinically or historically identified; therefore, all patients should be treated as though they are potentially infectious, and the CDC's standard precautions for infection control should be strictly followed. Implementation of infection control measures for patients with TB involves updating each patient's medical history, recognizing the signs and symptoms of TB, and following the guidelines of the CDC for infection control and the prevention of transmission of tuberculosis in health care facilities (see Appendix B).[71] These guidelines were updated in 2005 and address administrative, environmental, and respiratory protection controls for outpatient health care settings such as dental offices.[69] The CDC places most dental facilities in the low risk category for potential occupational exposure to TB. In keeping with this risk category, it recommends that each dental facility have a written TB control protocol that includes instrument reprocessing and operatory cleanup, as well as protocols for identifying, managing, and referring patients with active TB, and educating and training staff (Box 7-9). The CDC also recommends that baseline and periodic screening of dental care workers with PPD be provided to document any recent exposure, and that protocols be available that explain how the office assesses, manages, and investigates dental staff members with a positive result on PPD testing.[69]

Management of the patient infected with TB is based on potential infectivity status. The four infectivity categories are (1) active TB, (2) a history of TB, (3) a positive tuberculin test, and (4) signs or symptoms suggestive of TB (Box 7-10).

Patients with Clinically Active Sputum-Positive Tuberculosis. Patients with recently diagnosed, clinically active TB and positive sputum cultures should not be treated on an outpatient basis. Treatment is best rendered in a hospital setting with appropriate isolation, sterilization (mask, gloves, gown), and special engineering control (ventilation) systems and filtration masks. For greater detail, the clinician should refer to the CDC recommendations,[71] available at http://www.cdc.gov/mmwr/PDF/RR/RR4313.pdf. Also, because of the risk of TB transmission, treatment in the isolation room should be limited to urgent care, and a rubber dam should be used to minimize aerosolization of oropharyngeal microbes. After receiving chemotherapy for at least 2 to 3 weeks and after receiving confirmation from the physician that he or she is noninfectious and lacks any complicating factors, the patient may be treated on an outpatient basis in the same manner as for any normal, healthy person[72] (Box 7-11).

A child with active TB who is receiving chemotherapy usually can be treated as an outpatient, because bacilli are found only rarely in the sputum of young children. The child should be considered noninfectious unless a positive sputum culture has been obtained.[73] Reasons why a child with TB is considered noninfectious include the rarity of cavitary disease in children and their inability to cough up sputum effectively. In this context, defining exactly what age constitutes a "child" is difficult. As a general rule, children younger than 6 years of age who are receiving anti-TB drugs can be confidently treated. At the age of 6 years and beyond, some degree of concern is in order. The physician should be consulted before treatment is begun. Of greater concern in such cases is the TB status of family contacts of the patient, because the disease most likely was contracted from an infected adult. All family members who have had contact with the child should provide a history of skin testing and chest radiography to rule out the possibility of active disease. If such assurances are not obtained, the physician or health department should be contacted to ensure that proper preventive action is taken.

BOX 7-9 CDC Guidelines: *Tuberculosis (TB) Precautions for Use in Outpatient Dental Settings*

Administrative Controls

- Assign responsibility for managing TB infection control program.
- Conduct annual risk assessment.
- Develop written TB infection control policies for promptly identifying and isolating patients with suspected or confirmed TB for medical evaluation or urgent treatment.
- Ensure dental health care personnel are educated regarding the signs and symptoms of TB.
- Instruct patients to cover mouth when coughing and/or wear a surgical mask.
- Screen newly hired personnel for latent TB infection and disease.
- Postpone urgent dental treatment if TB is suspected or active.

Environmental Controls

- Use airborne infection isolation room to provide urgent treatment to patients with suspected or confirmed TB.
- Use high-efficiency particulate air filters or UV-germicidal irradiation in settings with high volume of patients with suspected or confirmed TB.
- Cover and clean and disinfect exposed patient area surfaces.
- Sterilize patient care items.

Respiratory Protection Controls

- Use respiratory protection (at least an N95 filtering face piece [disposable], N99 or N100 respirators) for exposed personnel when they are providing urgent dental treatment to patients with suspected or confirmed TB.
- Instruct TB patients to cover mouth when coughing and to wear a surgical mask.

CDC, Centers for Disease Control and Prevention; *UV,* Ultraviolet.
Data from Jensen PA, et al: CDC: Guidelines for preventing the transmission of Mycobacterium tuberculosis *in health-care settings, 2005,* MMWR Recomm Rep *54(RR-17):1-142, 2005.*

BOX 7-10 Principles of Dental Management for Patients with a History of Tuberculosis

Active Sputum-Positive Tuberculosis
- Consult with physician before treatment.
- Perform urgent care only; palliate urgent problems with medication if contained facility in a hospital environment is not available.
- Perform urgent care that requires the use of a handpiece (in patients older than 6 years) only in a hospital setting with isolation, sterilization (gloves, mask, gown), and special respiratory protection.
- Treat those less than 6 years of age as a normal patient (noninfectious after consultation with physician to verify status).
- Treat the patient who produces consistently negative sputum as for a normal patient (noninfectious—verify with physician).

Tuberculosis History Specifics
- Approach with caution; obtain thorough history of disease and its treatment duration, with appropriate review of systems.
- Obtain from patient a history of periodic chest radiographs and physical examination to rule out reactivation or relapse.
- Consult with physician, and postpone treatment with identification of any of the following:
  - Questionable adequacy of treatment time
  - Lack of appropriate medical follow-up evaluation since recovery
  - Sign or symptom of relapse
- Treat as for normal patient if present status is "free of clinically active disease."

Recent Conversion to Positive Tuberculin Skin Test
- Verify evaluation by physician to rule out active disease.
- Verify completion of drug therapy with isoniazid for 9 months .
- Treat as for a normal patient.

Signs or Symptoms Suggestive of Tuberculosis
- Refer to physician and postpone treatment.
- Treat as for patient with sputum-positive status if treatment is necessary.

BOX 7-11 General Guidelines[72] for Determining When a Patient with Pulmonary Tuberculosis (TB) Has Become Noninfectious During Therapy

- Likelihood of multidrug-resistant TB has been determined to be negligible.
- Patient has received standard multidrug anti-TB therapy for 2 to 3 weeks.
- Patient has demonstrated compliance with standard multidrug anti-TB treatment.
- Patient exhibits clinical improvement.
- Results of AFB testing on three consecutive sputum smears are negative.
- All close contacts of the patient have been identified, evaluated, advised, and, if indicated, started on treatment for latent TB infection.

AFB, Acid-fast bacilli.

Patients with a Past History of Tuberculosis. Fortunately, relapse is rare among patients who have received adequate treatment for the initial infection. This is not the case, however, in patients who have received inadequate treatment and in those who are immunosuppressed. Regardless of what type of treatment was received, any person with a history of TB requires an initial careful workup to investigate infectivity status before any dental treatment is contemplated. The dentist should obtain a medical history, including diagnosis and dates and type of treatment. Treatment duration of less than 18 months if treatment was provided in past decades, or less than 9 months if treatment was given recently, requires consultation with the physician to assess adequacy of the regimen used. Patients should provide a history of periodic physical examinations and chest radiographs to check for evidence of reactivation of the disease. Further consultation with the physician is advisable to verify current status. The patient who is found to be free of active disease and is not immunosuppressed may be treated with the use of standard precautions. A thorough review of systems is important with these patients, and referral to a physician is indicated if questionable signs or symptoms are present.

Patients with a Positive Tuberculin Test. A person with a positive result on skin testing for TB should be viewed as having been infected with mycobacteria. The patient should provide a history of being evaluated for active disease by physical examination and chest radiography. In the absence of clinically active disease, such patients have LTBI and are not considered infectious. A regimen of prophylactic isoniazid is administered for 9 months if they are considered to be at risk for disease progression (see Box 7-7). These patients may be treated in a normal manner with the use of standard precautions.

Patients with Signs or Symptoms Suggestive of TB. Any time a patient demonstrates unexplained, persistent signs or symptoms that may be suggestive of TB (e.g., dry nonproductive cough, pleuritic chest pain, fatigue, fever, dyspnea, hemoptysis, weight loss) or has a positive result on skin testing or IGRA and has not been given follow-up medical care, dental care should not be rendered, and the patient should be referred to a physician for evaluation. If a health care provider is exposed to TB, the provider should be evaluated for skin test conversion. Converters should be treated promptly with isoniazid.[66]

Adverse Effects of Drugs

Isoniazid, rifampin, and pyrazinamide therapy may cause hepatotoxicity and elevations in serum aminotransferases (Table 7-3). The prevalence of isoniazid-induced hepatitis is about 1% and increases with advancing age, daily alcohol intake, and previous

TABLE 7-3 Dental Treatment Considerations with Antituberculosis Drugs

Drug (Trade Name)	Adverse Effects	Dental Treatment Consideration(s)
Isoniazid (INH) (Laniazid, Nydrazid, Tubizid)	Hepatotoxicity; elevation in serum aminotransferase activity in 10-20% of patients*; rash, fever, peripheral neuropathy	Avoid acetaminophen Increases concentrations of other drugs (e.g., diazepam)
Rifampin (Rifadin, Rimactane)	Hepatotoxicity; gastrointestinal disturbances, flulike symptoms, thrombocytopenia, rash; turns urine red-orange	Increases incidence of infection, delayed healing, gingival bleeding; bidirectional interaction that decreases serum levels of diazepam, triazolam, erythromycin, clarithromycin (Biaxin), ketoconazole (Nizoral), itraconazole (Sporanox), fluconazole (Diflucan), and oral contraceptives
Pyrazinamide (generic)	Arthralgias, rash (photoallergy), hyperuricemia, gastrointestinal disturbances, arthralgias, and hepatitis	—
Ethambutol (Myambutol)	Decreased red-green color discrimination; reduced visual acuity; optic neuritis (rare)	—
Ethionamide (Trecator-SC)		—
Streptomycin (generic)	Ototoxicity, vestibular disturbances, infrequent renal toxicity, perioral numbness	Avoid concurrent use of aspirin
Amikacin (Amikin), Kanamycin (Kantrex), Capreomycin (Capastat)	Nephrotoxicity and ototoxicity	Avoid concurrent use of aspirin
Cycloserine	Neurotoxicity and hypersensitivity, vitamin deficiency	—
Aminosalicylic acid (Sodium P.A.S., Teebacin)	Gastrointestinal disturbances	—

*Greater risk of liver damage in persons older than 35 years of age; vitamin B_6 (pyridoxine) is recommended to counteract the potential for adverse effects of INH.

liver disease.[74] When serum aminotransferases are elevated in patients taking isoniazid, acetaminophen-containing medications should be avoided because of the increased potential for hepatotoxicity. Additional precautions regarding liver dysfunction are discussed in Chapter 10.

Rifampin induces cytochrome P-450 enzymes. As a result, the use of rifampin can lower plasma levels of oral contraceptives, diazepam, midazolam, clarithromycin (Biaxin), ketoconazole (Nizoral), itraconazole (Sporanox), and fluconazole (Diflucan). In addition, rifampin can cause leukopenia, hemolytic anemia, and thrombocytopenia, resulting in an increased incidence of infection, delayed healing, and gingival bleeding. Regimens that combine rifampin with pyrazinamide or isoniazid will increase the risks for hepatotoxicity and gastrointestinal and neurologic adverse events. Streptomycin should not be administered concurrently with aspirin because of the potential for increased ototoxicity.

Treatment Planning Modifications

Routine treatment must be delayed in patients who are infectious. Treatment may be resumed when patients become noninfectious (see Box 7-11).[72]

Oral Complications and Manifestations

TB manifests infrequently in the oral cavity. Oral lesions can occur at any age but most frequently are seen in men about 30 years of age and in children. The classic mucosal lesion is a painful, deep, irregular ulcer on the dorsum of the tongue. The palate, lips, buccal mucosa, and gingiva also may be affected. Mucosal lesions have been reported to be granular, nodular, or leukoplakic and sometimes painless. Extension into the jaws can result in osteomyelitis.[75] The cervical and submandibular lymph nodes may become infected with TB; this condition is called *scrofula*. The nodes become enlarged and painful (Figure 7-10), and abscesses may form with subsequent

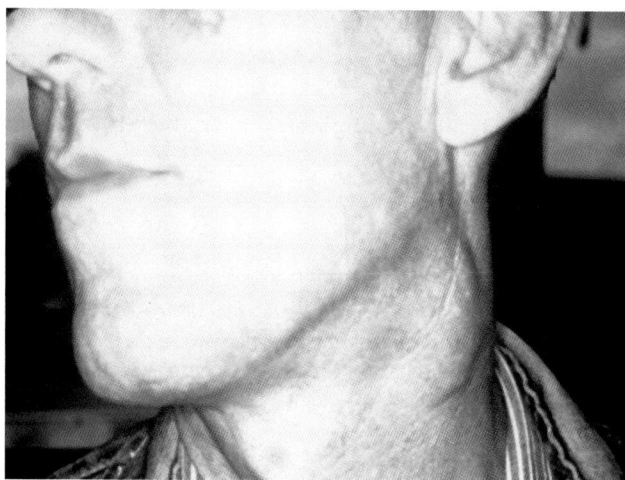

FIGURE 7-10 Tuberculosis of the cervical lymph nodes.

drainage.[76] Involvement of the salivary glands or temporomandibular joint is rare.[77,78]

Biopsy in addition to culture can be diagnostic if acid-fast bacilli are found. Resolution of the infectious oral lesion may result from treatment of TB with antituberculosis drugs. Pain is managed symptomatically (see Appendix C).

OCCUPATIONAL SAFETY AND HEALTH ASSOCIATION

Dentists should be aware that the Occupational Safety and Health Association (OSHA)[79] issued an enforcement guidance policy in 1993 to protect workers against exposure to *M. tuberculosis* and continues to mandate directives as public policy. Current policy mandates that employers provide a safe, healthful workplace and permit inspection for occupational exposure to TB in health care facilities when complaints are received from public sector employees. Employers who are found to be in violation of the requirements may be fined.

Since 1997, OSHA has mandated a specific policy regarding the risk of TB transmission based on CDC guidelines. Current policy can be viewed at http://www.osha.gov/SLTC/tuberculosis/index.html, which requires that dentists prepare a written exposure control plan, provide baseline skin test results and medical history, make medical management available after an exposure incident, provide medical removal protection if necessary, provide information and training to employees with exposure potential, comply with record-keeping requirements, and document any occupationally related tuberculosis infection. In addition, if respirators are deemed necessary to protect the health of an employee, the employer is required to establish and implement a written respiratory protection program. Periodic medical surveillance and respiratory protection are not required if the dental facility does not admit or treat patients with active TB, has not had a confirmed case of infectious TB within the past year, and is located in a county in which cases of active TB have not been reported within the previous 2 years. By contrast, stricter guidelines (i.e., isolation rooms for patients with suspected or confirmed infectious TB and use of ventilation equipment) are provided for instances in which employees may have been exposed to the exhaled air of a person with suspected or confirmed TB, or were exposed to a high-hazard procedure performed on a person who may have TB that has the potential to generate aerosols containing potentially infectious respiratory secretions. OSHA requires use of personal protective equipment to reduce employee exposure to hazards. To familiarize themselves with their legal responsibilities, dentists should visit the OSHA Web site at www.osha.gov/pls/oshaweb/owadisp.show_document?p_table=FEDERAL_REGISTER&p_id=13717 (29 CFR Part 1910).

REFERENCES

1. Anthonisen N: Chronic obstructive pulmonary disease. In Goldman L, Ausiello D, editors: *Cecil textbook of medicine*, ed 23, St. Louis, 2008, Saunders, pp 619-626.
2. Global Initiative for Chronic Obstructive Lung Disease (Rodriguez-Roisin R, et al, Executive Committee): *Pocket guide to COPD diagnosis, management, and prevention*, updated 2010 (available online): http://www.goldcopd.org/uploads/users/files/GOLD_Pocket_2010Mar31.pdf. Accessed on March 1, 2011.
3. Centers for Disease Control and Prevention: Deaths from chronic obstructive pulmonary disease—United States 2000-2005, *MMWR Morb Mortal Wkly Rep* 57:1229-1232, 2008.
4. Mannino DM, et al: Obstructive lung disease and low lung function in adults in the United States: data from the National Health and Nutrition Examination Survey, 1988-1994, *Arch Intern Med* 160:1683-1689, 2000.
5. American Lung Association: *Chronic obstructive pulmonary disease fact sheet, 2011* (website): http://www.lungusa.org/lung-disease/copd/resources/facts-figures/COPD-Fact-Sheet.html. Accessed on March 1, 2011.
6. Viegi G, et al: Definition, epidemiology and natural history of COPD, *Eur Respir J* 30:993-1013, 2007.
7. Rodarte J: Chronic bronchitis and emphysema. In Goldman L, Ausiello D, editors: *Cecil textbook of medicine*, ed 22, St. Louis, 2004, Saunders.
8. Anto JM, et al: Epidemiology of chronic obstructive pulmonary disease, *Eur Respir J* 17:982-994, 2001.
9. Soriano JB, et al: Patterns of comorbidities in newly diagnosed COPD and asthma in primary care, *Chest* 128:2099-2107, 2005.
10. Chan KM, Martinez FJ, Chang AC: Nonmedical therapy for chronic obstructive pulmonary disease, *Proc Am Thorac Soc* 6:137-145, 2009.
11. Barnes PJ: New therapies for chronic obstructive pulmonary disease, *Med Princ Pract* 19:330-338, 2010.
12. Abramson MJ, et al: COPDX: an update of guidelines for the management of chronic obstructive pulmonary disease with a review of recent evidence, *Med J Aust* 184:342-345, 2006.
13. Ramseier CA, et al: Consensus report: 2nd European Workshop on Tobacco Use Prevention and Cessation for Oral Health Professionals, *Int Dent J* 60:3-6, 2010.
14. Chandwani BP, et al: Smoking cessation in the dental setting: a practical approach, *Gen Dent* 58:318-323, 2010.

15. Vichitvejpaisal P, et al: Effect of severity of pulmonary disease on nitrous oxide washin and washout characteristics, *J Med Assoc Thai* 80:378-383, 1997.
16. Shakeri-Nejad K, Stahlmann R: Drug interactions during therapy with three major groups of antimicrobial agents, *Expert Opin Pharmacother* 7:639-651, 2006.
17. American Lung Association: *Asthma and children fact sheet* (website): http://www.lungusa.org/lung-disease/asthma/resources/facts-and-figures/asthma-children-fact-sheet.html. Accessed on March 1, 2011.
18. Masoli M, et al: The global burden of asthma: executive summary of the GINA Dissemination Committee report, *Allergy* 59:469-478, 2004.
19. Heraghty JL, Henderson AJ: Highlights in asthma 2005, *Arch Dis Child* 91:422-425, 2006.
20. Gibson PG, McDonald VM, Marks GB: Asthma in older adults, *Lancet* 376:803-813, 2010.
21. McDaniel M, Paxson C, Waldfogel J: Racial disparities in childhood asthma in the United States: evidence from the National Health Interview Survey, 1997 to 2003, *Pediatrics* 117:e868-e877, 2006.
22. Barnes PJ: Asthma. In Fauci AS, et al, editors: *Harrison's principles of internal medicine*, ed 17, New York, 2008, McGraw-Hill Medicine, pp 1596-1627.
23. Barnes PJ: Molecular mechanisms of antiasthma therapy, *Ann Med* 27:531-535, 1995.
24. Murphy DM, O'Byrne PM: Recent advances in the pathophysiology of asthma, *Chest* 137:1417-1426, 2010.
25. Mathison DA, Stevenson DD, Simon RA: Precipitating factors in asthma. Aspirin, sulfites, and other drugs and chemicals, *Chest* 87(1 Suppl):50S-54S, 1985.
26. Babu KS, Salvi SS: Aspirin and asthma, *Chest* 118:1470-1476, 2000.
27. U.S. Department of Health and Human Services: Warning on prescription drugs containing sulfites, *FDA Drug Bull* 17:2-3, 1987.
28. Barrios RJ, et al: Asthma: pathology and pathophysiology, *Arch Pathol Lab Med* 130:447-451, 2006.
29. Braman SS: The global burden of asthma, *Chest* 130(1 Suppl):4S-12S, 2006.
30. Malamed S: *Medical emergencies in the dental office*, ed 6, St. Louis, 2007, Mosby.
31. Elward KS, Pollart SM: Medical therapy for asthma: updates from the NAEPP guidelines, *Am Fam Physician* 82:1242-1251, 2010.
32. Abba AA: Exhaled nitric oxide in diagnosis and management of respiratory diseases, *Ann Thorac Med* 4:173-181, 2009.
33. National Heart, Lung, and Blood Institute, National Asthma Education and Prevention Program: *Expert panel report 3: guidelines for the diagnosis and management of asthma*, Bethesda, Md, 2007, U.S. Department of Health and Human Services, National Institutes of Health, National Heart, Lung, and Blood Institute, rev August.
34. Ernst P, et al: Risk of fatal and near-fatal asthma in relation to inhaled corticosteroid use, *JAMA* 268:3462-3464, 1992.
35. Rees J: Asthma control in adults, *BMJ* 332:767-771, 2006.
36. Di Domenico M, et al: Xolair in asthma therapy: an overview, *Inflamm Allergy Drug Targets* 10:2-12, 2010.
37. Suissa S, Ernst P: Albuterol in mild asthma, *N Engl J Med* 336:729, 1997.
38. Ulrik CS, Frederiksen J: Mortality and markers of risk of asthma death among 1,075 outpatients with asthma, *Chest* 108:10-15, 1995.
39. Mathew T, et al: Effect of dental treatment on the lung function of children with asthma, *J Am Dent Assoc* 129:1120-1128, 1998.
40. Schwartz HJ, et al: Metabisulfite sensitivity and local dental anesthesia, *Ann Allergy* 62:83-86, 1989.
41. Elnabtity MH, et al: Leukotriene modifiers in the management of asthma, *J Am Osteopath Assoc* 99(7 Suppl):S1-S6, 1999.
42. Lazarus SC: Clinical practice. Emergency treatment of asthma, *N Engl J Med* 363:755-764, 2010.
43. Bresolin D, et al: Mouth breathing in allergic children: its relationship to dentofacial development, *Am J Orthod* 83:334-340, 1983.
44. Kargul B, et al: Inhaler medicament effects on saliva and plaque pH in asthmatic children, *J Clin Pediatr Dent* 22:137-140, 1998.
45. Ryberg M, Moller C, Ericson T: Saliva composition and caries development in asthmatic patients treated with beta 2-adrenoceptor agonists: a 4-year follow-up study, *Scand J Dent Res* 99:212-218, 1991.
46. Reddy DK, Hegde AM, Munshi AK: Dental caries status of children with bronchial asthma, *J Clin Pediatr Dent* 27:293-295, 2003.
47. Diagnostic standards and classification of tuberculosis in adults and children, *Am J Respir Crit Care Med* 161(4 Pt 1):1376-1395, 2000.
48. Drugs for ambulatory asthma, *Med Lett Drugs Ther* 33:9-12, 1991.
49. Aziz MA, Wright A: The World Health Organization/International Union Against Tuberculosis and Lung Disease Global Project on Surveillance for Anti-Tuberculosis Drug Resistance: a model for other infectious diseases, *Clin Infect Dis* 41(Suppl 4):S258-S262, 2005.
50. *Global tuberculosis control—epidemiology, strategy, financing*. WHO Report 2009, Geneva, 2009, World Health Organization, (Publication WHO/HTM/TB/2009.411).
51. Centers for Disease Control and Prevention: *CDC fact sheet: tuberculin skin testing* (website): http://www.cdc.gov/tb/publications/factsheets/testing/skintesting.htm. Accessed on March 2, 2011.
52. Cantwell MF, et al: Epidemiology of tuberculosis in the United States, 1985 through 1992, *JAMA* 272:535-539, 1994.
53. Trends in tuberculosis—United States, 2008, *MMWR Morb Mortal Wkly Rep* 58:249-253, 2009.
54. Bradford WZ, Daley CL: Multiple drug-resistant tuberculosis, *Infect Dis Clin North Am* 12:157-172, 1998.
55. Jereb JA, et al: Tuberculosis morbidity in the United States: final data, 1990, *MMWR Surveill Summ* 40:23-27, 1991.
56. Fowler NO: Tuberculous pericarditis, *JAMA* 266:99-103, 1991.
57. Jung RS, et al: Trends in tuberculosis mortality in the United States, 1990-2006: a population-based case-control study, *Public Health Rep* 125:389-397, 2010.
58. Weir MR, Thornton GF: Extrapulmonary tuberculosis. Experience of a community hospital and review of the literature, *Am J Med* 79:467-478, 1985.
59. Salfinger M, Hale YM, Driscoll JR: Diagnostic tools in tuberculosis. Present and future, *Respiration* 65:163-170, 1998.
60. Wells CD: Global impact of multidrug-resistant pulmonary tuberculosis among HIV-infected and other immunocompromised hosts: epidemiology, diagnosis, and strategies for management, *Curr Infect Dis Rep* 12:192-197, 2010.
61. Kaufman E, et al: Intraligamentary injection of slow-release methylprednisolone for the prevention of pain after endodontic treatment, *Oral Surg Oral Med Oral Pathol* 77:651-654, 1994.
62. Holden M, Dubin MR, Diamond PH: Frequency of negative intermediate-strength tuberculin sensitivity in patients with active tuberculosis, *N Engl J Med* 285:1506-1509, 1971.
63. Centers for Disease Control and Prevention, Division of Tuberculosis Elimination: Module 2: Epidemiology of tuberculosis. In *Self-Study Modules on Tuberculosis, 1-5*, Atlanta, 1995, U.S. Department of Health and Human Services.

64. Mazurek GH, et al: Updated guidelines for using interferon gamma release assays to detect *Mycobacterium tuberculosis* infection—United States, 2010, *MMWR Recomm Rep* 59(RR-5):1-25, 2010.
65. Fair E, Hopewell PC, Pai M: International Standards for Tuberculosis Care: revisiting the cornerstones of tuberculosis care and control, *Expert Rev Anti Infect Ther* 5:61-65, 2007.
66. Centers for Disease Control and Prevention: *Tuberculosis fact sheets: treatment* (website): http://www.cdc.gov/tb/publications/factsheets/treatment.htm. Accessed on March 1, 2011.
67. Bacteriologic conversion of sputum among tuberculosis patients—United States, *MMWR Morb Mortal Wkly Rep* 34:747-750, 1985.
68. Ravikrishnan KP: Tuberculosis. How can we halt its resurgence? *Postgrad Med* 91:333-338, 1992.
69. Jensen PA, et al: Guidelines for preventing the transmission of *Mycobacterium tuberculosis* in health-care settings, 2005, *MMWR Recomm Rep* 54(RR-17):1-141, 2005.
70. Kaufmann SH: Future vaccination strategies against tuberculosis: thinking outside the box, *Immunity* 33:567-577, 2010.
71. Centers for Disease Control and Prevention: Guidelines for preventing the transmission of tuberculosis in health-care facilities, *MMWR Morb Mortal Wkly Rep* 43(RR-13):1-132, 1994.
72. Taylor Z, Nolan CM, Blumberg HM: Controlling tuberculosis in the United States. Recommendations from the American Thoracic Society, CDC, and the Infectious Diseases Society of America, *MMWR Recomm Rep* 54(RR-12):1-81, 2005.
73. Bass JB Jr, et al: Treatment of tuberculosis and tuberculosis infection in adults and children. American Thoracic Society and the Centers for Disease Control and Prevention, *Am J Respir Crit Care Med* 149:1359-1374, 1994.
74. Forget EJ, Menzies D: Adverse reactions to first-line antituberculosis drugs, *Expert Opin Drug Saf* 5:231-249, 2006.
75. Kakisi OK, et al: Tuberculosis of the oral cavity: a systematic review, *Eur J Oral Sci* 118:103-109, 2010.
76. Florio S, Ellis E 3rd, Frost DE: Persistent submandibular swelling after tooth extraction, *J Oral Maxillofac Surg*; 55:390-397, 1997.
77. Bhargava S, et al: Case report: tuberculosis of the parotid gland—diagnosis by CT, *Br J Radiol* 69:1181-1183, 1996.
78. Helbling CA, et al: Primary tuberculosis of the TMJ: presentation of a case and literature review, *Int J Oral Maxillofac Surg* 39:834-838, 2010.
79. Grosskurth H, et al: Impact of improved treatment of sexually transmitted diseases on HIV infection in rural Tanzania: randomised controlled trial, *Lancet* 346:530-536, 1995.

8

Smoking and Tobacco Use Cessation

The habitual use of tobacco by smoking (cigarettes, cigars, pipes) or as smokeless products (chewing tobacco, snuff) typically constitutes an addictive disease that continues to be a major public health problem. Smoking is the leading cause of preventable death and disease in the United States, resulting in an estimated 443,000 premature deaths per year and $193 billion in direct health care costs and lost productivity.[1] In addition, more than 8.6 million persons are disabled as a consequence of smoking-related diseases.[2] Smoking causes more than twice as many deaths as human immunodeficiency virus (HIV) infection and acquired immunodeficiency syndrome (AIDS), alcohol abuse, motor vehicle crashes, illicit drug use, and suicide combined.[3] On average, smokers die 10 years earlier than nonsmokers.[4]

With their perspective on the health of the oral cavity and upper airway, directly observed in routine clinical practice, dentists are in a unique position to provide assessment, advice, and referral for smoking cessation. This chapter summarizes current knowledge applicable to this role for the dental health professional, with content encompassing the following topics:

- The physical and psychological effects of smoking and tobacco use
- The basic principles involved in a smoking cessation program
- Approaches used for smoking cessation and the success rates for each
- Available nicotine replacement products and how they are used
- Drugs used in smoking cessation programs and how they are used
- The basics of counseling and other support for the patient who wishes to stop smoking

SYSTEMIC AND ORAL EFFECTS OF SMOKING

Cigarette smoking is a major risk factor for stroke, myocardial infarction, peripheral vascular disease, aortic aneurysm, and sudden death. It is the leading cause of lung disease, including chronic obstructive pulmonary disease (COPD), pneumonia, and lung cancer. It also is strongly linked to cancers of the mouth, esophagus, stomach, pancreas, cervix, kidney, colon, and bladder. Other effects include premature skin aging and an increased risk for cataracts. Cigar and pipe smokers are subject to addictive and general health risks similar to those for cigarette smokers, although pipe and cigar users typically do not inhale. Oral effects of smoking include squamous cell carcinoma (Figure 8-1), leukoplakia (Figure 8-2), nicotine stomatitis (Figure 8-3), smoker's melanosis, hairy tongue (Figure 8-4), and halitosis. Smoking increases the risk of failure of intraosseous implants and the risk of dry socket, and it also is associated with impaired wound healing.[5,6]

The adverse effects of smokeless tobacco consist primarily of addiction and pathologic changes in the oral mucosa, including squamous cell carcinoma, tobacco or snuff dipper's pouch (Figure 8-5), verrucous carcinoma (Figure 8-6), gingival recession (Figure 8-7), periodontitis, and necrotizing ulcerative gingivitis (Figure 8-8). The senses of taste and smell are diminished as well. Evidence suggests that smokeless tobacco use may be associated with adverse pregnancy outcomes and pancreatic cancer.[7,8]

Health care professionals must be vigilant in identifying those patients who use tobacco, with goals of encouraging them to stop smoking and assisting them in their efforts. Studies indicate that 70% of smokers want to quit smoking.[9] For every smoker who successfully quits, however, many more do not succeed. Tobacco dependence is a chronic condition that often requires repeated attempts at intervention. Smokers typically fail multiple attempts to quit before they achieve success.

SCOPE OF THE PROBLEM

It is estimated that approximately 20.6% (46 million) of adults older than 18 years of age in the United States are current smokers, and that of these, 78.1% (36.4 million) smoke every day.[10] Thus, in a dental practice of 2000 patients, approximately 400 of them will be smokers. The overall prevalence of cigarette smoking is lower than the 21.6% rate reported in 2003 and is significantly

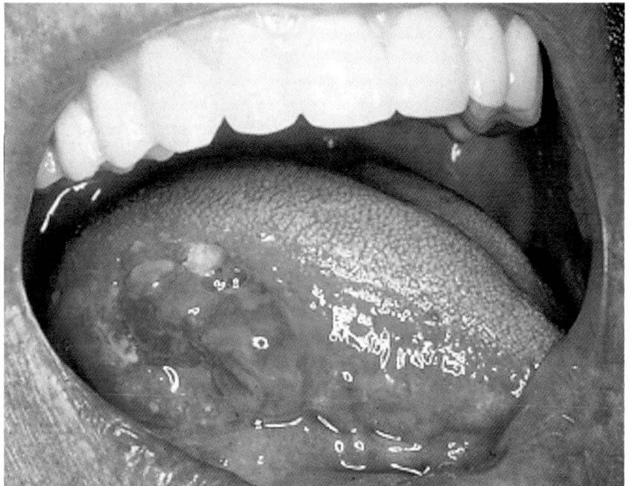

FIGURE 8-1 Squamous cell carcinoma of the tongue in a heavy cigarette smoker.

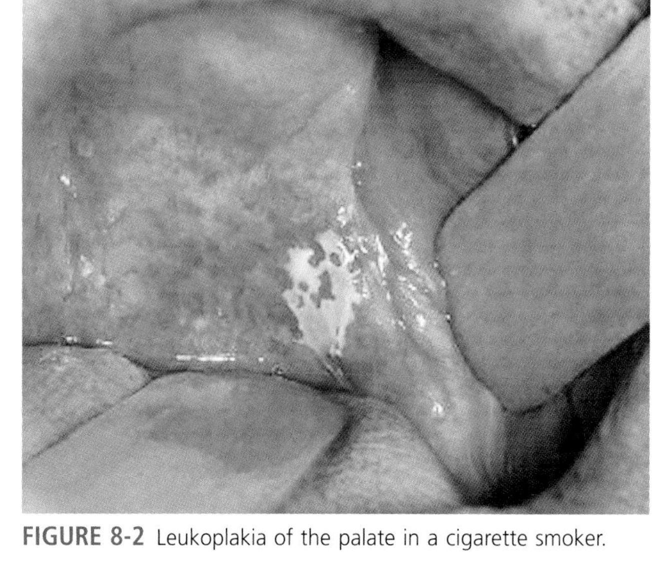

FIGURE 8-2 Leukoplakia of the palate in a cigarette smoker.

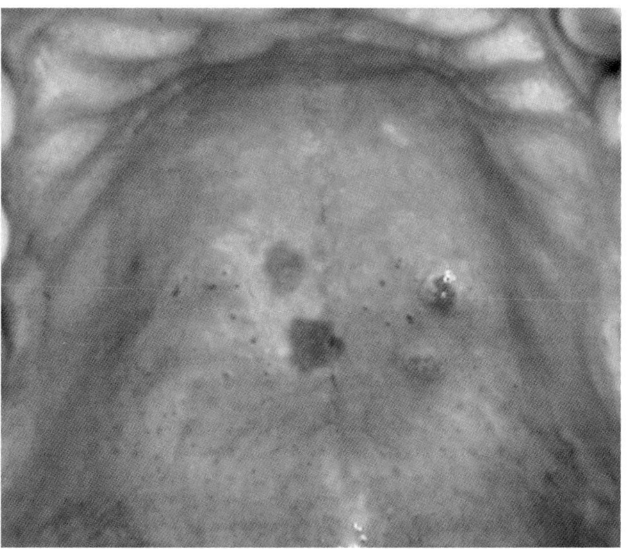

FIGURE 8-3 Severe nicotine stomatitis in a pipe smoker. Smoker's melanosis is evident in the palatal vault.

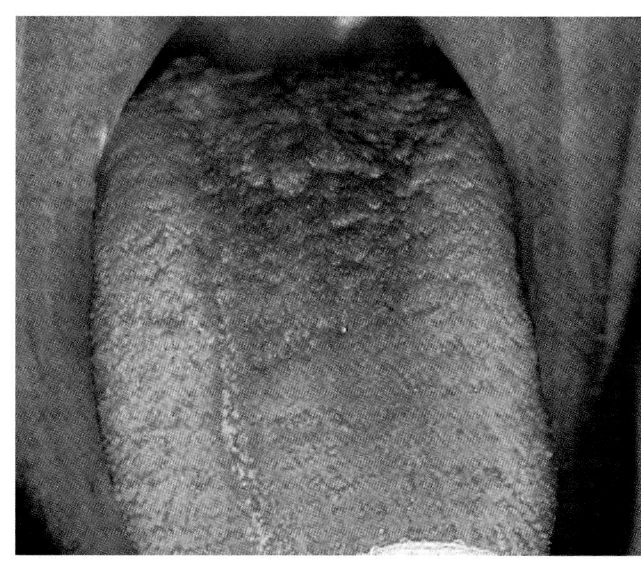

FIGURE 8-4 Brown hairy tongue in a cigarette smoker.

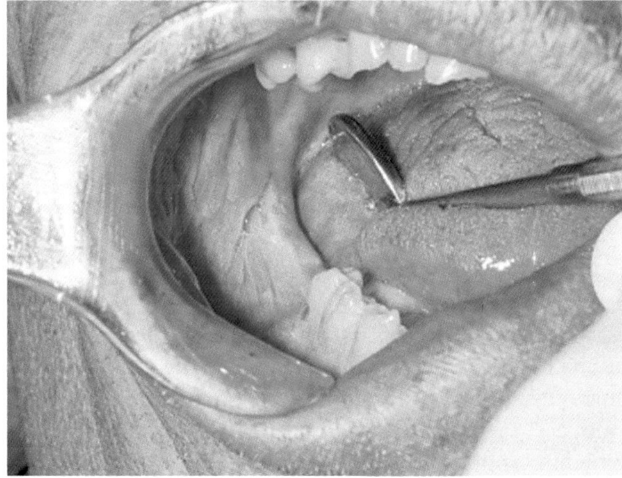

FIGURE 8-5 Tobacco pouch in the vestibule of a tobacco chewer. Note corrugated appearance of the vestibular mucosa.

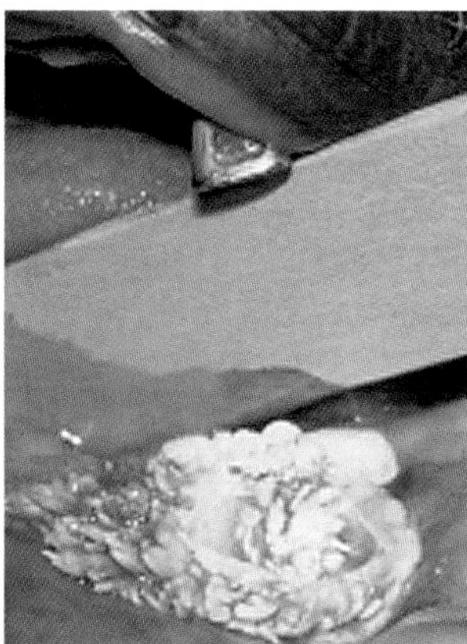

FIGURE 8-6 Verrucous carcinoma in a snuff user.

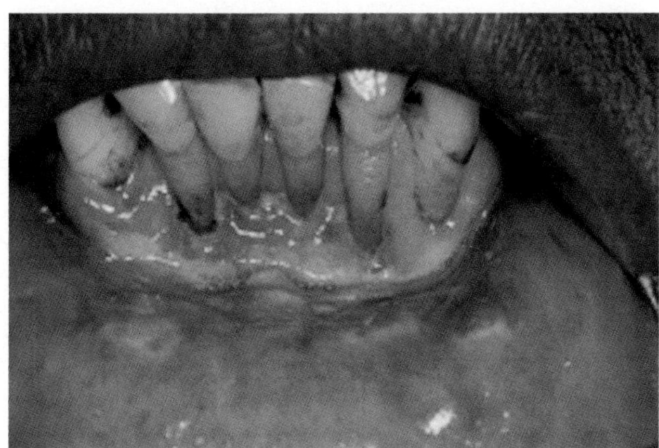

FIGURE 8-7 Gingival recession and leukoplakia in the area where snuff is held.

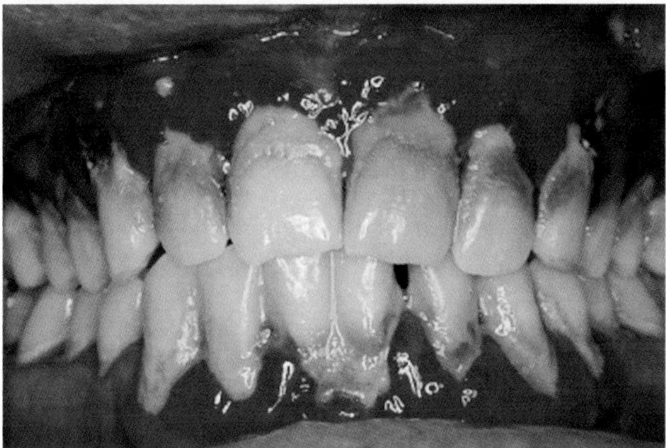

FIGURE 8-8 Necrotizing ulcerative gingivitis in a cigarette smoker.

lower than the 22.5% rate reported in 2002; however, these declines have stalled in the past 5 years, barely dropping from 20.9% in 2005 to 20.6% in 2009.[10] From 1993 through 2004, the percentage of daily smokers who smoked more than 25 cigarettes per day (CPD) (i.e., heavy smokers) decreased steadily, from 19.1% to 12.1%. The mean CPD count among daily smokers was 19.6 in 1993, falling to 16.8 in 2004. Although this trend is encouraging, the problem continues to be a serious public health issue.

The prevalence of current cigarette smoking varies substantially across population subgroups.[10] Current smoking rates are higher among men (23.5%) than among women (17.9%). Among racial and ethnic populations, Asians (12%) and Hispanics (14.5%) have the lowest prevalence of current smoking; multiracial persons have the highest (29.5%), followed by Native Americans and Native Alaskans (23.2%), non-Hispanic whites (22.1%), and non-Hispanic blacks (21.3%). By education level, current smoking is most prevalent among adults who have earned a graduate educational development (GED) diploma (49.1%) and lowest in those with a graduate degree (5.6%). Persons older than 65 years of age exhibit the lowest prevalence of current cigarette smoking (9.5%) among all adults. Current smoking prevalence is higher among adults who live below the poverty level (31.1%) than among those at or above the poverty level (19.4%). Smoking prevalence also varies significantly by state or other geographic area, ranging from 9.8% in Utah to 25.6% in Kentucky and West Virginia.

The use of smokeless tobacco is seen primarily in men and adolescent boys who are rural residents of southern and western states; in whites and Native Americans and Native Alaskans; and in persons with lower levels of education.[11] Prevalence is highest in Wyoming (9.1%), West Virginia (8.5%), and Mississippi (7.5%) and lowest in California (1.3%), the District of Columbia (1.5%), Massachusetts (1.5%), and Rhode Island (1.5%).[12] The use of smokeless tobacco became a national public health issue in the early to mid-1980s, when tobacco companies aggressively marketed their products by targeting young people. This practice was halted as a result of Congressional legislation and resulted in a gradual decline in prevalence, from 6.1% in 1987 to 4.5% in 2000. Of historical interest is the recommendation by some health care professionals that smokeless tobacco be promoted to cigarette smokers as a safer alternative for those who are having difficulty quitting smoking (harm reduction); current evidence questions the efficacy of such a practice.[13-15]

The economic impact of smoking is staggering. On a national level, the U.S. Public Health Service estimates a total annual cost of $50 billion for the treatment of patients with smoking-related disease, in addition to $47 billion in lost wages and productivity. For the individual smoker, the economic impact of smoking can be substantial, especially because as noted, smoking is more common among persons with limited financial resources. Smokers pay more for life and health insurance, the resale value of their cars and homes is decreased, and they have increased costs for dry cleaning, and of course medical and dental care. The cost of a pack of cigarettes varies, reflecting differences in excise taxes levied by states, counties, and cities, in addition to that imposed by the federal government.[16] The current federal excise tax is $1.01/pack. State-imposed cigarette tax ranges from a high of $2.75/pack (in New York) to a low of $0.07/pack (in South Carolina); the national average is $1.20/pack. Additional county and city taxes may add as much as $1.50 more (in New York City). States may have additional miscellaneous administrative fees. When all taxes and fees are taken into consideration, the average cost of a pack of cigarettes in the United States is higher than $5. Table 8-1 presents calculations of the average annual costs incurred by cigarette smokers, depending on how many packs are smoked per day and the cost of a pack of cigarettes. In comparison, the average daily costs for smoking cessation products are

TABLE 8-1 Annual Costs of Cigarette Smoking

Rate of Consumption	Annual Cost by Purchase Price		
	$4/Pack	$5/Pack	$6/Pack
1 pack/day	$1460	$1825	$2190
2 packs/day	$2920	$3350	$4380
3 packs/day	$4380	$5475	$6570

estimated to be $3.91 for the patch, $5.81 for the gum, $4.98 for the lozenges, and $4.30 for sustained-release bupropion.[17] These costs may vary, depending on the strengths used, and unlike cigarettes, which are purchased on a regular basis, these products will be used for only a limited period of time (several weeks or months). These cost comparisons should be brought forward when patients express concern about the cost of purchasing nicotine replacement products or medications.

BENEFITS OF QUITTING

People who quit smoking live longer than those who continue to smoke, because the chances for development of smoking-related fatal diseases begin to lessen immediately with cessation of smoking.[18] The extent to which a smoker's risk is reduced by quitting is dependent on several factors, including number of years as a smoker, number of cigarettes smoked per day, and presence or absence of disease at the time of quitting. Data show that persons who quit smoking before the age of 50 have half the risk of dying in the next 15 years compared with those who continue to smoke. Risks of dying of lung cancer are 22 times higher among male smokers and 12 times higher among female smokers than in those who have never smoked. The risk of dying of coronary heart disease for smokers is double that for lifetime nonsmokers, as is the risk of dying from a stroke. Smoking increases the risk for development of COPD by accelerating the age-related decline in lung function. Box 8-1 lists short-term and long-term benefits of smoking cessation.

BOX 8-1 Benefits of Quitting Smoking

Long-Term Benefits—Timeline*

- *20 minutes after quitting:* Heart rate drops.
- *12 hours after quitting:* Carbon monoxide level in the blood drops to normal.
- *2 weeks to 3 months after quitting:* Circulation improves and lung function increases.
- *1 to 9 months after quitting:* Coughing and shortness of breath decrease; cilia—tiny hairlike structures that move mucus out of the lungs—regain normal function, increasing the ability to handle mucus, clean the lungs, and reduce the risk of infection.
- *1 year after quitting:* The excess risk of coronary heart disease is half that of a smoker's.
- *5 years after quitting:* Stroke risk is reduced to that of a nonsmoker 5 to 15 years after quitting.
- *10 years after quitting:* The lung cancer death rate is about half that of a continuing smoker. Risks of cancer of the mouth, throat, esophagus, bladder, cervix, and pancreas decrease.
- *15 years after quitting:* The risk of coronary heart disease is that of a nonsmoker.

Short-Term Benefits—More Immediate Effects

- Quitting helps stop the damaging effects of tobacco on physical appearance, including:
  - Premature wrinkling of the skin
  - Bad breath
  - Stained teeth
  - Gum disease
  - Bad-smelling clothes and hair
  - Yellow fingernails
- Food tastes better.
- Sense of smell returns to normal.
- Ordinary activities (e.g., climbing stairs, light housework) no longer leave the patient out of breath.

**Data from 2004 Surgeon General's report*—The health consequences of smoking: Within 20 minutes of quitting. *U.S. Dept. of Health and Human Services. http://www.cdc.gov/tobacco/data_statistics/sgr/sgr_2004/posters/20mins.htm. Accessed November 17, 2011.*

ADDICTION TO NICOTINE

Smoking is a learned or conditioned behavior that is reinforced by the effects of nicotine.[19] Cigarettes promote this conditioning in that they allow precise dosing that can be repeated as often as necessary to avoid discomfort and produce maximal desired effects. In addition, smoking behavior is reinforced by and associated with common daily events such as awakening, eating, and socializing. Thus, these associations become almost unavoidable parts of smokers' lives.

Nicotine is a highly addictive drug that has been equated with heroin, cocaine, and amphetamine in terms of addiction potential and its effects on brain neurochemistry.[20,21] The addictive and behavioral effects of nicotine are complex and are due primarily to its action on dopaminergic pathways. The physiologic and behavioral effects of nicotine include increased heart rate, increased cardiac output, increased blood pressure, appetite suppression, a strong sense of pleasure and well-being, improved task performance, and reduced anxiety. Tolerance develops with repeated exposure, so that over time, it takes more and more nicotine to produce the same level of effect.

Nicotine is absorbed through the skin and the mucosal lining of the nose and mouth and by inhalation into the lungs. A cigarette is a very efficient delivery system for the inhalation of nicotine. Nicotine is rapidly distributed throughout the body after inhalation, reaching the brain in as little as 10 seconds. Mucosal absorption from smokeless tobacco is slower, but the effects are more sustained. Nicotine that is swallowed is not well absorbed in the stomach, because of the acidic environment. The effects of nicotine gradually diminish over 30 to 120 minutes; this produces withdrawal effects that may include agitation, restlessness, anxiety, difficulty concentrating, insomnia, hunger, and a conscious craving for the usual source of nicotine. The elimination half-life of nicotine is about 2 hours, which allows it to accumulate with repeated exposure to cigarettes throughout the day, with effects persisting for hours.[19] A typical smoker will take 10 puffs of every cigarette over a period of about 5 minutes that the cigarette is lit. Each cigarette delivers about 1 mg of nicotine. Thus, a person who smokes about 1½ packs (30 cigarettes) a day gets 300 hits of nicotine to the brain every day, each one within 10 seconds after a puff.[22] This repeated reinforcement is a strong contributor to the highly addictive nature of nicotine.

INTERVENTIONS FOR SMOKING CESSATION

Numerous interventions have been devised to encourage and assist the cessation of smoking and tobacco use. Public health measures include raising awareness of the dangers of smoking and tobacco use by airing public service annoucements on television or radio, increasing the price of cigarettes and other tobacco products, and banning smoking in public places. Individually directed methods of smoking cessation include the use of telephone quit lines, nicotine replacement therapy (NRT), and non-NRT pharmacotherapy with various medications, along with individual or group counseling.

Overall success rates for smoking cessation efforts are disappointingly low, and quitting is associated with high rates of relapse. The 1-year success rate for stopping "cold turkey" is about 5%. The use of telephone quit lines or brief counseling roughly doubles the chance of success, as does the use of any of the NRT products.[23] The 1-year success rate with bupropion is about 23%.[24] Varenicline appears to be as effective as bupropion.[25] NRT combined with bupropion improves the success rate to about 36%.[26] One study[27] reported a success rate of 38.5% when a combination of NRT plus bupropion was used, along with intensive counseling. Of interest, in one report, a program that used only intensive counseling yielded a success rate of 68%.[28] In general, the chance for success increases when more than one option is used, and counseling combined with NRT or medication significantly improves outcomes.[9]

On an individual basis, health care providers should ask their patients about smoking or tobacco use at each appointment, advise current users to quit, and assist those who express an interest in quitting. In 2008, the U.S. Department of Health and Human Services Public Health Service published an update of the earlier 2000 Clinical Practice Guidelines for Treating Tobacco Use and Dependence,[9] to aid health care professionals in helping their patients to quit smoking. These guidelines are based on the "5 As":

Asking patients about their tobacco use
Advising those who use tobacco to quit
Assessing the willingness of patients to make a quit attempt
Assisting in the quit attempt
Arranging for follow-up

The effectiveness of the 5 As initiative has been disappointing. Very few dentists or physicians are even aware of the 5 As, much less follow them.[29,30] Reasons most often cited by dentists for not incorporating smoking cessation services into their practices include time involved, lack of training, lack of reimbursement, lack of knowledge of available referral sources, and lack of patient education materials. In view of the poor outcomes with the 5 As approach, the following alternative approach has been suggested[17]:

- *Ask*
- *Advise*
- *Refer* (to an internal resource, an external resource, or a telephone quit line)

This approach requires the practitioner to be familiar with available referral sources.

INITIATING SMOKING CESSATION THERAPY

It should be made clear to patients that the dental office is a nonsmoking facility. Signs should be posted that clearly state this. No ash trays should be placed in the office. Dental health professionals should ask all patients about their use of tobacco. This can be easily accomplished by inclusion of tobacco use questions on the medical or dental history, followed by a brief interview. For patients who are current tobacco users, additional information, including the type of tobacco product used, the frequency of use, and the length of time the product has been used, should be ascertained. During the oral mucosa examination, mucosal changes associated with tobacco use should be noted and the patient should be advised of their presence and the association with tobacco use. Patients who use smokeless tobacco should be asked where they hold the tobacco in the mouth, and special attention should be paid to examination of that area. Any oral changes or concomitant systemic diseases that may be related to tobacco use should be discussed in that context, as motivation to quit smoking. Patients should then be asked whether they have ever considered quitting, and whether they would like to quit. They should be made aware that the dentist supports and encourages their quitting to improve their overall health and will assist them in their efforts to quit.

If a patient does not express the wish to quit, the dentist can point out the benefits of quitting as a potential method of motivating the patient. If the patient demonstrates resistance to further intervention, the subject should be dropped without subsequent "badgering." It generally is counterproductive to pursue the issue; however, patients can be reassured that if at any time they would like to quit, the dentist is available to provide appropriate support. At subsequent recall appointments, brief and tactful follow-up questioning can ascertain whether the patient has given any more thought to quitting smoking. If and when the patient indicates a readiness to quit, the practitioner has several options:

- Help to coordinate a cessation program for the patient, or designate another person (auxiliary) in the office to perform that function.
- Prescribe smoking cessation medications for the patient.
- Refer the patient to an outside smoking cessation program.
- Refer the patient to the primary care physician.
- Refer the patient to a counseling source, such as a telephone help line.

As described next, many options and resources are available to assist patients in the effort to quit smoking. Whether or how many of these interventions are implemented from the dental office will depend on how involved the practitioner wishes to become.

Patient Education Literature

To encourage and support tobacco use cessation, practitioners should have appropriate educational and motivational reading materials available for patients visiting the dental office. Posters can be placed on the walls of the waiting room and treatment areas. Brochures may be kept in the waiting room and in treatment areas as handouts for patients who express a desire to quit. Patient education materials are readily available from sources such as the American Cancer Society, the National Cancer Institute, and the Office of the Surgeon General. These materials can be ordered by telephone or through the agency's Web site (Box 8-2). Brochures or other handouts may be used to provide telephone quit line numbers or for referral to local smoking cessation programs or support groups. Practitioners also may wish to develop their own patient education materials.

Counseling

Even brief counseling, such as that occurring when a health care professional routinely asks about smoking and encourages quitting, has been shown to increase quit success rates. Telephone counseling help lines (quit lines) are now widely available and have been shown to double success rates over those reported with quitting "cold turkey." Help lines are available on national, regional, and state levels (see Box 8-2). Help lines provide the opportunity for the patient to speak to a counselor and can provide needed support, regardless of whether the person is considering quitting is attempting to quit, has successfully quit, or has relapsed. Group counseling can be especially effective by providing social support and encouragement from other people experiencing similar challenges.

Counseling typically consists of both cognitive and behavioral therapies. Cognitive therapy attempts to change the way a patient thinks about smoking, whereas behavioral therapy attempts to help the smoker avoid situations that might trigger the desire to smoke. Evidence has shown that the more intensive the counseling, the higher the success rate, and that when counseling is combined with other forms of therapy, such as nicotine replacement therapy (NRT) or pharmacotherapy, it is even more effective. Local, regional, and state health departments may be good sources for smoking cessation counseling and other programs.

BOX 8-2 Resources for Support Material

Telephone Help/Quit Lines

- 1-800-QUITNOW: Department of Health and Human Services national quit line
- 1-877-44-U-QUIT: National Cancer Institute dedicated quit smoking line
- 1-877-YES-QUIT: American Cancer Society quit line
- 1-800-4-CANCER: Cancer Information Service, National Cancer Institute

Helpful Web Sites

- www.surgeongeneral.gov/tobacco/
- www.smokefree.gov/
- www.nlm.nih.gov/medlineplus/smokingcessation.html
- www.cancer.gov/cancertopics/pdq/prevention/control-of-tobacco-use/HealthProfessional
- www.cdc.gov/tobacco/
- www.cancer.org/docroot/PED/content/PED_10_13X_Guide_for_Quitting_Smoking.asp

Nicotine Replacement Therapy

The rationale for nicotine replacement therapy (NRT) is to replace cigarettes or smokeless tobacco with a source of nicotine that does not have the tars and carbon monoxide of tobacco, and then gradually reduce the use of that replacement product to the point of abstinence. To prevent withdrawal symptoms, a smoker must maintain a baseline blood level of nicotine of about 15 to 18 ng/mL. Smoking one cigarette rapidly increases nicotine blood levels to 35 to 40 ng/mL, producing the "hit" or "rush" experienced with smoking; this level then gradually returns to baseline within about 25 to 30 minutes.

NRT attempts to provide a blood level that is adequate to prevent withdrawal symptoms without producing the "hit" or "rush" caused by the cigarette. The patient then gradually learns to accept progressively lower and lower blood nicotine levels and, finally, total abstinence.[22]

Five distinct types of nicotine replacement products are available that differ in cost, route of delivery, and efficiency of delivery of nicotine. These are the transdermal patch, gum, lozenges, the inhaler, and nasal spray (Table 8-2). All of these NRT products have been approved by the U.S. Food and Drug Administration (FDA) for smoking cessation. They all appear to be effective when included as part of a program of smoking cessation, and use of such products generally doubles the chance of success over that for quitting "cold turkey."[23] Selection of an NRT product is dependent on the number of cigarettes smoked per day, its potential adverse effects, and patient preference. Generally, the more dependent the patient is on nicotine, the higher the beginning doses that will be required, and the greater will be the need to

TABLE 8-2 Nicotine Replacement Products

Product	How Supplied	How Used	Adverse Effects	Advantages/ Disadvantages
Nicotine Transdermal Patches (OTC)				
Nicoderm CQ Nicorette Nicotrol, generic	7, 14, 21 mg 5, 10, 15 mg 5, 10, 15 mg	Start with patches of highest concentration; then use patches of progressively lower concentration over a 6- to 12-week period	Skin irritation, insomnia	Slow onset; takes 6 to 8 hours to reach peak blood level; cannot be readily titrated
Nicotine Gum (OTC)				
Nicorette, generic	Available in strengths of 2 mg and 4 mg	Not to be chewed as normal gum; should be chewed slightly and then "parked" in the vestibule; repeat chew-park sequence every 30 minutes; nicotine is absorbed through the mucosa; do not eat or drink for 15 minutes before using or while using; start with 8 to 24 pieces/day and gradually reduce over several weeks; maximum, 24/day	Mucosal irritation; indigestion	Quicker delivery than patch but not as quick as lozenge; produces less of a "rush" than is produced by cigarettes or lozenges
Nicotine Lozenges (OTC)				
Commit	Available in strengths of 2 mg and 4 mg	Strength required is determined by time to first cigarette in the morning; lozenge "parked" and moistened and allowed to dissolve in the mouth; start with 9 to 20/day and use progressively fewer per day over a 12-week period; do not eat or drink for 15 minutes before using or while using; maximum, 20/day	Gingival and throat irritation; indigestion	Peak blood levels in 20 to 30 minutes; 25% higher blood levels than gum; can be titrated as needed; very efficient; produces less of a rush than is caused by cigarettes but more of a rush than is produced by gum
Nicotine Nasal Spray (Prescription)				
Nicotrol NS	Supplied in a pump nasal spray bottle	One dose is a spray into each nostril; maximum of 40 doses per day is progressively decreased over 10 to 12 weeks	Nose and throat irritation	Fastest delivery system; provides the rush of cigarettes
Nicotine Inhaler (Prescription)				
Nicotrol Inhaler	Supplied as plastic cartridges; each cartridge provides 4 mg of nicotine (only 2 mg is absorbed)	Each inhaler contains 400 puffs; 80 puffs is equal to 1 cigarette; maximum, 16 cartridges/day; gradually decreased usage over several months	Mouth and throat irritation	Inefficient delivery system; expensive

OTC, Over-the-counter.

TABLE 8-3 Non–Nicotine Replacement Therapy Pharmacotherapeutic Agents

Drug	Dosage	Adverse Effects	Precautions/Advantages
Bupropion SR (Zyban)	150 mg daily for 3 days, then 150 mg twice a day for 2 to 3 months; begin 1 to 2 weeks before quit date and continue for at least 2 to 3 months	Dry mouth, insomnia	Contraindicated in patients with history of seizures or at risk for seizures; may prevent weight gain
Varenicline (Chantix)	Starting 1 week before quit date, 0.5 mg daily for 3 days, then 0.5 mg twice a day for 4 days, then 1.0 mg twice daily for 12 weeks	Nausea, insomnia, flatulence, headache; may cause mood changes, including depression and suicidal ideation	No clinically relevant drug interactions have been identified; may cause taste disturbance

titrate nicotine levels. For very dependent smokers, the combination of a patch with a shorter-acting product such as gum, lozenge, or nasal spray may be indicated. The combination of NRT with counseling also improves chances for success.

Non–Nicotine Replacement Therapy Pharmacotherapy

Another first-line, FDA-approved, non-NRT pharmacotherapeutic smoking cessation agent is slow-release bupropion, an atypical antidepressant that is thought to affect the dopaminergic and/or noradrenergic pathways involved in nicotine addiction. Bupropion is effective when used alone or in combination with an NRT product and/or counseling. An attractive feature of bupropion is that it may prevent weight gain, which is a common adverse effect of smoking cessation. It is contraindicated in patients with seizure disorders or in those who may be prone to seizures.

The most recently FDA-approved pharmacotherapeutic agent is varenicline. This novel medication is an $\alpha4\beta2$ nicotinic receptor partial agonist that stimulates dopamine and blocks nicotinic receptors, thereby preventing the reward and reinforcement associated with smoking.[31] This medication should be started 3 days before the target quit date and is taken for 12 weeks. It appears to be as effective as bupropion.[25] Reports of depression and suicidal ideation resulted in a change in product labeling; however, these effects have not been substantiated (Table 8-3).

Additional treatment strategies with less proven efficacy include the use of monoamine oxidase inhibitors, selective serotonin reuptake inhibitors, opioid receptor antagonists, bromocriptine, antianxiety drugs, nicotinic receptor antagonists, and glucose tablets. Various agents under investigation are partial nicotine agonists, anticonvulsants, inhibitors of the hepatic P-450 enzyme system, cannaboid-1 receptor antagonists, and nicotine vaccines.[32] Approaches to smoking cessation based in alternative or complementary medicine have been advocated; however, because of the lack of evidence of effectiveness, their use cannot be supported at this time.[33]

Reimbursement for Smoking Cessation Therapy

One of the reasons often cited by the dental health professional for not providing smoking cessation services is the lack of meaningful reimbursement for the time and effort required. This continues to be a problem in many states. Inconsistency has been noted in the coverage provided by managed care organizations and by state Medicaid and Medicare programs.

The decision to bill for smoking cessation services depends on the amount of time spent and the degree of involvement of the practitioner. In many instances, assessment, advice, and referral may occur within the context of the normal patient health history and examination; thus, the time specifically devoted to smoking cessation counseling is likely to be minimal, with such services covered by the normal examination fee. If more time is spent in actual counseling and monitoring of a patient's progress, billing for that service would certainly be appropriate.

If it is decided to bill for a separate procedure, the International Classification of Diseases (ICD)-9 code 305.1 (Tobacco Use Disorder: Tobacco Dependence) should be used. The Code for Dental Terminology (CDT) D1320 (Tobacco Counseling for the Control and Prevention of Oral Disease) is specifically designated for use by dental practitioners. Practitioners should check with individual programs and carriers to determine whether these services are covered.

REFERENCES

1. Centers for Disease Control and Prevention (CDC): Smoking-attributable mortality, years of potential life lost, and productivity losses—Uited States, 2000-2004, *MMWR Morb Mortal Wkly Rep* 57:1226-1228, 2008.
2. Schroeder S: Tobacco control in the wake of the 1998 master settlement agreement, *N Engl J Med* 350:293-301, 2004.
3. Centers for Disease Control and Prevention (CDC): Smoking attributable mortality, years of potential life lost, and productivity losses-United States 2000-2004, *MMWR Morb Mortal Wkly Rep* 57(45):1226-1228, 2008.
4. Doll R, et al: Mortality in relation to smoking: 50 years' observations on male British doctors, *BMJ* 328:1519, 2004.

5. Anner R, et al: Smoking, diabetes mellitus, periodontitis, and supportive periodontal treatment as factors associated with dental implant survival: a long-term retrospective evaluation of patients followed for up to 10 years, *Implant Dent* 19:57-64, 2010.
6. Noroozi AR, Philbert RF: Modern concepts in understanding and management of the "dry socket" syndrome: comprehensive review of the literature, *Oral Surg Oral Med Oral Pathol Oral Radiol Endod* 107:30-35, 2009.
7. Alguacil J, Silverman D: Smokeless and other noncigarette use and pancreatic cancer: a case-control study based on direct interviews, *Cancer Epidemiol Biomarkers Prev* 13:55-58, 2004.
8. England L, et al: Adverse pregnancy outcomes in snuff users, *Am J Obstet Gynecol* 189:939-943, 2003.
9. Fiore MC, Jaen CR, Baker TB: *Treating tobacco use and dependence: 2008 update. Clinical practice guideline*, Rockville, MD, 2008, U.S. Department of Health and Human Services, Public Health Service.
10. Centers for Disease Control and Prevention (CDC): Vital signs: current cigarette smoking among adults ≥18 years—United States 2009, *MMWR Morbid Mortal Wkly Rep* 59:1135-1140, 2010.
11. Nelson D, et al: Trends in smokeless tobacco use among adults and adolescents in the United States, *Am J Public Health* 96:897-905, 2006.
12. Centers for Disease Control and Prevention (CDC): State-specific prevalence of cigarette smoking and smokeless tobacco use among adults—United States, 2009, *MMWR Morbid Mortal Wkly Rep* 59:1400-1406, 2010.
13. Kozlowski L: Harm reduction, public health, and human rights: smokers have a right to be informed of significant harm reduction options, *Nicotine and Tob Res* 4(Suppl 2):S55-S60, 2002.
14. Klesges RC, et al: Tobacco use harm reduction, elimination, and escalation in a large military cohort, *Am J Public Health* 100:2487-2492, 2010.
15. Colilla SA: An epidemiologic review of smokeless tobacco health effects and harm reduction potential, *Regul Toxicol Pharmacol* 56:197-211, 2010.
16. Centers for Disease Control and Prevention (CDC): Federal and state cigarette excise taxes—United States, 1995-2009, *MMWR Morb Mortal Wkly Rep* 58:524-527, 2009.
17. Schroeder SA: What to do with a patient who smokes, *JAMA* 294:482-487, 2005.
18. U.S. Department of Health and Human Services: *The health benefits of smoking cessation: a report of the surgeon general, 1990*, DHHS Publication No. (CDC) 90-8416, Rockville, MD, 1990, Public Health Service, Centers for Disease Control, Office on Smoking and Health.
19. Dani JA, Harris RA: Nicotine addiction and comorbidity with alcohol abuse and mental illness, *Nat Neurosci* 8:1465-1470, 2005.
20. Benowitz NL: Neurobiology of nicotine addiction: implications for smoking cessation treatment, *Am J Med* 121(4 Suppl 1):S3-S10, 2008.
21. Jha P, et al: Tobacco addiction. In Jamison DT, et al, editors: *Disease control priorities in developing countries*, ed 2, Washington, DC, 2006, World Bank.
22. Cooper TM, Clayton RR: *The Cooper/Clayton method to stop smoking*, Lexington, KY, 2004, Institute for Comprehensive Behavioral Smoking Cessation.
23. Silagy C, et al: Nicotine replacement therapy for smoking cessation, *Cochrane Database Syst Rev* 3:CD000146, 2004.
24. Hurt RD, et al: A comparison of sustained-release bupropion and placebo for smoking cessation, *N Engl J Med* 337:1195-1202, 1997.
25. Cahill K, Stead LF, Lancaster T: Nicotine receptor partial agonists for smoking cessation, *Cochrane Database Syst Rev* 12:CD006103, 2010.
26. Jorenby DE, et al: A controlled trial of sustained-release bupropion, a nicotine patch, or both for smoking cessation, *N Engl J Med* 340:685-691, 1999.
27. Chatkin JM, et al: Abstinence rates and predictors of outcome for smoking cessation: do Brazilian smokers need special strategies? *Addiction* 99:778-784, 2004.
28. Willemse B, et al: High cessation rates of cigarette smoking in subjects with and without COPD, *Chest* 128:3685-3687, 2005.
29. Hu S, et al: Knowing how to help tobacco users. Dentists' familiarity and compliance with the clinical practice guideline, *J Am Dent Assoc* 137:170-179, 2006.
30. Johnson NW, Lowe JC, Warnakulasuriya KA: Tobacco cessation activities of UK dentists in primary care: signs of improvement, *Br Dent J* 200:85-89, 2006.
31. Corelli RL, Hudmon KS: Pharmacologic interventions for smoking cessation, *Crit Care Nurs Clin North Am* 18:39-51, xii, 2006.
32. Frishman WH, et al: Nicotine and non-nicotine smoking cessation pharmacotherapies, *Cardiol Rev* 14:57-73, 2006.
33. Dean AJ: Natural and complementary therapies for substance use disorders, *Curr Opin Psychiatry* 18:271-276, 2005.

9

Sleep-Related Breathing Disorders

SNORING AND OBSTRUCTIVE SLEEP APNEA

Sleep-related breathing disorders constitute a spectrum of clinical entities with variations in sleep structure, respiration, and blood oxygen saturation. The spectrum ranges from mild, intermittent snoring to severe obstructive sleep apnea (OSA) (Figure 9-1). *Obesity-hypoventilation syndrome* (formerly called Pickwickian syndrome) is the term used to describe a syndrome characterized by severe obesity, daytime hypoventilation, and sleep-disordered breathing.[1]

Snoring, upper airway resistance syndrome (UARS), and OSA are the main subjects of this chapter. All of these sleep-related breathing disorders are due to upper airway obstruction of variable degree, leading to resistance to airflow during respiration. Attempts to breathe continue despite the obstruction. A related disorder, central sleep apnea, is the cessation of breathing that is due to disruption of central nervous system ventilatory drive; this type of apnea usually is associated with an underlying medical problem such as heart failure and is not due to obstruction, so it is not included in this chapter.

Snoring may occur alone or may be due to a more significant airway impairment. Snoring is the result of vibration of the soft tissues of the upper airway, primarily during inspiration. Primary snoring is sometimes referred to as simple snoring or benign snoring. It occurs as an independent entity and is not associated with disrupted sleep or complaints of daytime sleepiness. Findings on an overnight sleep study, or polysomnogram (PSG), are normal. Snoring occurs without abnormal ventilation. UARS is a clinical entity midway between primary snoring and OSA that is characterized by snoring, complaints of daytime sleepiness, and fragmentation of sleep. A PSG demonstrates some increase in ventilatory efforts, but the impairment is not severe enough to be classified as OSA. OSA is characterized by loud snoring and excessive daytime sleepiness with episodes of complete cessation of breathing (apnea) or significantly decreased ventilation (hypopnea) due to airway obstruction during sleep, along with significant fragmentation of sleep architecture. A PSG demonstrates abnormalities in sleep architecture, ventilation, and blood oxygen saturation.

GENERAL DESCRIPTION

Epidemiology

Snoring is extremely common in both genders and in all age groups. It is reported to occur in nearly 50% of the adult population, with a higher prevalence among men.[2] Of note, however, estimates of its prevalence vary widely because detection methods rely heavily on subjective reports by bed partners or parents. Reported prevalence rates for snoring range between 5% and 86% in men and between 2% and 57% in women.[3] Evidence suggests that the frequency of snoring increases with age until about age 60, at which time a decrease occurs.[2] In children, snoring is common, with a reported prevalence of 10%.[4] It typically is associated with enlarged tonsils and adenoids, as well as obesity. Snoring also has been reported to increase markedly during pregnancy.[5,6]

The reported prevalence of OSA varies widely because of differences in assessment methods and in the number of abnormal respiratory events per hour used to define abnormality. It is estimated that about 2% to 4% of the adult population 30 to 60 years of age is affected by OSA; however, 9% of women and 24% of men have signs or symptoms suggestive of sleep-disordered breathing.[7] Different rates of occurrence have been reported for males and for females, with males affected more often. Variation among racial groups may be due to genetic differences. African Americans, Hispanics, and Asian Americans tend to have a somewhat higher prevalence than that in whites. About 3% of children are affected with OSA, with the highest prevalence reported between the ages of 2 and 5 years.[8]

Etiology and Pathophysiology

The underlying defect in sleep-related breathing disorders is an anatomically narrowed upper airway combined with pharyngeal dilator muscle collapsibility. The

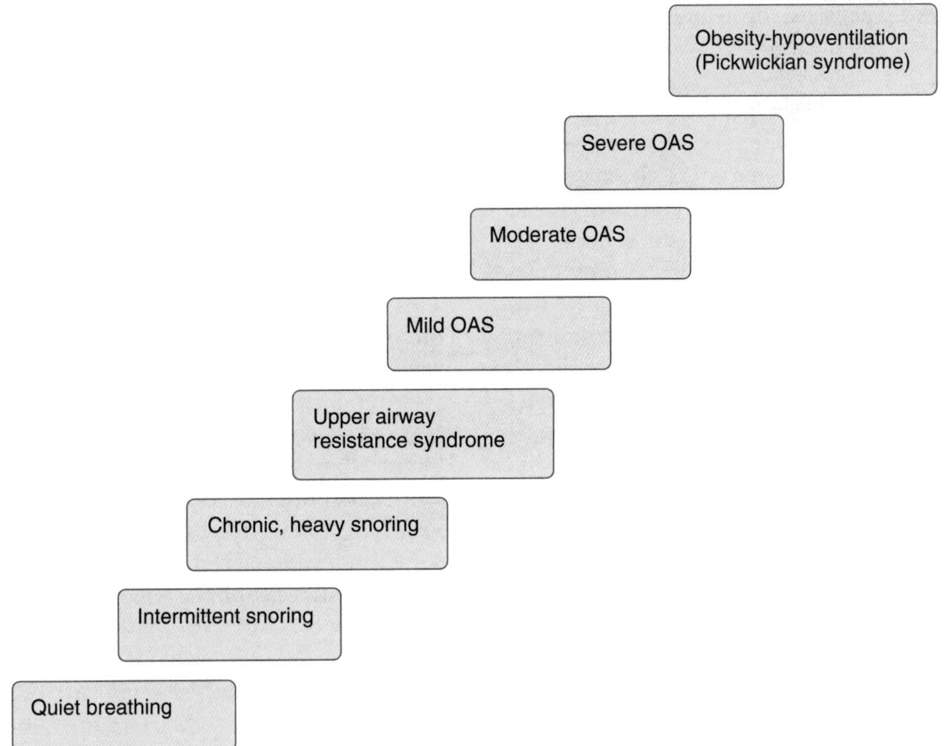

FIGURE 9-1 Clinical spectrum of sleep-related breathing disorders. *OSAS*, Obstructive sleep apnea syndrome. *(Redrawn from Phillips B, Naughton MT:* Fast facts: obstructive sleep apnea, *Oxford, 2004, Health Press Limited.)*

exact pathogenesis, however, is not well understood. Depending on the extent of narrowing, increased resistance to airflow may be clinically expressed as vibration of soft tissues (snoring), reduced ventilation (hypopnea), or complete obstruction (apnea).

Anatomic narrowing may occur at any site in the upper airway from the nasal cavity to the larynx. Within the nasal cavity, septal deviation and enlarged turbinates may cause narrowing. In the nasopharynx, hypertrophic adenoids and tonsils, an elongated soft palate, and an elongated and edematous uvula may be the cause. In the oropharynx, narrowing may be due to an enlarged tongue, retrognathia, excessive lymphoid tissue, palatine tonsils, or redundant parapharyngeal folds. The most common sites of airway narrowing or closure during sleep are the retropalatal and retroglossal regions.[9] Most patients with OSA have more than one site of narrowing.[10] It also has been demonstrated that the volume of the upper airway soft tissue structures (i.e., tongue, lateral pharyngeal walls, soft palate, parapharyngeal fat pads) is significantly greater in patients with OSA than in normal control subjects.[11] Factors that are thought to contribute to enlargement of the upper airway soft tissues in apneic patients include obesity, edema secondary to negative pressures, vibration trauma of the uvula, male gender, and possibly, genetics.[9] Other anatomic risk factors for narrowing of the upper airway include retrognathia, large tongue, long soft palate, and enlarged uvula, tonsils, and adenoids.

In addition to anatomic narrowing of the airway, an abnormal degree of collapsibility is observed in the pharyngeal dilator muscles surrounding the airway. Patency of the airway depends on a balance between air pressure within the airway and pressure outside of the airway exerted by the parapharyngeal musculature. Muscles that surround the airway receive phasic activation during inspiration and tend to promote a patent pharyngeal lumen by dilating the airway and stiffening the airway walls.[12] Normally, the intraluminal pressure exceeds the external pressure, and the airway remains patent during inhalation and exhalation. Normal function requires coordinated timing and activity of agonists and antagonists, and of individual muscles or groups of muscles. The cause of abnormal pharyngeal airway collapse is complex, involving both dynamic and static factors. These factors may include tissue volume, changes in the adhesive character of mucosal surfaces, changes in neck and jaw posture, decreased tracheal tug, effects of gravity, and decreased intraluminal pressure resulting from increased upstream resistance in the nasal cavity or pharynx.[9]

Complications and Outcomes

To appreciate the consequences of sleep-related breathing disorders, it is necessary to review the aspects of normal sleep. Normal sleep patterns vary with age but are nevertheless similar across patient groups; thus, for illustrative purposes, the sleep of young adults is discussed here. Normal sleep occurs in two phases: non–rapid eye movement (NREM) sleep and rapid eye movement (REM) sleep[13] (Table 9-1).

The phases of sleep are characterized by distinctive patterns on the electroencephalogram (EEG), as well as by the presence or absence of eye movements. NREM sleep occurs in three (or four) stages and generally is characterized by synchronous brain waves, mental inactivity, and physiologic stability (Figure 9-2). The NREM sleep state sometimes is referred to as "a quiet brain in a quiet body." Stage 1 NREM is a brief, transitional stage that lasts only a few minutes between wakefulness and sleep and from which the person can be easily aroused. Stage 2 NREM is the initial stage of true sleep, from which arousal is more difficult. The appearance of EEG waves called *sleep spindles,* or *K-complexes,* identifies this stage, which typically lasts 10 to 25 minutes. Stage 3 is characterized by the appearance on the EEG of high-voltage, high-amplitude slow waves that last for a few minutes and then undergo transition into stage 4, with more frequent and higher-amplitude slow waves. This stage lasts for 20 to 40 minutes. Stages 3 and 4 often are combined, and this combination is referred to as slow wave sleep (SWS).

TABLE 9-1 Percentage of Time Spent in the Various Stages of Sleep for Normal, Healthy Young Adults

Stage Plus EEG Characteristics	Percent of Sleep
Relaxed wakefulness	<5%
Non–rapid eye movement sleep (NREM)	
Stage 1: transitional; easy arousal	2-5%
Stage 2: sleep onset; K-complexes (sleep spindles)	45-55%
Stage 3: high-voltage, high-amplitude slow waves	3-8%
Stage 4: increased numbers of high-voltage slow waves	10-15%
Rapid eye movement sleep (REM)	20-25%
Associated with desynchronized brain waves on EEG, muscle atonia, bursts of rapid eye movement	

EEG, Electroencephalogram.

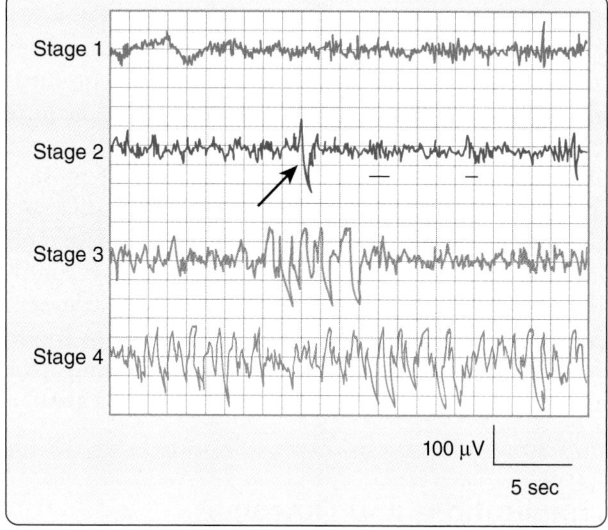

FIGURE 9-2 Electroencephalographic tracings of non–rapid eye movement (NREM) sleep stages. *(From Carskadon MA, Dement WC: Normal human sleep: an overview. In Kryger MH, Roth T, Dement WC, editors:* Principles and practice of sleep medicine, *ed 5, St. Louis, 2011, Saunders.)*

After a period of NREM sleep, a "lightening" occurs, marked by entry into REM sleep. REM sleep is very different from NREM sleep and is characterized by asynchronous brain waves, an active brain, and physiologic instability, and muscular inactivity. The REM sleeep state often is described as "an active brain in a paralyzed body." A key feature is the presence of periodic rapid movement of the eyes with low-voltage EEG waves resembling those typical of wakefulness (Figure 9-3). Variations in blood pressure, heart rate, and respiration occur, along with general muscle atonia and poikilothermia. Dreaming also occurs during REM sleep. Sleep normally is entered through NREM sleep and progresses to REM. Over the course of a night, sleep cycles between NREM and REM, with each cycle averaging about 90 minutes. Depending on the length of the sleep period, the sleeper typically passes through four to six cycles per night. The length of time in each stage varies, with NREM predominating in the earlier part of the night and REM predominating in the later part of the night (Figure 9-4). It is difficult to define the "normal" length of sleep because of multiple variables, including age, environment, circadian rhythm, and medication effects; however, most young adults report that they sleep an average of 7.5 hours per weeknight and 8.5 hours on weekend nights.[14]

To gain the restorative benefits of sleep, it is necessary to cycle through the normal stages of sleep. NREM sleep

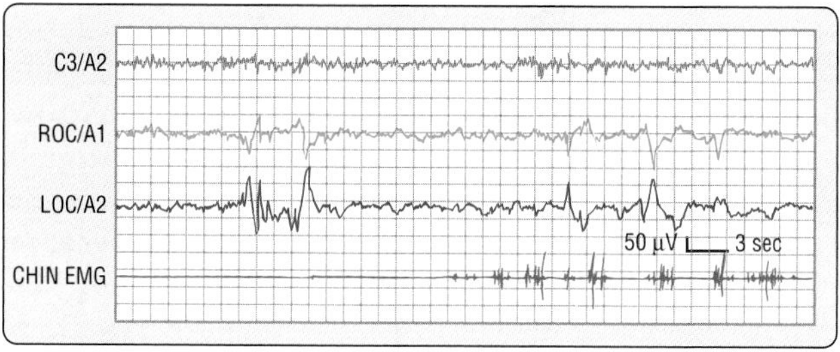

FIGURE 9-3 Phasic events in human rapid eye movement (REM) sleep. C3/A2 is an electrooculographic (EOG) lead. ROC/A1 is a lead from the outer canthus of the right eye, and LOC/A2 is another lead from the outer canthus of the left eye. Note the several bursts of activity in the eye lead tracings. *(From Carskadon MA, Dement WC: Normal human sleep: an overview. In Kryger MH, Roth T, Dement WC, editors:* Principles and practice of sleep medicine, *ed 5, St. Louis, 2011, Saunders.)*

provides physical restoration, whereas REM sleep provides psychic restoration. If such restoration does not occur because of sleep deprivation or sleep fragmentation, cognitive and physiologic disturbances will result. Within the spectrum of sleep-related breathing disorders, different outcomes may be seen. With *primary snoring*, the degree of airway resistance is such that vibration of the parapharyngeal soft tissues is the only result. No sleep fragmentation or disruption occurs, and no other impairment of airflow or oxygenation is noted. Generally accepted thought has been that primary snoring has no significant adverse health effects, but evidence now suggests that primary snoring may be a risk factor for type 2 diabetes, hypertension, carotid atherosclerosis, and stroke.[15-19]

With *OSA*, increasing resistance to airflow occurs to the point of partial (hypopnea) obstruction or complete (apnea) obstruction and the cessation of breathing, despite efforts to continue to breathe. Depending on the degree and duration of the obstruction, hypoxia, anoxia, and hypercarbia may occur. These changes lead to CNS arousal and transition to a lighter stage of sleep (stage 1 or 2), stimulating partial awakening, relief of the obstruction, and resumption of breathing. Depending on the frequency of arousals during the night, sleep can be fragmented (Figure 9-5). Sleep quality is poor, and the restorative benefits of sleep are not achieved, leading to a variety of cognitive and physiologic abnormalities.

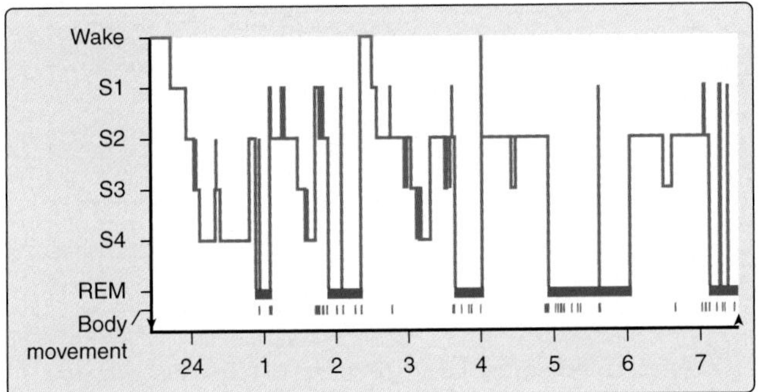

FIGURE 9-4 Histogram showing progression of sleep stages across a single night in a normal, healthy, young adult volunteer. *(From Carskadon MA, Dement WC: Normal human sleep: an overview. In Kryger MH, Roth T, Dement WC, editors:* Principles and practice of sleep medicine, *ed 5, St. Louis, 2011, Saunders.)*

Neurocognitive effects of OSA include sleepiness, decreased alertness, irritability, poor concentration, lack of libido, and memory loss. These deficits can lead to poor job performance, marital discord, interpersonal conflicts, and driving impairment. Up to 30% of traffic accidents involve sleepy drivers.[20] A systematic review investigating the relationship of crash risk and OSA found that drivers with OSA have a mean crash risk–to–OSA ratio of between 1.21 and 4.89.[21]

In addition to neurocognitive impairment, OSA is associated with numerous cardiovascular effects, including hypertension, stroke, congestive heart failure, pulmonary hypertension, and cardiac arrhythmia. OSA, which is now recognized as one of the treatable causes of hypertension,[22] also has been shown to significantly increase the risks of stroke and death.[23] Patients with OSA have two- to four-fold greater odds of experiencing complex arrhythmias over those without the sleep disorder.[24] It also is thought that treatment of OSA may increase the survival rate among patients with heart failure.[25] In addition, a relationship between OSA, obesity, and metabolic syndrome has been noted.[26] Recent data from the Sleep Heart Health Study provide evidence for an independent relationship among sleep apnea, glucose intolerance, and insulin resistance that may lead to type 2 diabetes.[27] Overall, the mortality rate from all causes is

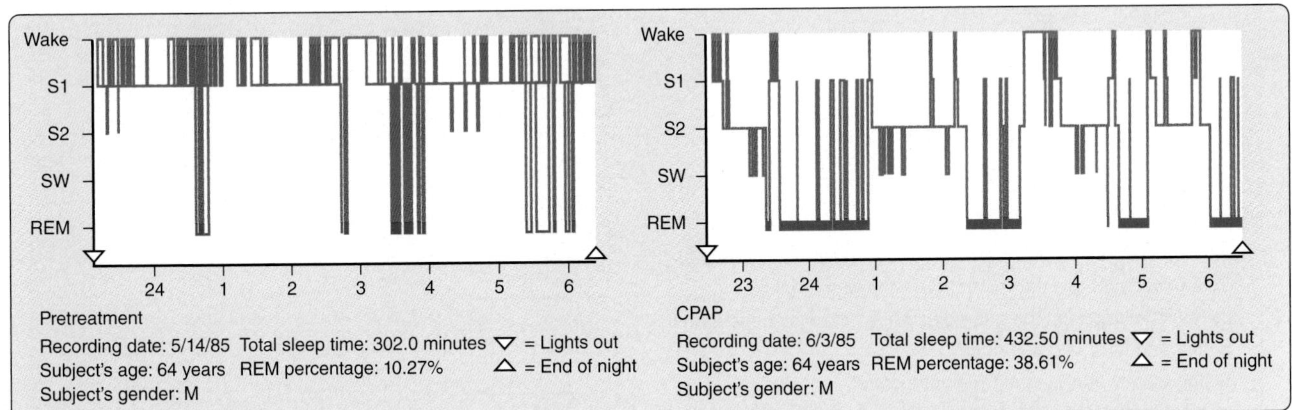

FIGURE 9-5 These sleep histograms show sleep study data for a 64-year-old male patient with obstructive sleep apnea syndrome. The *left graph* shows the sleep pattern before treatment. Note the absence of slow wave sleep (SWS), the preponderance of stage 1 (S1), and the very frequent disruptions. The *right graph* shows the sleep pattern in this patient during the second night of treatment with continuous positive airway pressure (CPAP). Note that sleep is much deeper (with more SWS) and more consolidated, and rapid eye movement (REM) sleep in particular is abnormally increased. The pretreatment REM percentage of sleep was only 10%, versus nearly 40% with treatment *(From Carskadon MA, Dement WC: Normal human sleep: an overview. In Kryger MH, Roth T, Dement WC, editors:* Principles and practice of sleep medicine, *ed 5, St. Louis, 2011, Saunders.)*

significantly increased among people with untreated OSA and is proportional to the severity.[28]

CLINICAL PRESENTATION

Signs and Symptoms

The signs and symptoms of sleep-related breathing disorders are those most often described by the bed partner or parent of a patient; they include snoring, snorting, gasping, and breath holding. Snoring is very common, as was previously indicated, and is the most common symptom in patients with OSA. However, most people who snore do not have OSA, but almost all patients with OSA snore. In the Wisconsin Sleep Cohort Study of subjects aged 30 to 60 years, 44% of men and 28% of women were habitual snorers, but only 4% of the men and 2% of the women had OSA.[29]

Snoring may be very loud and disruptive to other members of the household. When snoring is the only complaint, the problem most often is primary snoring. If snoring is accompanied by daytime sleepiness and no breathing changes during sleep, UARS must be considered. Snoring accompanied by snorting, choking, gasping, or a complete cessation of breathing is likely to be a sign of OSA. Of note, however, definitive diagnosis of sleep-related breathing disorders cannot be made on the basis of clinical signs and symptoms alone.

Complaints of excessive daytime sleepiness are common in patients with OSA but are not specific, and the problem may be multifactorial. A commonly used subjective measure of sleepiness is the Epworth Sleepiness Scale[30] (Figure 9-6). This assessment tool has been validated in clinical studies and correlates with objective measures of sleepiness. It is composed of eight questions or situations in which patients are asked how likely they are to fall asleep. Each question is answered on a scale of 0 to 3, with 0 meaning no likelihood of falling asleep and 3 indicating 100% likelihood of falling asleep in that situation. The maximum possible score is 24. A score

THE EPWORTH SLEEPINESS SCALE

Name: ____________________

Today's date: ____________________ Your age (years): ____________________

Your sex (male = M; female = F): ____________________

How likely are you to doze off or fall asleep in the following situations, in contrast to feeling just tired? This refers to your usual way of life in recent times. Even if you have not done some of these things recently try to work out how they would have affected you. Use the following scale to choose the *most appropriate number* for each situation:

0 = would *never* doze
1 = *slight* chance of dozing
2 = *moderate* chance of dozing
3 = *high* chance of dozing

Situation	Chance of dozing
Sitting and reading	________
Watching TV	________
Sitting, inactive in a public place (e.g., a theater or a meeting)	________
As a passenger in a car for an hour without a break	________
Lying down to rest in the afternoon when circumstances permit	________
Sitting and talking to someone	________
Sitting quietly after a lunch without alcohol	________
In a car, while stopped for a few minutes in the traffic	________

Thank you for your cooperation

FIGURE 9-6 Epworth Sleepiness Scale. *(Redrawn from Johns MW: A new method for measuring daytime sleepiness: the Epworth sleepiness scale,* Sleep *14:540-545, 1991.)*

greater than 10 is indicative of significant daytime sleepiness but is not specific for sleep-related breathing disorders. Other complaints that may be associated with OSA are nocturia or enuresis, mood changes, memory or learning difficulties, erectile dysfunction, morning headache, and dry mouth noted upon awakening.

Obesity is common among patients with OSA. Obesity increases the risk of OSA several-fold; the most marked effects are observed during middle age.[31] Approximately 70% of patients with OSA are obese.[32] One measure of obesity is the body mass index (BMI), which is calculated by dividing weight in kilograms by the height in meters squared. Adults with a BMI greater than 25 are considered overweight, and those with a BMI over 30 are considered to be obese. Of interest, however, is that neck circumference has been found to be more closely related to severity of OSA than is BMI.[33] A neck circumference greater than 17 inches (43 cm) in men and greater than 16 inches (41 cm) in women is predictive of OSA.[34] Along with obesity and collar size, other physical features associated with OSA include mandibular retrognathia, long soft palate, large edematous uvula, large tongue, tonsillar and adenoidal hypertrophy, and a high-arched palate. In summary, the most useful predictors of OSA are witnessed apneas, excessive daytime sleepiness, male gender, BMI above 30, and neck circumference greater than 17 and 16 inches, respectively, for men and women.

Laboratory Diagnosis

Definitive diagnosis of a sleep-related breathing disorder is made by polysomnography, in which the patient's brain waves, breathing, and other activity are recorded during sleep. As noted earlier, a polysomnogram (PSG) is an overnight sleep study that is performed in a laboratory setting (Figure 9-7). During the performance of a standard laboratory-based PSG, a technician who is present throughout the night records the activities of the patient during sleep. Multiple physiologic parameters are monitored and recorded on a computer. The components of a PSG typically include electroencephalogram (EEG) to monitor brain waves, electrooculogram (EOG) to monitor eye movements, electromyogram (EMG) to monitor jaw muscular activity and leg movements, electrocardiogram (ECG) to monitor heart rate and rhythm, pulse oximetry to monitor blood oxygen saturation, nasal thermistor monitoring of nasal airflow and CO_2 levels, and use of chest and abdominal strain gauges to track breathing efforts.

After all recording sensors are attached, the patient is allowed to go to sleep. Most contemporary sleep laboratories have sleeping rooms that are nicely decorated, resembling a normal bedroom. In addition to the sensors attached to the patient, an infrared camera often is used to enable the technician to watch patient movements, such as leg movements or sleep walking, or to relate sleeping position to periods of disturbed breathing. A microphone is present in the room to record snoring or other sounds, such as tooth grinding or sleep talking.

A typical PSG study encompasses the entire night and usually is sufficient to make a diagnosis, despite obvious questions about the "normality" of the night's sleep in such an environment. Often, a diagnosis can be made early in the course of the night, and a trial of therapy with positive airway pressure (PAP) will be attempted. This is called a *split-night study.* If no diagnosis is possible during the initial PSG, a second sleep study may be necessary to assess the effects of PAP. A computer recording of the entire night is produced; this tracing is scrutinized and interpreted by a qualified physician trained in sleep medicine, who then makes a diagnosis and recommends treatment (Figure 9-8).

Quantification of OSA severity is expressed by means of the *apnea-hypopnea index* (AHI) or the *respiratory disturbance index* (RDI). These two indices commonly are used interchangeably; however, there is a technical difference between the two. The AHI is scored by adding all of the apneic episodes together with all of the hypopneic episodes that occurred during the night and then dividing this total by the number of hours slept. The result is expressed as the number of respiratory events per hour. To calculate the RDI, respiratory effort–related arousals (RERAs) are added to the apneas and hypopneas. It is important to define these terms for use in characterizing the various sleep disorders. According to the American Academy of Sleep Medicine,[35] an *apnea* (apneic episode) is defined as the cessation or near-complete cessation (greater than 70% reduction) of airflow for a minimum of 10 seconds. *Hypopnea* is an episode of greater than 30% reduction in amplitude in thoracoabdominal movement or airflow from baseline, with a greater than 4% oxygen desaturation. *RERAs* are episodes that include a clear drop in respiratory airflow, increased respiratory effort, and a brief change in sleep state (arousal) but do not meet the criteria for an apnea or a hypopnea.

A diagnosis of OSA is made if the AHI or RDI is greater than 5/hour and symptoms of excessive daytime sleepiness, witnessed nocturnal apneas, or awakening with choking, breath holding, or gasping are noted. In quantifying the severity of OSA, some disagreement has been expressed; however, a commonly used classification defines an AHI of 0 to 5/hour as normal, 5 to 15/hour as mild, 15 to 30/hour as moderate, and greater than 30/hour as severe. Along with the AHI, the lowest point (nadir) of oxygen desaturation is reported. UARS is diagnosed in the presence of RERAs, an AHI less than 5/hour, and a complaint of excessive daytime sleepiness. Primary snoring is associated with completely normal findings on the PSG, with no complaint of excessive sleepiness in the presence of snoring.

Other aspects of the PSG that may be reported are total time spent in the various sleep stages, AHI for various sleep stages, and AHI for various sleep positions.

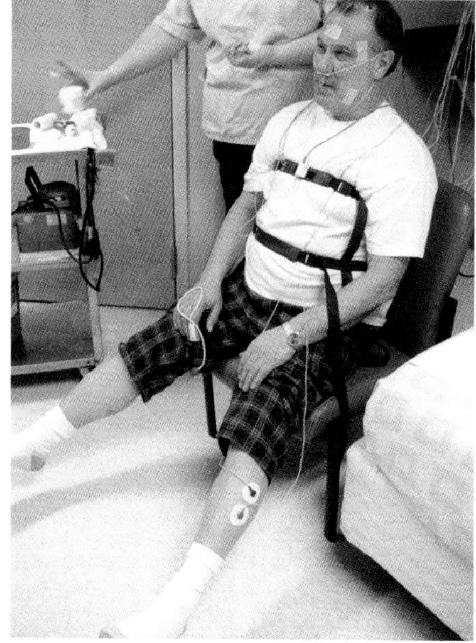

A

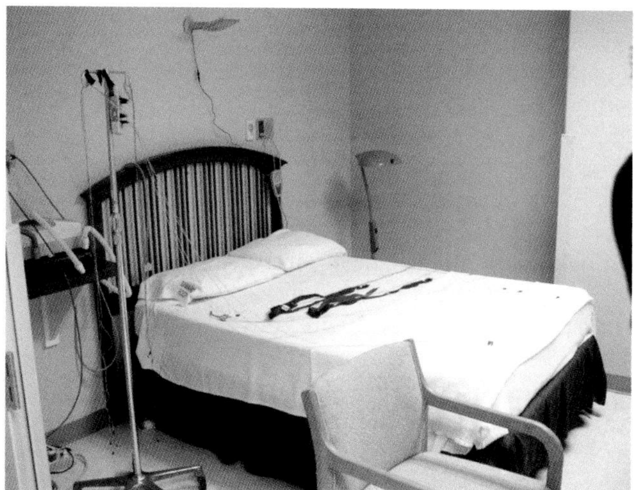

B

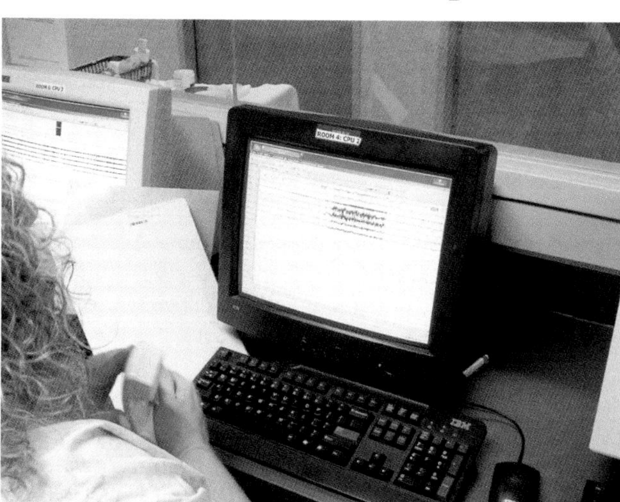

C

FIGURE 9-7 **A,** Patient being prepared for polysomnography study. Multiple recording leads are in place. **B,** Sleep laboratory/bedroom where the patient spends the night while being recorded. **C,** Sleep technician monitoring the computer printout of the polysomnogram.

In addition, a sleep histogram, which is a graph of the sleep pattern during the entire night that depicts cycling into and out of the various sleep stages, may be provided. Other tests that may be used include the *multiple sleep latency test* (MSLT), which assesses the ability to fall asleep, and the *maintenance of wakefulness test* (MWT), which assesses the ability to stay awake.

MEDICAL MANAGEMENT

The decision of when and how to treat sleep-related breathing disorders depends on the diagnosis and the severity of the disorder. Treatment of primary snoring is elective and essentially is a personal decision that is commonly motivated by the effects of snoring on a spouse or bed partner. Of interest, the snoring rarely disturbs the snorer. Parents of a child who snores often seek treatment out of concern for the health of the child. Patients who are given a diagnosis of UARS should receive treatment to alleviate the problems associated with snoring, as well as those resulting from sleep fragmentation and resultant sleepiness. UARS can progress, evolving into OSA over time. Patients who are given a diagnosis of OSA require treatment—not only to alleviate snoring and sleepiness but to prevent or treat the numerous adverse health effects associated with the disease. Even mild sleep apnea is associated with significant morbidity, which increases with severity.[29] An increased mortality rate is reported to be associated with an AHI greater than 20/hour.[36]

The treatment of OSA involves four different approaches: behavioral modification, positive airway

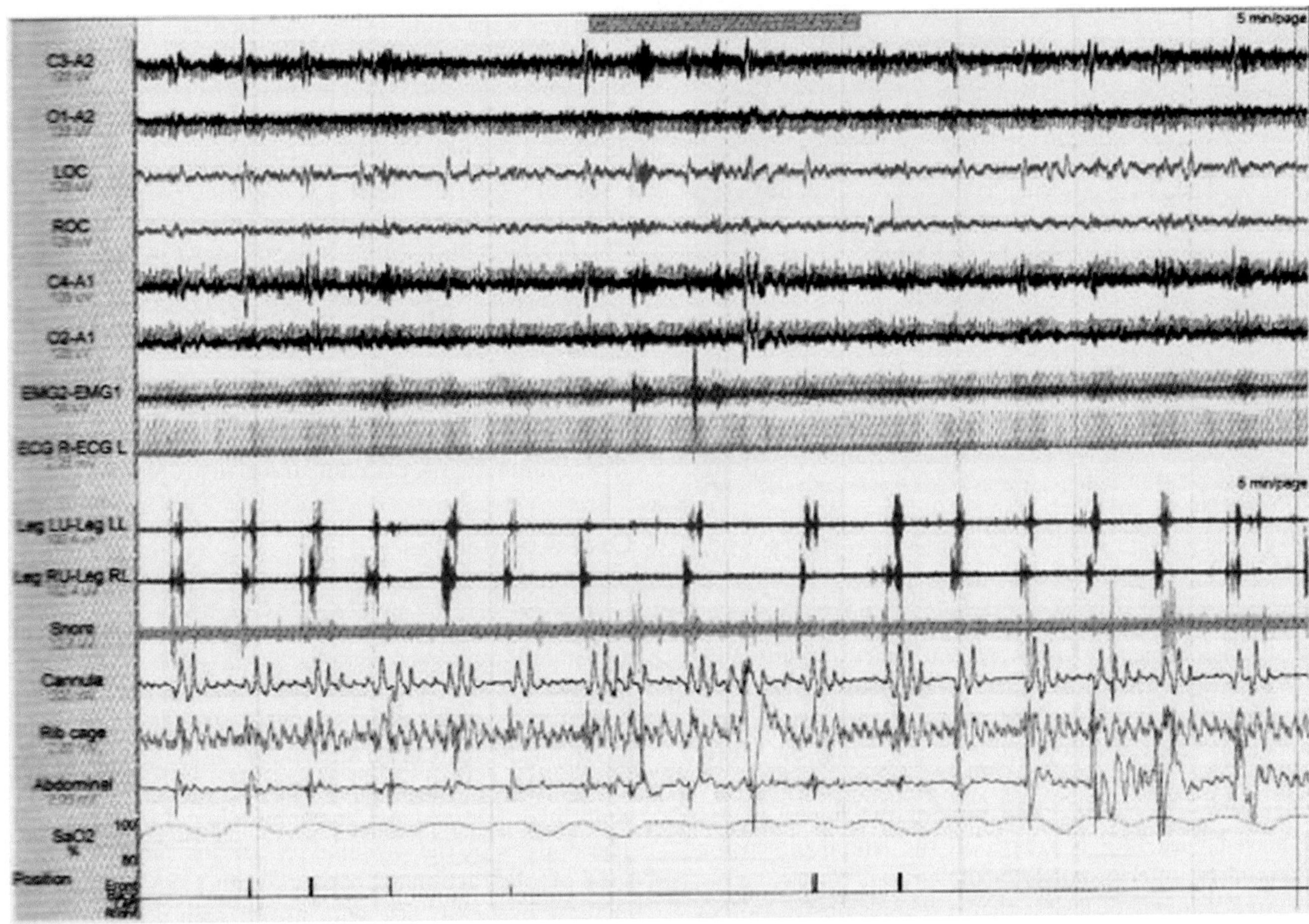

FIGURE 9-8 A 5-minute epoch of a polysomnogram. *C3-A2, O1-A2, C4-A1,* and *O2-A1* are electroencephalographic leads used to determine sleep stages. *LOC* and *ROC* designate eyelid leads at left and right outer canthi, respectively, for recording rapid eye movement. *EMG* tracing is an electromyogram of the chin used to record jaw movement. *ECG* tracing is an electrocardiogram that records heart rate and rhythm. *Leg LU* and *Leg RU* designate leads for recording leg movements. *Snore* tracing tracks subject's snoring. *Cannula* designates measurement of nasal airflow pressure. *Rib cage* tracing is a recording of rib cage movement. *Abdominal* tracing is a recording of abdominal movement. Sao_2 is blood oxygen saturation. *Position* tracing is a recording of body position. *(From Phillips B, Naughton M:* Fast facts: obstructive sleep apnea, *Oxford, 2004, Health Press Limited.)*

pressure (PAP) modalities, use of oral appliances, and surgery.

Behavioral Modification

Several measures may help to decrease or eliminate the signs or symptoms of sleep-related breathing disorders. Weight loss is one of the most effective measures that can be instituted. It has been shown that even modest weight loss can relieve mild sleep-related breathing disorders and in many cases may be curative.[37] Furthermore, independent of body habitus, regular aerobic exercise has been shown to be of clinical benefit in patients with OSA.[38] For patients with obstruction in the nasal cavity, nasal dilator strips may be helpful to physically open the nasal passages, as may the use of nasal decongestants or topical corticosteroids, or both. Many patients with OSA have positional apnea, with apneas occurring more frequently or with greater severity in the supine position.[39] For patients with position-dependent apnea, measures to prevent sleeping in a supine position may be helpful and include sewing a tennis ball into a pocket on the back of the pajamas, using a backpack-type device, and placement of pillows to maintain a side-sleeping posture. Alcohol, sedatives, or muscle relaxants near bedtime should be avoided. Patients who smoke should be encouraged to quit smoking, although the relationship between smoking and OSA remains unclear. Oral or nasal lubricants or sprays, as well as dietary supplements, magnets, hypnosis, and other treatment methods based in alternative and complementary medicine, have been purported to relieve snoring; however, credible evidence of effectiveness is lacking.

Positive Airway Pressure

The "gold standard" treatment for OSA is the delivery of positive airway pressure (PAP) to the patient's airway during sleep. This is accomplished with the use of an air compressor that is connected by tubing to a nasal or full

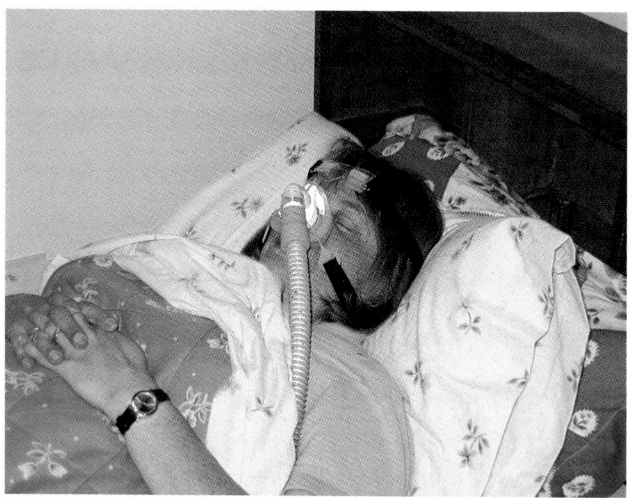

FIGURE 9-9 Patient using a positive airway pressure device with a nasal mask. *(Courtesy June Sorrenson, CRT, Lexington, Kentucky.)*

face mask attached to the patient's face (Figure 9-9). Room air is delivered under pressure to the patient's airway, where it acts in effect as a pneumatic stent, producing positive intraluminal pressure along the entire pharyngeal airway, thereby maintaining patency. Of interest in this context, dilation of the upper airway achieved with PAP is greater in the lateral dimension than in the anterior-posterior dimension.[40,41]

An advantage of PAP is that it relieves obstruction at all levels of the airway. Delivery of PAP may be accomplished using one of three modalities:

1. Continuous positive airway pressure (CPAP)
2. Bilevel positive airway pressure (BiPAP or BPAP)
3. Automatic (self-adjusting) positive airway pressure (APAP)

The air may be heated and humidified. CPAP provides air continuously throughout inspiration and exhalation at a single, set pressure, expressed in cm H_2O. BiPAP consists of two set pressures, with use of a higher pressure during inhalation and a lower pressure setting for during exhalation. With APAP, pressures vary continuously according to what is required at a particular moment to maintain airway patency. CPAP, the form most commonly used, is the least expensive. CPAP most is often titrated to an effective level during a PSG in the sleep laboratory, either as part of a split-night study or during a subsequent full-night study. Pressures typically are started at 3 to 5 cm H_2O and are gradually titrated upward, until all manifestations of OSA are eliminated. With CPAP, typical treatment pressures range between 5 and 15 cm H_2O.

In a review of PAP,[42] it was concluded that PAP was more effective than and eliminated respiratory disturbances and reduces AHI when compared with placebo, conservative management, or positional therapy. It also improves stage 3 and 4 sleep and decreases EEG arousals versus placebo. It significantly improves sleep architecture and sleep fragmentation, but these effects are not always consistent. In addition, daytime sleepiness may be decreased and neurobehavioral performance, psychological functioning, and quality of life may be improved. The impact on cardiovascular risk is mixed. Compliance with PAP has long been a problem, with only about 50% of patients who try it are able to tolerate it. Of those who do use PAP, the average patient uses it for only about 4 to 5 hours per night and for only about 5 nights per week.[42,43] Adverse effects with PAP are common and include mask leaks, skin ulceration or irritation under the mask, epistaxis, rhinorrhea, nasal congestion, sinus congestion, dry eyes, conjunctivitis, ear pain, and claustrophobia.

Oral Appliances

Oral appliances offer an attractive alternative for the management of sleep-related breathing disorders, (1) as a primary treatment option, (2) in patients who are unable to tolerate the use of PAP, or (3) in patients who refuse to use PAP. Oral appliances exert their effects by mechanically increasing the volume of the upper airway in the retropalatal and retroglossal areas, as has been confirmed by imaging and physiologic monitoring.[44] These areas of the oropharynx are the most common sites of obstruction in patients with OSA.[45] Expected increase in airway size with use of such devices would be greater in the retroglossal than in the retropalatal region, because they pull the tongue forward.[46,47] However, studies have shown that wearing oral appliances is associated with increased airway size in *both* the retropalatal and retroglossal regions, with increases occurring not only anteroposteriorly but in the lateral dimension as well.[47,48]

The two basic types of oral appliances are (1) mandibular advancement devices (MADs), which engage the mandible and reposition it (and indirectly, the tongue) in an anterior or forward position, and (2) tongue-retaining devices (TRDs), which directly engage the tongue and hold it in a forward position. Currently, more than 70 different types of OAs are available to treat snoring or obstructive sleep apnea. Less than half of them, however, have been approved by the U.S. Food and Drug Administration (FDA) for use in the treatment of OSA; the remainder have been approved only for snoring (Figure 9-10).

MADs most commonly are used to treat patients with sleep-related breathing disorders. They typically are made of acrylic resin and are composed of two pieces that cover the upper and lower dental arches (similar to retainers or athletic mouth guards) and are connected in such a way as to reposition and hold the mandible in a forward position. The parts may be fused together into a single (monoblock), nonadjustable appliance, or they may be connected in such a way as to allow some degree

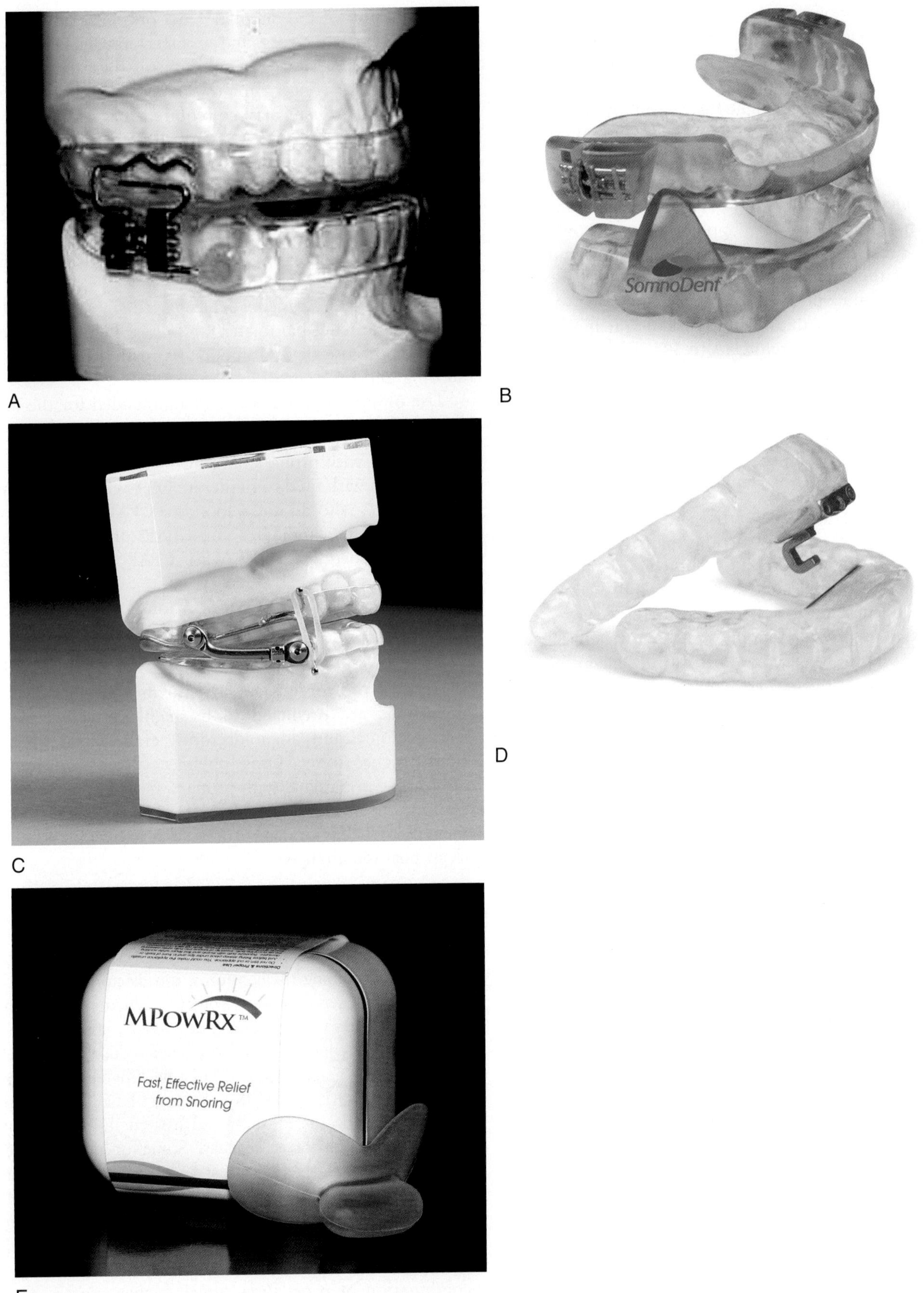

FIGURE 9-10 Examples of oral appliances used for the treatment of obstructive sleep apnea. **A,** Adjustable PM Positioner. **B,** SomnoDent MAS (Mandibular Advancement Splint). **C,** Modified Herbst appliance. **D,** TAP-T (Thornton Adjustable Positioner). **E,** MPowRX tongue retainer. *(**A,** Courtesy DSG Davis Dental Laboratory, Wyoming, Michigan. **B,** Courtesy Somnomed, Inc., Denton, Texas. **C** and **E,** Courtesy Great Lakes Orthodontics, Tonawanda, New York. **D,** Courtesy Airway Management, Inc., Dallas, Texas.)*

of mandibular movement and adjustability between the two pieces. TRDs generally are made of silicone in the shape of a bulb or cavity. The tongue is stuck into the bulb, which is then squeezed and released, producing a suction that holds the tongue forward in the bulb. Only one design of TRDs has been approved by the FDA for the treatment of OSA (see Figure 9-10, *E*). Studies have shown that TRDs provide treatment effects similar to those achieved with MADs.[49,50] Also available is another type of tongue displacement appliance that fits over one or both arches and depresses the tongue and guides it forward without moving the mandible as well.[51]

Numerous uncontrolled studies have reported various degrees of success with different types of oral appliances, ranging from 76% for mild OSA to 40% for more severe OSA.[52-57] Two large prospective studies of patients with OSA of a broad range of severity reported an average overall 1-year success rate (defined as AHI less than 10/hour) of 54%.[57,58] Two randomized, crossover, controlled trials with a total of 97 patients in whom adjustable appliances were used reported complete success (AHI less than 5/hour) or partial success (AHI reduced by more than 50% but with greater than 5/hour) in 63% of subjects.[59,60] A more recent comprehensive review of oral appliance trials found that the overall success rate with use of these devices as defined by the achievement of an AHI less than 10/hour was 52%.[44] It has been demonstrated, however, that with further advancement of the appliance during a follow-up PSG, the rate of complete success can be as high as 95%.[61] Of note, in a few patients, wearing an oral appliance may actually worsen the symptoms of OSA.[62-65]

Long-term compliance data for wearing oral appliances are lacking; however, reported rates for 1-year compliance range from 48% to 84%.[66,67] Available data suggest that compliance decreases somewhat over time, with compliance at 4 years reported at 62% to 76%.[58,68] A recent report found that 5.7 years after oral appliance treatment was begun, 64% of patients were still using their appliance, 93.7% wore it for longer than 4 hours a night, and 95% were satisfied with the outcome.[69]

Oral appliances generally are well tolerated, but adverse effects are common.[44] Fortunately, most such effects are minor and transient and resolve quickly on removal of the device. Commonly reported problems include temporomandibular (TM) joint pain, muscular pain, tooth pain, hypersalivation, TM joint sounds, dry mouth, gum irritation, and morning-after occlusal changes. Infrequently, a patient may develop jaw pain that may prevent use of the device. Of note, however, in a recent study of 34 patients, followed for 3 years, the intensity of TM disorder symptoms actually decreased in intensity, leading the investigators to conclude that long-term use of an oral appliance does not cause impairment to the TM joint.[70] Another study found that sleep bruxism is markedly decreased with the use of an oral appliance.[71] Persistent occlusal changes, including retroclination of the maxillary incisors, proclination of the mandibular incisors, and a posterior open bite, also have been reported.[72-74] Should any of these occur and be a matter of concern for the patient, orthodontic or restorative treatment may be required for correction.

When compared with CPAP, oral appliances are not as effective in reducing AHI; however, patients tend to prefer these devices over CPAP.[44] Very few studies have compared oral appliances with upper airway surgery (see further on); however, in two studies in which they were compared with uvulopalatopharyngoplasty, oral appliances were found to be superior.[75,76]

The American Academy of Sleep Medicine has recently published practice parameters and revised clinical guidelines for the use of oral appliances in the treatment of snoring and OSA.[77,78]

Use of an oral appliance is recommended for the following three categories of patients:

- Patients with primary snoring
- Patients with mild to moderate OSA who prefer OAs to CPAP, who do not respond to CPAP, who are not appropriate candidates for CPAP, or who do not obtain adequate relief with CPAP or behavioral measures
- Patients with severe OSA in whom an initial trial of CPAP has failed to correct the problem

Also of note, upper airway surgery may supersede the use of oral appliances in patients for whom such operations are predicted to be highly effective (e.g., tonsillectomy and adenoidectomy, craniofacial operations, tracheostomy). Oral appliances also are appropriate for use in patients with primary snoring who do not respond to, or are not appropriate candidates for, treatment with behavioral measures such as weight loss or sleep position change.

Surgical Approaches

A variety of surgical procedures have been advocated to treat OSA, including tracheostomy, tonsillectomy, adenoidectomy, nasal septoplasty, turbinate reduction, uvulopalatopharyngoplasty (UPPP), laser-assisted uvulopalatoplasty (LAUP), radiofrequency volumetric tissue reduction (RVTR), pillar implants, genioglossus advancement–hyoid myotomy and suspension (GAHMS), tongue base reduction, maxillary and mandibular advancement osteotomy (MMO), and bariatric surgery. Some of these procedures achieve relatively modest success rates when performed alone[79] (Figure 9-11). For example, with UPPP, the surgical procedure most commonly performed to correct OSA, the success rate is less than 50%.[80] With others, however, such as MMO or performance of a combination of procedures, much higher success rates are reported. The LAUP procedure was found not to be effective and is not recommended for treatment of OSA.[81]

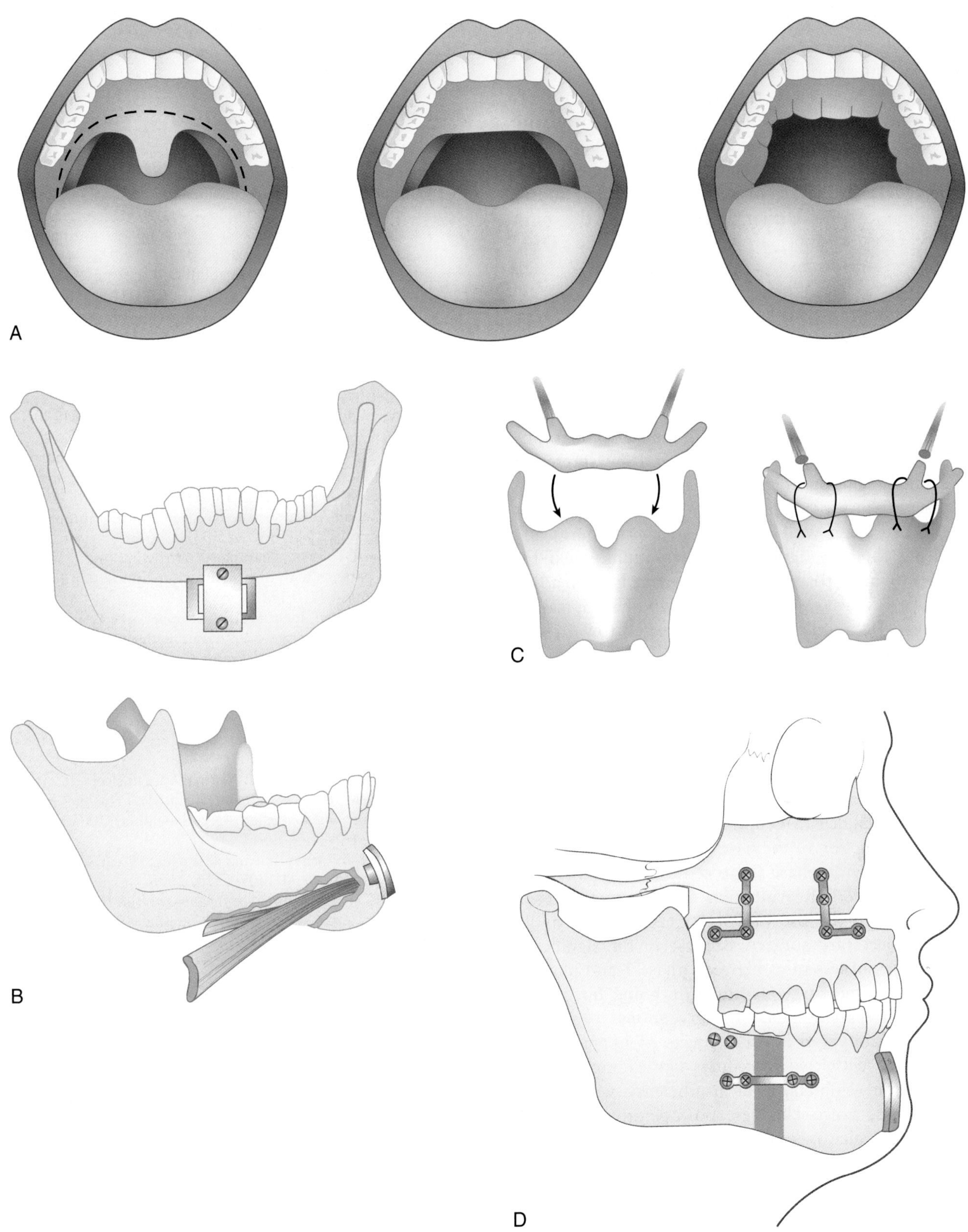

FIGURE 9-11 Surgical procedures of the upper airway used to treat obstructive sleep apnea. **A,** Uvulopalatopharyngoplasty (UPPP). **B,** Genioglossus advancement (GA). **C,** Hyoid myotomy and suspension (HMS). **D,** Maxillary and mandibular osteotomy (MMO). (***A,*** *Redrawn from Troell RJ, Strom CG: Surgical therapy for snoring,* Fed Practitioner *14:29-52, 1997.* ***B,*** *Redrawn from Fairbanks DNF, Fujita S, editors:* Snoring and obstructive sleep apnea, *ed 2, New York, 1994, Raven Press.* ***C,*** *Redrawn from Riley RW, Powell NB, Guilleminault C: Obstructive sleep apnea and the hyoid: a revised surgical procedure,* Otolaryngol Head Neck Surg *111:717-721, 1994.* ***D,*** *From Powell NB, Riley RW: Surgical management for obstructive sleep-disordered breathing. In Kryger MH, Roth T, Dement WC, editors:* Principles and practice of sleep medicine, *ed 5, St. Louis, 2011, Saunders.)*

Two forms of surgery are highly effective. Tracheostomy, which bypasses all obstruction in the entire upper airway, is almost uniformly effective in curing OSA. Its use is limited, however, in that it is unacceptable to most patients but may be used for the occasional patient with very severe OSA who is intolerant of CPAP and who requires urgent treatment.[81] Another predictably successful procedure is the removal of adenoids and tonsils in children. Adenotonsillar hypertrophy is the most common cause of upper airway obstruction (i.e., OSA) in children; adenotonsillectomy is curative in 75% to 100% of such cases.[82]

Because upper airway surgery is invasive and irreversible, efforts must be made to identify the site(s) of obstruction to determine which surgical approach should be used and to avoid unnecessary or ineffective surgery. A number of imaging techniques and laboratory modalities, including cephalometrics, computed tomography (CT) scanning, nasopharyngoscopy, and measurements of regional pharyngeal pressure, flow, and resistance, have been used for this purpose. A phased approach to surgery, beginning with less aggressive procedures and advancing to more aggressive interventions when the response to initial treatment is inadequate, is often advocated. The Powell-Riley protocol is a two-phase approach that advocates surgical treatment directed toward specific regions of obstruction during sleep.[83] Phase 1 procedures include nasal reconstruction, UPPP, GAHMS, and possibly, radiofrequency techniques directed to the soft palate or tongue. Reported success rates for phase 1 surgical procedures range between 42% and 75%.[84] If patients fail to improve after completion of phase 1, they become candidates for phase 2 surgery. Phase 2 procedures include MMO and possibly surgical or radiofrequency reduction of the base of the tongue. Reported success rates with phase 2 procedures range between 75% and 100%.[85] Reevaluation of patients after each procedure with the use of PSG is necessary to avoid further unnecessary surgery. Because of the significant difference in success rates between phase 1 and phase 2 procedures, some surgeons advocate going directly to MMO and bypassing phase 1 interventions.

Complications and adverse effects of upper airway surgery vary with the procedure. For example, UPPP may result in velopharyngeal insufficiency, velopharyngeal stenosis, voice changes, postoperative bleeding, postoperative airway obstruction, and death.[86] MMO and GAHMS may result in lip, cheek, or chin paresthesia or anesthesia, as well as tooth injury, postoperative bleeding, postoperative airway obstruction, and changes in facial appearance.

Inasmuch as obesity is a major risk factor for OSA, bariatric surgery has become a more commonly accepted treatment for patients with severe obesity. Morbid or severe obesity is defined as a BMI of 40 or greater.[87] In a large study, it was confirmed that surgically induced weight loss results in significant relief of clinical signs and symptoms associated with obesity-related OSA.[88]

REFERENCES

1. Mokhlesi B: Obesity hypoventilation syndrome: a state-of-the-art review, *Respir Care* 55:1347-1362, 2010.
2. Unhealthy sleep-related behaviors—12 states, 2009, *MMWR Morb Mortal Wkly Rep* 60:233-238, 2011.
3. Lindberg E, et al: A 10-year follow-up of snoring in men, *Chest* 114:1048-1055, 1998.
4. Ng DK, et al: An update on childhood snoring, *Acta Paediatr* 95:1029-1035, 2006.
5. Pien GW, et al: Changes in symptoms of sleep-disordered breathing during pregnancy, *Sleep* 28:1299-1305, 2005.
6. Venkata C, Venkateshiah SB: Sleep-disordered breathing during pregnancy, *J Am Board Fam Med* 22:158-168, 2009.
7. Young T, et al: The occurrence of sleep-disordered breathing among middle-aged adults, *N Engl J Med* 328:1230-1235, 1993.
8. Chang SJ, Chae KY: Obstructive sleep apnea syndrome in children: epidemiology, pathophysiology, diagnosis and sequelae, *Korean J Pediatr* 53:863-871, 2010.
9. Patil SP, et al: Adult obstructive sleep apnea: pathophysiology and diagnosis, *Chest* 132:325-337, 2007.
10. Morrison DL, et al: Pharyngeal narrowing and closing pressures in patients with obstructive sleep apnea, *Am Rev Respir Dis* 148:606-611, 1993.
11. Schwab RJ, et al: Identification of upper airway anatomic risk factors for obstructive sleep apnea with volumetric magnetic resonance imaging, *Am J Respir Crit Care Med* 168:522-530, 2003.
12. Series F: Upper airway muscles awake and asleep, *Sleep Med Rev* 6:229-242, 2002.
13. Silber MH, et al: The visual scoring of sleep in adults, *J Clin Sleep Med* 3:121-131, 2007.
14. Carskadon M, Dement W: Normal human sleep: an overview. In Kryger M, Roth T, Dement W, editors: *Principles and practice of sleep medicine*, ed 4, Philadelphia, 2005, Saunders, pp 13-23.
15. Lee SA, et al: Heavy snoring as a cause of carotid artery atherosclerosis, *Sleep* 31:1207-1213, 2008.
16. Neau JP, et al: Habitual snoring as a risk factor for brain infarction, *Acta Neurol Scand* 92:63-68, 1995.
17. Dunai A, et al: Cardiovascular disease and health-care utilization in snorers: a population survey, *Sleep* 31:411-416, 2008.
18. Kim J, et al: Snoring as an independent risk factor for hypertension in the nonobese population: the Korean Health and Genome Study, *Am J Hypertens* 20:819-824, 2007.
19. Lindberg E, et al: Snoring and daytime sleepiness as risk factors for hypertension and diabetes in women—a population-based study, *Respir Med* 101:1283-1290, 2007.
20. George CF: Sleepiness, sleep apnea, and driving: still miles to go before we safely sleep, *Am J Respir Crit Care Med* 170:927-928, 2004.
21. Tregear S, et al: Obstructive sleep apnea and risk of motor vehicle crash: systematic review and meta-analysis, *J Clin Sleep Med* 5:573-581, 2009.
22. Chobanian AV, et al: The Seventh Report of the Joint National Committee on Prevention, Detection, Evaluation, and Treatment of High Blood Pressure: the JNC 7 report, *JAMA* 289: 2560-2572, 2003.
23. Yaggi HK, et al: Obstructive sleep apnea as a risk factor for stroke and death, *N Engl J Med* 353:2034-2041, 2005.
24. Mehra R, et al: Association of nocturnal arrhythmias with sleep-disordered breathing: the Sleep Heart Health Study, *Am J Respir Crit Care Med* 173:910-916, 2006.

25. Javaheri S, Wexler L: Prevalence and treatment of breathing disorders during sleep in patients with heart failure, *Curr Treat Options Cardiovasc Med* 7:295-306, 2005.
26. Javaheri S: Sleep and cardiovascular disease: present and future. In Kryger M, Roth T, Dement W, editors: *Priciples and practice of sleep medicine*, ed 4, Philadelphia, 2005, Saunders, pp 1157-1160.
27. Punjabi NM, et al: Sleep-disordered breathing, glucose intolerance, and insulin resistance: the Sleep Heart Health Study, *Am J Epidemiol* 160:521-530, 2004.
28. Young T, et al: Sleep disordered breathing and mortality: eighteen-year follow-up of the Wisconsin sleep cohort, *Sleep* 31:1071-1078, 2008.
29. Young T, Peppard PE, Gottlieb DJ: Epidemiology of obstructive sleep apnea: a population health perspective, *Am J Respir Crit Care Med* 165:1217-1239, 2002.
30. Johns MW: Daytime sleepiness, snoring, and obstructive sleep apnea: the Epworth Sleepiness Scale, *Chest* 103:30-36, 1993.
31. Redline S: Age-related differences in sleep apnea: generalizability of findings in older populations. In Kuna S, Suratt P, Remmers J, editors: *Sleep and respiration in aging adults*, New York, 1991, Elsevier, pp 189-194.
32. Resta O, et al: Sleep-related breathing disorders, loud snoring and excessive daytime sleepiness in obese subjects, *Int J Obes Relat Metab Disord* 25:669-675, 2001.
33. Katz I, et al: Do patients with obstructive sleep apnea have thick necks? *Am Rev Respir Dis* 141(5 Pt 1):1228-1231, 1990.
34. Davies RJ, Ali NJ, Stradling JR: Neck circumference and other clinical features in the diagnosis of the obstructive sleep apnoea syndrome, *Thorax* 47:101-105, 1992.
35. American Academy of Sleep Medicine: *The international classification of sleep disorders, 2nd ed: diagnostic and coding manual*, Westchester, IL, 2005, American Academy of Sleep Medicine.
36. He J, et al: Mortality and apnea index in obstructive sleep apnea. Experience in 385 male patients, *Chest* 94:9-14, 1988.
37. Peppard PE, et al: Longitudinal study of moderate weight change and sleep-disordered breathing, *JAMA* 284:3015-3021, 2000.
38. Peppard PE, Young T: Exercise and sleep-disordered breathing: an association independent of body habitus, *Sleep* 27:480-484, 2004.
39. Oksenberg A, Silverberg DS: The effect of body posture on sleep-related breathing disorders: facts and therapeutic implications. *Sleep Med Rev* 2:139-162, 1998.
40. Kuna ST, Bedi DG, Ryckman CC: Effect of nasal airway positive pressure on upper airway size and configuration. *Am Rev Respir Dis* 138:969-975, 1988.
41. Schwab RJ, Goldberg AN: Upper airway assessment: radiographic and other imaging techniques, *Otolaryngol Clin North Am* 31:931-968, 1998.
42. Gay P, et al: Evaluation of positive airway pressure treatment for sleep related breathing disorders in adults, *Sleep* 29:381-401, 2006.
43. Phillips B, Kryger M: Management of obstructive sleep apnea. In Kryger M, Roth T, Dement W, editors: *Principles and practice of sleep medicine*, ed 4, Philadelphia, 2005, Saunders, pp 1109-1121.
44. Ferguson KA, et al: Oral appliances for snoring and obstructive sleep apnea: a review, *Sleep* 29:244-262, 2006.
45. Rama AN, Tekwani SH, Kushida CA: Sites of obstruction in obstructive sleep apnea, *Chest* 122:1139-1147, 2002.
46. Bennett LS, Davies RJ, Stradling JR: Oral appliances for the management of snoring and obstructive sleep apnoea, *Thorax* 53(Suppl 2):S58-S64, 1998.
47. Ryan CF, et al: Mandibular advancement oral appliance therapy for obstructive sleep apnoea: effect on awake calibre of the velopharynx, *Thorax* 54:972-977, 1999.
48. Liu Y, et al: Effects of a mandibular repositioner on obstructive sleep apnea, *Am J Orthod Dentofacial Orthop* 118:248-256, 2000.
49. Deane SA, et al: Comparison of mandibular advancement splint and tongue stabilizing device in obstructive sleep apnea: a randomized controlled trial, *Sleep* 32:648-653, 2009.
50. Lazard DS, et al: The tongue-retaining device: efficacy and side effects in obstructive sleep apnea syndrome, *J Clin Sleep Med* 5:431-438, 2009.
51. Singh GD, Keropian B, Pillar G: Effects of the full breath solution appliance for the treatment of obstructive sleep apnea: a preliminary study, *Cranio* 27:109-117, 2009.
52. Lowe AA, et al: Treatment, airway and compliance effects of a titratable oral appliance, *Sleep* 23(Suppl 4): S172-S178, 2000.
53. Marklund M, et al: The effect of a mandibular advancement device on apneas and sleep in patients with obstructive sleep apnea, *Chest* 113:707-713,1998.
54. Menn SJ, et al: The mandibular repositioning device: role in the treatment of obstructive sleep apnea, *Sleep* 19:794-800, 1996.
55. Pancer J, et al: Evaluation of variable mandibular advancement appliance for treatment of snoring and sleep apnea, *Chest* 116:1511-1518, 1999.
56. Pellanda A, Despland PA, Pasche P: The anterior mandibular positioning device for the treatment of obstructive sleep apnoea syndrome: experience with the Serenox, *Clin Otolaryngol Allied Sci* 24:134-141, 1999.
57. Yoshida K: Effects of a mandibular advancement device for the treatment of sleep apnea syndrome and snoring on respiratory function and sleep quality, *Cranio* 18:98-105, 2000.
58. Marklund M, Stenlund H, Franklin KA: Mandibular advancement devices in 630 men and women with obstructive sleep apnea and snoring: tolerability and predictors of treatment success, *Chest* 125:1270-1278, 2004.
59. Gotsopoulos H, et al: Oral appliance therapy improves symptoms in obstructive sleep apnea: a randomized, controlled trial, *Am J Respir Crit Care Med* 166:743-748, 2002.
60. Mehta A, et al: A randomized, controlled study of a mandibular advancement splint for obstructive sleep apnea, *Am J Respir Crit Care Med* 163:1457-1461, 2001.
61. Almeida FR, et al: Effect of a titration polysomnogram on treatment success with a mandibular repositioning appliance, *J Clin Sleep Med* 5:198-204, 2009.
62. Ferguson KA, et al: A short-term controlled trial of an adjustable oral appliance for the treatment of mild to moderate obstructive sleep apnoea, *Thorax* 52:362-368, 1997.
63. Hans MG, et al: Comparison of two dental devices for treatment of obstructive sleep apnea syndrome (OSAS), *Am J Orthod Dentofacial Orthop* 11:562-570, 1997.
64. Henke KG, Frantz DE, Kuna ST: An oral elastic mandibular advancement device for obstructive sleep apnea, *Am J Respir Crit Care Med* 161(2 Pt 1):420-425, 2000.
65. Schmidt-Nowara WW, Meade TE, Hays MB: Treatment of snoring and obstructive sleep apnea with a dental orthosis, *Chest* 99:1378-1385, 1991.
66. Clark GT, Sohn JW, Hong CN: Treating obstructive sleep apnea and snoring: assessment of an anterior mandibular positioning device, *J Am Dent Assoc* 131:765-771, 2000.
67. Fransson AM, et al: Effects of a mandibular protruding device on the sleep of patients with obstructive sleep apnea and snoring problems: a 2-year follow-up, *Sleep Breath* 7:131-141, 2003.
68. Ringqvist M, et al: Dental and skeletal changes after 4 years of obstructive sleep apnea treatment with a mandibular

advancement device: a prospective, randomized study, *Am J Orthod Dentofacial Orthop* 124:53-60, 2003.
69. de Almeida FR, et al: Long-term compliance and side effects of oral appliances used for the treatment of snoring and obstructive sleep apnea syndrome, *J Clin Sleep Med* 1:143-152, 2005.
70. Giannasi LC, et al: Systematic assessment of the impact of oral appliance therapy on the temporomandibular joint during treatment of obstructive sleep apnea: long-term evaluation, *Sleep Breath* 13:375-381, 2009.
71. Landry-Schonbeck A, et al: Effect of an adjustable mandibular advancement appliance on sleep bruxism: a crossover sleep laboratory study, *Int J Prosthodont* 22:251-259, 2009.
72. Almeida FR, et al: Long-term sequelae of oral appliance therapy in obstructive sleep apnea patients: Part 1. Cephalometric analysis, *Am J Orthod Dentofacial Orthop* 129:195-204, 2006.
73. Chen H, et al: Dental changes evaluated with a 3D computer-assisted model analysis after long-term tongue retaining device wear in OSA patients, *Sleep Breath* 12:169-178, 2008.
74. Chen H, et al: Three-dimensional computer-assisted study model analysis of long-term oral-appliance wear. Part 1: Methodology, *Am J Orthod Dentofacial Orthop* 134:393-407, 2008.
75. Walker-Engstrom ML, et al: 4-year follow-up of treatment with dental appliance or uvulopalatopharyngoplasty in patients with obstructive sleep apnea: a randomized study, *Chest* 121:739-746, 2002.
76. Wilhelmsson B, et al: A prospective randomized study of a dental appliance compared with uvulopalatopharyngoplasty in the treatment of obstructive sleep apnoea, *Acta Otolaryngol* 119:503-509, 1999.
77. Kushida CA, et al: Practice parameters for the treatment of snoring and obstructive sleep apnea with oral appliances: an update for 2005, *Sleep* 29:240-243, 2006.
78. Epstein LJ, et al: Clinical guideline for the evaluation, management and long-term care of obstructive sleep apnea in adults, *J Clin Sleep Med* 5:263-276, 2009.
79. Sundaram S, et al: Surgery for obstructive sleep apnoea, *Cochrane Database Syst Rev* 4:CD001004, 2005.
80. Maurer JT: Update on surgical treatments for sleep apnea, *Swiss Med Wkly* 139:624-629, 2009.
81. Aurora RN, et al: Practice parameters for the surgical modifications of the upper airway for obstructive sleep apnea in adults, *Sleep* 33:1408-1413, 2010.
82. Schechter MS: Technical report: diagnosis and management of childhood obstructive sleep apnea syndrome, *Pediatrics* 109:e69, 2002.
83. Powell NB: Contemporary surgery for obstructive sleep apnea syndrome, *Clin Exp Otorhinolaryngol* 2:107-114, 2009.
84. Riley RW, Powell NB, Guilleminault C: Obstructive sleep apnea syndrome: a surgical protocol for dynamic upper airway reconstruction, *J Oral Maxillofac Surg* 51:742-747, 1993.
85. Ryan CF: Sleep × 9: an approach to treatment of obstructive sleep apnoea/hypopnoea syndrome including upper airway surgery, *Thorax* 60:595-604, 2005.
86. Franklin KA, et al: Effects and side-effects of surgery for snoring and obstructive sleep apnea—a systematic review, *Sleep* 32:27-36, 2009.
87. Maciel Santos ME, et al: Obstructive sleep apnea-hypopnea syndrome—the role of bariatric and maxillofacial surgeries, *Obes Surg* 19:796-801, 2009.
88. Haines KL, et al: Objective evidence that bariatric surgery improves obesity-related obstructive sleep apnea, *Surgery* 141:354-358, 2007.

PART IV

Gastrointestinal Disease

CHAPTER

10

Liver Disease

Liver dysfunction may be attributed to a number of causes, including acquired infections and other pathologic conditions, as well as drug use. The patient with liver disease presents a significant management challenge for the dentist because the liver plays a vital role in metabolic functions, including the secretion of bile needed for fat absorption, conversion of sugar to glycogen, and excretion of bilirubin, a waste product of hemoglobin metabolism. Impairment of liver function can lead to abnormalities in the metabolism of amino acids, ammonia, protein, carbohydrates, and lipids (triglycerides and cholesterol). Many biochemical functions performed by the liver, such as synthesis of coagulation factors and drug metabolism, may be adversely affected in the dental patient with acute or chronic liver disease. Along with impaired drug metabolism, therefore, significant bleeding may be a problem to be addressed in the dental treatment plan.[1-5] In many cases, the liver dysfunction will continue to progress over time. Ultimately, serious end-stage liver dysfunction or cirrhosis may result.

Cirrhosis is the consequence of long-term damage to the liver tissues. This condition is irreversible and leads to fibrosis, resulting in jaundice, ascites, and portal hypertension, as well as significant liver dysfunction. The potential causes of viral hepatitis related cirrhosis are listed in Table 10-1. Obviously, liver disorders in persons presenting for treatment will be of significant clinical interest to the dentist in the context of the proper management of such patients.[1-5] In this chapter, the two most common liver disorders and main causes of cirrhosis, hepatitis and alcoholic liver disease, are presented.

HEPATITIS

Definition

Hepatitis is inflammation of the liver that may result from infectious or other causes. Examples of hepatitis with infectious causes are viral hepatitis and that associated with infectious mononucleosis, secondary syphilis, and tuberculosis. Approximately 15,000 people in the United States die each year of cirrhosis caused by viral hepatitis.[6,7] Also, noninfectious hepatitis can result from excessive or prolonged use of toxic substances: drugs (i.e., acetaminophen, alcohol, halothane, ketoconazole, methyldopa, and methotrexate) or, more commonly, alcohol.[2,7-10]

Since the several types of hepatitis have various degrees of impact on dental treatment, each is discussed separately in subsequent sections.

Viral hepatitis is a collective term describing liver inflammation or hepatitis caused by a group of several different viruses. Three viruses, hepatitis A virus (HAV), hepatitis B virus (HBV), and hepatitis C virus (HCV), cause most cases of viral hepatitis in the United States. Because hepatitis A is transmitted primarily in unsanitary conditions, the number of annual cases has declined significantly in the United States in recent years as a result of vaccination programs and food safety efforts.

Unlike HAV hepatitis, infections by HBV and HCV are bloodborne and/or often persist for years, resulting in ongoing (chronic) but usually asymptomatic liver inflammation and, in some cases, scarring (cirrhosis) that leads to liver failure and/or liver cancer. Chronic hepatitis is a major cause of liver cancer and chronic liver disease globally and in the United States.[2,11]

Epidemiology

Acute viral hepatitis is a common disease that affects 0.5% to 1% of persons in the United States each year. The annual incidence of acute hepatitis has been decreasing steadily since 1990, largely because of the use of hepatitis A and B vaccines and decrease in high-risk behaviors. In recent population-based surveys, viral causes of acute hepatitis were HAV in 37%, HBV in 45%, and HCV in 18% of cases. Worldwide, 480 million to 540 million persons are living with chronic viral hepatitis, with 350 million to 370 million infected with HBV and 130 million to 170 million infected with HCV.[2,12]

Chronic hepatitis causes considerable morbidity. Globally, an estimated 78% of primary liver cancer and 57% of liver cirrhosis are caused by chronic viral hepatitis, and about 1 million deaths from viral hepatitis occur each year.[10,13,14] Liver cancer is the fourth leading cause of death from cancer worldwide and the third leading cause among men. Recent liver cancer surveillance data indicate that long-term liver cancer incidence is increasing in the United States, with an average annual percentage increase of 3.5% per year between 2001 and 2006.[7,10,11,15] In the United States, acute infection leads to chronic viral hepatitis in 3.5 million to 5.3 million Americans.[7,10,11] The vast majority—an estimated 65% and 75%, for HBV and HCV, respectively—are not aware they are infected. In the absence of appropriate treatment, liver cirrhosis will develop in 15% to 40% of infected persons.[7,10,11]

The clinical manifestations of the five forms of viral hepatitis are quite similar, and the diseases can be distinguished from each other only by serologic assays.[6,7,11] The five known causes of acute hepatitis are hepatitis virus types A (HAV), B (HBV), C (HCV), D or delta (HDV), and E (HEV) (see Table 10-1). All except HBV are RNA viruses. Hepatitis A and hepatitis E are forms of *infectious* hepatitis; they are spread largely by the fecal-oral route, are associated with poor sanitary conditions, are highly contagious, occur in outbreaks as well as sporadically, and cause self-limited hepatitis only. Hepatitis B, hepatitis C, and hepatitis D are forms of *serum* hepatitis, are spread largely by parenteral routes and less commonly by intimate or sexual exposure, and are not highly contagious but instead occur sporadically and rarely cause outbreaks. They are capable of leading to chronic infection and, ultimately, to cirrhosis and hepatocellular carcinoma. Cases of an acute viral hepatitis–like syndrome that cannot be identified as being due to a known hepatitis virus have been reported; this syndrome has been called acute *non-A, non-B, non-C, non-D, non-E (non–A-E) hepatitis,* or *acute hepatitis of unknown cause.* Despite many attempts, the viral etiology of non–-A-E hepatitis remains unproved.[7,11]

Pathophysiology

The pathogenesis of the liver injury in viral hepatitis is not well understood. None of the five primary agents seems to be directly cytopathic, at least at levels of replication found during typical acute and chronic hepatitis. The timing and histologic appearance of hepatocyte injury in viral hepatitis suggest that immune responses, particularly cytotoxic T cell responses to viral antigens expressed on hepatocyte cell membranes, may be the major effectors of injury. Other proinflammatory cytokines, natural killer cell activity, and antibody-dependent cellular cytotoxicity also may play modulating roles in cell injury and inflammation during acute hepatitis virus infection. Recovery from hepatitis virus infection usually is accompanied by the appearance of rising titers of antibody against viral envelope antigens, such as anti-HAV, anti-HBs, anti-HCV-E1 and anti-HCV-E2, and anti-HEV; these antibodies may provide at least partial immunity to reinfection.[7,11]

Clinical Manifestations

The course of acute hepatitis is highly variable and ranges in severity from a transient, asymptomatic infection to severe or fulminant disease. The disease may be self-limited with complete resolution, run a relapsing course, or lead to chronic infection. In a typical, clinically apparent course of acute resolving viral hepatitis, the *incubation period* ranges from 2 to 20 weeks, as determined largely on the basis of the viral etiologic agent and exposure dose. During this phase, virus becomes detectable in blood, but serum aminotransferase and bilirubin levels are normal, and antibody is not detected.[7,11]

The *preicteric phase* of illness is marked by the onset of nonspecific symptoms such as fatigue, nausea, poor appetite, and vague right upper quadrant pain. Virus-specific antibody first appears during this phase. The preicteric phase typically lasts 3 to 10 days but may be of longer duration and even constitute the entire course of illness in patients with subclinical or anicteric forms of acute hepatitis. Viral titers generally are highest at this point, and serum aminotransferase levels start to increase.[7,11]

The onset of production of dark urine marks the *icteric phase* of illness, during which jaundice appears and symptoms of fatigue and nausea worsen. Typically, acute viral hepatitis rarely is diagnosed correctly before the onset of jaundice. If jaundice is severe, stool color lightens, often in association with pruritus. Other manifestations may include anorexia, dysgeusia, and weight loss. Physical examination usually shows jaundice and hepatic tenderness. In more severe cases, hepatomegaly and splenomegaly may be present. Serum bilirubin levels (total and direct) rise, and aminotransferase levels generally are higher than 10 times the upper limit of normal, at least at the onset. During the icteric, symptomatic phase, levels of hepatitis virus begin to decrease in serum and liver.[7,11]

The duration of clinical illness is variable; it typically lasts 1 to 3 weeks. Recovery is first manifested by return of appetite and is accompanied by resolution of the serum bilirubin and aminotransferase elevations and clearance of virus. *Convalescence* can be prolonged, however, before full energy and stamina return. Neutralizing antibodies usually appear during the icteric phase and rise to high levels during convalescence.[7,11]

Complications of acute viral hepatitis include chronic infection, fulminant hepatic failure, relapsing or cholestatic hepatitis, and extrahepatic syndromes. *Chronic hepatitis,* generally defined as illness of at least 6 months' duration, develops in approximately 2% to 7% of adults with hepatitis B and in 50% to 85% of adults with hepatitis C. Hepatitis B, C, and D infections are said to be chronic if viremia persists for more than 6 months, but chronicity can be suspected if viremia persists for 3 months after the onset of symptoms.[7,11]

TABLE 10-1 Most Common Agents of Acute Viral Hepatitis, with Associated Characteristics

Hepatitis Virus	Size (nm)	Genome	Spread*	Incubation Period (Days)	Fatality Rate	Chronicity Rate	Antibody	Diagnosis[†‡]
A (HAV)	27	RNA	Fecal-oral	15-45; mean, 25	1%	None	Anti-HAV	Anti-HAV IgG
B (HBV)	45	DNA	Parenteral	30-180; mean, 75	1%	2-7%	Anti-HBs	HBsAg (infectious) Anti-HBsAg (recovery) Anti-HBc (acute, persistently infected nonprotective) HBeAg (infectious) Anti-HBeAg (clearing/ cleared infection)
			Sexual				Anti-HBc Anti-HBe	
C (HCV)	60	RNA	Parenteral	15-150; mean, 50	<0.1%	50-85%	Anti-HCV	Anti-HCV (previous infection) HCV RNA (infectivity)
D (delta) (HDV)	40	RNA	Parenteral	30-150	2-10%	2-7%	Anti-HDV	Anti-HDV HD-Ag
			Sexual			50%		
E (HEV)	32	RNA	Fecal-oral	30-60	1%	None	Anti-HEV	Anti-HEV

HBc, Hepatitis B core; *HBeAg,* Hepatitis B e antigen; *HBsAg,* Hepatitis B surface antigen; *IgG,* Immunoglobulin G.

*With parenteral and sexual modes of transmission: Risk groups include intravenous drug users, health care workers, hemodialysis patients, persons of low socioeconomic status, sexual/household contacts of infected persons, persons with multiple sex partners, and patients with a history of transfusion before 1991.

The U.S. Food and Drug Administration (FDA) requires that all donated whole blood, transfusable components, and plasma for human blood use in the United States be subjected to serologic testing for syphilis, HBsAg, anti-HBc, anti-HCV, and anti-HIV. The current incidence of posttransfusion hepatitis B is approximately 0.002% per transfusion recipient.

A small number of cases of transmission of HAV through clotting factor concentrates also have been reported. *(Data from Centers for Disease Control and Prevention: Hepatitis A among persons with hemophilia who received clotting factor concentrate—United States, September–December 1995,* MMWR Morb Mortal Wkly Rep *45:29-32, 1996.)*

Acute liver failure or fulminant hepatitis occurs in 1% to 2% of patients with symptomatic acute hepatitis, perhaps most commonly with hepatitis B and hepatitis D and least commonly with hepatitis C. The disease is called *fulminant* if evidence of hepatic encephalopathy appears; however, the initial symptoms (changes in personality, aggressive behavior, or abnormal sleep patterns) may be subtle or misunderstood. The most reliable prognostic factor in acute hepatic failure is the degree of prolongation of the prothrombin time; other signs of poor prognosis are persistently worsening jaundice, ascites, and decreases in liver size. Serum aminotransferase levels and viral titers have little prognostic value and often decrease with worsening hepatic failure.[6,7,11] In a proportion of cases of acute hepatitis, a cholestatic pattern of illness consisting of prolonged and fluctuating jaundice and pruritus develops. Patients may experience one or more clinical relapses and may feel relatively well despite marked jaundice. Cholestatic hepatitis generally is benign and ultimately resolves.[7,11]

In 10% to 20% of patients with acute hepatitis, a *serum sickness–like syndrome* marked by variable combinations of rash, hives, arthralgias, and fever develops during the preicteric phase. This immune complex–like syndrome often is mistakenly attributed to other illnesses until the onset of jaundice, at which time the fever, hives, and arthralgias quickly resolve. Other extrahepatic manifestations of acute hepatitis are uncommon but may include severe headaches, encephalitis, aseptic meningitis, seizures, acute ascending flaccid paralysis, nephrotic syndrome, and seronegative arthritis.[7,11]

Diagnosis

Serologic tests are adequate for the diagnosis of acute viral hepatitis (Table 10-2), so liver biopsy is not recommended unless the diagnosis remains unclear and a therapeutic decision is needed. If biopsy is required, the histologic pattern in acute viral hepatitis is characterized by widespread parenchymal inflammation and spotty

Chronic Carrier State	Complications§ of the Liver	Associated Clinical Syndromes	Immunization: Passive	Immunization: Active
No	Rare		Immune globulin (0.02 mg/kg)	Harivax, Vaqta, Twinrix
Yes—90% risk of becoming carrier if infected as neonate; 25-50% risk if infected as infant; 5-10% risk if infected as adult	Yes—increased risk of cirrhosis and hepatocellular carcinoma (HCC) after 25-30 years of infection	Yes	Hepatitis B immune globulin (HBIg) (0.06 mg/kg)	Recombivax, Engerix,‖ Twinrix
Yes—risk of becoming carrier is 80-90%	Yes—10-fold increased risk of liver cirrhosis within 20 years; 1-5% of carriers develop HCC by 20 years, risk of HCC with chronic HCV infection exceeds risk with chronic HBV infection	Yes	Not available	None (difficult development because of the many genotypes)
Yes—carrier state in 20-70%	Yes		Not available	Yes—protected with Recombivax, Engerix‖, and Twinrix
No	Rare morbidity and mortality except in pregnant women		Not available	Genentech has applied for vaccine patent

†Diagnostic markers of viral hepatitis include elevation of aspartate aminotransferase, alanine aminotransferase, γ-glutamyl transferase, and white blood cell count and prolongation of prothrombin time.
‡*Preicteric phase:* anorexia, nausea, vomiting, fatigue, myalgia, malaise, fever. *Icterus:* jaundice, discolored stool, dark urine, hepatosplenomegaly, bleeding disorder. *Serum sickness–like features:* arthralgia, rash, angioedema (seen in 5% to 10% of patients).
§Risk for complications and severe liver disease increases with coinfection with HBV and HCV, and with chronic alcohol consumption.
‖Immunization is recommended for dental personnel.

TABLE 10-2 Serologic Diagnosis of Acute Hepatitis

Diagnosis	Screening Assays	Supplemental Assays
Hepatitis A	IgM anti-HAV	None needed
Hepatitis B	HBsAg, IgM anti-HBc	HBeAg, anti-HBe, HBV DNA
Hepatitis C	Anti-HCV by EIA	HCV RNA by PCR assay; anti-HCV by immunoblot analysis
Hepatitis D	HBsAg	Anti-HDV
Hepatitis E	History	Anti-HEV
Mononucleosis	History, white blood cell differential counts	Heterophile antibody
Drug-induced hepatitis	History	

EIA, Enzyme immunoassay; *HAV,* Hepatitis A; *HBc,* Hepatitis B core; *HBeAg,* Hepatitis B e antigen; *HBsAg,* Hepatitis B surface antigen; *HBV,* Hepatitis B; *HCV,* Hepatitis C; *HDV,* Hepatitis D; *HEV,* Hepatitis E; *IgM,* Immunoglobulin M; *PCR,* Polymerase chain reaction.

necrosis. Inflammatory cells are predominantly lymphocytes, macrophages, and histiocytes. Fibrosis is absent. Immunohistochemical stains for hepatitis antigens generally are negative during the acute disease, and there are no reliably distinctive anatomic features in the liver that separate the five viral forms of acute hepatitis from each other.[7,11]

Treatment

Although antiviral therapies have not been proved to be effective in prospective controlled trials, recent uncontrolled studies suggest that such therapies may be effective in acute hepatitis B and hepatitis C (see further on). However, several recommendations are applicable to the management of all patients with acute hepatitis. Bedrest and sensible nutrition are appropriate for patients who are symptomatic and jaundiced. Alcohol should be avoided until after convalescence. Sexual contacts should be limited until partners receive prophylaxis. In hepatitis A, all household contacts should be given immune globulin, and initiation of HAV vaccination is appropriate.

In hepatitis B, family members should be vaccinated, and hepatitis B immune globulin (HBIG) also should be given to recent sexual contacts. Patients in whom any signs of fulminant hepatic failure develop (prolongation of the prothrombin time, personality changes, confusion) should be considered for antiviral therapy and be evaluated quickly for possible liver transplantation (see Chapter 21). The success of transplantation for severe, acute viral hepatitis often depends on early referral and careful attention to all details of clinical care, with management provided by an experienced team of physicians. Follow-up evaluation for acute hepatitis should be adequate to show that resolution has occurred, particularly for patients with hepatitis C. Finally, and of greatest importance, all cases of acute hepatitis should be reported to the local or state health department as soon as possible after diagnosis.

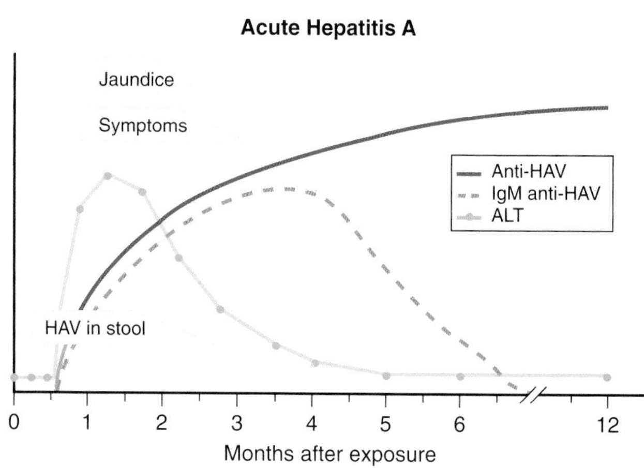

FIGURE 10-1 Serologic course of acute hepatitis A. *ALT*, Alanine aminotransferase; *HAV*, Hepatitis A virus. *(From Goldman L, Ausiello D, editors:* Cecil textbook of medicine, *ed 23, Philadelphia, 2008, Saunders.)*

HEPATITIS A

Epidemiology

Hepatitis A is highly contagious and is spread largely by the fecal-oral route, especially when sanitary conditions are poor. Hepatitis A has been decreasing in frequency in the United States but is still an important cause of acute liver disease worldwide. Acute hepatitis A can occur in sporadic as well as epidemic forms. Investigation of the source of infection reveals that most cases are due to direct person-to-person exposure and, to a lesser extent, to direct fecal contamination of food or water. Consumption of shellfish from contaminated waterways is a well-known but quite uncommon means of acquiring hepatitis A. Rare instances of spread of hepatitis A by blood transfusions and administration of pooled plasma products have been described. Groups at high risk for acquiring hepatitis A include travelers to developing areas of the world, children in day care centers (and secondarily their parents), men who have sex with men, injection drug users, hemophiliacs given plasma products, and residents and staff of institutions.[7,11]

Pathophysiology

HAV is a small RNA virus that belongs to the family Picornaviridae (genus *Hepatovirus*). The viral genome is 7.5 kilobases (kb) in length and has a single large open reading frame that encodes a polyprotein with structural and nonstructural components. The virus replicates largely in the liver and is assembled in the hepatocyte cytoplasm as a 27-nm particle with a single RNA genome and an outer capsid protein (HAVAg). The virus is secreted into bile and, to a lesser extent, serum. The highest titers of HAV are found in stool (10^6 to 10^{10} genomes per gram) during the incubation period and early symptomatic phase of illness.

Clinical Manifestations

The clinical course of typical acute hepatitis A (Figure 10-1) begins with an incubation period that usually is 15 to 45 days in duration (mean, 25 days). Jaundice occurs in 70% of adults infected with HAV but in smaller proportions of children. Antibody to HAV (anti-HAV [IgG antibody]), which develops in all patients infected with the virus, is first detectable shortly before the onset of symptoms; titers then rise to high levels, which persist for life. By contrast, IgM-specific anti-HAV arises early in the disease and persists for only 4 to 12 months. Severe and fulminant cases of hepatitis A can occur, particularly in elderly persons and in patients with preexisting chronic liver disease. Hepatitis A is the most common cause of relapsing cholestatic hepatitis.

Diagnosis

The diagnosis of acute hepatitis A is made by detection of IgM anti-HAV in the serum of a patient with the clinical and biochemical features of acute hepatitis. Testing for total anti-HAV is not helpful in diagnosis but is used to assess immunity to hepatitis A.[11]

Prevention

A safe and effective HAV vaccine is available and recommended for all children 1 year of age and older and for persons at increased risk for acquiring hepatitis A, including travelers to endemic areas of the world, men who have sex with men, and injection drug users. HAV vaccine also is recommended for all patients with chronic liver disease and recipients of pooled plasma products, such as hemophiliacs. Two formulations of HAV vaccine are available in the United States; both consist of inactivated hepatitis A antigen purified from cell culture.

Havrix (GlaxoSmithKline, Philadelphia, Pennsylvania) is recommended to be given as two injections 6 to 12 months apart in an adult dose of 1440 enzyme-linked immunosorbent assay (ELISA) units (1.0 mL) and in a pediatric (2 to 18 years of age) dose of 720 ELISA units (0.5 mL). Vaqta (Merck, West Point, Pennsylvania) is recommended to be given as two injections 6 to 18 months apart in an adult dose of 50 U (1.0 mL) and in a pediatric dose (1 to 18 years) of 25 U (0.5 mL). A combination HAV-HBV vaccine (Twinrix) (GlaxoSmith-Kline) also is available; this preparation is recommended for adults who require vaccination against both forms of hepatitis and is given in a three-injection schedule at 0, 1, and 6 months after exposure. HAV vaccines have an excellent safety record, with serious complications occurring in less than 0.1% of recipients. Seroconversion rates after HAV vaccine are greater than 95% but are lower among patients with chronic liver disease, human immunodeficiency virus (HIV) infection, and other conditions of immunocompromise.[16,17]

Treatment

No specific therapies have been shown to shorten or ameliorate the course of illness in hepatitis A. An important element of management should be prophylaxis for contacts. Persons with fulminant hepatitis should be referred early for possible liver transplantation.[16,18]

Prognosis

Acute hepatitis A is invariably a self-limited infection. The virus can persist for months, but this condition does not lead to chronic infection, chronic hepatitis, or cirrhosis.

HEPATITIS B

Epidemiology

Hepatitis B is spread predominantly by the parenteral route or by intimate personal contact. It is endemic in many areas of the world, such as Southeast Asia, China, Micronesia, and sub-Saharan Africa. Lesser rates occur in the Indian subcontinent and the Middle East. In the United States, hepatitis B is the most common cause of acute hepatitis, and chronic HVB infection affects approximately 0.5% of the population. Investigations of the source of infection reveal that most adult cases are due to sexual or parenteral contact. Hepatitis B is common in injection drug users, heterosexual persons with multiple sexual partners, and men who have sex with men. Blood transfusion and plasma products are now rarely infectious for hepatitis B because of the institution of routine screening of blood donations for hepatitis B surface antigen (HBsAg) and antibody to hepatitis B core antigen (HBcAg), anti-HBc (IgG antibody). Maternal-infant spread of hepatitis B is another important mode of transmission not only in endemic areas of the world but also in the United States among immigrants from these endemic areas. Routine screening of pregnant women and prophylaxis of newborns are now recommended. Intrafamilial spread of hepatitis B also can occur, although the mode of spread in this situation is not well defined. Unfortunately, lack of attention to standard (formerly universal) precautions and aseptic technique, especially the cleaning of shared medical devices, remains an important root cause of small outbreaks and sporadic cases of acute hepatitis B.[6,11]

Pathophysiology

HBV is a double-shelled, enveloped DNA virus belonging to the family Hepadnaviridae (genus *Orthohepadnavirus*). The viral genome consists of partially double-stranded DNA, is 3.2 kb in length, and possesses four partially overlapping open reading frames that encode the genes for HBsAg (*S* gene), HBcAg (*C* gene), HBV polymerase (*P* gene), and a small protein, HBxAg, that seems to have transactivating functions (*X* gene). The virus infects only humans and higher apes and replicates predominantly in hepatocytes and perhaps to a lesser extent in stem cells in the pancreas, bone marrow, and spleen. The clinical course of hepatitis B with serologic markers is depicted in Figure 10-2. During both acute and chronic infection, large amounts of HBsAg are detectable in serum, mostly in the form of incomplete 20-nm virus-like spherical and tubular particles. Persons who produce large amounts of HBV in serum typically also produce HBeAg—making HBeAg a surrogate marker for high levels of viral replication.[7,11]

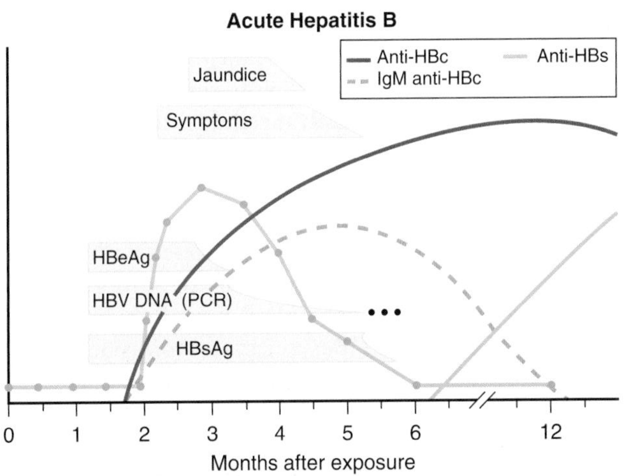

FIGURE 10-2 Serologic course of acute hepatitis B. *HBc*, Hepatitis B core; *HBeAg*, Hepatitis B e antigen; *HBs*, Hepatitis B surface; *HBsAg*, Hepatitis B surface antigen; *HBV*, Hepatitis B virus; *PCR*, Polymerase chain reaction. *(From Goldman L, Ausiello D, editors: Cecil textbook of medicine, ed 23, Philadelphia, 2008, Saunders.)*

Clinical Manifestations

The typical course of acute, self-limited hepatitis B begins with an incubation period of 30 to 150 days (mean, 75 days). During the incubation period, HBsAg, HBeAg, and HBV DNA (see Figure 10-2) become detectable in serum and rise to high titers, with the virus reaching titers of 10^8 to 10^{11} virions/mL. By the onset of symptoms, anti-HBc arises and serum aminotransferase levels are elevated. Jaundice appears in a third of adults with hepatitis B and in a lesser proportion of children. Generally, HBV DNA and HBeAg begin to fall at the onset of illness and may be undetectable at the time of peak clinical illness. HBsAg becomes undetectable and anti-HBs appears during recovery, several weeks to months after loss of HBsAg. Anti-HBs is a long-lasting antibody that is associated with immunity.[11,19,20]

Diagnosis

The diagnosis of acute hepatitis B can be made on the basis of finding HBsAg in the serum of a patient with the clinical and biochemical features of acute hepatitis. HBsAg also may be present as a result of chronic hepatitis B or the carrier state. Also, a patient with acute hepatitis and HBsAg in serum may have chronic hepatitis and a superimposed form of acute injury, such as acute hepatitis A or D or drug-induced liver disease. Testing for IgM anti-HBc (IgG antibody) is therefore helpful, because this antibody arises early and is lost within 6 to 12 months of the onset of illness. Testing for HBeAg, anti-HBe, HBV DNA, and anti-HBs generally is not helpful in the diagnosis of hepatitis B but may be valuable in assessing prognosis. Persons who remain HBV DNA– or HBeAg-positive (or both) at 6 weeks after the onset of symptoms are likely to be developing chronic hepatitis B. Loss of HBeAg or HBV DNA is a favorable serologic finding. Similarly, loss of HBsAg plus the development of anti-HBs denotes recovery.[7,11]

Hepatitis B also is an important cause of fulminant hepatitis. Factors associated with severe outcomes of acute hepatitis B include advanced age, female sex, and perhaps certain strains of virus. Some variants of HBV lack the ability to produce HBeAg because of a mutation in the precore region of the viral genome. These precore or HBeAg-negative mutants are associated with atypical forms of acute and chronic hepatitis B. Several clusters of severe or fulminant hepatitis B have been associated with infection with the HBeAg-negative forms of virus.[7,11]

Prevention

Vaccination against HBV is recommended for all newborns, children, and adolescents, as well as adults at risk for acquiring HBV, including health care and public safety workers with exposure to blood, injection drug users, men who have sex with men, persons at risk for sexually transmitted infections, people traveling internationally to endemic regions, and persons with close contact with patients who have chronic hepatitis B. Two formulations of HBV vaccine are available in the United States; both are made by recombinant techniques using cloned HBV *S* gene expressed in *Saccharomyces cerevisiae*. For adults, the recommended regimen is three injections of 1.0 mL (20 µg of Energix-B [GlaxoSmithKline][2,11] or 10 µg of Recombivax HB [Merck]) given intramuscularly in the deltoid muscle at 0, 1, and 6 months. Prevaccination screening for anti-HBs is not recommended except for adults in high-risk groups (e.g., persons born in endemic countries, injection drug users, men who have sex with men, and HIV-infected persons). Postvaccination testing for anti-HBs to document seroconversion is not recommended routinely except in persons whose subsequent clinical management depends on knowledge of their immune status, particularly health care and public safety workers. At present, booster doses are not recommended but may be appropriate for persons at high risk if titers of anti-HBs fall below what is considered protective (10 IU/mL).[7,11]

Postexposure prophylaxis with HBIG is recommended at birth for infants born to infected mothers and for persons with percutaneous exposure to a patient with hepatitis B. A single dose of HBIG (0.5 mL in newborns of infected mothers and 0.06 mL/kg in other settings and in adults) should be given as soon as possible after exposure, and HBV vaccination should be started immediately. HBIG is unlikely to provide benefit if the time since exposure is longer than 14 days; vaccine alone can be used in these circumstances. For patients who have had sexual or household contact with a person who has chronic hepatitis B, vaccination alone is appropriate; HBIG is recommended in addition for sexual exposure to a person with acute hepatitis B.[7,11,20]

Treatment

The use of antiviral therapy for acute hepatitis B is controversial. Regimens of interferon alfa and lamivudine are established therapies for chronic hepatitis B, but they have not been adequately evaluated for acute infection. In a small study, interferon alfa did not decrease the rate of chronicity or speed recovery. Uncontrolled observations with use of lamivudine in patients with fulminant and severe hepatitis B, however suggest that this therapy may ameliorate the course of infection. Because of the safety of lamivudine therapy and the unpredictable and potentially serious outcome with severe cases of acute hepatitis B, therapy with lamivudine (100 mg daily until the disease has resolved and results of HBsAg testing have become negative) is prudent for patients with signs or symptoms of fulminant liver disease (rising prothrombin time, severe jaundice), particularly if high levels of HBV DNA are present. Management of acute hepatitis B also should focus on avoidance of further hepatic injury and prophylaxis of contacts. The patient should be monitored by repeat testing for HBsAg and alanine aminotransferase levels 3 to 6 months later to determine whether chronic hepatitis B has developed.[11]

Prognosis

Chronic hepatitis B develops in 2% to 7% of adults infected with HBV, more commonly in men and in immunosuppressed persons. The risk of chronic infection also correlates with age. It occurs in 90% of newborns infected with HBV, in approximately 30% of infants, but in less than 10% of adults. Chronic hepatitis B is still the third or fourth most common cause of cirrhosis in the United States and is an important cause of liver cancer.[11]

HEPATITIS C

Epidemiology

Hepatitis C is spread predominantly by the parenteral route. At highest risk for contracting this disease are injection drug users and persons with multiple parenteral exposures. Sexual transmission of hepatitis C is uncommon. Prospective follow-up evaluation of spouses and sexual partners of patients with chronic hepatitis C shows the risk for sexual transmission to be low (less than 1% per year of exposure). Maternal-infant spread occurs in approximately 5% of cases, usually in infants whose mothers have high levels of HCV RNA in serum and have experienced a protracted delivery or early rupture of membranes. Other potential sources of HCV are needlestick accidents and either contamination or inadequate sterilization of reusable needles and syringes. There remain, however, many persons with chronic hepatitis C who were infected with the virus by these means in the past. Current studies of acute hepatitis C indicate that more than 60% of cases are attributable to injection drug use; 15% to 20% to sexual exposure (usually involving multiple sexual partners); and only a small proportion to maternal-infant spread, needlestick accidents, and iatrogenic causes. Approximately 10% of cases are not associated with any history of potential exposure and remain unexplained.[7,11]

Pathophysiology

HCV is an RNA virus that belongs to the family Flaviviridae (genus *Hepacivirus*). HCV originally was identified by molecular techniques, and the virus has not been well visualized. HCV probably circulates as a double-shelled enveloped virus, 50 to 60 nm in diameter. The genome is a positive-stranded RNA molecule; it is approximately 9.6 kb in length and contains a single large open reading frame encoding a large polyprotein that is posttranslationally modified into three structural and several nonstructural polypeptides. The structural proteins include two highly variable envelope antigens, E1 and E2, and the relatively conserved nucleocapsid protein C. HCV replicates largely in the liver and is detectable in serum in titers of 10^5 to 10^7 virions/mL during acute and chronic infection.[7,11]

Clinical Manifestations

The clinical course of acute hepatitis C (Figure 10-3) begins with an incubation period that ranges from 15 to 120 days (mean, 50 days). During the incubation period, often within 1 to 2 weeks of exposure, HCV RNA can be detected by sensitive assays such as those based on reverse transcriptase–polymerase chain reaction (PCR). HCV RNA persists until well into the clinical course of disease. Antibody to HCV (anti-HCV) arises late in the course of acute hepatitis C and may not be present at the time of onset of symptoms and serum aminotransferase elevations. If the hepatitis is self-limited, HCV RNA soon becomes undetectable in serum; in this situation, titers of anti-HCV generally are modest and eventually may fall to undetectable levels as well.[19,20]

Diagnosis

Diagnosis of acute hepatitis C generally is based on detection of anti-HCV in serum in a patient with the clinical and biochemical features of acute hepatitis. The clinical course of hepatitis C with serologic markers is depicted in Figure 10-3. In some patients, however, detectable levels of anti-HCV do not develop until weeks or months after the onset of illness, so retesting for anti-HCV during convalescence or direct tests for HCV RNA are necessary to exclude the diagnosis of acute hepatitis C in a patient who tests negative for all serologic markers.

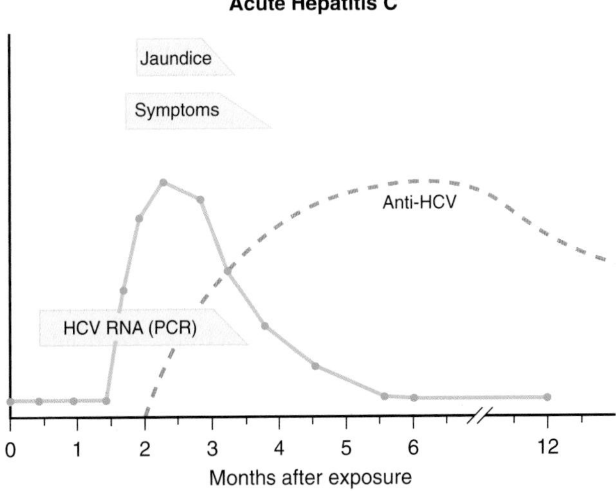

FIGURE 10-3 Serologic course of acute hepatitis C. *HCV*, Hepatitis C virus; *PCR*, Polymerase chain reaction. *(From Goldman L, Ausiello D, editors:* Cecil textbook of medicine, *ed 23, Philadelphia, 2008, Saunders.)*

Several commercial tests for HCV RNA are now licensed and are reliable in detecting HCV RNA at levels greater than 100 copies/mL. Tests that quantify the HCV RNA level also are available, but measuring viral levels is not clinically useful in diagnosis or monitoring of acute hepatitis C.[7,11]

Prevention

At present, there are no means of prevention of hepatitis C other than avoidance of high-risk behaviors and appropriate use of standard precautions. Injection drug use is currently the most common cause of newly acquired cases of hepatitis C. In this regard, needle exchange programs and education regarding the risks of drug use, including intranasal cocaine, and the risk of transmission from shared injection equipment are important.[3,10]

Accidental needlestick exposure is perhaps the most frequent issue in prevention of transmission. At present, neither immune globulin nor preemptive therapy with antiviral agents or interferon is recommended in this situation. Monitoring by means of determination of aminotransferase levels and HCV RNA and anti-HCV testing (at baseline and again at 1 and 6 months after exposure) is appropriate. This approach allows for early intervention and treatment.[7,11]

Treatment

Therapy with peginterferon alfa and ribavirin[21] has been shown to be beneficial in chronic hepatitis C—such therapy leads to sustained clearance of virus and resolution of disease in slightly more than 50% of cases. The role of therapy during acute infection is still unresolved. Because acute disease progresses to chronic infection in 50% to 85% of patients, the issue of early therapy often arises. Several studies have now documented that more than 90% of patients with acute hepatitis C treated with peginterferon with or without ribavirin for 24 weeks experience resolution of disease and sustained loss of HCV RNA.[2] The possible roles of HCV genotyping in guiding therapy and limiting therapy to 12 to 16 weeks in patients who become seronegative for HCV RNA within 4 weeks of starting therapy are currently under investigation.[11,22-24] In fact, a recent study by Poordad and co-workers found that the addition of boceprevir to standard therapy for HCV with peginterferon-ribavirin significantly increased the response in previously untreated adults with HCV infection. This line of research and therapy holds great promise for future treatment of hepatitis.[25]

Prognosis

The major complication of acute hepatitis C is the development of chronic hepatitis. The clinical course depicted in Figure 10-3 is not typical, because hepatitis C does not resolve in 50% to 85% of cases but rather progresses to chronic infection. In this situation, HCV RNA remains detectable, and aminotransferase levels generally remain elevated, often in a fluctuating pattern. In some instances, aminotransferase levels become normal despite persistence of viremia. Other complications include the development of immune complex phenomena and cryoglobulinemia, although these complications are more typical of chronic disease. Fulminant hepatitis resulting from HCV is rare; in several large surveys of acute liver failure, none of the cases could be attributed to HCV.[11]

HEPATITIS D

Epidemiology

Hepatitis D is linked to hepatitis B, and consequently its epidemiology is similar. HDV can be spread by the parenteral route and through sexual contact. People at greatest risk are chronic carriers of hepatitis B and persons who have repeated parenteral exposures. In the United States and Western Europe, delta hepatitis is most common in injection drug users and, before routine screening of blood donations, recipients of blood products, including persons with hemophilia and thalassemia. Delta hepatitis is endemic in the Amazon basin and central Africa and is common in some European and Mediterranean countries, including southern Italy, Greece, and eastern Europe.[11]

Pathophysiology

The hepatitis delta virus is a unique RNA virus that requires HBV for replication. The viral genome is a short, 1.7-kb circular single-stranded molecule of RNA that has a single open reading frame and a highly conserved, nontranslated region that resembles the self-replicating element of viroids. The single open reading frame encodes delta antigen, and RNA editing can vary the size of the molecule to produce either a small (195 amino acids) or large (214 amino acids) delta antigen. The small delta antigen promotes the replication of HDV RNA; the large delta antigen promotes viral assembly and secretion into serum as the mature 36-nm delta viral particle.[11]

Clinical Manifestations

Delta hepatitis occurs in two clinical patterns termed *coinfection* and *superinfection*. Delta coinfection is the simultaneous occurrence of acute HDV and acute HBV infections. Clinically and serologically it resembles acute hepatitis B but may manifest a second elevation in aminotransferase levels associated with the period of delta virus replication. The diagnosis of acute delta coinfection can be made in a patient with clinical features of acute hepatitis who has HBsAg, anti-HDV, and IgM anti-HBc in serum. Immunoassays for anti-HDV are commercially available and reliable, although antibody may appear late during the illness. In patients suspected of having delta hepatitis, repeat testing for anti-HDV during convalescence is appropriate.[7,11]

Diagnosis

Acute delta superinfection is the occurrence of acute HDV infection in a person with chronic hepatitis B or the HBsAg carrier state. The diagnosis of superinfection can be made in a patient with clinical features of acute hepatitis who has HBsAg and anti-HDV but no IgM anti-HBc in serum. Superinfection with HDV is more frequent than coinfection and is far more likely to lead to chronic delta hepatitis. Other tests that are helpful in making the diagnosis of ongoing HDV infection are determinations of serum HDV RNA (detectable by PCR assay) and HDV antigen (detectable by immunoblot analysis); both of these tests are currently research assays and not standardized. Delta antigen also can be detected readily in liver biopsy specimens[11] with immunohistochemical staining.

Prevention

Delta hepatitis can be prevented by preventing hepatitis B. The severity of delta hepatitis is another compelling rationale for routine hepatitis B vaccination in areas of the world where delta hepatitis is endemic. There are no means of prevention of delta hepatitis in a person who is already an HBsAg carrier; in this situation,[11] avoidance of further exposure is important.

Treatment

No specific therapies are available for acute delta hepatitis. Lamivudine and other anti-HBV agents are ineffective against HDV replication. Most cases of acute coinfection resolve; patients with superinfection should be treated when it is clear that chronic delta hepatitis has supervened.[2,11,21]

Prognosis

Delta hepatitis tends to be more severe than hepatitis B alone and is more likely to lead to fulminant hepatitis and to cause severe chronic hepatitis and ultimately cirrhosis.

HEPATITIS E

Epidemiology

Hepatitis E is responsible for epidemic and endemic forms of non-A, non-B hepatitis that occur in less-developed areas of the world. Large outbreaks have been described from India, Pakistan, China, northern and central Africa, and Central America. In studies from India and Egypt, hepatitis E has accounted for a high proportion of cases of sporadic acute hepatitis. In the United States and Western Europe, hepatitis E is rare, with most cases being imported or caused by zoonotic spread from swine or rats that harbor a similar virus. HEV is spread by the fecal-oral route, and most cases can be traced to exposure to contaminated water under poor hygienic conditions. Hepatitis E seems to be less contagious than hepatitis A, the other form of infectious hepatitis, and secondary cases are rare.[11]

Pathophysiology

HEV is a small nonenveloped, single-stranded RNA virus that is currently unclassified. The viral genome is 7.5 kb in length and encodes three open reading frames—the first, ORF1, for the nonstructural proteins responsible for viral replication; the second, ORF2, for the capsid protein (HEV antigen); and the third, ORF3, for a short protein of unknown function. The virus and HEV antigen can be detected in hepatocytes during acute infection. The highest levels of virus are detectable in stool during the incubation period of the disease. Viruses similar to HEV are found in other species, and strains found in domesticated swine may be infectious in humans.

Clinical Manifestations

The clinical course of hepatitis E resembles that of other forms of hepatitis. The incubation period is 15 to 60 days (mean, 35 days). The disease frequently is cholestatic, with prominence of bilirubin and alkaline phosphatase elevations. Hepatitis E also tends to be more severe than other forms of epidemic jaundice, with a fatality rate of 1% to 2% and a particularly high rate of acute liver failure in pregnant women. HEV virions and antigen can be detected in stool and liver during the incubation period and early symptomatic phase, but these tests are not practical methods of diagnosis. ELISAs for IgM and IgG antibody to HEV (anti-HEV) have been developed and are reactive in at least 90% of patients at the onset of clinical illness. These tests are neither generally available nor standardized, however. In addition, anti-HEV is found in 1% to 2% of the normal population, which may represent resolved subclinical cases of hepatitis E acquired during travel or as a result of exposure to livestock or other infected animals.[11,17]

Diagnosis

The diagnosis of hepatitis E should be considered in a patient with acute hepatitis who has recently traveled to an endemic area, particularly if tests for other forms of hepatitis are nonreactive. Detection of anti-HEV, particularly of the IgM subclass, is sufficient to make the diagnosis in this situation.[11,17]

Prevention and Treatment

There are no known means of prevention or treatment of hepatitis E. Immune globulin, even when prepared from plasma obtained from populations with a high rate of hepatitis E, does not seem to be effective. No specific modalities of treatment have been evaluated. Travelers (particularly pregnant women) to areas of the world where hepatitis E is endemic should be cautioned regarding drinking water and uncooked food. Recombinant vaccines against HEV have been developed and shown to be effective in animal models of hepatitis E. Efficacy trials of an HEV vaccine are now under way in endemic areas.[11]

DIFFERENTIAL DIAGNOSIS

The diagnostic approach to the patient with clinical features of acute hepatitis begins with a careful history for risk factors and possible exposure; for medication use, including herbal and over-the-counter drugs, and for alcohol use. The onset and progression of symptoms may give clues to the presence of other causes of liver or biliary tract disease, such as alcohol abuse or gallstones. Biochemical laboratory tests, including determinations of serum bilirubin, alanine and aspartate aminotransferases (ALT and AST), alkaline phosphatase (reported variously as ALP or alk phos), lactate dehydrogenase, albumin, and prothrombin time and a complete blood cell count (CBC), are valuable in defining whether the clinical picture is typical of acute hepatitis (high aminotransferases, normal or modest elevations in alkaline phosphatase and lactate dehydrogenase) or resembles that in obstructive jaundice or alcoholic liver disease. In atypical cases, an antinuclear antibody assay to evaluate for autoimmune hepatitis and a Venereal Disease Research Laboratory (VDRL) test to exclude secondary syphilis are needed. The presence of fever and atypical lymphocytosis points to mononucleosis. The presence of hemolysis should suggest Wilson disease. Serologic tests that are helpful in all cases of acute hepatitis are shown in Table 10-2.[11]

HEPATITIS NON–A-E

Epidemiology and Pathobiology

Cases of acute hepatitis that appear to be viral in etiology but cannot be attributed to any known virus are called *hepatitis non–A-E*. Various candidate viruses have been reported in association with this disease, including paramyxoviruses, togaviruses, and flaviviruses (GB virus C [GBV-C], hepatitis G virus, and TT virus), but none has been clearly linked to the clinical entity. In serologic surveys of cases of acute hepatitis in Western countries, 2% to 20% of cases cannot be attributed to any of the five known hepatitis viruses.

Clinical Manifestations

The clinical features of non–A-E hepatitis are similar to those of recognized forms of acute hepatitis. In most cases of non–A-E hepatitis, no clear source of exposure can be identified. Rare cases have been reported after blood transfusion. The absence of typical risk factors for viral hepatitis suggests that in some instances, non–A-E hepatitis may be due to nonviral causes, such as an autoimmune process, environmental exposure, or drugs.

Diagnosis

Non–A-E hepatitis is a diagnosis of exclusion.[17]

Treatment

There are no means of either treatment or prevention of non–A-E hepatitis.

Prognosis

The syndrome of non–A-E hepatitis has been particularly associated with the complications of acute liver failure and aplastic anemia. Hepatitis non–A-E is a more common cause of fulminant hepatic failure than both hepatitis A and hepatitis B combined and often accounts for 30% to 40% of cases. Chronic hepatitis develops in approximately a third of patients with non–A-E hepatitis, and cirrhosis ultimately develops in a small percentage.

OCCUPATIONAL TRANSMISSION

Little to no risk exists for transmission of HAV, HEV, and non–A-E hepatitis viruses from occupational exposure of dental health care workers to persons infected with these viruses. By contrast, risk for transmission of HBV is well recognized, and a lesser risk is present for HCV infection after occupational exposure to infected blood or body fluids containing infected blood. HCV is less infectious and less efficient in transmission than HBV. After percutaneous or other sharps injury in health care workers involving exposure to contaminated blood, the risk of contracting HBV infection is reported to range from 6% to 30%, with potential infectiousness correlating with presence of HBeAg in the serum (i.e., serum with HBeAg and HBsAg may be 10 times more infectious than serum with HBsAg alone). Recommendations for postexposure are presented in Table 10-3. Moreover, HBV can survive for at least 1 week in dried blood on environmental surfaces and contaminated needles and instruments. By contrast, the seroconversion rate for accidental blood

TABLE 10-3 Recommendations for Management After Accidental Exposure to Blood of a Person Infected with Hepatitis Virus

Infectivity Status of Source Person	Unvaccinated HCW	Vaccinated HCW,* Known Responder	Vaccinated HCW, Known Nonreceptor	Vaccinated HCW, Response Unknown
HBsAg-positive	1 dose of HBIG (0.06 mL/kg IM) as soon as possible (preferably within 24 hours) + initiate hepatitis B vaccine	No treatment	Administer 1 dose of HBIG + hepatitis B vaccine *or* 2 doses of HBIG, with second dose 1 month after the first	Test exposed worked for anti-HBsAg; with inadequate response (<10 mU/mL), 1 dose HBIG + hepatitis B vaccine booster dose
HBsAg-negative	Initiate hepatitis B vaccine series	No treatment	No treatment	No treatment
If unknown, not tested	Initiate hepatitis B vaccine series	No treatment	If known high-risk source, consider treating as for HBsAg-positive source	Test exposed worked for anti-HBsAg; with inadequate response, initiate revaccination

After a percutaneous or permucosal exposure, the blood of the source person (and of the exposed person) should be tested for HBsAg, anti-hepatitis C virus (HCV), and human immunodeficiency virus (HIV) antibody. Testing should be done in accordance with state laws and where appropriate pretest and posttest counseling is available. Currently, no treatment is available or recommended for occupational postexposure to HCV, hepatitis E virus (HEV), and non–A-E hepatitis viruses. *(Data from Centers for Disease Control: Recommendations for follow-up of health-care workers after occupational exposure to hepatitis C virus,* MMWR Morb Mortal Wkly Rep *46:603-606, 1997.)*

Also, current data suggest that a hepatitis A virus (HAV) percutaneous or permucosal exposure in an occupational setting is unlikely to result in transmission of HAV. Unvaccinated persons (younger than 2 years of age) recently exposed to HAV are advised to receive a single 0.02-mL/kg intramuscular injection of immune globulin according to the Advisory Committee on Immunization Practices recommendations. *(Data from Centers for Disease Control and Prevention: Prevention of hepatitis A through active or passive immunization: Recommendation of the the Advisory Committee on Immunization Practices,* MMWR Recomm Rep *48[RR-12]:1-31, 1999.)*

HBIG, Hepatitis B immune globulin; *HBsAg,* Hepatitis B surface antigen; *HCW,* Health care worker; *IM,* Intramuscular.

*Exposed worker vaccinated against hepatitis B virus.

Data from Centers for Disease Control and Prevention: Immunization of health-care workers: recommendations of the Advisory Committee on Immunization Practices (ACIP) and the Hospital Infection Control Practices Advisory Committee (HICPAC), MMWR Recomm Rep *46(RR-18):1-42, 1997.*

exposure to HCV is between 2% and 8%. By comparison, the risk of contracting HIV infection after a percutaneous or other sharps injury is 0.3%.[2,11]

The role of saliva in HBV or HCV transmission, except by percutaneous or permucosal routes, does not appear to be significant. During the past several decades, HBV transmission has been documented to occur from dental health care workers to dental patients.[9] Transmission of HCV from dental health care worker to patient has not been reported, but cardiac surgeons are recognized to have transferred this virus to several of their patients.[2,11]

PATHOPHYSIOLOGY AND COMPLICATIONS

Icterus (jaundice), the accumulation of bilirubin in the plasma, epithelium, and urine, is associated with hepatitis in approximately 70% of cases of HAV, approximately 30% of cases of HBV infection, and approximately 25% of cases of HCV and HEV. Bilirubin is a degradation product of hemoglobin and one of the major constituents of bile, to which it confers the characteristic yellowish color. Bilirubin normally is transported to the liver by way of the plasma. In the liver, it conjugates with glucuronic acid, and then it is excreted into the intestine, where it aids in the emulsification of fats and stimulates peristalsis. In the presence of liver disease, bilirubin tends to accumulate in the plasma as a consequence of decreased liver metabolism and transport. Jaundice usually becomes clinically apparent when the plasma level of bilirubin approaches 2.5 mg/100 mL (normal is less than 1 mg/100 mL). If the plasma bilirubin does not reach this level, the patient is anicteric (without jaundice)—thus explaining nonicteric hepatitis.[2,11] Most cases of viral hepatitis, especially types A and E, resolve without any complications. HBV, HCV, and HDV can persist and replicate in the liver when the virus is not completely cleared from the organ. Potential outcomes with hepatitis include recovery, persistent infection (or carrier state), dual infection, chronic active hepatitis, fulminant hepatitis, cirrhosis, hepatocellular carcinoma, and death. Dual infections and the chronic consumption of alcohol lead to more severe disease. Approximately 16,000 people die annually because of complications related to hepatitis infection.[2,11]

Fulminant Hepatitis

A serious complication of acute viral hepatitis is fulminant hepatitis, characterized by massive hepatocellular destruction and a mortality rate of approximately 80%.

The condition occurs more commonly among elderly persons and patients with chronic liver disease. Coinfection or superinfection with HBV and HDV or infection by a single hepatitis virus can cause fulminant disease. Mutant strains of these viruses have been proposed to be causative. In the United States, each year more than 100 persons die of fulminant hepatitis A and hepatitis E, and approximately 350 persons die of HBV-HDV–associated fulminant disease. HCV rarely causes fulminant hepatitis.[2,11]

Chronic Infection

Chronic infection (carrier state) is characterized by the persistence of low levels of virus in the liver and serum viral antigens (HBsAg, HBeAg, and HCVAg) for longer than 6 months without signs of liver disease. Persons with this condition potentially are infectious to others. The rate of carrier establishment varies depending on the virus, age, and health of the patient.[2,11] For example, approximately 50% to 90% of infants, 25% of children, and 6% to 10% of adults infected with HBV become carriers. By contrast, 70% to 90% of adults infected with HCV develop a persistent carrier state.[2,6,11] With both viruses, men and immunosuppressed persons are more commonly affected. Approximately 0.1% to 0.5% of the general population in the United States (more than 4 million persons) are carriers of HBV and/or HCV, whereas 5% to 15% of the populations of China, Southeast Asia, sub-Saharan Africa, most Pacific Islands, and the Amazon Basin are HBV carriers.[6,10] This marked difference reflects the endemicity of hepatitis B in these latter countries.

The carrier rate among dentists in the United States has decreased, but the risk is still estimated to be 3 to 10 times that in the general population. The highest HCV carrier rates (20%) are found among injection drug users and persons with hemophilia. Health care workers show an approximately 1% to 2% prevalence. The lowest rates of anti-HCV are found among blood donors, with about 0.5% to 1.0% being positive. Approximately 2% to 5% of acute coinfections of HBV and HDV result in chronic infections. Superinfections are more frequent than coinfections and result in a chronic carrier state in more than 70% of persons.[2,6,11] The carrier state may persist for decades or cause liver disease by progressing to chronic active hepatitis.

Chronic active hepatitis is characterized by active virus replication in the liver, HBsAg and HBeAg or HCVAg in the serum, signs and symptoms of chronic liver disease, persistent hepatic cellular necrosis, and elevation of liver enzymes for longer than 6 months. Approximately 3% to 5% of patients infected with HBV, 25% of HBV carriers, and 40% to 50% of those infected with HCV develop chronic active hepatitis.[22,23] HBV- and HCV-related chronic liver destruction and the resulting fibrosis lead to cirrhosis in approximately 20% of cases of chronic hepatitis. Approximately 1% to 5% of these patients develop primary hepatocellular carcinoma. An estimated 4000 persons die each year from HBV-related cirrhosis, 10,000 die from HCV-related cirrhosis, and more than 800 die from HBV- and HCV-related liver cancer. The correlation with liver cancer is 30 to 100 times stronger for chronic carriers than for uninfected persons and is particularly strong in some selected Asian populations.[22,23]

Liver cancer, primarily hepatocellular carcinoma, is the third leading cause of death from cancer worldwide and the ninth leading cause of cancer deaths in the United States.[24] Chronic HBV and HCV infections account for an estimated 78% of global cases of hepatocellular carcinoma.[24] The average annual incidence rate of hepatocellular carcinoma for 2001 to 2006 was 3.0 per 100,000 persons and increased significantly from 2.7 per 100,000 persons in 2001 to 3.2 in 2006, with an average annual percentage change in incidence rate (APC) of 3.5%. The largest increases in incidence rates for hepatocellular carcinoma were among whites (APC = 3.8), blacks (APC = 4.8), and persons aged 50 to 59 years (APC = 9.1).[24] The data demonstrate a continuation of long-term increases in incidence of hepatocellular carcinoma and persistent relevant racial or ethnic disparities. Development of viral hepatitis services, including screening with care referral for persons chronically infected with HBV or HCV, full implementation of vaccine-based strategies to eliminate hepatitis B, and improved public health surveillance, is needed to help reverse the trend in hepatocellular carcinoma.[24]

Clinical Presentation

After an incubation phase that varies with the infecting virus, approximately 10% of hepatitis A, 60% to 70% of hepatitis C, and 70% to 90% of hepatitis B cases are asymptomatic. When manifestations occur, the clinical features of acute viral hepatitis are similar and are discussed together. Many of the signs and symptoms are common to many viral illnesses and may be described as flulike. This clinical picture is especially characteristic of the early, or prodromal, phase. Patients classically exhibit three phases of acute illness.[2,6,11]

The *prodromal (preicteric) phase* usually precedes the onset of jaundice by 1 or 2 weeks and consists of abdominal pain, anorexia, intermittent nausea, vomiting, fatigue, myalgia, malaise, and fever. With hepatitis B, 5% to 10% of patients demonstrate serum sickness–like manifestations including arthralgia or arthritis, rash, and angioedema.[2,6,11]

The *icteric phase* is heralded by the onset of clinical jaundice, manifested by a yellow-brown cast to the conjunctivae, skin, oral mucosa, and urine. Many of the nonspecific prodromal symptoms may subside, but gastrointestinal manifestations (e.g., anorexia, nausea, vomiting, right upper quadrant pain) may increase, especially early in this phase. Hepatomegaly and splenomegaly frequently are noted. This phase lasts 2 to 8 weeks and is part of the clinical course in at least 70% of patients infected with HAV, 30% of those acutely infected with HBV, and 25% to 30% of patients acutely infected with HCV.[22,23]

During the *convalescent* or *recovery (posticteric) phase,* symptoms disappear, but hepatomegaly and abnormal liver function values may persist for a variable period. This phase can last for weeks or months, with recovery times for hepatitis B and hepatitis C generally longer. The usual sequence is recovery (clinical and biochemical) within approximately 4 months after the onset of jaundice. HBV infrequently is associated with clinical syndromes, including polyarteritis nodosa, glomerulonephritis, and leukocytoclastic vasculitis. Coagulopathy, encephalopathy, cerebral edema, and fulminant hepatitis are rare.[2,6,11] Chronic hepatitis is associated with liver abnormalities but often is asymptomatic for 10 to 30 years. Nonspecific symptoms of chronic hepatitis C (loss of weight, easy fatigue, sleep disorder, difficulty in concentrating, right upper quadrant pain, and liver tenderness) may not appear until hepatic fibrosis, cirrhosis, or hepatocellular carcinoma are present. The hepatic damage is caused by both the cytopathic effect of the virus and the inflammatory changes secondary to immune activation. Extrahepatic immunologic disorders associated with chronic HCV infection result from the production of autoantibodies and include immune complex–mediated disease (vasculitis, polyarteritis nodosa), autoimmune disorders (rheumatoid arthritis, glomerulonephritis, thrombocytopenic purpura, thyroiditis, pulmonary fibrosis), and two immunologic disorders: lichen planus and Sjögren-like syndrome (lymphocytic sialadenitis). If these diseases or signs of advanced liver disease (bleeding esophageal varices, ascites, jaundice, spider angioma, dark urine) develop, testing for chronic hepatitis is recommended.[2,6,11] HDV infection often results in severe acute hepatitis or rapidly progressive chronic liver disease. Coinfection usually results in transient and self-limiting disease, whereas superinfection more often results in severe clinical disease, indicated by sudden exacerbation, in a chronic carrier of HBV.[2,6,11]

LABORATORY FINDINGS

The standard battery of tests that are most helpful in assessing liver disease includes determinations of total and direct bilirubin, albumin, prothrombin time, and the serum enzymes ALT, AST, and alkaline phosphatase. Interpretation of these results in concert with careful history taking and a physical examination may suggest a specific type of liver injury, allowing a directed evaluation, risk assessment for surgical procedures, and estimation of prognosis.[7] Bilirubin is a breakdown product of heme (ferroprotoporphyrin IX). Hyperbilirubinemia may be the result of overproduction of bilirubin through excessive breakdown of hemoglobin; impaired hepatocellular uptake, conjugation, or excretion of bilirubin; or regurgitation of unconjugated and conjugated bilirubin from damaged hepatocytes or bile ducts. The presence of conjunctival icterus suggests a total serum bilirubin level of at least 3.0 mg/dL.[7]

Aminotransferases

The serum aminotransferases (also called transaminases), the most sensitive markers of acute hepatocellular injury, have been used to identify liver disease since the 1950s. ALT (formerly serum glutamate-pyruvate transaminase [SGPT]) and AST (formerly serum glutamate-oxaloacetate transaminase [SGOT]) catalyze the transfer of the α-amino groups of alanine and L-aspartic acid, respectively, to the α-keto group of ketoglutaric acid. AST, present in cytosol and mitochondria, is widely distributed throughout the body; it is found, in order of decreasing concentration, in liver, cardiac muscle, skeletal muscle, kidney, brain, pancreas, lung, leukocytes, and erythrocytes. Increases in serum values of the aminotransferases reflect either damage to tissues rich in these enzymes or changes in cell membrane permeability that allow ALT and AST to leak into serum; hepatocyte necrosis is not required for the release of aminotransferases, and the degree of elevation of the aminotransferases does not correlate with the extent of liver injury.[7]

Alkaline Phosphatase

The term *alkaline phosphatase* applies generally to a group of isoenzymes distributed widely throughout the body. The isoenzymes of greatest clinical importance in adults are in the liver and bone, because these organs are the major sources of serum alkaline phosphatase. Hepatobiliary disease leads to increased serum alkaline phosphatase levels through induced synthesis of the enzyme and leakage into the serum, a process mediated by bile acids.[7] A low serum alkaline phosphatase level may be observed in patients with Wilson disease, especially those presenting with fulminant hepatitis and hemolysis, possibly because of reduced activity of the enzyme owing to displacement of the cofactor zinc by copper.[7] The serum transaminases, AST[26] and ALT,[17] are sensitive indicators of liver injury and acute viral hepatitis, with ALT being a more specific indicator. Also useful in the diagnosis of hepatitis are elevated levels of serum bilirubin, alkaline phosphatase (heat fraction), γ-glutamyl transpeptidase (GGT), and lactate dehydrogenase; an increased white blood cell count; and prolongation of the prothrombin time. Antigen-antibody serologic tests are required for identifying the viral agent and in distinguishing among acute, resolved, and chronic infections.[7,27]

PREVENTION

Prevention Through Active Immunization

The risk of viral hepatitis is reduced by receiving active immunization. At present, two vaccines are available for HAV, two vaccines are available for HBV, one vaccine (Twinrix) is available for combination hepatitis A and B, and one vaccine (Comvax) is available for hepatitis B and *Haemophilus influenzae* type b (in combination with *Neisseria meningitidis* OMPC) in infants. The hepatitis A vaccine was first approved for use in the United States in 1995. Harivax and Vaqta are the formalin-inactivated whole virus vaccines used specifically to prevent HAV infection. The hepatitis A virus vaccines are safe, highly immunogenic, and recommended for patients 2 years of age and older.[16]

The vaccine originally was derived from pooled donor plasma; however, this form is no longer available. The two vaccines licensed for prevention of HBV infection (Engerix-B and Recombivax HB) are produced by recombinant DNA technology. These vaccines are administered in three doses over a 6-month period and produce an effective antibody response in more than 90% of adults and 95% of infants, children, and adolescents. The conversion rate is based on data obtained for injections given in the deltoid muscle, because injections administered in the buttocks resulted in development of effective antibody titers in only 81% of recipients. Adverse effects with all three vaccines include soreness at the injection site, fever, chills, flulike symptoms, arthralgia, and rarely neuropathy. No risk for development of viral infection in association with use of these vaccines, including the original plasma-derived vaccine, has been documented.[6,20,26,28]

The duration of immunity and the need for booster doses remain controversial. Current information based on experience with the plasma-derived HBV indicates that immunity remains effective for more than 10 years. Current guidelines published by the Centers for Disease Control and Prevention (CDC) Advisory Committee on Immunization Practices recommend booster doses only for persons who did not respond to the primary vaccine series.[6,20,28]

During the decade after vaccine licensure, vaccination of target populations of persons at high risk for contracting HBV infection became the accepted approach to prevention (Box 10-1). At the top of the list are health care workers, including dentists, for whom inoculation with the vaccine is strongly recommended. Implementation of a posttesting strategy is important for identifying persons who are nonresponders.[6,20,28]

A strategy to interrupt HBV transmission in all age groups was developed in 1991 and updated in 1995. The current strategy includes (1) prevention of perinatal HBV infection, (2) routine vaccination of all infants, and (3) vaccination of selected adolescents and adults not vaccinated as infants. Implementation of this strategy also eventually should control hepatitis D in parallel with control of hepatitis B.[6,20,26,28]

BOX 10-1 Persons at Substantial Risk for Hepatitis B Who Should Receive Vaccine

Individuals with occupational risk
Health care workers
Public safety workers
Clients and staff of institutions for the developmentally disabled
Hemodialysis patients
Recipients of certain blood products
Household contacts and sex partners of HBV carriers
Adoptees from countries where HBV infection is endemic
International travelers
Illicit drug users
Sexually active homosexual and bisexual men (men who have sex with men)
Sexually active heterosexual men and women (who have multiple partners)
Inmates of long-term correctional facilities

HBV, Hepatitis B virus.
Data from the Centers for Disease Control and Prevention: Hepatitis B information for health professionals *(website): http://www.cdc.gov/hepatitis/HBV/index.htm. Accessed September 15, 2011.*

Prevention Through Passive Immunization

Treatment of viral hepatitis can be accomplished by administering early postexposure immune globulins or postexposure hepatitis B vaccine (see earlier under "Prevention Through Active Immunization"). Immune serum globulin is derived from a pool of antibodies collected from human plasma that is free of HBsAg, HCV, and HIV. This sterile solution contains antibodies against both hepatitis A and hepatitis B. Another type of immune globulin is called *hepatitis B immune globulin* (HBIG). It is specially prepared from preselected plasma that is high in titers of anti-HBs. Administration of both immune globulin and HBIG is safe, but they interact adversely with live attenuated vaccines (i.e., measles-mumps-rubella [MMR] vaccine) if given within 5 months of each other.[6,20,26,28]

TREATMENT

As with many viral diseases, therapy basically is palliative and supportive. Bed rest and fluids may be prescribed, especially during the acute phase. A nutritious and high-calorie diet is advised. Alcohol and drugs metabolized by the liver are not to be ingested. Viral antigen and ALT levels should be monitored for 6 months to determine whether the hepatitis is resolving. Chronic hepatitis rarely resolves spontaneously. Standard therapy for patients with chronic hepatitis is administration of interferon (alfa-2b) (3 to 10 million units given three times weekly for 6 months to 1 year). Newer modalities have used the pegylated form of interferon (peginterferon), with better sustained virologic response.[21,29-31] Interferon therapy normalizes ALT levels in up to 17% of patients infected with HDV, 30% of those infected with HCV, and 40% of those infected with HBV and reduces the risk for development of hepatocellular carcinoma. Response is better when interferon is initiated early in the course of the disease. Treatment costs, however, are high, and only 10% to 30% of patients achieve long-term remission. Adverse effects (fatigue, flulike symptoms, and bone marrow suppression) are common, and up to 15% experience significant side effects that result in the discontinuation of treatment. The addition of lamuvidine (a nucleoside analogue active against HBV) or ribavirin (a guanosine analogue active against HCV) gains a virologic response in an additional 15% to 25%.[21,29-31] Ribavirin (1000 mg daily) also is an effective agent for treatment but has many side effects and adverse interactions.[11] More recent clinical trials have indicated that telaprevir is effective for treating hepatitis C that previously has been ineffectively treated with other agents.[32] Depending on the severity of the liver damage (as determined by laboratory tests or live biopsy, combination therapy is recommended.[11] Corticosteroids usually are reserved for patients with fulminant hepatitis. Liver transplantation is a last resort for patients who develop cirrhosis (see Chapter 21).[33]

DENTAL MANAGEMENT

Treatment Considerations in Specific Patient Groups

The identification of potential or actual carriers of HBV, HCV, and HDV is problematic, because in most instances carriers cannot be identified by history. The inability to identify potentially infectious patients extends to HIV infection and other sexually transmitted diseases. Therefore, all patients with a history of viral hepatitis must be managed as though they were potentially infectious (Box 10-2).

The recommendations for infection control practice in dentistry published by the CDC and the American Dental Association have become the standard of care to prevent cross-infection in dental practice (see Appendix B).[34] These organizations strongly recommend that all dental health care workers who provide patient care receive vaccination against hepatitis B virus and implement standard precautions during the care of all dental patients. In addition, Occupational Safety and Health Administration (OSHA) standards require employers to offer hepatitis B vaccine for free to employees occupationally exposed to blood or other potentially infectious materials. No recommendations exist for immunization against the other hepatitis viruses.[3,4,6,20,28]

Patients with Active Hepatitis. No dental treatment other than urgent care (absolutely necessary work) should be rendered for a patient with active hepatitis unless the patient has attained clinical and biochemical recovery (see Box 10-2). Urgent care should be provided only in an isolated operatory with strict adherence to standard precautions (see Appendix B). Aerosols should be minimized and drugs that are metabolized in the liver avoided as much as possible (Box 10-3). If surgery is necessary, a preoperative prothrombin time and bleeding time should be obtained and abnormal results discussed with the physician. The dentist should refer the patient who has acute hepatitis for medical diagnosis and treatment.[6,28]

Patients with a History of Hepatitis. Most carriers of HBV, HCV, and HDV are unaware that they have had hepatitis. An explanation is that many cases of hepatitis B and hepatitis C apparently are mild, subclinical, and nonicteric. such cases may be essentially asymptomatic or resemble a mild viral disease and therefore go undetected. Thus, the only practical method of protection from exposure to potential infection associated with providing dental care for persons with undiagnosed hepatitis, or with other undetected infectious diseases, is to adopt a strict program of clinical asepsis for all patients (see Appendix B). In addition, use of the hepatitis B vaccine further decreases the threat of hepatitis B infection. Inoculation of all dental personnel with hepatitis B vaccine is strongly urged.

For those patients who provide a positive history of hepatitis, additional historical information occasionally can be of some help in determining the type of disease.[6,20,28]

An additional aspect of a prudent approach to provision of clinical care for patients with a history of hepatitis of unknown type is to use the clinical laboratory to screen for the presence of HBsAg or anti-HCV. Such screeening may be indicated even in persons who specifically indicate which type of hepatitis they had, because information provided in patient histories of this type is unreliable 50% of the time.

Patients at High Risk for HBV or HCV Infection. Several groups are at unusually high risk for HBV and HCV infection (see Box 10-1). Screening for HBsAg and anti-HCV is recommended in persons who fit into one or more of these categories unless they are already known to be seropositive. Even if a patient is found to be a carrier, no modifications in treatment approach theoretically would be necessary. Information derived from such screening may nevertheless be of benefit in certain situations. If a patient is found to be a carrier, this knowledge could be of extreme importance for the modification of lifestyle. In addition, the patient might have undetected chronic active hepatitis, which could lead to bleeding complications or drug metabolism problems. Finally, if an accidental needlestick or puncture wound occurs during treatment and the dentist is not vaccinated (or antibody titer status is unknown), knowing whether the

BOX 10-2 Dental Management
Considerations in Patients with Liver Disease

P

Patient Evaluation/Risk Assessment (see Box 1-1)

- Evaluation is directed at determining the nature, severity, control, and stability of disease.

Potential Issues/Factors of Concern

A	
Analgesics	Nonsteroidal antiinflammatory drugs (NSAIDs), including aspirin, and acetaminophen, as well as codeine and meperidine, should be avoided or their use very limited in persons who have end-stage liver disease.
Antibiotics	Antibiotic prophylaxis is not recommended; however, patients who have severe liver disease may be more susceptible to infection. Selection of antibiotic agent is based on risk and severity of dental infection. Avoid use of metronidazole and vancomycin
Anesthesia	Higher doses may be required to achieve adequate anesthesia in presence of alcoholic liver disease. Knowledge of current liver function is important to establish proper dosages. Epinephrine (1:100,000, in a dose of no more than two carpules) in local anesthetics generally is not associated with any problems, but patients should be monitored closely.
Anxiety	Use anxiety/stress reduction techniques as needed, but avoid benzodiazepines.
Allergy	No issues.
B	
Breathing	No issues.
Bleeding	Excessive bleeding may occur in the patient with end-stage liver disease. Most such patients will have reductions in coagulation factors and thrombocytopenia, so they are at greater risk for postsurgical bleeding; they may need vitamin K and/or platelet or clotting factor replacement.
Blood pressure	Monitor blood pressure, because it may be significantly increased with portal hypertension in patients with end-stage liver disease.
C	
Chair position	No issues.
Consultation	Once the patient is under good medical management, the dental treatment plan is unaffected. However, consultation with the patient's physician to establish the level of control and to identify bleeding tendencies and altered drug metabolism is recommended as part of the management program.
D	
Devices	No issues.
Drugs	Because many medications are metabolized in the liver, certain drugs may need to be avoided or reduced in dosage. Limit or avoid use of acetaminophen, aspirin, ibuprofen, codeine, meperidine, diazepam, barbiturates, metronidazole, and vancomycin. Refer to a good drug reference. The use of epinephrine or other pressor amines (in gingival retraction cord or to control bleeding) must be limited, especially if portal hypertension is present.
E	
Equipment	No issues.
Emergencies and urgent care	For patient with severe liver disease who requires urgent care, consider treating in special care clinic or hospital. After consulting with physician, provide limited care only for pain control, treatment of acute infection, or control of bleeding until condition improves.
F	
Follow-up	It is important to follow up with the patient post-operatively to be certain that there are no complications.

patient was HBsAg- or HCV-positive would be of extreme importance in determining the need for HBIG, vaccination, and follow-up medical care.

Patients Who Are Hepatitis Carriers. If a patient is found to be a hepatitis B carrier (HBsAg-positive) or has a history of hepatitis C, standard precautions (see Appendix A) must be followed to prevent transmission of infection. In addition, some hepatitis carriers may have chronic active hepatitis, leading to compromised liver function and interference with hemostasis and drug metabolism. Physician consultation and laboratory screening of liver function are advised to determine current status and future risks.

Patients with Signs or Symptoms of Hepatitis. Any patient who has signs or symptoms suggestive of hepatitis should not receive elective dental treatment but instead should be referred immediately to a physician (Table 10-4). Necessary emergency dental care can be provided by using an isolated operatory and minimizing aerosol production.[9]

Drug Administration

No special drug considerations are needed for a patient who has completely recovered from viral hepatitis. If the patient has chronic active hepatitis, however, or is a carrier of HBsAg or HCV and has impaired liver function, the dosage for drugs metabolized by the liver should be decreased, or such drugs avoided if possible, as advised by the patient's physician (see Box 10-2). As a guideline, drugs metabolized in the liver should be considered for diminished dosage when one or more of the following factors are present (see Table 10-4): Child-Pugh classification as well as the Model of End-Stage Liver Disease (MELD) system: (1) elevation of aminotransferase levels to greater than four times normal, (2) elevation of serum bilirubin above 35 mM/L or 2 mg/dL, (3) serum albumin levels less than 35 g/L, and (4) signs of ascites, encephalopathy, and malnutrition. Many drugs commonly used in dentistry are metabolized principally by the liver, but in other than the most severe cases of hepatic disease, these drugs can be used, although in limited amounts (see Box 10-3). A one-procedure dose of three cartridges of 2% lidocaine (120 mg) is considered to represent a relatively limited amount of drug.[4,9]

BOX 10-3 Dental Drugs Metabolized Primarily by the Liver

Local Anesthetics*
Lidocaine (Xylocaine)
Mepivacaine (Carbocaine)
Prilocaine (Citanest)
Bupivacaine (Marcaine)

Analgesics
Aspirin†
Acetaminophen (Tylenol, Datril)†
Codeine‡
Meperidine (Demerol)‡
Ibuprofen (Motrin)†

Sedatives
Diazepam (Valium)‡
Barbiturates‡

Antibiotics
Ampicillin
Tetracycline
Metronidazole§
Vancomycin§

*Most of these agents appear to be safe for use in patients with liver disease when given in appropriate amounts.
†Limit dose or avoid if severe liver disease (acute hepatitis and cirrhosis) or hemostatic abnormalities are present.
‡Limit dose or avoid if severe liver disease (acute hepatitis and cirrhosis) or encephalopathy is present, or if taken with alcohol.
§Avoid if severe liver disease (acute hepatitis and cirrhosis) is present.

Treatment Planning Modifications

Treatment planning modifications are not required for the patient who has recovered from hepatitis.

Oral Manifestations and Complications

A problem that may be associated with chronic hepatitis and significant liver damage (or cirrhosis) is abnormal bleeding (see Chapter 24). The bleeding problem can be the result of abnormal synthesis of blood clotting factors, abnormal polymerization of fibrin, inadequate fibrin stabilization, excessive fibrinolysis, or thrombocytopenia associated with splenomegaly that accompanies chronic liver disease. Before any surgery is undertaken, a platelet count should be performed to determine whether platelet replacement may be required before surgery and should be discussed with the patient's physician (see Chapter 24).[4,9,20,28,35-39]

Chronic viral hepatitis increases the risk for hepatocellular carcinoma. This malignancy rarely metastasizes to the jaw (less than 30 cases had been reported in the jaws as of this writing). However, the incidence of hepatocellular carcinoma is on the rise in the United States. Oral metastases primarily manifest as hemorrhagic expanding masses located in the premolar and ramus region of the mandible.[28,38,39]

TABLE 10-4 The Two Most Commonly Used Scoring Systems in Grading Cirrhosis

1. Child-Pugh-Turcotte (CPT) Score (Range, 5-15)			
	Points Ascribed		
Parameter	1	2	3
Ascites	None	Grade 1-2 (or easy to treat)	Grade 3-4 (or refractory)
Hepatic encephalopathy	None	Grade 1-2 (or induced by a precipitant)	Grade 3-4 (or spontaneous)
Billrubin (mg/dL)	<2	2-3	>3
Albumin (g/dL)	>3.5	2.8-3.5	<2.8
Prothrombin time (seconds > control) *or*	<4	4-6	>6
INR	<1.7	1.7-2.3	>2.3
CPT Classification			
Child A: score of 5-6			
Child B: score of 7-9			
Child C: score of 10-15			
2. Model of End-Stage Liver Disease (MELD) Score (Range, 6-40)			
Score = $[0.957 \times \ln$ creatine (mg/dL) $+ 0.378 \times \ln$ bilirubin (mg/dL) $+ 1.12 \times \ln$ INR $+ 0.643] \times 10$			

INR, International normalized ratio; *ln*, Natural logarithm.

POSTEXPOSURE PROTOCOLS FOR HEALTH CARE WORKERS

To reduce the risk of transmission of hepatitis viruses, the CDC has published postexposure protocols for percutaneous or permucosal exposures to blood. Implementation of the protocol is dependent on the virus present in the source person and the vaccination status of the exposed person (e.g., a dental health care worker) (see Tables 10-2 and 10-3).[26]

The CDC guidelines for exposures involving HBV outline protocols for both vaccinated and unvacccinated persons. For example, a vaccinated health care worker who sustains a needlestick or puncture wound contaminated with blood from a patient known to be HBsAg-positive should be tested for an adequate titer of anti-HBs if those levels are unknown. If the levels are inadequate, the worker should immediately receive an injection of HBIG and a vaccine booster dose. (The risk of contracting HBV infection from a sharps injury in health care workers from HBV carriers may approach 30%.) If the antibody titer is adequate, however, nothing further is required. If an unvaccinated person sustains an inadvertent percutaneous or permucosal exposure to hepatitis B, immediate administration of HBIG and initiation of the vaccine are recommended.[26]

Although no postexposure protocol or vaccine is available yet for HCV infection, current CDC guidelines include the following recommendations: (1) The source person should receive baseline testing for anti-HCV; (2) exposed persons should receive baseline and follow-up testing at 6 months for anti-HCV and liver enzyme activity; (3) anti-HCV enzyme immunoassay positive results should be confirmed by recombinant immunoblot assay (RIBA); (4) postexposure prophylaxis with immunoglobulin or antiviral agents should be avoided; and (5) health care workers should be educated regarding the risk and prevention of blood-borne infections.[26]

EXPOSURE CONTROL PLAN

With respect to hepatitis viruses, OSHA mandates that all employers maintain an exposure control plan and protect their employees from the hazards of bloodborne pathogens by using standard precautions and providing the following as a minimum: (1) hepatitis B vaccinations to employees, (2) postexposure evaluation and follow-up, (3) record-keeping for exposure data, (4) generic blood-borne pathogens training, and (5) personal protective equipment, made available at no cost. All dentists should be familiar with OSHA's compliance directive "Enforcement Procedures for the Occupational Exposure to Bloodborne Pathogens" (CPL 02-02-069; available at http://www.osha.gov/pls/oshaweb/owadisp.show_document?p_table=DIRECTIVES&p_id=257).

ALCOHOLIC LIVER DISEASE

Definition

The exact effect of alcohol on the liver was not known until researchers demonstrated that alcohol is hepatotoxic and its metabolite, acetylaldehyde, is fibrinogenic. Alcohol consumption in large or chronic amounts contributes to disease and injury. The quantity and the duration of alcohol ingestion required to produce cirrhosis are not clear. However, the typical alcoholic with cirrhosis has a history for at least 10 years of daily consumption of a pint or more of whiskey, or several quarts of wine, or an equivalent amount of beer.[5,7,31,40-42] A relationship exists between excessive alcohol ingestion and liver dysfunction, leading to end-stage liver disease or cirrhosis. Also implicated in the pathogenesis of alcoholic liver disease are *cytokines.* Alcohol-induced influx of endotoxin (lipopolysaccharides) from the gut into the portal circulation can activate Kupffer cells, leading to enhanced chemokine release. Chemokines, in turn, directly and indirectly damage liver hepatocytes. Curiously, only 10% to 15% of heavy alcohol users ever develop cirrhosis, a fact probably explained by hereditary, nutrition, and biochemical differences between individual patients.[5,7,31,41-45]

The lack of treatment of alcohol abuse leads to significant morbidity and mortality rates. Chapter 30 discusses the dental patient with alcohol abuse. Current figures indicate that over 100,000 persons die annually in the United States as a consequence of alcohol abuse, and more than 20% of all hospital admissions are alcohol-related. Cirrhosis is a sequela of alcohol abuse and the 10th leading cause of death among adults in the United States. In addition, ethanol alone or with other drugs such as benzodiazepines probably is responsible for more toxic overdose deaths than those attributable to any other agent.[5,7,31,40-42]

Pathophysiology and Complications

Alcohol has a deleterious effect on neural development, the corticotropin-releasing hormone system, metabolism of neurotransmitters, and the function of neurotransmitter receptors. As a result, the acetylcholine and dopaminergic systems are impaired, causing sensory and motor disturbances (e.g., peripheral neuropathies). Prolonged abuse of alcohol contributes to malnutrition (folic acid deficiency), anemias, and decreased immune function. Increased mortality rates have been noted for men who consume more than three drinks daily.*

The pathologic effects of alcohol on the liver are expressed as one of three disease entities. These conditions may exist alone but commonly appear in

*References 5, 7, 31, 40-42, 46, 47.

combination. The earliest change seen in alcoholic liver disease is so-called *fatty liver,* characterized by presence of a fatty infiltrate. The hepatocytes become engorged with fatty lobules and distended, with enlargement of the entire liver. No other structural changes usually are noted. This condition may emerge after only moderate usage of alcohol for a brief time; however, it is considered completely reversible.[5,7,31,40-42]

A second and more serious form of alcoholic liver disease is *alcoholic hepatitis.* This diffuse inflammatory condition of the liver is characterized by destructive cellular changes, some of which may be irreversible. The irreversible changes can lead to necrosis. Nutritional factors may play a significant role in the progression of this disease. For the most part, alcoholic hepatitis is considered a reversible condition; however, it can be fatal if damage is widespread.*

The third and most serious form of alcoholic liver disease is *cirrhosis,* which generally is considered an irreversible condition characterized by progressive fibrosis and abnormal regeneration of liver architecture in response to chronic injury or insult (i.e., prolonged and heavy use of ethanol) (Figure 10-4). Cirrhosis results in the progressive deterioration of the metabolic and excretory functions of the liver, ultimately leading to hepatic failure. Hepatic failure is manifested by myriad of health problems. Some of the more important of these are esophagitis, gastritis, and pancreatitis, which contribute to generalized malnutrition, weight loss, protein deficiency (including coagulation factors), impairment of urea synthesis and glucose metabolism, endocrine disturbances, encephalopathy, renal failure, portal hypertension, and jaundice. Accompanying portal hypertension is the development of ascites and esophageal varices (Figure 10-5). In some patients with cirrhosis, blood from bleeding ulcers and esophageal varices is incompletely metabolized to ammonia, which travels to the brain and contributes to encephalopathy. In addition, chronic large consumption of ethanol can result in dementia and psychosis (Wernicke and Korsakoff syndromes), cerebellar degeneration, upper alimentary tract cancer and liver cancer, and hematopoietic changes.[41,44,48]

Classically, severe alcoholic steatohepatitis (formerly called "alcoholic hepatitis") is characterized by the sudden development of tender hepatomegaly, jaundice, and fever in an person who has been drinking heavily. Often, the illness is associated with a flu-like prodrome that includes malaise, anorexia, and weakness. These symptoms sometimes prompt reduced alcohol ingestion, which in turn may precipitate an alcohol withdrawal syndrome (see Chapter 30). Some affected persons require hospitalization because of decompensated liver disease or associated conditions such as alcohol withdrawal syndrome, gastrointestinal bleeding, infection,

A

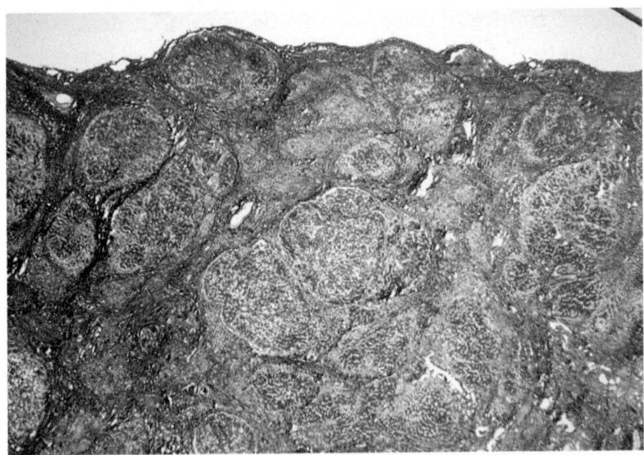

B

FIGURE 10-4 Photomicrographs showing liver architecture. A, Normal liver. **B,** Liver in alcoholic cirrhosis. (***A,*** *From Klatt EC: In* Robbins & Cotran atlas of pathology, *ed 2, Philadelphia, 2010, Saunders.* ***B,*** *From Kumar V, et al, editors:* Robbins basic pathology, *ed 8, Philadelphia, 2007, Saunders.*)

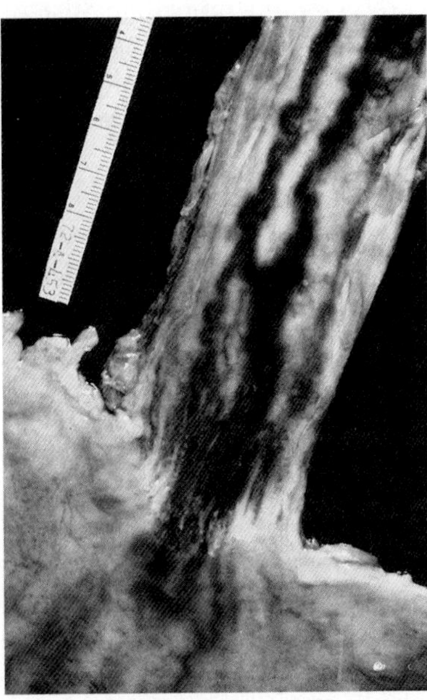

FIGURE 10-5 Gross specimen of esophageal varices from an alcoholic patient. (*Courtesy A. Golden, Lexington, Kentucky.*)

*References 5, 7, 31, 40-42, 44, 46, 47.

or pancreatitis. Although most people gradually recover during early abstinence, others deteriorate despite abstinence and aggressive management of their associated problems.[11]

Bleeding tendencies are a significant feature in advanced liver disease. The basis for the diathesis is in part a deficiency of coagulation factors, especially the prothrombin group (factors II, VII, IX, and X). These factors all rely on vitamin K as a precursor for production (see Chapter 24). Vitamin K is absorbed from the large intestine and stored in the liver, where it is converted into an enzymatic cofactor for the carboxylation of prothrombin complex proteins. Widespread hepatocellular destruction as seen in cirrhosis decreases the liver's storage and capacity for conversion of vitamin K, leading to deficiencies of the prothrombin-dependent coagulation factors. In addition to these deficiencies, thrombocytopenia may be caused by hypersplenism secondary to portal hypertension and to bone marrow depression. Anemia and leukopenia also may result from toxic effects of alcohol on the bone marrow and nutritional deficiencies. Accelerated fibrinolysis also is seen.[5,7,31,40-42]

The combination of hemorrhagic tendencies and severe portal hypertension (which causes thrombocytopenia as a consequence of sequestration of platelets in the spleen) sets the stage for episodes of gastrointestinal bleeding, epistaxis, ecchymoses, or ruptured esophageal varices. Most patients with advanced cirrhosis die of complications of hepatic coma, often precipitated by massive hemorrhage from esophageal varices or intercurrent infection.[41,44]

Ethanol abuse predisposes the person engaging in such behaviors to infection by several mechanisms. The liver's resident cell population in patients with alcoholism is exposed to high concentrations of ethanol. The Kupffer cells, representing more than 80% of tissue macrophages in the body, become impaired with continued bathing of the liver sinusoids in alcohol. Alcohol-induced impairment of Kupffer cell function and T cell responses result in increased risk of infection. Although cirrhosis generally is considered to be an end-stage condition, some evidence suggests that at least partial reversibility of the process is possible with complete and permanent removal of the offending agent during the early phase of cirrhosis.[5,7,31,40-42]

Clinical Presentation

The behavioral and physiologic effects of alcohol depend on the amount of intake, its rate of increase in plasma, concomitant use of other drugs or concurrent medical problems, and the past experience with alcohol. Chronic heavy alcohol intake can result in clinically significant cognitive impairment (even when the affected person is sober) or distress. The pattern displayed usually is one of intermittent relapse and remission. If the dependency problem is allowed to progress untreated, the development of other psychiatric problems (anxiety, antisocial behavior, and affective disorders) is not uncommon, with the emergence of alcohol amnestic disorder, in which the patient is unable to learn new material or to recall known material, in some cases. Alcoholic blackouts also may be a feature. In some patients, alcohol-induced dementia and severe personality changes develop.

Clinically, with the possible exception of enlargement, no visible manifestations of a fatty liver are present, and the diagnosis usually is made incidentally in conjunction with evaluation for another illness. The clinical presentation of alcoholic hepatitis often is nonspecific and may include features such as nausea, vomiting, anorexia, malaise, weight loss, and fever. More specific findings include hepatomegaly, splenomegaly, jaundice, ascites, ankle edema, and spider angiomas. With advancing disease, encephalopathy and hepatic coma may ensue, ending in death.[41,44]

Alcoholic cirrhosis may remain asymptomatic for many years until sufficient destruction of the liver parenchyma has occurred to produce clinical evidence of hepatic failure. Ascites, spider angiomas (Figure 10-6), ankle edema, and jaundice may be the earliest manifestations, but frequently hemorrhage from esophageal varices is the initial sign. The hemorrhagic episode may herald rapid progression to hepatic encephalopathy, coma, and death. Other, less specific signs of alcoholic liver disease include anemia, purpura, ecchymoses, gingival bleeding, palmar erythema, nail changes, and parotid gland enlargement (known as sialadenosis)[5,7,31,40-42] (Figure 10-7).

Laboratory Findings

Laboratory findings in alcoholic liver disease range in significance from minimal abnormalities caused by a fatty liver to manifestations of alcoholic hepatitis and

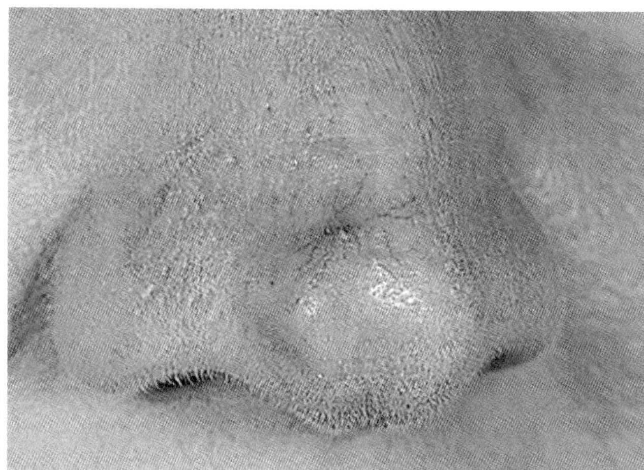

FIGURE 10-6 Spider angioma. (*From Swartz MH:* Textbook of physical diagnosis, *ed 6, Philadelphia, 2010, Saunders.*)

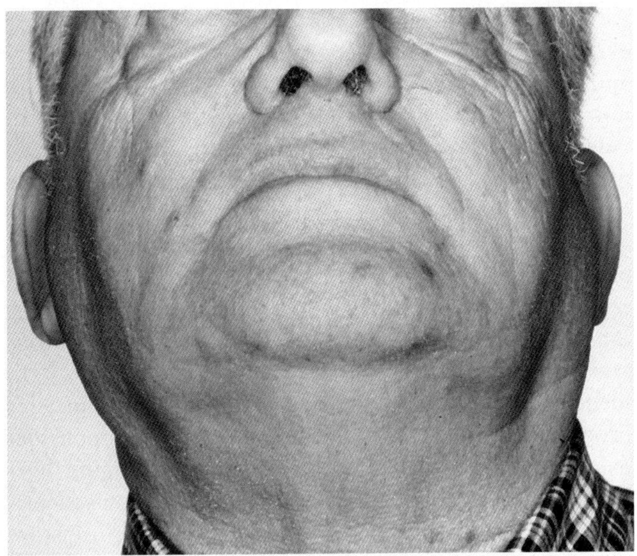

FIGURE 10-7 Painless enlargement of the parotid glands associated with alcoholism. (*Courtesy Valerie Murrah, Chapel Hill, North Carolina.*)

cirrhosis. Liver abnormalities cause elevations of bilirubin, alkaline phosphatase, AST, ALT, GGT, amylase, uric acid, triglyceride, and cholesterol levels. Leukopenia (or leukocytosis) or anemia often is present. A simple screen for alcoholism can be performed using a sequential Mult-Analyzer-20 and CBC with differential. Elevated blood levels of GGT and mean corpuscular volume are highly suggestive of alcoholism, whereas an AST/ALT ratio of at least 2 is 90% predictive of alcoholic liver disease. The carbohydrate-deficient transferrin test also is used to screen for and monitor clinical status in alcohol dependency.[5,7,31,40-42]

Alcoholic liver disease also leads to deficiencies of clotting factors reflected as elevations in the prothrombin time and partial thromboplastin time. Thrombocytopenia may be present owing to hepatosplenomegaly, causing a decreased platelet count. Increased fibrinolytic activity may be evidenced by a prolonged thrombin time or a decreased euglobulin clot lysis time (see Chapter 24).[5,7,31,40-42]

Medical Management

Treatment of patients with alcoholism consists of three basic steps. The first and second steps consist of identification and intervention, respectively. A thorough physical examination is performed to evaluate organ systems that could be impaired. This assessment includes a search for evidence of liver failure, gastrointestinal bleeding, cardiac arrhythmia, and glucose or electrolyte imbalance. Hemorrhage from esophageal varices and hepatic encephalopathy require immediate treatment. Ascites mandates measures to control fluids and electrolytes, alcoholic hepatitis often is treated with glucocorticoids, and infection or sepsis is managed with antimicrobial agents. During this phase, the patient may refuse to accept the diagnosis and often will deny that a problem exists (see Chapter 30).[5,7,31,40-42]

The third step is to manage the central nervous system depression caused by the rapid removal of the ethanol. Administration of a benzodiazepine, such as diazepam or chlordiazepoxide, with gradual decrease in serum levels of the drug occurring over a 3- to 5-day period, alleviates alcohol withdrawal symptoms. The beta blockers clonidine and carbamazepine are more recent additions to the pharmacotherapeutic management of withdrawal.[5,7,31,40-42]

Once treatment of withdrawal has been completed, the patient is educated about the disease of alcoholism. The education program should include teaching family members and friends to stop protecting the patient from the problems caused by alcohol. Attempts are made to help the patient with alcoholism achieve and maintain a high level of motivation toward abstinence. Other interventions are aimed at helping the patient with alcoholism to readjust to life without alcohol and to reestablish a functional lifestyle. The drug disulfiram has been used for some patients during alcohol rehabilitation. Disulfiram inhibits aldehyde dehydrogenase causing accumulation of acetaldehyde blood levels and thus sweating, nausea, vomiting, and diarrhea when taken with ethanol. Naltrexone (an opioid antagonist) and acamprosate (an inhibitor of the γ-aminobutyric acid [GABA] system) may be used to decrease the amount of alcohol consumed or shorten the period during which alcohol is used in cases of relapse. Untreated disease that progresses to cirrhosis requires alcohol withdrawal and management of any complications that arise. End-stage cirrhosis cannot be reversed and is remedied only by liver transplantation (see Chapter 21).[7]

Dental Management

Treatment Considerations. In addition to the aforementioned considerations, three major areas of concern in providing dental treatment (see Box 10-2) for a patient with alcoholism are recognized: (1) bleeding tendencies, (2) unpredictable metabolism of certain drugs, and (3) risk of spread of infection. A CBC with differential and determinations of AST and ALT, bleeding time, thrombin time, and prothrombin time are sufficient to screen for potential problems. Abnormal laboratory values, on a background of suggestive findings on the clinical examination or a positive history, constitute the basis for referral to a physician for definitive diagnosis and treatment. A patient with untreated alcoholic liver disease is not a candidate for elective, outpatient dental care and should be referred to a physician. Once good medical management has been instituted and the patient appears stable, dental care may be provided after consultation with the physician.[4,5,36,49-51]

If a patient provides a history of alcoholic liver disease or alcohol abuse, the physician should be consulted to verify the patient's current status, medications, laboratory values, and contraindications to medications, surgery, or other treatment. In cases in which the patient has not been seen by a physician within the past several months, screening laboratory tests should be ordered, including CBC with differential and determinations of AST and ALT, platelet count, thrombin time, and prothrombin time, before invasive procedures are undertaken. Precautionary measures to minimize the risk for bleeding (see Chapter 24), including a prothrombin time test that is particularly sensitive to deficiency of factor VII, also are indicated. Bleeding diatheses should be managed in conjunction with the physician and may entail use of local hemostatic agents, fresh frozen plasma, vitamin K, platelets, and antifibrinolytic agents. Hemostatic measures are particularly important when major invasive or traumatic procedures are performed in a patient who has been assigned an American Society of Anesthesiologists (ASA) category of III or higher and exhibits signs of jaundice, ascites, or clubbing of the fingers, or with alcoholic liver disease of Child-Pugh class B or C or MELD grade of moderate-severe (see Table 10-4).[52,53]

A second area of concern in patients with alcoholic liver disease is the unpredictable metabolism of drugs. This concern is two-fold: In mild to moderate alcoholic liver disease, significant enzyme induction is likely to have occurred, leading to an increased tolerance of local anesthetics, sedative and hypnotic drugs, and general anesthesia. Thus, larger-than-normal doses of these medications may be required to obtain the desired effects.[4,5,36]

Also, with more advanced liver destruction, drug metabolism may be markedly diminished, potentially leading to an increased or unexpected effect. For example, if acetaminophen is used in usual therapeutic doses in chronic alcoholism, or if acetaminophen is taken with alcohol during a fasting state, severe, fatal hepatocellular disease may result. The dentist should exercise caution in use of the drugs listed in Box 10-3 when treating patients with chronic alcoholism. The dose may need to be adjusted (e.g., half the regular adult dose may be appropriate if cirrhosis or alcoholic hepatitis is present), or a specific agent or class of drugs may be contraindicated as advised by the patient's physician. Once again, presence of more than one of the following findings is suggestive that drug metabolism will be impaired: aminotransferase levels elevated to higher than four times normal, serum bilirubin level elevated above 35 mM/L (2 mg/dL), serum albumin level less than 35 g/L, and signs of ascites, encephalopathy, or malnutrition (see Table 10-4).[4,5,36]

A third area of concern is risk for infection or spread of infection in the patient who has alcoholic liver disease. Risk increases with surgical procedures or trauma, which can introduce oral microorganisms into the blood circulation, with less efficient elimination by the reticuloendothelial system owing to impaired cellular function. Although patients who have alcoholic liver disease exhibit reduced reticuloendothelial functional capacity and altered cell-mediated immune function, studies do not indicate that antibiotic prophylaxis should be provided before invasive dental procedures in the absence of an ongoing infection. Despite the lack of evidence, recommendations exist in the literature for the use of antibiotic prophylaxis for these patients. Antibiotic prophylaxis is not needed if oral infection is absent. Of greater concern is the risk for spread of a preexisting infection, because bacterial infections are more serious and sometimes fatal in patients with liver disease.[4,5,36] To identify patients likely to respond poorly to invasive procedures and infections, the clinician should consider using one of the assessment formulas for staging liver disease (i.e., Child-Pugh or MELD classification scheme) (see Table 10-4) as well as identifying whether a history of bacterial infections (e.g., spontaneous bacterial peritonitis, pneumonia, bacteremia) exists. Consultation with the patient's physician regarding the use of antibiotics should be considered for persons with moderate to severe disease (Child-Pugh class B or C—characterized by ascites, encephalopathy, elevated bilirubin levels, or increase in systolic blood pressure). Antibiotics should be provided when infection is present and unlikely to resolve without such treatment.[37,41,44,47,53-55]

Treatment Planning Modifications

Patients with cirrhosis tend to have more plaque, calculus, and gingival inflammation than patients without the condition. This seems to be the case in any patient who is a substance abuser and is related to oral neglect, rather than to any inherent property of the abused substance. As indicated by the degree of neglect and extent of caries and periodontal disease, the dentist should not provide extensive care until the patient demonstrates an interest in and ability to care for the dentition.[56]

Liver enzyme induction and central nervous system effects of alcohol in patients with alcoholism can require use of increased amounts of local anesthetic or additional anxiolytic procedures. Appointments with these patients may therefore require more than the scheduled time if this manifestation was not anticipated.

Oral Complications and Manifestations

Poor hygiene and neglect (as evidenced by caries) are prominent oral manifestations of chronic alcoholism. In addition, a variety of other abnormalities may be found (Box 10-4). Patients with cirrhosis have been reported to have impaired gustatory function and are malnourished. Nutritional deficiencies can result in glossitis and loss of tongue papillae, along with angular or labial cheilitis, which may be complicated by concomitant candidal infection. Vitamin K deficiency, disordered hemostasis, portal hypertension, and splenomegaly (causing thrombocytopenia) can result in spontaneous gingival bleeding and mucosal ecchymoses and petechiae. In some instances, unexplained gingival bleeding has been the initial complaint of alcoholic patients. Also, a sweet,

BOX 10-4 Features Suggestive of Advanced Alcoholic Liver Disease

Systemic Complications

Traumatic or unexplained injuries (driving under the influence, bruises, cuts, scars, broken teeth)
Attention and memory deficits
Slurred speech
Spider angiomas
Jaundice (sclerae, mucosa)
Peripheral edema (edematous puffy face, ankle edema)
Ascites
Palmar erythema, white nails or transverse pale band on nails
Ecchymoses, petechiae, or prolonged bleeding
Failure to fulfill role obligations at work, school, home (e.g., missed dental appointments)
Increased levels of bilirubin, aminotransferases, alkaline phosphatase, and γ-glutamyl transpeptidase; increased mean corpuscular volume

Oral Complications

Poor oral hygiene
Oral neglect—caries, gingivitis, periodontitis
Glossitis
Angular or labial cheilosis
Candidiasis
Gingival bleeding
Oral cancer
Petechiae
Ecchymoses
Jaundiced mucosa
Parotid gland enlargement
Alcohol (sweet musty) breath odor
Impaired healing
Bruxism
Dental attrition
Xerostomia

musty odor to the breath is associated with liver failure, as is jaundiced mucosal tissue.[9,31,36]

A bilateral, painless hypertrophy of the parotid glands, termed sialadenosis, is a frequent finding in patients with cirrhosis. The enlarged glands are soft and nontender and are not fixed to the overlying skin. The condition appears to be caused by a demyelinating polyneuropathy that results in abnormal sympathetic signaling, abnormal acinar protein secretion, and acinar cytoplasmic swelling. In sialadenosis, the parotid ducts remain patent and produce clear salivary flow.[11,31,35,41]

Alcohol abuse and tobacco use are strong risk factors for the development of oral squamous cell carcinoma, and as with all patients, the dentist must be aggressive in the detection of unexplained or suspicious soft tissue lesions (especially leukoplakia, erythroplakia, or ulceration) in chronic alcoholics. Sites with a marked predilection for development of oral squamous cell carcinoma include the lateral border of the tongue and the floor of the mouth (see Chapter 26).

REFERENCES

1. Friedman LF, Keefe FA, editors: *Handbook of liver disease*, Amsterdam, 2005, Elsevier, p 496.
2. Ghany M, Hoofnagle JH: Approach to the patient with liver disease. In Fauci B, et al, editors: *Harrison's principles of internal medicine*, ed 17, New York, 2008, McGraw-Hill.
3. Firriolo FJ: Dental management of patients with end-stage liver disease, *Dent Clin North Am* 50:563-590, vii, 2006.
4. Golla K, Epstein JB, Cabay RJ: Liver disease: current perspectives on medical and dental management, *Oral Surg Oral Med Oral Pathol Oral Radiol Endod* 98:516-521, 2004.
5. Friedlander AH: Alcohol use and dependence, *J Am Dent Assoc* 134:731-740, 2003.
6. Centers for Disease Control and Prevention: Surveillance for acute viral hepatitis—United States, 2006, *MMWR Surveill Sum* 57(SS-2):289-299, 2008.
7. Feldman M: Liver disease. In Feldman M, Scharschmidt BF, Sleisenger MH, editors: *Sleisenger & Fordtran's gastrointestinal and liver disease: pathophysiology/diagnosis/ management*, ed 9, St. Louis, 2010, Saunders, pp 1911-1991.
8. Miyake Y, et al: Clinical features of autoimmune hepatitis diagnosed based on simplified criteria of the International Autoimmune Hepatitis Group, *Dig Liver Dis* 42:210-215, 2010.
9. Friedman LS: Surgery in the patient with liver disease, *Trans Am Clin Climatol Assoc* 121:192-204, 2010.
10. Fassio E: Hepatitis C and hepatocellular carcinoma, *Ann Hepatol* 9(suppl):119-122, 2010.
11. Bergasa, Nora V: Approaches to the patient with liver disease. In Goldman L, Ausiello D, editors: *Cecil textbook of medicine*, ed 23, Philadelphia, 2008, Saunders, pp 1087-1256.
12. Centers for Disease Control and Prevention: *Hepatitis B information for health professionals* (website): http://www.cdc.gov/hepatitis/HBV/index.htm. Accessed September 15, 2011.
13. Weismuller TJ, et al: Multicentric evaluation of model for end-stage liver disease-based allocation and survival after liver transplantation in Germany—limitations of the "sickest first" concept, *Transpl Int* 24:91-99, 2011.
14. Hansen L, Sasaki A, Zucker B: End-stage liver disease: challenges and practice implications, *Nurs Clin North Am* 45:411-426, 2010.
15. Watanabe T, et al: Features of hepatocellular carcinoma in cases with autoimmune hepatitis and primary biliary cirrhosis, *World J Gastroenterol* 15:231-239, 2009.
16. American Academy of Pediatrics Committee on Infectious Diseases: Hepatitis A vaccine recommendations, *Pediatrics* 120:189-199, 2008.
17. Dalton HR, et al: Hepatitis E: an emerging infection in developed countries, *Lancet Infect Dis* 8:698-709, 2008.
18. Advisory Committee on Immunization Practices (ACIP) Centers for Disease Control and Prevention (CDC): Update: Prevention of hepatitis A after exposure to hepatitis A virus and in international travelers. Updated recommendations of the Advisory Committee on Immunization Practices (ACIP), *MMWR Morb Mortal Wkly Rep* 56:1080-1084, 2007.
19. Fujiwara A, et al: Fibrosis progression rates between chronic hepatitis B and C patients with elevated alanine aminotransferase levels, *J Gastroenterol* 43:484-491, 2008.
20. Obika M, et al: Hepatitis B virus DNA in liver tissue and risk for hepatocarcinogenesis in patients with hepatitis C virus-related chronic liver disease. A prospective study, *Intervirology* 51:59-68, 2008.
21. Pareja E, et al: New alternatives to the treatment of acute liver failure, *Transplant Proc* 42:2959-2961, 2010.
22. Recommended infection-control practices for dentistry, 1993. Centers for Disease Control and Prevention, *MMWR Recomm Rep* 42(RR-8):1-12, 1993.

23. Vinayek R: Acute and chronic hepatitis. In Stein JA, editor: Internal medicine, ed 5, vol 1, St. Louis, 1998, Mosby, p 876.
24. Centers for Disease Control and Prevention: Hepatocellular carcinoma—United States, 2001-2006, *MMWR Morb Mortal Wkly Rep* 59:517-520, 2010.
25. Poordad F, et al: Boceprevir for untreated chronic HCV genotype 1 infection, *N Engl J Med* 364:1195-1204, 2011.
26. Mast EE, et al: A comprehensive immunization strategy to eliminate transmission of hepatitis B virus infection in the United States: recommendations of the Advisory Committee on Immunization Practices (ACIP) part 1: immunization of infants, children, and adolescents, *MMWR Recomm Rep* 54:1-23, 2005.
27. Pratt DS, Kaplan MM: Evaluation of abnormal liver-enzyme results in asymptomatic patients, *N Engl J Med* 342:1266-1271, 2000.
28. Resende VL, et al: Concerns regarding hepatitis B vaccination and post-vaccination test among Brazilian dentists, *Virol J* 7:154, 2010.
29. Zeuzem P: Peginterferon alfa-2a in patients with chronic hepatitis C, *N Engl J Med* 343:1666-1669, 2000.
30. Miranda-Mendez A, Lugo-Baruqui A, Armendariz-Borunda J: Molecular basis and current treatment for alcoholic liver disease, *Int J Environ Res Public Health* 7:1872-1888, 2010.
31. McCullough AJ, O'Shea RS, Dasarathy S: Diagnosis and management of alcoholic liver disease, *J Dig Dis* 12:257-262, 2011.
32. McHutchinson J, et al: Telaprevir for previously treated hepatitis C, *N Engl J Med* 362:1292-1301, 2010.
33. Zeuzem P: Perinterferon alfa2a in patients with chronic hepatitis, *N Engl J Med* 343:581-586, 2000.
34. Infection control recommendations for the dental office and the dental laboratory. ADA Council on Scientific Affairs and ADA Council on Dental Practice, *J Am Dent Assoc* 127:672-680, 1996.
35. Ojha J, et al: Xerostomia and lichenoid reaction in a hepatitis C patient treated with interferon-alpha: a case report, *Quintessence Int* 39:343-348, 2008.
36. Brennan MT, et al: Utility of an international normalized ratio testing device in a hospital-based dental practice, *J Am Dent Assoc* 139:697-703, 2008.
37. Tarantino G, Savastano S, Colao A: Hepatic steatosis, low-grade chronic inflammation and hormone/growth factor/adipokine imbalance, *World J Gastroenterol* 16:4773-4783, 2010.
38. Severi T, et al: Tumor initiation and progression in hepatocellular carcinoma: risk factors, classification, and therapeutic targets, *Acta Pharmacol Sin* 31:1409-1420, 2010.
39. Sanyal AJ, Yoon SK, Lencioni R: The etiology of hepatocellular carcinoma and consequences for treatment, *Oncologist* 15(Suppl 4):14-22, 2010.
40. Rehm J, Kanteres F, Lachenmeier DW: Unrecorded consumption, quality of alcohol and health consequences, *Drug Alcohol Rev* 29:426-436, 2010.
41. Stickel F, Seitz HK: Alcoholic steatohepatitis, *Best Pract Res Clin Gastroenterol* 24:683-693, 2010.
42. Katoonizadeh A, et al: Early features of acute-on-chronic alcoholic liver failure: a prospective cohort study, *Gut* 59:1561-1569, 2010.
43. Singh DK, et al: Comparison of clinical, biochemical and histological features of alcoholic steatohepatitis and non-alcoholic steatohepatitis in Asian Indian patients, *Indian J Pathol Microbiol* 53:408-413, 2010.
44. Stokkeland K, Ebrahim F, Ekbom A: Increased risk of esophageal varices, liver cancer, and death in patients with alcoholic liver disease, *Alcohol Clin Exp Res* 34:1993-1999, 2010.
45. Sozio MS, Liangpunsakul S, Crabb D: The role of lipid metabolism in the pathogenesis of alcoholic and nonalcoholic hepatic steatosis, *Semin Liver Dis* 30:378-390, 2010.
46. Yerian L: Histopathological evaluation of fatty and alcoholic liver diseases, *J Dig Dis* 12:17-24, 2011
47. Vega AB, et al: [Prolonged fever and jaundice in a patient with alcoholic liver disease.] *Gastroenterol Hepatol* 33:574-577, 2010.
48. Podolsky DK: Cirrhosis of the liver. In Wilson JD, et al, editors: *Harrison's principles of internal medicine*, ed 12, New York, 1991, McGraw-Hill, p 1567.
49. Cohen JI, Nagy LE: Pathogenesis of alcoholic liver disease: interactions between parenchymal and non-parenchymal cells, *J Dig Dis* 12:3-9, 2011.
50. Beier JI, Arteel GE, McClain CJ: Advances in alcoholic liver disease, *Curr Gastroenterol Rep* 13:56-64, 2011.
51. Amini M, Runyon BA: Alcoholic hepatitis 2010: a clinician's guide to diagnosis and therapy, *World J Gastroenterol* 16:4905-4912, 2010.
52. Albers I, et al: Superiority of the Child-Pugh classification to quantitative liver function tests for assessing prognosis of liver cirrhosis *Scand J Gastroenterol* 24:269-274, 1989.
53. Gex L, Bernard C, Spahr L: [Child-Pugh, MELD and Maddrey scores.] *Rev Med Suisse* 6:1803-1804, 1806-1808, 2010.
54. Varma V, Webb K, Mirza DF: Liver transplantation for alcoholic liver disease, *World J Gastroenterol* 16:4377-4393, 2010.
55. Topcheeva ON: [Hepatic osteodystrophy in patients with liver cirrhosis.] *Eksp Klin Gastroenterol* 6:89-94, 2010.
56. Lindroth J: Management of acute dental pain in the recovering alcoholic, *Oral Surg Oral Med Oral Pathol Oral Radiol Endod* 95:492-497, 2003.

CHAPTER 11

Gastrointestinal Disease

Gastrointestinal diseases such as peptic ulcer disease, inflammatory bowel disease, and pseudomembranous colitis are common and may affect the delivery of dental care. When a patient who has one of these conditions presents for treatment, several areas of clinical importance require consideration by the dental practitioner. The dentist must be cognizant of the patient's condition, must monitor for symptoms indicative of initial disease or relapse, and must be aware of drugs that interact with gastrointestinal medications or that may aggravate these conditions. In addition, oral manifestations of gastrointestinal disease are not uncommon, so the dentist also must be familiar with oral patterns of disease.

PEPTIC ULCER DISEASE

DEFINITION

A peptic ulcer is a well-defined break in the gastrointestinal mucosa (greater than 3 mm in diameter, as defined by many industry-sponsored studies) that results from chronic acid or pepsin secretions and the destructive effects of and host response to *Helicobacter pylori*. Peptic ulcers develop principally in regions of the gastrointestinal tract that are proximal to acid and pepsin secretions (Figure 11-1). The first portion of the duodenum is the location of most ulcers in Western populations, whereas gastric ulcers are more frequent in Asia.[1] The upper jejunum rarely is involved. Peptic ulcer disease usually is chronic and focal in distribution; only approximately 10% of patients have multiple ulcers.

EPIDEMIOLOGY

Incidence and Prevalence

Peptic ulcer disease is one of the most common human ailments, once affecting up to 15% of the population in industrialized countries. Current estimates suggest that 5% to 10% of the world population is affected, and 350,000 new cases are diagnosed annually in the United States.[2-6] The incidence of peptic ulceration peaked between 1900 and 1950 and progressively decreased thereafter. The decline in northern Europe and the United States may be the result of decreased cigarette and aspirin consumption, increased use of vegetable cooking oils (a rich source of raw materials for synthesis of prostaglandins, which have cytoprotective properties), and better sanitation leading to fewer *H. pylori* infections.[7] The disease affects 5% to 7% of northern Europeans and accounts for about 200,000 hospitalizations annually in the United States. Peptic ulcers are rare in Greenlander Eskimos, southwestern Native Americans, Australian aborigines, and Indonesians.[2]

Peak prevalence of peptic ulceration has shifted to the elderly population.[5] Until the 1980s, the male-to-female ratio in the United States was 2:1, but current data approximate this ratio at 1:1.[8] First-degree relatives have a three-fold greater risk of developing the disease.[5] Persons who smoke and are heavy drinkers of alcohol are more prone to development of the disease. An association with blood type O also is recognized. A higher prevalence is seen among patients with hyperparathyroidism and hypersecretory states (e.g., renal dialysis, Zollinger-Ellison syndrome, mastocytosis). Use of nonsteroidal antiinflammatory drugs (NSAIDs), including aspirin, for longer than 1 month is associated with an annual rate of 2% to 4% for gastrointestinal bleeding or ulcer complications in patients who ingest these drugs.[9,10]

The disease is rare in children, with only 1 in 2500 pediatric hospital admissions attributable to peptic ulceration.[11] When a peptic ulcer is diagnosed in a child younger than 10 years of age, the condition most often is associated with an underlying systemic illness, such as severe burn injury or other major trauma.[12] Most deaths that result from peptic ulcer disease occur in patients older than 65 years of age. An average dental practice of 2000 adult patients is predicted to serve about 100 patients with peptic ulcer disease.

Etiology

Peptic ulcers result when the balance between aggressive factors that are potentially destructive to the gastrointestinal mucosa and defensive factors that usually are protective of the mucosa is disrupted (Figure 11-2). The

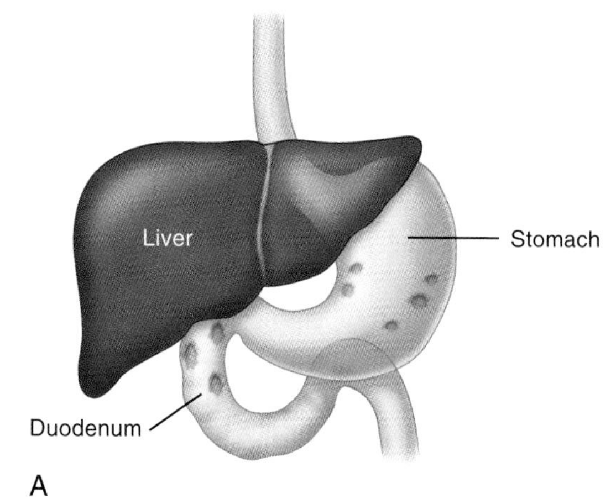

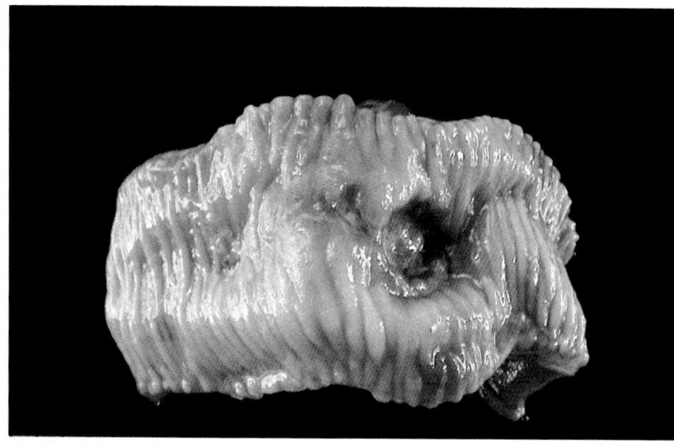

FIGURE 11-1 **A,** Location of peptic ulceration (*shaded areas*). *Darker-stippled areas* are higher-risk sites. **B,** Peptic ulcer of the duodenum. (***B,*** *From Kumar V, Abbas A, Fausto N, editors:* Robbins & Cotran pathologic basis of disease, *ed 7, Philadelphia, 2005, Saunders. Courtesy Robin Foss, University of Florida–Gainesville.)*

primary aggressive factor is *H. pylori* (formerly *Campylobacter pylori*). This organism is present in 60% to 90% of duodenal ulcers and in 50% to 70% of gastric ulcers.[1,13] Use of NSAIDs is the second most common cause of peptic ulcer disease. Other aggressive factors include acid hypersecretion, cigarette smoking, and psychological and physical stress.[14,15] Cytomegalovirus infection is a rare cause noted in human immunodeficiency virus (HIV)-positive patients.[16,17] Non-NSAID, non–*H. pylori* peptic ulcers are infrequent and occur more often in elderly persons.

H. pylori is a microaerophilic, gram-negative, spiral-shaped motile bacillus with 4 to 6 flagella.[18] *H. pylori* was first reported to reside in the antral mucosa by Marshall and Warren.[19] The organism is an adherent but noninvasive bacterium that resides at the interface between the surface of the gastric epithelium and the overlying mucous gel. It produces a potent urease that hydrolyzes urea to ammonia and carbon dioxide. This urease may protect bacteria from the immediate acidic environment by increasing local pH while damaging mucosa through generation of its byproduct, ammonia. Upregulation of cyclooxygenase-2 (COX-2), chemotaxis of neutrophils, and the cellular immune response are involved in the local tissue damage that subsequently occurs.

Humans are the only known hosts of *H. pylori.* This bacterium infects 0.5% of adults annually—a rate that has been declining since the early 1990's.[20,21] *H. pylori* is acquired primarily during childhood, possibly as a result of entry from the oral cavity via contaminated food and poor sanitary habits. The organism resides in the oral cavity,[22] from which it probably descends to

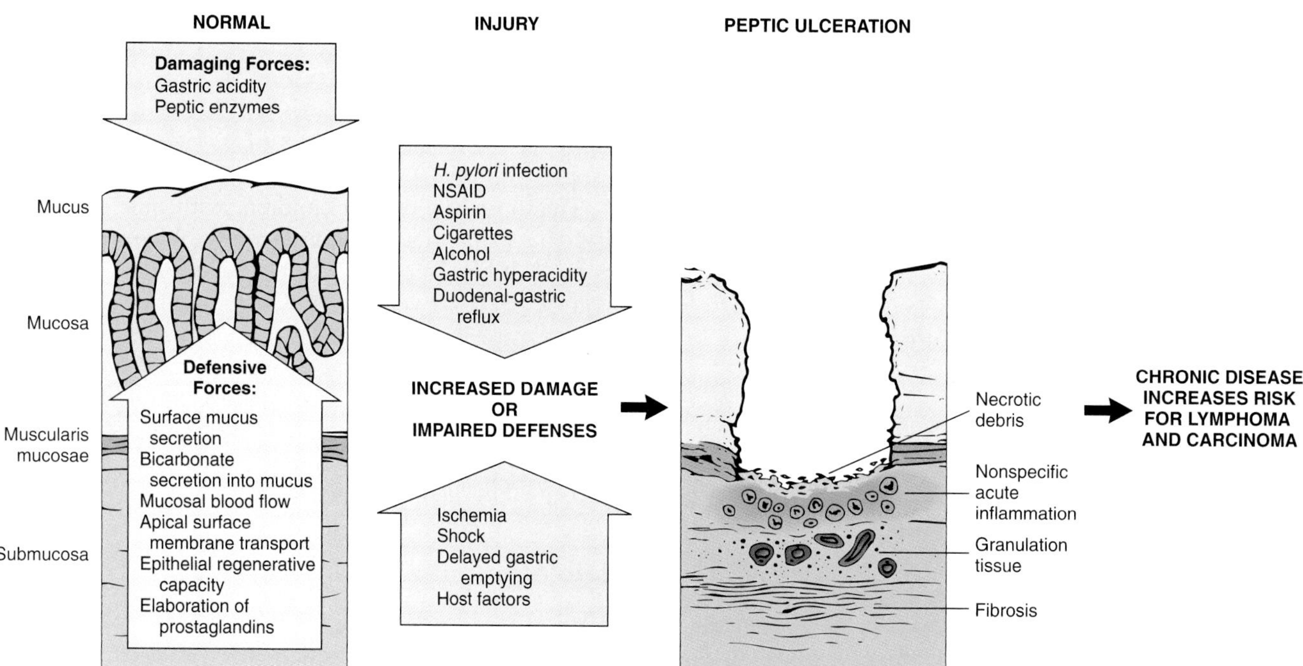

FIGURE 11-2 Complex interplay of aggressive and defensive factors involved in the formation of peptic ulcer disease. *(Modified from Kumar V, Abbas A, Fausto N, editors:* Robbins & Cotran pathologic basis of disease, *ed 7, Philadelphia, 2005, Saunders.)*

colonize the gastric mucosa. *H. pylori* can persist in the stomach indefinitely, and infection with the bacterium remains clinically silent in most affected persons.[23] The rate of *H. pylori* acquisition is higher in developing than in developed countries. In developing countries, 80% of the population carries the bacterium by the age of 20 years, whereas in the United States, only 20% of 20-year-olds are infected. The prevalence of infection among African Americans and Hispanics is twice that for whites in the United States.[24] Infection is correlated with lower socioeconomic status, contaminated drinking water, and familial overcrowding, especially during childhood. Approximately 20% of infected persons go on to develop peptic ulcer disease,[15] suggesting that other physiologic and psychological (stress) factors are required for presentation of this disease.[25]

Use of NSAIDs is an etiologic factor in 15% to 20% of cases of peptic ulcer.[1,10] These drugs directly damage mucosa, reduce mucosal prostaglandin production, and inhibit mucus secretion. Ulcers caused by NSAIDs are located more often in the stomach than in the duodenum. Risk with NSAID use increases with age older than 60 years, high-dosage long-term therapy, use of NSAIDs with long plasma half-lives (e.g., piroxicam) rather than those with short half-lives (i.e., ibuprofen), and concomitant use of alcohol, corticosteroids, anticoagulants, or aspirin.[26] Use of orally administered nitrogen-containing bisphosphonate drugs (aledronate, risedronate) for the treatment of osteoporosis and immunosuppressive medications such as mycophenolate is associated with development of esophageal and gastric ulcers.[1,27]

Pathophysiology and Complications

Ulcer formation is the result of a complex interplay of aggressive and defensive factors (see Figure 11-2). Resistance to acidic breakdown normally is provided by mucosal resistance, mucus and prostaglandin production, blood flow, bicarbonate secretion, and ion carrier exchange. Additional resistance is gained from the actions of antibacterial proteins such as lysozyme, lactoferrin, interferon, and α-defensin, or cryptdin.

Under normal circumstances, food stimulates gastrin release, gastrin stimulates histamine release by enterochromaffin-like cells in the stomach, and parietal cells secrete hydrogen ions and chloride ions (hydrochloric acid). Vagal nerve stimulation, caffeine, and histamine also are stimulants of parietal cell secretion of hydrochloric acid.[28] Aggressive factors include vagal overactivity and agents and events that enhance the release of pepsin, gastrin, and histamine. Physical and emotional stress, obsessive-compulsive behavior, parasitic infections, and drugs such as caffeine, high-dose corticosteroids, and phenylbutazone enhance hypersecretion of stomach acid. Alcohol and NSAIDs are directly injurious to gastric mucosa. Alcohol alters cell permeability and can cause cell death. NSAIDs including aspirin disrupt mucosal resistance by impairing prostaglandin production and denaturing mucous glycoproteins. Hyperparathyroidism enhances gastrin secretion, and renal dialysis does not adequately remove circulating gastrin. Smoking tobacco and family history are risk factors independent of gastric acid secretion for peptic ulcer disease.[8,29] Tobacco smoke, similar to other aggressive factors, can affect gastric mucosa by reducing levels of nitric oxide,[30] which is important for stimulating mucus secretion and maintaining mucosal blood flow.[31]

H. pylori is strongly associated with peptic ulcer disease[32]; however, the mechanism whereby infection with *H. pylori* results in peptic ulcer disease is not completely understood. Current evidence suggests that *H. pylori* causes inflammation of the gastric mucosa by producing proteases and increasing gastrin release by G cells, which leads to increased gastric acid production, acute gastritis, and eventually ulcer formation.[33-35] Complications associated with peptic ulcer disease vary with the degree of destruction of the gastrointestinal epithelium and supporting tissues. Superficial ulcers are characterized by the presence of necrotic debris, fibrin and subjacent inflammatory infiltrate, granulation tissue, and fibrosis. Ulcers that penetrate through the fibrotic tissue into the muscularis layer (muscularis mucosae) can perforate into the peritoneal cavity (peritonitis) or into the head of the pancreas. Arteries or veins in the muscularis layer may be eroded by ulcers, giving rise to hemorrhage (a bleeding ulcer), anemia, and potential shock. Untreated ulcers often heal by fibrosis, which can lead to pyloric stenosis, gastric outlet obstruction, dehydration, and alkalosis. Complications are more common in elderly people, and approximately 5% of those with duodenal ulcers die annually as a result of such complications.[36]

H. pylori is associated with the development of a low-grade gastric mucosa–associated lymphoid tissue lymphoma.[37] Accordingly, *H. pylori* has been classified by the World Health Organization (WHO) as a definite (class I) human carcinogen.[38]

Peptic ulcers rarely undergo carcinomatous transformation. Ulcers of the greater curvature of the stomach have a greater propensity for malignant degeneration than do those of the duodenum. Evidence that long-term use of proton pump inhibitors (PPIs) increases the risk for atrophic gastritis and stomach cancer remains controversial; however, the eradication of *H. pylori* halts progression of atrophic gastritis and may lead to regression of atrophy.[39-41]

CLINICAL PRESENTATION

Signs and Symptoms

Although many patients with active peptic ulcer report no ulcer symptoms, most experience epigastric pain that is long-standing (several hours) and sharply localized. The pain is described as "burning" or "gnawing" but may be "ill-defined" or "aching." The discomfort of a duodenal ulcer manifests most commonly on an empty stomach, usually 90 minutes to 3 hours after eating, and frequently awakens the patient in the middle of the night. Ingestion of food, milk, or antacids provides rapid relief in most cases. In contrast, patients with gastric ulcers are unpredictable in their response to food; in fact, eating may precipitate abdominal pain. Symptoms associated with peptic ulceration tend to be episodic and recurrent. Epigastric tenderness often accompanies the condition.

Changes in the character of pain may indicate the development of complications. For example, increased discomfort, loss of antacid relief, or pain radiating to the back may signal deeper penetration or perforation of the ulcer. Protracted vomiting a few hours after a meal is a sign of gastric outlet (pyloric) obstruction. Melena (bloody stools) or black tarry stools indicate blood loss due to gastrointestinal hemorrhage.

Laboratory Findings

A peptic ulcer is diagnosed primarily by fiberoptic endoscopy and laboratory testing for *H. pylori.* Endoscopy affords the opportunity for visualization, access for biopsy, and therapeutic procedures if bleeding is present. During endoscopy, a biopsy of the marginal mucosa adjacent to the ulcer is performed to confirm the diagnosis and rule out malignancy. A rapid urease test is then performed to detect the bacterial product urease in the mucosal biopsy specimen. Microscopic analysis of biopsied tissue prepared with Giemsa, acridine orange, and Warthin-Starry stains is effective in the microscopic detection of *H. pylori* (Figure 11-3). Culture of the organism is reserved for cases in which antimicrobial resistance is suspected, because the technique is tedious, difficult, and no more sensitive than routine histologic analysis.

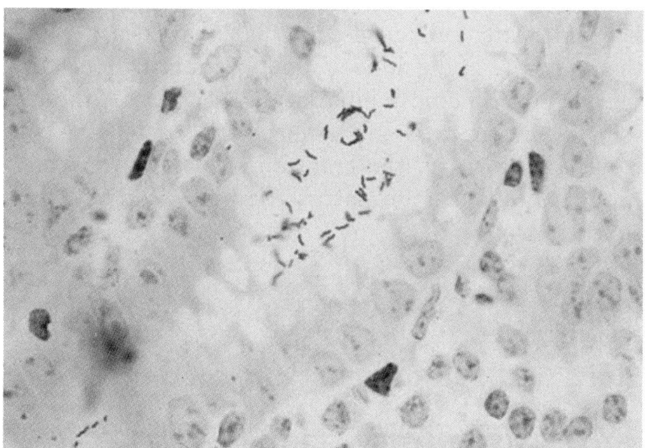

FIGURE 11-3 *Helicobacter pylori* organisms (*dark rods*) evident in the lumen of the intestine. (Warthin-Starry stain.) *(Courtesy Eun Lee, Lexington, Kentucky.)*

Nonendoscopic laboratory tests include urea breath tests (UBTs), serologic tests, and, less commonly, *H. pylori* stool antigen tests. A UBT is a highly sensitive, noninvasive test that involves the ingestion of urea labeled with carbon-13 (^{13}C) or carbon-14 (^{14}C). Degradation of urea by the bacillus releases ^{13}C or ^{14}C in expired carbon dioxide.[42] These tests are advantageous because they indirectly measure the presence of *H. pylori* before treatment and its eradication after treatment. Serologic testing is useful in determining current or past infection but is limited in documenting the eradication of *H. pylori,* because antibody titers persist after the organism has been eliminated. Upper gastrointestinal imaging is infrequently performed, because it lacks the sensitivity of biopsy.

MEDICAL MANAGEMENT

Most patients with peptic ulcer disease suffer for several weeks before going to a doctor for treatment. If the peptic ulcer is confined and uncomplicated and *H. pylori* is not present, antisecretory drugs are administered (Table 11-1). If the patient is infected with *H. pylori,* inhibitors of gastric acid secretion and antimicrobial agents are recommended.[43] Combination therapy is recommended because antisecretory drugs, such as histamine H_2 receptor antagonists and PPIs, provide rapid relief of pain and accelerate healing, and antibiotics are effective in eradicating *H. pylori.* Combination treatment accelerates healing and produces an ulcer-free state in 92% to 99% of treated patients.[39,40]

Four-drug treatment regimens, including a PPI plus three antimicrobials (clarithromycin, metronidazole or tinidazole, and amoxicillin), or a PPI plus a bismuth plus tetracycline and metronidazole, provide the best results for persons with a peptic ulcer and *H. pylori* infection (Box 11-1). This four-drug regimen is recommended over the previously standard triple therapy (a PPI, amoxicillin, and clarithromycin) because of increasing antibiotic resistance.[44] Therapy is given for 10 to 14 days, and eradication of infection should be confirmed afterward.

Prior to 2000, more than 50% of patients with peptic ulcer disease experienced recurrences after treatment. Such recurrence was likely because regimens consisting solely of antisecretory drugs were the treatment of choice; however, these drugs alone do not eradicate *H. pylori* infection and are noncurative of peptic ulcer disease. Eradication of *H. pylori* with antibiotic treatment reduces the rate of recurrence of peptic ulceration by 85% to 100%.[43,45] Reemergence of an ulcer usually is traced to the persistence of *H. pylori* after treatment because of inappropriate drug choice, discontinuance of drug therapy, lack of behavior modification, or bacterial resistance.[1]

In all patients who undergo peptic ulcer therapy, ulcerogenic factors (e.g., use of alcohol, aspirin or other NSAIDs, and corticosteroids; consumption of foods that aggravate symptoms and stimulate gastric acid secretion; persistent stress) should be eliminated to accelerate healing and limit the occurrence of relapse. Patients benefit from smoking cessation, in that perforation rates are higher in smokers, and continued smoking results in a higher relapse rate after treatment and lower rates of eradication of *H. pylori*.[46] When *H. pylori* is successfully eradicated, cigarette smoking does not appear to increase the risk of recurrence.[47]

Elective surgical intervention (e.g., dissection of the vagus nerves from the gastric fundus) largely has been abandoned in the management of peptic ulcer disease. Today, surgery is reserved primarily for complications of peptic ulcer disease such as significant bleeding (when unresponsive to coagulant endoscopic procedures), perforation, and gastric outlet obstruction. On occasions when peptic ulcer disease is associated with hyperparathyroidism and parathyroid adenoma, surgical removal of the affected gland is the treatment of choice. Resolution of gastrointestinal disease occurs after abnormal endocrine function is terminated. Prototype protein-based vaccines against *H. pylori* continue to be investigated.[48]

BOX 11-1 Antimicrobial Regimens for the Treatment of Helicobacter Pylori Infection in Peptic Ulcer Disease

First-Line Therapy*

- Proton pump inhibitor (*or* ranitidine bismuth citrate) twice daily *plus* 3 antimicrobials:
  - Clarithromycin 500 mg twice daily *plus*
  - Metronidazole 500 mg twice daily *or* tinidazole 500 mg twice daily *plus*
  - Amoxicillin 1000 mg twice daily

Alternative First-Line Therapy*

- *Quadruple therapy:* proton pump inhibitor twice daily, bismuth subsalicylate/subcitrate 120 mg four times daily, plus metronidazole 500 mg twice daily, tetracycline 500 mg four times daily

*Medications are given for 10 to 14 days. Clinicians are advised to select drugs on the basis of the presence or absence of antibiotic resistance.
Data from Rimbara E, Fischbach LA, Graham DY: Optimal therapy for Helicobacter pylori, Nat Rev Gastroenterol Hepatol *8:79-88, 2011.*

DENTAL MANAGEMENT

Medical Considerations

The dentist must identify intestinal symptoms through a careful history that is taken before dental treatment is initiated, because many gastrointestinal diseases, although they are chronic and recurrent, remain undetected for long periods. This history includes a careful review of medications (e.g., aspirin and other NSAIDs, oral anticoagulants) and level of alcohol consumption that may result in gastrointestinal bleeding. If gastrointestinal symptoms are suggestive of active disease, a medical referral is needed. Once the patient returns from the physician and the condition is under control, the dentist should update current medications in the dental record, including the type and dosage, and should follow physician guidelines. Further, periodic physician visits should be encouraged to afford early diagnosis and cancer screenings for at-risk patients.

TABLE 11-1 Antisecretory Drugs

Class	Drug	Trade Name	Dental Management Considerations
Histamine H_2 receptor antagonists	Cimetidine	Tagamet	Delayed liver metabolism of benzodiazepines; reversible joint symptoms with preexisting arthritis
	Ranitidine	Zantac	—
	Famotidine	Pepcid	Anorexia, dry mouth
	Nizatidine	Axid	Potentially increased serum salicylate levels with concurrent aspirin use
Proton pump inhibitors	Omeprazole—rapid release form	Prilosec, Zegarid	May reduce absorption of ampicillin, ketoconazole, and itraconazole; may increase the concentration of benzodiazepines, warfarin, and phenytoin
	Lansoprazole	Prevacid	May reduce absorption of ampicillin, ketoconazole, and itraconazole; may increase the concentration of warfarin
	Pantoprazole	Protonix, Protium	May reduce absorption of ampicillin, ketoconazole, and itraconazole; may increase the concentration of warfarin
	Rabeprazole	Aciphex	May reduce absorption of ampicillin, ketoconazole, and itraconazole; may increase the concentration of clarithromycin and warfarin
	Esomeprazole	Nexium	May reduce absorption of ampicillin, ketoconazole, and itraconazole; may increase the concentration of benzodiazepines, warfarin, and phenytoin
Prostaglandins*	Misoprostol	Cytotec	Diarrhea, cramps

*Not a first-line drug for treating patients with peptic ulcer. Used in the prevention of peptic ulcer and in users of nonsteroidal antiinflammatory drugs (NSAIDs).

Of primary importance are the impact and interactions of certain drugs prescribed to patients with peptic ulcer disease (Box 11-2). In general, the dentist should avoid prescribing aspirin, aspirin-containing compounds, and other NSAIDs to patients with a history of peptic ulcer disease because of the irritative effects of these drugs on the gastrointestinal epithelium. Acetaminophen and compounded acetaminophen products are recommended instead. If NSAIDs are used, a cyclooxygenase-2–selective inhibitor (e.g., celecoxib [Celebrex]) given in combination with a PPI or misoprostol (Cytotec), 200 µg 4 times per day—a prostaglandin E_1 analogue—is advised for short-term use to reduce the risk of gastrointestinal bleeding.[49-51] Analgesic selection should be based on patient risk factors (previous gastrointestinal bleeding, advanced age, use of alcohol, anticoagulants, or steroids), and the lowest dose for the shortest period to achieve the desired effect should be prescribed. Histamine H_2 receptor antagonists and sucralfate are not beneficial selections because they do

BOX 11-2 Dental Management
Considerations in Patients with Gastrointestinal (GI) Disease

P

Patient Evaluation/Risk Assessment (see Box 1-1)

- Evaluate and determine whether GI disease or comorbid conditions exist.
- Obtain medical consultation if patient's disease is poorly controlled, if signs or symptoms appear suggesting an undiagnosed condition, or if the diagnosis is uncertain.

Potential Issues/Factors of Concern

A

Analgesics	Avoid prescribing aspirin, aspirin-containing compounds, and other nonsteroidal antiinflammatory drugs (NSAIDs) for patients with a history of peptic ulcer disease or inflammatory bowel disease (IBD). Use acetaminophen-containing products or celecoxib (Celebrex) in combination with a proton pump inhibitor or misoprostol (Cytotec).
Antibiotics	Selection of antibiotics for oral infections may be influenced by recent use of antibiotics for peptic ulcer disease; certain drugs can increase the risk of intestinal flareup in a patient with inflammatory bowel disease. Avoid long-term use of antibiotics, especially in elderly and debilitated persons, to minimize risk of pseudomembranous colitis. Monitor for signs or symptoms (diarrhea, GI distress) suggestive of pseudomembranous colitis or disease worsening. Contact patient's physician if GI symptoms worsen while patient is on antibiotics, so that alternative therapies can be initiated.
Anesthesia	No issues.
Anxiety	Intraoperative sedation can be provided by an oral, inhalation, or intravenous route.
Allergy	No issues.

B

Bleeding	Use of acid-blocking drugs and proton pump inhibitors can enhance the blood levels of warfarin (Coumadin). Obtain complete blood count if medication profile increases patient risk for anemia, leukopenia, or thrombocytopenia.
Blood pressure	No issues.

C

Chair position	Chair position should be based on patient comfort relative to the GI disorder.

D

Devices	No issues.
Drugs	Lower doses of diazepam, lidocaine, or tricyclic antidepressants may be required if the patient is taking acid-blocking drugs, such as cimetidine, which decreases the metabolism of some dentally prescribed drugs and enhances the duration of action of these medications. Proton pump inhibitors may reduce absorption of select antibiotics and antifungals. Monitor effects of immunosuppressant medications. If patient has recently taken corticosteroids, dosage modification generally is not needed; however, clinician should evaluate the need for supplemental steroids as indicated by health status, level of anxiety/fear, presence of infection, and dental procedure (see Box 15-2).

E

Equipment	No issues.
Emergencies and urgent care	No issues.

F

Follow-up	Schedule appointments during periods of remission. Be flexible in scheduling appointments; disease flareups can be unpredictable. Shorter appointments may be necessary. Increased risk for medical complications could affect scheduling—for example: • Peptic ulcer disease is more likely in patients older than 65 years of age and those with previous history of ulcer complications, prolonged use of NSAIDs, and concomitant use of anticoagulants, corticosteroids, or bisphosphonates. • IBD flareups are more likely when patient is reporting symptoms and has a fever. • Pseudomembranous colitis is more likely in patients older than 65 years of age and those with history of recent hospitalization or taking broad-spectrum antibiotics (clindamycin, cephalosporins, ampicillin) or multiple antibiotics, or with HIV-seropositive status associated with immune suppression. • Patients with ulcerative colitis are at increased risk for colon cancer.

not appear to protect patients from NSAID-induced complications.[52]

Acid-blocking drugs, such as cimetidine, decrease the metabolism of certain dentally prescribed drugs (i.e., diazepam, lidocaine, tricyclic antidepressants) and enhance the duration of action of these medications (see Table 11-1). Under such circumstances, dosing of anesthetics, benzodiazepines, and antidepressants that are metabolized in the liver may require adjustment. Antacids also impair the absorption of tetracycline, erythromycin, oral iron, and fluoride, thereby preventing attainment of optimal blood levels of these drugs. To avoid this problem, antibiotics and dietary supplements should be taken 2 hours before or 2 hours after antacids are ingested.

Routine dental treatment may be provided during medical therapy for peptic ulceration; however, the decision should be based on patient comfort and convenience. Should antibiotics become necessary to treat a dental infection during the course of peptic ulcer disease therapy, the choice of antibiotics may be altered as required by the patient's current medications.

Treatment Planning Modifications

H. pylori is found in dental plaque and may serve as a reservoir of infection and reinfection along the alimentary tract.[22,53] Good oral hygiene measures and periodic scaling and prophylaxis may be useful in reducing the spread of this organism. The need for rigorous hygiene measures should be explained to the patient, and consideration given to laboratory detection of oral organisms in patients who have a history of peptic ulcer disease and are symptomatic or are experiencing recurrences. Routine dental care requires no other modifications in technique for patients with peptic ulcer disease.

Oral Complications and Manifestations

The use of systemic antibiotics for peptic ulcer disease may result in *fungal overgrowth* (candidiasis) in the oral cavity. The dentist should be alert to identifying oral fungal infections, including median rhomboid glossitis, in this patient population (Figure 11-4). A course of antifungal agents (see Appendix C) should be prescribed to resolve the fungal infection.

Vascular malformations of the lip and *erosion of the enamel* are two less common oral manifestations of peptic ulcer disease. The former have been reported to range in size from a small macule (microcherry) to a large venous pool, and they typically occur in older men with peptic ulcer disease.[54] Enamel erosion is the result of persistent regurgitation of gastric juices into the mouth when pyloric stenosis occurs (Figure 11-5). The finding of such erosion combined with a history of reflux indicates that the patient must be evaluated by a physician.

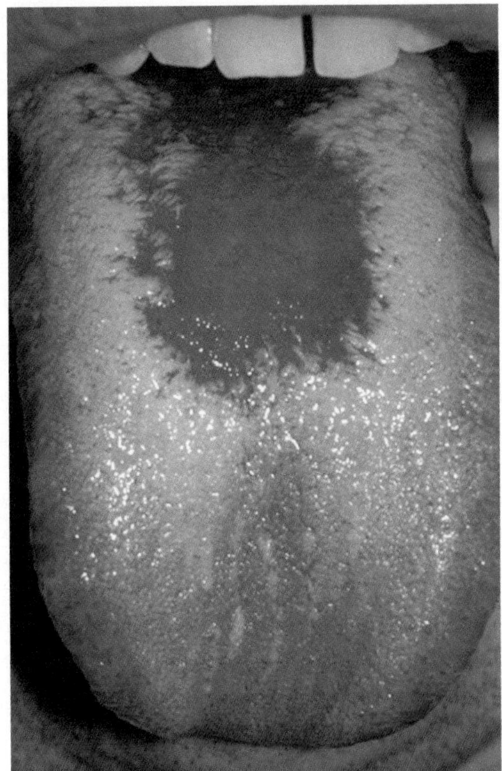

FIGURE 11-4 Median rhomboid glossitis caused by antibiotic use.

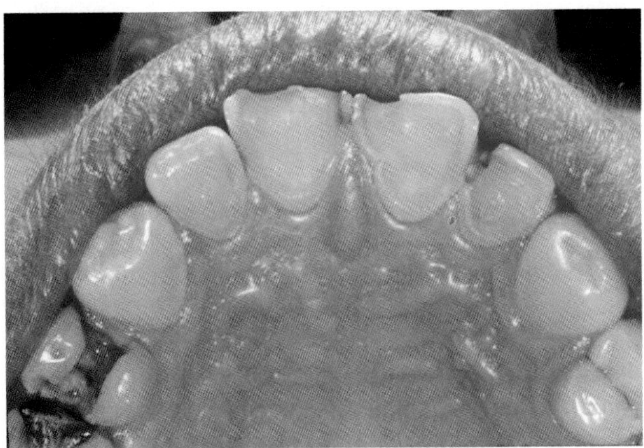

FIGURE 11-5 Perimylolysis. Destruction of palatal enamel of maxillary incisors in a patient with persistent regurgitation.

Medications taken by patients for the treatment of peptic ulcer disease can produce oral manifestations. PPIs can alter taste perception. Cimetidine and ranitidine may have a toxic effect on bone marrow; infrequently, they cause anemia, agranulocytosis, or thrombocytopenia. Mucosal ulcerations may be a sign of agranulocytosis, whereas anemia may manifest as mucosal pallor, and thrombocytopenia as gingival bleeding or petechiae. Xerostomia has been associated with the use of famotidine and anticholinergic drugs, such as propantheline (Pro-Banthine). A chronic dry mouth renders the patient susceptible to bacterial infection (caries and periodontal disease) and fungal disease (candidiasis). Erythema multiforme has been associated with the use of cimetidine, ranitidine, omeprazole, and lansoprazole.

INFLAMMATORY BOWEL DISEASE

DEFINITION

Inflammatory bowel disease (IBD) is a term encompassing two idiopathic diseases of the gastrointestinal tract: ulcerative colitis and Crohn's disease. The main criteria that separate the two diseases are the site and extent of tissue involvement; thus, it is logical to consider these clinical entities together. *Ulcerative colitis* is a mucosal disease that is limited to the large intestine and rectum. In contrast, *Crohn's disease* is a transmural process (involving the entire thickness of the bowel wall) that may produce "patchy" ulcerations at any point along the alimentary canal from the mouth to the anus but most commonly involves the terminal ileum.

EPIDEMIOLOGY

Incidence and Prevalence

The incidence and prevalence of IBD vary widely by race and geographic location. Occurrence is much higher among Jews and whites than in blacks, and it is considerably higher in the United States and Europe than in Africa and Asia, although the incidence is rising in Asia.[55] Fifteen to 30 new cases of IBD per 100,000 people are diagnosed annually in the United States, Australia, and Europe,[56,57] and currently a total of 580,000 persons in the United States are affected.[55] Peak age at onset is 20 to 40 years (young adulthood). However, a second incidence peak for Crohn's disease has been noted between the ages of 55 and 65 years. Children are known to develop IBD, and the incidence in this population is rising.[58] Ulcerative colitis affects men and women equally, whereas Crohn's disease has a slight predilection for women. A 10-fold increased risk of disease in first-degree relatives of patients strongly suggests that genetic factors are involved.[59] Environment factors also are contributory: Crohn's disease occurs more often in nonsmokers, whereas smoking protects against ulcerative colitis.[16] Breast-feeding also appears to reduce the risk of IBD.[60] In the average general dentistry practice with 2000 adult patients, approximately 5 adults are predicted to have IBD.

Etiology

Ulcerative colitis and Crohn's disease are inflammatory diseases of unknown cause that are generally thought to be associated with immune dysfunction in response to environmental factors in genetically susceptible persons. Several genetic susceptibility genes have been identified, including *Nod2*, interleukin (IL)-23 receptor gene, tumor necrosis factor (TNF) superfamily (TNFSF15) gene, and Toll-like receptor (TLR)-4 gene. Mutations in these genes impair the immune response, thereby contributing to inefficient recognition and clearing of bacteria and cell degradation products by intestinal epithelium and leading to inflammation and increased permeability of the intestinal wall.[59,61] At present, no specific enteric microbe has been determined to be responsible for inducing the proinflammatory responses observed in IBD.

Pathophysiology and Complications

Ulcerative Colitis. Ulcerative colitis is an inflammatory reaction that resembles an atypical T_H2 response. The disease targets the large intestine and is characterized by remissions and exacerbations. It starts in the colon-rectum region and may spread proximally to involve the entire large intestine and the ileum. Histopathologic findings include edema, vascular congestion, distorted cryptic architecture, and monocellular infiltration. Persistent disease causes epithelial erosions and hemorrhage, pseudopolyp formation, crypt abscesses, and submucosal fibrosis. Chronic deposition of fibrous tissue may lead to fibrotic shortening, thickening, and narrowing of the colon.

Ulcerative colitis usually is a lifelong disease, and progression to its more severe forms predisposes affected persons to toxic dilatation (toxic megacolon) and dysplastic changes (carcinoma) of the intestine. *Toxic megacolon* is the result of disease extension through deep muscular layers. The colon dilates because of weakening of the wall, and intestinal perforation then becomes likely. Associated fever, electrolyte imbalance, and volume depletion are reported. *Carcinoma of the colon* is 10 times more likely in patients with ulcerative colitis than in the general population.[62] Likelihood of malignant transformation increases with proximal extension of involvement and with long-standing disease (longer than 8 to 10 years), at a rate of 0.5% to 2% per year.[62,63]

Crohn Disease. Crohn disease is a chronic, relapsing idiopathic disease that is characterized by segmental distribution of intestinal ulcers (so-called skip lesions) interrupted by normal-appearing mucosa. Although the distal ileum and the proximal colon are affected most frequently, any portion of the bowel may be involved. In gross specimens, the intestine displays sharply delimited regions of thickened bowel wall, irregular glandular openings, mucosal fissuring, ulcerations, erosions, and benign strictures (Figure 11-6). With chronic disease, the intestinal mucosa takes on a nodular or "cobblestone" appearance as a result of dense inflammatory infiltrates and submucosal thickening. Transmural involvement of

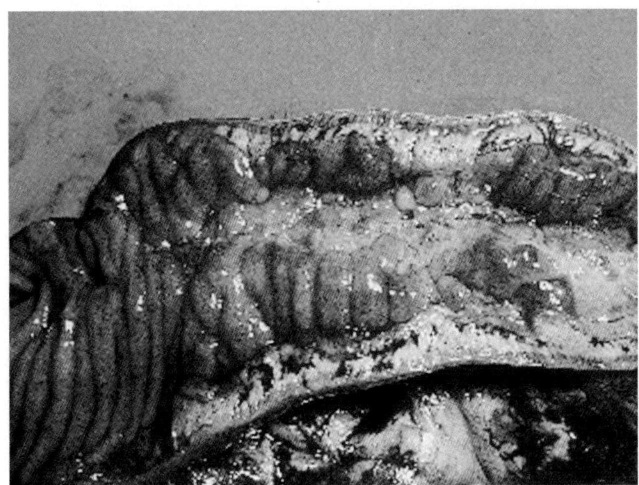

A

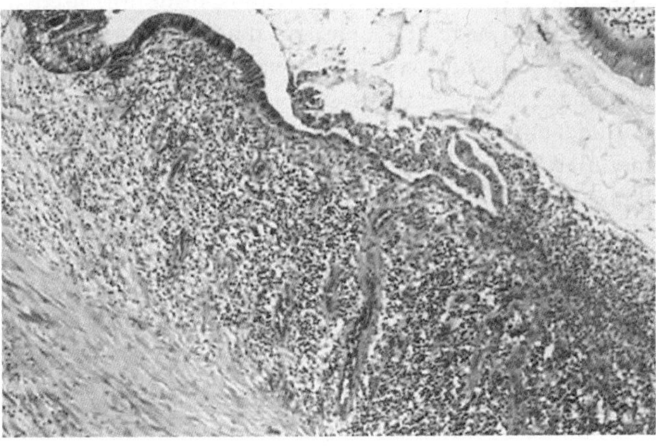

B

FIGURE 11-6 **A,** Crohn's disease that exhibits ulceration of the intestinal mucosa. **B,** Low-power micrograph showing ulcerated intestinal mucosa of Crohn's disease with dense inflammatory infiltrate. *(**A,** From Allison MC, et al:* Inflammatory bowel disease, *London, 1998, Mosby.)*

the intestinal wall and noncaseating epithelioid granulomas of the intestine and mesenteric lymph nodes are classic features of the disease. As a result, the mesentery thickens and fixes the intestine in one position. Mesenteric fat tissue contributes numerous immune-regulating adipokines that influence the disease process.[64]

At the microscopic level, ulcerative colitis and Crohn disease are characterized by infiltrative lesions of the bowel wall that contain activated inflammatory cells (neutrophils and macrophages), immune-based cells (lymphocytes and plasma cells), and noncaseating granulomas. In Crohn's disease, the immune cells attracted to the region produce increased levels of proinflammatory mediators such as interleukin-1 (IL-1), IL-23, TNF, and interferon-γ—consistent with the view that the disease is a T_H1 response–like condition.[65] Crohn's disease is further characterized by defects in mucosal immunity and in the mucosal barrier that result in increased intestinal permeability, increased adherence of bacteria, and decreased expression of defensins.[66] The clinical course in Crohn's disease consists of remissions and relapses; relapses are more common in persons who smoke tobacco. Unremitting disease is complicated by small bowel stenosis and fistula formation. Most patients who have Crohn's disease require at least one operation for their condition.[67] Long-standing colonic Crohn's disease increases the risk for the development of colorectal cancer.

CLINICAL PRESENTATION

Signs and Symptoms

Ulcerative Colitis. Patients with ulcerative colitis experience three prominent symptoms: (1) attacks of diarrhea, (2) rectal bleeding (or bloody diarrhea), and (3) abdominal cramps. Onset may be sudden or insidious, but in most cases the disease continues along a chronic intermittent course. Dehydration, fatigue, weight loss, and fever caused by malabsorption of water and electrolytes frequently accompany the condition. Extraintestinal manifestations may include arthritis, erythema nodosum or pyoderma gangrenosum, eye disorders such as iritis and uveitis, and growth failure. Although many patients enjoy long periods of remission, less than 5% remain symptom-free over a 10-year period; about 50% experience a relapse in any given year.[63,68,69]

Crohn's Disease. Initial manifestations of Crohn's disease consist of recurrent or persistent diarrhea (often without blood), abdominal pain or cramping, anorexia, and weight loss. Unexplained fever, malaise, arthritis, uveitis, and features related to malabsorption often emerge next. However, symptoms vary from patient to patient according to the site and extent of involved tissue, with three major patterns recognized: (1) disease of the ileum and cecum, (2) disease confined to the small intestine, and (3) disease confined to the colon. Variability in symptoms and the episodic pattern contribute to the average 3-year delay in diagnosis from onset of symptoms.[65] Intestinal complications from chronic inflammatory damage include transmural fibrosis, intestinal fissuring, and formation of fistulas or abscesses. These complications are common; 70% to 80% of patients require surgery within their lifetime. Malabsorption is an additional complication that can result in a striking degree of weight loss, growth failure, anemia, and clubbing of the fingers. Reduced bone mineral density (i.e., osteoporosis) also results from malabsorption and chronic corticosteroid use. Extraintestinal manifestations (e.g., peripheral arthritis, erythema nodosum, aphthous, episcleritis, hepatic complications) occur in about 25% of patients.

Laboratory Findings

The diagnosis of IBD is based primarily on clinical findings, results of endoscopy and biopsy, and observations on histolopathologic examination of intestinal mucosa. Abdominal radiographic imaging, including computed tomography and magnetic resonance enterography, and stool examinations also may provide supportive evidence.[70]

Ulcerative colitis is characterized by friable, granular, erythematous, and eroded mucosa of the colon, with regions of edema and chronic inflammation seen on endoscopic and microscopic examinations. Crohn's disease, in contrast, features patchy erosions and ulcerations, with noncaseating granulomas that can arise in any part of the gastrointestinal tract. Blood tests in IBD may show anemia (deficiencies of iron, folate, or vitamin B_{12}) caused by malabsorption, decreased levels of serum total protein and albumin (as a result of malabsorption), inflammatory activity (evidenced as elevated erythrocyte sedimentation rate and increased C-reactive protein titer), and an elevated platelet count, in conjunction with a negative microbial stool sample.

MEDICAL MANAGEMENT

Ulcerative colitis and Crohn's disease can be managed, but not cured, by an array of drugs. Antidiarrheal and antiinflammatory medications (e.g., sulfasalazine, 5-aminosalicylic acid [ASA], corticosteroids) generally are first-line drugs.[68,69] Immunosuppressive agents and antibiotics are used as second-line drugs. Third-line approaches for management of Crohn's disease in persons who are refractory to steroid treatment include monoclonal antibody (infliximab [Remicade]) active against TNF[68,71] and surgical resection to remove the diseased portion of the colon. Supportive therapy that includes bed rest, dietary manipulation, and nutritional supplementation often is required. Dietary intervention with fish oil supplements may be beneficial to persons with Crohn's disease.[72]

Drugs containing 5-aminosalicylic acid (5-ASA) remain the mainstay of treatment for ulcerative colitis and play a small role in management of Crohn's disease.[73] These drugs—sulfasalazine, mesalamine (Asacol [Procter & Gamble Pharmaceuticals, Cincinnati, Ohio], Pentasa [Shire US Inc., Wayne, Pennsylvania], olsalazine, and balsalazide—are covalently bound to 5-ASA, which is released when cleaved by colonic bacteria.[74,75] The released 5-ASA delivers local antiinflammatory effects within the intestine. Because use of sulfasalazine is associated with adverse effects (nausea, headache, fever, arthralgia, rash, anemia, agranulocytosis, cholestatic hepatitis) and because this agent is not well delivered past the proximal bowel, controlled-release oral formulations of 5-ASA (mesalamine, olsalazine, and balsalazide) that dissolve in the distal ileum and colon are used; rectal suppositories or enemas also are used. Of note, 5-ASA drugs are potentially nephrotoxic, so physician monitoring of renal function is advised.

Corticosteroids often are combined with sulfasalazine to induce remission in patients who are moderately to severely ill. Steroids are not prescribed for maintenance therapy because several adverse effects are associated with long-term use. When severe attacks produce abdominal tenderness, dehydration, fever, vomiting, and severe bloody diarrhea, the patient should be hospitalized, and parenteral corticosteroids administered. After about 2 weeks, or once a satisfactory response is achieved, oral steroids are substituted for parenteral steroids, and the dosage is gradually reduced until the drug is no longer needed.

Immunomodulator drugs such as azathioprine (Imuran), and its metabolite 6-mercaptopurine are used in patients who have active disease that is unresponsive to corticosteroids and in corticosteroid-dependent patients to reduce the amount of steroid needed, and to limit dose-dependent adverse effects of steroids.[73] Immunomodulators may be given for years; however their use is limited by their toxicity (flulike symptoms, leukopenia, pancreatitis, hepatitis, and life-threatening infections). Intravenous administration of cyclosporine, an immunosuppressant, also has been used to heal fistulas caused by ulcerative colitis and Crohn disease.[63] Bone marrow and hematopoietic stem cell transplantation has been associated with permanent remission.[76,77]

Infliximab (anti-TNF monoclonal antibody) is used for severe disease (more than one relapse per year) that is refractory to other drugs and for maintenance of remission.[78] It is an expensive drug that is given as a single 2-hour infusion specifically for Crohn's disease.[32] Infusions generally are performed at 8- to 12-week intervals.[79] Infliximab demonstrates greater efficacy and a lower rate of side effects when given in combination with azathioprine.

Antibiotics (metronidazole or ciprofloxacin) have been used for treatment of active Crohn's disease (e.g., abscesses) and to maintain remission. They also are used after surgery when toxic colitis develops, or when fever and leukocytosis are present. Additional medications such as opioids, cromolyn sodium, and supplemental iron sometimes are used for their different effects, as required: antidiarrheal, anti–mast cell release, and treatment of anemia, respectively.

Surgery is recommended for severe cases of IBD that do not respond to corticosteroids, and to manage serious complications (e.g., massive hemorrhage, obstruction, perforation, toxic megacolon, carcinomatous transformation). Total proctocolectomy with ileostomy is the standard but infrequent treatment for intractable ulcerative colitis. Approximately 70% of patients with Crohn's disease require some form of surgery, and 40% have recurrent disease, thus necessitating additional resections.

DENTAL MANAGEMENT

Medical Considerations

The dentist should evaluate the patient with IBD to determine the severity and level of control of the condition. Patients who have less than four bowel movements per day with little or no blood, no fever, few symptoms, and a sedimentation rate below 20 mm/hour are considered to have mild disease and can receive dental care in the dentist's office. Patients with moderate disease (i.e., between mild and severe) or severe disease—the latter defined as having six or more bowel movements per day with blood, fever, anemia, and a sedimentation rate higher than 30 mm/hour—are poor candidates for dental care and should be referred to their physician.

Patients with IBD are likely to be taking antiinflammatory drugs, corticosteroids, or immunomodulators, which can have an impact on dental care. The use of antiinflammatory drugs and the involvement of the intestinal tract suggest that aspirin and other NSAIDs are to be avoided. Acetaminophen may be used alone or in combination with opioids. Alternatively, cotherapy with a COX-2 inhibitor (celecoxib) and a PPI can provide pain relief and simultaneous protection of the gastrointestinal mucosa. A careful drug history should be obtained to avoid prescribing additional opioids to patients who take these medications to manage their intestinal pain (Box 11-2).

Antibiotics can be prescribed to patients with IBD who have dental infections; some antibiotics, however, can promote overgrowth of *Clostridium difficile,* leading to symptomatic flares and diarrhea (see next section). Although data on specific antibiotics and flares in this patient population are lacking, clindamycin and penicillins have documented association with pseudomembranous colitis. Dentists who provide antibiotics are encouraged to minimize the use of clindamycin, if possible, and should advise the patient to report a symptomatic flare (diarrhea), so that the physician can be alerted to check for *C. difficile,* with consequent modification of therapy as appropriate.

The use of a steroid drug by a patient with IBD can be of clinical concern because corticosteroids can suppress adrenal function and reduce the ability of the patient to withstand stress. Current recommendations are that the patient take the usual daily dose of corticosteroids before the dental appointment and that the dentist provide adequate pain and anxiety control (see Box 15-2). Supplemental corticosteroids may be required in rare circumstances if the patient's health is poor, infection is present, the patient is fearful, and major surgery is being performed (see Chapter 15).

Immunosuppressors (azathioprine and 6-mercaptopurine) are associated with development of pancytopenia in approximately 5% of patients. In addition, a thorough head and neck examination should be performed in patients who take immunosuppressants, because of their increased risk for lymphoma and infection (e.g., infectious mononucleosis, recurrent herpes). Presence of fever without an obvious causative illness in this select population mandates prompt referral to the physician.

Treatment Planning Modifications

The severity, clinical course, and ultimate prognosis with IBD are highly variable and can have an impact on routine dental care. Most patients with IBD experience intermittent attacks, with asymptomatic remissions between attacks. Patients often require physical rest and emotional support throughout the disease, because anxiety and depression may be severe. Only urgent dental care is advised during acute exacerbations of gastrointestinal disease. The clinician can assess current disease severity by taking the patient's temperature and through a brief review of symptoms to ascertain the number of diarrheal bowel movements occurring per day and whether blood is present in the stool.

Elective dental procedures should be scheduled during periods of remission when complications are absent and a feeling of well-being has returned. Flexibility in appointment scheduling may be required because of the unpredictability of the disease. When elective surgical procedures are scheduled for patients with IBD who take sulfasalazine, the dentist should review preoperatively the patient's systemic health and obtain a complete blood count with differential and bleeding times. This preoperative assessment can be important, because in addition to the immunosuppressive effects of IBD medications, sulfasalazine is associated with pulmonary, nephrotic, and hematologic abnormalities (i.e., a variety of anemias, leukopenia, and thrombocytopenia).

Oral Complications and Manifestations

Several oral complications have been associated with IBD. Aphthous–like lesions occur in up to 20% of patients with ulcerative colitis (Figure 11-7). Oral lesions erupt generally during gastrointestinal flareups. The ulcers are mildly painful and may be of the major or minor variety. They typically are located on the alveolar, labial, and buccal mucosa, as well as the soft palate, uvula, and retromolar trigone, and they may be difficult to distinguish from aphthous lesions. Granularity or presence of irregular margins may be helpful in the diagnosis.

Pyostomatitis vegetans also can affect patients with ulcerative colitis and may aid in the diagnosis. To date, fewer than 60 cases have been reported in the literature.[80-82] This form of stomatitis produces raised papillary, vegetative projections or pustules on an erythematous base of the labial mucosa, gingiva, and palate (Figure 11-8). The tongue rarely is involved. Without treatment, the initial erythematous appearance worsens,

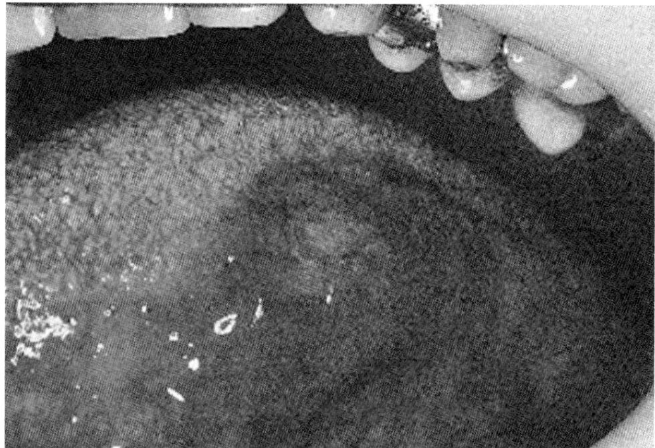

FIGURE 11-7 Oral ulceration associated with ulcerative colitis. *(From Allison MC, et al:* Inflammatory bowel disease, *London, 1998, Mosby.)*

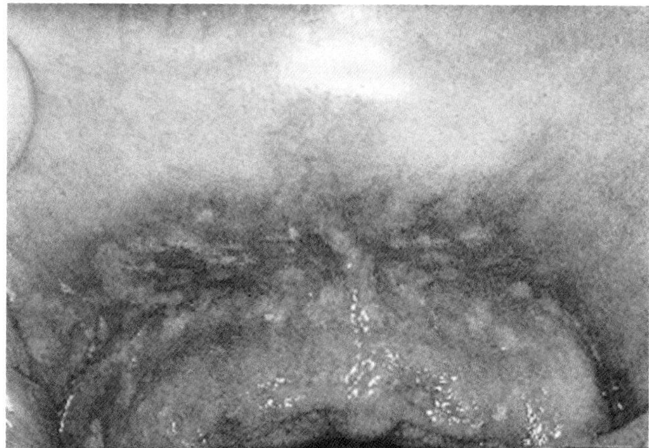

FIGURE 11-8 Pyostomatitis vegetans. Pustular raised lesions of palate in a patient with ulcerative colitis. *(From Allison MC, et al:* Inflammatory bowel disease, *London, 1998, Mosby.)*

with eventual degeneration into an ulcerative and suppurative mass. Treatment of both the aphthous-like lesions and pyostomatitis vegetans requires medical control of the colitis. Oral lesions that persist after anti-inflammatory drug therapy typically respond to repeated topical steroid applications. The vegetative growths can be eradicated by surgical means.

Unique oral manifestations of Crohn's disease occur in approximately 20% of patients and may precede the diagnosis of gastrointestinal disease by several years. Features include atypical mucosal ulcerations and diffuse swelling of the lips and cheeks (orofacial granulomatosis). Oral ulcers appear as linear mucosal ulcers with hyperplastic margins or papulonodular "cobblestone" proliferations of the mucosa, often in the buccal vestibule and on the soft palate. Oral lesions are intermittent, but chronically present. They become symptomatic when intestinal disease is exacerbated.[83] Similar to the oral lesions associated with ulcerative colitis, oral ulcerations of Crohn's disease resolve when the gastrointestinal state is medically controlled. Topical steroids are beneficial during symptomatic phases.

Use of sulfasalazine has been associated with toxic effects on bone marrow, resulting in anemia, agranulocytosis, or thrombocytopenia, which can manifest as a bald tongue, an oral infection, or bleeding, respectively. Corticosteroid use can result in osteopenia, which may involve the alveolar bone. Additional information on the oral management of these abnormalities is found in Appendix C.

PSEUDOMEMBRANOUS COLITIS

DEFINITION

Pseudomembranous colitis is a severe and sometimes fatal form of colitis that results from the overgrowth of *Clostridium difficile* in the large colon. Overgrowth results from the loss of competitive anaerobic gut bacteria, most commonly through the use of broad-spectrum antibiotics, but it also can result from heavy metal intoxication, sepsis, and organ failure. The causative organism, *C. difficile,* produces and releases potent enterotoxins that induce colitis and diarrhea. Rarely, other pathogenic microbes may cause pseudomembranous colitis.[84]

EPIDEMIOLOGY

Incidence and Prevalence

Pseudomembranous colitis is the most common nosocomial infection of the gastrointestinal tract. The incidence is about 50 cases per 100,000 persons in the United States, and it is rising.[84,85] Reported incidence varies with type and frequency of antibiotic exposure. No gender predilection exists; however, the disease is most common in elderly persons, patients in hospitals and nursing homes, those who receive tube feeding, and those with suppressed immune systems.[85,86] Infants and young children rarely are affected.

Etiology

C. difficile, the causative agent in 90% to 99% of pseudomembranous colitis cases, is a gram-positive, spore-forming anaerobic rod that has been found in sand, soil, and feces. Spores may survive on contaminated surfaces for months and are relatively resistant to many disinfectants. *C. difficile* colonizes the gut in 2% to 3% of asymptomatic adults and up to 50% of elderly persons.[87] Risk of disease increases in areas where spores are inhaled (e.g., hospitals, farmyards) and when broad-spectrum antibiotics are in prolonged use. The most frequently offending antimicrobial agents are broad-spectrum agents and those that target anaerobic flora of the colon. Highest risk is associated with clindamycin

(2% to 20% of usage) or ampicillin or amoxicillin (5% to 9% of usage) and third-generation cephalosporins (less than 2% of usage). Macrolides, penicillins, trimethoprim-sulfamethoxazole (Bactrim, Septra), and tetracycline are involved less frequently, and aminoglycosides, antifungal agents, metronidazole, and vancomycin are rarely causative. In general, oral antibiotics are more often causative then parenteral antibiotics.[84,88]

Pathophysiology

As commensal intestinal bacteria are eliminated, *C. difficile* overgrows and produces enzymes that mediate tissue degradation, as well as two toxins, A and B, that bind to intestinal mucosal cells, resulting in cytoskeletal disaggregation and altered vascular permeability, respectively. As cells (enterocytes) die, fluid is lost, and microscopic and macroscopic pseudomembranes form in the distal colon. Mild disease is characterized by antiinflammatory lesions, whereas severe disease manifests with large, coalescent plaques and extensive denuded areas (Figure 11-9). Histopathologic findings include epithelial necrosis, distended goblet cells, leukocyte infiltration of the lamina propria, and pseudomembranous plaques consisting of inflammatory cells, mucin, fibrin, and sloughed mucosal cells.

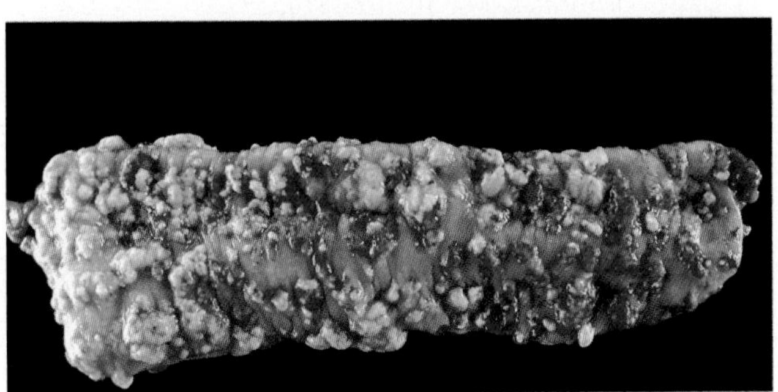

A

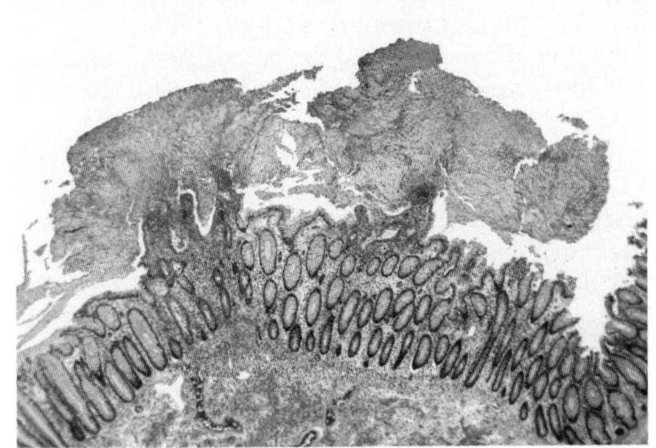

B

FIGURE 11-9 Pseudomembranous colitis from *Clostridium difficile* infection. **A,** Gross photograph showing plaques of yellow fibrin and inflammatory debris adhering to a reddened colonic mucosa. **B,** Low-power micrograph showing superficial erosion of the mucosa and adherent pseudomembrane of fibrin, mucus, and inflammatory debris. *(From Kumar V, et al, editors:* Robbins & Cotran pathologic basis of disease, *ed 8, Philadelphia, 2010, Saunders.)*

CLINICAL PRESENTATION

Signs and Symptoms

Although the course of illness can be variable, diarrhea is the most common presenting manifestation of pseudomembranous colitis. In mild cases, the stool is watery and loose. In severe cases, bloody diarrhea is accompanied by abdominal cramps, tenderness, and fever. Diarrhea often begins within the first 4 to 10 days of antibiotic administration but may develop 1 day to 8 weeks after drug administration. Severe dehydration, metabolic acidosis, hypotension, peritonitis, and toxic megacolon are serious complications of untreated disease.

Laboratory Findings

Pseudomembranous colitis is associated with leukocytosis, leukocyte-laden stools, and a stool sample positive for *C. difficile* or one of its toxins, as determined by tissue culture assay or enzyme immunoassay. Colonic yellow-white pseudomembranes that are 5 to 10 mm in diameter often are visible on colonoscopy or sigmoidoscopy.

MEDICAL MANAGEMENT

First-line treatment of pseudomembranous colitis involves discontinuing use of the inciting antimicrobial agent, along with introducing an antibiotic that will eradicate the toxin-producing *C. difficile.* In patients with mild disease, cessation of the offending antibiotic is all that may be needed. In moderate disease, oral metronidazole (Flagyl) (500 mg three times a day for 10 to 14 days) is recommended. Vancomycin (125 to 500 mg four times a day for 10 to 14 days) or rifaximin is recommended for patients whose disease is unresponsive to metronidazole.[89,90] However, *C. difficile* spores can survive treatment, and relapse occurs in about 20% of patients. Hydration and intravenous fluids are provided to correct electrolyte and fluid imbalances.

DENTAL MANAGEMENT

Medical Considerations

The practitioner should be cognizant that the use of some systemic antibiotics—especially clindamycin, ampicillin, and cephalosporins—is associated with a higher risk of pseudomembranous colitis in elderly, debilitated patients and in those with a previous history of pseudomembranous colitis (see Box 11-2). Risk increases with higher doses, longer duration of administration, and greater number of antimicrobials used. The decision to use an antibiotic and the duration of use should be based on sound clinical judgment that these drugs are indeed necessary and should not be prescribed in a cavalier manner. The dentist also should be aware that pseudomembranous colitis has not been reported after short-term use of clindamycin in the American Heart Association (AHA) prophylactic regimen.

TREATMENT PLANNING MODIFICATIONS

Elective dental care should be delayed until after pseudomembranous colitis has resolved.

Oral Complications and Manifestations

The use of systemic antibiotics for the treatment of patients with pseudomembranous colitis can result in fungal overgrowth (candidiasis) in the oral cavity (see Figure 11-4).

REFERENCES

1. Yuan Y, Padol IT, Hunt RH: Peptic ulcer disease today, *Nat Clin Pract Gastroenterol Hepatol* 3:80-89, 2006.
2. Lam SK: Aetiological factors of peptic ulcer: perspectives of epidemiological observations this century, *J Gastroenterol Hepatol* 9(Suppl 1):S93-S98, 1994.
3. Lam SK: Differences in peptic ulcer between East and West, *Baillieres Best Pract Res Clin Gastroenterol* 14:41-52, 2000.
4. Shaheen NJ, et al: The burden of gastrointestinal and liver diseases, 2006, *Am J Gastroenterol* 101:2128-2138, 2006.
5. Sonnenberg A, Everhart JE: The prevalence of self-reported peptic ulcer in the United States, *Am J Public Health* 86:200-205, 1996.
6. van Kerkhoven LA, et al: Open-access upper gastrointestinal endoscopy a decade after the introduction of proton pump inhibitors and *Helicobacter pylori* eradication: a shift in endoscopic findings, *Digestion* 75:227-231, 2007.
7. Hollander D, Tarnawski A: Is there a role for dietary essential fatty acids in gastroduodenal mucosal protection? *J Clin Gastroenterol* 13(Suppl 1):S72-S74, 1991.
8. Leoci C, et al: Incidence and risk factors of duodenal ulcer. A retrospective cohort study, *J Clin Gastroenterol* 20:104-109, 1995.
9. Derry S, Loke YK: Risk of gastrointestinal haemorrhage with long term use of aspirin: meta-analysis, *BMJ* 321:1183-1187, 2000.
10. McCarthy D: Nonsteroidal anti-inflammatory drug-related gastrointestinal toxicity: definitions and epidemiology, *Am J Med* 105:3S-9S, 1998.
11. Drumm B, et al: Peptic ulcer disease in children: etiology, clinical findings, and clinical course, *Pediatrics* 82(3 Pt 2):410-414, 1988.
12. Sherman PM: Peptic ulcer disease in children. Diagnosis, treatment, and the implication of *Helicobacter pylori*, *Gastroenterol Clin North Am* 23:707-725, 1994.
13. Walsh JH, Peterson WL: The treatment of *Helicobacter pylori* infection in the management of peptic ulcer disease, *N Engl J Med* 333:984-991, 1995.
14. Euler AR, Byrne WJ, Campbell MF: Basal and pentagastrin-stimulated gastric acid secretory rates in normal children and in those with peptic ulcer disease, *J Pediatr* 103:766-768, 1983.
15. Borum ML: Peptic-ulcer disease in the elderly, *Clin Geriatr Med* 15:457-471, 1999.
16. Russel MG, et al: Inflammatory bowel disease: is there any relation between smoking status and disease presentation? European Collaborative IBD Study Group, *Inflamm Bowel Dis* 4:182-186, 1998.
17. Varsky CG, et al: Prevalence and etiology of gastroduodenal ulcer in HIV-positive patients: a comparative study of 497 symptomatic subjects evaluated by endoscopy, *Am J Gastroenterol* 93:935-940, 1998.
18. Graham DY: *Helicobacter pylori* infection in the pathogenesis of duodenal ulcer and gastric cancer: a model, *Gastroenterology* 113:1983-1991, 1997.
19. Marshall BJ, Warren JR: Unidentified curved bacilli in the stomach of patients with gastritis and peptic ulceration, *Lancet* 1:1311-1315, 1984.
20. Nakajima S, et al: Changes in the prevalence of *Helicobacter pylori* infection and gastrointestinal diseases in the past 17 years, *J Gastroenterol Hepatol* 25(Suppl 1):S99-S110, 2010.
21. Tan VP, Wong BC: *Helicobacter pylori* and gastritis: untangling a complex relationship 27 years on, *J Gastroenterol Hepatol* 26(Suppl 1):42-45, 2010.
22. Shames B, et al: Evidence for the occurrence of the same strain of *Campylobacter pylori* in the stomach and dental plaque, *J Clin Microbiol* 27:2849-2850, 1989.
23. Dooley CP, et al: Prevalence of *Helicobacter pylori* infection and histologic gastritis in asymptomatic persons, *N Engl J Med* 321:1562-1566, 1989.
24. Malaty HM, et al: *Helicobacter pylori* in Hispanics: comparison with blacks and whites of similar age and socioeconomic class, *Gastroenterology* 103:813-816, 1992.
25. Levenstein S: Peptic ulcer at the end of the 20th century: biological and psychological risk factors, *Can J Gastroenterol* 13:753-759, 1999.
26. Zullo A, et al: Bleeding peptic ulcer in the elderly: risk factors and prevention strategies, *Drugs Aging* 24:815-828, 2007.
27. Lanza FL, et al: Endoscopic comparison of esophageal and gastroduodenal effects of risedronate and alendronate in postmenopausal women, *Gastroenterology* 119:631-638, 2000.
28. Scott DR, et al: Actions of antiulcer drugs, *Science* 262:1453-1454, 1993.
29. Kikendall JW, Evaul J, Johnson LF: Effect of cigarette smoking on gastrointestinal physiology and non-neoplastic digestive disease, *J Clin Gastroenterol* 6:65-79, 1984.
30. Maity P, et al: Smoking and the pathogenesis of gastroduodenal ulcer—recent mechanistic update, *Mol Cell Biochem* 253:329-338, 2003.
31. Chan FK, Leung WK: Peptic-ulcer disease, *Lancet* 360:933-941, 2002.
32. Huang JQ, Sridhar S, Hunt RH: Role of *Helicobacter pylori* infection and non-steroidal anti-inflammatory drugs in peptic-ulcer disease: a meta-analysis, *Lancet* 359:14-22, 2002.
33. Peterson WL: *Helicobacter pylori* and peptic ulcer disease, *N Engl J Med* 324:1043-1048, 1991.
34. Peterson WL, et al: Acid secretion and serum gastrin in normal subjects and patients with duodenal ulcer: the role of *Helicobacter pylori*, *Am J Gastroenterol* 88:2038-2043, 1993.
35. Laine L, Shah A, Bemanian S: Intragastric pH with oral vs intravenous bolus plus infusion proton-pump inhibitor therapy in patients with bleeding ulcers, *Gastroenterology* 134:1836-1841, 2008.
36. Ahsberg K, et al: Hospitalisation of and mortality from bleeding peptic ulcer in Sweden: a nationwide time-trend analysis, *Aliment Pharmacol Ther* 33:578-584, 2011.
37. Zucca E, et al: Molecular analysis of the progression from *Helicobacter pylori*-associated chronic gastritis to

mucosa-associated lymphoid-tissue lymphoma of the stomach, *N Engl J Med* 338:804-810, 1998.
38. Schistosomes, liver flukes and *Helicobacter pylori*. IARC Working Group on the Evaluation of Carcinogenic Risks to Humans. Lyon, 7-14 June 1994, *IARC Monogr Eval Carcinog Risks Hum* 61:1-241,1994.
39. Klinkenberg-Knol EC, et al: Long-term omeprazole treatment in resistant gastroesophageal reflux disease: efficacy, safety, and influence on gastric mucosa, *Gastroenterology* 118:661-669, 2000.
40. Hansson LE: Risk of stomach cancer in patients with peptic ulcer disease, *World J Surg* 24:315-320, 2000.
41. Malfertheiner P: *Helicobacter pylori*—a timeless source of lessons and research initiatives, *Helicobacter* 12(Suppl 2):85-89, 2007.
42. Ozturk E, et al: A new, practical, low-dose 14C-urea breath test for the diagnosis of *Helicobacter pylori* infection: clinical validation and comparison with the standard method, *Eur J Nucl Med Mol Imaging* 30:1457-1462, 2003.
43. Malfertheiner P, et al: Current concepts in the management of *Helicobacter pylori* infection: the Maastricht III Consensus Report, *Gut* 56:772-781, 2007.
44. Rimbara E, Fischbach LA, Graham DY: Optimal therapy for *Helicobacter pylori* infections, *Nat Rev Gastroenterol Hepatol* 8:79-88, 2011.
45. Forbes GM, et al: Duodenal ulcer treated with *Helicobacter pylori* eradication: seven-year follow-up, *Lancet* 343:258-260, 1994.
46. Korman MG, et al: Influence of cigarette smoking on healing and relapse in duodenal ulcer disease, *Gastroenterology* 85:871-874, 1983.
47. Borody TJ, et al: Smoking does not contribute to duodenal ulcer relapse after *Helicobacter pylori* eradication, *Am J Gastroenterol* 87:1390-1393, 1992.
48. Permin H, Andersen LP: Inflammation, immunity, and vaccines for *Helicobacter* infection, *Helicobacter* 10(Suppl 1):21-25, 2005.
49. Lai KC, et al: Celecoxib compared with lansoprazole and naproxen to prevent gastrointestinal ulcer complications, *Am J Med* 118:1271-1278, 2005.
50. Chan FK, et al: Combination of a cyclo-oxygenase-2 inhibitor and a proton-pump inhibitor for prevention of recurrent ulcer bleeding in patients at very high risk: a double-blind, randomised trial, *Lancet* 369:1621-1626, 2007.
51. Wolfe MM, Lichtenstein DR, Singh G: Gastrointestinal toxicity of nonsteroidal antiinflammatory drugs, *N Engl J Med* 340:1888-1899, 1999.
52. Ehsanullah RS, et al: Prevention of gastroduodenal damage induced by non-steroidal anti-inflammatory drugs: controlled trial of ranitidine, *BMJ* 297:1017-1021, 1988.
53. Nguyen AM, el-Zaatari FA, Graham DY: *Helicobacter pylori* in the oral cavity. A critical review of the literature, *Oral Surg Oral Med Oral Pathol Oral Radiol Endod* 79:705-709, 1995.
54. Gius JA, et al: Vascular formations of the lip and peptic ulcer, *JAMA* 183:725-729, 1963.
55. Loftus EV Jr: Clinical epidemiology of inflammatory bowel disease: incidence, prevalence, and environmental influences, *Gastroenterology* 126:1504-1517, 2004.
56. Jacobsen BA, et al: Increase in incidence and prevalence of inflammatory bowel disease in northern Denmark: a population-based study, 1978-2002, *Eur J Gastroenterol Hepatol* 18:601-606, 2006.
57. Wilson J, et al: High incidence of inflammatory bowel disease in Australia: a prospective population-based Australian incidence study, *Inflamm Bowel Dis* 16:1550-1556, 2010.
58. Benchimol EI, et al: Epidemiology of pediatric inflammatory bowel disease: a systematic review of international trends, *Inflamm Bowel Dis* 17:423-439, 2011.
59. Schirbel A, Fiocchi C: Inflammatory bowel disease: established and evolving considerations on its etiopathogenesis and therapy, *J Dig Dis* 11:266-276, 2010.
60. Rigas A, et al: Breast-feeding and maternal smoking in the etiology of Crohn's disease and ulcerative colitis in childhood, *Ann Epidemiol* 3:387-392, 1993.
61. Gaya DR, et al: New genes in inflammatory bowel disease: lessons for complex diseases? *Lancet* 367:1271-1284, 2006.
62. Lukas M: Inflammatory bowel disease as a risk factor for colorectal cancer, *Dig Dis* 28:619-624, 2010.
63. Ghosh S, Shand A, Ferguson A: Ulcerative colitis, *BMJ* 320:1119-1123, 2000.
64. Batra A, Zeitz M, Siegmund B: Adipokine signaling in inflammatory bowel disease, *Inflamm Bowel Dis* 15:1897-1905, 2009.
65. Rogler G, Andus T: Cytokines in inflammatory bowel disease, *World J Surg* 22:382-389, 1998.
66. Cobrin GM, Abreu MT: Defects in mucosal immunity leading to Crohn's disease, *Immunol Rev* 206:277-295, 2005.
67. Becker JM: Surgical therapy for ulcerative colitis and Crohn's disease, *Gastroenterol Clin North Am* 28:371-390, viii-ix, 1999.
68. Katz JA: Management of inflammatory bowel disease in adults, *J Dig Dis* 8:65-71, 2007.
69. Carter MJ, Lobo AJ, Travis SP: Guidelines for the management of inflammatory bowel disease in adults, *Gut* 53(Suppl 5):V1-V16, 2004.
70. Ali S, Tamboli CP: Advances in epidemiology and diagnosis of inflammatory bowel diseases, *Curr Gastroenterol Rep* 10:576-584, 2008.
71. Chaparro M, et al: Long-term durability of infliximab treatment in Crohn's disease and efficacy of dose "escalation" in patients losing response, *J Clin Gastroenterol* 45:113-118, 2011.
72. Ruggiero C, et al: Omega-3 polyunsaturated fatty acids and immune-mediated diseases: inflammatory bowel disease and rheumatoid arthritis, *Curr Pharm Des* 15:4135-4148, 2009.
73. Kornbluth A, Sachar DB: Ulcerative colitis practice guidelines in adults: American College of Gastroenterology Practice Parameters Committee, *Am J Gastroenterol* 105:501-523, 2010.
74. Ludwig D, Stange EF: Treatment of ulcerative colitis, *Hepatogastroenterology* 47:83-89, 2000.
75. Peppercorn MA: Advances in drug therapy for inflammatory bowel disease, *Ann Intern Med* 112:50-60, 1990.
76. Annaloro C, Onida F, Lambertenghi Deliliers G: Autologous hematopoietic stem cell transplantation in autoimmune diseases, *Expert Rev Hematol* 2:699-715, 2009.
77. Kashyap A, Forman SJ: Autologous bone marrow transplantation for non-Hodgkin's lymphoma resulting in long-term remission of coincidental Crohn's disease, *Br J Haematol* 103:651-652, 1998.
78. Reenaers C, Louis E, Belaiche J: Current directions of biologic therapies in inflammatory bowel disease, *Therap Adv Gastroenterol* 3:99-106, 2010.
79. Colombel JF, et al: Infliximab, azathioprine, or combination therapy for Crohn's disease, *N Engl J Med* 362:1383-1395, 2010.
80. Soriano ML, et al: Pyodermatitis-pyostomatitis vegetans: report of a case and review of the literature, *Oral Surg Oral Med Oral Pathol Oral Radiol Endod* 87:322-326, 1999.
81. Ruiz-Roca JA, Berini-Aytes L, Gay-Escoda C: Pyostomatitis vegetans. Report of two cases and review of the literature, *Oral Surg Oral Med Oral Pathol Oral Radiol Endod* 99:447-454, 2005.
82. Femiano F, et al: Pyostomatitis vegetans: a review of the literature, *Med Oral Patol Oral Cir Bucal* 14:E114-E117, 2009.

83. Lourenco SV, et al: Oral manifestations of inflammatory bowel disease: a review based on the observation of six cases, *J Eur Acad Dermatol Venereol* 24:204-207, 2010.
84. Surawicz CM: Antibiotic-associated diarrhea and pseudomembranous colitis: are they less common with poorly absorbed antimicrobials? *Chemotherapy* 51(Suppl 1):81-89, 2005.
85. McFarland LV: Renewed interest in a difficult disease: *Clostridium difficile* infections—epidemiology and current treatment strategies, *Curr Opin Gastroenterol* 25:24-35, 2009.
86. McDonald LC, Owings M, Jernigan DB: *Clostridium difficile* infection in patients discharged from U.S. short-stay hospitals, 1996-2003, *Emerg Infect Dis* 12:409-415, 2006.
87. Fekety R: Pseudomembranous colitis. In Goldman L, Ausiello D, editors: *Cecil textbook of medicine*, ed 22, Philadelphia, 2004, Saunders.
88. Salkind AR: *Clostridium difficile:* an update for the primary care clinician, *South Med J* 103:896-902, 2010.
89. Cohen SH, et al: Clinical practice guidelines for *Clostridium difficile* infection in adults: 2010 update by the Society for Healthcare Epidemiology of America (SHEA) and the Infectious Diseases Society of America (IDSA), *Infect Control Hosp Epidemiol* 31:431-455, 2010.
90. Garey KW, et al: Rifamycin antibiotics for treatment of *Clostridium difficile*–associated diarrhea, *Ann Pharmacother* 42:827-835, 2008.

PART V

Genitourinary Disease

12

Chronic Kidney Disease and Dialysis

Chronic kidney disease (CKD) and its ultimate result, kidney failure, is a worldwide problem that continues to increase in prevalence.[1] CKD is associated with many serious medical problems; thus, the dentist will need to recognize the clinical status of patients with this condition and must be cognizant of the possible adverse outcomes, as well as the principles of proper management. Progressive kidney disease can result in reduced renal function, with effects on multiple organ systems. Potential manifestations include anemia, abnormal bleeding, electrolyte and fluid imbalance, hypertension, drug intolerance, and skeletal abnormalities that can affect the delivery of dental care. In addition, patients who have severe and progressive disease may require artificial filtration of the blood through dialysis or kidney transplantation (see Chapter 21). This chapter reviews the current knowledge on CKD and presents principles for dental management.

The kidneys have several important functions: They regulate fluid volume and the acid/base balance of plasma; excrete nitrogenous waste; synthesize erythropoietin, 1,25-dihydroxycholecalciferol, and renin; are responsible for drug metabolism; and serve as the target organ for parathormone and aldosterone. Under normal physiologic conditions, 25% of the circulating blood perfuses the kidney each minute. The blood is filtered through a complex series of tubules and glomerular capillaries within the *nephron,* the functional unit of the kidney (Figure 12-1). Ultrafiltrate, the precursor of urine, is produced in nephrons at a rate of about 125 mL/min[2].

DEFINITION

CKD is a progressive loss of renal function that persists for 3 months or longer.[3] It results from direct damage to nephrons or from progressive, chronic bilateral deterioration of nephrons. CKD results in uremia and kidney failure and can lead to death. The National Kidney Foundation defines a five-stage classification system for CKD based on the glomerular filtration rate (GFR)[4,5] (Table 12-1). *Stage 1* is characterized by normal or only slightly increased GFR associated with some degree of kidney damage. This stage usually is asymptomatic, with a slight (10% to 20%) decline in renal function. *Stage 2* is marked by a mildly decreased GFR. *Stage 3* is evidenced as a moderately decreased GFR, with loss of 50% or more of normal renal function. *Stage 4* is defined by a severely decreased GFR. *Stage 5* is reflected by *renal failure,* wherein 75% or more of the approximately 2 million nephrons have lost function. With disease progression (stages 2 through 5), nitrogen products accumulate in the blood, and the kidneys perform fewer excretory, endocrine, and metabolic functions, with eventual loss of the ability to maintain normal homeostasis. The resultant clinical syndrome—caused by renal failure, retention of excretory products, and interference with endocrine and metabolic functions—is called *uremia.* Sequelae involve multiple organ systems, with cardiovascular, hematologic, neuromuscular, endocrine, gastrointestinal, and dermatologic manifestations. The rate of destruction and the severity of disease depend on the underlying causative disorders and contributing factors, with diabetes and hypertension recognized as the primary etiologic diseases.[2,6]

EPIDEMIOLOGY

Incidence and Prevalence

More than 26 million people (an estimated 11% of the adult population) in the United States have some form of kidney disease.[1] The early stages of CKD (stages 1 to 3) tend to be asymptomatic and constitute 96.5% of the disease.[7,8] Each year, more than 100,000 new cases of kidney failure are diagnosed, and more than 526,000 people have end-stage renal disease (ESRD).[7] The prevalence of CKD is increasing by approximately 4% per year, most rapidly in patients over age 65 and in those who have diabetes and hypertension.[6] CKD is diagnosed more commonly in men; African, Native, and Asian Americans; and those between the ages of 45 and 64 years. More than 90% of patients with kidney failure are older than 18 years of age. Approximately 86,000 Americans die annually as a result of kidney failure;

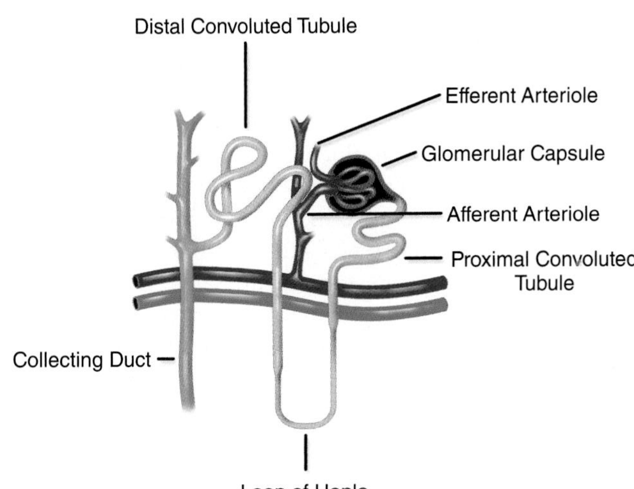

FIGURE 12-1 The nephron. *(Courtesy Matt Hazzard, University of Kentucky.)*

TABLE 12-1 Classification of Stages of Chronic Kidney Disease (CKD) and Associated Comorbid Conditions

CKD Stage	Description	GFR (mL/min/1.73 m^2)	Frequency of Comorbid Conditions
1	Kidney damage with normal or ↑ GFR	≥90	Anemia 4%, HTN 40%, DM 9%
2	Kidney damage with normal or mild ↓ GFR	60-89	Anemia 7%, HTN 40%, DM 13%
3	Moderate ↓ GFR	30-59	Anemia 7%, HTN 55%, DM 20%, HPT >50%
4	Severe ↓ GFR	15-29	Anemia >30%, HTN >75%, DM 30%, HPT >50%
5	Kidney failure—end-stage renal disease (ESRD)	<15 (or dialysis)	Anemia >70%, HTN >75%, DM 40%, HPT >50%

DM, Diabetes mellitus; *GFR,* Glomerular filtration rate; *HPT,* Hyperparathyroidism; *HTN,* Hypertension.
Data from Mitch WE: Chronic kidney disease. In Goldman L, Ausiello D, editors: Cecil medicine, *ed 23, Philadelphia, 2008, Saunders, pp 921-930; Pendse S, Singh AK: Complications of chronic kidney disease: anemia, mineral metabolism, and cardiovascular disease,* Med Clin North Am *89:549-561, 2005; National Kidney Foundation: K/DOQI Clinical practice guidelines for chronic kidney disease: evaluation, classification, and stratification,* Am J Kidney Dis *39:S1-S266, 2002; Whaley-Connell AT, et al: Diabetes mellitus in CKD: Kidney Early Evaluation Program (KEEP) and National Health and Nutrition and Examination Survey (NHANES) 1999-2004,* Am J Kidney Dis *51(4 Suppl 2):S21-S29, 2008.*

cardiovascular system–related disease is the cause of death for most. An average dental practice that treats 2000 adults is likely to include 220 patients with physiologic evidence of chronic kidney disease.[1,3] CKD also has well-known associations with cardiovascular disease, diabetes, and aging. For example, in 14% of persons with hypertension without diabetes, 20% of persons with diabetes, and 25% of persons older than 70 years of age, laboratory findings are consistent with stage 3 or higher CKD.[7,9]

Etiology

ESRD is caused by conditions that destroy nephrons. The four most common known causes of ESRD are diabetes mellitus (37%), hypertension (24%), chronic glomerulonephritis (16%), and polycystic kidney disease (4.5%). Other common causes, in decreasing order, are systemic lupus erythematosus, neoplasm, urologic disease, and acquired immunodeficiency syndrome (AIDS) nephropathy.[2] Hereditary and environmental factors such as amyloidosis, congenital disease, hyperlipidemia, immunoglobulin A nephropathy, and silica exposure also contribute to the disease.

Pathophysiology and Complications

Deterioration and destruction of functioning nephrons are the underlying pathologic processes of renal failure. The nephron includes the glomerulus, tubules, and vasculature. Various diseases affect different segments of the nephron at first, but the entire nephron eventually is affected. For example, hypertension affects the vasculature first, whereas glomerulonephritis affects the glomeruli first. Once lost, nephrons are not replaced. However, because of compensatory hypertrophy of the remaining nephrons, normal renal function is maintained for a time. During this period of relative renal insufficiency, homeostasis is preserved. The patient remains asymptomatic and demonstrates minimal laboratory abnormalities such as a diminished GFR. Normal function is maintained until greater than 50% of nephrons are destroyed. Subsequently, compensatory mechanisms are overwhelmed, and the signs and symptoms of uremia appear. In terms of morphology, the end-stage kidney is markedly reduced in size, scarred, and nodular[2] (Figure 12-2).

A patient in early renal failure may remain asymptomatic, but physiologic changes invariably develop as the disease progresses. Such changes result from the loss of nephrons. Renal tubular malfunction causes the sodium pump to lose its effectiveness, and sodium excretion occurs. Along with sodium, excessive amounts of dilute urine are excreted, which accounts for the polyuria that is commonly encountered.[2]

Patients with advanced renal disease develop uremia, which is uniformly fatal if not treated. Failing kidneys

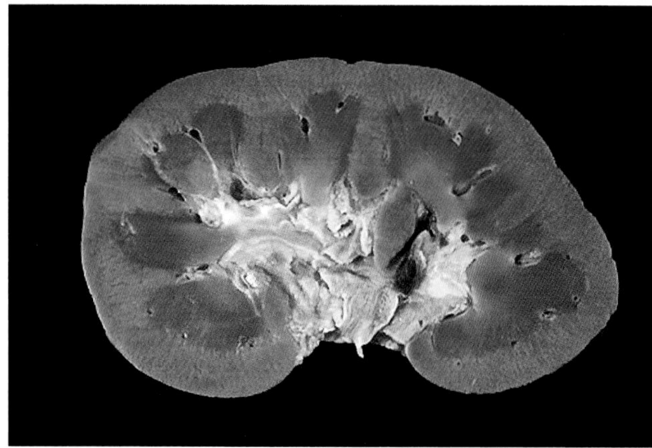

A

B

FIGURE 12-2 Gross renal anatomy. **A,** A normal kidney. **B,** Atrophic kidneys from a patient with chronic glomerulonephritis. *(From Klatt EC: Robbins and Cotran atlas of pathology, ed 2, Philadelphia, 2010, Saunders.)*

are unable to concentrate and filter the intake of sodium, which contributes to the drop in urine output, development of fluid overload, hypertension, and risk for severe electrolyte disturbances (sodium depletion and hyperkalemia—higher-than-normal levels of potassium) and cardiac disease. These cardiovascular system–related events cause approximately half of the deaths occurring annually among patients with ESRD.[2,10]

The buildup of nonprotein nitrogen compounds in the blood, mainly urea, as a consequence of loss of glomerular filtration function, is called *azotemia*. Level of azotemia is measured as blood urea nitrogen (BUN). Acids also accumulate because of tubular impairment. The combination of waste products serves as a substrate for the development of metabolic acidosis, the major result of which is ammonia retention. In the later stages of renal failure, acidosis causes nausea, anorexia, and fatigue. Patients may hyperventilate to compensate for the metabolic acidosis. With acidosis superimposed on ESRD, adaptive mechanisms already are taxed beyond normal levels, and any increase in demand can lead to serious consequences. For example, sepsis or a febrile illness can result in profound acidosis and may be fatal.[2]

Patients with ESRD demonstrate several hematologic abnormalities, including anemia, leukocyte and platelet dysfunction, and coagulopathy. Anemia, caused by decreased erythropoietin production by the kidney, inhibition of red blood cell production and hemolysis, bleeding episodes, and shortened red cell survival, is one of the most familiar manifestations of ESRD. Most of these effects result from unidentified toxic substances in uremic plasma and from other factors.[2] Host defense is compromised by nutritional deficiencies, leukocyte dysfunction, depressed cellular immunity, and hypogammaglobulinemia. This diminished capacity leads to diminished granulocyte chemotaxis, phagocytosis, and bactericidal activity, making affected persons more susceptible to infection.[9]

Hemorrhagic diatheses, characterized by tendency toward abnormal bleeding and bruising, are common in patients with ESRD and are attributed primarily to abnormal platelet aggregation and adhesiveness, decreased platelet factor 3, and impaired prothrombin consumption. Defective platelet production also may play a role. Platelet factor 3 enhances the conversion of prothrombin to thrombin by activated factor X.[9]

The cardiovascular system is affected by athero- and arteriosclerosis and arterial hypertension—the latter due to sodium chloride (NaCl) retention, fluid overload, and inappropriately high renin levels. Congestive heart failure and hypertrophy of the left ventricle, which may compromise coronary artery blood flow, are relatively common developments. These complications, along with electrolyte disturbances, put patients with ESRD at increased risk for sudden death due to myocardial infarction.[11]

A variety of bone disorders are seen in ESRD; these are collectively referred to as *renal osteodystrophy*. Decreased kidney function results in decreased 1,25-dihydroxyvitamin D production, which leads to reduced intestinal absorption of calcium (thereby contributing to hypocalcemia). With advanced CKD, renal phosphate excretion drops, and results in increased levels of serum phosphorus. Excess phosphorus causes serum calcium to be deposited in bone (osteoid), leading to a decreased serum calcium level and weak bones. In response to low serum calcium, the parathyroid glands are stimulated to secrete parathormone (PTH). This results in secondary hyperparathyroidism. PTH has three main functions:

- Inhibiting the tubular reabsorption of phosphorus
- Stimulating renal production of the vitamin D necessary for calcium metabolism
- Enhancing vitamin D absorption within the intestine

High levels of PTH are sustained, however, because in ESRD the failing kidney does not synthesize 1,25-dihydroxycholecalciferol, the active metabolite of vitamin D; thus, calcium absorption in the gut is inhibited. PTH activates tumor necrosis factor and interleukin-1, which mediate bone remodeling, calcium mobilization from bones, and increased excretion of phosphorus, potentially leading to formation of renal and metastatic calcifications. Levels of fibroblast growth factor 23 (FGF-23), a key regulator of phosphorus and vitamin D metabolism, also increase and result in inhibition of osteoblast maturation and matrix mineralization.[12] The progression of osseous changes is as follows: *osteomalacia* (increased unmineralized bone matrix), followed by *osteitis fibrosa* (bone resorption with lytic lesions and marrow fibrosis) (Figure 12-3), and finally, *osteosclerosis* of variable degree (enhanced bone density) (Figure 12-4). With renal osteodystrophy in children, bone growth is impaired, along with a tendency for spontaneous fractures with slow healing, myopathy, aseptic necrosis of the hip, and extraosseous calcifications.

CLINICAL PRESENTATION

Clinical features of renal failure are listed in Box 12-1. Although the type and extent of manifestations vary with severity and the particular patient, they must be recognized in the context of the patient's overall physical status. Also, the effects of renal failure often are widespread and can involve multiple systems (e.g., more than 40% of patients with ESRD also have diabetes, and more than 15% have concurrent hypertension).[2]

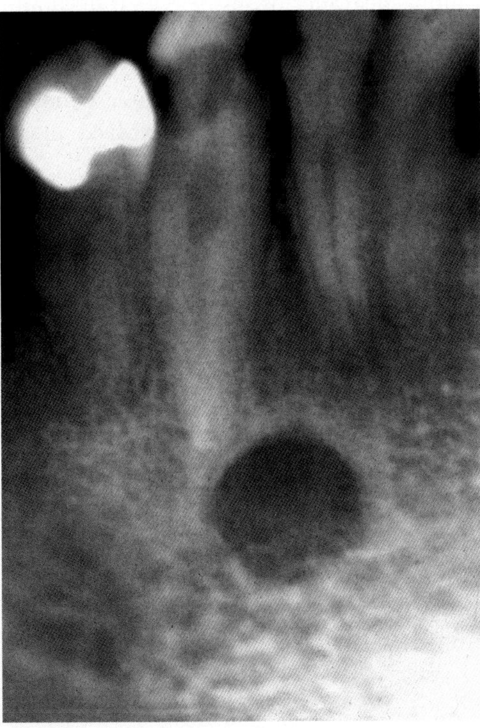

FIGURE 12-3 Lytic lesion in the anterior mandible of a patient with hyperparathyroidism. *(Courtesy L.R. Bean, Lexington, Kentucky.)*

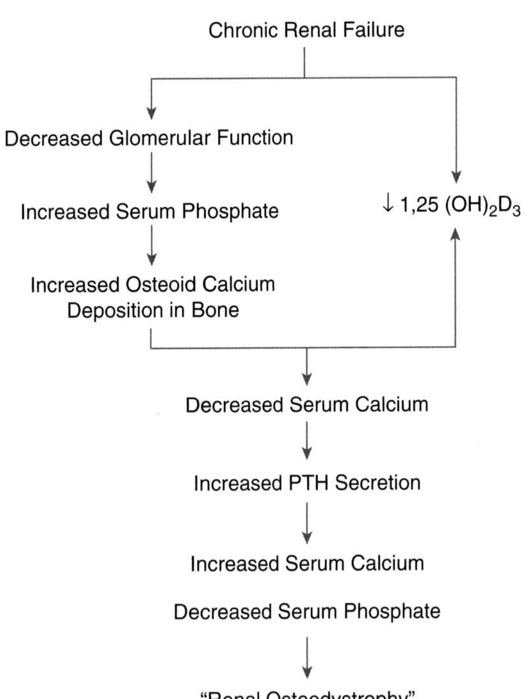

FIGURE 12-4 Summary of changes that result in renal osteodystrophy.

BOX 12-1 Clinical Features of Chronic Renal Failure

Cardiovascular
Hypertension, congestive heart failure
Cardiomyopathy, pericarditis
Accelerated atherosclerosis

Gastrointestinal
Anorexia, nausea and vomiting
Peptic ulcer and gastrointestinal bleeding
Hepatitis, peritonitis

Neuromuscular
Weakness and lassitude, drowsiness
Headaches, disturbance of vision
Sensory disturbances—peripheral neuropathy
Seizures, muscle cramps, coma

Dermatologic
Pruritus, bruising, pallor
Hyperpigmentation, uremic frost

Hematologic
Bleeding, anemia
Lymphopenia and leukopenia
Splenomegaly and hypersplenism

Immunologic
Prone to infections

Metabolic
Thirst, nocturia and polyuria
Insulin resistance, glycosuria, metabolic acidosis
Raised serum blood urea nitrogen, creatinine, lipids, and uric acid
Electrolyte disturbances, secondary hyperparathyroidism

Signs and Symptoms

Patients with CKD may show few clinical signs or symptoms until the condition progresses to stage 3. At this stage and beyond, patients may complain of a general ill feeling, fatigue, headaches, nausea, loss of appetite, and weight loss. With further progression, anemia, leg cramps, insomnia, and nocturia often develop. The anemia produces pallor of the skin and mucous membranes and contributes to the symptoms of lethargy and dizziness. Hyperpigmentation of the skin is characterized by a brownish-yellow appearance caused by the retention of carotene-like pigments normally excreted by the kidney. These pigments also may cause profound pruritus. An occasional finding is a whitish coating on the skin of the trunk and arms produced by residual urea crystals left when perspiration evaporates ("uremic frost").[2]

Patients with renal failure are more likely to experience bone pain and to develop gastrointestinal signs and symptoms such as anorexia, nausea, and vomiting, generalized gastroenteritis, and peptic ulcer disease. Uremic syndrome commonly causes malnutrition and diarrhea. Patients demonstrate mental slowness or depression and become psychotic in later stages. They also may exhibit signs of peripheral neuropathy and muscular hyperactivity (twitching). Convulsions may be a late manifestation that directly correlates with the degree of azotemia. Additional findings may include stomatitis manifested by oral ulceration and candidiasis (Figure 12-5), or parotitis. A urine-like odor to the breath may be detected.[9,13]

Because of the bleeding diatheses that accompany ESRD, hemorrhagic episodes are not uncommon, particularly occult gastrointestinal bleeding. In patients who receive dialysis, however, benefits include improved control of uremia and less severe bleeding. Skin manifestations include ecchymoses, petechiae, purpura, and gingival or mucous membrane bleeding (e.g., epistaxis).

Cardiovascular manifestations of ESRD include hypertension, congestive heart failure (shortness of breath, orthopnea, dyspnea on exertion, peripheral edema), and pericarditis.[2,9]

Laboratory Findings

The diagnosis of kidney disease is based on history, physical evidence, laboratory evaluation, and, in select disorders, imaging and biopsy. GFR, urinalysis, BUN, serum creatinine, creatinine clearance, electrolyte measurements, and protein electrophoresis are used to monitor disease progress. The most basic test of kidney function is urinalysis, with special emphasis on specific gravity and the presence of protein. The principal marker of kidney damage is persistent protein in the urine, whereas GFR is the best measure of overall kidney function.[14]

Figure 12-6 illustrates common laboratory features associated with the stages of CKD. Table 12-2 lists specific laboratory values indicative of renal function and dysfunction. The serum creatinine level is a measure of muscle breakdown and filtration capacity of the nephron. The creatinine concentration is proportional to the glomerular filtration and can be measured in serum as well as urine. The creatinine clearance compares the creatinine concentrations in blood and urine (in a 24-hour urine collection). BUN is a commonly used indicator of kidney function, however, it is not as specific as creatinine clearance or serum creatinine level.[2]

As renal failure develops, the patient often remains asymptomatic until the GFR drops below 20 mL/minute, the creatinine clearance drops below 20 mL/minute, and the BUN is above 20 mg/dL. In fact, uremic syndrome is rare before the BUN concentration exceeds 60 mg/dL. Other tests used to monitor kidney disease include determinations of serum electrolytes involved in acid-base

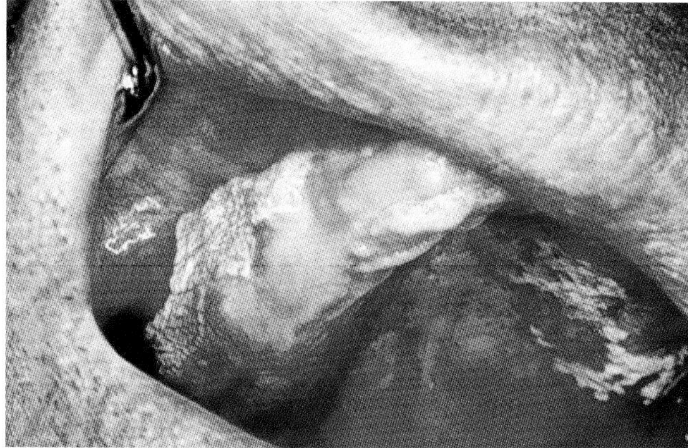

FIGURE 12-5 Oral candidiasis in a patient with end-stage renal disease.

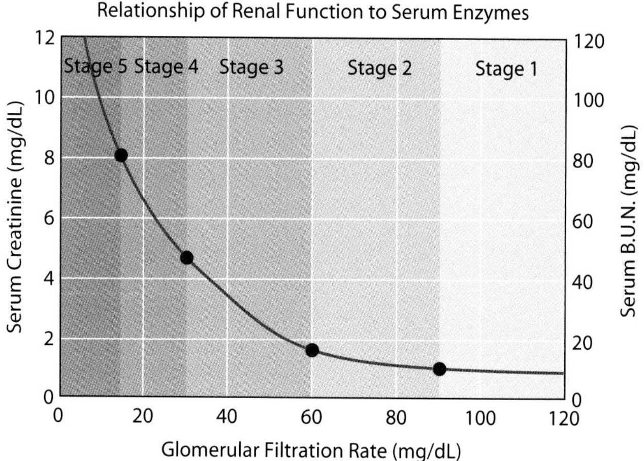

FIGURE 12-6 Relationship of renal function to serum enzymes. *(Courtesy Matt Hazzard, University of Kentucky.)*

TABLE 12-2 Laboratory Values for the Assessment of Renal Function and Failure

Laboratory Test	Reference Value	Indicator of Renal Insufficiency (Stages II-IV)	Indicator of Renal Failure (Stage V)
Urine			
Creatinine clearance	85-125 mL/min (women) 97-140 mL/min[28] (men)	50-90 mL/min	*Moderate:* 10-50 mL/min; *severe:* <10 mL/min
Glomerular filtration rate	100-150 mL/min	15-89 mL/min	*Moderate:* <15 mL/min; *severe:* <10 mL/min
Serum			
Blood urea nitrogen	8-18 mg/dL (3-6.5 mmol/L)	20-30 mg/dL	*Moderate:* 30-50 mg/dL; *severe:* >50 mg/dL
Creatinine	0.6-1.20 mg/dL	2-3 mg/dL	*Moderate:* 3-6 mg/dL; *severe:* >6 mg/dL

Secondary indicators of renal function. *Normal reference values:* calcium, 8.2-11.2 mg/dL; chloride, 95-103 mmol/L; inorganic phosphorus, 2.7-4.5 mg/dL; potassium, 3.8-5 mmol/L; sodium, 136-142 mmol/L; total carbon dioxide for venous blood, 22-26 mmol/L.
Adapted from National Kidney Foundation: K/DOQI clinical practice guidelines for chronic kidney disease: evaluation, classification, and stratification, Am J Kidney Dis *39:S1-S266, 2002; De Rossi SS, Glick M: Dental considerations for the patient with renal disease receiving hemodialysis,* J Am Dent Assoc *127:211-219, 1996; and Zachee P, Vermylen J, Boogaerts MA: Hematologic aspects of end-stage renal failure,* Ann Hematol *69:33-40, 1994.*

regulation and calcium and phosphorus metabolism (see Table 12-2), complete blood count, and bone density measures.[2]

MEDICAL MANAGEMENT

Conservative Care

The National Kidney Foundation published clinical practice guidelines for the management of CKD.[5] The goals of treatment are to retard the progress of disease and to preserve the patient's quality of life. A conservative approach, which may be adequate for prolonged periods, is recommended for stage 1 and stage 2 disease. Conservative care involves decreasing the retention of nitrogenous waste products and controlling hypertension, fluids, and electrolyte imbalances. These improvements are accomplished by dietary modifications including instituting a low-protein diet and limiting fluid, sodium, and potassium intake. Comorbid conditions such as diabetes, hypertension, congestive heart failure, and hyperparathyroidism are corrected or controlled during the earliest stage possible. Anemia, malnutrition, and bone disease (e.g., hyperparathyroidism) typically are managed beginning in stage 3. By stage 4, care by a nephrologist is recommended, and preparations for renal replacement therapy begin. In stage 5, dialysis is started. Renoprotective strategies for slowing progression of CKD and addressing comorbid conditions are summarized in Table 12-3.[8,15]

Dialysis

Dialysis is a medical procedure that artificially filters blood. Dialysis becomes necessary when the number of nephrons diminishes to the point that azotemia is unpreventable or uncontrollable. The initiation of dialysis is an individual patient decision that becomes important when the GFR drops below 30 mL/minute/1.73 m^2. More than 368,000 people receive dialysis in the United States, at a cost of more than $7 billion a year. The procedure can be accomplished by peritoneal dialysis or hemodialysis.[4,15,16]

Peritoneal dialysis is performed on more than 36,000 Americans. It may be provided as continuous cyclic peritoneal dialysis (CCPD) or chronic ambulatory peritoneal dialysis (CAPD). With both modalities, a hypertonic solution is instilled into the peritoneal cavity through a permanent peritoneal catheter. After a time, the solution and dissolved solutes (e.g., urea) are drawn out. The older method, CCPD, also known as automated peritoneal dialysis (APD), uses a machine to perform three to five dialysate exchanges while the patient sleeps (for 8 to 10 hours). During the day, excretory fluids accumulate in the patient's abdomen until dialysis is repeated that evening.[16,17]

CAPD is the more commonly used procedure. Dialysis performed using this method (Figure 12-7) requires shorter exchange periods of 30 to 45 minutes, 4 to 5 times per day. Exchanges are performed manually, with instillation of 1.5 to 3 L of dialysate into the peritoneal cavity. The catheter is sealed, and every 3 to 6 hours the dialysate is allowed to drain into a bag strapped to the patient, and new dialysate is instilled by gravity. CAPD allows the patient more freedom than CCPD. However, both methods allow patients to perform routine functions between exchanges (e.g., walking, working).[15]

The advantages of peritoneal dialysis are its relatively low initial cost, ease of performance, reduced likelihood of infectious disease transmission, and absence of requirement for anticoagulation. Disadvantages include the need for frequent sessions, risk of peritonitis

TABLE 12-3 Renoprotective Strategies for Slowing Progression of Chronic Kidney Disease and Addressing Comorbid Conditions

Parameter	Goal	Intervention
Lifestyle modifications	Smoking cessation, achieving ideal body weight, regularly exercising	Counseling, exercise program, medical appointments every 3-6 months
Lipid lowering	LDL <100 mg/dL	Dietary counseling, statins
Blood pressure control (mm Hg)	<130/80 for proteinuria with excretion less than 1 g protein/day; <125/75 for proteinuria with excretion greater than 1 g/day	ACE inhibitors, ARBs, sodium, restriction, diuretics, beta blockers
Dietary protein and potassium restriction	0.6-0.8 g/kg/day and 40-70 mEq/day, respectively	Dietary counseling
Reduction in proteinuria	<0.5 g/day	ACE inhibitors, ARBs
Glycemic control	$HgbA_{1c}$ <7%	Dietary counseling, oral hypoglycemic agents, insulin
Anemia	Hemoglobin 11-12 g/dL	Recombinant human erythropoietin (epoetin alfa or darbepoetin alfa)
Secondary hyperparathyroidism	PTH: stage 3: 35-70 pg/mL; stage 4: 70-110 pg/mL; stage 5: 150-300 pg/mL	Low-phosphate diet + use of nonaluminum phosphate binders (e.g., calcium carbonate) + vitamin D analogue

ACE, Angiotensin-converting enzyme; *ARBs*, Angiotensin receptor blockers; *$HgbA_{1c}$*, Hemoglobin A_{1c}; *LDL*, Low-density lipoprotein; *PTH*, Parathyroid hormone.
Adapted from Carey WD, editor: Cleveland Clinic: current clinical medicine, *ed 2, St. Louis, 2010, Saunders; and Abboud H, Henrich WL: Clinical practice. Stage IV chronic kidney disease,* N Engl J Med *362:56-65, 2010.*

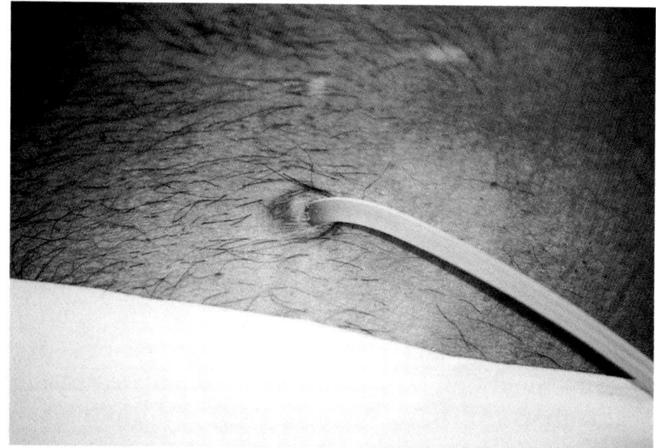

FIGURE 12-7 Chronic ambulatory peritoneal dialysis catheter site in the abdominal wall. *(From Lewis SM, et al, editors:* Medical surgical nursing, *ed 8, St. Louis, 2011, Mosby. Courtesy Mary Jo Holechek, Baltimore, Maryland.)*

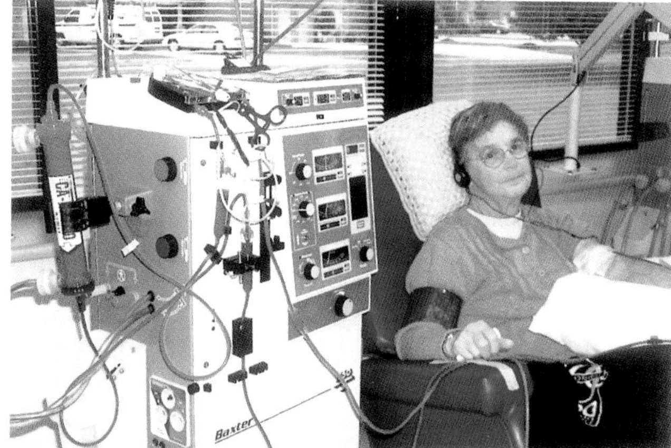

FIGURE 12-8 Patient undergoing hemodialysis. *(From Ignatavicius D, Workman ML:* Medical-surgical nursing: patient-centered collaborative care, *ed 6, St. Louis, 2010, Saunders.)*

(approximately one case per patient every 1.5 years), frequent association with abdominal hernia, and significantly lower effectiveness than that for hemodialysis. Its principal use is in patients in acute renal failure or those who require only occasional dialysis.

Most dialysis patients (80%) in the United States receive hemodialysis. Hemodialysis is the method of choice when azotemia occurs and dialysis is needed on a long-term basis. Treatments are performed every 2 or 3 days, depending on need. Usually 3 to 4 hours is required for each session (Figure 12-8). Hemodialysis consumes an enormous amount of the patient's time and is extremely confining. However, between dialysis sessions, patients lead a relatively normal life.[18]

More than 80% of the people who receive hemodialysis in the United States do so through a permanent and surgically created arteriovenous graft or fistula, usually placed in the forearm. Access is achieved by cannulation of the fistula with a large-gauge needle (Figure 12-9). Approximately 18% of patients receive dialysis through a temporary or permanent central catheter while permanent access site is healing, or when all other access options have been exhausted. Patients are "plugged in" to the hemodialysis machine at the fistula or graft site, and blood is passed through the machine, filtered, and returned to the patient. Heparin usually is administered during the procedure to prevent clotting.[19]

Although hemodialysis is a lifesaving technique, dialysis provides only about 15% of normal renal function,

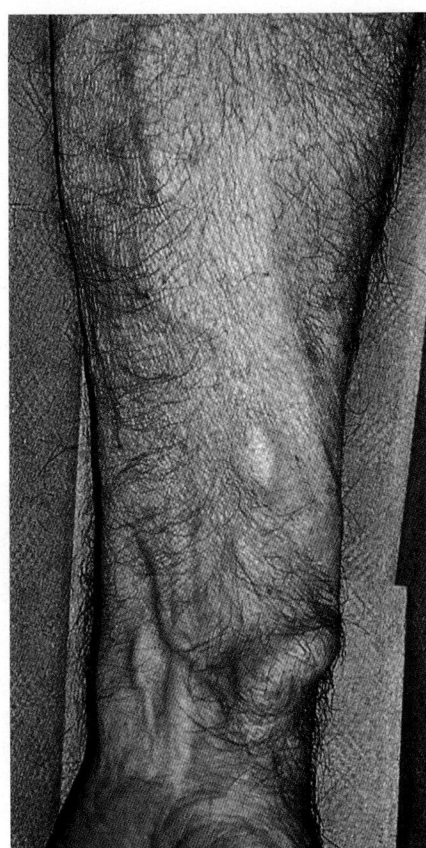

FIGURE 12-9 Site of a surgically created arteriovenous fistula, with subsequent dilation and hypertrophy of the veins. *(From Kumar P, Clark ML: Kumar and Clark's clinical medicine, ed7, Edinburgh, 2009, Saunders.)*

and complications develop as a result of the procedure. Serum calcium concentrations require close regulation that is achieved using calcium supplements, active forms of vitamin D (i.e., calcitriol, alfacalcidol, paricalcitol, or doxercalciferol), or dialysate that contains calcium.[5] Improper blood levels contribute to muscle tetany and oversecretion of parathyroid hormone. Dialysis-related amyloidosis is common in persons on dialysis for more than 5 years as a consequence of deposition of proteins present in the blood on joints and tendons, causing pain and stiffness. Anemia is a common feature of renal failure and dialysis, and is treated with recombinant human erythropoietin. The risk of hepatitis B, hepatitis C, and human immunodeficiency virus (HIV)[20] infections is increased because dialyzers usually are disinfected—not sterilized—between uses, and patients usually have multiple blood exposures. A 2002 national survey reported that among patients maintained on hemodialysis, the prevalence of hepatitis B surface antigen positivity (carriers of hepatitis B) was 1.0%; of hepatitis C seropositive status, 7.8%; and of HIV seropositivity, 1.5%. Although all three viruses constitute a reservoir of potential infection, only hepatitis B virus and hepatitis C virus have been reported to be transmitted nosocomially in dialysis centers in the United States.[17,21]

Infection of the arteriovenous fistula is always a possibility and can result in septicemia, septic emboli, infective endarteritis, and infective endocarditis. *Staphylococcus aureus* is the most common cause of vascular access infection and related bacteremia in these patients. The risk of fistula infection from surgical procedures (e.g., urogenital, oral surgical, dental) is not precisely known but is considered to be low. A related concern is risk for infection and antibiotic-resistant infection. Of note, rates of tuberculosis and vancomycin- and methicillin-resistant infections are higher among patients maintained on long-term hemodialysis than in the general public.[17]

As with all patients with ESRD, drugs that are metabolized primarily by the kidney or that are nephrotoxic must be avoided in patients receiving dialysis.

Another problem associated with dialysis is abnormal bleeding. Patients with ESRD also have bleeding tendencies secondary to altered platelet aggregation and decreased platelet factor 3. Hemodialysis is associated with the additional problem of platelet destruction by mechanical trauma of the procedure. Aluminum contamination of the dialysate water may interfere with heme synthesis, contributing to the development of anemia and osteomalacia.[18] Also, the process of hemodialysis may activate prostaglandin I_2 (prostacyclin), which can reduce platelet aggregation. The 1-year survival rate for patients on dialysis is 79%. The 5-year survival rate has increased to 34%. An alternative to long-term dialysis is renal transplantation (see Chapter 21). This approach has obvious advantages but also is associated with a significant number of problems.

DENTAL MANAGEMENT

Patient Under Conservative Care

Medical Considerations. The National Kidney Foundation's guidelines recommend that high-risk groups (i.e., patients with diabetes and hypertension) be screened for CKD. Thus, medical referrals should be made for screening when diabetes and hypertension are present and when other known risk factors are present (e.g., patients who are obese, smoke, have cardiovascular disease, or have family members with ESRD). With CKD graded below stage 3, problems generally do not arise in the provision of outpatient dental care if the patient's disease is well controlled and conservative medical care is being provided. With CKD of stage 4 or higher, consultation with the patient's physician is suggested before dental care is provided. If the patient is in advanced stages of failure or has another comorbid condition (e.g., diabetes mellitus, hypertension, systemic lupus erythematosus), or if electrolyte imbalance is present, dental care may best be provided after physician consultation in a hospital-like setting. Deferral of treatment may be required until the status of the patient has been ascertained and the CKD is adequately controlled (Box 12-2).

If dental treatment is to be provided on an outpatient basis, blood pressure should be closely monitored before and during the procedure (see Chapter 3). Patients should be informed that good control of blood pressure will benefit both kidney and overall health. Because of the potential for bleeding problems, if an invasive procedure is planned, the patient should undergo pretreatment screening for bleeding disorders, and a platelet count should be obtained (see Chapter 24). Hematocrit level and hemoglobin count also should be obtained for assessment of the status of anemia. Any abnormal values should be discussed with the physician. Few problems are encountered with nonhemorrhagic dental procedures when the hematocrit level is above 25%. If bleeding is anticipated, hematocrit levels can be raised with use of erythropoietin under the guidance of the physician. A less desirable option is red blood cell transfusion, which carries the risks of sensitization and bloodborne infection. If an orofacial infection occurs, aggressive management with the use of culture and sensitivity testing and appropriate antibiotics is necessary.

When surgical procedures are undertaken, meticulous attention to good surgical technique is necessary to decrease the risks of excessive bleeding and infection.

BOX 12-2 Dental Management

Considerations in Patients with End-Stage Renal Disease Under Conservative Care

P

Patient Evaluation/Risk Assessment (see Box 1-1)

- Evaluate and determine whether renal disease exists.
- Obtain medical consultation if patient's disease is poorly controlled, if signs and symptoms point to an undiagnosed condition, or if the diagnosis is uncertain.

Potential Issues/Factors of Concern

A	
Analgesics	Dosage adjustment likely when glomerular filtration rate (GFR) is <60. Avoid long-term use of nonsteroidal antiinflammatory drugs (NSAIDs) in chronic kidney disease (CKD). Avoid narcotics in CKD because these drugs can cause prolonged sedation and respiratory depression.
Antibiotics	Dosage adjustments likely when GFR is <60. Aggressively manage orofacial infections with culture and sensitivity testing and antibiotics. Consider hospitalization for severe infection or major procedures. A loading dose may be required when infection and CKD are concurrent.
Anesthetics (local)	Dosage adjustment generally is not required.
Antianxiety	No dosage adjustment for single-dose benzodiazepines is necessary.
B	
Bleeding	Screen for bleeding disorder before invasive procedures. Pay meticulous attention to good surgical technique. Excessive bleeding may occur in the patient with untreated or poorly controlled CKD. Have topical anticoagulants available for use.
Blood pressure	Monitor blood pressure closely, because hypertension is common in CKD. Refer patient for physician evaluation if pressure is elevated.
C	
Chair position	If patient is on antihypertensive medication, assist person to regain equilibrium in upright position before exiting dental chair.
D	
Devices	No issues.
Drugs (interactions, allergies, or supplementation)	Adjust dosage of drugs metabolized by the kidney when GFR is <60, per Table 12-1. Avoid nephrotoxic drugs (aminoglycosides, acetaminophen in high doses, acyclovir, aspirin, and other NSAIDs).
E	
Emergencies	Minimize risk for emergencies by avoiding invasive procedures and long appointments if disease is unstable (poorly controlled) or advanced (CKD stage 3 or higher).

Receiving Hemodialysis

P

Patient Evaluation/Risk Assessment (see Box 1-1)

- Same as for conservative care recommendations.
- Also determine liver function status and assess for presence of opportunistic infection in these patients because of increased risk for development of carrier state with hepatitis B and C viruses and human immunodeficiency virus.[20]

Potential Issues/Factors of Concern

- Same as for conservative care recommendations, plus the following issues:

A	
Antibiotics	Consider antimicrobial prophylaxis if abscess is present (based on guidelines—see Box 12-4).
D	
Day of appointment	Avoid dental care on day of treatment (especially within first 6 hours afterward); best to treat on day after.
Devices	Avoid blood pressure cuff and intravenous medications in arm with shunt.
Drugs (interactions, allergies, or supplementation)	Consider corticosteroid supplementation if indicated (see Table 15-2).
F	
Follow up	Patients who have had CKD should be contacted to ensure that the postoperative course proceeds without complications.

When invasive procedures are planned for a patient with CKD above stage 3, the dentist should consult with the physician to assess the need for antibiotics. Alterations in drug dosage may be needed, depending on the amount of renal function retained.

Taking large doses of corticosteroids (e.g., 10 mg or more daily of prednisone or equivalent), as often prescribed for medical management of ESRD, may lead to the development of adrenal insufficiency. To avoid an adrenal crisis in patients on such regimens, the dental clinician should ensure that the usual corticosteroid dose is taken before surgical procedures and will need to monitor the patient closely during the postsurgical phase of care (see Chapter 15).[22]

A major concern in the treatment of a patient with ESRD is the potential for toxic effects on the kidney and other adverse effects associated with drug therapy related to dental problems. Some drugs are excreted primarily by the kidney; moreover, certain agents are inherently nephrotoxic. As a general rule, drugs excreted by the kidney are eliminated two-fold less efficiently when the GFR drops to 50 mL/minute and thus may reach toxic levels at lower GFR. In such circumstances, drug dosage needs to be reduced and timing of administration must be prolonged. Nephrotoxic drugs such as acyclovir, aminoglycosides, aspirin and other nonsteroidal antiinflammatory drugs (NSAIDs), and tetracycline require special dosage adjustments. Acetaminophen also is nephrotoxic and may cause renal tubular necrosis at high doses, but it probably is safer than aspirin in these patients because it is metabolized in the liver.[23]

The frequency and dosage of dental drug administration require adjustment during advanced CKD for reasons besides nephrotoxicity and renal metabolism. For example, (1) a low serum albumin value reduces the number of binding sites for circulating drugs, thereby enhancing drug effects; (2) uremia can modify hepatic metabolism of drugs (increasing or decreasing clearance)[24]; (3) antacids can affect acid-base or electrolyte balance, further complicating uremic effects on electrolyte balance; (4) larger initial doses may be required in the presence of substantial edema or ascites, whereas smaller initial doses may be required if dehydration or severe debilitation is present; and (5) aspirin and other NSAIDs potentiate uremic platelet defects, so these antiplatelet agents may need to be avoided if invasive procedures are performed[25] (Table 12-4).

Although nitrous oxide and diazepam are antianxiety agents that require little modification for use in patients with ESRD, the hematocrit or hemoglobin concentration should be measured before intravenous sedation to ensure adequate oxygenation. Drugs that depress the central nervous system (barbiturates, narcotics) are best avoided in the presence of uremia because the blood-brain barrier may not be intact, so that excessive sedation may result. In particular, meperidine should be avoided in patients with CKD because its metabolite can accumulate, leading to seizures. When the hemoglobin concentration is below 10 g/100 mL, general anesthesia is not recommended for patients with ESRD.[26]

The risk of a bleeding diathesis in patients with uremia dictates that local (topical thrombin, microfibrillar collagen, suture) or systemic (desmopressin 0.3 μg/kg in 50 mL saline over 30 minutes, or 3 μg/kg nasally) hemostatic agents be available during dental surgical procedures. Conjugated estrogens are helpful when longer duration of action is required; however, 1 week of therapy usually is needed to guarantee efficacy. High-purity plasma-derived products such as cryoprecipitate (a plasma derivative rich in factor VIII, fibrinogen, and fibronectin) are less frequently used hemostatic alternatives. Platelet transfusions are used infrequently because of the associated risk of immunogenic sensitization.[27]

Oral Complications and Manifestations. Box 12-3 lists some of the common oral manifestations of chronic renal failure.[13] A common sign is pallor of the oral mucosa related to anemia. Red-orange discoloration of the cheeks and mucosa associated with pruritus and deposition of carotene-like pigments appears when renal filtration is decreased. Salivary flow may be diminished, resulting in xerostomia and parotid infections.[28] Candidiasis is more frequent when salivary flow is diminished. Patients frequently complain of an altered or metallic taste, and saliva is altered in composition, has a higher pH, and may have a characteristic ammonia-like odor, which results from a high urea content.[29,30] Poor oral hygiene, gingivitis, and periodontal disease are more common in patients with stage 3 or higher CKD.[28,31]

In severe renal failure, uremic stomatitis may be present. Early changes typically include red, burning mucosa covered with gray exudates and later by frank ulceration. Adherent white patches called *uremic frost* caused by urea crystal deposition are more common on the skin but may be seen on the oral mucosa. These mucosal changes are generally associated with BUN levels greater than 55 mg/dL. Bleeding tendencies are

BOX 12-3 Oral Manifestations of Chronic Kidney Failure

- Pallor of oral mucosa
- Xerostomia
- Pigmentation of oral mucosa
- Parotid infections
- Dysgeusia
- Candidiasis
- Petechiae and ecchymosis of oral mucosa
- Enamel hypoplasia
- Osteodystrophy (radiolucent jaw lesions)
- Uremic stomatitis*

*Noted in severe end-stage renal disease.

Data from Proctor R, et al: Oral and dental aspects of chronic renal failure, J Dent Res *84:199-208, 2005.*

TABLE 12-4 Drug Adjustments in Chronic Renal Disease

Drug	Route of Elimination/ Metabolism	Removed by Dialysis	Dosage Adjustment for Renal Failure*				Supplement Dose After Hemodialysis
				GFR (mL/min)			
			Method	*30-50*	*10-29*	*<10*	
Analgesic							
Aspirin	Liver[15] (kidney)	Yes		100%	100%	Avoid	Yes
Acetaminophen	Liver	*HD:* Yes *PD:* No	I	100%	100%	q8h	No
Ibuprofen (Motrin)	Liver	?	—	100%	100%	100%	No
Propoxyphene† (Darvon)	Liver[5] (kidney)	No	D	100%	100%	Avoid	No
Codeine	Liver	?	D	75%	75%	50%	No
Meperidine‡ (Demerol)	Liver	?	D	75%	75%	50%	No
Anesthetic							
Lidocaine (Xylocaine)	Liver[5] (kidney)	No	—	100%	100%	100%	N/A
Antimicrobial							
Acyclovir (Zovirax)	Kidney	Yes	I, D	100% q8h	100% q12-24h	50% q24h	Yes
Amoxicillin, Penicillin V	Kidney[37]	No	I	q8h	q8-12h	q24h	Yes
Cephalexin (Keflex)	Kidney	Yes	I	q6-8h	q8-12h	q12-24h	Yes
Clindamycin (Cleocin)	Liver	No	D	100%	100%	100%	No
Erythromycin	Liver	No	—	100%	100%	100%	No
Ketoconazole (Nizoral)	Liver	No	—	100%	100%	100%	No
Metronidazole (Flagyl)	Liver[5]	Yes		100%	100%	100%	Yes (HD)
Tetracycline† (Doxycycline)	Kidney[37]	No	I	q8-12h	q12-24h	q24h	No
Benzodiazepine							
Diazepam (Valium),‡ triazolam (Halcion)	Liver	?	D	100%	100%	100%	No
Corticosteroid							
Dexamethasone	Local site and liver		—		No adjustment		No

*100% means no dosage adjustment required.
†Tetracyclines and aminoglycosides are nephrotoxic and should be avoided in CKD. Nafcillin, clindamycin, and ceftriaxone do not need dosage adjustment during CKD. Note: NSAIDs can aggravate sodium retention and edema: full-dose aspirin can aggravate coagulopathy.
‡Active metabolites can accumulate in renal failure; reduce dose if drug will be given longer than a few days.
D, Dosage reduction; *I,* Interval extension between doses; *GFR,* Glomerular filtration rate; *HD, Hemodialysis; PD,* Peritoneal dialysis.
Modified from Aronoff GR, et al: Drug prescribing in renal failure: dosing guidelines for adults and children, *ed 5, Philadelphia, 2007, American College of Physicians.*

evident as petechiae and ecchymoses on the labial and buccal mucosa, soft palate, and margins of the tongue, and as gingival bleeding[29] (Figure 12-10).

Oral mucosa lesions including ulcers, lichen planus or lichenoid-like lesions, hairy tongue, hairy leukoplakia, and pyogenic granulomas have been noted with increased frequency in patients with chronic renal failure.[13] The clinical appearance of these lesions at presentation is similar to such lesions in persons with normal renal function, and treatment is similar albeit drug dosages may require modification based on renal function.

Tooth-specific changes also may be seen. Enamel hypoplasia is evident when ESRD begins at an early age. In the developing dentition, red-brown discoloration

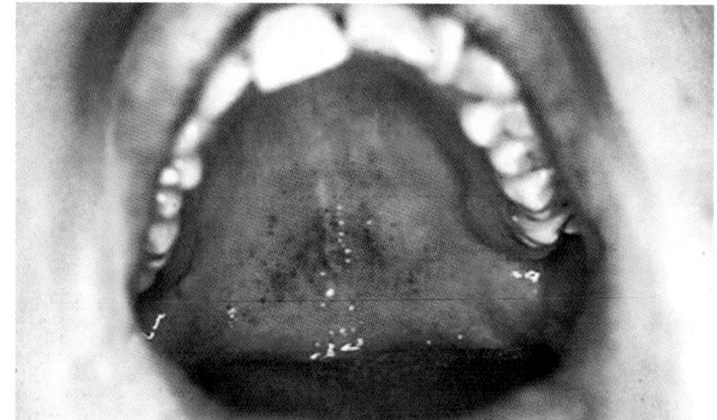

FIGURE 12-10 Palatal petechiae in a patient with end-stage renal disease.

and a slight delay in eruption have been reported. Tooth erosion from persistent vomiting may be seen. Also, pulp narrowing or obliteration has been documented.[32] Caries, however, is not a feature because salivary urea inhibits the metabolic end products of bacterial plaque and increases the buffering capacity of saliva, thus preventing a drop in pH sufficient to attain cariogenic levels.[13]

Specific osseous changes of the jaws accompany chronic renal failure. The most classically described osseous change is the triad of loss of lamina dura, demineralized bone (resulting in a "ground glass" appearance), and localized radiolucent jaw lesions (central giant cell granulomas, also called brown tumors), the latter from secondary hyperparathyroidism. Other osseous findings include widened trabeculations, loss of cortication, calcified extraction sites (so-called socket sclerosis), and metastatic calcifications within the skull.[13]

Patients with CKD who take calcium channel blocker hypotensive medication as well as renal transplant recipients who are taking cyclosporine may exhibit gingival enlargement. The clinical presentation is similar to that caused by phenytoin (Dilantin).

Treatment Planning Modifications. Persons with CKD often exhibit evidence of poor oral hygiene, low salivary flow, and unmet dental needs. In these patients, the goal of restoring dental health must address these factors while balancing their medical needs. Oral hygiene instruction and frequent periodic recall appointments are important for the maintenance of long-term oral health. Meticulous oral hygiene, frequent professional prophylaxis, and antiplaque measures (chlorhexidine or triclosan rinses) also will help to reduce the effects of drug-induced gingival enlargement in transplant recipients taking cyclosporine. Once an acceptable level of oral hygiene has been established, no contraindication exists to routine dental care, provided that proper attention is paid to the systemic health of the patient.

Patient Receiving Dialysis

Medical Considerations. Peritoneal dialysis presents no additional problems in dental management. However, this is not the case with patients who are receiving hemodialysis (see Box 12-2). The arteriovenous fistula surgically created for the dialysis procedure in these patients is susceptible to infection (endarteritis) and may become a source of bacteremia, resulting in infective endocarditis. Infective endocarditis has been associated with hemodialysis even in the absence of preexisting cardiac defects.[33,34] Although the risk factors for infective endocarditis in this setting have not been fully established, altered host defenses, altered cardiac output and mechanical stresses, and bacterial seeding and growth on the shunt are recognized as important.

Infective endocarditis occurs in 2% to 9% of patients receiving hemodialysis. This rate is significantly higher than that reported in persons with rheumatic heart disease. Most such infections are secondary to spread of staphylococcal infections that develop at the site of the graft, fistula, or catheter. Approximately 10% to 17% of cases are caused by organisms that can arise from the oral cavity (*Streptococcus viridans,* lactobacillus).[34] The following devices are considered to place the patient at increased risk for bacterial seeding over that associated with primary arteriovenous fistulas: dual-lumen cuffed venous catheters and polytetrafluoroethylene grafts, newly placed grafts, and long-term catheters. On the basis of an apparently low risk,[33] the American Heart Association (AHA) 2003 guidelines[35] do not include a recommendation for prophylactic antibiotics before invasive dental procedures are performed on patients with intravascular access devices to prevent endarteritis or infective endocarditis, except if an abscess is being incised and drained (Box 12-4). This position also is supported by systematic reviews of the literature.[36-38]

The clinician should be aware of other cardiovascular considerations in patients undergoing hemodialysis. For example, the arm that contains the arteriovenous shunt should be protected from application of the blood pressure cuff, blood drawing, and the introduction of intravenous medications. An inflated blood pressure cuff or tourniquet may potentially collapse the shunt, rendering it useless. Likewise, the complication of phlebitis from intravenous medications can produce a clot that may jeopardize the shunt.

Comorbid conditions such as cardiovascular disease and diabetes are common in patients receiving dialysis. Moreover, approximately 40% of patients on dialysis have congestive heart failure, and 39% of them die of cardiovascular complications each year.[39] These patients often take several medications to control hypertension, diabetes, congestive heart failure, or hypercoagulability (i.e., anticoagulation). Dental care must be provided only when the patient is medically stable, and treatment

BOX 12-4 Antibiotic Prophylaxis Recommendations for Use with Existing Nonvalvular Cardiovascular Devices

- Antibiotic prophylaxis is *not* routinely recommended after device placement for patients who undergo dental, respiratory, gastrointestinal, or genitourinary procedures.
- Antibiotic prophylaxis *is* recommended for patients with these devices if they undergo incision and drainage of infection at other sites (e.g., abscess) or replacement of an infected device.
- Antibiotic prophylaxis *is* recommended for patients with residual leak after device placement for attempted closure of the leak associated with patent ductus arteriosus, atrial septal defect, or ventricular septal defect.

Adapted from Baddour LM, et al: Nonvalvular cardiovascular device-related infections, Circulation *108:2015-2031, 2003.*

should be planned with an understanding of the required medications and the appropriate dental precautionary measures (see Chapters 3, 4, 6, and 24).[26]

Hemodialysis tends to aggravate bleeding tendencies through physical destruction of platelets and the associated use of heparin. Therefore, determination of the status of hemostasis is important before oral surgery is performed. Screening tests, such as the activated partial thromboplastin time (aPTT) and platelet count, should be ordered. Patients at higher risk are those with elevated values on these laboratory tests and a history of gastrointestinal bleeding (see Chapter 24). Although increased risk for bleeding is anticipated in these patients, several management modifications can be used to reduce the chance of serious bleeding:

- Providing dental treatment at the optimum time, usually on the day after hemodialysis, because on the day of dialysis, patients typically are fatigued and may have a tendency to bleed. The activity of heparin lasts for 3 to 6 hours after infusion, and delay of treatment is prudent until that medication is eliminated from the bloodstream.
- Obtaining primary closure and, as needed, using pressure and hemostatic agents. Such agents include thrombin, oxidized cellulose, chitosan, desmopressin, and tranexamic acid (see Chapter 24).
- Performing major surgical procedures on the day after the end of the week of hemodialysis treatment to provide additional time for clot retention before dialysis is resumed. For example, for a patient on a Monday-Wednesday-Friday weekly hemodialysis regimen, surgery performed on Saturday allows an additional day for clot stabilization before hemodialysis is resumed on Monday of the following week.
- Contacting the nephrologist, as indicated, to request that the heparin dose be reduced or eliminated during the first hemodialysis session after the surgical procedure. Of note, hemodialysis can be performed without heparin when hemostasis and clot retention are especially critical.
- Administering protamine sulfate (usually by a physician) if immediate care is necessary. This agent will block the anticoagulant effects of heparin.

Patients who are dependent on long-term dialysis, especially those with diabetes, are prone to infection. In addition, rates of tuberculosis and vancomycin- and methicillin-resistant infections are higher among such patients than in the general public. Thus, efforts should be directed at identifying orofacial manifestations of these infections and eliminating oral sources of infection. Patients with active tuberculosis should not receive dialysis until the disease is rendered inactive (see Chapter 7). Selection of antibiotics for hemodialysis patients with oral infections should be prudent and based on appropriate criteria.

Patients who undergo hemodialysis also can benefit from periodic testing for hepatitis viruses and HIV, because vaccination or antiviral agents can be administered to reduce the risk of complications with these diseases. The dentist should be aware that a negative test result in the past is not predictive of their current status. Patients may have acquired the disease since they were last tested, or they may be carriers of other infectious viruses (e.g., Epstein-Barr virus, cytomegalovirus) that can cause hepatic injury (see Chapter 10) or immune deficiency. Accordingly, the use of standard infection control procedures is warranted for dental procedures performed in all patients.

Patients who are carriers of hepatitis viruses from infection during hemodialysis may have altered hepatic function. Liver function should be assessed before hemorrhagic procedures are performed (see Chapter 10).

The dentist should be aware that hemodialysis removes some drugs from the circulating blood; this may shorten the duration of effect of prescribed medications. The chance that a given drug will be dialyzed is governed by four factors: (1) molecular weight and size, (2) degree of protein binding,[24] (3) volume of drug distribution, and (4) endogenous drug clearance. For example, larger-molecule (more than 500 daltons) drugs are poorly dialyzed. Drugs removed during hemodialysis are those with low capacity for binding to plasma proteins. However, uremia may greatly alter the normal degree of protein binding. A drug such as phenytoin that normally is highly protein-bound exhibits lower plasma protein binding during uremia and is available to a greater extent for dialysis removal. Drugs with high lipid affinity exhibit high tissue binding and are not available for dialysis removal. Finally, efficient liver clearing of a drug greatly reduces the effect of dialysis treatment. Dosage amounts and intervals should be adjusted in accordance with advice from the patient's physician (see Table 12-4).

Oral Complications and Manifestations. Hemodialysis reverses many of the severe oral pathologic changes associated with ESRD. However, uremic odor, dry mouth, taste change, and tongue and mucosal pain are signs and symptoms that persist in many of these patients. Petechiae, ecchymoses, higher plaque and calculus indices, and lower levels of salivary secretion are more common among patients undergoing hemodialysis than among healthy patients. Secondary hyperparathyroidism along with the associated osseous changes in the jaws has been reported in up to 92% of patients receiving hemodialysis.[13]

Patient with Renal Transplant

Patients who have a transplanted kidney may have special management needs, including the need for corticosteroids or antibiotic prophylaxis and the need for management of oral infection and gingival overgrowth caused by cyclosporine therapy (see Chapter 21).

REFERENCES

1. Collins AJ, et al: Excerpts from the U.S. Renal Data System 2009 annual data report, *Am J Kidney Dis* 55(1 Suppl 1):S1-S420, A6-A7, 2009.
2. Mitch WE: Chronic kidney disease. In Goldman L, Ausiello D, editors: *Cecil medicine*, ed 23, Philadelphia, 2008, Saunders, pp 921-930.
3. Levey AS, et al: National Kidney Foundation practice guidelines for chronic kidney disease: evaluation, classification, and stratification, *Ann Intern Med* 139:137-147, 2003.
4. National Kidney Foundation: K/DOQI Clinical practice guidelines for chronic kidney disease: evaluation, classification, and stratification, *Am J Kidney Dis* 39:S1-S266, 2002.
5. National Kidney Foundation: K/DOQI clinical practice guidelines for bone metabolism and disease in chronic kidney disease, *Am J Kidney Dis* 42(4 Suppl 3):S1-S201, 2003.
6. Incidence of end-stage renal disease attributed to diabetes among persons with diagnosed diabetes—United States and Puerto Rico, 1996-2007, *MMWR Morb Mortal Wkly Rep* 59:1361-1366, 2010.
7. United States Renal Data System: *USRDS 2010 annual data report. In Atlas of chronic kidney disease and end-stage renal disease in the United States*, Bethesda, MD, 2010, National Institutes of Health, National Institute of Diabetes and Digestive and Kidney Diseases.
8. Carey WD, editor: *Cleveland Clinic: current clinical medicine*, ed 2, St. Louis, 2010, Saunders.
9. Bargman JM, Skorecki K: Chronic kidney disease. In Fauci AS, et al, editors: *Harrison's principles of internal medicine*, ed 17, New York, 2008, McGraw-Hill, pp 1761-1771.
10. Pun PH, et al: Chronic kidney disease is associated with increased risk of sudden cardiac death among patients with coronary artery disease, *Kidney Int* 76:652-658, 2009.
11. Pendse S, Singh AK: Complications of chronic kidney disease: anemia, mineral metabolism, and cardiovascular disease, *Med Clin North Am* 89:549-561, 2005.
12. Wesseling-Perry K: FGF-23 in bone biology, *Pediatr Nephrol* 25:603-608, 2010.
13. Proctor R, et al: Oral and dental aspects of chronic renal failure, *J Dent Res* 84:199-208, 2005.
14. Keane WF, Eknoyan G: Proteinuria, albuminuria, risk, assessment, detection, elimination (PARADE): a position paper of the National Kidney Foundation, *Am J Kidney Dis* 33:1004-1010, 1999.
15. National Kidney & Urologic Diseases Information Clearinghouse (NKUDIC): *Treatment methods for kidney failure: peritoneal dialysis, NIH Publication No. 06-4688*, Bethesda, MD, 2010, National Institute of Diabetes and Digestive and Kidney Diseases (NIDDK).
16. Uribarri J: Past, present and future of end-stage renal disease therapy in the United States, *Mt Sinai J Med* 66:14-19, 1999.
17. Finelli L, et al: National surveillance of dialysis-associated diseases in the United States, 2002, *Semin Dial* 18:52-61, 2005.
18. Tokoff-Rubin N: Treatment of irreversible renal failure. In Goldman L, Ausiello D, editors: *Cecil medicine*, ed 23, Philadelphia, 2008, Saunders, pp 936-947.
19. Liu KD, Chertow GM: Dialysis in the treatment of renal failure. In Fauci AS, et al, editors: *Harrison's principles of internal medicine*, ed 17, New York, 2008, McGraw-Hill, pp 1772-1776.
20. Russel MG, et al: Inflammatory bowel disease: is there any relation between smoking status and disease presentation? European Collaborative IBD Study Group, *Inflamm Bowel Dis* 4:182-186, 1998.
21. Tokars JI, et al: National surveillance of dialysis-associated diseases in the United States, 1997, *Semin Dial* 13:75-85, 2000.
22. Marik PE, Varon J: Requirement of perioperative stress doses of corticosteroids: a systematic review of the literature, *Arch Surg* 143:1222-1226, 2008.
23. Aronoff GR, et al: *Drug prescribing in renal failure*, Philadelphia, 2007, American College of Physicians.
24. Plantinga LC, et al: Prevalence of chronic kidney disease in U.S. adults with undiagnosed diabetes or prediabetes, *Clin J Am Soc Nephrol* 5:673-682, 2010.
25. Gabardi S, Abramson S: Drug dosing in chronic kidney disease, *Med Clin North Am* 89:649-687, 2005.
26. De Rossi SS, Glick M: Dental considerations for the patient with renal disease receiving hemodialysis, *J Am Dent Assoc* 127:211-219, 1996.
27. Lockhart PB, et al: Dental management considerations for the patient with an acquired coagulopathy. Part 1: Coagulopathies from systemic disease, *Br Dent J* 195:439-445, 2003.
28. Gavalda C, et al: Renal hemodialysis patients: oral, salivary, dental and periodontal findings in 105 adult cases, *Oral Dis* 5:299-302, 1999.
29. Kho HS, et al: Oral manifestations and salivary flow rate, pH, and buffer capacity in patients with end-stage renal disease undergoing hemodialysis, *Oral Surg Oral Med Oral Pathol Oral Radiol Endod* 88:316-319, 1999.
30. Tomas I, et al: Changes in salivary composition in patients with renal failure, *Arch Oral Biol* 53:528-532, 2008.
31. Kshirsagar AV, et al: Periodontal disease is associated with renal insufficiency in the Atherosclerosis Risk In Communities (ARIC) study, *Am J Kidney Dis* 45:650-657, 2005.
32. Davidovich E, et al: Pathophysiology, therapy, and oral implications of renal failure in children and adolescents: an update, *Pediatr Dent* 27:98-106, 2005.
33. Goodman JS, et al: Bacterial endocarditis as a possible complication of chronic hemodialysis, *N Engl J Med* 280:876-877, 1969.
34. Robinson DL, et al: Bacterial endocarditis in hemodialysis patients, *Am J Kidney Dis* 30:521-524, 1997.
35. Baddour LM, et al: Nonvalvular cardiovascular device-related infections, *Circulation* 108:2015-2031, 2003.
36. Lockhart PB, et al; The evidence base for the efficacy of antibiotic prophylaxis in dental practice, *J Am Dent Assoc* 138:458-474, 2007.
37. Oliver R, et al: Antibiotics for the prophylaxis of bacterial endocarditis in dentistry, *Cochrane Database Syst Rev* 4:CD003813, 2008.
38. Termine N, et al: Antibiotic prophylaxis in dentistry and oral surgery: use and misuse, *Int Dent J* 59:263-270, 2009.
39. de Jager DJ, et al: Cardiovascular and noncardiovascular mortality among patients starting dialysis, *JAMA* 302:1782-1789, 2009.

CHAPTER

13

Sexually Transmitted Diseases

Sexually transmitted diseases (STDs) continue to be a major health problem worldwide and, in many instances, are on the increase. In the United States, some of the highest rates of infection occur in adolescents and young adults. More than 25 STDs have been identified and are listed in Table 13-1. Current estimates predict that more than 65 million Americans are infected with one or more STDs, and 19 million new infections occur annually.[1] The morbidity and mortality associated with STDs vary, with clinical consequences ranging from minor inconvenience or irritation to severe disability and death. The diagnosis of an STD also has psychosocial effects.

STDs have important implications for clinical practice in dentistry:

- STDs are transmitted by intimate interpersonal contact, which can result in oral manifestations. Dental health professionals need to be cognizant of these manifestations as a basis for referral of patients for proper medical treatment.
- Some STDs can be transmitted by direct contact with lesions, blood, or saliva, and because many affected persons may be asymptomatic, the dentist should approach all patients as though disease transmission were possible and must adhere to standard precautions.
- A single STD is accompanied by additional STDs in about 10% of cases, and STD-associated genital ulceration increases the risk for human immunodeficiency virus (HIV) infection.[1-3]
- Pathogens responsible for STDs can exhibit antimicrobial resistance, thus proper treatment is essential.[1,4]
- Some STDs are incurable, but all are preventable.
- Patient interaction with dental health care workers can be an important component of STD control by providing opportunities for diagnosis, education, and information regarding access to treatment.

Although most STDs have the potential for oral infection and transmission, discussion in this chapter is limited to gonorrhea, syphilis, and select human herpesvirus and human papillomavirus infections, because these entities are of special interest or importance in the provision of dental care and serve to illustrate basic principles. Chapters 10 and 18 present information about hepatitis B and HIV infections.

GONORRHEA

DEFINITION

Gonorrhea is an STD of worldwide distribution that is caused by *Neisseria gonorrhoeae*. It produces symptoms in men that usually cause them to seek treatment soon enough to prevent serious sequelae, but maybe not soon enough to prevent transmission to others. Infections in women often do not produce recognizable symptoms until complications have emerged. Because gonococcal infections among women frequently are asymptomatic, an important component of gonorrhea control in the United States continues to be the screening of women who are at high risk for STDs. Of note, patients infected with *N. gonorrhoeae* often are coinfected with *Chlamydia trachomatis*.

EPIDEMIOLOGY

Incidence and Prevalence

Gonorrhea is the second most commonly reported infectious disease and STD in the United States, behind chlamydial infection. An estimated 700,000 new cases are reported each year in the United States, and about half of these are reported to the Centers for Disease Control and Prevention (CDC).[1,5] The reported incidence of gonorrhea in 2009 (i.e., 111 cases per 100,000 persons) was the lowest ever reported in the United States and was significantly lower than the incidence in the mid-1970s, when more than 1 million cases were reported.[5,6]

Humans are the only natural hosts for this disease, and its occurrence is worldwide. Gonorrhea is transmitted almost exclusively by sexual contact, whether genital–genital, oral–genital, or rectal–genital. The primary sites of infection are the genitalia, the anal canal, and the pharynx.

Gonorrhea can occur at any age, although it is seen most commonly in sexually active teenagers and young

TABLE 13-1 Sexually Transmitted Diseases

Disease	Pathogen
Acquired immunodeficiency syndrome (AIDS)	Human immunodeficiency virus (HIV)[55]
Amebiasis	*Entamoeba histolytica*
Bacterial vaginosis	*Bacteroides* spp., *Mobiluncus* spp.
Chancroid	*Haemophilus ducreyi*
Condyloma acuminatum (genital warts)	Human papillomavirus (HPV-6, HPV-11)
Cytomegalovirus infection	Cytomegalovirus
Enterobiasis	*Enterobius vermicularis*
Epididymitis, mucopurulent cervicitis, lymphogranuloma venereum, nongonococcal urethritis, pelvic inflammatory disease, Reiter's syndrome	*Chlamydia trachomatis*
Epididymitis, gonorrhea, mucopurulent cervicitis, pelvic inflammatory disease	*Neisseria gonorrhoeae*
Genital herpes	Herpes simplex viruses (HSV-1, HSV-2)
Giardiasis	*Giardia lamblia*
Granuloma inguinale (donovanosis)	*Calymmatobacterium granulomatis*
Hepatitis B	Hepatitis B virus (HBV)
Molluscum contagiosum	Poxvirus
Nongonococcal urethritis, nonspecific vaginitis	*Trichomonas vaginalis*
Nongonococcal urethritis	*Ureaplasma urealyticum*
Pediculosis	*Pediculus pubis*
Salmonellosis	*Salmonella* spp.
Shigellosis	*Shigella* spp.
Streptococcal infection	Group B streptococci
Syphilis	*Treponema pallidum*
Vulvovaginal candidiasis	*Candida* spp., *Torulopsis* spp.

adults (8.5 per 1000 in the 15- to 29-year-old age group) and in the South. Rates of infection are similar in men and women, but differ by racial background. African Americans and Hispanics have 20.5 times higher rates of gonorrhea than whites.[5] Risk factors other than age include young age at first sexual experience, multiple sexual partners, low level of education, low socioeconomic status, and living in an urban setting.[1,5] At the current rate of infection, an average dental practice of 2000 adult patients can expect to provide care for 2 patients with gonorrhea.

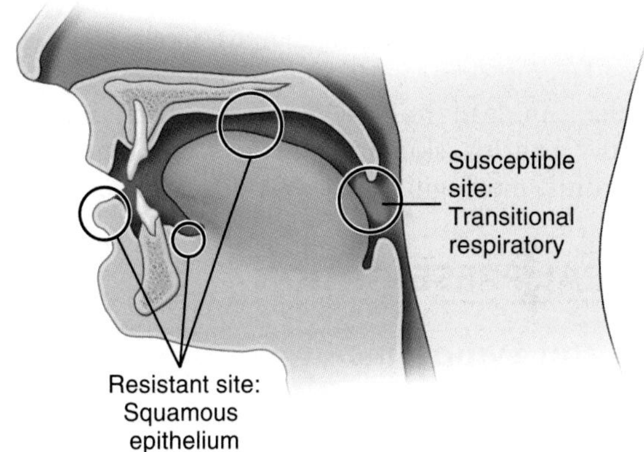

FIGURE 13-1 Areas of relative epithelial susceptibility to infection by *Neisseria gonorrhoeae* within the oral cavity.

Etiology

Gonorrhea is caused by *N. gonorrhoeae,* a gram-negative intracellular diplococcus. *N. gonorrhoeae* is an aerobic microbe that replicates easily in warm, moist areas and preferentially requires high humidity and specific temperature and pH for optimum growth. It is a fragile bacterium that is readily killed by drying, so it is not easily transmitted by fomites. It develops resistance to antibiotics rather easily, and many strains have become resistant to penicillin, tetracycline, and quinolones.

PATHOPHYSIOLOGY AND COMPLICATIONS

N. gonorrhoeae infects columnar epithelium (as found in the mucosal lining of the urethra and cervix) and transitional epithelium (as in the oropharynx and rectum), whereas stratified squamous epithelium (skin and mucosal lining of the oral cavity) generally is resistant to infection.[7] This anatomic susceptibility explains the occurrence of rectal, pharyngeal, and tonsillar infections and the relative infrequency of oral infection, and the fact that there are no reported cases of gonorrhea occurring in the skin of the fingers. Figure 13-1 depicts the areas of relative epithelial susceptibility to *N. gonorrhoeae* infection in the oral cavity and oropharynx.

Infection in men usually begins in the anterior urethra. The bacteria invade epithelial tissues and are engulfed within polymorphonuclear leukocytes, leading to cytokine production and purulent discharge.[7] The infection may remain localized or may extend to the posterior urethra, bladder, epididymis, prostate, or seminal vesicles. It spreads by means of lymphatics and blood vessels. Gonococcemia, although infrequent (occurring in 1% to 2% of cases), may occur and results in dissemination of the disease to distant body sites. Epididymitis is another complication of infection that can lead to infertility.

Infection in women occurs most commonly in the cervix and the urethra. Invasion of cervical epithelium can be associated with the production of a purulent exudate but more often leads to an ascending infection of the endometrium, fallopian tubes, ovaries, and pelvic peritoneum. The ascending infection is a common cause of pelvic inflammatory disease (PID), which affects about 1 million women each year in the United States.[1] PID can be symptomatic or asymptomatic and may contribute to tubal scarring and infertility or ectopic pregnancy. Disseminated gonorrhea also can occur, with varying frequency. Vertical transmission accounts for a small percentage of cases of gonorrhea in the United States. If the infection goes untreated, it can cause blindness or joint infection in infants.

In both genders, gonorrhea of the rectum may occur after anal–genital intercourse or through direct anal contamination from genital lesions. Infection of the pharynx and oral cavity is predominantly seen in women and homosexual men after fellatio. It also occasionally is seen after cunnilingus.

Widespread dissemination is more likely in infected persons lacking select complement proteins. The gonococcemia can lead to variety of disorders, including migratory arthritis, skin and mucous membrane lesions, endocarditis, meningitis, PID, and pericarditis.

CLINICAL PRESENTATION

Signs and Symptoms

In men, symptoms usually occur after an incubation period of 2 to 5 days, although they may take as long as 30 days to appear. The most common findings include a mucopurulent (white, yellow, or green) urethral discharge, burning pain on urination, urgency, and frequency. Tenderness and swelling of the meatus may occur.

In women, a significant percentage of cases may be asymptomatic or only minimally symptomatic. Symptomatic infection may demonstrate vaginal or urethral discharge, dysuria with frequency and urgency, and burning pain when urinating. Backache and abdominal pain also may be present.

Approximately 50% of women and 1% to 3% of men are asymptomatic or only mildly symptomatic. This is unfortunate because patients may not seek medical care for their problem and as a result constitute a large reservoir of infection.

Gonococcal infection of the anal canal commonly is less intense than genital infection, but similar signs and symptoms, including a copious purulent discharge, soreness, and pain, may be noted.

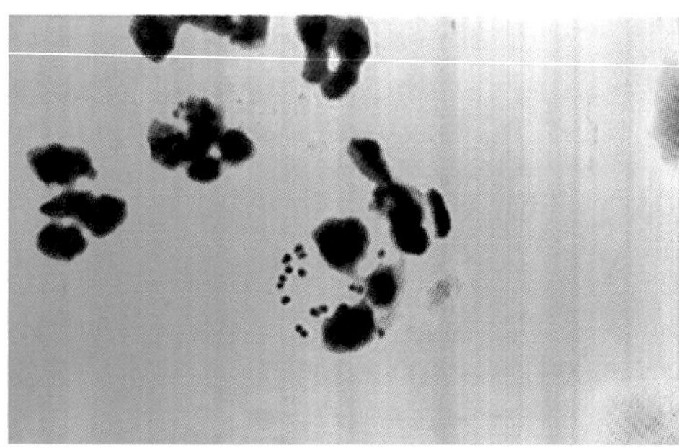

FIGURE 13-2 Smear demonstrates gram-negative diplococci within a leukocyte. *(Courtesy University of Iowa, Iowa City, Iowa, and Gary E. Kaiser, PhD, The Community College of Baltimore County, Baltimore, Maryland)*

Within the oral cavity, the pharynx is most commonly affected.[8] Pharyngeal infection is reported to occur in 3% to 7% of heterosexual men, 10% to 20% of heterosexual women, and 10% to 25% of homosexual men.[9] It usually is seen as an asymptomatic infection with diffuse, nonspecific inflammation or as a mild sore throat. The likelihood of transmission of pharyngeal gonorrhea to the genitalia seems much less than that of genital–genital transmission.[10,11] Of significance, however, is the fact that *N. gonorrhoeae* has been cultured in expectorated saliva from two thirds of patients with oropharyngeal gonorrhea.[10]

Gonococcal stomatitis or oral gonorrhea is uncommon; case reports in the literature are limited.[9,12-15] Acute temporomandibular joint arthritis caused by disseminated gonococcal infection from a genital site has been described.[16]

Laboratory Findings

Laboratory diagnosis of a genital *N. gonorrhoeae* infection can be made based on the finding of gram-negative diplococci within polymorphonuclear leukocytes in a smear of urine or of purulent discharge in symptomatic mean (Figure 13-2). In women and asymptomatic men, nucleic acid amplification testing (NAAT) of urine is recommended because of its high sensitivity and specificity, and it can be used to simultaneously test for *C. trachomatis*.[1,17] Culture is also available for diagnosis of *N. gonorrhoeae* from rectal and pharyngeal specimens. In suspected cases of oropharyngeal gonorrhea, because other species of *Neisseria* are normal inhabitants of the oral cavity, NAAT is more specific than a gram stain.

MEDICAL MANAGEMENT

The CDC recommendations[1] offer several choices for the treatment of uncomplicated gonococcal infection of the cervix, urethra, and rectum. The single-dose regimens are: injectable ceftriaxone 250 mg (intramuscularly [IM]) in a single dose) or oral cefixime 400 mg in a single dose. Alternatively, a single-dose of injectable cephalosporin plus azithromycin 1 gram orally or doxycycline 100 mg a day for 7 days is recommended. Since patients infected with *N. gonorrhoeae* are often coinfected with *Chlamydia trachomatis* dosing regimens that include either azithromycin 1 g given orally in a single dose, or doxycycline 100 mg orally two times a day for 7 days is recommended. For patients who cannot take ceftriaxone, spectinomycin (2 g IM) or azithromycin 2 g are recommended alternatives. A very low (0.8%) treatment failure rate has been reported with ceftriaxone-doxycycline in the United States, and follow-up cultures are not considered essential unless symptoms persist. After antibiotic therapy is begun, infectiousness is diminished rapidly (within a matter of hours).[11,17] Infections detected after treatment are generally the result of reinfection by a sexual partner—not treatment failure. Due to widely disseminated quinolone-resistant strains (QRNs) quinolones are no longer recommended for treatment of gonorrhea.

The clinician should be aware that gonococcal pharyngitis is more difficult to eradicate than infections at urogenital and anorectal sites.[17] Few antimicrobial regimens can reliably cure such infections more than 90% of the time, and IM cefixime 250 mg plus azithromycin 1 g single oral dose or doxycycline 100 mg a day for 7 days is recommended.[1] As with all STDs, all sex partners of patients who have *N. gonorrhoeae* infection should be assessed and treated.

SYPHILIS

DEFINITION

Syphilis is an acute and chronic STD, caused by *Treponema pallidum,* that produces skin and mucous membrane lesions in the *acute phase* and bone, visceral, cardiovascular, and neurologic disease in the *chronic phase.* The variety of systemic manifestations associated with the later stages of syphilis resulted in its historical designation as the "great imitator" disease. As with gonorrhea, humans are the only known natural hosts for syphilis. The primary site of syphilitic infection is the genitalia, although primary lesions also occur extragenitally. Syphilis remains an important infection in contemporary medicine because of the morbidity it causes, and because it enhances the transmission of HIV.[18]

EPIDEMIOLOGY

Incidence and Prevalence

Syphilis is the fifth most frequently reported STD in the United States today, surpassed only by chlamydial infection, gonorrhea, salmonellosis, and AIDS. In 1990, the incidence of primary and secondary syphilis reached 50,223 cases.[5] The number of cases of primary and secondary syphilis dropped to 6,000 in 2000. Since then, the rate has been steadily climbing. In 2009, almost 13,997 cases were reported, a rate of decline of 4.6 cases per 100,000 population.[4,5,19] A disproportionately high number of cases continue to occur in the South and among Hispanic and non-Hispanic African American men and women. Syphilis occurs more commonly in persons aged 25 to 39 years. Its incidence in males is greater than in females, with a ratio of almost 6 : 1.[19]

Congenital syphilis occurs when the fetus is infected in utero by an infected mother. In 2008, a total of 431 cases of congenital syphilis were reported to the CDC. This represents a rate of 10.1 per 100,000 live births—higher than the 8.2 cases per 100,000 live births in 2005—but still a dramatic decline from the peak of 107.3 cases per 100,000 live births in 1991.[19]

Etiology

The etiologic agent of syphilis is *Treponema pallidum,* which is a slender, fragile anaerobic spirochete. It is transmitted predominantly sexually, including by oral–genital and rectal–genital contact with contaminated sores. However, transmission also can occur through nonsexual means such as kissing, blood transfusion, or accidental inoculation with a contaminated needle. Indirect transmission by fomites is possible but uncommon, because the organism survives for only a short time outside the body.[1,20] *T. pallidum* is easily killed by heating, drying, disinfecting, and using soap and water. The organism is difficult to stain, except with use of certain silver impregnation methods. Demonstration is best done with darkfield microscopy on a fresh specimen.

Pathophysiology

Available evidence suggests that *T. pallidum* does not invade completely intact skin; however, it can invade intact mucosal epithelium and gain entry through minute abrasions or at the hair follicles. Within a few hours after invasion, bacterial spread to the lymphatics and the bloodstream occurs, resulting in early widespread dissemination of the disease. The early response to bacterial invasion consists of endarteritis and periarteritis.[20] The risk of transmission is during the primary, secondary, and early latent stages of disease, but not in late syphilis.[21] Overall, patients are most infectious during the first 2 years of the disease.

CLINICAL PRESENTATION

Signs and Symptoms

Manifestations and descriptions of syphilis are classically divided according to stages of the disease, with each stage having its own specific signs and symptoms related

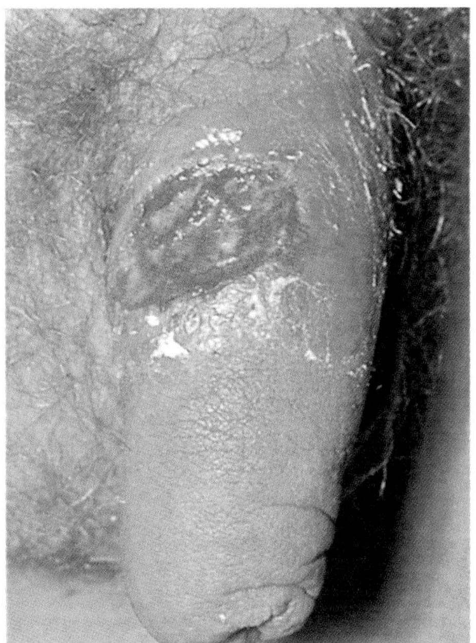

FIGURE 13-3 Primary syphilis: Chancre of the penis. *(From Swartz MH: Textbook of physical diagnosis, ed 6, Philadelphia, Saunders, 2010.)*

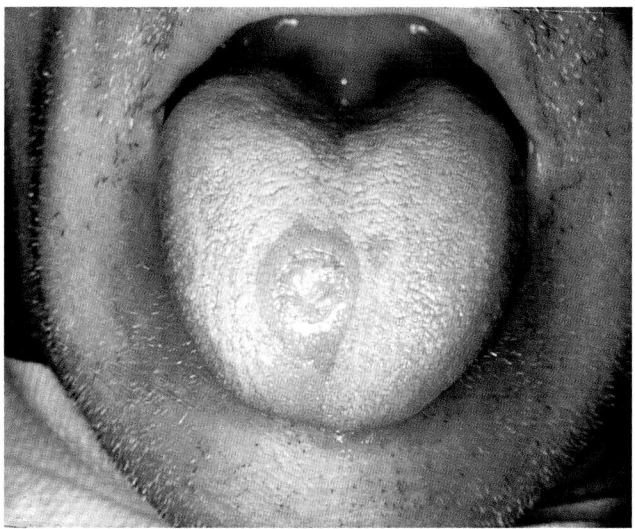

A

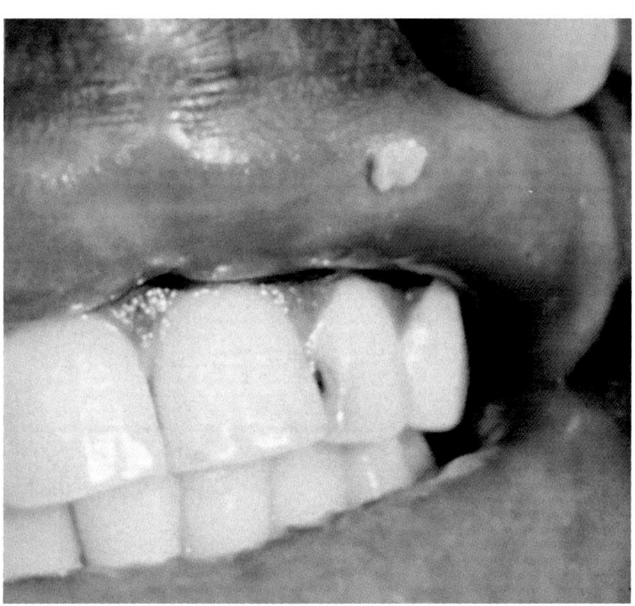

B

FIGURE 13-4 **Primary Syphilis. A,** Chancre on tongue seen in primary syphilis. **B,** Extragenital chancre of the lip. *(**A,** From Ibsen DAC, Phelan JA:* Oral pathology for the hygienist, *ed 5, St. Louis, Saunders, 2009.)*

to disease duration and antigen-antibody responses. The stages are primary, secondary, latent, tertiary, and congenital. Of note, many infected persons do not develop symptoms for years, yet remain at risk for late complications if the infection is not treated.

Primary Syphilis. The classic manifestation of primary syphilis is the chancre, a solitary firm, round, granulomatous lesion that develops at the site of inoculation with the infectious organism. The chancre usually occurs within 2 to 3 weeks (range, 10 to 90 days) after exposure (Figure 13-3). Patients are infectious, however, before it appears. The lesion begins as a small papule and enlarges to form a surface erosion or ulceration that commonly is covered by a yellowish hemorrhagic crust and teems with *T. pallidum*. It typically is painless. Associated with the chancre are enlarged, painless, hard regional lymph nodes. The chancre usually subsides in 3 to 6 weeks without treatment, leaving variable scarring in the form of a healed papule.[20,22] The genitalia, oral cavity (lips, tongue), fingers, nipples, and anus are common sites for chancres. Figure 13-4 shows examples of extragenital syphilitic chancres (lip and tongue). If adequate treatment is not provided, the infection progresses to secondary syphilis.

Secondary Syphilis. The manifestations of secondary syphilis appear 6 to 8 weeks after initial exposure. The chancre may or may not have completely resolved by this time. The symptoms and signs of secondary syphilis include fever, arthralgia and malaise, generalized lymphadenopathy, and patchy hair loss and develop in 80% of patients. Generalized eruptions of the skin and mucous membranes also occur (Figure 13-5, *A*) and include condyloma lata or wart-like growths on the genitalia. The papules of the rash are well demarcated and reddish brown and have a predilection for the palms and soles; they typically are not itchy. Oral manifestations of secondary syphilis include pharyngitis, papular lesions, erythematous or grayish-white erosions (mucous patches) (see Figure 13-5, *B*), irregular linear erosions, and, rarely, parotid gland enlargement. The lesions of skin and mucous membranes are highly infectious.[20,22] Without treatment, clinical manifestations of secondary syphilis ultimately resolve; however, infection progresses to latent or the tertiary stages.

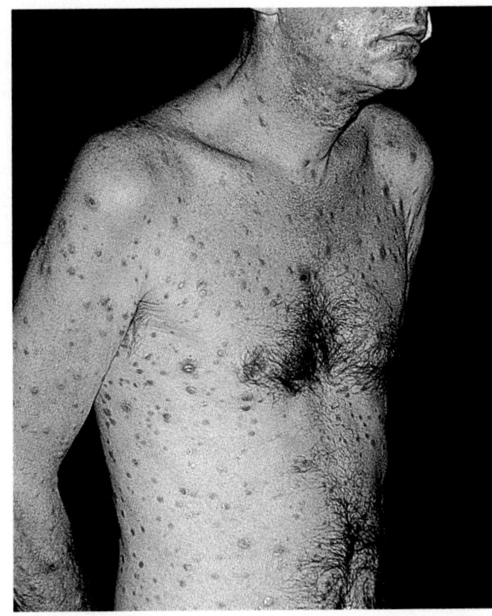

A

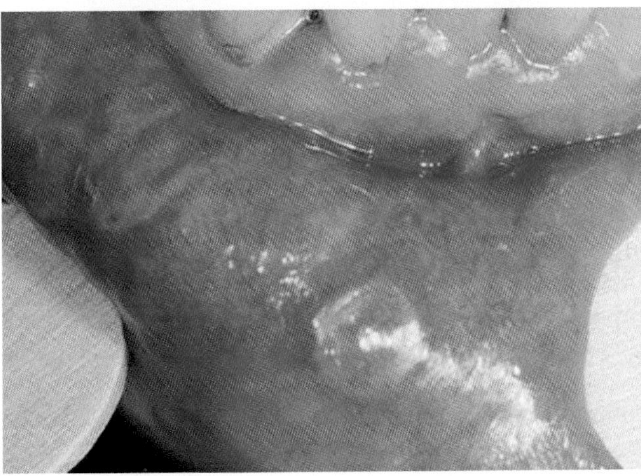

B

FIGURE 13-5 Lesions of Secondary Syphilis. A, Profuse papular rash. **B,** Mucous patch of the lower lip *(**A,** From Habif TP, et al: Skin disease: diagnosis and treatment, ed 3, St. Louis, 2011, Mosby.)*

Latent Syphilis. Latent syphilis is defined as an untreated infection in which the patient displays seroreactivity but no clinical evidence of disease. This stage of the infection is divided into early latent syphilis (disease acquired within the preceding year) and late latent syphilis (disease present for longer than 1 year) or latent syphilis of unknown duration. During the first 4 years of latent syphilis, patients may exhibit mucocutaneous relapses and are considered infectious. After 4 years, relapses do not occur, and patients are considered noninfectious (except for blood transfusions and pregnant women).[7,22] The latent stage may last for many years or, in fact, for the remainder of the person's life. In some untreated patients, however, progression to tertiary syphilis occurs.

Tertiary (Late) Syphilis. The tertiary (late) stage occurs in roughly 1/3 of untreated persons, generally several years after disease onset.[23] It is the destructive stage of the disease that involves mucocutaneous, osseous, and visceral structures). Signs and symptoms of this stage do not occur until years after the initial infection.

More than 80% of manifestations of tertiary syphilis are essentially vascular in nature and result from an obliterative endarteritis. Cardiovascular syphilis most commonly manifests as an aneurysm of the ascending aorta.

The benign tertiary stage of syphilis is classically characterized by the formation of gummas. These localized nodular, tender lesions may involve the skin, mucous membranes, bone, nervous tissue, and/or viscera. They are thought to be the end result of a delayed hypersensitivity reaction. Pathologically, they consist of an inflammatory granulomatous lesion with a central zone of necrosis. Gummas are not infectious but can be destructive.

The oral lesions of tertiary syphilis consist of diffuse interstitial glossitis and the gumma. Interstitial glossitis should be considered a premalignant condition. The tongue may appear lobulated and fissured with atrophic papillae, resulting in a bald-appearing and wrinkled surface. Leukoplakia frequently is present. The oral gumma is a rare lesion that most commonly involves the tongue and palate. It appears as a firm tissue mass with central necrosis. Palatal gummas may perforate into the nasal cavity or maxillary sinus.

Neurosyphilis can occur during any stage of syphilis. It can produce a meningitis-like syndrome, Argyll Robertson pupils (which react to accommodation but not to light), altered tendon reflexes, general paresis, tabes dorsalis (degeneration of dorsal columns of the spinal cord and sensory nerve trunks), difficulty in coordinating muscle movements, cognitive dysfunction or insanity.

Congenital Syphilis. Syphilis or its sequelae occur in the newborn if the mother is infected while carrying the child. The disease is transmitted to the fetus in utero, usually after the 16th week, because before this time, the placenta prevents transmission of bacteria. The disease persists worldwide because a substantial number of women do not receive serologic testing for syphilis during pregnancy, or they may undergo testing too late in pregnancy to receive prenatal care.[24] Physical manifestations vary according to the time of infection. The sequelae of early infection include osteochondritis, periostitis (frontal bossing of Parrot), rhinitis, rash, and ectodermal changes. Syphilis contracted during late pregnancy may involve bones, teeth (see "Oral Manifestations"), eyes, cranial nerves, viscera, skin, and mucous membranes. A classic triad of congenital syphilis known as *Hutchinson's triad* includes interstitial keratitis of the cornea, eighth nerve deafness, and dental abnormalities, including Hutchinson's incisors (Figure 13-6) and mulberry molars.

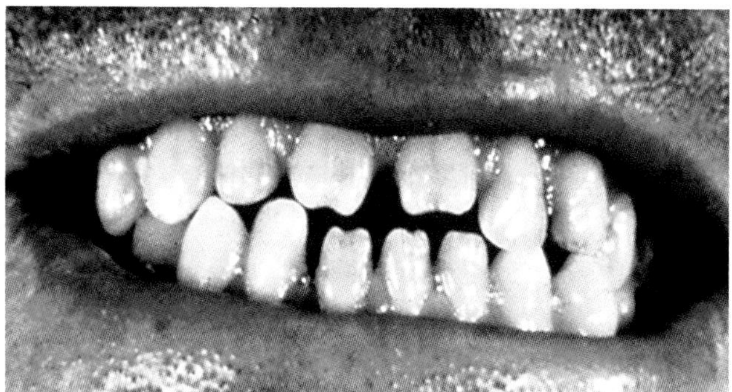

FIGURE 13-6 Congenital syphilis: Hutchinson's teeth.

Laboratory Findings

T. pallidum has never been cultured successfully on any type of medium; therefore, the definitive diagnosis of syphilis is made from a positive darkfield microscopic examination or on the basis of direct immunofluorescent antibody tests on fresh lesion exudates. Darkfield examination yields consistently positive findings only during primary and early secondary stages. Definitive diagnosis of oral lesions by this method is difficult, because other species of *Treponema* are indigenous to the oral cavity.

Syphilis typically is diagnosed by a two-step process involving a nonspecific (screening) antibody test, followed by a treponeme-specific test. Screening antibody tests of blood also are known as serologic tests for syphilis (STS). These tests are of two basic types, indirect and direct, and are differentiated by the types of antibodies they measure.

Screening Serologic Tests for Syphilis: Nontreponemal Tests—VDRL and RPR. Standard screening tests for syphilis consist of the Venereal Disease Research Laboratory (VDRL) slide test, the rapid plasma reagin (RPR) test, and the automated reagin test (ART). These indirect, nontreponemal serologic tests are designed to detect the presence of an antibody-like substance called *reagin* that is produced when *T. pallidum* reacts with various body tissues. They are equally valid. A disadvantage of reaginic tests is the occasional biologic false-positive result that can occur.

Nontreponemal tests produce titers (reported quantitatively as serologic dilutions [e.g., 1:2, 1:4, 1:8]) that usually correlate with disease activity. Results are consistently positive and the highest titers are obtained between 3 and 8 weeks after the appearance of the primary chancre. In primary syphilis, nontreponemal tests usually revert to negative within 12 months after successful treatment. In secondary syphilis, up to 24 months may be required for the patient to become seronegative. Occasionally, a patient will remain seropositive for life, or will test positive in the presence of an associated infection or condition (false-positive). With tertiary syphilis, many patients remain seropositive for life.[1]

Confirmatory Serologic Tests for Syphilis: Treponemal Tests (FTA-ABS and MHA-TP). Treponemal tests are designed to detect the specific antibody produced against treponemes that cause syphilis, yaws, and pinta.[7,22] These tests are more specific than reaginic tests but less sensitive. Thus, they typically are performed after a positive VDRL or RPR. The fluorescent treponemal antibody (FTA) test, fluorescent treponemal antibody absorption (FTA-ABS) test, and *T. pallidum* particle agglutination test (TP-PA) are examples. Treponemal antibody titers wane over time but remain positive in about 80% of patients, regardless of treatment. Thus, they should not be used to assess response to treatment.[1] Polymerase chain reaction (PCR) for specific treponemal DNA sequences may be helpful in confirming the diagnosis when other studies are inconclusive.

MEDICAL MANAGEMENT

Parenteral injection of long-acting benzathine penicillins (e.g., penicillin G, 2.4 million U IM in a single dose) remains the recommended treatment for primary, secondary, or early latent syphilis. Additional doses for 3 weeks are recommended for patients who have had syphilis for longer than a year (late latent). Alternative drugs for patients allergic to penicillin include oral doxycycline (100 mg orally two times a day for 2 weeks), tetracycline (500 mg orally four times a day for 2 weeks), or azithromycin.[1] Testing for HIV serostatus and treatment of sexual partners also are recommended. After completing treatment, patients should be retested at 6 and 12 months to monitor for seroconversion status. A low failure rate has been reported in the treatment of syphilis. An important aspect to note in the management of syphilis is that, as with gonorrhea, infectiousness is reversed rapidly, probably within a matter of hours, on initiation of appropriate antibiotic treatment.[22]

The Jarisch-Herxheimer reaction is an acute febrile reaction that frequently is accompanied by chills, myalgias, hyperventilation, and headache that occur within 24 hours after initiation of therapy for syphilis. It occurs most often (i.e., in 50% patients) after treatment for early syphilis.

Congenital syphilis is best managed through implementation of preventive measures. This approach requires that all pregnant women be screened for syphilis by serologic testing at the first prenatal visit. If results are positive, the expectant mother should be treated with penicillin and retested at the 28th week and again at delivery. Infants born to seroreactive mothers should be assessed by means of clinical, radiographic, and laboratory tests of blood and cerebrospinal fluid (CSF) for VDRL. If results prove the disease or suggest that syphilis is highly probable, then infants should be treated with intravenous penicillin G for at least 10 days. The treatment response for congenital and tertiary stages of syphilis is limited by the extent of damage already incurred.

GENITAL HERPES

DEFINITION

Genital herpes is a life-long viral disease of the genitalia that is caused by one of two closely related types of herpes simplex virus (HSV)—HSV-1 and HSV-2. Most genital herpes infections are caused by HSV-2. The disease consists of acute and recurrent phases and is associated with high rates of subclinical infection and asymptomatic viral shedding. The prevalence of genital herpes has increased by 30% since the late 1970s.[25]

EPIDEMIOLOGY

Incidence and Prevalence

Genital herpes is an important STD worldwide. Its exact incidence in the United States is unknown because it is not a reportable disease, and most persons have not been diagnosed because their disease is mild or asymptomatic. An estimated 50 million people, or more than 25% of persons 12 years of age and older, in the United States are infected.[1,25] An estimated 1.6 million new cases of HSV-2 occur annually in the United States.[26,27] The prevalence in developing countries is between 40% and 60%.[27] About 70% to 95% of first-episode cases of genital herpes are caused by HSV-2, whereas up to 30% in some series are caused by HSV-1.[1] Prevalence rates in women (25%) and in African Americans (46%) are reportedly higher than those in men (20%) and in whites (18%).[25] Most persons infected with HSV-2 have not been diagnosed with genital herpes thus enhancing its transmission.

Etiology

HSV belongs to a family of eight human herpesviruses that includes cytomegalovirus, Epstein-Barr virus (EBV), varicella-zoster virus (VZV), human herpesvirus type 6 (HHV-6), human herpesvirus type 7 (HHV-7), and Kaposi sarcoma–associated herpesvirus (HHV-8). HSV-1 is the causative agent of most herpetic infections that occur above the waist, especially on the mucosa of the mouth (herpetic gingivostomatitis, herpes labialis), nose, eyes, brain, and skin. Infection with HSV-1 is extremely common; most adults demonstrate antibodies to this virus. It is thought that many primary infections with HSV-1 are subclinical and thus are never known to the infected person. Transmission usually occurs through close contact, such as touching or kissing, and transfer of infective saliva. HSV-1 also is transmitted by sexual contact. Airborne droplet infection has not been well demonstrated, although it is possible.[28] Autoinoculation from contact with face, fingers, eyes, and genitalia is a persistent clinical problem.

HSV-2 is the causative agent of most herpes infections that occur below the waist, such as in or around the genitalia (genital herpes). HSV-2 is transmitted predominantly by sexual contact but also may be passed nonsexually. Its primary mode of transmission is through an asymptomatic viral shedder. HSV-2 can be transmitted to a newborn from an infected mother.

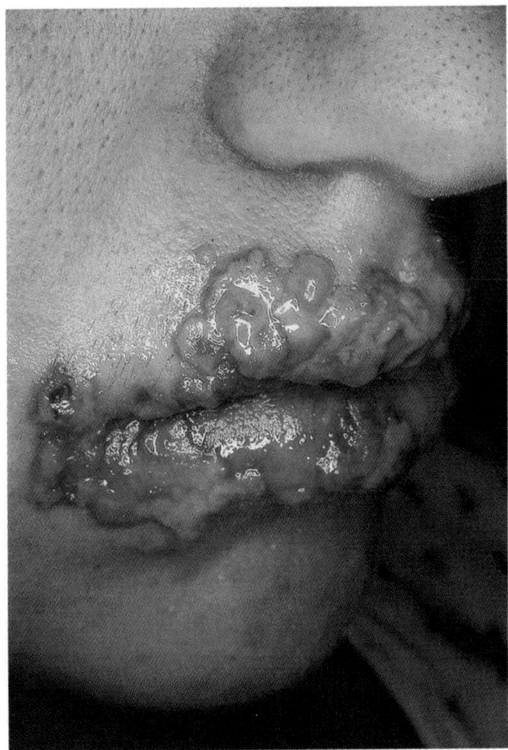

FIGURE 13-7 Primary herpes simplex type 2 occurring in the oral cavity documented by laboratory testing. *(From Sapp JP, et al: Contemporary oral and maxillofacial pathology, ed 2, St. Louis, 2004, Mosby.)*

Although the primary site of occurrence of HSV-1 is above the waist and of HSV-2 below the waist, each infection may occur at either site and in fact can be inoculated from one site to the other (Figure 13-7). Furthermore, the two types cannot be differentiated on basis of skin lesions and other clinical manifestations.

Pathophysiology and Complications

The pathologic processes of herpesvirus infections HSV-1 and HSV-2 are essentially identical; thus, the lesions of skin and mucous membranes are identical. Infection arises from intimate contact with a lesion or infective fluid (e.g., saliva). Epithelial cells are invaded, and viral replication occurs. Characteristic cellular changes include ballooning degeneration, intranuclear inclusion bodies, and the formation of multinucleated giant cells. With cellular destruction come inflammation and increasing edema, which result in formation of a papule that progresses to a fluid-filled vesicle. These vesicles rupture, leaving an ulcerated or crusted surface.

Lymphadenopathy and viremia are prominent features. In normal persons, the primary infection is contained by usual host defenses and runs its course within 10 to 20 days. However, spread to other epidermal sites (e.g., herpetic whitlow [infection of the fingers], keratoconjunctivitis [eyes]) and in neonates during childbirth has been documented. In rare cases, infants and immunosuppressed persons can develop systemic (meningitis) and widespread infection that may result in significant morbidity and death.

During the epithelial infection, progeny enter the ends of local peripheral neurons and migrate up the axon to the regional ganglion (HSV-1 primarily in the trigeminal, and HSV-2 primarily in the sacral), where they reside for the life of the host. After stimulation such as trauma, sunlight, menses, or intercourse, the virus can reactivate, migrate down the axon, and produce recurrent infection. Of the two HSV serotypes that can infect the sacral ganglia, HSV-2 is more efficient in reactivating and producing recurrent genital lesions, whereas HSV-1 may pose a greater risk for neonatal herpes.[29] Also, immune suppression increases the risk for more frequent and severe recurrences.

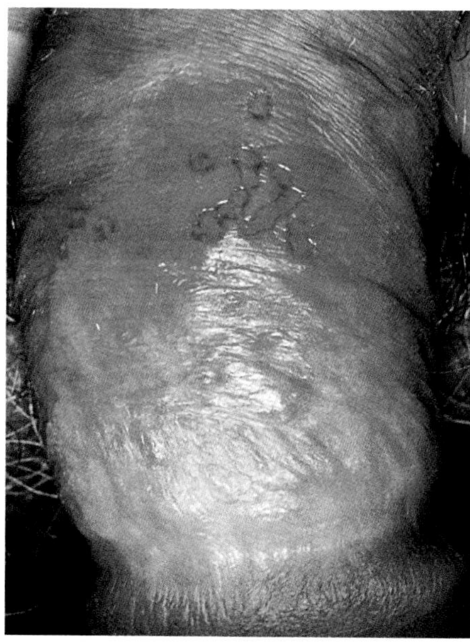

FIGURE 13-8 Recurrent herpes simplex virus infection of the foreskin. *(From Habif TP, et al:* Skin disease: diagnosis and treatment, *ed 3, St. Louis, 2011, Mosby.)*

CLINICAL PRESENTATION

Signs and Symptoms

Most (about 60%) new cases of HSV-2 infection are asymptomatic[27]; newly acquired cases are asymptomatic more frequently in men than in women. After an incubation period of 2 to 7 days, lesions (i.e., papules, vesicles, ulcers, crusts, and fissures) of primary genital herpes may appear. In women, both internal and external genitalia may be involved, as well as the perineal region and the skin of the thighs and buttocks. In men, the external genitalia is typically involved, as may the skin of the inguinal area. Lesions in moist areas tend to ulcerate early, are painful, and may be associated with dysuria. Lesions on exposed dry areas tend to remain pustular or vesicular and then crust over. Painful regional lymphadenopathy accompanies the primary infection, along with headache, malaise, myalgia, and fever. Clinical manifestations subside in about 2 weeks, and healing occurs in 3 to 5 weeks.

Outbreaks of recurrent genital herpes typically occur 2 to 6 times per year and generally are less severe and more localized than the primary infection. Recurrences frequently are precipitated by menstruation, intercourse, or immunosuppression. A *prodrome* of localized itching, tingling, paresthesia, pain, and burning may be noted and is variably followed by a vesicular eruption (Figure 13-8). Healing occurs in 10 to 14 days. Constitutional symptoms generally are absent. Between recurrences, infected persons shed virus intermittently and asymptomatically from the genital tract.

HSV-1 and HSV-2 lesions are highly infectious, promoting transmission to other people, or to other sites on the body. Orogenital contact may result in spread from the source to the oral cavity or genitals of the sexual partner. The infectious period of herpetic lesions is considered to extend until the crusting stage. Therefore, all herpetic lesions (i.e., papular, vesicular, pustular, and ulcerative) before completion of crusting should be assumed to be infectious.

Laboratory Findings

Cytologic examination of a smear (Tzanck preparation) taken from the base of a herpetic lesion reveals typical features, including ballooning degeneration of cells, intranuclear inclusion bodies, and multinucleated (fused) giant cells. However, cytologic evaluation is nonspecific and less sensitive than viral culture. Diagnosis is best established by swabbing an infected secretion or ulcer and isolating the virus by cell culture or amplifying its sequences by PCR. Cultured virus is identified by staining the infected cells for HSV antigen with the use of immunofluorescence or immunoperoxidase. PCR is particularly helpful when neurologic symptoms develop and cerebrospinal fluid is sampled. Serologic detection of antibodies to HSV-1 glycoprotein G1 or HSV-2 glycoprotein G2 aids in diagnosis and management (e.g., counseling the patient about the potential for recurrences and transmission).[1]

MEDICAL MANAGEMENT

Management of patients with a first clinical episode of genital herpes includes antiviral therapy and counseling regarding the natural history of genital herpes, sexual and perinatal transmission, and ways to reduce transmission. Current CDC recommendations[1] call for the use of

BOX 13-1 Oral Regimens Recommended by the Centers for Disease Control and Prevention for the Treatment of Genital Herpes*

Primary Episode*
- Acyclovir 400 mg orally three times a day for 7-10 days, *or*
- Acyclovir 200 mg orally five times a day for 7-10 days, *or*
- Famciclovir 250 mg orally three times a day for 7-10 days, *or*
- Valacyclovir 1 g orally twice a day for 7-10 days

Recurrent Infection
- Acyclovir 400 mg orally three times a day for 5 days, *or*
- Acyclovir 200 mg orally five times a day for 5 days, *or*
- Acyclovir 800 mg orally twice a day for 2-5 days, *or*
- Famciclovir 125 mg orally twice a day for 5 days, *or*
- Famciclovir 500 mg once, then 250 mg twice daily for 2 days
- Famciclovir 1000 mg twice daily for 1 day
- Valacyclovir 500 mg orally twice a day for 5 days, *or*
- Valacyclovir 1 g orally once a day for 5 days

Daily Suppressive Therapy
- Acyclovir 400 mg twice daily, *or*
- Famciclovir 250 mg twice a day, *or*
- Valacyclovir 500 mg once a day, *or*
- Valacyclovir 1† g once a day

*NOTE: Treatment may be extended if healing is incomplete after 10 days of therapy. Higher dosages of acyclovir (e.g., 400 mg orally five times a day) were used in treatment studies of first-episode herpes proctitis and first-episode oral infection. However, comparative studies with respect to genital herpes have not been performed. Valacyclovir and famciclovir probably also are effective for acute herpes simplex virus proctitis or oral infection, but clinical experience is lacking.[20]

†Higher doses may be required for patients who have more than 10 recurrences per year.

acyclovir (Zovirax), famciclovir (Famvir), or valacyclovir (Valtrex). All three are nucleoside analogue drugs that act as DNA chain terminators during virus replication in infected cells. Some of these agents are available in oral, topical, and intravenous formulations. Topical acyclovir therapy is substantially less effective than systemic drug administration, and its use is not recommended for genital herpes. Systemic antiviral drug therapy can shorten the duration, frequency, and symptoms of outbreaks and can reduce the frequency of asymptomatic shedding and the risk of transmission.[30] Antiviral agents do not eliminate the virus from the latent state, however, nor do they affect subsequent risk, frequency, or severity of recurrence after drug use is discontinued. Antiviral drugs are most effective when given for prevention at least 1 day within appearance of symptoms, whether for primary or recurrent disease. Current treatment recommendations are addressed in Box 13-1.[1] These protocols also may be used for oral infection. Intravenous antiviral agents (cidofovir [Vistide] and foscarnet [Foscavir]) are reserved for severe or complicated infections and may be required for immunosuppressed patients.

Daily suppressive antiviral therapy can be implemented for patients with frequent recurrences (more than five recurrences per year). Suppressive therapy reduces the frequency of recurrence by 70% to 80% among persons who experience six or more recurrences per year and reduces asymptomatic viral shedding between outbreaks.[1] Suppressive therapy has not been associated with emergence of clinically significant acyclovir resistance among immunocompetent patients. Because the frequency of recurrence tends to diminish over time in many patients, current recommendations include discussing periodically the possibility of discontinuing suppressive therapy to reassess the need for continued therapy.

Acyclovir, famciclovir, and valacyclovir have been assigned pregnancy category C, B, and B, respectively, by the U.S. Food and Drug Administration (FDA). Accordingly, famciclovir and valacyclovir are considered relatively safe to administer to pregnant women.[31]

INFECTIOUS MONONUCLEOSIS

DEFINITION

Although not classically defined as an STD, infectious mononucleosis is discussed in this chapter because transmission occurs through intimate personal contact. Infectious mononucleosis is an infection that is caused, in at least 90% of cases, by EBV, a lymphotropic herpesvirus. Other viruses also may produce features of acute infectious mononucleosis. Infectious mononucleosis produces the classic clinical triad of fever, pharyngitis, and bilateral symmetrical cervical lymphadenopathy. Transmission of the virus occurs primarily by way of the oropharyngeal route during close personal contact (i.e., intimate kissing). Children, adolescents, and young adults are affected most commonly. About 40% of asymptomatic herpesvirus-seropositive adults carry EBV in their saliva on any given day.[32]

EPIDEMIOLOGY

Incidence, Prevalence, and Etiology

More than 90% of adults worldwide have been infected with EBV. In the United States, about 50% of 5-year-old children and 70% of college freshmen have evidence of previous EBV infection.[33,34] The peak age of acquisition in the United States is reportedly 15 to 19 years.[35] The annual incidence in this adolescent age group is 3.4 to 6.7 cases per 1000 persons. Incidence has been reported as 30 times higher in whites than in blacks in the United States.[33] No gender predilection has been noted. Having numerous sexual partners increases the risk for acquisition of EBV.

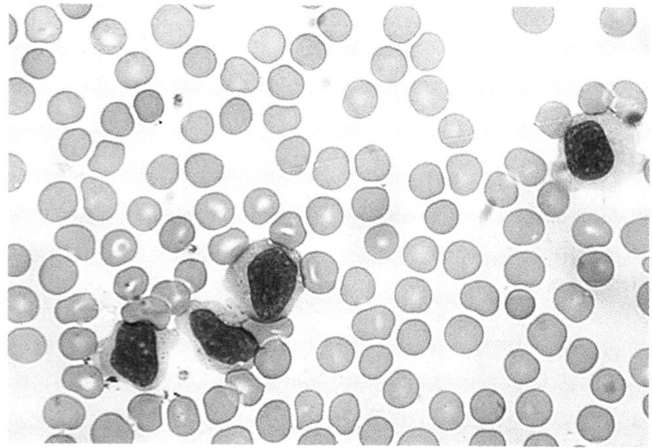

FIGURE 13-9 Atypical lymphocytes in infectious mononucleosis. *(From Kumar V, Abbas A, Fausto N, editors:* Robbins & Cotran's pathologic basis of disease, *ed 8, Philadelphia, 2010, Saunders.)*

Pathophysiology

EBV is a lymphotropic herpesvirus that is transmitted primarily through close personal contact (i.e., intimate kissing) and exposure to infected saliva and oropharyngeal secretions. Infrequently, it is transmitted through shared infected drinks, eating utensils, or infected blood products. Incubation time is 30 to 50 days. A prodromal period of 3 to 5 days precedes the clinical phase, which lasts 7 to 20 days. During the *prodromal phase,* the virus infects oropharyngeal epithelial cells and spreads to B lymphocytes in the tonsillar crypts. Infected B lymphocytes circulate through the reticuloendothelial system, triggering a marked lymphocytic response. In infectious mononucleosis, large, reactive lymphocytes expand from 1% to 2% to 10% to 40% of the circulating white blood cells. These expanded T lymphocytes are reactive to the EBV-infected B lymphocytes (Figure 13-9).[34] The combination of reactive lymphocytes, the cytokines they produce, and the B cell–produced (heterophile) antibodies directed against EBV antigens contributes to the clinical manifestation of the acute infection. Hepatosplenomegaly develops in about 40% to 50% of patients, self-limiting hepatitis develops in about 10%, splenic rupture occurs in 0.1% to 0.2% of all cases, and death is a rare outcome.[34,36] After the acute infection, the EBV remains latent in B lymphocytes for the life of the host and is shed in the saliva. EBV is an effective transforming agent and is associated with the development of lymphomas and nasopharyngeal.

CLINICAL PRESENTATION

Signs and Symptoms

Infectious mononucleosis usually is asymptomatic when found in children; however, about 50% of infected young adults develop symptoms. Fever, sore throat, tonsillar enlargement, lymphadenopathy, malaise, and fatigue are the predominant features. About a third of patients demonstrate palatal petechiae during the first week of the illness, and about 30% of patients develop an exudative pharyngitis.[34,37,38] Generalized skin rash and petechiae of the lips are seen in about 10% of cases, and in sexually active persons genital ulcers may be present. The liver and spleen can enlarge, and become tender and inflamed. Symptoms tend to dissipate within 3 weeks of onset, and the majority recovers without apparent sequelae.

Laboratory Findings

The diagnosis is made on the basis of signs and symptoms and a laboratory profile characterized by marked lymphocytosis (e.g., 50% lymphocytes [primarily T lymphocytes]) with at least 10% atypical lymphocytes on a peripheral blood smear (see Figure 13-9) and a positive heterophile antibody test. Heterophile antibodies are immunoglobulin M (IgM) antibodies that bind (agglutinate) to antigens different from the antigen that induced them, such as erythrocytes from nonhuman (sheep, horses) species.[42] This process forms the basis for the Monospot (Meridian Bioscience, Inc., Cincinnati, Ohio) rapid latex agglutination test. Symptomatic patients in whom a heterophile antibody test is negative should be retested in 7 to 10 days, because this test can be insensitive during the first week. If the second test is negative, tests for viral capsid antigen (VCA) IgG and VCA IgM antibody and EBV nuclear antigen (EBNA) should be performed.[38] These tests are more specific but costly. If test results are positive, the patient has heterophile-negative infectious mononucleosis. A few patients with the classic disease description may be heterophile antibody-negative and EBV IgM-negative. In these patients, tests for cytomegalovirus (CMV), *Toxoplasma gondii,* HHV-6, HIV, and adenovirus should be performed.[33,38] Once EBV-associated mononucleosis has been diagnosed, EBV copy numbers in the blood can be used to monitor the severity and progression of the infection.[39]

MEDICAL MANAGEMENT

Although a number of antiviral drugs can inhibit EBV replication in culture, no drug is yet licensed for clinical treatment of EBV infection. The lack of effective antivirals results from the fact that mononucleosis is largely due to the immune response. However, a recent study of 20 young adults with infectious mononucleosis, showed that valacyclovir can decrease the level of EBV oropharyngeal shedding and reduce the number and severity of symptoms.[40]

Nevertheless until larger studies are performed, treatment of patients with infectious mononucleosis remains symptomatic and supportive with bed rest, fluids, acetaminophen or nonsteroidal anti-inflammatory agents for pain control, and gargling and irrigation with saline solution or lidocaine to relieve throat symptoms. Vigorous activity is to be avoided for at least 3 weeks to reduce the risk of rupture of an enlarged spleen. In some patients with severe toxic exudative pharyngotonsillitis, pharyngeal edema and upper airway obstruction, or seizures, a short course of prednisone may be given. About 20% of patients with symptomatic infectious mononucleosis have concurrent beta-hemolytic streptococcal pharyngotonsillitis and should be treated with penicillin V, if they are not allergic to penicillin. Ampicillin should be avoided because at least 90% of patients develop a hypersensitivity skin rash when treated with this drug.[1,38] Most persons feel better and return to normal activities within a month.

HUMAN PAPILLOMAVIRUS INFECTION

DEFINITION

Human papillomaviruses (HPVs) are small, double-stranded, nonenveloped DNA viruses that infect and replicate in epithelial cells. More than 100 genotypes of HPV have been identified, and more than 40 types are known to be sexually transmitted and to affect anogenital epithelium.[1] Each HPV subtype exhibits preferential anatomic sites of infection and a propensity for altering epithelial growth and replication. The spectrum of disease that is induced is dependent on the type of HPV infection, location, and immune response. Subtypes of HPV have been classified as high-risk, intermediate-risk, or low-risk types. *Low-risk* HPVs (HPV-6, -11) produce benign proliferative lesions of mucocutaneous structures. *Intermediate-risk* HPVs are oncogenic. *High-risk* HPV types (HPV-16, -18) are strongly associated with dysplasia and carcinoma of the uterine and anal tract and other mucosal sites.[41,42] Table 13-2 lists HPV-associated lesions.

TABLE 13-2 Human Papillomavirus (HPV)-Associated Oral Mucosa Lesions

Lesion	Most Common HPV Types
Condyloma acuminatum	6, 11
Epithelial dysplasia, carcinoma in situ, squamous cell carcinoma	2, 16, 18
Focal epithelial hyperplasia (Heck's disease)	13, 32
Lichen planus	11, 16
Oral bowenoid papulosis	6, 11, 16
Squamous papilloma	6, 11
Verruca plana	3, 10
Verruca vulgaris	2, 4, 6, 11, 16
Verrucous carcinoma	2, 6, 11, 16, 18

EPIDEMIOLOGY

Incidence and Prevalence

HPV infections are one of the three most common STDs in the United States. An estimated 20 million people in the United States have genital HPV infection,[1] which can be transmitted through sexual contact.[45] Although the exact incidence of HPV infection remains unknown, because HPV-induced diseases is not a reportable STD and most cases are asymptomatic or subclinical, it is estimated that more than 6 million new infections occur every year in the United States,[1] and up to 40% of sexually active persons are infected with the virus.[43,44] The infection is more common among African American women than white women. The highest rates of infection are in persons between 19 and 26 years of age.[44] Approximately 1% of sexually active adults in the United States have visible genital warts.[45] The lifetime number of sexual partners is the most important risk factor that has been identified for the development of genital warts.[46,47]

Etiology

Genital HPV can be transmitted by direct contact during sexual intercourse or passage of a fetus through an infected birth canal, or by autoinoculation. Genital lesions usually appear after an incubation period of 3 weeks to 8 months. The most common manifestation of HPV replication is the venereal wart, or condyloma acuminatum. HPV types 6 and 11 are the subtypes most frequently associated with condyloma acuminatum.[48] Less commonly, HPV type 2 has been identified in condylomata.

Pathophysiology

HPV is transmitted through mucosa, skin-to-skin, or sexual contact. The virus replicates in the nuclei of epithelial cells and increases the turnover of infected cells, or it remains episomally in a latent state. Benign types such as HPV-6 and -11 have a strong tendency to induce epithelial hyperplasia and wart-like growths. High-risk HPV types (HPV-16 and -18) have a propensity to induce dysplasia and malignant transformation. HPV types 31, 33, 35, 39, 45, 51, 52, 54, 56, and 58 are considered intermediate for inducing carcinoma. Persistent oncogenic HPV infection is the strongest risk factor for the development of precancer and cancer, with HPV DNA detected in 99.7% of cervical cancers. Smoking is also a contributory cofactor.

CLINICAL PRESENTATION

Signs and Symptoms

Most persons infected with HPV are asymptomatic, and the infection clears on its own. Visible genital warts caused by HPV-6 or -11 typically are diagnosed as condyloma acuminatum. These growths are seen in sexually active persons and arise in warm, moist, intertriginous areas such as the anogenital skin and mouth, where friction and microabrasion allow entrance of the pathogen. Condylomata appear as small, soft, exophytic papillomatous growths (Figure 13-10, *A*). The irregular-appearing surface has been described to resemble a head of cauliflower; the base is sessile. The borders are raised and rounded. The color varies, ranging from pink to dusky gray. Lesions often are multiple and recurrent and can coalesce to form large, pebbly warts. Most condylomata are asymptomatic; however, patients may report itching, irritation, pain, or bleeding as a result of manipulation or trauma. During pregnancy, condylomata may enlarge as the result of increased vascularity. Condylomata can occur on the vagina, anus, mouth (see Figure 13-10, *B*), pharynx, or larynx and may appear weeks or months after the onset of infection.

HPV types 16, 18, 31, 33, and 35 have an infrequent association with genital warts and a more common association with dysplasia and carcinoma of the cervix. These intermediate and high-risk HPV types also contribute to the development of squamous intraepithelial neoplasia (Bowen's disease) of the genitalia.

Laboratory Findings

HPV does not grow in cell culture, and serologic tests are not routinely performed, in part because 90% of infected persons become HPV-seronegative within 2 years. Therefore, lesions of condyloma acuminatum should be biopsied and examined microscopically, if the clinical diagnosis is uncertain. The microscopic appearance consists of a sessile base, with raised epithelial borders, a thick spinous spinosum layer (acanthosis), and hyperkeratosis. Identification of HPV within the lesion confirms the diagnosis. This is achieved with the use of FDA-approved tests that use RNA probes to detect viral DNA specific to HPV genotypes (see Figure 13-10, C). Viral subtyping can be important for determining risk for carcinogenesis when cervical tissue and an abnormal Papanicolaou smear are involved (see Chapter 26 under "Cervical Cancer").

MEDICAL MANAGEMENT

The HPV vaccine (Gardasil) was introduced in 2006. This quadrivalent vaccine is 95% to 100% effective in preventing infection with HPV types 6, 11, 16, and 18. Shortly after, a bivalent vaccine (Cervarix) was introduced. It protects against HPV types 16 and 18.[49] Both vaccines have been approved for use in girls and women aged 9 to 26 years and is administered in a 3-shot regimen over a 6-month period. Gardasil is also offered to young men.[1] These vaccines are highly effective for preventing infection by high-risk HPV types, thereby curtailing the major risk for cervical cancer associated

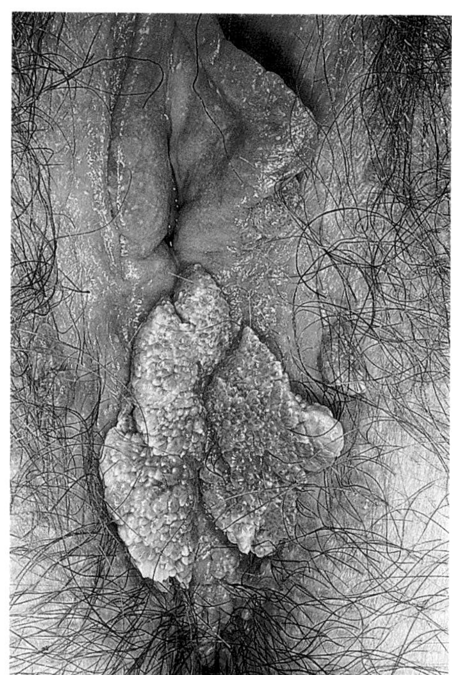

A

B

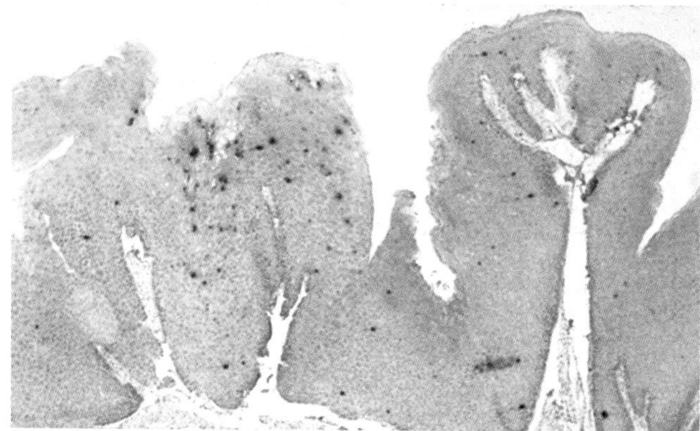

C

FIGURE 13-10 Human Papillomavirus (HPV) Infections. A, Large, cauliflower-like wart of the vagina. **B,** Dome-shaped HPV-induced lesions of the soft palate and retromolar trigone. **C,** In situ hybridization showing HPV DNA as indicated by dark purple stains in the epithelium of a condyloma acuminatum. *(**A,** From Habif TP, et al:* Skin disease: diagnosis and treatment, *ed 3., St. Louis, 2011, Mosby.)*

with these types. They are most beneficial if administered before the onset of sexual activity. Of note, they have not been shown to eliminate or cure HPV infection, and they do not work against all HPV types.

HPV-induced genital warts can be completely removed with chemicals, antiviral drugs, or surgery. The best response is attained with small warts that have been present for less than 1 year. The CDC[1] recommends podofilox 0.5% (Condylox) as the medication of first choice. It causes necrosis by arresting cells in mitosis. This patient-applied medication should be used twice a day for 3 days, with no treatment given for the next 4 days and the cycle repeated up to four times. Alternatively, the patient may apply imiquimod (Aldara) 5% cream at bedtime, three times per week or sinecatechins 15% ointment. Most warts dissipate within 3 months. Other available therapies include surgery (excision, cryotherapy, laser), weekly provider-applied podophyllin 10% to 25% in tincture of benzoin, or bichloroacetic/trichloroacetic acid 80% to 90%. Topical and intralesional therapy with 5-fluorouracil, an antimetabolite, has resulted in a greater than 60% response rate,[50] and cidofovir is an antiviral that yields an effective response. Intralesional interferon is an option, but it is rarely recommended because of cost and adverse effects. Recurrences are common despite the use of first-line therapies (in about 10% to 25% of cases, generally within 3 months), even when the entire lesion, including the base, is removed. As with all STDs, treatment should include the patient's sexual partner to avoid reinfection, as well as counseling regarding methods for reducing transmission. Without treatment, lesions may enlarge and spread. Spontaneous regression occurs in about 20% of patients.[44]

DENTAL MANAGEMENT

Medical Considerations

The dental management of patients with an STD begins with identification. The obvious goal is to identify all people who have active disease in order to limit the spread of the infection and the adverse outcomes of disease progression. Unfortunately, this is not possible in every case, because some persons will not provide a history or may not demonstrate significant signs or symptoms suggestive of their disease. The inability of clinicians to identify potentially infectious patients applies to other diseases as well, such as HIV infection and viral hepatitis. Therefore, it is necessary for all patients to be managed as though they were infectious. The U.S. Public Health Service, through the CDC, has published recommendations for standard precautions to be followed in controlling infection in dentistry that have become the standard for preventing cross-infection[51] (see Appendix B). Strict adherence to these recommendations will, for all practical purposes, eliminate the danger of disease transmission between dentist and patient.

BOX 13-2 Dental Management of the Patient Who Has a Sexually Transmitted Disease (STD)

P: Patient Evaluation and Risk Assessment (see Box 1-1)

- Evaluate and determine whether an STD exists.
- Obtain medical consultation if undiagnosed or uncertain.

Potential Issues or Concerns

Reduce risk of transmission using standard infection control procedures*

- **Gonorrhea**—Little threat of transmission to dentist; oral lesions are possible
- **Syphilis**—Untreated primary and secondary lesions infectious; blood also is potentially infectious
- **Genital herpes**—Little threat of transmission to dentist; oral lesions (possible from autoinoculation) are infectious and can recur after trauma or stress
- **HPV infection**—Little threat of transmission to dentist; oral lesions are possible

Followup: Persons with sexually transmitted disease (STD) are at risk for human immunodeficiency virus [6] infection—testing is advised. Also, new cases of syphilis, gonorrhea, and acquired immunodeficiency syndrome (AIDS) should be reported to the local/state health department.

*Because many patients with an active STD (as well as with other infectious diseases such as AIDS and hepatitis B) cannot be identified by the dentist, all patients should be considered potentially infectious and should be managed with the use of standard precautions. Preventive measures should be implemented that include patient education, as well as evaluation, treatment, and counseling of sexual partners.

Even though these procedures are followed, several aspects of disease transmission specific to particular STDs warrant consideration. Box 13-2 presents a summary of such dental considerations.

Gonorrhea. The patient with (nonoral) gonorrhea poses little threat of disease transmission during dental procedures. This limited infectivity reflects the specific requirements for transmission as well as the early reversal of infectiousness with the institution of antibiotics. Patients in this category can receive dental care within days of beginning antibiotic treatment.

Syphilis. Lesions of untreated primary and secondary syphilis are infectious, as are the patient's blood and saliva. Even after treatment has begun, its absolute effectiveness cannot be determined except through conversion of the positive result on serologic testing to negative; however, early reversal of infectiousness is expected after antibiotic treatment has been initiated. The time required for this conversion varies, ranging from a few months to longer than a year. Therefore, patients who are currently under treatment or who have a positive STS result after receiving treatment should be viewed as potentially infectious. Still, any necessary dental care may be provided with adherence to standard precautions, unless oral lesions are present. Dental treatment can commence once oral lesions have been successfully treated.

Genital Herpes. Localized uncomplicated genital herpes infection poses no problem for the dentist. In the absence of oral lesions, any necessary dental work may be provided. If oral lesions are present, elective treatment should be delayed until lesions scab over, to avoid inadvertent inoculation of adjacent sites. Antiviral agents may be required to prevent recurrence after dental treatment has been provided.

Infectious Mononucleosis. Patients with infectious mononucleosis may come to the dentist because of oral signs and symptoms. Clinical findings of fever, sore throat, petechiae, and cervical lymphadenopathy necessitate further assessment to establish a diagnosis of the underlying condition. Screening clinical laboratory tests can be ordered by the dentist (complete blood count [CBC], heterophil [Monospot] antibody test, and EBV antigen testing), or the patient may be referred to a physician for evaluation and treatment. Routine dental treatment should be delayed for about 4 weeks until the patient has recovered, the patient's liver is capable of normal metabolism of drugs, and the blood count, spleen, and immune system have returned to normal.

Human Papillomavirus Infection. Although presence of genital condylomata acuminata does not affect dental management, oral warts are infectious, and standard precautions apply during oral dental procedures. The presence of oral lesions necessitates referral to a physician to rule out genital lesions in the patient or any sexual partner. Excisional biopsy or antivirals is recommended for HPV oral lesions.

Patients with a History of Sexually Transmitted Disease

Patients who have had an STD should be assessed carefully. They are at increased risk for additional STDs and recurrent infection. The clinician should ensure that adequate treatment was provided for any previous infection and that new infections have not developed. Special attention should be given to unexplained lesions of the oral, pharyngeal, or perioral tissues. Also, a review of systems may reveal urogenital symptoms. Patients with a history of gonorrhea or syphilis should report a history of antibiotic therapy. Patients treated for syphilis should receive a periodic STS for 1 year to monitor conversion of results from positive to negative. Adequate medical follow-up care should have been provided; if it was not, consultation and referral to a physician should be considered.

Patients with Signs, Symptoms, or Oral Lesions Suggestive of a Sexually Transmitted Disease

In patients who have signs or symptoms that suggest an STD, or who have unexplained oral or pharyngeal lesions, further assessment is indicated. The index of suspicion should be higher if the patient is between 15 and 29 years of age and has risk factors such as being an urban dweller, being single, and belonging to a lower socioeconomic group. Any patient who has unexplained lesions should be questioned about possible relationship of the lesions to past sexual activity and should be advised to seek medical care. Herpetic lesions in or around the oral cavity should be recognizable. Patients with oral herpes lesions should not receive routine dental care but should be given palliative treatment only. For a severe primary oral infection or for infectious mononucleosis, the patient may require specific therapy and referral to a physician.

Treatment Planning Modifications

No modifications in the technical treatment plan are required for a patient with an STD. No adverse interactions have been reported between the usual antibiotics or drugs used to treat STDs and drugs commonly used in dentistry. No drugs are contraindicated. Patients with Hutchinson's incisors due to congenital syphilis may request aesthetic repair of affected anterior teeth.

Reporting to State Health Officials

Dentists should be aware of local statutory requirements regarding reporting STDs to state health officials. Syphilis, gonorrhea, and AIDS are diseases that must be reported in every state. Local health departments and state STD programs are sources of information regarding this issue.

Oral Manifestations

Gonorrhea. The presentation of oral gonorrhea is infrequent, nonspecific, and varied—that is, it may range from acute and severe ulceration with a pseudomembranous coating to slight or diffuse erythema of the oropharynx. Lesions of oral gonorrhea may closely resemble the lesions of erythema multiforme, bullous or erosive lichen planus, or herpetic gingivostomatitis, and have been reported to cause necrosis of the interdental papillae, lingual edema, edematous tissues that bleed easily, vesiculations, and a pseudomembrane that is nonadherent and leaves a bleeding surface on removal. Lesions may be solitary or widely disseminated. Lesions usually develop within 1 week of contact with an infected person; often, a history of fellatio is reported.[8,52] With involvement of the oropharynx, patients report a sore throat, and the mucosa becomes fiery red, with tiny pustules and an itching and burning sensation (Figure 13-11). Symptoms also include an increased salivation, bad taste, fetid breath, fever, and submandibular lymphadenopathy. When the tonsils become involved, they are invariably enlarged and inflamed, with or without a yellowish exudate. The patient may be asymptomatic or

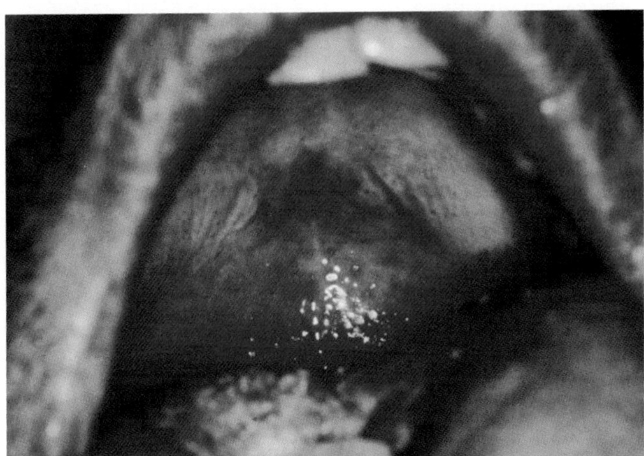

FIGURE 13-11 Gonococcal infection of the oral pharynx.

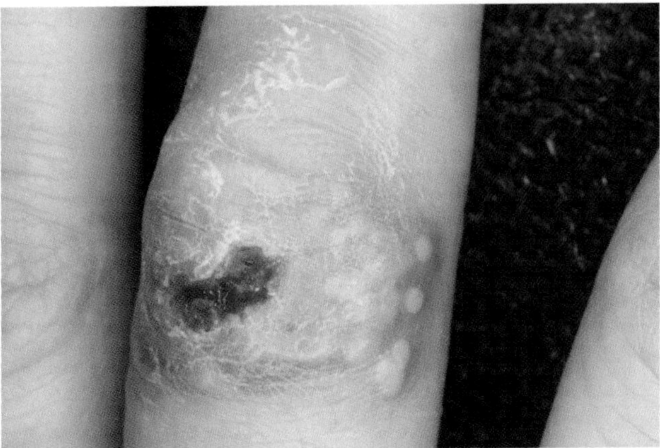

FIGURE 13-12 Herpetic whitlow. *(From Ibsen DAC, Phelan JA: Oral pathology for the hygienist, ed 5, St. Louis, 2009, Saunders. Courtesy Susan Rod Graham.)*

incapacitated, with limited oral function (eating, drinking, talking), depending on the degree of inflammation. Diagnosis of oral lesions should be attempted with a smear and Gram stain, followed by confirmatory tests.

The initial step in treatment is to ensure that the patient is under the care of a physician and is receiving proper antimicrobial therapy. Thereafter, treatment of oral lesions is symptomatic (see Appendix C). The patient should be assured that oral infection will resolve with the use of appropriate antibiotics.

Syphilis. Syphilitic chancres and mucous patches usually are painless, unless they become secondarily infected. Both of these lesions are highly infectious. The chancre begins as a round papule that erodes into a painless ulcer with a smooth grayish surface (see Figure 13-4). Size can range from a few millimeters to 2 to 3 cm. A key feature is lymphadenopathy that may be unilateral. The intraoral mucous patch often appears as a slightly raised, asymptomatic papule(s) with an ulcerated or glistening surface. The lips, tongue, and buccal or labial mucosa may be affected. Both the chancre and the mucous patch (see Figure 13-5) regress spontaneously with or without antibiotic therapy, although chemotherapy is required to eradicate the systemic infection. The gumma is a painless lesion that may become secondarily infected. It is noninfectious and frequently occurs on and destroys the hard palate. Interstitial glossitis, the result of contracture of the tongue musculature after healing of a gumma, is viewed as a premalignant lesion. Oral manifestations of congenital syphilis include peg-shaped permanent central incisors with notching of the incisal edge (Hutchinson's incisors) (see Figure 13-6), defective molars with multiple supernumerary cusps (mulberry molars), atrophic glossitis, a high-arched and narrow palate, and perioral rhagades (skin fissures).

Genital Herpes. HSV-1–induced ulcers are more common in the oral cavity than are those caused by HSV-2; however, these lesions cannot be differentiated clinically, and both should be treated similarly with antiviral agents (see Box 13-1 and Appendix C). Oral and perioral herpetic lesions are infectious during the papular, vesicular, and ulcerative stages, and elective dental treatment should be delayed until the herpetic lesion has completely healed. Dental manipulation during these infectious stages poses risks of (1) inoculation to a new site on the patient, (2) development of infection in the dental care worker, and (3) aerosol or droplet inoculation of the conjunctivae of the patient or of dental personnel. Once the lesion has crusted, it can be considered to be relatively noninfectious.

A problem of particular concern to dentists is herpetic infection of the fingers or nail beds contracted by dermal contact with a herpetic lesion of the lip or oral cavity of a patient. The infection is called a *herpetic whitlow,* or a *herpetic paronychia* (Figure 13-12). It is serious, debilitating, and recurrent. Herpetic whitlow can be triggered to recur by trauma or vibration from operating dental handpieces. Also, asymptomatic HSV shedding at oral or nonoral sites can trigger erythema multiforme, a mucocutaneous eruption characterized by "target" papules and ulcers that results from an immune response to the virus.

Infectious Mononucleosis. Head, neck, and oral manifestations of infectious mononucleosis include fever, severe sore throat, palatal petechiae, and cervical lymphadenopathy. Lymph nodes in the anterior and posterior cervical chain often are enlarged and tender to palpation. After recovery, EBV is associated with the development of oral hairy leukoplakia, a benign entity, as well as Hodgkin and non-Hodgkin lymphomas.

Human Papillomavirus Infection. Condylomata acuminata commonly occur on the ventral tongue, gingiva, labial mucosa, and palate (see Figure 13-10, *B*). Transmission occurs by direct contact with infected anal, genital, or oral sites, or by self-inoculation. Lesions can be surgically excised, chemically removed with podophyllin, or laser-ablated. Caustic chemicals such as podophyllin are to be used with great caution to avoid damage to adjacent uninfected tissue, and should be rinsed off several hours after application. In addition, high-speed evacuation should be used during laser therapy to avoid inhalation of the virion-laden plume which can lead to laryngeal condylomata.[53]

The dentist also should be cognizant that a condyloma identified in children raises the suspicion for sexual child abuse when autoinoculation by hand-to-genital contact, nonsexual contact, or maternal fetal transmission has been ruled out. Failure to report signs of an STD to state health officials is a legal offense in some states. Tonsillar and base of the tongue squamous cell carcinomas are associated with high-risk HPVs.[54]

REFERENCES

1. Workowski KA, Berman S: Sexually transmitted diseases treatment guidelines, 2010, *MMWR Recomm Rep* 59(RR-12):1-110, 2010.
2. 2009 Sexually Transmitted Diseases Surveillance. http://www.cdc.gov/std/stats09/tables/21b.htm. Accessed March 14, 2011.
3. Gwanzura L, McFarland W, Alexander D, Burke RL, Katzenstein D: Association between human immunodeficiency virus and herpes simplex virus type 2 seropositivity among male factory workers in Zimbabwe, *J Infect Dis* 177(2):481-484, 1998.
4. Deguchi T, Nakane K, Yasuda M, Maeda S: Emergence and spread of drug resistant Neisseria gonorrhoeae, *J Urol* 184(3):851-858; quiz 1235, 2010.
5. Centers for Disease Control and Prevention: Trends in Sexually Transmitted Diseases in the United States: 2009 National Data for Gonorrhea, Chlamydia and Syphilis. http://www.cdc.gov/std/stats09/trends.htm. Accessed March 7, 2011.
6. STD Statistics for the USA. http://www.avert.org/std-statistics-america.htm. Accessed March 14, 2011.
7. McAdam AJ, Sharpe AH: Infectious diseases. In Kumar V, Abbas AK, Fausto N, Aster J, editors. *Robbins and Cotran's pathologic basis of disease.* 8th ed. Philadelphia, 2010, W.B. Saunders.
8. Balmelli C, Gunthard HF: Gonococcal tonsillar infection–a case report and literature review, *Infection* 31(5):362-365, 2003.
9. Escobar V, Farman AG, Arm RN: Oral gonococcal infection, *Int J Oral Surg* 13(6):549-554, 1984.
10. Summary of notifiable diseases, United States. 1990, *MMWR Morb Mortal Wkly Rep* 39(53):1-61, 1991.
11. Giunta JL, Fiumara NJ: Facts about gonorrhea and dentistry, *Oral Surg Oral Med Oral Pathol* 62(5):529-531, 1986.
12. Jamsky RJ, Christen AG: Oral gonococcal infections. Report of two cases, *Oral Surg Oral Med Oral Pathol* 53(4):358-362, 1982.
13. Kohn SR, Shaffer JF, Chomenko AG: Primary gonococcal stomatitis, *JAMA* 219(1):86, 1972.
14. Merchant HW, Schuster GS: Oral gonococcal infection, *J Am Dent Assoc* 95(4):807-809, 1977.
15. Schmidt H, Hjorting-Hansen E, Philipsen HP: Gonococcal stomatitis, *Acta Derm Venereol* 41:324-327, 1961.
16. Chue PW: Gonococcal arthritis of the temporomandibular joint, *Oral Surg Oral Med Oral Pathol* 39(4):572-577, 1975.
17. Van Dyck E, Ieven M, Pattyn S, Van Damme L, Laga M: Detection of Chlamydia trachomatis and Neisseria gonorrhoeae by enzyme immunoassay, culture, and three nucleic acid amplification tests, *J Clin Microbiol* 39(5):1751-1756, 2001.
18. Grosskurth H, Mosha F, Todd J, Mwijarubi E, Klokke A, Senkoro K, et al: Impact of improved treatment of sexually transmitted diseases on HIV infection in rural Tanzania: randomised controlled trial, *Lancet* 346(8974):530-536, 1995.
19. Syphilis Surveillance Profiles and Annual Reports - All Years. http://www.cdc.gov/std/Syphilis/syphilis-stats-all-years.htm. Accessed March 14, 2011.
20. McAdam AJ, Sharpe AH: Infectious diseases. In Kumar V, Abbas AK, Fausto N, editors. *Robbins and Cotran's pathologic basis of disease.* Philadelphia, 2009, W.B. Saunders.
21. Lowhagen GB: Syphilis: test procedures and therapeutic strategies, *Semin Dermatol* 9(2):152-159, 1990.
22. Little JW: Syphilis: an update, *Oral Surg Oral Med Oral Pathol Oral Radiol Endod* 100(1):3-9, 2005.
23. Hook EW, 3rd, Marra CM: Acquired syphilis in adults, *N Engl J Med* 326(16):1060-1069, 1992.
24. Southwick KL, Guidry HM, Weldon MM, Mert KJ, Berman SM, Levine WC: An epidemic of congenital syphilis in Jefferson County, Texas, 1994-1995: inadequate prenatal syphilis testing after an outbreak in adults, *Am J Public Health* 89(4):557-560, 1999.
25. Fleming DT, McQuillan GM, Johnson RE, Nahmias AJ, Aral SO, Lee FK, et al: Herpes simplex virus type 2 in the United States, 1976 to 1994, *N Engl J Med* 337(16):1105-1111, 1997.
26. Armstrong GL, Schillinger J, Markowitz L, Nahmias AJ, Johnson RE, McQuillan GM, et al: Incidence of herpes simplex virus type 2 infection in the United States, *Am J Epidemiol* 153(9):912-920, 2001.
27. Langenberg AG, Corey L, Ashley RL, Leong WP, Straus SE: A prospective study of new infections with herpes simplex virus type 1 and type 2. Chiron HSV Vaccine Study Group, *N Engl J Med* 341(19):1432-1438, 1999.
28. Nahmias AJ, Roizman B: Infection with herpes-simplex viruses 1 and 2. 3, *N Engl J Med* 289(15):781-789, 1973.
29. Brown ZA, Wald A, Morrow RA, Selke S, Zeh J, Corey L: Effect of serologic status and cesarean delivery on transmission rates of herpes simplex virus from mother to infant, *JAMA* 289(2):203-209, 2003.
30. Corey L, Wald A, Patel R, Sacks SL, Tyring SK, Warren T, et al: Once-daily valacyclovir to reduce the risk of transmission of genital herpes, *N Engl J Med* 350(1):11-20, 2004.
31. Physician desk reference. http://www.pdr.net/. Accessed March 14, 2011.
32. Miller CS, Avdiushko SA, Kryscio RJ, Danaher RJ, Jacob RJ: Effect of prophylactic valacyclovir on the presence of human herpesvirus DNA in saliva of healthy individuals after dental treatment, *J Clin Microbiol* 43(5):2173-2180, 2005.
33. Ebell MH: Epstein-Barr virus infectious mononucleosis, *Am Fam Physician* 70(7):1279-1287, 2004.
34. Godshall SE, Kirchner JT: Infectious mononucleosis. Complexities of a common syndrome, *Postgrad Med* 107(7):175-179, 83-4, 86, 2000.
35. Crawford DH, Macsween KF, Higgins CD, Thomas R, McAulay K, Williams H, et al: A cohort study among university students: identification of risk factors for Epstein-Barr virus seroconversion and infectious mononucleosis, *Clin Infect Dis* 43(3):276-282, 2006.
36. Lawee D: Mild infectious mononucleosis presenting with transient mixed liver disease: case report with a literature review, *Can Fam Physician* 53(8):1314-1316, 2007.
37. Auwaerter PG: Infectious mononucleosis in middle age, *JAMA* 281(5):454-459, 1999.
38. Luzuriaga K, Sullivan JL: Infectious mononucleosis, *N Engl J Med* 362(21):1993-2000, 2010.
39. Balfour HH, Jr., Holman CJ, Hokanson KM, Lelonek MM, Giesbrecht JE, White DR, et al: A prospective clinical study of Epstein-Barr virus and host interactions during acute infectious mononucleosis, *J Infect Dis* 192(9):1505-1512, 2005.

40. Balfour HH, Jr., Hokanson KM, Schacherer RM, Fietzer CM, Schmeling DO, Holman CJ, et al: A virologic pilot study of valacyclovir in infectious mononucleosis, *J Clin Virol* 39(1):16-21, 2007.
41. Forcier M, Musacchio N: An overview of human papillomavirus infection for the dermatologist: disease, diagnosis, management, and prevention, *Dermatol Ther*; 23(5):458-476, 2010.
42. Brown TJ, Yen-Moore A, Tyring SK: An overview of sexually transmitted diseases. Part II, *J Am Acad Dermatol* 41(5 Pt 1):661-677; quiz 78-80, 1999.
43. Koutsky L: Epidemiology of genital human papillomavirus infection, *Am J Med* 102(5A):3-8, 1997.
44. Ault KA: Epidemiology and natural history of human papillomavirus infections in the female genital tract, *Infect Dis Obstet Gynecol* 2006(Suppl):40470, 2006.
45. Wiley D, Masongsong E: Human papillomavirus: the burden of infection, *Obstet Gynecol Surv* 61(6 Suppl 1):S3-S14, 2006.
46. Cates W, Jr: Estimates of the incidence and prevalence of sexually transmitted diseases in the United States. American Social Health Association Panel, *Sex Transm Dis* 26(4 Suppl):S2-S7, 1999.
47. Munk C, Svare EI, Poll P, Bock JE, Kjaer SK: History of genital warts in 10,838 women 20 to 29 years of age from the general population. Risk factors and association with Papanicolaou smear history, *Sex Transm Dis* 24(10):567-572, 1997.
48. Ahmed AM, Madkan V, Tyring SK: Human papillomaviruses and genital disease, *Dermatol Clin* 24(2):157-165, vi, 2006.
49. Moscicki AB: HPV vaccines: today and in the future, *J Adolesc Health* 43(4 Suppl):S26-S40, 2008.
50. Swinehart JM, Skinner RB, McCarty JM, Miller BH, Tyring SK, Korey A, et al: Development of intralesional therapy with fluorouracil/adrenaline injectable gel for management of condylomata acuminata: two phase II clinical studies, *Genitourin Med* 73(6):481-487, 1997.
51. Cleveland JL, Bond WW: Recommended infection-control practices for dentistry, 1993, *MMWR Morb Mortal Wkly Rep* 42(RR-8):1-12, 1993.
52. Chue PW: Gonorrhea–its natural history, oral manifestations, diagnosis, treatment, and prevention, *J Am Dent Assoc* 90(6):1297-1301, 1975.
53. Hallmo P, Naess O: Laryngeal papillomatosis with human papillomavirus DNA contracted by a laser surgeon, *Eur Arch Otorhinolaryngol* 248(7):425-427, 1991.
54. Syrjanen S, Lodi G, von Bultzingslowen I, Aliko A, Arduino P, Campisi G, et al: Human papillomaviruses in oral carcinoma and oral potentially malignant disorders: a systematic review, *Oral Dis* 17(Suppl 1):58-72, 2011.
55. Russel MG, Volovics A, Schoon EJ, van Wijlick EH, Logan RF, Shivananda S, et al: Inflammatory bowel disease: is there any relation between smoking status and disease presentation? European Collaborative IBD Study Group, *Inflamm Bowel Dis* 4(3):182-186, 1998.

PART VI

Endocrine and Metabolic Disease

14

Diabetes Mellitus

BACKGROUND AND DEFINITIONS

Diabetes mellitus is a group of metabolic diseases characterized by high blood glucose levels (hyperglycemia) and the inability to produce and/or use insulin. The disease is defined by abnormal blood glucose levels and utilization and is classified by the American Diabetes Association into four general types (Box 14-1).[1] The four types are determined by the underlying mechanism, each demonstrating different levels of glycemia (Figure 14-1).

Type 1 diabetes is primarily the result of pancreatic beta cell destruction and is characterized by insulin deficiency. *Type 2 diabetes* is characterized by insulin resistance and relative insulin deficiency. The broad category of *other specific types* (see Box 14-1) comprises more than 56 pathologic conditions that are attributed to genetic defects in beta cell function, as well as diseases or infections that cause diabetes. *Gestational diabetes* is abnormal glucose tolerance that first appears or is detected during pregnancy. In addition, there are two types of *prediabetes:* impaired glucose tolerance and impaired fasting glucose. Persons who have abnormal blood glucose levels that are not high enough to be classified as diabetes are assigned a diagnosis of prediabetes.

Diabetes affects persons of all ages and is a chronic condition. Persistent hyperglycemia leads to metabolic and vascular complications as well as a variety of clinical neuropathies that are costly to manage.[2,3] The vascular complications include premature macrovascular disease and serious microvascular disease. The metabolic component involves the elevation of blood glucose associated with alterations in lipid protein metabolism, resulting from a relative or absolute lack of insulin. Maintenance of good glycemic control can prevent or retard the development of microvascular complications of diabetes. The vascular component includes an accelerated onset of nonspecific atherosclerosis and a more specific microangiopathy that particularly affects the eyes and kidneys. Retinopathy and nephropathy are eventual complications in nearly every person with chronic diabetes. These complications result in serious morbidity.[4]

Diabetes mellitus is of great importance to dentists, because dentists are in a position as members of a health care team to detect many new cases of this disease. Also, dentists must be able to render care to patients already under medical management for their disease without endangering their well-being. A crucial aspect of care of the dental patient who has diabetes is determination of the level of disease severity and the level of glycemic control, as well as the presence of complications from diabetes, so that appropriate dental treatment can be provided. Essential to this determination is knowledge of the patient's blood glucose level at the time that dental treatment is provided.

Incidence and Prevalence

More than 240 million persons worldwide have diabetes mellitus, and health officials estimate that this figure will exceed 300 million within the next 10 years.[5,6] Nearly 26 million Americans, representing 8.3% of the entire population, are living with diabetes. Of these, 7 million cases have not been diagnosed. In 2009, 1.9 million new cases of diabetes were diagnosed among adults in the United States. The disease affects 16.1% of Native Americans and Alaska Natives, 12.6% blacks, 11.8% Hispanics, and 7.1% of whites. Diabetes mellitus accounts for about 71,000 deaths per year and is the seventh most common cause of death in the United States.[7-9]

Type 2 disease is the most prevalent type of diabetes mellitus. Of patients with diabetes in the United States, 90% to 95% have type 2 disease. The incidence of type 2 diabetes increases with age, and is primarily an adult disease. In contrast, type 1 diabetes occurs in 0.3% of Americans but is more than four times more prevalent than type 2 diabetes in persons younger than 20 years of age. Currently, there are about 23 million persons with type 2 disease (90%), 2.6 million with type 1 disease (10%), 79 million who have prediabetes, and approximately 12% of the general population in the United States who have impaired glucose tolerance. It is estimated that about 210,000 people younger than 20 years of age have diabetes (0.26% of all people in this age group). The vast majority of undiagnosed cases of diabetes are of the type 2 variety.[8,10,11]

The prevalence of diabetes mellitus has increased more than six-fold in the United States over the past several decades. The major reason for the dramatic increase is the obesity epidemic—especially in relation to type 2 diabetes. Recent reports indicate that more than 60% of patients with type 2 diabetes are obese at the time of diagnosis, and more than two thirds of U.S.

adults are overweight or obese. Obesity is a major factor in the continual rise in the number of cases of diabetes in the United States.[12] Obesity in American youth contributes to the rising number of cases in this segment of the population. Other factors associated with the increasing prevalence of diabetes are the increasing population, increasing life expectancy, and increasing number of affected persons who are having children who will pass on the disease.[4,10,12]

BOX 14-1	Current Classification of Diabetes

Type 1	• Beta cell destruction, usually leading to absolute insulin deficiency
	  • Immune-mediated: presence of islet cell or insulin antibodies that identify the autoimmune process, leading to beta cell destruction
	  • Idiopathic: no evidence of autoimmunity

Type 2	• Insulin resistance with relative insulin deficiency/insulin secretory defect with insulin resistance
Other specific types	• Genetic defects of beta cell function or insulin action, diseases of exocrine pancreas, endocrinopathies, drug- or chemical-induced diabetes, infections, uncommon forms of immune-mediated diabetes, other genetic syndromes • Impaired fasting glucose (impaired glucose tolerance) • Abnormalities of fasting glucose (abnormal glucose tolerance)
Gestational	• Any degree of abnormal glucose tolerance during pregnancy diabetes

Data from American Diabetes Association: Standards of Care—2011, Diabetes Care *34(Suppl 1):S11-S61, 2011.*

Etiology

Diabetes results from several pathogenic processes ranging from autoimmune destruction of pancreatic beta cells in type 1 diabetes to abnormalities that cause insulin resistance (type 2 diabetes). Type 1 diabetes is thought to be the result of genetic, autoimmune, and environmental factors. The genetic component is demonstrated by data showing concordance rates of 30% to 40% amongst identical twins. HLA genes on chromosome 6 are linked to type 1 diabetes. Autoantibodies against beta cell constituents are present in 85% to 90% of patients with type 1 diabetes, and destruction of beta cells is modulated by T cells. Viral infections (mumps, rubella, and coxsackievirus infection) are suggested environmental factors that could trigger the autoimmune response associated with type 1 disease. About 10% to 15% of cases of type 1 diabetes are of unknown etiology (i.e., idiopathic).[1,4]

Type 2 diabetes has genetic, environmental, and aging components. Positive family history confers a lifetime risk of 38% to the offspring if one parent is affected, and 60% if both parents are affected.[13] Identical twin concordance rates approach 100%.[4] The peroxisome proliferator-activated receptor γ (PPARγ) gene, which has a key role in regulation of adipogenic differentiation, is a candidate gene of type 2 diabetes, however the disease is likely multigenic. Together the genetic and environmental factors contribute to defects in insulin receptor function, insulin receptor signal transduction,

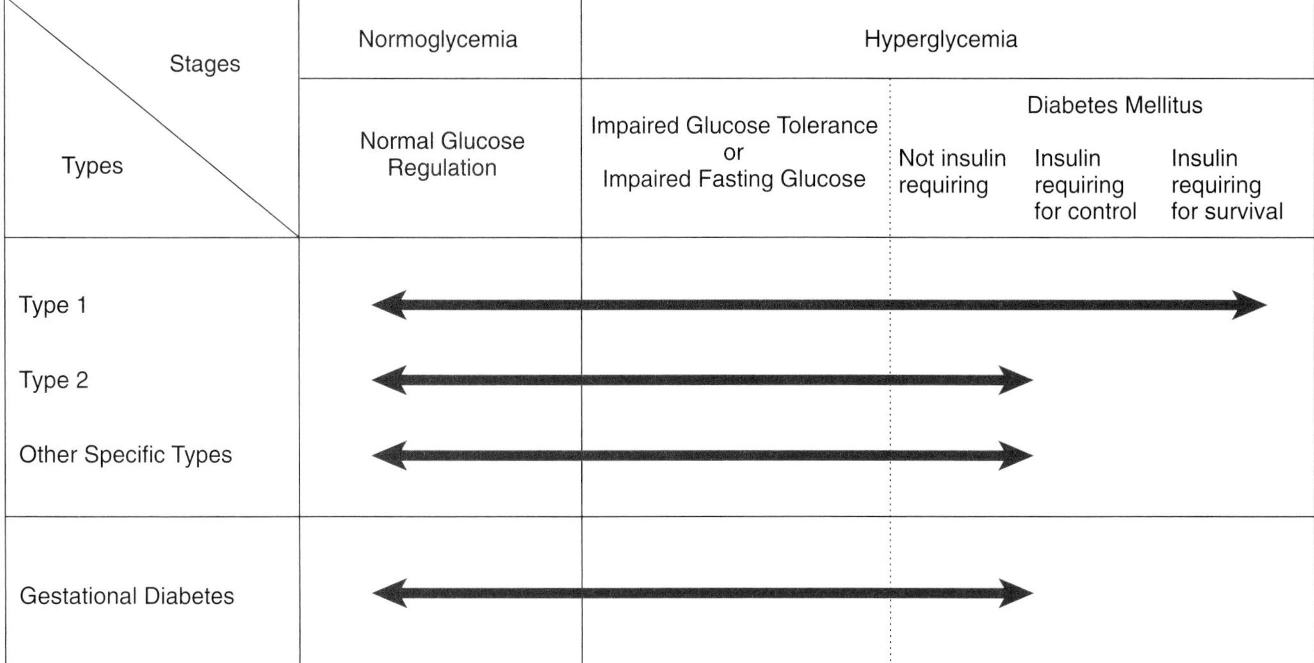

FIGURE 14-1 Disorders of glycemia: etiologic types, stages, and requirements for insulin. Range of glycemic control are indicated by *arrows. (From the American Diabetes Association: Diagnosis and classification of diabetes mellitus,* Diabetes Care *34(Suppl 1):S62-69, 2011.)*

insulin secretion, glucose transport and phosphorylation, glycogen synthesis, glucose oxidation that contribute to insulin resistance, and accelerated endogenous glucose production. Obesity and lack of physical activity are the primary environmental factors involved in the pathogenesis of type 2 diabetes.[1,13,14]

Other specific types of diabetes can be caused by specific gene defects, endocrine conditions such as primary destruction of islet cells through inflammation, cancer, surgery, hyperpituitarism, or hyperthyroidism. Iatrogenic disease that occurs after steroid administration is a known cause.

Gestational diabetes mellitus occurs in 5% to 7% of pregnant women during pregnancy. Obesity during pregnancy is a known risk factor for the condition. After childbirth, the mother's glycemic control usually returns to normal, but these women have an increased risk of developing diabetes within 5 to 10 years. Gestational diabetes enhances the risk for loss of the fetus and is associated with increased size of surviving fetuses. Insulin resistance is the suggested underlying etiopathogenic mechanism. A genetic basis may play a role; however, the underlying genetic factors have not yet been identified.[15,16]

Pathophysiology and Complications

Persistent elevated blood glucose levels put persons at risk for diabetes. In fact, about 11% of people with prediabetes who were followed annually developed overt diabetes each year during the average 3 years of follow-up.[17] An overview of the pathophysiologic processes involved is presented next.

Glucose is rapidly taken up by the pancreatic beta cell and serves as the most important stimulus for insulin secretion. Insulin remains in circulation for only several minutes (half-life [$t_{1/2}$], 4 to 8 minutes); it then interacts with target tissues (e.g., muscle, liver, fat cells) and binds with cell surface insulin receptors. Secondary intracellular messengers are activated and interact with cellular effector systems, including enzymes and glucose transport proteins. Lack of insulin or deficient action of insulin leads to abnormalities in carbohydrate, fat, and protein metabolism (i.e, increased production of glucose from glycogen, fat, and protein). This combination of underutilization and overproduction of glucose attained through glycogenolysis and fat metabolism results in glucose accumulation in the tissue fluids and in blood[18] (Figure 14-2).

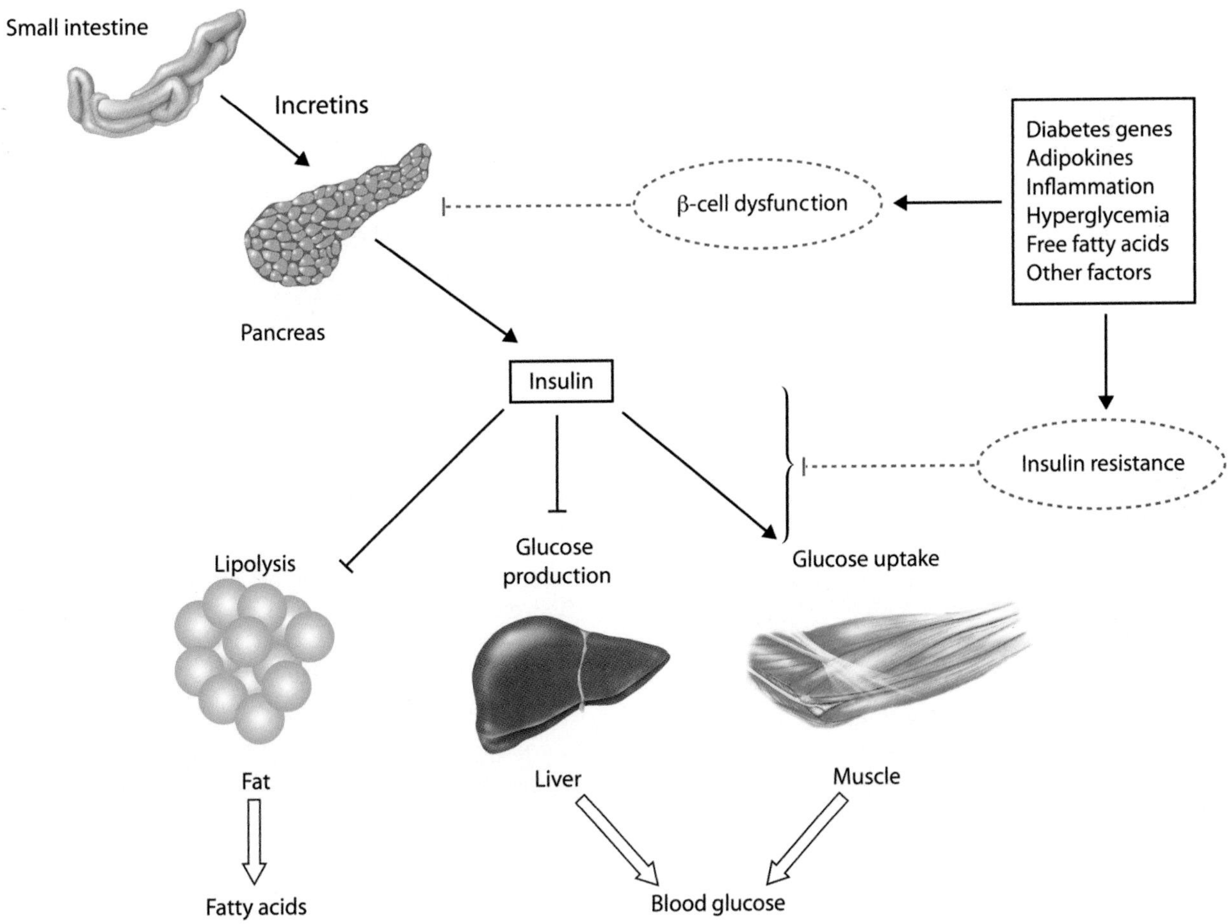

FIGURE 14-2 Pathophysiology of hyperglycemia and target tissues. *(Courtesy Mary Lous Cahal, University of Kentucky.)*

Hyperglycemia leads to glucose excretion in the urine, which results in increased urinary volume. The increase in fluid lost through urine may lead to dehydration and loss of electrolytes. With type 2 diabetes, prolonged hyperglycemia can lead to significant losses of fluid in the urine. When this type of severe dehydration occurs, urinary output drops, and a hyperosmolar nonketotic coma may result. This condition is seen most often in elderly persons with type 2 diabetes.[18]

Lack of glucose utilization by many cells of the body leads to cellular starvation. The patient often increases intake of food but in many cases still loses weight. If these events continue to progress, the person with type 1 diabetes develops metabolic acidosis. For a time, the body may be able to maintain the pH at nearly normal levels, but as the buffer system and respiratory and renal regulators fail to compensate, body fluids become more acidic (i.e., pH falls). Severe acidosis will lead to coma and death if it is not identified and treated. The primary manifestations of diabetes—hyperglycemia, ketoacidosis, and vascular wall disease—contribute to the inability of patients with uncontrolled diabetes to fight infection and to characteristic poor wound healing. The end results of these effects, as well as others yet to be identified, are that the patient with uncontrolled diabetes is rendered much more susceptible to infection, the patient's ability to deal with an infection once it has been established is reduced, and healing of traumatic and surgical wounds is delayed.[18,19]

Patients with diabetes demonstrate significant effects of the disease on long-term survival, which is affected by the type of diabetes, age at diagnosis, and compliance with therapy (Table 14-1). Few deaths occur among patients diagnosed before the age of 30 years. However, in persons diagnosed before age 40, less than half are still alive by age 55. In a recent study of 3589 diabetics, the 10-year survival rate still remained below 65%.[20] In addition to decreasing life expectancy by at least 5 to 10 years, the complications of diabetes mellitus lead to significant signs and symptoms that impair the quality of life.[21,22]

Complications of diabetes are related to the level of hyperglycemia and pathologic changes that occur within the vascular system and the peripheral nervous system (Box 14-2). The vascular complications result from microangiopathy and atherosclerosis. The mechanisms by which hyperglycemia may lead to microvascular and atherosclerotic complications include increased accumulation of polyols through the aldose reductase pathway, advanced glycation end products, and increased production of vascular endothelial cell growth factor (VEGF).[23] Vessel changes include thickening of the intima, endothelial proliferation, lipid deposition, and accumulation of *para*-aminosalicylic acid–positive material. These changes can be seen throughout the body but have particular clinical importance when they occur within the retina and the small vessels of the kidney.[4,24]

Retinopathy occurs in all forms of diabetes. It consists of nonproliferative changes (microaneurysms, retinal hemorrhages, retinal edema, and retinal exudates) and proliferative changes (neovascularization, glial proliferation, and vitreoretinal traction) and is the leading cause of blindness in the United States. The incidence of blindness in all persons with diabetes is 0.2% per year; it is 0.6% per year for diabetic patients with retinopathy. Proliferative retinopathy is most common among patients with type 1 diabetes; a much lower incidence is seen among those with type 2 diabetes. Cataracts occur at an earlier age and with greater frequency in those with type 1 diabetes. The typical cataract, senile cataract, is identified in 59% of persons with diabetes aged 35 to 55 years but in only 12% of those without the disease. Young people with diabetes are prone to the development of metabolic cataracts. The risk that a person with diabetes will become blind is 20 times greater than that for the general population.[4,25]

TABLE 14-1 Expected Years of Additional Life in Persons with and without Diabetes Compared With Given-Age Cohorts

Attained Age of Diabetic (Years)	Expected Years Additional Life in Nondiabetic	Expected Years Additional Life in Diabetic	Years Lost Because of Diabetes
10	61.5	44.3	17.2
20	51.9	36.1	13.8
30	42.5	30.1	12.4
40	33.3	23.7	9.6

BOX 14-2 Complications of Diabetes Mellitus (DM)

Metabolic disturbances: ketoacidosis and hyperosmolar nonketotic coma (type 2 diabetes)
Cardiovascular: accelerated atherosclerosis (coronary heart disease[1]); two thirds have high blood pressure; risk for stroke and heart disease death is 2 to 4 times higher among people with DM
Eyes: retinopathy, cataracts; DM is leading cause of new cases of blindness among adults
Kidney: diabetic nephropathy; DM is leading cause of renal failure
Extremities: ulceration and gangrene of feet; DM is leading cause of non–accident-related leg and foot amputations
Diabetic neuropathy: dysphagia, gastric distention, diarrhea, impotence, muscle weakness or cramps, numbness, tingling, deep burning pain
Early death: DM is the seventh leading cause of death in the United States, most commonly due to cardiovascular disease

Data from Centers for Disease Control and Prevention. National diabetes fact sheet: national estimates and general information on diabetes and prediabetes in the United States, 2011. Atlanta, GA: U.S. Department of Health and Human Services, Centers for Disease Control and Prevention, 2011.

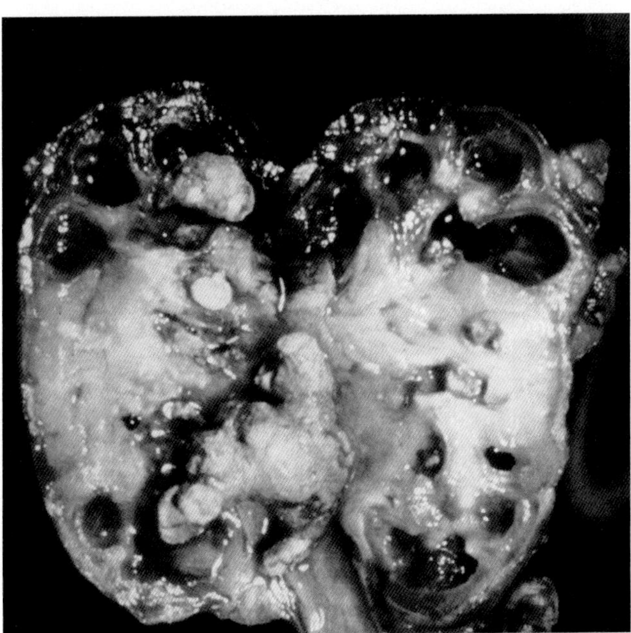

FIGURE 14-3 Diabetic nephropathy: cross section of kidney. *(Courtesy Richard Estensen, MD, Minneapolis, Minnesota.)*

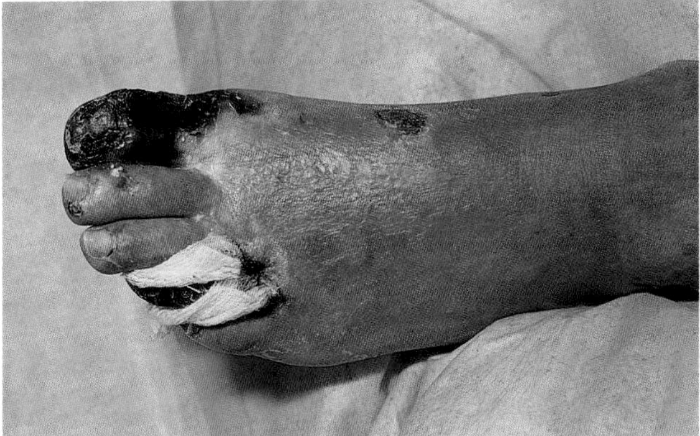

FIGURE 14-4 Diabetic gangrene of the feet. *(From Swartz MH:* Textbook of physical diagnosis: history and examination, *ed 6, Philadelphia, 2010, Saunders.)*

Diabetics are 25 times more likely to acquire end-stage renal disease than persons without diabetes.[12] Diabetic nephropathy leads to end-stage renal disease in 30% to 40% of patients with type 1 diabetes (Figure 14-3) and in 5% of patients with type 2 diabetes. However, because type 2 diabetes is much more common than type 1, the number of persons with renal failure is the same for the two types of diabetes. Renal failure is the leading cause of death in patients with type 1 diabetes. Of all patients who undergo dialysis, 37% have diabetes. Microangiopathy in the kidney usually involves the capillaries of the glomerulus.[8,26,27]

Macrovascular disease (atherosclerosis) occurs earlier and is more widespread and more severe in persons with diabetes. In patients with type 1 diabetes, atherosclerosis seems to develop independent of microvascular disease (microangiopathy). Hyperglycemia plays a role in the evolution of atherosclerotic plaques. Persons with uncontrolled diabetes have increased levels of low-density lipoprotein (LDL) cholesterol and reduced levels of high-density lipoprotein (HDL) cholesterol. Attainment of normal glycemia often improves the LDL-to-HDL ratio.[2]

A major determinant of the morbidity associated with poor glycemic control in diabetes is accelerated atherosclerosis. Atherosclerosis increases the risks of ulceration and gangrene of the feet (Figure 14-4), hypertension, renal failure, coronary insufficiency, myocardial infarction, and stroke. The most common cause of death in patients with type 2 diabetes is myocardial infarction. By age 60, a third of all persons with diabetes die of complications from coronary heart disease (CHD). Women with diabetes treated with insulin are at higher risk for CHD than non–insulin-treated women. This is not true for insulin-treated men. Also, diabetics are at a two- to four-fold greater risk for myocardial infarction and stroke than in persons without the disease, and a person with diabetes has less chance of surviving a myocardial infarction than that typical for a nondiabetic person.[2,7,28]

In the extremities, diabetic neuropathy may lead to muscle weakness, muscle cramps, a deep burning pain, tingling sensations, and numbness. In addition, tendon reflexes, two-point discrimination, and position sense may be lost. Some cases of oral paresthesia and burning tongue are caused by this complication.[4,29-31]

Diabetic neuropathy also may involve the autonomic nervous system. Esophageal dysfunction may cause dysphagia, stomach involvement may cause a loss of motility with massive gastric distention, and involvement of the small intestine may result in nocturnal diabetic diarrhea. Sexual impotence and bladder dysfunction also may occur. Diabetic neuropathy is common with type 1 and type 2 diabetes and may occur in more than 50% of patients. Neuropathy progresses over time in type 2 diabetes, and this increase may be greater in patients with hypoinsulinemia.[4,29-31]

Diabetes is associated with skin rashes, deposits of fat in the skin (xanthoma diabeticorum), decubitus ulcerations, poor wound healing, and gangrenous extremities. The relative risk that patients with diabetes will require amputation of an extremity because of diabetic complications is more than 40 times that of normal persons. Recent data show that more than 65,000 amputations are performed annually in patients with diabetes mellitus. This number represents more than 60% of all non-traumatic amputations.[8]

The severity of complications of diabetes is largely dependent on the level of glycemic control.[32] In one longitudinal study conducted over a period of more than 17 years, scientists demonstrated that diabetic patients with good glycemic control (hemoglobin A_{1c} levels below 7%) had 42% fewer systemic complications and 57% fewer deaths than those reported for patients with diabetes and poorly controlled hyperglycemia (HbA1c levels above 8%).[2] Thus, a strong case can be made for early diagnosis and appropriate glycemic control to prevent or reduce progression of complications.

CLINICAL PRESENTATION

Signs and Symptoms

In patients with type 1 diabetes, the onset of symptoms is sudden and acute, often developing over days or weeks. Typically the diagnosis is made in nonobese children or young adults less than 40 years of age; however it may occur at any age. Signs and symptoms include polydipsia, polyuria, polyphagia, weight loss, loss of strength, marked irritability, recurrence of bed wetting, drowsiness, malaise, and blurred vision. Patients also may present with ketoacidosis, which if severe is accompanied by vomiting, abdominal pain, nausea, tachypnea, paralysis, and loss of consciousness.[4]

Type 2 diabetes generally occurs after age 40 and more often affects obese individuals. The onset of symptoms in type 2 diabetes usually is insidious, and the cardinal manifestations and symptoms (polydipsia, polyuria, polyphagia, weight loss, and loss of strength) are less commonly seen.[1,4] The signs and symptoms of type 1 and type 2 diabetes are summarized in Table 14-2 and Box 14-3.

Other signs and symptoms related to the complications of diabetes include skin lesions, cataracts, blindness, hypertension, chest pain, and anemia. The rapid onset of myopia in an adult is highly suggestive of diabetes mellitus.

TABLE 14-2 Clinical Features of Type 1 and Type 2 Diabetes

Feature	Type 1	Type 2
Frequency, % of person with diabetes	5-10	90-95
Age at onset (years)	15	40 and over
Body build	Normal or thin	Obese
Severity	Extreme	Mild
Insulin	Almost all	25% to 30%
Plasma glucagons	High, suppressible	High, resistant
Oral hypoglycemic agents	Few respond	50% respond
Ketoacidosis	Common	Uncommon
Complications	90% in 20 years	Less common
Rate of clinical onset	Rapid	Slow
Stability	Unstable	Stable
Genetic locus	Chromosome 6	Chromosomes 2, 7, 12, 13, 17
HLA and abnormal autoimmune reactions	Present	Not present
Insulin receptor defects	Usually not found	Often found

HLA, Human leukocyte antigen.

Laboratory Findings

The American Diabetes Association recommends screening tests for diabetes mellitus for all persons who are 45 years of age and older, and for persons with risk factors such as obesity, family history, belonging to an ethnic or minority group at risk for diabetes, the combination of low HDL cholesterol and high triglycerides, high blood pressure, or gestational diabetes, and for women who have delivered large babies (weighing more than 9 lb at birth) or who have had spontaneous abortions or stillbirths, or have signs and symptoms of diabetes or its complications. For persons older than age 45, screening should occur routinely at 3-year intervals. Most screenings for diabetes involve evaluation for undiagnosed type 2 diabetes.[1]

The diagnostic criteria for diabetes relies on the plasma glucose level, either (1) at a random sampling, (2) after fasting, or (3) after a 75-g glucose test (oral glucose tolerance test, OGGT). Alternatively, the glycosylated hemoglobin test can be used. The American Diabetes Association criteria for diabetes are presented in Table 14-3.[1]

The primary diagnostic criterion for *impaired fasting glucose* is fasting plasma glucose levels of 100 to 125 mg/dL and for *impaired glucose tolerance* (IGT) is 140 to 199 mg/dL at 2 hours in the OGTT (Table 14-4).[1]

Blood Glucose Determination. Measurements of glucose are critical to the diagnosis and management of diabetes. Most glucose assays use enzymatic methods, based on either glucose dehydrogenase, glucose oxidase (coupled to ferricyanide) or glucose hexokinase. Of note, levels of blood glucose are influenced by the source of blood (venous versus capillary), the age of the patient, the nature of the diet, the physical activity level of the

BOX 14-3 Early Clinical Manifestations of Diabetes

Type 1
- *Cardinal signs/symptoms (common):* polydipsia, polyuria, polyphagia, weight loss, loss of strength
- *Other signs/symptoms:* recurrence of bed wetting, repeated skin infections, marked irritability, headache, drowsiness, malaise, dry mouth

Type 2
- *Cardinal signs/symptoms* (much less common): polydipsia, polyuria, polyphagia, weight loss, loss of strength
- *Frequent signs/symptoms:* slight weight loss or gain, gastrointestinal upset, nausea, urination at night, vulvar pruritus, blurred vision, decreased vision, paresthesias, dry flushed skin, loss of sensation, impotence, postural hypotension

TABLE 14-3 Diagnostic Criteria for Diabetes Mellitus*

1. FPG ≥126 mg/dL (7.0 mmol/L) on two occasions. Fasting is defined as no caloric intake for at least 8 hours. This fasting glucose value is consistently associated with the risk for retinopathy.

OR

2. Symptoms and signs of diabetes plus casual (random) plasma glucose concentration ≥200 mg/dL (11.1 mmol/L). *Casual* is defined as obtained at any time of day without regard to time since last meal. Many patients do not have obvious symptoms. The cardinal manifestations of diabetes include polyuria, polydipsia, and unexplained weight loss.

OR

3. 2-hour postload glucose ≥200 mg/dL (11.1 mmol/L) during an OGTT. The test should be performed as described by the WHO, using a glucose load containing the equivalent of 75 g anhydrous glucose dissolved in water.*

OR

4. Glycosylated hemoglobin (by A1C assay) ≥6.5%

*Oral glucose tolerance testng generally is not recommended in clinical practice.

FPG, Fasting plasma glucose; *OGTT*, Oral glucose tolerance test.; *WHO*, World Health Organization.

Data from Executive summary: standards of medical care in diabetes—2010: current criteria for the diagnosis of diabetes, Diabetes Care *33:S4-S10, 2010; Diagnosis and classification of diabetes mellitus,* Diabetes Care *33(Suppl 1):S62-S69, 2010; International Expert Committee Report on the Role of the A1C Assay in the Diagnosis of Diabetes,* Diabetes Care *32:1327-1334, 2009.*

TABLE 14-4 Categories of Increased Risk for Diabetes (Prediabetes)

Fasting Plasma Glucose Level (FPG)	2-Hour (75-g) Oral Glucose Tolerance Test (OGTT)		
	<140 mg/dL	**140-199 mg/dL**	**>200 mg/dL**
<100 mg/dL	Normal	IGT	Diabetes mellitus
100-125 mg/dL	IFG	IGT and IFG	Diabetes mellitus

Impaired fasting glucose (IFG): FPG levels 100-125 mg/dL

Impaired glucose tolerance (IGT): 2-hour values in the OGTT of 140-199 mg/dL

Data from the American Diabetes Association: Diagnosis and classification of diabetes mellitus, Diabetes Care 34(Suppl 1):S62-69, 2011.

patient, and the method used to measure the amount of sugar present in the blood sample. Abnormalities in diet (e.g., diet poor in carbohydrate for several days) can lead to misdiagnoses. To minimize this possibility, the diet should contain at least 250 to 300 g of carbohydrate on each of the 3 days before testing. Patients whose blood glucose level is going to be assessed should not participate in excessive physical activity, because exercise tends to lower blood glucose levels.[33,34]

Oral Glucose Tolerance Test. The OGTT reflects how quickly glucose is cleared from the blood—taking in consideration the rate of absorption, uptake by tissues, and excretion in urine. Glucose load is usually given as Glucola, which contains 75 g of glucose in a 7–fl oz bottle. Venous blood samples are drawn from the arm just before and most often at 2 hours after ingestion of the glucose. Urine samples also are collected at each interval. The most characteristic alterations seen in diabetes are an increased fasting blood glucose (126 mg/100 mL or higher), an increased peak value (200 mg/100 mL or higher), and a delayed return to normal in the 2-hour sample. Hypoglycemia may develop in persons with early, mild diabetes 3 to 5 hours after ingestion of glucose. For this reason, some physicians extend the glucose tolerance test period to 5 hours for some patients. Urine samples should not contain glucose at any point during the test.[35]

Glycohemoglobin. The extent of glycosylation of hemoglobin A (a nonenzymatic addition of glucose) that results in formation of HbA_{1c} (i.e., glycated hemoglobin) in red blood cells is used to detect and assess the long-term level (and control) of hyperglycemia in patients with diabetes (Table 14-5). The laboratory test to determine HbA_{1c} is known as the A1C assay. This assay measures the amount of sugar attached to Hb; levels increase in the presence of hyperglycemia. The A1C reflect glucose levels in the blood over the preceding 2 to 3 months. In health, patients should have HbA_{1c} levels less than 6%. In well-controlled diabetes, the level should stay below 7%, without the occurrence of clinically significant hypoglycemia.[35] The level of hyperglycemia as indicated by the A1C assay may reach as high as 20% in some cases of uncontrolled diabetes. Patients do not have to fast before they undergo testing, which is useful in monitoring progress of the disease. It is now standard practice to measure HbA_{1c} levels at least twice a year in patients whose treatment goals are being met (and who have stable glycemic control), and quarterly in patients whose treatment has changed or whose goals are not being met. Complications from diabetes are accelerated in patients with elevated HbA_{1c}. Therefore, monitoring is particularly important for those patients who are not monitoring their blood glucose at home on a regular basis.[35]

Urinary Glucose and Acetone. Determination of urinary glucose and acetone is of limited value in detecting overt diabetes.

Medical Management

Diabetes mellitus is not a curable disease; however, strict glycemic control established through regular monitoring reduces vascular and ocular complications.[1,12] Hence, the guidelines published by the American Diabetes Association target outcomes focused on glycemic control modified nutrient intake and weight reduction (as appropriate), blood pressure control, and a favorable lipid profile (Tables 14-5 and 14-6). For most patients a flexible treatment plan is devised that includes healthy food choices, physical activity recommendations, along with the use of

TABLE 14-5 Goals for Risk Factor Management in Patients with Diabetes

Risk Factor	Goal of Therapy	Recommending Body(ies)
Nutrition and obesity	Monitored carbohydrate intake; restrict alcohol, sodium, protein intake Weight loss to achieve ideal body weight	ADA, AHA, and NHLBI's ATP III, OEI, JNC VI, OEI (NHLBI)
Physical inactivity	Exercise prescription depending on patient's status	ADA
Cigarette smoking	Complete cessation	ADA
Blood pressure	<130/85 mm Hg <130/80 mm Hg	JNC VI (NHLBI) ADA
LDL cholesterol level	<100 mg/dL	ATP III (NHLBI), ADA
Triglyceride level 200-499 mg/dL	Non-HDL cholesterol level <130 mg/dL	ATP III (NHLBI)
HDL cholesterol level <40 mg/dL	Raise HDL (no set goal)	ATP III (NHLBI)
Prothrombotic state	Low-dose aspirin therapy (patients with CHD and other risk factors)	ADA
Glucose	Hemoglobin A_{1C} <7%	ADA

ADA, American Diabetes Association; *AHA,* American Heart Association; *ATP III,* National Cholesterol Education Program Adult Treatment Panel III; *BMI,* Body mass index; *CHD,* Coronary heart disease; *HDL,* High-density lipoprotein; *JNC VI,* Sixth Report of the Joint National Committee on Prevention, Evaluation, and Treatment of High Blood Pressure; *LDL,* Low-density lipoprotein; *NHLBI,* National Heart, Lung, and Blood Institute; *OEI,* Obesity Education Initiative Expert Panel on Identification, Evaluation, and Treatment of Overweight and Obesity in Adults.

Adapted from Grundy SM, et al: Prevention Conference VI: diabetes and cardiovascular disease: executive summary: conference proceeding for health care professionals from a special writing group of the American Heart Association, Circulation *105:2231-2239, 2002.*

oral hypoglycemic medications, insulin injections and insulin pumps (Box 14-4). These therapies generally are provided over many years. Management also involves medications to address the vascular, kidney and ocular complications, including antihypertensive drugs such as angiotensin-converting enzyme (ACE) inhibitors that reduce blood pressure, slow the decline of overall renal function, and reduce progression to diabetic neuropathy.[35] If standard therapies fail, pancreas and kidney transplantation or transplantation of pancreatic islet cells into the recipient's liver are options. However, transplantations are associated with a number of complications (see Chapter 21) including the lack of sufficient number of organ donors and less than 60% survival at 10 years.[36]

TABLE 14-6 American Diabetes Association (ADA) and American College of Endocrinology (ACE): Targets for Glycemia Management

Parameter	Normal	ADA*	ACE
Premeal plasma glucose (mg/dL)	<100 (mean ~90)	90-130	<110
Postprandial plasma glucose* (mg/dL)	<140	<180	<140
A_{1C}	4-6%	<7%	<6.5%

The ADA further recommends: (1) goals should be individualized; (2) certain populations (children, pregnant women, and elderly) require special considerations; (3) less intensive goals may be indicated in patients with severe or frequent hypoglycemia; (4) as indicated by epidemiologic analysis, more stringent glycemic goals (i.e., a normal A_{1C} assay result, <6%) may further reduce complications at the cost of increased risk of hypoglycemia; and (5) postprandial glucose may be targeted if A_{1C} goals are not met despite reaching preprandial glucose goals.

*Postprandial glucose measurements should be made 1 to 2 hours after the beginning of the meal, generally representing peak levels in patients with diabetes.

Adapted from American Diabetes Association: Standards of medical care in diabetes, Diabetes Care *27:S15-S35, 2004; and American College of Endocrinologists: American College of Endocrinology consensus statement on guidelines for glycemic control,* Endocr Pract *8(Suppl 1):5-11, 2002.*

BOX 14-4 Medical Management of Diabetes Mellitus

Type 1 Diabetes

- Diet and physical activity
- Insulin
  - Conventional
  - Multiple injections
  - Continuous infusion
  - Pancreatic transplantation (see Chapter 21)

Type 2 Diabetes

- Diet and physical activity
- Oral hypoglycemic agents
- Insulin plus oral hypoglycemic agents
- Insulin

In this section, discussion is limited to the common forms of diabetes, type 1 and type 2. Support for the management guidelines comes in large part from two large trials—the Diabetes Control and Complications Trial (DCCT) and the United Kingdom Prospective Diabetes Study (UKPDS).[12,35] In these trials, early and intensive therapy was advocated in which fasting blood glucose levels were targeted to be 70 to 120 mg/100 mL; postprandial blood glucose levels 180 mg/100 mL; and HbA_{1c} levels approximating the mean value in normal subjects. First steps were to manage blood glucose levels with diet and physical activity. If these methods failed, hypoglycemic agents were used (oral hypoglycemic agents, then insulin injections). The results of the DCCT indicated significant improvement in diabetic status and reduction of diabetic complications across the board.[37-39]

Pharmacologic Treatment of Type 1 Diabetes

Patients with type 1 diabetes are treated with some form of insulin.[40] In most cases, insulin is injected subcutaneously. Insulin therapies were first introduced in 1922 and for more than 60 years relied on animal insulins obtained from bovine or porcine pancreatic extracts, because of the similarity in amino acid structure to human insulin. However, the use of animal insulins was complicated by incomplete purification and tendency to induce the formation of antiinsulin antibodies. Now, human insulin is the only form of insulin sold in North America. Highly purified animal insulins are available because of cost in other countries.[40] Today, many patients wear an external programmable insulin pump used to deliver insulin by subcutaneous injection.

The type of insulin selected for use is based on the speed of onset, peak affect, and duration of action (Table 14-7). Insulins are characterized as either rapid-acting, short-acting, intermediate-acting, or long-acting preparations. Rapid-acting and short-acting preparations are used at meals (for bolus delivery), and intermediate-acting and long-acting insulins serve as basal insulins.[40,41]

TABLE 14-7 Insulin Preparations Classified by Pharmacodynamic Profile

	Onset of Action (hr)	Peak Action (hr)	Duration of Action (hr)
Rapid-Acting			
Insulin aspart	0.25-0.5	0.5-2.5	≤5
Insulin lispro	<0.25	1-3	3-5
Short-Acting			
Regular (soluble)	0.5-1	2-4	5-8
Intermediate-Acting			
NPH (Isophane)	1-2	2-8	14-24
Lente (insulin zinc suspension)	1-2	3-10	20-24
Long-Acting			
Ultralente	0.5-3	4-20	20-36
Insulin glargine	2-4	No pronounced peak	20-24
Insulin detemir	1	6-8	6-23
Premixed Combinations			
50% NPH, 50% regular	0.5-1	Dual (~4)	14-24
70% NPH, 30% regular	0.5-1	Dual (~4)	14-24
70% NPA, 30% aspart	<0.25	Dual (~3)	14-24
75% NPL, 25% lispro	<0.25	Dual (~4)	14-24

NPA, Neutral protamine aspart; *NPL*, Neutral protamine lispro. Both NPA and NPL are stable premixed combinations of intermediate- and short-acting insulins.

Data from Wolfsdorf JI, Weinstein DA: Management of diabetes in children. In DeGroot LJ, Jameson JL: Endocrinology, *ed 5, Philadelphia, 2006, Saunders; and Inzucchi SE, Sherwin RS: Diabetes mellitus. In Goldman L, Ausiello D, editors:* Cecil medicine, *ed 23, Philadelphia, 2008, Saunders.*

Two *rapid-acting insulin* analogues are available: *lispro* and *aspart.* Lispro is a human insulin analogue that has reversed the amino acids at positions 28 and 29 (lysine and proline) in the β chain. This change allows for more rapid absorption than regular (short-acting) insulin and effects beginning within 10 to 15 minutes of administration. Lispro acts similarly to monomeric human insulin, mimicking the normal prandial insulin surge in response to carbohydrate ingestion. Insulin aspart has a single amino acid substitution (aspartic acid for proline residue at position 28 of the β chain). It has a pharmacokinetic profile similar to that of lispro—both lasting for only 3 to 4 hours.[40,41]

Regular human insulin acts in about 30 minutes; thus, it is given about 30 minutes before a meal. It has a short duration of action (approximately 5 to 8 hours). It is used to blunt postprandial glucose elevations (after consumption of large meals), and is given during glucose elevations that occur during illness. In comparison with regular (short-acting) insulin, rapid-acting insulins are more convenient because they can be given just before eating.

The *intermediate-* and *longer-acting human insulins* were developed to delay their absorption after injection to mimic the basal insulin secretion seen in nondiabetic persons. *Neutral protamine Hagedorn* (NPH) insulin, first introduced in 1946, consists of a suspension of insulin complexed with protamine and zinc to delay its absorption. Another intermediate-acting insulin is *lente,* a crystalline suspension of insulin with zinc and acetate (see Table 14-7). NPH and lente show a substantial variation in subcutaneous absorption and are no longer widely available.[40,41]

Long-acting human insulins (Ultralente, glargine [Lantus], detemir) are to provide smooth basal insulin profiles. They take effect within 8 hours and reach peak effect 16 to 24 hours. The duration of effect can last more than 36 hours. Ultralente consists of a zinc suspension of insulin and is no longer widely available, because its effects may wane before 24 hours. Newer long-acting analogues, such as insulin *glargine,* which consists of two modifications to human insulin (two arginines added to the carboxyl terminus of the β chain and replacement of asparagine by glycine at position A21), and *detemir,* which has had the β30 amino acid of human insulin removed and a 14-carbon aliphatic fatty acid acylated to the B29 amino acid, show consistently delayed absorption and prolonged duration of activity.[40,41]

Premixed human insulin or premixed insulin analogues are available. Commonly used mixtures include NPH–regular 70/30, insulin lispro protamine suspension–insulin lispro 75/25, and insulin aspart protamine suspension–insulin aspart 70/30.[4,42]

Pramlintide, a noninsulin product, also is approved for the treatment of patients with type 1 and type 2 diabetes who have failed to achieve targets for glucose control despite optimal insulin therapy.[4] Additional detail on this agent is presented further on and in Table 14-8.

In some patients, CD3 antibody therapy can be added to slow the autoimmune attack and reduce insulin requirements.[4,43]

Insulin Regimens and Delivery. Insulin regimens for type 1 diabetics may be classified as conservative, intensive, or continuous insulin infusion with pumps. These regimens attempt to mimic physiologic insulin secretion through appropriate meal and basal insulin replacement. The choice generally is determined by patient factors, such as lifestyle, finances, and personal preference.[40,41]

A conservative approach can be taken in the early stages of type 1 diabetes when some degree of beta cell function is still intact. Here, two daily subcutaneous abdominal injections consisting of a mixture of intermediate-acting and short-or rapid-acting are given one before breakfast and one before dinner.[4,35] A problem with this approach is that the peak glucose-lowering effect of the evening intermediate-acting insulin injection is around 3 AM which can induce severe hypoglycemia.

Successful management often requires intensive (multidose) injections throughout the day with self-monitoring finger sticks (120 minutes after meals) to ensure proper glucose levels are maintained. These regimens often utilize two to three rapid-acting insulin injections with one (or two) intermediate or one long-acting insulin injection. Delivery is by needle injection using either disposable syringes or pen-and-cartridge devices. The needle and its injection site are changed every 48 to 72 hours to reduce the risk of infection. Of note, rapid- and short-acting insulin and basal (intermediate- and long-acting) insulins that are being taken at the same time can be drawn into the same syringe, with the exception of glargine, which cannot be mixed with other insulins.[35]

External insulin pumps with a real-time glucose sensor are available. The pumps are worn around the waist and provide continuous subcutaneous infusion of rapid-acting (or less frequently short-acting) insulin through a catheter inserted into the subcutaneous tissue of the abdominal wall[35,44,45] (Figure 14-5). The pump is programmed to deliver insulin continuously at a specified rate to meet the patient's basal insulin needs. For meal coverage, the patient uses the pump to deliver a specified bolus of insulin before eating. The major limitation is the cost of pump and necessary supplies (tubing), which must be changed every 48 to 72 hours. There is also a small risk of infection at the insertion site of the catheter. Finally, pump malfunction or catheter disruption can lead rapidly to hyperglycemia or ketoacidosis.

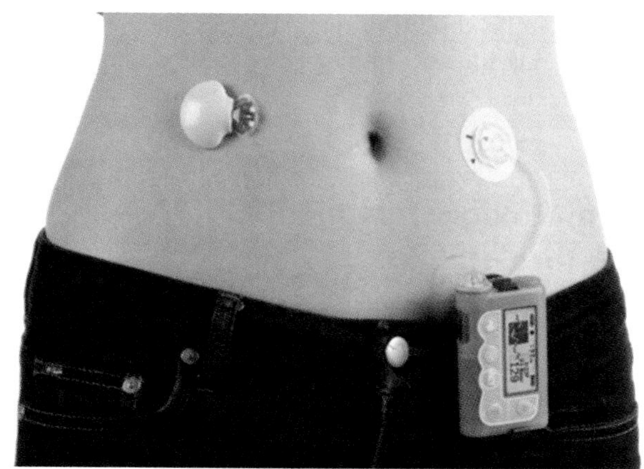

FIGURE 14-5 MiniMed Paradigm REAL-Time Revel System. The insulin pump is small and can be worn under clothing or on a belt. It delivers insulin through a tube or cannula (infusion set) that is inserted into the subcutaneous tissue. The pump can be disconnected for bathing, swimming, or changing clothes. A small sensor for glucose is inserted into the subcutaneous tissue using an automatic insertion device. Sensor data is sent to a transmitter that is attached to the skin with a waterproof adhesive patch. The transmitter sends data to the insulin pump using wireless technology. The sensor and tube (new tubing) from the pump must be relocated every 3 days to minimize the risk of infection obstruction of the tube. *(Courtesy Medtronics, Inc., Diabetes, Minneapolis, Minnesota.)*

Alternative routes of delivery of insulin continue to be of great interest. Options explored include nasal, pulmonary, oral, transdermal, and peritoneal delivery of insulin. These options have had only limited success to date.[5] The first inhaled version of insulin, Exubera (Pfizer Inc.), which became available in 2006, was withdrawn from the market in 2007 for lack of demand.[46,47] Implantable intraperitoneal insulin pumps (Medtronic Inc.) are now being used in Europe, with placement of more than 181 devices since 1995. They are in clinical trial and may soon be commercially available in the United States.[48] These implantable insulin pumps are placed directly into the abdominal subcutaneous tissues, with a catheter inserted directly into the peritoneal cavity. Insulin secretion is regulated by the patient from a handset, which signals the pump by way of the catheter to deliver insulin on demand. The pump reservoir holds a 2- to 3-month supply of insulin.

Treatment of Type 2 Diabetes

The management of type 2 diabetes involves lifestyle interventions, drug therapy, and control of risk factors for cardiovascular disease.[35] This includes control of blood glucose levels, blood pressure, lipid levels, and aspirin (antiplatelet) therapy, as indicated.[2] Most patients with type 2 diabetes under medical care are treated with one or more pharmacologic agents. If monotherapy is

TABLE 14-8 Noninsulin Antidiabetic Drugs

Class Drug	Mechanism of Action (Target Tissue)	Principal Adverse Effects	Drug Interaction(s)
Sulfonylureas *Administer 30 minutes before meals*			
First-Generation Chlorpropamide (Diabenese, Insulase) Acetohexamide (Dymelor) Tolazamide (Tolinase) Tolbutamide (Orinase)	Enhance insulin secretion (beta cells)	Hypoglycemia, weight gain, hyperinsulinemia	Salicylates and ketoconazole increase hypoglycemia
Second-Generation Glipizide (Glucotrol, Glucotrol XL) Glyburide (Micronase, Glynase, DiaBeta) Glimepiride (Amaryl)	Enhance insulin secretion (beta cells)	Hypoglycemia, weight gain, hyperinsulinemia	Corticosteroids decrease action
Biguanides *Administer with meals* Metformin (Foramet)	Reduce glucose production*	Gastrointestinal disturbances (abdominal pain, nausea, diarrhea), lactic acidosis	—
Gamma-Glucosidase Inhibitors *Administer just before meals* Acarbose (Precose) Miglitol (Glyset)	Delay carbohydrate digestion (gut)	Gastrointestinal disturbances (abdominal pain, nausea, diarrhea), liver function test elevation	—
Thiazolidinediones Glitazones *Administer with meals* Pioglitazone (Actos) Rosiglitazone (Avandia)	Improves insulin sensitivity (fat, muscle)	Headache, weight gain, flatulence Causes/exacerbates heart failure, decreased hemoglobin/hematocrit	—
Glinides *Administer 15 minutes before meals* Repaglinide (Prandin) Nateglinide (Starlix)	Enhance insulin secretion (beta cells)	Hypoglycemia (less than sulfonylureas), weight gain, hyperinsulinemia, hypersensitivity, increased uric acid levels	Increased risk of hypoglycemia with salicylates, nonselective beta blockers, NSAIDs Metabolism may be inhibited by azoles, erythromycin
Incretin (GLP-1) Analogues *Administer 15 minutes before meals* Exenatide (Byetta) *Injected subcutaneously* Liraglutide (Victoza) *Injected subcutaneously*	Enhance insulin secretion (beta cells), delay gastric emptying (gut), suppress prandial glucagon secretion	Gastrointestinal adverse effects (nausea, vomiting, diarrhea)	—
Amylin Analogue *Administer before meals* Pramlintide (Symlin) *Injected subcutaneously*	Aids absorption of glucose by slowing gastric emptying (gut), promotes satiety (hypothalamic receptors)	Gastrointestinal disturbances, headache	Avoid anticholinergics that alter gastrointestinal motility Can delay absorption of oral medications; administer oral hypoglycemic agents 1-2 hr after Symlin
Dipeptidyl Peptidase-4 Inhibitors *Administer once daily regardless of meals* Linagliptin (Tradjenta)	Inhibits enzymatic breakdown of GLP-1 and GIP; increases insulin secretion; decreases glucagon secretion (pancreas)	Runny nose, headache	Hypoglycemia may occur when combined with insulin or sulfonylurea drugs
Saxagliptin (Onglyza) Sitagliptin (Januvia)		Peripheral edema Headache	—
Combination Drugs Some combination drugs include glyburide and metformin (Glucovance), glipizide and metformin (Metaglip), and pioglitazone hydrochloride and glimepiride (Duetact).			

*Data from Dungan KM, Buse JB: Management of Type 2 Diabetes Mellitus. In Jameson JL, Degroot LJ (eds): Endocrinology, ed 6, 2010, Saunders.

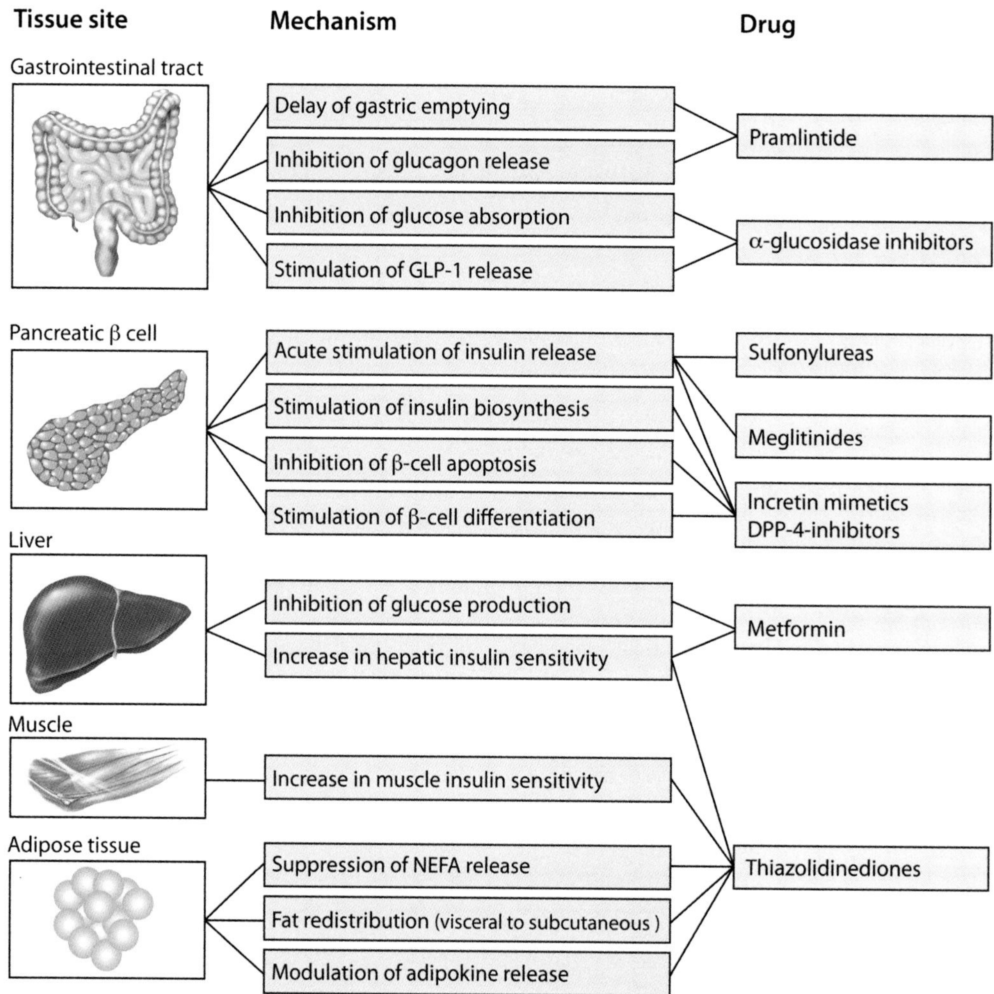

FIGURE 14-6 Antidiabetic agents used to treat hyperglycemia according to site and mechanism of action. *NEFA*, Non-esterified ("free" or unsaturated) fatty acids; *GLP=1*, Glucagon-like peptide-1. *(Courtesy Medtronics, Inc., Diabetes, Minneapolis, Minnesota.)*

insufficient, additional agents are used to achieve glycemic control. Injectable drugs (exenatide and pramlintide and insulin) are used to treat type 2 diabetes when oral agents alone fail to provide adequate glycemic control (see Table 14-8).[4,35,49]

Drug Treatment of Type 2 Diabetes. There are four classes of drugs used to treat type 2 diabetes: insulin sensitizers, insulin secretagogues, drugs that slow the absorption of carbohydrates in the gut, and incretins (see Table 14-8). The largest class is sulfonylurea drugs, which are secretagogues. Figure 14-6 illustrates the subclasses and their site and mechanism of action.

Oral Agents

Insulin Sensitizers. Insulin sensitizers can have their primary action in the liver or in peripheral tissues.

Primary Action in Liver: Biguanides. Metformin (Glucophage) is the only biguanide available in the United States. Its major action is to suppress hepatic glucose output and gluconeogenesis. Its main pharmacologic advantage is that it lowers blood glucose levels without increasing insulin levels, so it is not associated with significant risk of hypoglycemia. It also enhances insulin sensitivity of muscle and fat and has weight-neutral effects. A rare complication is lactic acidosis. An extended-release metformin formulation (Glucophage XR) provides effective and well-tolerated glycemic control with once-daily dosing.[4,50]

Primary Action in Peripheral Tissues: Thiazolidinediones. Thiazolidinediones (TZDs), also referred to as glitazones, are agonists of peroxisome proliferator-activated receptor gamma (PPARγ)—a family of nuclear transcription factors. This class of drugs decrease insulin resistance primarily by making muscle and adipose cells more sensitive to insulin, and they mildly decrease hepatic glucose production. Glycemic control develops over several weeks to months along with improvement in insulin sensitivity and reduction of free fatty acid levels. Two drugs, pioglitazone (Actos) and rosiglitazone (Avandia), from this class are on the market for use in the United States. They are well tolerated but cause weight gain and fluid retention. TZDs should not be used in patients with active liver disease or elevated alanine aminotransferase levels greater than 2.5 times the upper limit of normal.[4,51]

Insulin Secretagogues. Insulin secretagogues are agents that bind to the sulfonylurea receptor on the plasma membrane of pancreatic beta cells, causing insulin secretion from the pancreas. The major clinical differences between these agents is the duration of action and subtle variations in their hypoglycemic potential.[4]

Sulfonylureas have been available since the 1950s. They are the most cost-effective glucose-lowering agents on the market. They have a slow onset of action and variable duration of action—but can cause hypoglycemia. First- and second-generation sulfonylureas are listed in Table 14-8. The more recent, second-generation agents are more potent and have fewer adverse effects and drug interactions than those typical for first-generation drugs. The extended-release glipizide and glimepiride are preferred, because they can be dosed once daily and have a relatively low risk of hypoglycemia and weight gain.[4] Side effects include weight gain and, much less commonly, GI upset, rashes, purpura, and pruritus. Rare adverse effects are leukopenia, thrombocytopenia, hemolytic anemia, and cholestasis.

Glinides. Glinides—repaglinide (Prandin) and nateglinide (Starlix)—increase the secretion of insulin in the presence of glucose in a manner similar to that for the sulfonylureas; however, they are more rapid in action and of shorter duration. They are dosed with each meal and provide good postprandial control of glucose. Lesser degrees of hypoglycemia and weight gain are associated with glinides than with sulfonylureas.[4]

Alpha-Glucosidase Inhibitors (AGIs). AGIs inhibit the enzyme α-glucosidase at the brush border of the intestinal epithelium, thus blocking the absorption of carbohydrates in the small intestine. They are administered with the first bite of a carbohydrate-containing meal and limit postprandial hyperglycemia without causing hypoglycemia. Two AGI drugs are marketed in the United States, acarbose (Precose) and miglitol (Glyset). Their use has been limited by frequent GI complaints, the need to administer the drugs at the beginning of each meal, only modest reduction in HbA_{1c} levels, and limited effect on fasting glucose levels.[4,52]

Fixed Combination Pills. Several combinations of oral hypoglycemic agents are available. Two combinations of a sulfonylurea and a biguanide on the market are Glucovance (glyburide plus metformin) and Metaglip (glipizide plus metformin). Other combinations include Avandamet (rosiglitazone plus metformin), Actosplus MET (pioglitazone plus metformin), and Prandimet (metformin plus repaglinide).[53]

Dipeptidyl Peptidase-4 Inhibitors. Recent oral agents available for the management of type 2 diabetes include the dipeptidyl peptidase-4 (DPP-4) inhibitors. These drugs block the enzyme responsible for the breakdown of incretins (see under "Injectable Agents," next). Agents such as sitagliptin (Januvia) have been shown to provide good glycemic control in monotherapy or combined with metformin.[4,54]

Injectable Agents

Insulin. Patients with type 2 diabetes with failing beta cell function may require insulin therapy to gain tighter glycemic control. The human and animal insulins and analogues are discussed earlier under "Pharmacologic Treatment of Type 1 Diabetes."

Incretin Mimetics. Incretins are a group of GI hormones that increase insulin release from beta cells in the pancreas. They also inhibit glucagon secretion and slow absorption of carbohydrates. The incretin effect (increased insulin response) is modulated by two incretin hormones, glucagon-like peptide-1 (GLP-1) and glucose-dependent insulinotropic polypeptide (GIP). Both are located in the epithelium of the small intestine and together account for up to 60% of the postprandial insulin secretion. The incretin response is defective or diminished in type 2 diabetes.[55,56]

Currently, four drugs that target the incretin pathway are available for use in management of type 2 diabetes. Exenatide (Byetta) is an incretin GLP-1 mimetic and a synthetic form of exendin 4, a hormone found in the saliva of the Gila monster. Exenatide is injected subcutaneously. It can be used as monotherapy or as adjunctive therapy; when used with a sulfonylurea, it can cause hypoglycemia.[57] Liraglutide also is a GLP-1 agonist that is long-acting and has the advantage of once-daily injectable dosing.[58] Sitagliptin (Januvia) and saxagliptin (Onglyza) are inhibitors of dipeptidyl peptidase-4 (DDP-4), the enzyme responsible for degradation of incretin hormones (GLP-1 and GIP). DDP-4 inhibitors are taken orally, are generally well tolerated and do not cause hypoglycemia.[59,60]

Amylinomimetics. Another more recently developed approach to type 2 diabetes treatment is the use of an analogue of human amylin. Amylin is cosecreted from beta cells of the pancreas with insulin and modulates gastric emptying. It has an incretin effect that prevents postprandial rise in serum glucagon and also suppresses appetite. Pramlintide (Symlin), a synthetic form of amylin, is approved only as an adjunct to insulin therapy. It is administered subcutaneously by separate injection (it cannot be mixed with insulin) just before meals. Insulin dosage must be adjusted on the basis of blood glucose monitoring.[61,62]

Insulin Shock

Patients who are treated with insulin must closely adhere to their diet. If they fail to eat in accordance with their diabetes management plan (consumption of adequate calories at proper intervals) but continue to take their regular insulin injections, they may experience a hypoglycemic reaction caused by an excess of insulin (insulin shock). A hypoglycemic reaction also may be due to an overdose of insulin or an oral hypoglycemic agent, particularly sulfonylurea drugs. Reaction or shock caused by excess insulin usually occurs in three well-defined

BOX 14-5 Signs and Symptoms of Insulin Reaction

Mild Stage
- Hunger
- Weakness
- Tachycardia
- Pallor
- Sweating
- Paresthesias

Moderate Stage
- Incoherence
- Uncooperativeness
- Belligerence
- Lack of judgment
- Poor orientation

Severe Stage
- Unconsciousness
- Tonic or clonic movements
- Hypotension
- Hypothermia
- Rapid, thready pulse

stages, each more severe and dangerous than the one preceding it (Box 14-5).

Mild Stage. The mild stage, which is the most common, is characterized by hunger, weakness, trembling, tachycardia, pallor, and sweating; paresthesias may be noted on occasion. It may occur before meals, during exercise, or when food has been omitted or delayed.

Moderate Stage. In the moderate stage, because blood glucose drops substantially, the patient becomes incoherent, uncooperative, and sometimes belligerent or resistant to reason or efforts at restraint; judgment and orientation are defective. The chief danger during this stage is that patients may injure themselves or someone else (e.g., if the affected person is driving).

Severe Stage. Complete unconsciousness with or without tonic or clonic muscular movements occurs during the severe stage. Most of these reactions take place during sleep, after the first two stages have gone unrecognized. Onset of this stage also may occur after exercise or after the ingestion of alcohol, if earlier signs have been ignored. Sweating, pallor, rapid and thready pulse, hypotension, and hypothermia may be present.

The reaction to excessive insulin can be corrected by giving the patient sweetened fruit juice or anything with sugar in it (cake icing). Patients in the severe stage (unconsciousness) are best treated with an intravenous glucose solution; glucagon or epinephrine may be used for transient relief.

DENTAL MANAGEMENT

Medical Considerations

Any dental patient whose condition remains undiagnosed but who has the cardinal signs and symptoms of diabetes (i.e., polydipsia, polyuria, polyphagia, weight loss, and weakness) should be referred to a physician for diagnosis and treatment. Patients with findings that may suggest diabetes (headache, dry mouth, marked irritability, repeated skin infection, blurred vision, paresthesias, progressive periodontal disease, multiple periodontal abscesses, loss of sensation) should be referred to a clinical laboratory or to a physician for screening tests, to determine if diabetes mellitus type 1 or type 2 or another type of diabetes is responsible for their symptoms.

Today, patients are able to readily monitor their blood glucose level with the use of a personal blood glucose monitoring device (e.g., Glucometer or Glucowatch). Patients with an estimated fasting blood glucose level of 126 mg/100 mL or higher should be referred to a physician for medical evaluation and treatment, if indicated. Those with a 2-hour postprandial blood glucose level of 200 mg/100 mL or higher also should be referred.[63,64]

In one study, fasting blood glucose was determined as part of the initial dental examination in a total of 97 patients (mean age, 57.7 years); 28 patients (28.9%) were found to be hyperglycemic (blood glucose levels greater than 130 mg/100 mL; mean, 174.8 ± 40.8 mg/100 mL), and two were noted to be hypoglycemic (blood glucose less than 70 mg/100 mL). These findings illustrate that patients with diabetes presenting for dental care commonly are not under good glycemic control.[65]

Patients who are obese, who are older than 45 years of age, or who have close relatives with diabetes should be screened routinely (at least at 3-year intervals) for any indication of hyperglycemia that may reveal the onset of diabetes. Women who have given birth to large babies (birth weight greater than 9 lb) or who have had multiple spontaneous abortions or stillbirths also should be screened once a year for diabetes.[63,64]

All patients with diagnosed diabetes must be identified by history, and the type of medical treatment they are receiving must be established (Box 14-6). The type of diabetes (type 1, type 2, other) should be determined, and the presence of complications noted. Patients who are being treated with insulin should be asked how much insulin they use and how often they inject themselves each day. They also should be asked whether they monitor their own blood glucose and if so, by which method, how often, and the value of the most recent level. The frequency of insulin reactions and when the last one occurred should be ascertained. The frequency of visits to the physician should be established, as should the timing and results of the last A_{1C} test. Whether the patient performs self-monitoring of blood glucose levels should be determined. The specific glucose monitoring system and regimen used by the patient should be identified. This information will provide additional input on the severity of diabetes and the level of control that has been attained.

Vital signs also serve as a guide to the control and management of disease in the diabetic patient. Patients with abnormal pulse rate and rhythm and/or elevated blood pressure should be approached with a measure of caution. Functional capacity is important for

BOX 14-6 Clinical Detection of the Patient with Diabetes

Patient with Known Diabetes

1. Detection by history:
   a. Are you diabetic?
   b. What medications are you taking?
   c. Are you being treated by a physician?
2. Establishment of severity of disease and degree of "control":
   a. When were you first diagnosed as diabetic?
   b. What was the level of the last measurement of your blood glucose?
   c. What is the usual level of blood glucose for you?
   d. How are you being treated for your diabetes?
   e. How often do you have insulin reactions?
   f. How much insulin do you take with each injection, and how often do you receive injections?
   g. How often do you test your blood glucose?
   h. When did you last visit your physician?
   i. Do you have any symptoms of diabetes at the present time?

Patient with Undiagnosed Diabetes

1. History of signs or symptoms of diabetes or its complications
2. High risk for developing diabetes:
   a. Presence of diabetes in a parent
   b. Giving birth to one or more large babies (greater than 9 lb)
   c. History of spontaneous abortions or stillbirths
   d. Obesity
   e. Age older than 40 years
3. Referral or screening test for diabetes

determination of the severity and level of control of diabetes and should be part of the patient's evaluation prior to dental treatment. Overall poor functional capacity (i.e., less than 4 metabolic equivalent levels [METs]) increases the risk of complications during and after dental treatment. The risk for serious cardiovascular events increases substantially in patients with diminished functional capacity to less than 4 METs—that is, those who have difficulty completing normal daily physical activities (see Chapter 1). These patients should be approached with caution.[63,64]

Patients with type 2 diabetes who have no evidence of complications and whose disease is under good medical control, as determined by consultation with the patient's physician, require little or no special attention when receiving dental treatment, unless they develop a significant dental or oral infection that is possibly accompanied by swelling or fever. In contrast, patients with complications such as renal disease or cardiovascular disease may require specific alterations in dental management. Those who are treated with insulin or who are not under good medical management also require special attention (Box 14-7). This typically involves consultation with the patient's physician.

Patients who have not seen their physician for a long time, who have had frequent episodes of insulin shock, or who report signs and symptoms of diabetes may have disease that is unstable. These patients should be referred to their physician for evaluation, or the physician should be consulted to establish the patient's current status.

Some patients with type 1 diabetes who are being treated with large doses of insulin experience periods of extreme hyperglycemia and hypoglycemia (brittle diabetes), even when given the best of medical management. For these patients, close consultation with the physician is required before any dental treatment is started.

A major goal in the dental management of patients with diabetes who are being treated with insulin is to prevent insulin shock during the dental appointment. Patients should be told to take their usual insulin dosage and to eat normal meals before the appointment, which usually is best scheduled in the morning. When such a patient arrives, the dentist should confirm that the patient has taken insulin and has eaten breakfast. In addition, patients should be instructed to tell the dentist whether at any time during the appointment they are experiencing symptoms of an insulin reaction. A source of sugar such as orange juice, cake icing, or non-diet soft drink must be available in the dental office to be given to the patient if symptoms of an insulin reaction develop (see Box 14-7 and see Appendix A).

Any patient with diabetes who is going to undergo extensive periodontal or oral surgery procedures other than single simple extractions should be given special dietary instructions for after surgery. It is important that the total caloric content and the protein-carbohydrate-fat ratio of the diet remain the same, so that control of the disease and proper blood glucose balance are maintained. The patient's physician should be consulted about dietary recommendations for the postoperative period. One suggestion is to have the patient use a blender to prepare his or her usual diet so that it can be ingested with minimum discomfort; alternatively, special food supplements in a liquid form may be used. The physician also may alter the patient's insulin regimen according to ability to eat properly, and according to the extent of the surgery to be performed.

A protocol for intravenous sedation often involves fasting before the appointment (i.e., nothing by mouth after midnight); using only half the usual insulin dose; and then supplementing with intravenous glucose during the procedure. Patients with well-controlled diabetes may be given general anesthesia, if necessary. However, management with local anesthetics is preferable especially in outpatient office settings.[63,64]

Patients who have brittle diabetes (in which control is very difficult to achieve) or who require a high dosage of insulin (in type 1 diabetes) may be at increased risk for postoperative infection. However, prophylactic antibiotics usually are not indicated. If the patient develops an infection, appropriate systemic antibiotics may be given.

An acute dental or oral infection in a patient with diabetes is a potential significant management problem

BOX 14-7 Dental Management
Considerations in the Patient with Diabetes

P

Patient Evaluation/Risk Assessment (see Box 1-1)

- Evaluate and determine whether diabetes exists.
- Obtain medical consultation if glycemic control is poor, or if signs and symptoms point to an undiagnosed problem, or if the diagnosis is uncertain. If diabetes is well controlled,* all routine dental procedures can be performed without special precautions. Morning appointments usually are best.

Potential Issues/Factors of Concern

A	
Analgesics	Avoid use of aspirin and other NSAIDs in patients taking sulfonylureas, because these can worsen hypoglycemia.
Antibiotics	Prophylactic antibiotics generally are not required. Antibiotics may be prescribed for a patient with brittle (very difficult to control) diabetes for whom an invasive procedure is planned but whose oral health is poor and the fasting plasma glucose exceeds 200 mg/dL. Manage infections aggressively by incision and drainage, extraction, pulpotomy, warm rinses, and antibiotics.
Anesthesia	No issues if diabetes is well controlled. For diabetic patients with concurrent hypertension or history of recent myocardial infarction, or with a cardiac arrhythmia, dose of epinephrine should be limited to no more than two cartridges containing 1:100,000 epinephrine.
Anxiety	No issues.
Allergy	No issues.
B	
Bleeding	For surgical issues, see "Notes on Surgery," below. Thrombocytopenia is a rare adverse effect associated with sulfonylureas.
Breathing	No issues.
Blood pressure	Monitor blood pressure, because diabetes is associated with hypertension.
C	
Chair position	No issues.
Cardiovascular	Confirm cardiovascular status. Beta blocker drugs can exacerbate hypoglycemia in patients taking sulfonylureas.
D	
Devices	Insulin pump may be worn by patient. Ensure attached and working properly. Antibiotic prophylaxis is not needed.
Drugs	Patient advised to take usual insulin dosage and normal meals on day of dental appointment; information confirmed with patient at appointment.
Drug interactions	See Table 14-8.
E	
Equipment	Use office glucometer to ensure good glucose control.
Emergencies/urgencies	Advise patient to inform dentist or staff if symptoms of insulin reaction occur during dental visit. Have glucose source (orange juice, soda, cake icing) available; give to the patient if symptoms of insulin reaction occur.
F	
Follow-up	Routine and periodic follow-up evaluation is advised for patients who have diabetes. Inspect for oral lesions as a way to monitor for disease progression. Poor periodontal health is associated with poor glycemic control.

Notes on Surgery

If extensive surgery is needed:

- Consult with patient's physician concerning dietary needs during postoperative period.
- If diabetes is not well controlled (i.e., fasting blood glucose <70 mg/dL or >200 mg/dL and comorbidities [post-MI, renal disease, congestive heart failure, symptomatic angina, old age, cardiac dysrrhythmia, cerebrovascular accident] present, and blood pressure >180/110 mm Hg, or functional capacity <4 metabolic equivalents):
    - Provide appropriate emergency care only.
    - Request referral for medical evaluation, management, and risk factor modification.
  - If patient is symptomatic, seek IMMEDIATE referral.
  - If patient is asymptomatic, request routine referral.

NOTE: special precautions may be needed for patients with complications of diabetes, renal disease, or heart disease.

*Well-controlled: fasting blood glucose between 70 mg/dL and 200 mg/dL and no complications (i.e., post MI, renal disease, congestive heart failure, symptomatic angina, old age, cardiac dysrrhythmia, cerebrovascular accident), blood pressure <180/110 mm Hg, and functional capacity >4 metabolic equivalents.

(Box 14-8). Management will be even more difficult in patients who take a high insulin dosage and those who have type 1 diabetes. Infection often leads to loss of control over the diabetic condition; as a result, infection is not well handled by the body's defenses, as it would be in the normal patient. Patients with brittle diabetes (e.g., necessitating a high dosage of insulin) may require hospitalization for adequate management of an infection. The patient's physician should be consulted and should become a partner during this period.[63,64]

Risk for infection in patients with diabetes is, in theory, directly related to fasting blood glucose levels,

BOX 14-8 Dental Management of the Patient with Diabetes and Acute Oral Infection

1. Non–insulin-controlled patients may require insulin; consultation with physician is indicated.
2. Insulin-controlled patients usually require increased dosage of insulin; consultation with physician is indicated.
3. Patient with brittle diabetes or receiving high insulin dosage should have culture(s) taken from the infected area for antibiotic sensitivity testing.
   a. Culture is sent for testing.
   b. Antibiotic therapy is initiated.
   c. In cases of poor clinical responses to the first antibiotic, a more effective antibiotic is selected according to sensitivity test results.
4. Infection should be treated with the use of standard methods:
   a. Warm intraoral rinses
   b. Incision and drainage
   c. Pulpotomy, pulpectomy, extractions
   d. Antibiotics

presence of infecting organisms, and invasiveness of dental procedures. As indicated by data for general surgery procedures, if the fasting blood glucose level is below 206 mg/100 mL, increased risk is not predicted. However, if fasting blood glucose level is between 207 and 229 mg/100 mL, the risk is predicted to be increased by 20% if surgical procedures are being performed. Additionally, if fasting blood glucose level rises to above 230 mg/100 mL, an 80% increase risk of infection postoperatively has been reported.[66,67] Although these studies predict risk based on non-oral surgical procedures, dentists should be aware of the level of glycemic control in patients undergoing complex oral surgical procedures, because of the predicted increased risk of infection. Judicious monitoring and appropriate use of antibiotics should be considered in the management of these patients.[63]

The basic aim of treatment in this setting is to simultaneously cure the oral infection and restore control of the patient's blood glucose level. Patients who are receiving insulin usually require additional insulin, which should be prescribed by their physician. Non–insulin-controlled patients may need more aggressive medical management of their diabetes, which may include insulin, during this period. The dentist should treat the infection aggressively by incision and drainage, extraction, pulpotomy, warm rinses, and antibiotics. Antibiotic sensitivity testing is recommended for patients with brittle diabetes and for those who require a high insulin dosage for control. For these patients, penicillin therapy can be initiated. Then, if the clinical response is poor, a more effective antibiotic can be selected on the basis of results of antibiotic sensitivity testing. Attention also should be paid to the patient's electrolyte balance and to fluid and dietary needs.[63]

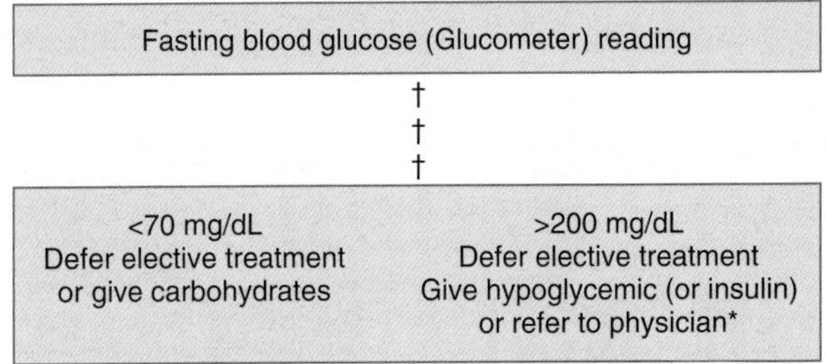

*Oral hypoglycemic agent prescribed by patient's physician.

FIGURE 14-7 Decision-making diagram for the dental treatment of patients with diabetes according to blood glucose (Glucometer) reading.

Local Anesthetics and Epinephrine

For most patients with diabetes, routine use of local anesthetic with 1:100,000 epinephrine is well tolerated. Of note, however, epinephrine has a pharmacologic effect that is opposite that of insulin, so blood glucose could rise with the use of epinephrine. In diabetic patients with hypertension, history of recent myocardial infarction, or cardiac arrhythmia, caution may be indicated with use of epinephrine. Guidelines for these patients are similar to those for patients with cardiovascular conditions and may be even stricter for those with diabetes and cardiovascular conditions, who have functional capacity below 4 METs. Obviously, diabetic patients may fluctuate between these states, from time to time, and from appointment to appointment (see Box 14-7).[63,68]

Treatment Planning Modifications

The patient with diabetes who is receiving good medical management and demonstrates good glycemic control without serious complications such as renal disease, hypertension, or coronary atherosclerotic heart disease can undergo any indicated dental treatment. If diabetes is under good control, even cardiac transplantation can be safely performed.[2]

In patients with diabetes who have serious medical complications, however, the plan of dental treatment may need to be altered (see Chapters 3, 4, 5, 6, and 13). Studies have indicated that many dental patients with diabetes are not under good glycemic control. Elevated fasting blood glucose levels render the dental patient more susceptible to complications. Another concern is that the patient experiences too much glycemic control (hypoglycemia), resulting in low blood glucose levels (below 70 mg/dL). This situation also must be recognized and managed appropriately (Figure 14-7). Therefore, careful and continuous monitoring of the patient's physical status is mandatory.[65]

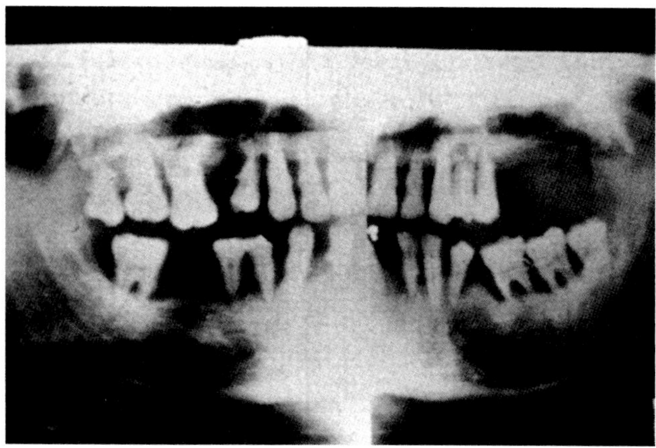

FIGURE 14-8 Panoramic radiograph of a young adult with severe, progressive periodontitis. After positive screening for diabetes, the patient was referred to a physician, and the diagnosis of diabetes mellitus was established. The patient required insulin treatment.

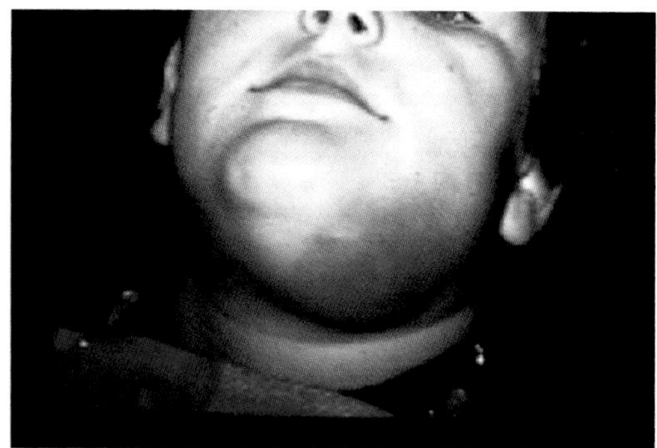

A

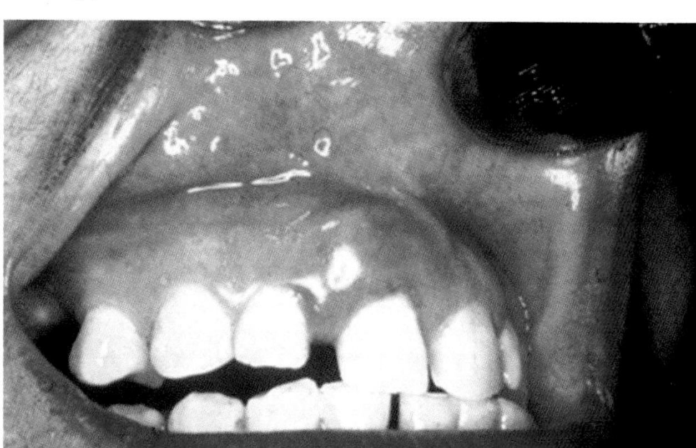

B

FIGURE 14-9 **A,** Patient with cellulitis resulting from a mandibular tooth abscess. **B,** Periodontal abscess in a patient with multiple abscesses. After evaluation by a physician, the diagnosis of diabetes was established.

Oral Complications and Manifestations

Oral complications of poorly controlled diabetes mellitus may include xerostomia; bacterial, viral, and fungal infections (including candidiasis); poor wound healing; increased incidence and severity of caries; gingivitis and periodontal disease; periapical abscesses; and burning mouth symptoms. Oral findings in patients with uncontrolled diabetes most likely relate to excessive loss of fluids through urination, altered response to infection, microvascular changes, and possibly, increased glucose concentrations in saliva.[69-71]

The effects of hyperglycemia lead to increased amounts of urine, which deplete the extracellular fluids and reduce the secretion of saliva, resulting in dry mouth. A high percentage of patients with diabetes present with xerostomia and low levels of salivary calcium, phosphate, and fluoride.[72,73] Saliva glucose levels are elevated in persons with uncontrolled and controlled diabetes.[74,75] Several studies have reported increased incidence and severity of gingival inflammation, periodontal abscess, and chronic periodontal disease in diabetic patients[69,71-76] (Figures 14-8 and 14-9).

Diabetes results in enhanced inflammatory responses, depressed wound healing and small blood vessel changes that contribute to increased risk for periodontitis. Thus it is not surprising that adults with uncontrolled diabetes have more severe manifestations of periodontal disease than do adults without diabetes. As a group, patients with controlled diabetes appear to have more severe periodontal disease than do those without it, but the differences are not great.[69-71,77] The time relationship between the occurrence of the diabetic state and the onset of periodontal disease has yet to be established. However, periodontal disease is clearly a complication of type 1 and type 2 diabetes, and the association cannot be explained solely by increased supragingival plaque accumulations.[69-71,77,78] Periodontal disease found in these young adults (older than 30 years of age) usually is asymptomatic and typically remains undetected. Overall, periodontal disease is more severe and more frequent in patients with poorly controlled diabetes.[69-71,77]

Caries appears to be more significant in patients with diabetes who have poor glycemic control.[75] Oral fungal infections, including candidiasis and the more rare mucormycosis (Figures 14-10 and 14-11), may be noted in the patient with uncontrolled diabetes. The general consensus is that healing is delayed in persons with uncontrolled diabetes, and that they are more prone to various oral infections after undergoing surgical procedures.[79-81] Treatment recommendations for these infections are found in Appendix C.

Oral lesions are more common in patients with diabetes. A significantly higher percentage of oral lesions, especially candidiasis, traumatic ulcers, lichen planus, and delayed healing, have been noted in patients with type 1 diabetes, as compared with a control population. Altered immune system function contributes to the appearance of these lesions in diabetes.[63,80,82]

Diabetic neuropathy may lead to oral symptoms of paresthesias and tingling, numbness, burning, or pain

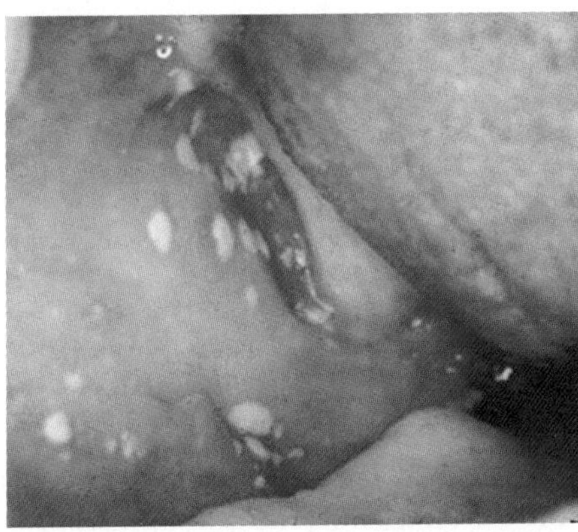

FIGURE 14-10 Oral candidiasis in a patient with diabetes. The multiple small white lesions on the buccal mucosa were easily scraped off. Cytologic study and cultures confirmed the clinical impression of infection by *Candida albicans*.

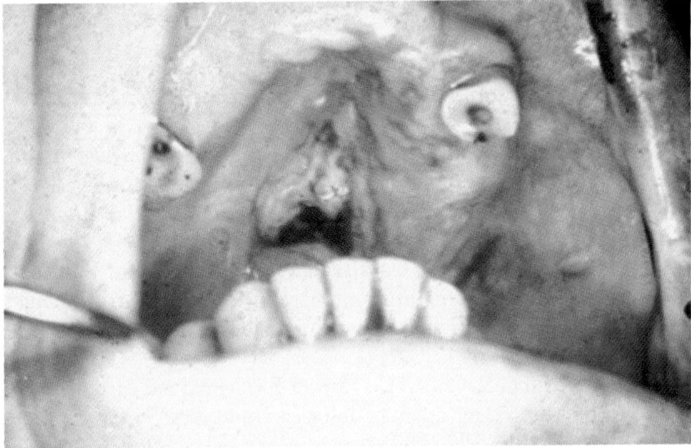

FIGURE 14-11 Tan-dark brown lesion involving the palate in a patient with diabetes. Cultures established the diagnosis of mucormycosis, a serious fungal infection that may occur in patients with systemic diseases such as diabetes or cancer. Treatment usually includes control of diabetes, surgical excisions of the lesion, and administration of antibiotics and potent antifungals.

caused by pathologic changes involving nerves in the oral region. Diabetes has been associated with oral burning symptoms. Early diagnosis and treatment of diabetes may lead to regression of these symptoms, but in long-standing cases, the changes may be irreversible.[83]

Metformin is associated with a metallic taste.[84]

REFERENCES

1. American Diabetes Association: Diagnosis and classification of diabetes mellitus, *Diabetes Care* 34(Suppl 1):S62-S69, 2010.
2. Nathan DM, et al: Intensive diabetes treatment and cardiovascular disease in patients with type 1 diabetes, *N Engl J Med* 353:2643-2653, 2005.
3. Stolar M: Glycemic control and complications in type 2 diabetes mellitus, *Am J Med* 123(3 Suppl):S3-S11, 2010.
4. Inzucchi SE, Sherwin RS: Diabetes mellitus, type 1 and type 2. In Goldman L, Ausiello D, editors: *Cecil medicine*, ed 23, Philadelphia, 2008, Saunders, pp 1727-1766.
5. Wild S, et al: Global prevalence of diabetes: estimates for the year 2000 and projections for 2030, *Diabetes Care* 27:1047-1053, 2004.
6. International Diabetes Federation: *Prevalence estimates of diabetes mellitus (DM), 2010* (article online), http://www.diabetesatlas.org/content/prevalence-estimates-diabetes-mellitus-dm-2010; accessed on May 11, 2011.
7. *National diabetes statistics, 2011* (article online), http://diabetes.niddk.nih.gov/dm/pubs/statistics/#fast; accessed on May 11, 2011.
8. *Diabetes statistics* (article online), http://www.diabetes.org/diabetes-basics/diabetes-statistics; accessed on May 11, 2011.
9. *Get the facts on diabetes* (article online), http://www.cdc.gov/Features/DiabetesFactSheet/; accessed on May 11, 2011.
10. Geiss LS, et al: Changes in incidence of diabetes in U.S. adults, 1997-2003, *Am J Prev Med* 30:371-377, 2006.
11. Colagiuri S: Epidemiology of prediabetes, *Med Clin North Am* 95:299-307, vii, 2011.
12. Karam JG, McFarlane SI: Update on the prevention of type 2 diabetes, *Curr Diab Rep* 11:56-63, 2011.
13. Stumvoll M, Goldstein BJ, van Haeften TW: Type 2 diabetes: principles of pathogenesis and therapy, *Lancet* 365:1333-1346, 2005.
14. Dedoussis GV, Kaliora AC, Panagiotakos DB: Genes, diet and type 2 diabetes mellitus: a review, *Rev Diabet Stud* 4:13-24, 2007.
15. Greene MF, Solomon CG: Gestational diabetes mellitus—time to treat, *N Engl J Med* 352:2544-2546, 2005.
16. Lambrinoudaki I, Vlachou SA, Creatsas G: Genetics in gestational diabetes mellitus: association with incidence, severity, pregnancy outcome and response to treatment, *Curr Diabetes Rev* 6:393-399, 2010.
17. *Prediabetes FAQs* (article online), http://www.diabetes.org/diabetes-basics/prevention/pre-diabetes/pre-diabetes-faqs.html; accessed on May 11, 2011.
18. Diabetes: definition and pathophysiology. In Beaser RS, Joslin Diabetes Center Staff, editors: *Joslin's diabetes deskbook: a guide for primary care providers*, ed 2, Philadelphia, 2007, Lippincott Williams & Wilkins, pp 1-23.
19. Blakytny R, Jude E: The molecular biology of chronic wounds and delayed healing in diabetes, *Diabet Med* 23:594-608, 2006.
20. Eliasson M, Talback M, Rosen M: Improved survival in both men and women with diabetes between 1980 and 2004—a cohort study in Sweden, *Cardiovasc Diabetol* 7:32, 2008.
21. Leal J, Gray AM, Clarke PM: Development of life-expectancy tables for people with type 2 diabetes, *Eur Heart J* 30:834-839, 2009.
22. Pera PI: Living with diabetes: quality of care and quality of life, *Patient Prefer Adherence* 5:65-72, 2011.
23. Mironidou-Tzouveleki M, Tsartsalis S, Tomos C: Vascular endothelial growth factor (VEGF) in the pathogenesis of diabetic nephropathy of type 1 diabetes mellitus, *Curr Drug Targets* 12:107-114, 2011.
24. Tomkin GH: Atherosclerosis, diabetes and lipoproteins, *Expert Rev Cardiovasc Ther* 8:1015-1029, 2010.
25. Aiello LP: Angiogenic pathways in diabetic retinopathy, *N Engl J Med* 353:839-841, 2005.
26. Mlynarski WM, et al: Risk of diabetic nephropathy in type 1 diabetes is associated with functional polymorphisms in RANTES receptor gene (CCR5): a sex-specific effect, *Diabetes* 54:3331-3335, 2005.
27. Cavallerano JD, Stanton RM: Microvascular complications. In Beaser RS, Joslin Diabetes Center Staff, editors: *Joslin's diabetes deskbook: a guide for primary care providers*, ed 2, Philadelphia, 2007, Lippincott Williams & Wilkins, pp 429-458.
28. Beaser RS, Johnstone M: Macrovascular complications. In Beaser RS, Joslin Diabetes Center Staff, editors: *Joslin's*

diabetes deskbook: a guide for primary care providers, ed 2, Philadelphia, 2007, Lippincott Williams & Wilkins, pp 459-478.
29. Tesfaye S, et al: Vascular risk factors and diabetic neuropathy, *N Engl J Med* 352:341-350, 2005.
30. Bloomgarden ZT: Clinical diabetic neuropathy, *Diabetes Care* 28:2968-2974, 2005.
31. Freeman R: Diabetic neuropathy. In Beaser RS, Joslin Diabetes Center Staff, editors: *Joslin's diabetes deskbook: a guide for primary care providers*, ed 2, Philadelphia, 2007, Lippincott Williams & Wilkins, pp 481-504.
32. Genuth S: Insights from the diabetes control and complications trial/epidemiology of diabetes interventions and complications study on the use of intensive glycemic treatment to reduce the risk of complications of type 1 diabetes, *Endocr Pract* 12(Suppl 1):34-41, 2006.
33. Monitoring diabetes. In Beaser RS, Joslin Diabetes Center Staff, editors: *Joslin's diabetes deskbook: a guide for primary care providers*, ed 2, Philadelphia, 2007, Lippincott Williams & Wilkins, pp 465-466.
34. Khan MI, Weinstock RS: Carbohydrates. In McPherson RA, Pincus MR, editors: *Henry's clinical diagnosis and management by laboratory methods*, ed 21, Philadelphia, 2007, Saunders, pp 185-190.
35. American Diabetes Association: Standards of medical care in diabetes—2011, *Diabetes Care* 34(Suppl 1):S11-S61, 2011.
36. White SA, Shaw JA, Sutherland DE: Pancreas transplantation, *Lancet* 373:1808-1817, 2009.
37. Chrisholm DJ: The Diabetes Control and Complications Trial (DCCT). A milestone in diabetes management, *Med J Aust* 159:721-723, 1993.
38. The relationship of glycemic exposure (HbA_{1c}) to the risk of development and progression of retinopathy in the diabetes control and complications trial, *Diabetes* 44:968-983, 1995.
39. Stratton IM, et al: Association of glycaemia with macrovascular and microvascular complications of type 2 diabetes (UKPDS 35): prospective observational study, *BMJ* 321:405-412, 2000.
40. Joshi SR, Parikh RM, Das AK: Insulin—history, biochemistry, physiology and pharmacology, *J Assoc Physicians India* 55(Suppl):19-25, 2007.
41. Beaser RS: Using insulin to treat diabetes—general principles. In Beaser RS, Joslin Diabetes Center Staff, editors: *Joslin's diabetes deskbook: a guide for primary care providers*, ed 2, Philadelphia, 2007, Lippincott Williams & Wilkins, pp 249-280.
42. Qayyum R, Greene L: AHRQ's comparative effectiveness research on premixed insulin analogues for adults with type 2 diabetes: understanding and applying the systematic review findings, *J Manag Care Pharm* 17(3 Suppl):S3-S19, 2011.
43. Chatenoud L: Immune therapy for type 1 diabetes mellitus—what is unique about anti-CD3 antibodies? *Nat Rev Endocrinol* 6:149-157, 2010.
44. Reznik Y: Continuous subcutaneous insulin infusion (CSII) using an external insulin pump for the treatment of type 2 diabetes, *Diabetes Metab* 36:415-421, 2010.
45. Pickup J: Insulin pumps, *Int J Clin Pract Suppl* 166:16-19, 2010.
46. Inhaled insulin (Exubera), *Med Lett Drugs Ther* 48:57-58, 2006.
47. Baran MK, Godoy AT: What went wrong? A retrospective on Exubera, *Adv Nurse Pract* 16:53-54, 77, 2008.
48. Bruttomesso D, et al: Closed-loop artificial pancreas using subcutaneous glucose sensing and insulin delivery and a model predictive control algorithm: preliminary studies in Padova and Montpellier, *J Diabetes Sci Technol* 3:1014-1021, 2009.
49. Jones MC: Therapies for diabetes: pramlintide and exenatide, *Am Fam Physician* 275:1831-1835, 2007.
50. Jabbour S, Ziring B: Advantages of extended-release metformin in patients with type 2 diabetes mellitus, *Postgrad Med* 123:15-23, 2011.
51. Derosa G: Efficacy and tolerability of pioglitazone in patients with type 2 diabetes mellitus: comparison with other oral antihyperglycaemic agents, *Drugs* 70:1945-1961, 2010.
52. Cheng AY, Fantus IG: Oral antihyperglycemic therapy for type 2 diabetes mellitus, *CMAJ* 172:213-226, 2005.
53. Nyenwe EA, et al: Management of type 2 diabetes: evolving strategies for the treatment of patients with type 2 diabetes, *Metabolism* 60:1-23, 2011.
54. Shomali M: Add-on therapies to metformin for type 2 diabetes, *Expert Opin Pharmacother* 12:47-62, 2011.
55. Drucker DJ, Nauck MA: The incretin system: glucagon-like peptide-1 receptor agonists and dipeptidyl peptidase-4 inhibitors in type 2 diabetes, *Lancet* 368:1696-1705, 2006.
56. Verspohl EJ: Novel therapeutics for type 2 diabetes: incretin hormone mimetics (glucagon-like peptide-1 receptor agonists) and dipeptidyl peptidase-4 inhibitors, *Pharmacol Ther* 124:113-138, 2008.
57. Yoo BK, Triller DM, Yoo DJ: Exenatide: a new option for the treatment of type 2 diabetes, *Ann Pharmacother* 40:1777-1784, 2006.
58. Peterson GE, Pollom RD: Liraglutide in clinical practice: dosing, safety and efficacy, *Int J Clin Pract Suppl* 64:35-43, 2010.
59. Schwartz SL: Treatment of elderly patients with type 2 diabetes mellitus: a systematic review of the benefits and risks of dipeptidyl peptidase-4 inhibitors, *Am J Geriatr Pharmacother* 8:405-418, 2010.
60. Norris SL, et al: Drug class review: newer drugs for the treatment of diabetes mellitus: final report, *Drug Class Reviews* (serial online), http://www.ncbi.nlm.nih.gov/books/NBK10611/; accessed on May 12, 2011.
61. VanDeKoppel S, Choe HM, Sweet BV: Managed care perspective on three new agents for type 2 diabetes, *J Manag Care Pharm* 14:363-380, 2008.
62. Nogid A, Pham DQ: Adjunctive therapy with pramlintide in patients with type 1 or type 2 diabetes mellitus, *Pharmacotherapy* 26:1626-1640, 2006.
63. Miley DD, Terezhalmy GT: The patient with diabetes mellitus: etiology, epidemiology, principles of medical management, oral disease burden, and principles of dental management, *Quintessence Int* 36:779-795, 2005.
64. Fiske J: Diabetes mellitus and oral care, *Dent Update* 31:190-196, 198, 2008.
65. Rhodus NL, Vibeto BM, Hamamoto DT: Glycemic control in patients with diabetes mellitus upon admission to a dental clinic: considerations for dental management, *Quintessence Int* 36:474-482, 2005.
66. Golden SH, et al: Perioperative glycemic control and the risk of infectious complications in a cohort of adults with diabetes, *Diabetes Care* 22:1408-1414, 1999.
67. Guvener M, et al: Perioperative hyperglycemia is a strong correlate of postoperative infection in type II diabetic patients after coronary artery bypass grafting, *Endocr J* 49:531-537, 2002.
68. Brown RS, Rhodus NL: Epinephrine and local anesthesia revisited, *Oral Surg Oral Med Oral Pathol Oral Radiol Endod* 100:401-408, 2005.
69. Aren G, et al: Periodontal health, salivary status, and metabolic control in children with type 1 diabetes mellitus, *J Periodontol* 74:1789-1795, 2003.
70. Campus G, et al: Diabetes and periodontal disease: a case-control study, *J Periodontol* 76:418-425, 2005.
71. Lalla E, et al: Oral disease burden in northern Manhattan patients with diabetes mellitus, *Am J Public Health* 98(9 Suppl):S91-S94, 2008.

72. Borges BC, et al: Xerostomia and hyposalivation: a preliminary report of their prevalence and associated factors in Brazilian elderly diabetic patients, *Oral Health Prev Dent* 8:153-158, 2010.
73. Jawed M, et al: Dental caries in diabetes mellitus: role of salivary flow rate and minerals, *J Diabetes Complications* 25:183-186, 2011.
74. Panchbhai AS, Degwekar SS, Bhowte RR: Estimation of salivary glucose, salivary amylase, salivary total protein and salivary flow rate in diabetics in India, *J Oral Sci* 52:359-368, 2010.
75. Twetman S, et al: Caries incidence in young type 1 diabetes mellitus patients in relation to metabolic control and caries-associated risk factors, *Caries Res* 36:31-35, 2002.
76. Thorstensson H: Periodontal disease in adult insulin-dependent diabetics, *Swed Dent J Suppl* 107:1-68, 1995.
77. Iacopino AM: Periodontitis and diabetes interrelationships: role of inflammation, *Ann Periodontol* 6:125-137, 2001.
78. Shlossman M, et al: Type 2 diabetes mellitus and periodontal disease, *J Am Dent Assoc* 121:532-536, 1990.
79. Iatta R, et al: Rare mycoses of the oral cavity: a literature epidemiologic review, *Oral Surg Oral Med Oral Pathol Oral Radiol Endod* 108:647-655, 2009.
80. Belazi M, et al: Candidal overgrowth in diabetic patients: potential predisposing factors, *Mycoses* 48:192-196, 2005.
81. Lee DH, et al: Risk factors of surgical site infection in patients undergoing major oncological surgery for head and neck cancer, *Oral Oncol* 47:528-531, 2011.
82. Marsot-Dupuch K, Quillard J, Meyohas MC: Head and neck lesions in the immunocompromised host, *Eur Radiol* 14(Suppl 3):E155-E167, 2004.
83. Rhodus NL, Carlson CR, Miller CS: Burning mouth (syndrome) disorder, *Quintessence Int* 34:587-593, 2003.
84. Lee AJ: Metformin in noninsulin-dependent diabetes mellitus, *Pharmacotherapy* 16:327-351, 1996.

15

Adrenal Insufficiency

BACKGROUND

The adrenal glands are small (6 to 8 g) endocrine glands located bilaterally at the superior pole of each kidney. Each gland contains an outer cortex and an inner medulla. The adrenal medulla functions as a sympathetic ganglion and secretes catecholamines, primarily epinephrine, whereas the adrenal cortex secretes several steroid hormones with multiple actions (Figure 15-1).

The adrenal cortex makes up about 90% of the gland and consists of three zones. The outer zone is the zona glomerulosa. The middle zone is the zona fasciculata, and the innermost zone is the zona reticularis. The cortex manufactures three classes of adrenal steroids: glucocorticoids, mineralocorticoids, and androgens. All are derived from cholesterol and share a common molecular nucleus. The predominant hormone of the zona glomerulosa is aldosterone, a mineralocorticoid. Aldosterone regulates physiologic levels of sodium and potassium and is relatively independent of pituitary gland feedback. The zona fasciculata secretes glucocorticoids, and the zona reticularis secretes androgens, or sex hormones.[1,2]

Cortisol, the primary glucocorticoid, has several important physiologic actions on metabolism, cardiovascular function, the immune system, and for maintaining homeostasis during periods of physical or emotional stress.[1] Cortisol acts as an insulin antagonist (Figure 15-2), increasing blood levels and peripheral use of glucose by activating key enzymes involved in hepatic gluconeogenesis and inhibiting glucose uptake in peripheral tissues (i.e., skeletal muscles). In adipose tissue, cortisol activates lipolysis, resulting in the release of free fatty acids into circulation. Cortisol increases blood pressure by potentiating the vasoconstrictor action of catecholamines and angiotensin II on the kidney and vasculature.[2,3] Its antiinflammatory action is modulated by its inhibitory action on (1) lysosome release, (2) prostaglandin production, (3) eicosanoid and cytokine release, (4) endothelial cell expression of intracellular and extracellular adhesion molecules (ICAMs and ECAMs, respectively) that attract neutrophils, and (5) leukocyte function. Cortisol also activates osteoclasts and inhibits osteoblasts.

Regulation of cortisol secretion occurs through activity of the hypothalamic-pituitary-adrenal (HPA) axis (Figure 15-3). Central nervous system afferents mediating circadian rhythm and responses to stress stimulate the hypothalamus to release corticotropin-releasing hormone (CRH), which stimulates the production and secretion of adrenocorticotropic hormone (ACTH) by the anterior pituitary. ACTH then stimulates the adrenal cortex to produce and secrete cortisol. Plasma cortisol levels are increased within a few minutes after stimulation. Circulating levels of cortisol inhibit the production of CRH and ACTH, thus completing a negative feedback loop.[2]

Cortisol secretion normally follows a diurnal pattern. Peak levels of plasma cortisol occur around the time of waking in the morning and are lowest in the evening and night[2] (Figure 15-4). This pattern is reversed in a person who habitually works nights and sleeps during the day. The normal secretion rate of cortisol over a 24-hour period is approximately 20 mg.[1,2,4] During periods of stress, the HPA axis is stimulated, resulting in increased secretion of cortisol. Anticipation of surgery or an athletic event usually is accompanied by only minimal increases in cortisol secretion. However, surgery itself is one of the most potent activators of the HPA axis.[2,5,6] Also, various stressors such as trauma, illness, burns, fever, hypoglycemia, and emotional upset (e.g., anxiety) can trigger this effect.[7] The most pronounced response is noted in the immediate postoperative period. However, this can be reduced by morphine-like analgesics, benzodiazepines, or local anesthesia, suggesting that the pain response mechanism increases the requirement for cortisol.[8-10]

Synthetic glucocorticoids (cortisol-like drugs) are used in the treatment of many diseases (e.g., rheumatoid arthritis, systemic lupus erythematosus, asthma, hepatitis, inflammatory bowel disease, dermatoses, mucositis) and can affect adrenal function. Glucocorticoids are used on a long-term basis in patients during immunosuppressive therapy for organ transplantation and joint replacement. In dentistry, corticosteroids may be used during the perioperative period for the reduction of pain, edema, and trismus after oral surgical and endodontic

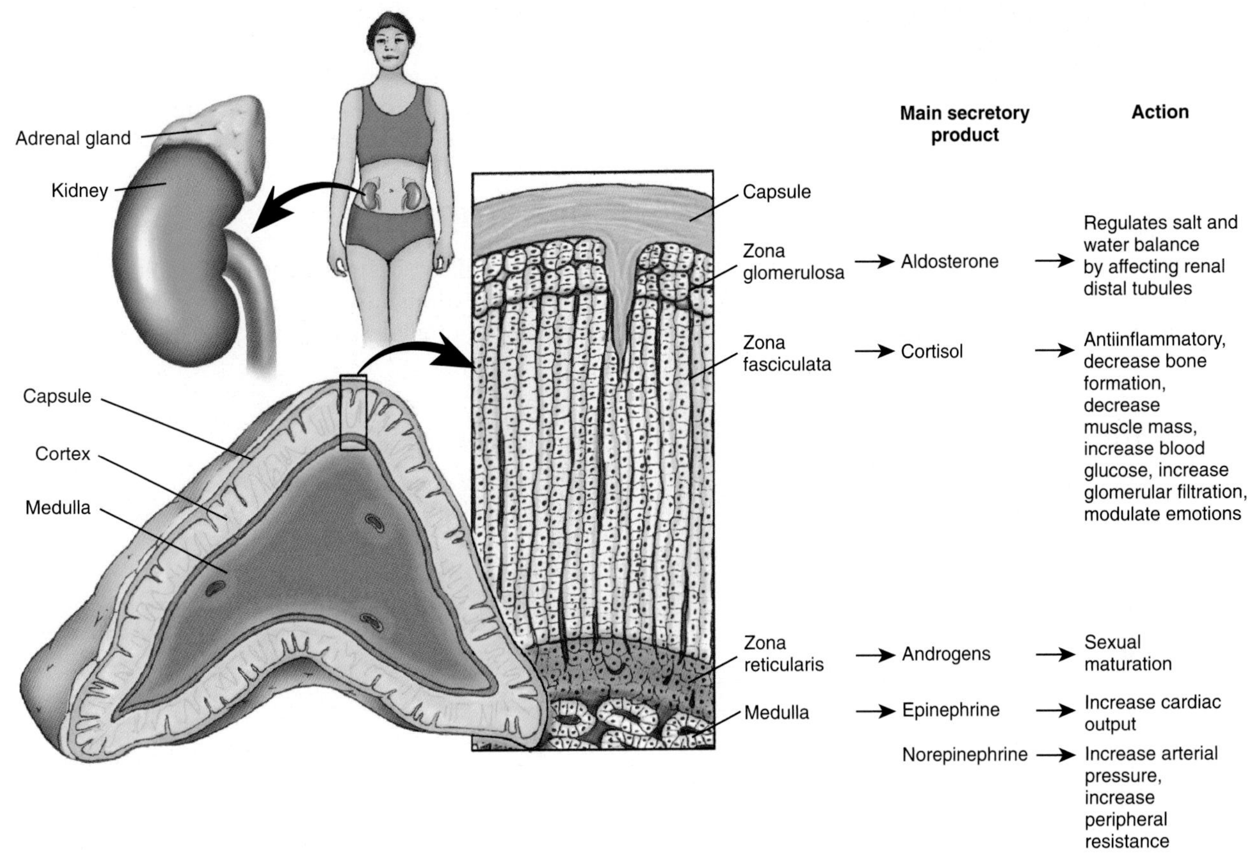

FIGURE 15-1 Structure of the adrenal gland, representative zones, and their main secretory products and physiologic actions. (*Adapted from Thibodeau GA, Patton KT:* Anatomy and physiology, *ed 7, St. Louis, 2010, Mosby.*)

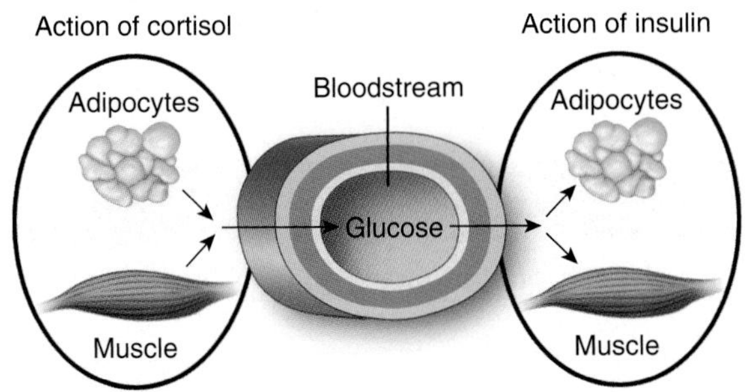

FIGURE 15-2 Effects of cortisol and insulin on glucose in the bloodstream.

procedures.[11,12] Many synthetic glucocorticoids are available, and they differ in potency relative to cortisol and in their duration of action (Table 15-1).

Mineralocorticoids

Aldosterone is the primary mineralocorticoid secreted by the adrenal cortex. It is essential to sodium and potassium balance and to the maintenance of extracellular fluid (i.e., intravascular volume). Its actions occur primarily on the distal tubule and the collecting duct of the kidney, where it promotes sodium and water retention, and potassium excretion. Aldosterone secretion is

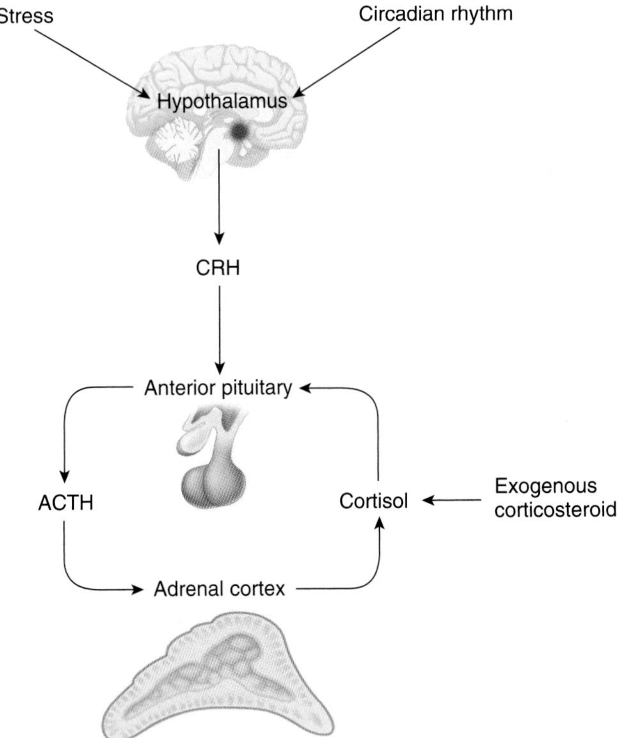

FIGURE 15-3 Hypothalamic-pituitary-adrenal axis and the regulation of cortisol secretion.

regulated by the renin-angiotensin system, ACTH, and plasma sodium and potassium levels. Aldosterone secretion is stimulated by a fall in renal blood pressure, which results from decreased intravascular volume or a sodium imbalance.[2] The drop in volume and/or pressure causes renin release from the kidney which activates angiotensinogen to form angiotensin I and II. Angiotensin II, in turn, stimulates secretion of aldosterone from the adrenal cortex. When blood pressure rises, renin-angiotensin release diminishes, serving as a negative feedback loop that inhibits additional production of aldosterone (Figure 15-5).

Adrenal Androgens

Dehydroepiandrosterone (DHEA) is the principal androgen secreted by the adrenal cortex. The effects of adrenal androgens are the same as those of testicular androgens (i.e., masculinization and the promotion of protein anabolism and growth). The activity of the adrenal androgens, however, is only about 20% that of the testicular androgens and is of relatively minor physiologic importance.[2] Estrogen precursors are secreted from the zona reticularis of the adrenal cortex.

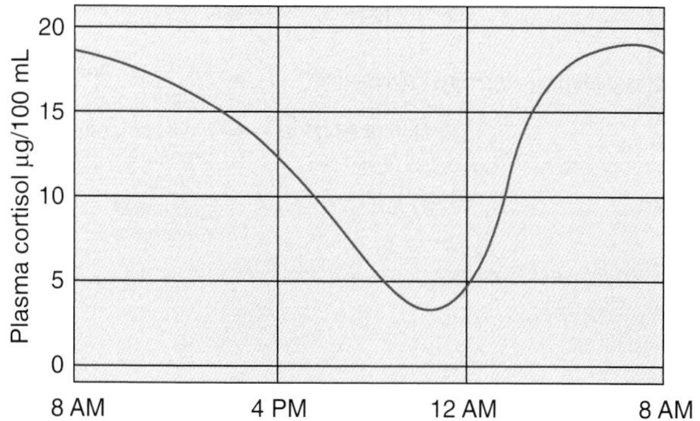

FIGURE 15-4 Normal pattern of cortisol secretion over a 24-hour period.

DEFINITION

Disorders of the adrenal glands can result in overproduction (hyperadrenalism) or underproduction (hypoadrenalism or adrenal insufficiency) of adrenal products.

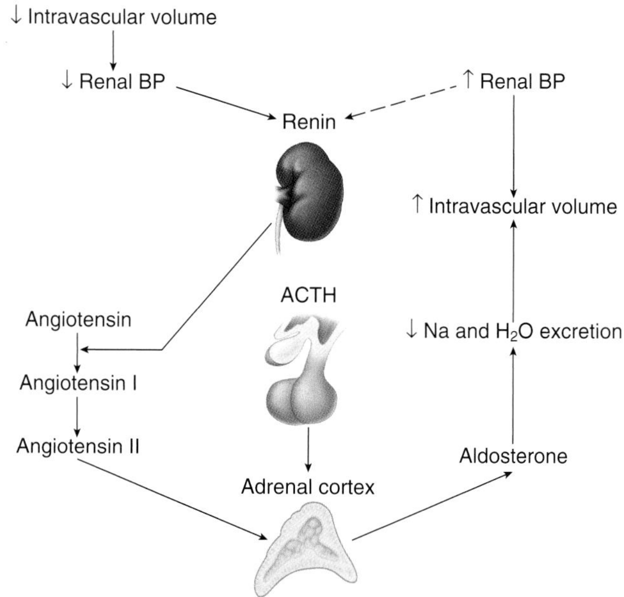

FIGURE 15-5 Regulation of aldosterone secretion.

TABLE 15-1 Glucocorticoids and Their Relative Potency

Compound	Antiinflammatory Potency	Mineralocorticoid Potency	Equivalent Dose* (mg)
Short-Acting (<12 Hours)			
Cortisol	1	2	20
Hydrocortisone	0.8	2	20
Intermediate-Acting (12-36 Hours)			
Prednisone	4	1	5
Prednisolone	4	1	5
Triamcinolone	5	0	4
Methylprednisolone	5	0.5	4
Fludrocortisone	15	200	1.4
Long-Acting (>36 Hours)			
Betamethasone	25	0	0.75
Dexamethasone	25	0	0.75
Inhaled			
Beclometasone dipropionate	8 puffs 4 times a day equals 14 mg oral prednisone once a day	—	—

NOTE: Fluticasone propionate is roughly twice as potent as beclometasone dipropionate and budesonide. Data from Barnes N: Relative safety and efficacy of inhaled corticosteroids, *J Allergy Clin Immunol* 101:S460-S464, 1998.

*Approximate.

Data from Schimmer BP, Parker KL: In Brunton LL, et al, editors: Goodman and Gilman's the pharmacological basis of therapeutics, *ed 11, New York, 2006, McGraw-Hill; and Kroenberg HM, et al:* Williams textbook of endocrinology, *ed 11, Philadelphia, 2008, Saunders.*

Hyperadrenalism results from excessive secretion of adrenal cortisol, mineralocorticoids, androgens, or estrogen, in isolation or combination. The most common type of overproduction is due to glucocorticoid excess; when this is caused by pathophysiologic processes, the condition is known as *Cushing's disease.*[1]

Adrenal insufficiency is divided into two categories: primary and secondary. Primary adrenocortical insufficiency, also known as *Addison's disease,* is characterized by destruction of the adrenal cortex with resulting deficiency of all of the adrenocortical hormones. The more common form, secondary adrenocortical insufficiency, may be the consequence of hypothalamic or pituitary disease, critical illness, or the administration of exogenous corticosteroids, with a deficiency of primarily cortisol. Both types of insufficiency downregulate adrenal production of cortisol. Inasmuch as abnormalities of adrenal function can render the patient medically compromised, these conditions are of significant concern in clinical practice.

EPIDEMIOLOGY

Incidence and Prevalence

Adrenal insufficiency occurs in 90 to 110 per 1 million persons of all ages, and diagnosis peaks in the fourth decade of life.[13] Secondary adrenocortical insufficiency is about 2 to 3 times more common than primary adrenal insufficiency, and diagnosis peaks in the sixth decade.[14] Both conditions are more common in women. Approximately 5% of adults in the United States use corticosteroids on a chronic basis and thus are at risk for secondary adrenocortical insufficiency. A dental practice serving 2000 adults can expect to encounter 100 patients who use corticosteroids or who have potential adrenal abnormalities.

Etiology

Primary adrenocortical insufficiency is caused by progressive destruction of the adrenal cortex, usually because of autoimmune disease, chronic infectious disease (tuberculosis, human immunodeficiency virus [HIV] infection, cytomegalovirus infection, and fungal infection) or malignancy. The condition also may result from hemorrhage, sepsis, adrenalectomy, drugs, or genetic mutations (e.g., familial glucocorticoid deficiency).[14-16]

Secondary adrenocortical insufficiency is a far more common problem and may be caused by structural lesions of the hypothalamus or pituitary gland (e.g., tumor), administration of exogenous corticosteroids, or less commonly, administration of specific drugs (e.g., desferrioxamine in the treatment of thalassemia) or a critical illness (burns, trauma, systemic infection).[17] Suppression of the HPA axis by exogenous or endogenous glucocorticoids is the most common cause of secondary adrenal insufficiency. The secretion of cortisol is directly dependent on the level of circulating ACTH. As plasma cortisol level increases, the production of ACTH decreases by virtue of negative feedback to the pituitary and the hypothalamus. With the administration of corticosteroids, the feedback system senses the elevated plasma steroid levels and inhibits ACTH production, which in turn suppresses adrenal production of cortisol (see Figure 15-3). The result is partial adrenal insufficiency. The production of aldosterone, because it is ACTH-independent, is not appreciably affected.

Pathophysiology and Complications

The major hormones of the adrenal cortex are cortisol and aldosterone. Addison's disease is caused by the lack of these compounds. Lack of cortisol results in impaired metabolism of glucose, fat, and protein, as well as hypotension, increased ACTH secretion, impaired fluid excretion, excessive pigmentation, and an inability to tolerate stress. The relationship between corticosteroids and response to stress involves the maintenance of vascular reactivity to vasoactive agents and the maintenance of normal blood pressure and cardiac output. Aldosterone deficiency results in an inability to conserve sodium and eliminate potassium and hydrogen ions, leading to hypovolemia, hyperkalemia, and acidosis.[1,2]

Chronic excessive use of glucocorticoids can result in clinical features mimicking those of Cushing's disease. This collection of clinical features of glucocorticoid excess is known as *Cushing's syndrome.* This condition results from high levels of cortisol altering the proteins, carbohydrate and fat metabolism, the effects of insulin and vasculature homeostasis.

Corticosteroids that are topically applied or repeatedly locally injected or inhaled are rare inducers of adrenal suppression by absorption through the skin, subjacent tissues, or pulmonary alveoli.[18] Although the amount of topical steroid required to treat small, noninflamed areas probably does not cause significant suppression, prolonged treatment of large inflamed areas may be a cause for concern, especially if occlusive dressings are used with highly potent steroids.[19-21] Similar comments may be made regarding the use of inhaled corticosteroids, if they are given in frequent and high doses.[22,23] Doses above 400 to 500 μg/day in children or 800 to 1000 μg/day of beclomethasone dipropionate equivalent in adults (depending on body mass) generally are considered to represent the cutoff point, indicating that adrenal suppression is probable.[23-25]

Once corticosteroid administration has ceased, the HPA axis regains its responsiveness, and normal ACTH and cortisol secretion eventually resumes. The time required to regain normal adrenal responsiveness is thought to range from days to months. However, studies from a large review[26] demonstrated a return to stress stimulation of HPA function within 14 days, despite the fact that supraphysiologic doses were given for a month or longer.

CLINICAL PRESENTATION

Signs and Symptoms

Hypoadrenalism. Signs and symptoms of the adrenal insufficiency are the result of deficiencies of adrenocortical hormones and often are nonspecific, leading to delays in diagnosis. Clinical evidence of deficiency generally appears only after 90% of the adrenal cortices have been destroyed.

Primary adrenal insufficiency (Addison's disease) produces signs and symptoms that relate to a deficiency of aldosterone and cortisol. The most common complaints are weakness, fatigue, abdominal pain, and hyperpigmentation of the skin and mucous membranes (Figure 15-6). Hypotension, anorexia, salt craving, myalgia, hypoglycemia, and weight loss are additional commonly associated features. If a patient with Addison's disease is challenged by stress (e.g., illness, infection, surgery), an *adrenal crisis* may be precipitated.[27] This medical emergency evolves over a few hours and manifests as severe exacerbation of the patient's condition, including sunken eyes, profuse sweating, hypotension, weak pulse, cyanosis, nausea, vomiting, weakness, headache, dehydration, fever, dyspnea, myalgias, arthralgia, hyponatremia, and eosinophilia. If not treated rapidly, the patient may develop hypothermia, severe hypotension, hypoglycemia, confusion, and circulatory collapse that can result in death.[1,2]

Secondary adrenal insufficiency caused by long-term corticosteroid administration may cause a partial insufficiency that is limited to glucocorticoids. The condition usually does not produce any symptoms unless the patient is significantly stressed and does not have adequate circulating cortisol during times surrounding stress. In this event, an adrenal crisis is possible. However, an adrenal crisis in a patient with secondary adrenal suppression is rare and tends not to be as severe as that seen with primary adrenal insufficiency, because aldosterone secretion is normal. Thus, hypotension, dehydration, and shock are seldom encountered.[2]

Hyperadrenalism. Adrenal hyperfunction can produce four syndromes that are dependent on the adrenal product that is in excess—androgen, estrogen, mineralocorticoid, and cortisol. Androgen-related disorders are rare and primarily affect the reproductive organs. Mineralocorticoid excess (primary aldosteronism) is associated with hypertension, hypokalemia, and dependent edema (see Chapter 3). The most common form of hyperadrenalism is due to glucocorticoid excess (endogenous or exogenous), and it leads to a syndrome known as Cushing's syndrome. This syndrome classically produces weight gain, a broad and round face ("moon facies") (Figure 15-7), a "buffalo hump" on the upper

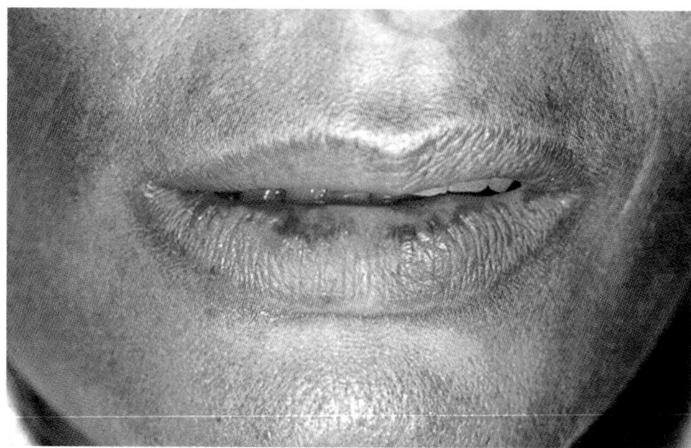

A

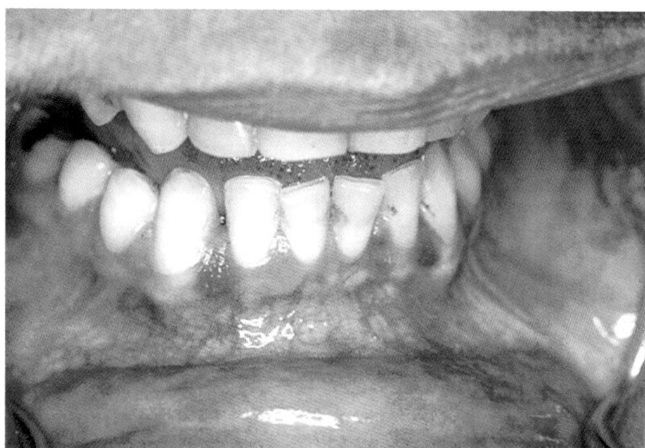

B

FIGURE 15-6 Patient with Addison's disease. Note bronzing of the skin with pigmentation of the lip (**A**) and the oral mucosa (**B**).

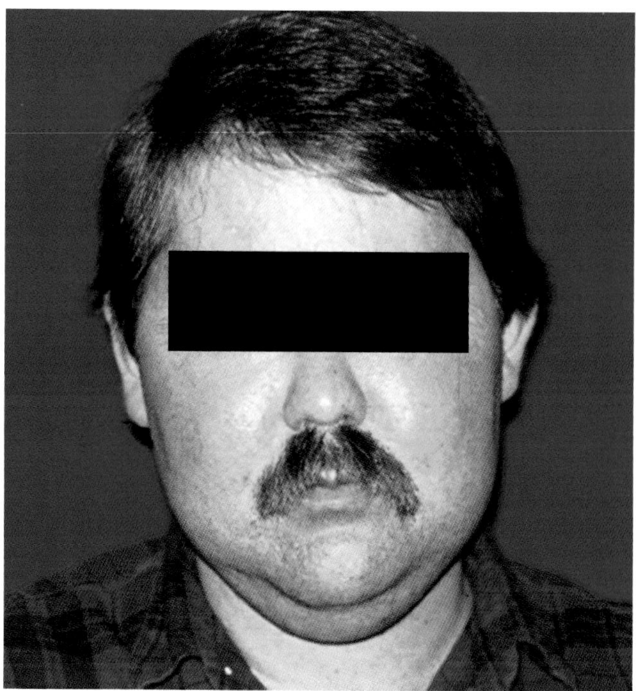

FIGURE 15-7 "Moon-shaped face": A clinical manifestation of Cushing's disease.

back, abdominal striae, hypertension, hirsutism, and acne. Other findings may include glucose intolerance (e.g., diabetes mellitus), heart failure, osteoporosis and bone fractures, impaired healing, and psychiatric disorders (mental depression, mania, anxiety disorders, cognitive dysfunction, and psychosis).[21] Long-term steroid use also may increase risks for insomnia, peptic ulceration, cataract formation, glaucoma, growth suppression, and delayed wound healing.

Laboratory Findings

Laboratory assessment for adrenal insufficiency generally is initiated with a provocative stimulation test of the HPA axis. These tests include the synthetic ACTH (cosyntropin) stimulation test, the CRH test, and the dexamethasone suppression test. The ACTH stimulation test is the most reliable and most commonly used test of the three. It is carried out by injecting a synthetic ACTH hormone, such as cosyntropin, either at 1 μg in the physiologic low-dose test or at 250 μg in the conventional-dose short test. Blood is collected 30 minutes and 60 minutes after injection to determine stimulated cortisol levels. A positive response (i.e., an increase in plasma cortisol level after ACTH administration) is indicative of adrenal reserve and function. A subnormal test response (60-minute cortisol level less than 18 μg/dL) is suggestive of adrenal insufficiency, but has limited correlation with the patient's clinical ability to respond to stress.[28]

Intact adrenocortical reserve can also be assessed by measuring cortisol levels in either urine, plasma, and saliva. Of the three, saliva is considered the most sensitive. The test usually is performed as an early-morning sample at the time of maximal secretion (range, 10 to 20 μg/dL). Samples procured in the late afternoon typically yield lower values (3 to 10 μg/dL) owing to the effects of circadian rhythm. Clinicians also should be aware that cortisol levels vary in response to diet, stress, and sleep pattern.[29,30]

To evaluate the entire HPA axis, the insulin tolerance test is used. This test however, is costly and unpleasant for the patient, because the insulin bolus induces severe hypoglycemia, and constant medical supervision is required.[31] Imaging of the adrenal gland and pituitary gland is recommended if malignancy, infiltrative disease, or hemorrhage is suspected.

MEDICAL MANAGEMENT

Primary Adrenal Insufficiency

The primary medical needs of the addisonian patient are (1) management of the adrenal disease (e.g., elimination of the infectious agent or malignant disease) and (2) hormonal replacement therapy. Glucocorticoid replacement is accomplished at levels that correspond to normal physiologic output of the adrenal cortex, usually about 20 to 30 mg of hydrocortisone or cortisone acetate per day, with a range of 12.5 to 50 mg daily. Cortisone 30 mg daily or prednisone 7.5 mg daily provides adequate substitution therapy. Current practice recommends that half to two thirds of the dose be given in the morning and one third in the later afternoon, to reflect the normal diurnal cycle. Mineralocorticoid replacement is accomplished by daily administration of fludrocortisone (0.05 to 0.2 mg). Patients also are encouraged to ingest adequate sodium and to monitor their blood pressure closely.[14] Although patients with Addison's disease can lead essentially normal lives with appropriate treatment, the need for supplemental glucocorticoids during periods of illness, trauma, or stress continues indefinitely. Target dose levels are 25 to 75 mg of hydrocortisone the day of minor to moderate surgery and 100 to 150 mg on the day of major surgery and the day after (Table 15-2).[32,33] These target doses are based on the cortisol responses elicited by surgery, as explained below.

TABLE 15-2 Recommendations for Steroid Supplementation During Surgery*

Procedure	Target Dose: Primary Adrenal Insufficiency†	Target Dose: Secondary Adrenal Insufficiency‡
Routine dentistry	None	None
Minor surgery	25 mg hydrocortisone equivalent, preoperatively on the day of surgery	Daily therapeutic dose
Moderate surgical stress	50-75 mg on day of surgery and up to 1 day after Return to preoperative glucocorticoid dose on postoperative day 2	Daily therapeutic dose
Major surgical stress	100-150 mg per day of hydrocortisone equivalent given for 2 to 3 days After preoperative dose, 50 mg hydrocortisone IV every 8 hours after the initial dose for the first 48 to 72 hours after surgery	Daily therapeutic dose

*Guidelines based on patient's adrenal insufficiency status; however, requirements could increase if the patient's health is poor, if concurrent fear/anxiety or infection that is poorly managed is present, and if major surgery is being performed. Frequent monitoring of blood pressure during the first 8 hours postoperatively is recommended.

†*Data from Salem M, et al: Perioperative glucocorticoid coverage. A reassessment 42 years after emergence of a problem,* Ann Surg *219:416-425, 1994.*

‡*Data from Marik PE, Varon J: Requirement of perioperative stress doses of corticosteroids: a systematic review of the literature,* Arch Surg *143:1222-1226, 2008. Supplemental doses can be provided if signs or symptoms of adrenal insufficiency (e.g., hypotension, abdominal pain, fatigue) appear.*

Surgery causes increased plasma corticosteroid levels during and after operations.[5] Plasma cortisol levels peak at 2- to 10-fold above baseline between 4 and 10 hours after the operation.[34,35] The level of response is based on the magnitude of the surgery and whether general anesthesia is used. Postoperative pain is also contributory to elevated cortisol requirements. Kehlet[6] and others estimate that adults secrete 75 to 200 mg a day in response to major surgery and 50 mg a day during minor procedures. Cortisol levels usually return to baseline within 24 to 48 hours of surgery.[5,32,36,37] Urine levels of cortisol metabolites, however, have been shown to remain increased for 3 to 6 days after the surgery.[35]

Secondary Adrenal Insufficiency

Secondary adrenal insufficiency may result from destructive hypothalamic-pituitary disorders or long-term steroid use. For hypothalamic-pituitary disorders, treatment involves correcting the ACTH-dependent disorder and replacing the missing glucocorticoid. In patients who take corticosteroids on a chronic basis, physicians may be challenged in trying to balance the beneficial effects of steroids with their unwanted adverse effects. Steroids are prescribed in the management of nonendocrine, inflammatory, and autoimmune disorders for their anti-inflammatory and immunosuppressive properties. Selection is based on potency, route of administration, duration of action, and anticipated adverse effects. The goal is to achieve resolution of disease symptoms while minimizing adverse effects.

Depending on the condition, dosages generally are targeted to be the same as or less than the daily replacement dose of the preparation used. For example, hydrocortisone usually is dispensed at about 20 mg/day, prednisone or prednisolone at 5 mg/day, and dexamethasone at 0.3 to 0.5 mg/day (see Table 15-1). Such regimens given as a morning dose are less suppressive. Higher and divided daily doses are more suppressive and usually take at least 3 weeks to result in clinical manifestation of glucocortiocoid deficiency. A method for minimizing the adverse effects of long-term systemic steroid therapy is the *alternate-day regimen*. This method consists of giving steroids in the morning every other day instead of daily, but at a higher dose to maintain an elevated serum level. The alternate-day regimen allows the adrenal gland to function normally during the off day and thus does not tend to cause adrenal axis suppression. A *tapered dosage* schedule often is implemented for the discontinuation of steroid usage, but this approach may not be necessary in many cases.[38]

The need for additional (i.e., supplemental) corticosteroids for patients taking daily or alternate-day steroids to prevent adrenal crisis during and after surgery has been a concern ever since Fraser and colleagues[39] reported in 1952 that a patient who had taken cortisone for 8 months experienced refractory hypotension at the end of a routine surgical procedure and died 3 hours later. A similar case was reported a year later.[40] The general consensus for several decades was that "at-risk" patients who take corticosteroids should be provided supplemental steroids during periods of stress, trauma, or illness.[32] More recent evidence, however, has led to revised recommendations (see Table 15-2). The new recommendations, based on evidence-based reviews, suggest that only patients with primary adrenal insufficiency receive supplemental doses of steroid, whereas those with secondary adrenal insufficiency who take daily corticosteroids, regardless of the type of surgery, should receive only their usual daily dose of corticosteroid before the surgery.[41,42] The rationale for these new recommendations is that the vast majority of patients who take daily equivalent or lower doses of steroid (e.g., mean dose of 5 to 10 mg prednisone daily) on a long-term basis for conditions such as renal transplantation or rheumatoid arthritis maintain adrenal function and do not experience adverse outcomes after minor or even major surgical procedures.[38,43-47] In addition, patients who took 5 to 50 mg prednisone daily for several years who had their glucocorticoid medications discontinued within a week before surgery have withstood general surgical procedures without the development of adrenal crisis.[5,36,44,45] Clinicians should recognize that major surgery generally is performed in hospital-like environments, in which close monitoring of blood pressure and fluid balance helps to ensure minimal adverse events during the postsurgical period. Thus, the recommendations listed in Table 15-2 include good operative and postoperative monitoring.

Inasmuch as the recommendations in Table 15-2 serve as guidelines, clinicians should be aware that the need for corticosteroid supplementation also can be influenced by factors that may complicate the postsurgical course and exacerbate adrenal insufficiency. These factors include the overall physical status of the patient including level of pain, liver dysfunction, febrile illness, sepsis, fluid loss, nausea and vomiting, and drugs taken.[39] Clinicians are advised to monitor the patient for these conditions and to select medications carefully. Drugs that can lower plasma cortisol levels include general anesthetics, midazolam, barbiturates, aminoglutethimide (an adrenolytic), etomidate (an anesthetic agent), ketoconazole, and inducers of hepatic cytochrome P-450 oxygenases (e.g., phenytoin, barbiturates, rifampin) that accelerate degradation of cortisol.[43,48,49] Also of note, the action of oral anticoagulants can be potentiated (resulting in increased risk of bleeding) by the intravenous administration of high-dose methylprednisolone.[50,51]

Adrenal Crisis

A rare and potentially life-threatening outcome in spite of steroid supplementation is acute adrenal insufficiency (adrenal crisis). This condition requires timely diagnosis and immediate treatment, including intravenous injection of a glucocorticoid—usually a 100-mg hydrocortisone bolus—and fluid and electrolyte replacement. Intramuscular injection results in slow absorption and is not preferred for emergency treatment. After the initial bolus, 50 mg hydrocortisone is administered IV slowly every 6 to 8 hours for 24 hours, for a typical total dose of 100 to 200 mg per 24 hours; along with fluid replacement, vasopressors, continuous infusion of saline, and correction of hypoglycemia, if needed. Resolution of the precipitating event or condition also is required.

DENTAL MANAGEMENT

In developing recommendations for dental patients with adrenal disease, the dentist must consider the type and degree of adrenal dysfunction and the dental procedure planned. Patients with hyperadrenalism or who take corticosteroids for prolonged periods have an increased likelihood of having hypertension, diabetes, delayed wound healing, osteoporosis, and peptic ulcer disease. To minimize the risk of an adverse outcome, blood pressure should be taken at baseline and monitored during dental appointments. Blood glucose levels should be determined and invasive procedures should be performed during periods of good glucose control. Follow-up appointments should be arranged to assess proper wound healing. Because osteoporosis has a relationship with periodontal bone loss, implant placement and bone fracture, periodic measures of periodontal bone loss are indicated, and measures should be instituted that promote bone mineralization and avoid extensive neck manipulation if osteoporosis is severe. Because of the risk of peptic ulceration, postoperative analgesics for long-term steroid users should not include aspirin and other nonsteroidal antiinflammatory drugs (NSAIDs).

Evidence indicates that the vast majority of patients with secondary adrenal insufficiency may undergo routine dental treatment without the need for supplemental glucocorticoids.[34,36,45,46,52] Patients at risk for adrenal crisis are those who undergo stressful surgical procedures and have no or extremely low adrenal function because of primary or severe secondary adrenal insufficiency.

Risk assessment for primary or secondary adrenal insufficiency should be determined by performing a thorough medical history and physical examination. A past or present history of tuberculosis, histoplasmosis, or HIV infection increases the risk for primary adrenal disease (insufficiency) in that opportunistic infectious agents may attack the adrenal glands. In addition, adrenal crisis is more likely in patients with malignancy or major traumatic injury, or in adrenally deficient patients who have a severe infection, discontinue treatment, or simply do not take their glucocorticoid before a stressful surgical procedure.

Although biochemical testing (i.e., ACTH stimulation test) can be helpful in identifying those who may have primary adrenal insufficiency, it is generally not recommended for patients taking glucocorticoids. In the latter, test results do not necessarily reflect how patients will react clinically or whether an adverse reaction will occur.[5,26,30] In primary adrenal insufficiency, a low ACTH stimulation test result (levels below 18 μg/dL achieved after administration of 250 mg of cosyntropin) demonstrating inadequate adrenal cortical function indicates that supplemental steroids should be provided if surgical procedures are planned.

The two major factors influencing the recommendation for supplemental corticosteroids are the type of adrenal insufficiency and the level and type of stress. Currently, only patients with primary adrenal insufficiency are recommended to receive supplementation, and this recommendation applies only when surgery is being performed and/or in the management of a dental or systemic infection (see Table 15-2).[41,44,47,53-57] Patients with secondary adrenal insufficiency and those who take daily or alternate-day corticosteroids have enough exogenous and endogenous cortisol to handle routine dental procedures and surgery, if their usual steroid dose (or parenteral dose equivalent) is taken the morning of the procedure.[41] Thus, the recommendation is for patients to take their usual daily dose of steroid within 2 hours of the surgical procedure, and that the surgeon, anesthetist, and nurses be advised of possible complications associated with the patient's adrenal state. Routine dental procedures do not stimulate cortisol production at levels comparable with those that occur at the time of surgery and do not require supplementation, even in patients with controlled primary adrenal insufficiency.[52,58] Patients undergoing surgery should be closely monitored for blood and fluid loss and for hypotension during the postoperative period. If hypotension appears during monitoring, intravenous fluids are to be given and additional doses of corticosteroid considered if fluid replacement fails to rectify the blood pressure. Patients are returned to their usual glucocorticoid dosage as soon as their vital signs are stabilized.

Additional measures recommended to minimize the risk of adrenal crisis associated with surgical stress are shown in Box 15-1. Surgery should be scheduled in the morning when cortisol levels are highest. Proper stress reduction should be provided because fear and anxiety increase cortisol demand. Nitrous oxide–oxygen inhalation and benzodiazepine sedation[8,59] are helpful in minimizing stress and reducing cortisol demand.[35] In contrast, reversal of and recovery from general anesthesia and extubation, and not the trauma of surgery itself, are major determinants of secretion of ACTH, cortisol, and epinephrine.[59,60] Thus, general anesthesia increases glucocorticoid demand for these patients. Barbiturates also should be used cautiously because these drugs enhance the metabolism of cortisol and reduce blood levels of

BOX 15-1 Dental Management
Considerations in Patients with Possible Adrenal Insufficiency

P

Patient Evaluation/Risk Assessment (see Box 1-1)

- Evaluate and determine whether primary adrenal sufficiency or secondary adrenal insufficiency exists.
- Obtain medical consultation if condition is poorly controlled (e.g., acute infection), if clinical signs and symptoms point to an undiagnosed problem, or if diagnosis is uncertain.

Potential Issues/Factors of Concern

A	
Analgesics	Provide good postoperative pain control to avoid adrenal crisis.
Antibiotics	No issues.
Anesthesia	Provide adequate operative and postoperative anesthesia; routine use of epinephrine (1:100,000) is appropriate. Consider using long-acting local anesthetics (e.g., bupivacaine) at the end of the procedure to provide longer postoperative pain control. General anesthesia increases glucocorticoid demand and could render an adrenal-insufficient patient susceptible to adrenal crisis; therefore use cautiously.
Anxiety	Anxiety and stress increase the risk of adrenal crisis, if adrenal insufficiency present. Use anxiety/stress reduction techniques as needed.
Allergy	No issues.
B	
Bleeding	Minimize blood loss.
Blood pressure	Monitor blood pressure throughout stressful and invasive procedures. Postoperative monitoring for at least 8 hours is recommended for procedures involving more than moderate surgery. If blood pressure drops below 100/60 mm Hg and the patient is unresponsive to fluid replacement and vasopressive measures, administer supplemental steroids.
C	
Chair position	Hypotension (e.g., from severe adrenal insufficiency) may dictate a supine position. Otherwise, normal chair position can be used.
D	
Devices	No issues.
Drugs	Provide steroid supplementation for primary adrenal insufficiency during surgical procedures or infection (see Table 15-2). Provide usual morning corticosteroid dose for patients who have secondary adrenal insufficiency and are undergoing surgical procedures. Use barbiturates with caution, because they increase the metabolism of cortisol and reduce blood levels of cortisol. Also, discontinue inhibitors of corticosteroid production (e.g., ketoconazole metyrapone, aminoglutethimide) at least 24 hours before surgery, with the consent of the patient's physician.
E	
Equipment	Have emergency medical kit readily available.
Emergencies	Acute adrenal crisis is a medical emergency. Call 911. Apply wet/ice packs, assess and monitor vital signs, start intravenous saline solution, inject 100 to 300 mg IV of hydrocortisone, start intravenous infusion of glucose solution, and transport patient to emergency medical facility.
F	
Follow-up	Postsurgery patients should be monitored for good fluid balance and adequate blood pressure during the first 24 hours. Communicate with the patient at the end of the appointment and within 4 hours postoperatively to determine whether features of weak pulse, hypotension, dyspnea, myalgias, arthralgia, ileus, and fever are present. Signs and symptoms of adrenal crisis dictate transport to a hospital for emergency care.

Surgical procedures lasting longer than 1 hour are more stressful than shorter procedures and are considered major surgery. Major surgery should be performed with the consideration for the need of steroid supplementation based on the overall health status of the patient. In addition, inadequate pain and anxiety control in the perioperative period increases the risk of adrenal crisis. Performance of major surgical procedures in a hospital environment is recommended to afford adequate patient monitoring during the postoperative phase.

cortisol.[49,61,62] In addition, inhibitors of corticosteroid production (e.g., ketoconazole metyrapone, aminoglutethimide) should be discontinued at least 24 hours before surgery, with the consent of the patient's physician.

Surgeries that last longer than 1 hour are more stressful than shorter surgeries and should be considered major surgical procedures that can require the need for steroid supplementation. Blood and fluid volume loss exacerbate hypotension, thereby increasing the risk for development of adrenal insufficiency–like symptoms. Thus, methods of reducing blood loss are important in this setting. Likewise, a fasting state can contribute to hypoglycemia which can mimic features of an adrenal crisis, but does not require glucocorticoids for resolution. Patients who take anticoagulants are at increased risk for postsurgical bleeding and hypotension. In addition, inadequate pain control during the postoperative period increases the risk of adrenal crisis. Clinicians should provide good postoperative pain control by means of long-acting local anesthetics (e.g., bupivacaine) given at the end of the procedure.

Monitoring of blood pressure throughout the procedure is critical for recognition of the development of an adrenal crisis. During surgery, blood pressure should be evaluated at 5-minute intervals and before the patient leaves the office. A systolic blood pressure below 100 mm Hg or a diastolic pressure at or below 60 mm Hg represents hypotension. A diagnosis of hypotension dictates that the clinician must take corrective action. This would include proper patient positioning (i.e., head lower than feet), fluid replacement, administration of vasopressors, and evaluation for signs of adrenal dysfunction versus hypoglycemia. Immediate treatment during an adrenal crisis requires the administration of 100 mg of hydrocortisone or 4 mg of dexamethasone IV and immediate transportation to a medical facility.

Inasmuch as significant cortisol increases generally are not seen before or during the operation but are increased in the postoperative period, approximately 1 to 5 hours after the procedure commensurate with the pain response,[34,44,54,63] and the rise in cortisol levels is blunted by the use of analgesics and midazolam,[8,34] good pain control with local anesthesia and analgesics is recommended for these patients.

Treatment Planning Modifications

Dental treatment of a patient with undiagnosed and untreated adrenal insufficiency should be delayed until the patient has been medically stabilized. Otherwise, treatment modifications are not required for patients with well-controlled adrenal disorders.

Oral Complications and Manifestations

In primary adrenal insufficiency, diffuse or focal brown macular pigmentation of the oral mucous membranes is a common finding (see Figure 15-6). Pigmentation of sun-exposed skin often follows the appearance of oral pigmentation and is accompanied by lethargy. Patients with secondary adrenal insufficiency may be prone to delayed healing and may have increased susceptibility to infection.

REFERENCES

1. Williams GD, Dluhy RG: Disorders of the adrenal cortex. In Fauci AS, et al, editors: *Harrison's principles of internal medicine*, ed 17, New York, 2009, McGraw-Hill, pp 2247-2268.
2. Stewart PM: The adrenal cortex. In Kronenberg HM, et al, editors: *Williams textbook of endocrinology*, ed 11, Philadelphia, 2008, Saunders, pp 445-504.
3. Collins S, Caron MG, Lefkowitz RJ: Beta-adrenergic receptors in hamster smooth muscle cells are transcriptionally regulated by glucocorticoids, *J Biol Chem* 263:9067-9070, 1988.
4. Annetta M, et al: Use of corticosteroids in critically ill septic patients: a review of mechanisms of adrenal insufficiency in sepsis and treatment, *Curr Drug Targets* 10:887-894, 2009.
5. Chernow B, et al: Hormonal responses to graded surgical stress, *Arch Intern Med* 147:1273-1278, 1987.
6. Kehlet H: *Clinical course and hypothalamic-pituitary-adrenocortical function in glucocorticoid-treated surgical patients*, Copenhagen, 1976, FADL's Forlag.
7. Cooper MS, Stewart PM: Corticosteroid insufficiency in acutely ill patients, *N Engl J Med* 348:727-734, 2003.
8. Jerjes W, et al: Midazolam in the reduction of surgical stress: a randomized clinical trial, *Oral Surg Oral Med Oral Pathol Oral Radiol Endod* 100:564-570, 2005.
9. George JM, et al: Morphine anesthesia blocks cortisol and growth hormone response to surgical stress in humans, *J Clin Endocrinol Metab* 38:736-741, 1974.
10. Raff H, et al: Inhibition of the adrenocorticotropin response to surgery in humans: interaction between dexamethasone and fentanyl, *J Clin Endocrinol Metab* 65:295-298, 1987.
11. Gersema L, Baker K: Use of corticosteroids in oral surgery, *J Oral Maxillofac Surg* 50:270-277, 1992.
12. Kaufman E, et al: Intraligamentary injection of slow-release methylprednisolone for the prevention of pain after endodontic treatment, *Oral Surg Oral Med Oral Pathol* 77:651-654, 1994.
13. Willis AC, Vince FP: The prevalence of Addison's disease in Coventry, UK, *Postgrad Med J* 73:286-288, 1997.
14. Arlt W, Allolio B: Adrenal insufficiency, *Lancet* 361:1881-1893, 2003.
15. Shenker Y, Skatrud JB: Adrenal insufficiency in critically ill patients, *Am J Respir Crit Care Med* 163:1520-1523, 2001.
16. Bornstein SR: Predisposing factors for adrenal insufficiency, *N Engl J Med* 360:2328-2339, 2009.
17. Al-Elq AH, Al-Saeed HH: Endocrinopathies in patients with thalassemias, *Saudi Med J* 25:1347-1351, 2004.
18. Hameed R, Zacharin MR: Cushing syndrome, adrenal suppression and local corticosteroid use, *J Paediatr Child Health* 42:392-394, 2006.
19. Coskey RJ: Adverse effects of corticosteroids: I. Topical and intralesional, *Clin Dermatol* 4:155-160, 1986.
20. Patel L, et al: Adrenal function following topical steroid treatment in children with atopic dermatitis, *Br J Dermatol* 132:950-955, 1995.
21. Plemons JM, Rees TD, Zachariah NY: Absorption of a topical steroid and evaluation of adrenal suppression in patients with erosive lichen planus, *Oral Surg Oral Med Oral Pathol* 69:688-693, 1990.
22. Hanania NA, Chapman KR, Kesten S: Adverse effects of inhaled corticosteroids, *Am J Med* 98:196-208, 1995.
23. Molimard M, et al: Inhaled corticosteroids and adrenal insufficiency, *Drug Saf* 31:769-774, 2008.
24. Kelly HW, Nelson HS: Potential adverse effects of the inhaled corticosteroids, *J Allergy Clin Immunol* 112:469-478, 2003.
25. Toogood JH, et al: Personal observations on the use of inhaled corticosteroid drugs for chronic asthma, *Eur J Respir Dis* 65:321-338, 1984.
26. Glick M: Glucocorticosteroid replacement therapy: a literature review and suggested replacement therapy, *Oral Surg Oral Med Oral Pathol* 67:614-620, 1989.
27. Hahner S, et al: Epidemiology of adrenal crisis in chronic adrenal insufficiency: the need for new prevention strategies, *Eur J Endocrinol* 162:597-602, 2010.
28. Dorin RI, Qualls CR, Crapo LM: Diagnosis of adrenal insufficiency, *Ann Intern Med* 139:194-204, 2003.
29. Findling JW, Raff H: Screening and diagnosis of Cushing's syndrome, *Endocrinol Metab Clin North Am* 34:385-402, ix-x, 2005.
30. Wallace I, Cunningham S, Lindsay J: The diagnosis and investigation of adrenal insufficiency in adults, *Ann Clin Biochem* 46:351-367, 2009.
31. Grinspoon SK, Biller BM: Clinical review 62: Laboratory assessment of adrenal insufficiency, *J Clin Endocrinol Metab* 79:923-931, 1994.
32. Salem M, et al: Perioperative glucocorticoid coverage. A reassessment 42 years after emergence of a problem, *Ann Surg* 219:416-425, 1994.

33. Perry RJ, McLaughlin EA, Rice PJ: Steroid cover in dentistry: recommendations following a review of current policy in UK dental teaching hospitals, *Dent Update* 30:45-47, 2003.
34. Banks P: The adreno-cortical response to oral surgery, *Br J Oral Surg* 8:32-44, 1907.
35. Thomasson B: Studies on the content of 17-hydroxycorticosteroids and its diurnal rhythm in the plasma of surgical patients, *Scand J Clin Lab Invest* 11(Suppl 42):1-180, 1959.
36. Kehlet H, Binder C: Adrenocortical function and clinical course during and after surgery in unsupplemented glucocorticoid-treated patients, *Br J Anaesth* 45:1043-1048, 1973.
37. Udelsman R, Holbrook NJ: Endocrine and molecular responses to surgical stress, *Curr Probl Surg* 31:653-720, 1994.
38. Shapiro R, et al: Adrenal reserve in renal transplant recipients with cyclosporine, azathioprine, and prednisone immunosuppression, *Transplantation* 49:1011-1013, 1990.
39. Fraser CG, Preuss FS, Bigford WD: Adrenal atrophy and irreversible shock associated with cortisone therapy, *JAMA* 149:1542-1543, 1952.
40. Lewis L, et al: Fatal adrenal cortical insufficiency precipitated by surgery during prolonged continuous cortisone treatment, *Ann Intern Med* 39:116-126, 1953.
41. Marik PE, Varon J: Requirement of perioperative stress doses of corticosteroids: a systematic review of the literature, *Arch Surg* 143:1222-1226, 2008.
42. Yong SL, et al: Supplemental perioperative steroids for surgical patients with adrenal insufficiency, *Cochrane Database Syst Rev* 4:CD005367, 2009.
43. Jasani MK, et al: Cardiovascular and plasma cortisol responses to surgery in corticosteroid-treated R.A. patients, *Acta Rheumatol Scand* 14:65-70, 1968.
44. Plumpton FS, Besser GM, Cole PV: Corticosteroid treatment and surgery. 2. The management of steroid cover, *Anaesthesia* 24:12-18, 1969.
45. Bromberg JS, et al: Stress steroids are not required for patients receiving a renal allograft and undergoing operation, *J Am Coll Surg* 180:532-536, 1995.
46. Friedman RJ, Schiff CF, Bromberg JS: Use of supplemental steroids in patients having orthopaedic operations, *J Bone Joint Surg Am* 77:1801-1806, 1995.
47. Singh N, et al: Acute adrenal insufficiency in critically ill liver transplant recipients. Implications for diagnosis, *Transplantation* 59:1744-1745, 1995.
48. Lehtinen AM, Hovorka J, Widholm O: Modification of aspects of the endocrine response to tracheal intubation by lignocaine, halothane and thiopentone, *Br J Anaesth* 56:239-246, 1984.
49. Oyama T, et al: Adrenocortical function related to thiopental-nitrous oxide-oxygen anesthesia and surgery in man, *Anesth Analg* 50:727-731, 1971.
50. Oliver R, et al: Antibiotics for the prophylaxis of bacterial endocarditis in dentistry, *Cochrane Database Syst Rev* 4:CD003813, 2008.
51. Costedoat-Chalumeau N, et al: Potentiation of vitamin K antagonists by high-dose intravenous methylprednisolone, *Ann Intern Med* 132:631-635, 2000.
52. Miller CS, Little JW, Falace DA: Supplemental corticosteroids for dental patients with adrenal insufficiency: reconsideration of the problem, *J Am Dent Assoc* 132:1570-1579, 2001.
53. Milenkovic A, et al: Adrenal crisis provoked by dental infection: case report and review of the literature, *Oral Surg Oral Med Oral Pathol Oral Radiol Endod* 110:325-329, 2010.
54. Ziccardi VB, et al: Precipitation of an Addisonian crisis during dental surgery: recognition and management, *Compendium* 13:518, 1992.
55. Broutsas MG, Seldin R: Adrenal crisis after tooth extractions in an adrenalectomized patient: report of case, *J Oral Surg* 30:301-302, 1972.
56. Cawson RA, James J: Adrenal crisis in a dental patient having systemic corticosteroids, *Br J Oral Surg* 10:305-309, 1973.
57. Scheitler LE, et al: Adrenal insufficiency: report of case, *Spec Care Dentist* 4:22-24, 1984.
58. Miller CS, et al: Salivary cortisol response to dental treatment of varying stress, *Oral Surg Oral Med Oral Pathol Oral Radiol Endod* 79:436-441, 1995.
59. Hempenstall PD, et al: Cardiovascular, biochemical, and hormonal responses to intravenous sedation with local analgesia versus general anesthesia in patients undergoing oral surgery, *J Oral Maxillofac Surg* 44:441-446, 1986.
60. Udelsman R, et al: Responses of the hypothalamic-pituitary-adrenal and renin-angiotensin axes and the sympathetic system during controlled surgical and anesthetic stress, *J Clin Endocrinol Metab* 64:986-994, 1987.
61. Parnell AG: Adrenal crisis and the dental surgeon, *Br Dent J* 116:294-298, 1964.
62. Siker ES, Lipschitz E, Klein R: The effect of preanesthetic medications on the blood level of 17-hydroxycorticosteroids, *Ann Surg* 143:88-91, 1956.
63. Shannon IL, et al: Stress in dental patients. II. The serum free 17-hydroxycorticosteroid response in routinely appointed patients undergoing simple exodontia, *Oral Surg Oral Med Oral Pathol* 15:1142-1146, 1962.

16

Thyroid Diseases

Thyroid disease in a patient who presents for dental treatment is a cause for concern on several fronts. Undiagnosed or poorly controlled disorders of the thyroid can be expected to compromise outcomes with otherwise perfectly appropriate dental management plans. Detection of early signs and symptoms of such disorders during the dentist's initial assessment, however, can lead to referral of the patient for medical evaluation and treatment. In some instances, such intervention may be lifesaving, whereas in others, quality of life can be improved and complications of certain thyroid disorders avoided, particularly in the context of delivery of dental care.

The focus of this chapter is on disorders involving hyperfunction of the gland (hyperthyroidism or thyrotoxicosis), hypofunction of the gland (hypothyroidism or myxedema or cretinism), thyroiditis, and the detection of lesions that may be cancerous (Table 16-1). In an average dental practice of 2000 patients, an estimated 20 to 150 patients will have a thyroid disorder.

THYROID GLAND

LOCATION

The thyroid gland, which is located in the anterior portion of the neck just below and bilateral to the thyroid cartilage, develops from the thyroglossal duct and portions of the ultimobranchial body[1,2] (Figure 16-1). It consists of two lateral lobes connected by an isthmus. A superior portion of glandular tissue, or a pyramidal lobe, can be identified. Thyroid tissue may be found anywhere along the path of the thyroglossal duct, from its origin (midline posterior portion of the tongue) to its termination (thyroid gland, in the neck).[1,2] In rare cases, the entire thyroid lies within the anterior mediastinal compartment; in most people, however, remnants of the duct atrophy and disappear.[1,2] The thyroglossal duct passes through the region of the developing hyoid bone, and remnants of the duct may become enclosed or surrounded by bone.[2,3] Ectopic thyroid tissue may secrete thyroid hormones or may become cystic (Figure 16-2) or neoplastic.[2,4] In a few people, the only functional thyroid tissue is found in these ectopic locations.[2]

The parathyroid glands develop from the third and fourth pharyngeal pouches and become embedded within the thyroid gland.[5] Neural crest cells from the ultimobranchial body give rise to thyroid medullary C cells, which produce calcitonin, a calcium-lowering hormone.[2,6] These C cells are found throughout the thyroid gland.[2,6]

ENLARGEMENT AND NODULES OF THE THYROID GLAND

Generalized enlargement of the thyroid gland, referred to as a *goiter,* may be diffuse (Figure 16-3) or nodular (Figure 16-4), and the goiter may be functional or nonfunctional.[1,7,8] On a functional basis, thyroid enlargement can be divided into three types: primary goiter (simple goiter and thyroid cancer), thyrostimulatory secondary goiters (Graves' disease and congenital hereditary goiter), and thyroinvasive secondary goiters (Hashimoto's thyroiditis, subacute painful thyroiditis, Riedel's thyroiditis, and metastatic tumors to the thyroid). Simple goiter accounts for about 75% of all thyroid swellings.[7] Most of these goiters are nonfunctional and thus do not cause hyperthyroidism. The goiter of Graves' disease is associated with hyperthyroidism.[1,7] Hashimoto's thyroiditis leads to hypothyroidism and thyroid enlargement.[7] By contrast, patients with enlargement due to subacute thyroiditis experience a transient period of hyperthyroidism.[7] Nodules found in the thyroid may be hyperplastic nodules, adenomas, or carcinomas. Hyperplastic nodules and adenomas can be functional

TABLE 16-1 Etiology of Thyroid Conditions

Thyroid Condition	Causes
Hyperthyroidism	Primary thyroid hyperfunction Grave's disease Toxic multinodular goiter Toxic adenoma Secondary thyroid hyperfunction Pituitary adenoma—TSH secretion Inappropriate TSH secretion (pituitary) Trophoblastic hCG secretion Without thyroid hyperfunction Hormonal leakage—subacute thyroiditis Thyroid hormone use (factitia) Bovine thyroid in ground beef Metastatic thyroid cancer Iatrogenic (overdosage of thyroid hormone)
Hypothyroidism (cretinism, myxedema)	Primary atrophic hypothyroidism Insufficient amount of thyroid tissue *Destruction of tissue by autoimmune process* Hashimoto's thyroiditis (atrophic and goitrous) Graves' disease—end-stage *Destruction of tissue by iatrogenic procedures* ^{131}I therapy Surgical thyroidectomy External radiation to thyroid gland *Destruction of tissue by infiltrative process* Amyloidosis, lymphoma, scleroderma Defects of thyroid hormone biosynthesis Congenital enzyme defects Congenital mutations in TSH receptor Iodine deficiency of excess Drug-induced: thionamides, lithium, others Agenesis or dysplasia Secondary hypothyroidism Pituitary Panhypopituitarism (neoplasm, irradiation, surgery) Isolated TSH deficiency Hypothalamic Congenital Infection Infiltration (sarcoidosis, granulomas) Transient hypothyroidism Silent and subacute thyroiditis Thyroxine withdrawal Generalized resistance to thyroid hormone
Thyroiditis	Acute suppurative Subacute painful Subacute painless Hashimoto's Chronic fibrosing (Riedel's)
Thyroid neoplasms	Adenomas Carcinomas Others

hCG, Human chorionic gonadotropin; *TSH,* Thyroid-stimulating hormone.

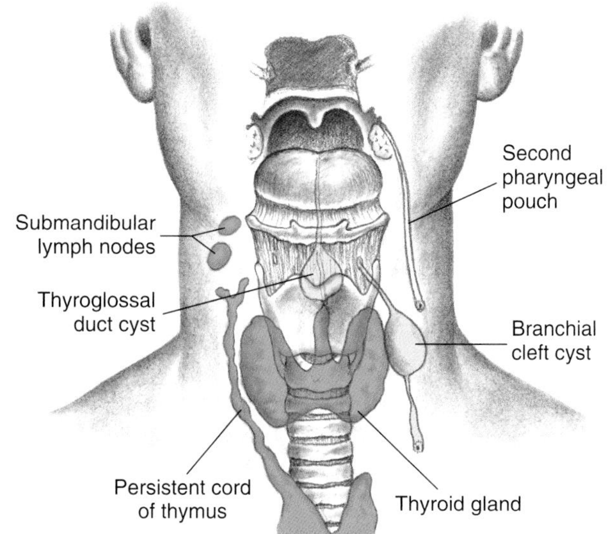

FIGURE 16-1 Thyroglossal duct cyst and branchial cleft cyst development. (*From Seidel HM, et al:* Mosby's guide to physical examination, *ed 7, St. Louis, 2011, Mosby.*)

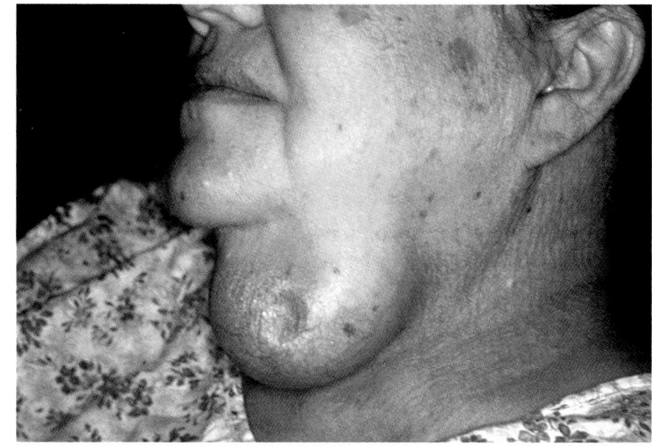

FIGURE 16-2 Thyroglossal duct cyst.

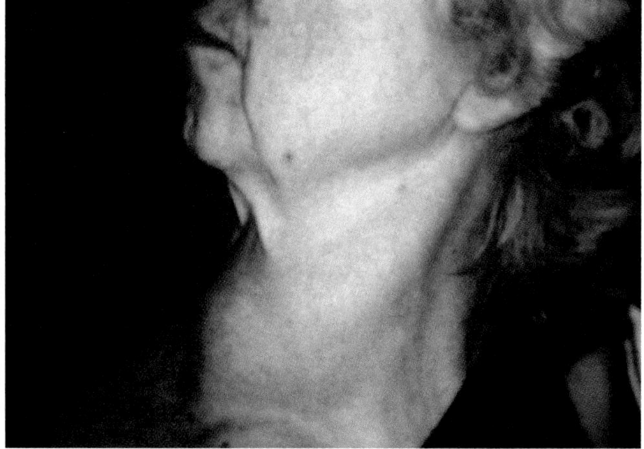

FIGURE 16-3 Diffuse enlargement of the thyroid gland due to Graves' disease (goiter).

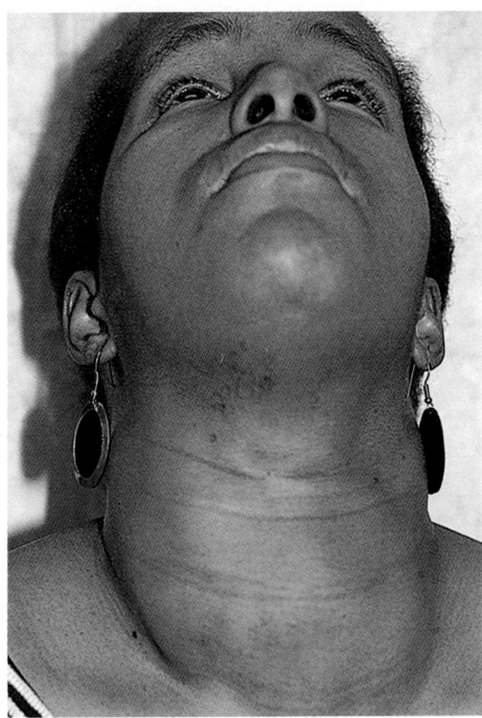

FIGURE 16-4 Multinodular goiter. (*From Swartz MH:* Textbook of physical diagnosis: history and examination, *ed 6, Philadelphia, 2010, Saunders.*)

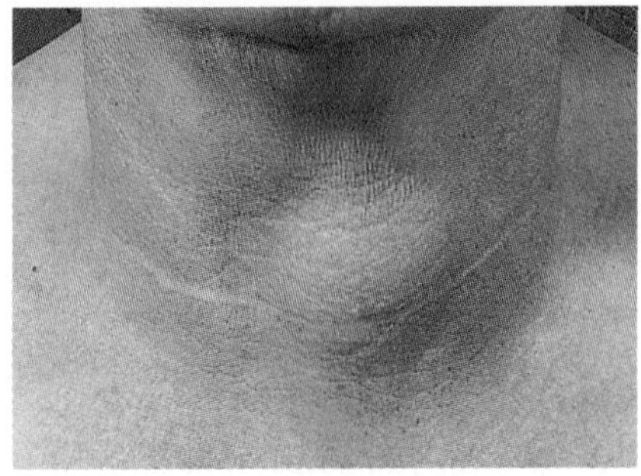

A

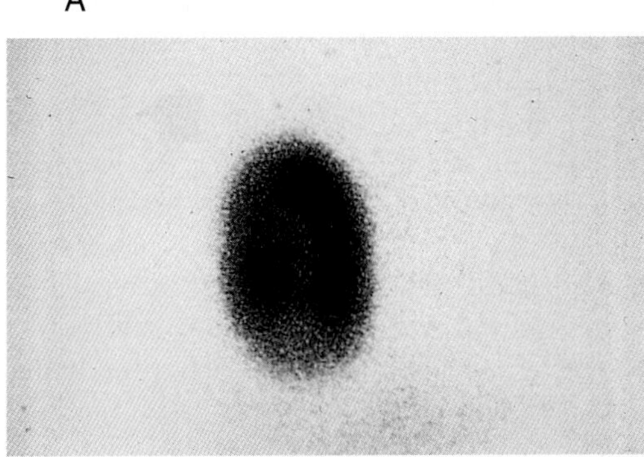

B

FIGURE 16-5 A, Toxic adenoma of the thyroid gland causing hyperthyroidism. **B,** Toxic adenoma in the right thyroid demonstrated with the use of Tc-pertechnetate scanning. (*From Forbes CD, Jackson WF:* Color atlas and text of clinical medicine, *ed 3, Edinburgh, 2003, Mosby.*)

(Figure 16-5) or nonfunctional. Most carcinomas are nonfunctional.[1,7,9] Thyroid cancer most often manifests as a single nodule but can arise as multiple lesions or, in rare cases, can occur within a benign goiter.[1,7,9]

FUNCTION OF THE THYROID GLAND

The thyroid gland secretes three hormones: thyroxine (T_4), triiodothyronine (T_3), and calcitonin.[8,10,11] Thyroxine and triiodothyronine collectively, they are termed *thyoid hormone.* Thyroid hormone influences the growth and maturation of tissues, cell respiration, and total energy expenditure. This hormone is involved in the turnover of essentially all substances, vitamins, and hormones.[8,10,11]

Most thyroid actions (metabolic and developmental) are mediated through activity of nuclear receptors that are tissue site–specific.[8] Thyroid receptors work by altering gene expression in response to changes in thyroid hormone concentrations (mostly T_3). This alteration in gene transcription profile is believed to account for most of the observed physiologic effects of thyroid hormones, although there are also actions of thyroid hormones that do not involve transcription.[11] Thyroid hormone increases oxygen consumption, thermogenesis, and expression of the low-density lipoprotein (LDL) receptor, resulting in accelerated LDL cholesterol degradation. In myocardium, T_3 increases myocyte contractility and relaxation by altering myosin heavy chain and sarcoplasmic reticulum adenosine triphosphatase (ATPase). In the cardiac conducting system, T_3 increases the heart rate by altering sinoatrial node depolarization and repolarization. Other physiologic effects of thyroid hormone include increased mental alertness, ventilatory drive, gastrointestinal motility, and bone turnover. During fetal development, thyroid hormone plays a critical role in brain development and skeletal maturation.[1]

Calcitonin is involved, along with parathyroid hormone and vitamin D, in regulating serum calcium and phosphorus levels and skeletal remodeling. (This hormone and its actions are considered further in Chapter 12.)[8,10,11]

Epidemiology

Incidence and Prevalence. Graves' disease occurs in up to 2% of women and 0.2% of men. Graves' disease is rare before adolescence; the usual age at presentation is between 20 and 50 years, although it does occur in elderly persons.[7,12] Congenital hypothyroidism is present in about 1 in 4000 newborns. Most cases (80% to 85%) are due to thyroid gland dysgenesis, and developmental abnormalities are twice as common in girls. The annual incidence rate of autoimmune hypothyroidism is 4 cases per 1000 women and 1 per 1000 men. Prevalence increases with age, and mean age at diagnosis is 60 years.

Subclinical hypothyroidism is diagnosed in 6% to 8% of women (10% in women over 60 years of age) and 3% of men.[13]

Subacute painful thyroiditis accounts for 5% of all medical consultations regarding thyroid disorders, and is three times more common in women than men. Subacute painless thyroiditis occurs in patients with underlying autoimmune thyroid disease and is reported in up to 5% of women 3 to 6 months after pregnancy. In these circumstances it is called *postpartum thyroiditis.* Riedel's thyroiditis is a rare form of chronic thyroiditis that typically occurs in middle-aged women. Acute suppurative thyroiditis is rare.[1,7,12,13]

Thyroid nodules can be found in about 5% of the adult population in the United States.[1,7,9] The frequency of cancer in solitary thyroid nodules has been reported to be about 1% to 5%.[1,7,9] During the past 10 years or so, the incidence of thyroid cancer has increased at a rate of about 5% per year.[9,14] In 2007, 434,000 people (96,000 men and 338,000 women) were living with thyroid cancer.[15] For 2010, the National Cancer Institute estimated a total of 44,670 new cases of thyroid cancer, with about 1690 deaths.[16]

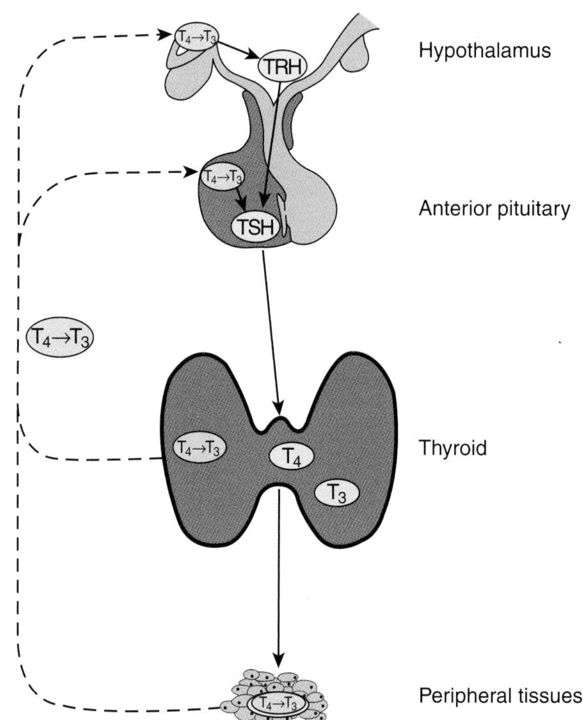

FIGURE 16-6 Hypothalamic-Pituitary-Thyroid Axis. *Solid lines* correspond to stimulatory effects, and *dotted lines* depict inhibitory effects. Conversion of T_4 to T_3 in the pituitary and the hypothalamus is mediated by 5′-deiodinase type II. This event also is important throughout the central nervous system, thyroid, and muscle. 5′-Deiodinase type I (propylthiouracil-sensitive) plays a major role in liver, kidney, and thyroid function. *TRH,* Thyrotropin-releasing hormone; *TSH,* Thyroid-stimulating hormone. (*Redrawn from DeGroot LJ, Jameson JL:* Endocrinology, *ed 5, vol 2, Philadelphia, 2006, Saunders.*)

Pathophysiology and Etiology

Blood levels of T_4 and T_3 are controlled through a servofeedback mechanism mediated by the hypothalamic-pituitary-thyroid axis (Figure 16-6). Increased or decreased metabolic demand appears to be the main modifier of the system. Drugs, illness, thyroid disease, and pituitary disorders may affect control of this balance.[7,8,11,17] Studies also show that age has some effect on the system.

Under normal conditions, thyrotropin-releasing hormone (TRH) is released by the hypothalamus in response to external stimuli (e.g., stress, illness, metabolic demand, low levels of T_3 and, to a lesser extent, T_4). TRH stimulates the pituitary to release thyroid-stimulating hormone (TSH), which causes the thyroid gland to secrete T_4 and T_3. T_4 and T_3 also have a direct influence on the pituitary. High levels turn off the release of TSH, and low levels turn it on. In the blood, T_4 and T_3 are almost entirely bound to plasma proteins.[7,8,11,17]

Binding plasma proteins consist of thyroxine-binding globulin (TBG), transthyretin, and thyroid-binding albumin (TBA). Small amounts of T_3 and T_4 are bound to high-density lipoproteins.[1] The most important thyroid hormone–binding serum protein is TBG, which binds about 70% of T_4 and 75% to 80% of T_3.[1] Only 0.02% to 0.03% of free thyroxine (FT_4) and about 0.3% of free triidothyroxine (FT_3) is found in plasma.[1,7]

Low T_4 and T_3 plasma levels often are found in ill and medicated older persons. Protein abnormalities can affect total T_4 and T_3 levels. Illness can reduce the conversion of T_4 to T_3. Drugs and illness also can affect free levels of T_4 and T_3. The main age-related change seen in much older individuals is a fall in T_3 due to the reduced peripheral conversion of T_4 to T_3.[18]

Antibodies to various structures within the thyroid are associated with autoimmune diseases of the thyroid. Graves' disease and Hashimoto's thyroiditis have such an association. Three autoantibodies are most often involved in autoimmune thyroid disease: TSH receptor antibodies (TSHRAb), thyroid peroxidase antibodies (TPoAb), and thyroglobulin antibodies (TgAb).[19] TSHRAb are not found in the general population but are present in 80% to 95% of patients with Graves' disease and in 10% to 20% of those with autoimmune thyroiditis. Most TSHRAb in Graves' disease are stimulating antibodies, which stimulate the release of thyroid hormone. However, blocking antibodies to the TSH receptor (TSHR-blocking Ab) also are found, which block the release of thyroid hormone. The ratio of these TSH receptor antibodies determines the clinical status of the patient and the functional status of the thyroid gland.[12,19]

TgAb are found in about 10% to 20% of the general population. These antibodies are present in 50% to 70% of patients with Graves' disease and in 80% to 90% of those with autoimmune thyroiditis.[7,12,19] TPoAb are found in 8% to 27% of the general population. About 50% to 80% of patients with Graves' disease have these antibodies. TPoAb are found in 90% to 100% of patients with autoimmune thyroiditis.[7,12,19]

Laboratory Tests

Direct tests of thyroid function involve the administration of radioactive iodine. Measurement of thyroid radioactive iodine uptake (RAIU) is the most common of these tests. ^{131}I has been used for this test, but ^{123}I is preferred because it exposes the patient to a lower radiation dose. RAIU, which is measured 24 hours after administration of the isotope, varies inversely with plasma iodide concentration and directly with the functional status of the thyroid. In the United States, normal 24-hour RAIU is 10% to 30%. RAIU discriminates poorly between normal and hypothyroid states. Values above the normal range usually indicate thyroid hyperfunction.[1,7,8,20]

Several tests are available that measure thyroid hormone concentration and binding in blood. Highly specific and sensitive radioimmunoassays are used most often to measure serum T_4 and T_3 concentrations and rarely to measure reverse T_3 (rT_3) concentration. The normal range for T_4 is 64 to 154 nmol/L (5 to 12 µg/dL). The normal range for T_3 is 1.2 to 2.9 nmol/L (80 to 190 ng/dL).[20] Elevated levels usually indicate hyperthyroidism, and lower levels usually indicate hypothyroidism. Free hormone levels usually correlate better with the metabolic state than do total hormone levels.[8,20]

Measurement of basal serum TSH concentration is useful in the diagnosis of hyperthyroidism and hypothyroidism. Very sensitive methods, such as immunoradiometric or chemiluminescent techniques, are now available to measure serum TSH. The normal range for TSH is 0.5 to 4.5 mIU/L (µIU/mL). In cases of hyperthyroidism, the TSH level is almost always low or nondetectable. Higher levels indicate hypothyroidism[8,20] (Table 16-2).

Other tests used in selected cases include the TSH stimulation test, the T_3 suppression test, and radioassay techniques for measuring TSHRAb, TSHR-blocking Ab, TPoAb, and TgAb.[8,20] A thyroid scan commonly is used to localize thyroid nodules and to locate functional ectopic thyroid tissue. ^{123}I or ^{99}Tc (technetium) is injected, and a scanner localizes areas of radioactive concentration. This technique allows for the identification of nodules 1 cm or larger. When a pinhole thyroid scan is used, 2- to 3-mm lesions may be detected.[7,20-22]

Ultrasonography may be used to detect thyroid lesions. Nodules 1 to 2 mm in size can be identified. This technique also is used to distinguish solid from cystic lesions, to measure the gland, and to guide needles for aspiration of cysts or for biopsy of thyroid masses. Computed tomography (CT) and magnetic resonance imaging (MRI) are helpful mainly in the postoperative management of patients with thyroid cancer. These forms of imaging also are used for the preoperative evaluation of larger lesions of the thyroid (greater than 3 cm in diameter) that extend beyond the gland into adjacent tissues.[7,20-22]

TABLE 16-2 Laboratory Tests

Test	Normal Range	Interpretation
Radioactive iodine uptake (RIU)	5-30%	*Elevated:* hyperthyroidism *Decreased:* hypothyroidism
Thyroid-stimulating hormone (TSH)	0.5-4.5 mIU/L	*Elevated:* hypothyroidism *Suppressed:* hyperthyroidism
Total serum T_4 (TT_4)	5-12 µg/dL 64-154 nmol/L	*High:* hyperthyroidism *Low:* hypothyroidism
Free T_4 (FT_4)	1.0-3.0 ng/dL 13-39 pmol/L	*Increased:* hyperthyroidism *Decreased:* hypothyroidism
Total serum T_3 (TT_3)	1.2-2.9 nmol/L 80-190 ng/dL	*High:* hyperthyroidism *Low:* hypothyroidism
Free T_3 (FT_3)	0.25-0.65 ng/dL 3.8-10 nmol/L	*Increased:* hyperthyroidism *Decreased:* hypothyroidism

THYROTOXICOSIS (HYPERTHYROIDISM)

Etiology, Pathophysiology, and Complications

The term *thyrotoxicosis* refers to an excess of T_4 and T_3 in the bloodstream. This excess may be the result of production by ectopic thyroid tissue, multinodular goiter, or thyroid adenoma or may be associated with subacute thyroiditis (painful and painless), ingestion of thyroid hormone (thyrotoxicosis factitia) or of foodstuffs containing thyroid hormone, or pituitary disease involving the anterior portion of the gland (see Table 16-1). In this section, the signs and symptoms, laboratory tests, treatment, and dental considerations for the patient with Graves' disease are considered in detail; this disease serves as a model for other conditions that can result in similar clinical manifestations. Of note, multinodular goiter, ectopic thyroid tissue, and neoplastic causes of hyperthyroidism are rare compared with toxic goiter.[1,8,12]

Graves' disease is an autoimmune disease in which thyroid-stimulating immunoglobulins bind to and activate thyrotrophic receptors, causing the gland to grow and stimulating the thyroid follicles to increase the synthesis of thyroid hormone.[1,8,12] The chief risk factors for Graves' disease are genetic mutations (i.e., in susceptibility genes for CD40, cytotoxic T lymphocyte antigen [CTLA-4], thyroglobulin, TSH receptor, and PTPN22[12]) and female gender, in part because of modulation of the autoimmune response by estrogen. This disorder is much more common in women (with a male-to-female ratio of 10 : 1) and may manifest during puberty or pregnancy, or at menopause (see Figure 16-3). Genetic predisposition along with emotional stress such as severe fright or separation from loved ones has been reported to be associated with its onset. The disease may occur in a cyclic pattern and may then "burn itself out" or continue in an active state.[1,8,12]

Clinical Presentation

Signs and Symptoms. Direct and indirect effects of excessive thyroid hormones contribute to the clinical picture in Graves' disease. The most common symptoms and signs are nervousness, fatigue, rapid heartbeat or palpitations, heat intolerance, and weight loss (Table 16-3). These manifestations are reported in more than 50% of all diagnosed patients. With increasing age, weight loss and decreased appetite become more common, and irritability and heat intolerance are less common. Atrial fibrillation is rare in patients younger than 50 years of age but occurs in approximately 20% of older patients. The patient's skin is warm and moist and the complexion rosy; the patient may blush readily. Palmar erythema may be present, profuse sweating is common, and excessive melanin pigmentation of the skin is evident in many patients; however, pigmentation of the oral mucosa has not been reported. In addition, the patient's hair becomes fine and friable, and the nails soften.[1,8,12]

Graves' ophthalmopathy, which is identified in approximately 50% of patients, is characterized by edema and inflammation of the extraocular muscles, as well as an increase in orbital connective tissue and fat. Ophthalmopathy is an organ-specific autoimmune process that is strongly linked to Graves' hyperthyroidism. Although hyperthyroidism may be successfully treated, ophthalmopathy often produces the greatest long-term disability for patients with this disease. Figures 16-7 and 16-8 demonstrate the changes associated with ophthalmopathy (eyelid retraction, proptosis, periorbital edema, chemosis, and bilateral exophthalmos). This disease may progress to visual loss through exposure keratopathy or compressive optic neuropathy.[23,24]

Most thyrotoxic patients show eye signs not related to the ophthalmopathy of Graves' disease as well. These signs (i.e., stare with widened palpebral fissures, infrequent blinking, lid lag, jerky movements of the lids, and failure to wrinkle the brow on upward gaze) result from sympathetic overstimulation and usually clear when thyrotoxicosis is corrected.[23,24]

Another complication, which is found in about 1% to 2% of patients with Graves' disease, is dermopathy

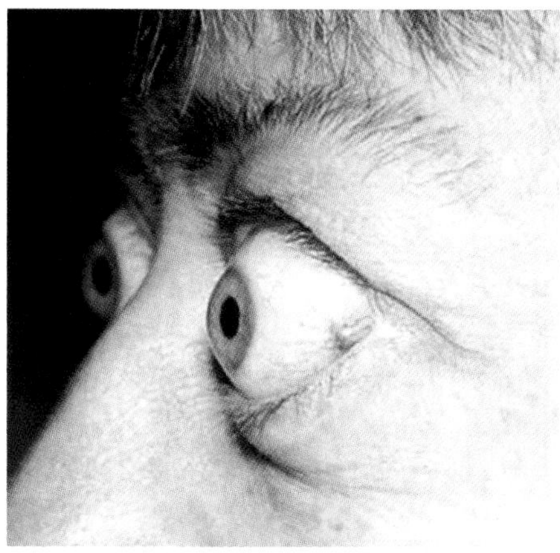

A

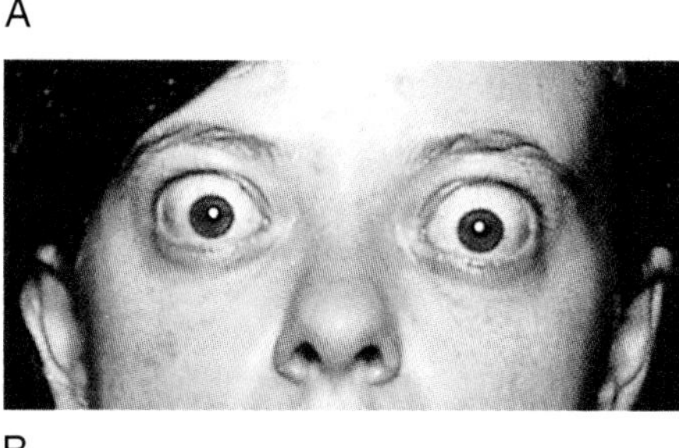

B

FIGURE 16-7 Eyelid changes in Graves' disease. **A,** Lid retraction is a common eye sign in Graves' disease. It is recognized when the sclera is visible between the lower margin of the upper lid and the cornea. **B,** Proptosis in Graves' disease results from enlargement of muscles and fat within the orbit as a result of mucopolysaccharide infiltration. (***A,*** *From Goldman L, Ausiello D:* Cecil textbook of medicine, *ed 23, Philadelphia, 2008, Saunders.* ***B,*** *From Seidel H:* Mosby's guide to physical examination, *4th ed 4, St. Louis, 1999, Mosby.*)

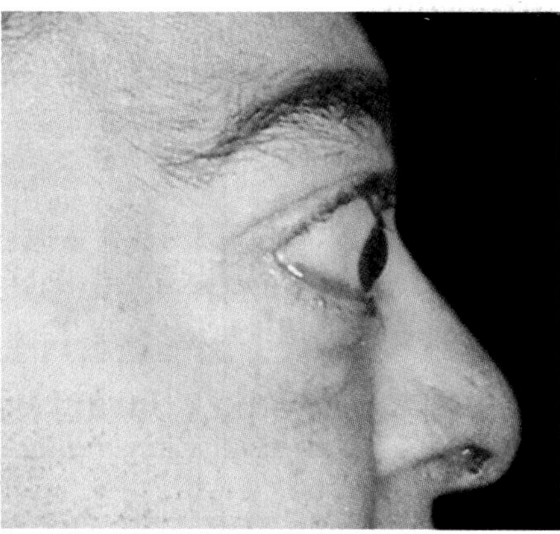

FIGURE 16-8 Exophthalmos of Graves' disease can be unilateral or bilateral. The forward protrusion of the globe results from an increase in volume of the orbital contents. (*From Stein HA, Stein RM, Freeman MI:* The ophthalmic assistant: a text for allied and associated ophthalmic personnel, *ed 8, Philadelphia, 2006, Mosby.*)

(Figure 16-9). In focal areas of the skin, hyaluronic acid and chondroitin sulfate concentrations in the dermis are increased. This may occur as the result of lymphokine activation of fibroblasts. Accumulation causes compression of the dermal lymphatics and nonpitting edema.

TABLE 16-3 Clinical Findings and Treatment of Thyroid Disorders

Condition	Signs and Symptoms	Laboratory Tests	Treatment
Hyperthyroidism	*Skeletal*—osteoporosis *Cardiovascular*—palpitations, tachycardia, arrhythmias, hypertension, cardiomegaly, congestive heart failure, angina, MI *GI*—weight loss, increased appetite, pernicious anemia *CNS*—anxiety, restlessness, sleep disturbances, emotional lability, impaired concentration, weakness, tremors (hands, fingers, tongue) *Skin*—erythema, thin fine hair, areas of alopecia, soft nails *Eyes*—retraction of upper lid, exophthalmos, corneal ulceration, ocular muscle weakness *Other*—increased risk for diabetes, decreased serum cholesterol level, increased risk for thrombocytopenia, sweating	T_4—elevated T_3—elevated *TSH*—none or very decreased *TBG*—elevated *Normal range*: T_4—5-12 μg/dL or 64-154 nmol/L T_3—80-190 ng/dL or 1.2-2.9 nmol/L *TSH*—0.5-4.5 mIU/L *TBG*—1-25 ng/mL	Antithyroid agents: Propylthiouracil Carbimazole Methimazole Radioactive iodine Subtotal thyroidectomy Propranolol: for adrenergic component in thyrotoxicosis (sweating, tremor, and tachycardia)
Hypothyroidism	*Musculoskeletal*—arthritis, muscle cramps *Cardiovascular*—shortness of breath, hypotension, slow pulse *GI*—constipation, anorexia, nausea or vomiting *CNS*—mental and physical slowness, sleepiness, headache *General*—dry, thick skin/dry hair; fatigue; edema (puffy hand, face, eyes), cold intolerance; hoarseness; weight gain	T_4—decreased T_3—decreased *TSH*—elevated *TBG*—decreased	Sodium levothyroxine (Synthyroid, LT_4) or sodium liothyronine (Leotrix, LT_3)
Thyroiditis	*Hashimoto's*—rubbery firm goiter, hypothyroidism develops later	Later in disease: T_4, T_3, and *TBG* are decreased, *TSH* becomes elevated	Thyroid hormone, surgery in rare cases (compression of vital tissues)
	Subacute painful—enlarged, firm, tender gland, pain that may radiate to ear or jaw	Hyperthyroid returning to euthyroid status	Aspirin, prednisone, propranolol for symptoms of thyrotoxicosis
	Acute suppurative—pain, tenderness in gland, fever, malaise	Euthyroid	Incision and drainage, appropriate antibiotics
	Chronic fibrosing—hard, fixed, enlarged gland	Usually remains euthyroid hypothyroid status can occur	Usually none, surgery if vital tissues compressed, thyroid hormone
	Subacute painless—firm, nontender, enlarged gland	Hyperthyroid for 5 to 6 months, returning to euthyroid status	Propranolol for symptoms of thyrotoxicosis

CNS, Central nervous system; *GI*, Gastrointestinal; T_3, Triiodothyronine; T_4, Tetraiodothyronine (thyroxine); *TBG*, Thyroid-binding globulin; *TSH*, Thyroid-stimulating hormone.
Data from references 1, 8, 12, 13, 26.

Early lesions contain a lymphocytic infiltrate. Nodular and plaque formation may occur in chronic lesions. These lesions are most common over the anterolateral aspects of the shin. Patients with dermopathy almost always develop severe ophthalmopathy.[1,12,23,24]

Thyroid acropachy is another rare manifestation of Graves' disease. This feature is associated with presence of TgAbs (Figure 16-10). It is characterized by clubbing and soft tissue swelling of the last phalanx of the fingers and toes. The overlying skin often is discolored and thickened. Subperiosteal new bone formation occurs, along with glycosaminoglycan deposits in the skin. The pathogenesis of thyroid acropachy is unknown.[12]

Increased metabolic activity caused by excessive hormone secretion increases circulatory demand; increases in stroke volume and heart rate often are noted, in addition to widened pulse pressure, resulting in palpitations. Supraventricular cardiac dysrhythmias develop in many patients. Congestive heart failure may occur and often is somewhat resistant to the effects of digitalis. Patients with untreated or incompletely treated thyrotoxicosis are highly sensitive to the actions of epinephrine or other pressor amines, so the use of these agents is contraindicated in this setting. Once good medical management has been instituted, however, administration of these agents can be resumed.[1,12,23]

Dyspnea not related to the effects of congestive heart failure may occur in some patients. The respiratory effect is caused by reduction in vital capacity related to weakness of the respiratory muscles. Weight loss,

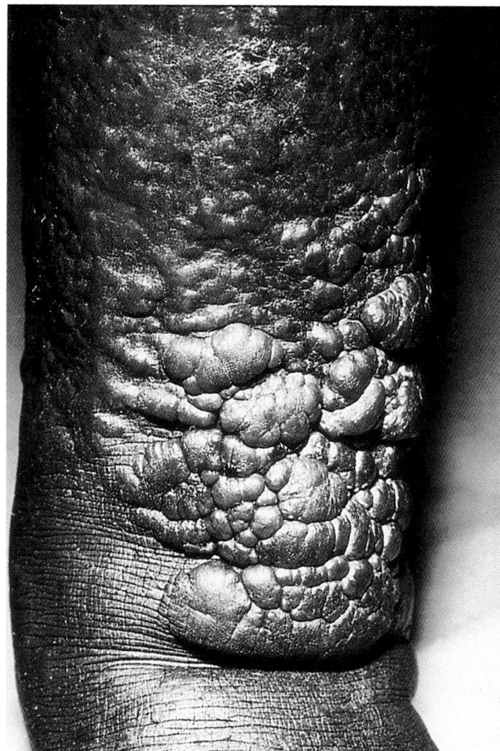

FIGURE 16-9 Infiltrative dermopathy seen in Graves' disease. Hyperpigmented, nonpitting induration of the skin of the legs usually is found in the pretibial area (pretibial myxedema). Lesions are firm, and clear edges can be seen. (*From Melmed S, et al:* Williams textbook of endocrinology, *ed 12, Philadelphia, 2011, Saunders. Courtesy Dr. Andrew Werner, New York, New York.*)

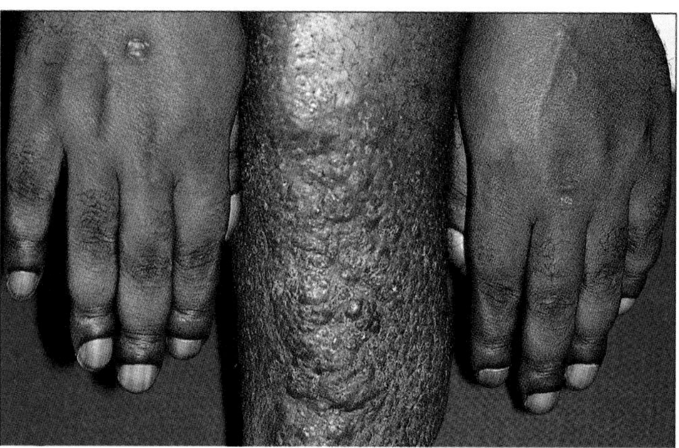

FIGURE 16-10 Thyroid acropachy. Thyroid acropachy is an extreme manifestation of autoimmune thyroid disease. It presents with digital clubbing, swelling of digits and toes, and periosteal reaction of extremity bones. (*From James WD, Berger T, Elston DMD:* Andrews' diseases of the skin, *ed 11, London, 2011, Saunders.*)

despite an increased appetite, is a common finding in younger patients. Stools are poorly formed, and the frequency of bowel movements is increased. Anorexia, nausea, and vomiting are rare but when they occur may herald the onset of thyroid storm. Gastric ulcers are rare in patients with thyrotoxicosis. Many of these patients have achlorhydria, and about 3% develop pernicious anemia.[1,12,23]

Thyrotoxic patients tend to be nervous and often show a great deal of emotional lability, losing their tempers easily and crying often; severe psychiatric reactions may occur. Patients cannot sit still and are always moving. A tremor of the hands and tongue, along with lightly closed eyelids, often is present; in addition, generalized muscle weakness may lead to easy fatigability (see Table 16-3).[1,12,23]

The effect of excessive thyroid hormone production on mineral metabolism is complex and not well understood. However, thyrotoxic patients have increased excretion of calcium and phosphorus into their urine and stools, and radiographs show increased bone loss. Hypercalcemia occurs sometimes, but serum levels of alkaline phosphatase usually are normal. Bone age in young patients is advanced (see Chapter 12).[1,12,23] Glucose intolerance and, rarely, diabetes mellitus may accompany hyperthyroidism. Patients with diabetes who are treated with insulin require an increased dose of insulin if they develop Graves' disease.[23] Individual red blood cells (RBCs) in patients with thyrotoxicosis usually are normal; however, the RBC mass is enlarged, to carry the additional oxygen needed for increased metabolic activities. In addition to the increased total numbers of circulating RBCs, the bone marrow reveals erythroid hyperplasia, and requirements for vitamin B_{12} and folic acid are increased. White blood cell (WBC) count may be decreased because of a reduction in the number of neutrophils, whereas the absolute number of eosinophils may be increased. Enlargement of the spleen and lymph nodes occurs in some patients. The platelets and the clotting mechanism usually are normal, but thrombocytopenia has been reported.[1,12,23] Increased metabolic activity associated with thyrotoxicosis leads to increased secretion and breakdown of cortisol; however, serum levels remain within normal limits.

Laboratory Findings. T_4, T_3, TBG, and TSH tests can be used to screen for hyperthyroidism. Current practice, however, is to screen patients suspected of being hyperthyroid by means of the TSH serum assay and measurement or estimation of the free T_4 concentration. A low TSH level and a high free T_4 concentration are classically combined in hyperthyroidism (see Tables 16-2 and 16-3). Some patients are hyperthyroid with a low TSH level and a normal free T_4 concentration, but they have an elevated free T_3 level. A few patients have normal or elevated TSH and high free T_4. These patients usually are found to have a TSH-secreting pituitary adenoma or thyroid hormone resistance syndrome.[1,12,23]

Medical Management

Treatment of patients with thyrotoxicosis may involve antithyroid agents that block hormone synthesis, iodides, radioactive iodine, or subtotal thyroidectomy (Box

BOX 16-1 Treatment of Thyrotoxicosis

Severe Thyrotoxicosis

Propylthiouracil (PTU) 100 to 150 mg every 8 hours; in some cases, PTU 200 to 300 mg every 6 hours. With decrease in symptoms, the PTU dosage can be lowered. As improvement continues, can switch to once-a-day methimazole (MMI) 2.5 to 5.0 mg once per day for 12 to 24 months.

Moderate Thyrotoxicosis

Start with methimazole (MMI), which is 10 times more potent than propylthiouracil (PTU). MMI also has longer intrathyroid residence time but does not inhibit conversion of T_4 to T_3 as PTU does. Start with 20 to 30 mg once per day. Within 4 to 6 weeks the patient will be euthyroid. Reduce dosage to 2.5 to 5 mg/day for 12 to 24 months. Relapses are frequent, and drug side effects may complicate treatment.

^{131}I Therapy

^{131}I therapy is the most common form of treatment in the United States. Antithyroid drugs are given first to make the patient euthyroid. The antithyroid medicine is stopped for 3 to 5 days; then 6000 to 8000 rad dosage of ^{131}I is given. More than 80% of the patients are cured with a single dose of ^{131}I. Delayed control of thyrotoxicosis and lower efficacy are typical with large goiters.

Surgery

Patient must be euthyroid before surgery is performed, usually achieved with one of the antithyroid drugs (PTU or MMI). Subtotal thyroidectomy is the treatment of choice. Hypoparathyroidism occurs in 0.9% to 2.0% of cases and recurrent laryngeal nerve damage is found in 0.1% to 2.0% of cases. Bleeding, infection, and anesthetic complications can occur. Results in a fast correction of thyrotoxicosis but at a high cost.

Data from references 1, 8, 12.

BOX 16-2 Side Effects of Antithyroid Drugs*

Severe

Agranulocytosis (0.2% to 0.5%)

Only rare cases reported
Hepatitis (can result in hepatic failure)
Cholestatic jaundice
Thrombocytopenia

Hypoprothrombinemia

Aplastic anemia
Lupus-like syndrome with vasculitis
Hypoglycemia (insulin antibodies)

Less Severe

Most Frequent (1% to 5%)

Rash
Urticaria
Arthralgia
Decreased leukocyte level (drop in white blood cell counts by 2-3 × 10^3)
Fever

Less Frequent

Arthritis
Diarrhea
Decreased sense of taste

*Propylthiouracil and methimazole.
Data from Goldman L, Ausiello D, editors: Cecil textbook of medicine, *ed 23, Philadelphia, 2008, Saunders.*

16-1). The antithyroid agents most often used in the United States are propylthiouracil and methimazole, both of which inhibit thyroid peroxidase and thus the synthesis of thyroid hormone. Propylthiouracil also blocks extrathyroidal deiodination of T_4 to T_3. Carbimazole is the drug of choice in the United Kingdom, and propylthiouracil is the drug of choice in North America. The usual duration of treatment ranges up to 18 months. Antithyroid agents may cause a mild leukopenia, but drug therapy is not stopped unless the WBC count is more severely depressed. In rare cases, agranulocytosis may occur (Box 16-2). If sore throat, fever, or mouth ulcers develop, most physicians advise the patient to stop the antithyroid medication and have a WBC count performed.[1,12,23]

Administration of radioactive iodine is the preferred initial treatment for patients with Graves' disease in North America. This agent is contraindicated in pregnant women and in those who are breast feeding. Radioactive iodine can induce or worsen ophthalmopathy, particularly in smokers. Weetman[23] recommends antithyroid drug treatment for patients younger than 50 years of age at their first episode of Graves' disease; radioactive iodine is recommended for those older than 50 years of age. The main adverse effect associated with radioactive iodine treatment is hypothyroidism. The incidence of cancer is unchanged or slightly reduced in patients treated with radioactive iodine, but the risk of death from thyroid cancer and possibly other cancers is slightly increased. Patients with severe hyperthyroidism should be treated with an antithyroid drug for 4 to 8 weeks before radioactive iodine therapy is initiated. This approach reduces the slight risk of thyrotoxic crisis if radioactive iodine was given initially.[1,12,23]

Subtotal thyroidectomy is preferred by some patients with a large goiter and is indicated in those with a coexistent thyroid nodule whose nature is unclear. The patient is first treated with an antithyroid drug until euthyroidism is achieved. Then, inorganic iodide is administered for 7 days before surgery. In major centers, hyperthyroidism is cured in more than 98% of cases, and low rates of operative complications are reported. Postoperative hypothyroidism becomes more frequent as the accumulated effects of multiple surgical treatments result in near-total thyroidectomy.[23]

If exophthalmos is present, it follows a course independent of the therapeutic metabolic response to antithyroid treatment modalities and usually is irreversible. The adrenergic component in thyrotoxicosis can be managed with β-adrenergic antagonists such as propranolol. Propranolol alleviates adrenergic manifestations such as sweating, tremor, and tachycardia.[1,12,23]

Management of Thyrotoxic Crisis. Patients with thyrotoxicosis who are untreated or incompletely treated may develop thyrotoxic crisis, a serious but fortunately rare complication of abrupt onset that may occur at any age. Thyrotoxic crisis occurs in less than 1% of patients hospitalized for thyrotoxicosis.[1,12,23] Most patients who develop thyrotoxic crisis have a goiter, wide pulse pressure, eye signs, and a long history of thyrotoxicosis. Precipitating factors include infection, trauma, surgical emergencies, and operations. Early signs and symptoms of extreme restlessness, nausea, vomiting, and abdominal pain have been reported; fever, profuse sweating, marked tachycardia, cardiac arrhythmias, pulmonary edema, and congestive heart failure soon develop. The patient appears to be in a stupor, and coma may follow. Severe hypotension develops, and death may occur. These reactions appear to be associated, at least in part, with adrenal cortical insufficiency.[1,12,23] Immediate treatment for the patient in thyrotoxic crisis consists of large doses of antithyroid drugs (200 mg of propylthiouracil), potassium iodide, propranolol (to antagonize the adrenergic component), hydrocortisone (100 to 300 mg), dexamethasone (2 mg orally every 6 hours, to inhibit release of hormone from the gland and peripheral conversion of T_4 to T_3), intravenous (IV) glucose solution, vitamin B complex, wet packs, fans, and ice packs. Cardiopulmonary resuscitation is sometimes needed.[1,12,23]

Thyrotoxicosis Factitia. Thyrotoxicosis that results from the ingestion, usually chronic, of excessive quantities of thyroid hormone is referred to as *thyrotoxicosis factitia*. This condition usually occurs in patients with underlying psychiatric disease, or in persons such as nurses and physicians who have access to the medication. In other cases, patients may not be aware that they are taking the hormone or some other thyroid-active agent (e.g., iodocasein) as part of a weight reduction program.[1,7,12]

Other Causes of Thyrotoxicosis. Thyrotoxicosis has been reported to occur in patients who ate ground beef containing large quantities of bovine thyroid. Functional ectopic thyroid tissue also can cause thyrotoxicosis. Thyroid tissue may be found in ovarian teratomas (struma ovarii). In rare cases, hyperfunctioning metastases of follicular carcinoma may cause thyrotoxicosis.[1,7,12]

THYROIDITIS

DEFINITION

Thyroiditis is inflammation of the thyroid gland, which may occur for a variety of reasons. Five types of thyroiditis have been identified: Hashimoto's, subacute painful, subacute painless, acute suppurative, and Riedel's (Table 16-4).[1,7,25-27] Radiation therapy and drugs such as lithium, interleukin-2, interferons, and amiodarone also may cause thyroiditis iatrogenically.[1,7,25-27] In some cases (subacute painful thyroiditis), inflammation may result from transient hyperthyroidism due to follicle damage and release of preformed thyroid hormone.[25] By contrast, Hashimoto's thyroiditis (chronic autoimmune thyroiditis) results in progressive hypothyroidism.[1,7,25-27]

Because Hashimoto's thyroiditis is the most common type of thyroiditis, it is discussed next in greater detail.

CLINICAL PRESENTATION—HASHIMOTO'S THYROIDITIS

Hashimoto's thyroiditis is the most common cause of primary hypothyroidism in the United States.[25] It is an autoimmune disorder that manifests most often as an asymptomatic diffuse goiter. High titers of circulating thyroid autoantibodies and thyroid antigen–specific T cells are observed. It usually affects young and middle-aged women. It also can occur in men, although much less commonly (it is three to four times more frequent in women), and in persons of any age.[25] By the time the diagnosis has been established, most patients are hypothyroid. A family history of Hashimoto's thyroiditis or other autoimmune thyroid disorder often is reported.[1,7,25-27] It may be associated with other autoimmune diseases such as pernicious anemia and type 1 diabetes mellitus.[1,7,25-27]

Signs and Symptoms

Goiter is the clinical hallmark of Hashimoto's thyroiditis (Figure 16-11). The goiter usually is moderate in size and rubbery firm in consistency, and it moves freely with swallowing. In cases of sudden onset, the clinical picture suggests subacute thyroiditis with pain. Patients may be euthyroid during early phases of the disease. Early in the disease course, the thyroid becomes enlarged and firm and may have a nodular consistency. Over time, most patients develop hypothyroidism as lymphocytes replace functioning tissue. In a few cases, the patient develops transient hyperthyroidism, to be followed later by hypothyroidism.[1,7,19,27]

Laboratory Findings

Early in the course of Hashimoto's disease, the patient is euthyroid, but TSH level is often slightly increased and RAIU is increased. Increasing titers of autoantibodies are found early in the disease; anti-TPoAb and anti-TgAb are the most important from a clinical standpoint. Fine needle biopsy of the thyroid gland at this stage helps to confirm the diagnosis. Later in the disease, serum levels of T_4 and T_3 start to fall, and the level of TSH continues to increase. At this stage the patient is hypothyroid and requires treatment with hormone replacement.[1,7,19,27]

TABLE 16-4 Thyroiditis

Type	Cause	Clinical Findings	Thyroid Function	Treatment
Hashimoto thyroiditis	Autoimmune-related	Goiter—moderate in size, rubbery, firm	Euthyroid early Few cases with transient hyperfunction Hypothyroidism develops in most cases	Thyroid hormone In rare cases of compression of vital tissues, surgery is indicated
Subacute painful thyroiditis	Possible viral infection	Enlarged, firm, tender, gland with pain that may radiate to ear, jaw, or occipital region	Hyperthyroidism with return to euthyroid state	Aspirin Prednisone Propranolol for symptoms of thyrotoxicosis
Acute suppurative thyroiditis	Bacterial infection	Pain and tenderness in gland; fever, malaise; skin over the gland warm and red	Euthyroid	Incision and drainage, appropriate antibiotics
Chronic fibrosing thyroiditis (Riedel's)	Unknown	Enlarged gland that is stony hard and fixed to surrounding tissues	Usually remain euthyroid but in some cases hypothyroidism may occur	Usually none; if vital structures are compressed, surgery is indicated; thyroid hormone
Subacute painless thyroiditis (postpartum thyroiditis)	Not established but related to autoimmune thyroid disease	Enlarged gland that is firm and nontender; may occur in women 5 to 6 months after pregnancy	Hyperthyroidism for 5 to 6 months, then return to euthyroid state	Propranolol for symptoms of thyrotoxicosis

Data from references 1, 7, 26.

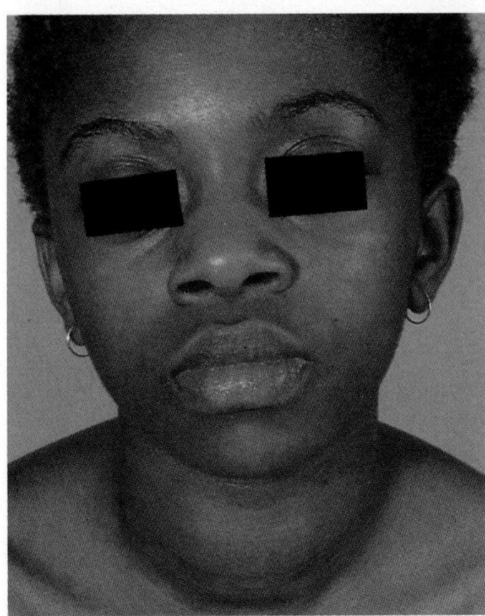

FIGURE 16-11 Hashimoto's disease is the most common cause of goitrous hypothyroidism. The initial lesion consists of a diffuse goiter, and the patient may be euthyroid. Later, the patient becomes hypothyroid, and very late in the disease, the gland atrophies. (*From Forbes CD, Jackson WF:* Color atlas and text of clinical medicine, *ed 3, Edinburgh, 2003, Mosby.*)

MEDICAL MANAGEMENT

Early in the course of the disease, patients with Hashimoto's disease have small goiters, are asymptomatic, and do not require treatment. Patients with larger goiters or mild hypothyroidism are treated with thyroid hormone replacement. More recent goiters usually respond by decreasing in size. Long-standing goiters often do not respond to hormone treatment. In these cases, unsightly goiters or those compressing adjacent structures may be managed surgically after an attempt has been made to decrease their size with the use of hormone therapy. Patients with full-blown hypothyroidism require hormone replacement treatment.[1,7,13,19,27]

HYPOTHYROIDISM

DEFINITION

The causes of hypothyroidism can be divided into four main categories (see Table 16-1): primary atrophic, secondary, transient, and generalized resistance to thyroid hormone. Up to 95% of cases of hypothyroidism are caused by primary and goitrous hypothyroidism. Acquired impairment of thyroid function affects about 2% of adult women and about 0.1% to 0.2% of adult men in North America.[1,7,8,13] Hypothyroidism may be congenital or acquired. Permanent hypothyroidism occurs about once in every 4000 live births in the United States. Transient hypothyroidism occurs in 1% to 2% of newborns. Most infants with permanent congenital hypothyroidism have thyroid dysgenesis—that is, ectopic, hypoplastic, or thyroid agenesis. The acquired form may follow thyroid gland or pituitary gland failure and commonly is due to irradiation of the thyroid gland (radioactive iodine), surgical removal, and excessive antithyroid drug therapy. However, some occur with no identifiable cause.[1,7,8,13]

Subclinical hypothyroidism is a prevalent condition that is characterized by elevated serum TSH concentration and normal serum FT_4 and T_3.[13] It occurs in about 75 of 1000 women and in 28 of 1000 men. It is most common in women and older adults and may be caused by chronic autoimmune thyroiditis, postpartum thyroiditis, ^{131}I therapy, thyroidectomy, or antithyroid drugs. Subclinical hypothyroidism secondary to chronic autoimmune thyroiditis has a predictable clinical course.[13] Spontaneous return to normal TSH values occurs in 5% to 6% of cases. Progression to overt hypothyroidism occurs at a rate of about 5% per year. Some patients report fatigue, weight gain, poor memory, poor ability to concentrate, and depressed feelings.[13]

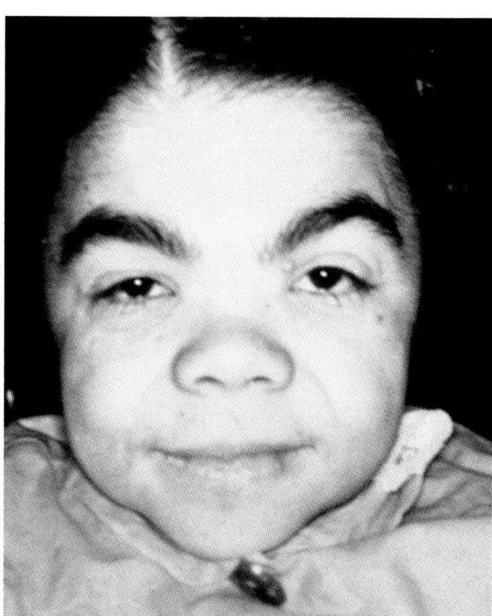

FIGURE 16-12 Cretinism.

CLINICAL PRESENTATION

Signs and Symptoms

Neonatal cretinism is characterized by dwarfism; overweight; well-recognized facial features consisting of a broad, flat nose, wide-set eyes, thick lips, and a large protruding tongue; poor muscle tone; pale skin; stubby hands; retarded bone age; delayed eruption of teeth; malocclusions; a hoarse cry; an umbilical hernia; and mental retardation (Figure 16-12). All of these abnormalities can be prevented by early detection and treatment.

The onset of hypothyroidism in older children and adults (Figure 16-13) is manifested by characteristic changes in physical appearance: a dull expression, puffy eyelids, alopecia of the outer third of the eyebrows, palmar yellowing, dry and rough skin, and dry, brittle, and coarse hair, along with increased size of the tongue. Other features include slowing of physical and mental activity, slurred and hoarse speech, anemia, constipation, increased sensitivity to cold, increased capillary fragility, weight gain, muscle weakness, and deafness (see Table 16-3).

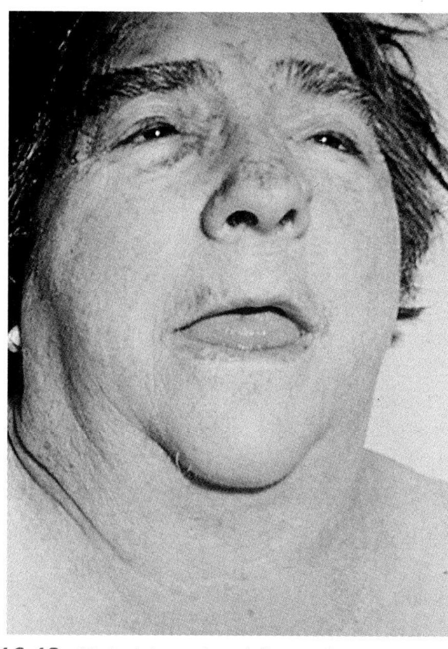

FIGURE 16-13 Clinical hypothyroidism. Characteristic nonpitting edematous changes are evident in the skin of the face. Note the dry skin, puffy facial appearance, and coarse hair. (*Courtesy Paul W. Ladenson, MD, The Johns Hopkins University and Hospital, Baltimore, Maryland. In Seidel HM, et al:* Mosby's guide to physical examination, *ed 7, St. Louis, 2011, Mosby.*)

Accumulation of subcutaneous fluid (intracellularly and extracellularly) usually is not as pronounced in patients with pituitary myxedema as it is in those with primary (thyroid) myxedema. Serum cholesterol levels are elevated in thyroid myxedema and are closer to normal values in patients with pituitary myxedema. Untreated patients with severe myxedema may develop hypothyroid coma, which usually is fatal. T_4, T_3, TBG, and TSH tests are used to screen for hypothyroidism.[1,7,8,13] Results that indicate hypothyroidism are shown in Table 16-3.

MEDICAL MANAGEMENT

Patients with hypothyroidism are treated with synthetic preparations that contain sodium levothyroxine (LT_4) or sodium liothyronine (LT_3).[1,7,8,13] The usual prescribed dose of sodium levothyroxine for patients of ideal body weight is 75 to 100 μg per day. In hypothyroid patients receiving warfarin or other related oral anticoagulants, treatment with T_4 may cause further prolongation of prothrombin time, associated with risk for hemorrhage. In addition, hypothyroid patients with diabetes with a decreased need for insulin or sulfonylureas may become hyperglycemic when treated with T_4.[1,7,8,13]

Congestive heart failure may occur in severe cases of myxedema. Levothyroxine therapy can correct this condition (Figure 16-14). The treatment of hypothyroid children with levothyroxine can result in a dramatic reversal of the associated clinical changes (Figure 16-15).

Patients with untreated hypothyroidism are sensitive to the actions of narcotics, barbiturates, and tranquilizers, so these drugs must be used with caution. Smoking can worsen the disease. Stressful situations such as cold, operations, infections, or trauma may precipitate a hypothyroid (myxedema) coma in untreated hypothyroid patients. This condition is noted for severe myxedema, bradycardia, and severe hypotension. Myxedematous coma occurs most often in severely hypothyroid elderly persons. It is more common during the winter months and carries a high mortality rate. Hypothyroid coma is treated by parenteral levothyroxine (T_4) and steroids; the patient is covered to conserve heat. Hypertonic saline and glucose may be required to alleviate dilutional hyponatremia and occasional hypoglycemia, respectively.[1,7,8,13]

THYROID CANCER

DEFINITION

Three main histologic types of thyroid cancer have been identified: differentiated, medullary, and anaplastic. Differentiated cancers are subdivided into papillary, follicular, mixed, and Hürthle cell carcinomas[1,7,9] (Table 16-5). In addition, primary lymphomas may occur in the thyroid gland, and other cancers may metastasize to the thyroid. An important neoplastic syndrome, multiple endocrine neoplasia type 2 (MEN2), involves the thyroid gland. MEN2 consists of medullary thyroid carcinoma (MTC), pheochromocytoma in 50% of cases, and parathyroid hyperplasia or adenoma in 10% to 35% of cases.[28] In rare cases, cancer from other locations may metastasize to the thyroid gland.[29] The kidney is the most common site of origin for metastasis to the thyroid gland; other sites include cancer of the breast and lung, and melanoma.[28,29]

Etiology and Clinical Findings

External radiation to the cervical region is believed to be one cause of thyroid cancer.[9] Children who underwent thymic irradiation are at increased risk for this neoplasm. Teenagers with acne that was treated by irradiation also are at greater risk for thyroid cancer. Patients with other types of neck cancer treated with irradiation are at increased risk for thyroid cancer.[28] External medical diagnostic radiation can add to the risk for thyroid cancer; however, dental radiographs do not appear to add to this burden.[28] Radiation delivered to the thyroid from internal sources and diagnostic or

TABLE 16-5 Classification of Thyroid Cancer

Type (Histologic)	Frequency (%)	10-Year Survival Rate (%)
Differentiated—papillary	75-80	>90
Differentiated—follicular	8-10	80
Differentiated—Hürthle cell	1	70
Anaplastic	1-5	< 2
Medullary	5-8	40
Lymphoma	1-5	45
Metastases to the thyroid	<1	Determined by primary

Data from references 1, 7, 9, 30, 31.

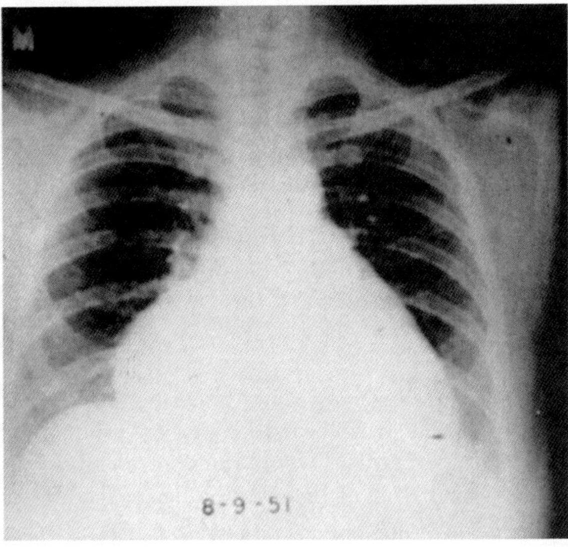

A

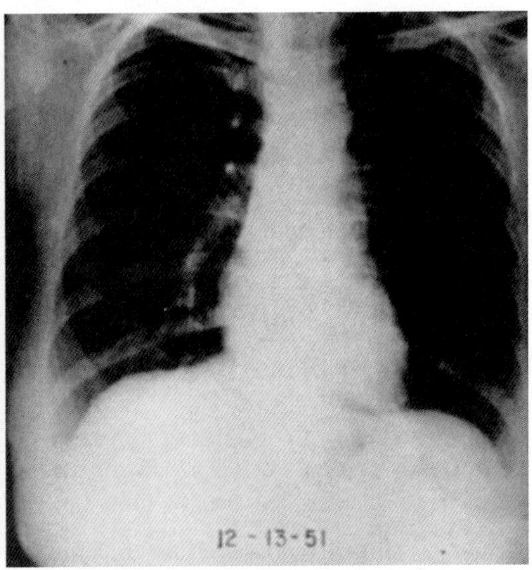

B

FIGURE 16-14 **A,** Radiograph showing enlargement of the heart in a patient with heart failure due to myxedema. **B,** After treatment with thyroid hormone, the radiograph shows a return to normal heart size. (*From Melmed S, et al:* Williams textbook of endocrinology, *ed 12, Philadelphia, 2011, Saunders.*)

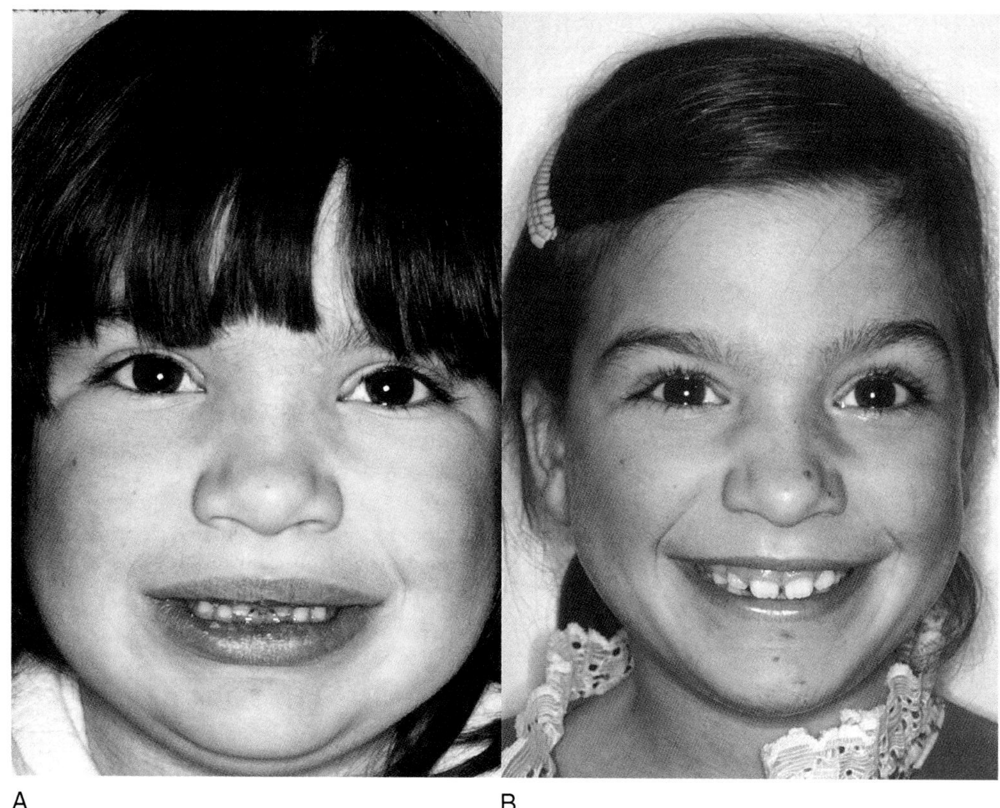

FIGURE 16-15 **A,** A 9-year-old girl with severe hypothyroidism. **B,** The same patient 1 year after treatment with thyroid hormone replacement. Note the return to normal facial appearance. (*From Neville B, et al:* Oral and maxillofacial pathology, *ed 3, St. Louis, 2009, Saunders.*)

therapeutic doses of ^{131}I have not been associated with an increased risk for thyroid cancer.[9] Environmental factors such as high dietary iodine intake (associated with papillary cancer) or a very low iodine intake (associated with follicular cancer) appear to increase the risk for thyroid cancer.[28] A genetic factor is suggested by an increased risk for thyroid cancer when a family member has had thyroid cancer or MEN2.[1,7,9,28,30] In some cases, no risk factor can be identified.

On physical examination, manifestations of thyroid malignancy, including firm consistency of the nodule, irregular shape, fixation to underlying or overlying tissue, and suspicious regional lymphadenopathy.[1,7,9,28,30] Signs and symptoms that may be associated with thyroid cancer include a lump in the region of the gland, a dominant nodule(s) in multinodular goiter, a hard painless mass, fixation to adjacent structures, enlarged cervical lymph nodes, a rapidly growing mass, hemoptysis, dysphagia, stridor, and hoarseness.[28]

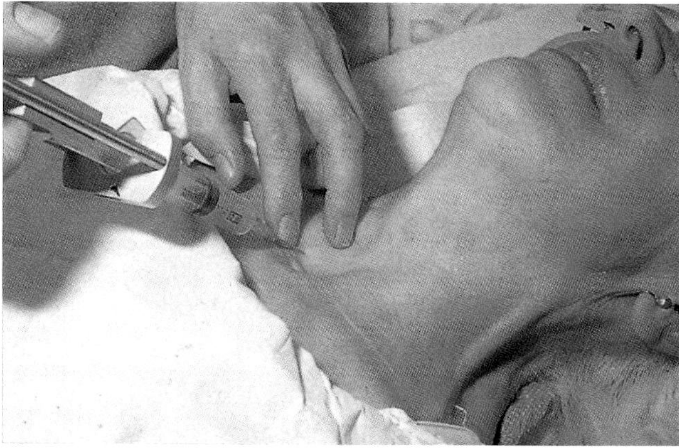

FIGURE 16-16 Fine needle aspiration of a thyroid nodule is the investigation of choice in a patient with a solitary nodule of the thyroid. (*From Forbes CD, Jackson WF:* Color atlas and text of clinical medicine, *ed 3, Edinburgh, 2003, Mosby.*)

DIAGNOSIS

The cornerstone for the diagnosis of thyroid nodules is ultrasonography and fine needle aspiration biopsy (FNAB).[1,7,9,28,30] Clinically detected nodules should be evaluated by ultrasonography. Hypoechoic nodules should be submitted for FNAB (Figure 16-16). Ultrasound imaging also can be used in cases of nonpalpable nodules, to guide FNAB. Overall rates of sensitivity and specificity for FNAB of thyroid nodules exceed 90% in iodine-sufficient areas.[1,7,9,28,30] FNAB is easy to perform and safe; very few complications have been reported.[28] The key to accuracy of the technique is to obtain an adequate specimen. This usually involves obtaining three to six aspirated samples, which should contain at least five or six groups of 10 to 15 well-preserved cells.[28] Nodules found in patients living in iodine-deficient areas may require surgical removal before a diagnosis can be established.[28]

TREATMENT

For most papillary carcinomas, surgery is the indicated treatment.[7,9,30,31] Options include lobectomy and total thyroidectomy. The recurrence rate is higher for lobectomy, but complications are fewer.[28] Radioiodine ablation of residual thyroid tissue does not improve survival but does allow for interpretation of thyroglobulin levels.[28] Radioiodine ablation is useful in metastatic disease and locally invasive disease, and in cases in which cervical lymph nodes cannot be resected.[28] Suppression of levothyroxine can be used to limit thyrotropin stimulation of tumor growth, but adverse effects may be difficult for the patient to tolerate.[28]

Treatment of follicular carcinomas involves surgery followed by radioiodine ablation and lifelong thyrotropin suppression achieved through levothyroxine replacement therapy.[7,9,30,31] Initial surgery may consist of thyroid lobectomy or total thyroidectomy.[28] Other available options for minimally invasive disease include lobectomy and levothyroxine suppression of thyrotropin secretion alone; if cancer recurs, the rest of the thyroid is surgically removed, and radioiodine scanning for recurrence or radioiodine ablation of remaining thyroid tissue is performed.[28]

Hürthle cell cancers and medullary carcinomas are treated by total thyroidectomy with cervical lymph node dissection.[7,9,30,31] Patients with medullary carcinoma should undergo regular monitoring of serum calcitonin for evidence of recurrence.[28] The main objective of treatment for patients with anaplastic carcinomas is to control symptoms and relieve airway obstruction.[28] Any combination of surgery, external beam radiotherapy, and chemotherapy may be used. At best, however, these treatments occasionally may add several months to the life span.[28] External beam radiotherapy is used to manage bone pain caused by metastases.[28]

Complications associated with total or subtotal thyroidectomy are hypoparathyroidism, recurrent laryngeal nerve damage, hemorrhage, and general risks associated with surgery.[7,9,30,31] Complications of external beam radiotherapy include damage to the spinal cord, skin damage, and mucosal ulceration.[28] Complications associated with chemotherapy include nausea and vomiting, mucosal damage, hair loss, infection, and bleeding (see Chapter 26).[28]

PROGNOSIS

The prognosis for differentiated cancers is based on age of the patient, metastases, and extent and size of the lesion. The best outlook is projected for young people with localized cancers that are smaller than 2 cm.[9] Overall 10-year survival rates for papillary carcinoma are 80% to 90%; for follicular carcinoma, 65% to 75%; and for medullary carcinoma, 60% to 70%.[28] Involvement of cervical nodes predicts recurrence in older patients (older than 45 years) but does not predict overall survival. In patients with distant metastases of a differentiated carcinoma, the long-term survival rate is 43%. The prognosis for anaplastic carcinoma is very poor, and 5-year survival is rare (see Table 16-5).[28]

DENTAL MANAGEMENT

Clinical Examination

Examination of the thyroid gland should be included as part of a head and neck examination performed by the dentist.[32,33] The anterior neck region should be inspected for indications of old surgical scars, and the posterior dorsal region of the tongue should be examined for a nodule, which could represent lingual thyroid tissue. Also, the area just superior and lateral to the thyroid cartilage should be palpated for the presence of a pyramidal lobe. Although difficult to detect, the normal thyroid gland can be palpated in many patients.[32] It may feel rubbery and may be more easily identified by having the patient swallow during the examination. As the patient swallows, the thyroid rises; lumps in the neck that may be associated with it also rise (move superiorly). Nodules in the midline area of the thyroglossal duct move upward with protrusion of the patient's tongue.[32]

An enlarged thyroid gland caused by hyperplasia (goiter) feels softer than the normal gland. Adenomas and carcinomas involving the gland are firmer on palpation and are usually seen as isolated swellings. In patients with Hashimoto's disease or Riedel's thyroiditis, the gland is much firmer than normal (see Table 16-4).[32]

If a diffuse enlargement of the thyroid is detected, auscultation should be used to examine for a systolic or continuous bruit that can be heard over the hyperactive gland of thyrotoxicosis or Graves' disease as a result of engorgement of the gland's vascular system.

MEDICAL CONSIDERATIONS

Thyrotoxicosis

The dentist should be aware of the clinical manifestations of thyrotoxicosis, so that undiagnosed or poorly treated disease can be detected and the patient referred for medical evaluation and treatment (see Table 16-3). Such timely intervention originating in the dental office can help reduce the morbidity and mortality rates associated with thyrotoxicosis.[32,33] In addition, thyrotoxicosis is associated with higher risk for adverse consequences of dental treatment (Box 16-3).

BOX 16-3 Medical Problems Potentially Encountered in or Associated with Dental Treatment of the Patient with Undiagnosed or Poorly Controlled Thyroid Disease

Hyperthyroidism

Adverse interaction with epinephrine
Life-threatening cardiac arrhythmias
Congestive heart failure
Complications of underlying cardiovascular pathologic conditions
Thyrotoxic crisis can be precipitated by:
- Infection
- Surgical procedures

Hypothyroidism

Exaggerated response to CNS depressants:
- Sedatives
- Narcotic analgesics

Myxedematous coma can be precipitated by:
- CNS depressants
- Infection
- Surgical procedures

CNS, Central nervous system.

Patients with untreated or poorly treated thyrotoxicosis are susceptible to developing an acute medical emergency called *thyrotoxic crisis,* which is another important reason for detection and referral. Clinical manifestations include restlessness, fever, tachycardia, pulmonary edema, tremor, sweating, stupor, and finally, coma and death, if treatment is not provided. Of note, dental surgery performed in these patients may precipitate a thyrotoxic crisis. In addition, acute oral infection also has been associated with such events. If a crisis occurs, the dentist should be able to recognize the features, begin emergency treatment, and seek immediate medical assistance (Box 16-4). The patient can be cooled with cold towels, given an injection of hydrocortisone (100 to 300 mg), and started on an intravenous infusion of hypertonic glucose (if equipment is available). Vital signs must be monitored, and cardiopulmonary resuscitation initiated, if necessary. Immediate medical assistance should be sought, and when available, other measures such as antithyroid drugs and potassium iodide may be started.[1,12,32]

Although the role of chronic infection and thyrotoxicosis is unclear, these conditions should be treated as in any other patient. Once the disorder has been identified and the patient referred for medical management, oral foci of infection can be treated. Patients with extensive dental caries or periodontal disease, or both, can be treated after medical management of the thyroid problem has been instituted.

The use of epinephrine or other pressor amines (in local anesthetics or gingival retraction cords, or to control bleeding) must be avoided in the untreated or poorly treated thyrotoxic patient. However, the well-managed (euthyroid) thyrotoxic patient with thyroid disease requires no special consideration in this regard and may be given normal concentrations of these vasoconstrictors.[32] Care must be taken with patients whose disease is being controlled with nonselective beta blockers. When epinephrine is given to these patients, it is possible that blood pressure can be increased through inhibition of the vasodilatory action of epinephrine attained through blocking of β_2-receptors.[33] Clinical experience has shown that small amounts of epinephrine can be used safely in these patients. Use of more concentrated preparations of epinephrine (as in retraction cords and preparations used to control bleeding) should be avoided (see Chapter 3).

Adverse reactions to propylthiouracil include agranulocytosis and leukopenia (see Box 16-2). If these should occur, the patient is at risk for serious infection. The physician should monitor the patient for these adverse reactions. The dentist can consult with the patient's physician or can order a complete blood count to rule out the presence of these complications before undertaking surgical procedures. It has been reported that propylthiouracil can induce sialolith formation. This drug also can increase the anticoagulant effects of warfarin. Aspirin and other nonsteroidal antiinflammatory drugs (NSAIDs) can increase the amount of circulating T_4, making control of thyroid disease more difficult.[33]

Once the thyrotoxic patient is under good medical management, the dental treatment plan can proceed without alteration. If acute oral infection occurs, however, consultation with the patient's physician is recommended as part of the management program (see Box 16-4).[32] Box 16-3 lists the medical concerns the dentist should be aware of regarding the hyperthyroid patient.

Hypothyroidism

In general, the patient with mild symptoms of untreated hypothyroidism is not in danger when receiving dental therapy. Central nervous system (CNS) depressants, sedatives, or narcotic analgesics may cause an exaggerated response in patients with mild to severe hypothyroidism (see Box 16-4). These drugs must be avoided in all patients with severe hypothyroidism and must be used with care (reduced dosage) in patients with mild hypothyroidism; however, a few patients with untreated severe symptoms of hypothyroidism may be in danger if dental treatment is rendered (see Box 16-3). This is particularly true of patients with poorly controlled disease who have infection and elderly persons with myxedema. A myxedematous coma can be precipitated by CNS depressants, surgical procedures, and infections; thus, once again, the major concern of dental management of patients with this condition is detection and referral for medical management before any dental treatment is rendered (see Box 16-4).[1,13,34] If myxedema coma should

BOX 16-4 Dental Management
Considerations in the Patient with Thyroid Disease

P

Patient Evaluation/Risk Assessment (see Box 1-1)

- Evaluate and determine whether a hyper, hypo-, or euthyroid condition exists.
- Obtain medical consultation if poorly controlled or undiagnosed problem, or if uncertain.

Potential Issues/Factors of Concern

Hyperthyroid Patient

A

Analgesics	Aspirin and other NSAIDs can increase the amount of circulating T_4, making control of thyroid disease more difficult. Use appropriately.
Antibiotics	Crofloxacin should not be taken simultaneously with levothyroxine, because the antibiotic appears to decrease absorption of the thyroid hormone.
Anesthesia	Avoid using epinephrine in local anesthetics in untreated or poorly controlled patients.
Anxiety	Patients with untreated or poorly controlled disease may appear very anxious.
Allergy	Look for signs and symptoms of allergic reaction in patients treated with antithyroid medications (propylthiouracil or methimazole).

B

Bleeding	Excessive bleeding may occur in patients with untreated or poorly controlled disease owing to thrombocytopenia, which fortunately is not a common finding.
Breathing	No issues.
Blood pressure	Monitor blood pressure as it may be elevated in patients with untreated or poorly controlled disease.

C

Chair position	No issues.
Cardiovascular	Patients with untreated or poorly controlled disease may be subject to arrhythmias.

D

Devices	No issues.
Drugs	The use of epinephrine or other pressor amines (gingival retraction cords, or to control bleeding) must be avoided in the untreated or poorly treated thyrotoxic patient. Common side effects of the antithyroid drugs (methimazole and propylthiouracil) are rash, pruritus, fever, and arthralgias. Agranulocytosis and hepatitis are rare but serious complications of the antithyroid drugs.

E

Equipment	No issues.
Emergencies	Patients taking antithyroid drugs who develop fever, sore throat, or oral ulcerations should seek urgent medical care (possible agranulocytosis). Patients who develop jaundice and abdominal pain (possible hepatitis) should seek urgent medical care.
	Thyrotoxic crisis occurring in the dental office: Seek medical aid; vital signs must be monitored and cardiopulmonary resuscitation initiated if necessary; apply wet packs or ice packs; inject 100 to 300 mg of hydrocortisone, intravenous glucose solution; administer propylthiouracil; transport patient to emergency medical facilities.

F

Follow-up:	Routine, unless patient develops complications.

Hypothyroid Patient

A

Analgesics	Avoid CNS depressants such as narcotics, barbiturates. and sedatives in patients with poorly controlled disease.
Antibiotics	In patients with poorly controlled as well as well-controlled disease, treat acute infection aggressively using appropriate antibiotics and incision and drainage when indicated.
Anesthesia	No issues.
Anxiety	Avoid CNS depressants such as narcotics, barbiturates, and sedatives in patients with poorly controlled disease.
Allergy	No issues.

B

Bleeding	No issues.
Breathing	No issues.
Blood pressure	No issues.

C

Chair position	No issues.
Cardiovascular	No issues.

D

Devices	No issues.
Drugs	Phenytoin, phenobarbital, carbamazepine, and rifampin should be used with care, because they increase the metabolism of thyroid replacement drugs. Ferrous sulfate, calcium carbonate, and aluminum hydroxide can interfere with thyroxine absorption (thyroxine doses should be separated from ingestion of these substances by 4 or more hours).

E

Equipment	No issues.
Emergencies	*Myxedema coma*: Seek medical aid; vital signs must be monitored and cardiopulmonary resuscitation initiated if necessary, cover patient to conserve body heat; inject 100 to 300 mg of hydrocortisone, thyroxine (1.8 µg/kg daily with a 500-µg loading dose), intravenous saline, and glucose; transport to medical emergency facility.

F

Follow-up	Routine, unless patient develops complications.

occur, the dentist should call for medical aid; while waiting for this assistance, the dentist can inject 100 to 300 mg of hydrocortisone, cover the patient to conserve heat, and apply cardiopulmonary resuscitation (CPR) as indicated. Once medical aid becomes available, parental levothyroxine is administered, and intravenous hypertonic saline and glucose are given as needed.

Patients with less severe forms of hypothyroidism should be identified when possible, because their quality of life can be greatly improved with medical treatment. With detection early in childhood, permanent mental retardation can be avoided with appropriate medical management. In addition, oral complications of delayed eruption of teeth, malocclusion, enlarged tongue, and skeletal retardation can be prevented through early detection and medical treatment.

Once the hypothyroid patient is under good medical care, no special problems in terms of dental management remain, except for the need to address malocclusion and the enlarged tongue, if they are present.

Thyroid Cancer

Palpation and inspection of the thyroid gland should be included as part of the routine head and neck examination performed by the dentist. If thyroid enlargement is noted, even though the patient may appear euthyroid (i.e., has normal thyroid function), a referral should be made for medical evaluation before dental treatment is rendered. A diffuse enlargement may represent a simple goiter, subacute thyroiditis, or chronic thyroiditis. The patient may be hyperthyroid, hypothyroid, or euthyroid. Isolated nodules may turn out to be an adenoma or carcinoma. Growing nodules in diffusely enlarged glands or in glands with multinodular involvement may be manifestations of thyroid carcinoma and must be evaluated by a physician.[35]

ORAL COMPLICATIONS AND MANIFESTATIONS

Thyrotoxicosis

In children, the teeth and jaws develop rapidly, and premature loss of deciduous teeth with early eruption of permanent teeth is common. Euthyroid infants of hyperthyroid mothers have been reported to have erupted teeth at birth. A few patients with thyrotoxicosis have been found to have a lingual "thyroid," consisting of thyroid tissue below the area of the foramen cecum.[32,33]

If the dentist detects a lingual tumor in a euthyroid patient, a physician should examine the patient before the mass is surgically removed (Figure 16-17). This usually is done with radioactive iodine scanning.[32,36] Osteoporosis involving the alveolar bone may be an associated feature, and development of dental caries and periodontal disease may occur rapid in these patients.

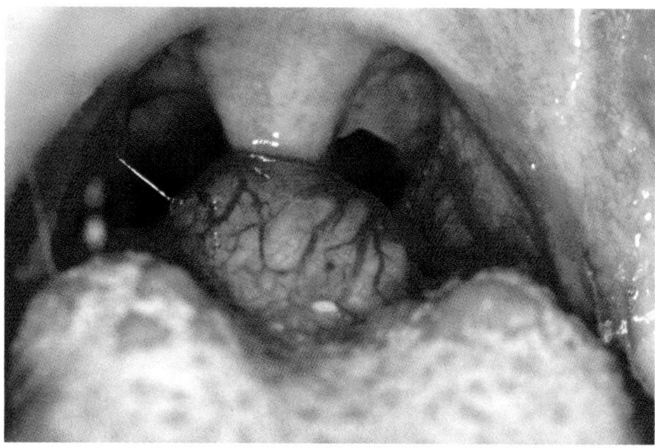

A

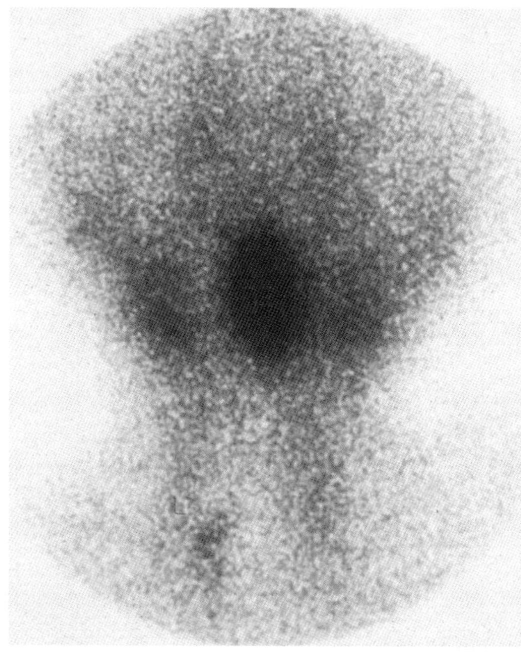

B

FIGURE 16-17 **A,** Lingual thyroid nodule in a 4-year-old girl. **B,** Thyroid scan of the nodule. *(From Neville BW, et al:* Oral and maxillofacial pathology, *ed 3, St. Louis, 2009, Saunders.)*

Hypothyroidism

Infants with cretinism may present with thick lips, enlarged tongue, and delayed eruption of teeth with resulting malocclusion. The only specific oral change manifested in adults with acquired hypothyroidism is an enlarged tongue.[34,36] A recent study reported the coexistence of hypothyroidism and burning mouth syndrome; however, this relationship needs to be further defined.[37]

Thyroiditis

The pain associated with subacute painful thyroiditis may radiate to the ear, jaw, or occipital region. Hoarseness and dysphagia may be accompanying features. Patients may report palpitations, nervousness, and lassitude. On palpation, the thyroid is enlarged, firm, often nodular, and usually very tender.[1,26,34]

Radioactive Iodine

Radioactive iodine (RAI) used to treat hyperthyroid conditions and thyroid cancer is associated with acute and long-term risks and side effects. Acute risks include salivary gland swelling and pain and loss of taste. Longer-term complications include recurrent sialoadenitis, hyposalivation, xerostomia, mouth pain, and dental caries.[38] Grewal and associates[39] reported that 39% (102) of a cohort of 262 patients treated with RAI ablation for thyroid cancer developed salivary gland side effects in the first year after treatment. Persistent side effects were noted in 5% (13) of the patients at 7 years after treatment (see Chapter 26 and Appendix C for management of xerostomia).

Thyroid Disease and Lichen Planus

A study from Finland reported by Siponen and colleagues[40] suggested a possible association with thyroid disease and lichen planus. On this basis, the investigators call for further investigation involving other populations and into the possible mechanisms that could be involved with such an association.

REFERENCES

1. Ladenson P, Kim M: Thyroid. In Goldman L, Ausiello D, editors: *Cecil medicine*, ed 23, Philadelphia, 2008, Saunders, pp 1698-1712.
2. DeFelice M, DiLauro R: Anatomy and development of the thyroid. In Jameson JL, DeGroot LJ, editors: *Endocrinology: adult and pediatric*, Philadelphia, 2010, Saunders, pp 1342-1361.
3. Mazzaferri EL: The thyroid. In Mazzaferri EL, editor: *Endocrinology*, ed 3, New York, 1986, Medical Examination Publishing.
4. Marinovic D, et al: Ultrasonographic assessment of the ectopic thyroid tissue in children with congenital hypothyroidism, *Pediatr Radiol* 34:109-113, 2004.
5. Jameson JL, Weetman AP: Diseases of the thyroid gland. In Kasper DL, et al, editors: *Harrison's online principles of medicine*, ed 16, New York, 2005, McGraw-Hill, pp 2104-2127.
6. Larsen PW, Davies TF: Hypothyroidism and thyroiditis. In Larsen PR, et al: editors: *Williams textbook of endocrinology*, ed 10, Philedelphia, 2003, WB Saunders, pp 415-465.
7. Jameson JL, Weetman AP: Disorders of the thyroid gland. In Fauci AS, et al, editors: *Harrison's principles of internal medicine*, ed 17, New York, 2008, McGraw-Hill, pp 2224-2246.
8. Skugor M, Fleseriu M: Hypothyroidism and hyperthyroidism. In Carey WD, et al, editors: *Current clinical medicine 2009—Cleveland Clinic*, Philadelphia, 2009, Saunders, pp 431-439.
9. Pacini F, et al: Thyroid neoplasia. In Jameson JL, DeGroot LJ, editors: *Endocrinology: adult and pediatric*, Philadelphia, 2010, Saunders, pp 1668-1701.
10. Germain DLS: Thyroid hormone metabolism. In Jameson JL, DeGroot LJ, editors: *Endocrinology: adult and pediatric*, Philadelphia, 2010, Saunders, pp 1409-1422.
11. Webb P, et al: Mechanisms of thyroid hormone action. In Jameson JL, DeGroot LJ, editors: *Endocrinology: adult and pediatric*, Philadelphia, 2010, Saunders, pp 1423-1443.
12. Marino M: Graves' disease. In Jameson JL, DeGroot LJ, editors: *Endocrinology: adult and pediatric*, Philadelphia, 2010, Saunders, pp 1527-1558.
13. Wiersinga WM: Hypothyroidism and myxedema coma. In Jameson JL, DeGroot LJ, editors: *Endocrinology: adult and pediatric*, Philadelphia, 2010, Saunders, pp 1607-1622.
14. Schlurnberger MJ, Filetti S, Hay ID: Benign and malignant nodular thyroid disease. In Larsen PR, et al, editors: *Williams textbook of endocrinology*, ed 10, Philadelphia, 2003, WB Saunders, pp 465-491.
15. Altekruse SF, et al: *SEER cancer statistics review, 1976-2007*, Bethesda, Md, 2010, National Cancer Institute.
16. Thyroid cancer, Washington, DC, 2010, National Institutes of Health.
17. Dumont JE, et al: Thyroid regulatory factors. In Jameson JL, DeGroot LJ, editors: *Endocrinology: adult and pediatric*, Philadelphia, 2010, Saunders, pp 1384-1409.
18. Germain DLS: Thyroid hormone metabolism. In DeGroot LJ, Jameson JL, editors: *Endocrinology*, ed 5, Philadelphia, 2006, Saunders, pp 1861-1873.
19. Weetman AP: Autoimmune thyroid disease. In Jameson JL, DeGroot LJ, editors: *Endocrinology: adult and pediatric*, Philadelphia, 2010, Saunders, pp 1512-1526.
20. Weiss RE, Refetoff S: Thyroid function testing. In Jameson JL, DeGroot LJ, editors: *Endocrinology: adult and pediatric*, Philadelphia, 2010, Saunders, pp 1444-1492.
21. Blum M: Thyroid imaging. In DeGroot LJ, Jameson JL, editors: *Endocrinology*, ed 5, Philadelphia, 2006, Saunders, pp 1963-1979.
22. Blum M: Thyroid imaging. In Jameson JL, DeGroot LJ, editors: *Endocrinology: adult and pediatric*, Philadelphia, 2010, Saunders, pp 1493-1512.
23. Weetman AP: Graves' disease, *N Engl J Med* 343:1236-1248, 2000.
24. Burch HB, Bahn RS: Graves' ophthalmopathy. In Jameson JL, DeGroot LJ, editors: *Endocrinology: adult and pediatric*, Philadelphia, 2010, Saunders, pp 1559-1571.
25. Saver DF, et al: *Thyroiditis* (series online), http://www.firstconsult.com/thyroiditis, Elsevier, 2004; accessed on March 5, 2010.
26. Guimaraes VC: Subacute and Riedel's thyroiditis. In Jameson JL, DeGroot LJ, editors: *Endocrinology: adult and pediatric*, Philadelphia, 2010, Saunders, pp 1595-1606.
27. Lazarus JH: Chronic (Hashimoto's) thyroiditis. In Jameson JL, DeGroot LJ, editors: *Endocrinology: adult and pediatric*, Philadelphia, 2010, Saunders, pp 1583-1593.
28. Saver DF, et al: *Thyroid carcinoma* (series online), http://www.firstconsult.com/thyroid_carcinoma, Elsevier, 2004; accessed on March 5, 2010.
29. Wood K, Vini L, Harmer C: Metastases to the thyroid gland: the Royal Marsden experience, *Eur J Surg Oncol* 30:583-588, 2004.
30. Weigel RJ, Macdonald JS, Haller D: Cancer of the endocrine system. In Abeloff MD, et al, editors. *Clinical oncology*, ed 3, London, 2004, Churchill Livingstone, pp 1612-1621.
31. McHenry CR: Thyroid cancer. In Rakel RE, Bope ET, editors: *Conn's current therapy*, ed 53, Philadelphia, 2006, Saunders.
32. Little JW: Thyroid disorders: part I, hyperthyroidism, *Oral Surg Oral Med Oral Path Oral Radiol Endod* 101:276-284, 2006.
33. Pinto A, Glick M: Management of patients with thyroid disease: oral health considerations, *J Am Dent Assoc* 133:849-858, 2002.
34. Little JW: Thyroid disorders: part II, hypothyroidism and thyroiditis, *Oral Surg Oral Med Oral Path Oral Radiol Endod* 102:148-153, 2006.

35. Little JW: Thyroid disorders: Part III, thyroid neoplasms, *Oral Surg Oral Med Oral Path Oral Radiol Endod* 102:275-280, 2006.
36. Neville BW, et al: *Oral and maxillofacial pathology*, ed 2, Philadelphia, 2002, WB Saunders.
37. Femiano F, et al: Burning mouth syndrome and burning mouth in hypothyroidism: proposal for a diagnostic and therapeutic protocol, *Oral Surg Oral Med Oral Pathol Oral Radiol Endod* 105:e22-e27, 2008.
38. Lee SL: Complications of radioactive iodine treatment of thyroid carcinoma, *J Natl Compr Canc Netw* 8:1277-1287, 2010.
39. Grewal RK, et al: Salivary gland side effects commonly develop several weeks after initial radioactive iodine ablation, *J Nucl Med* 50:1605-1610, 2009.
40. Siponen M, et al: Association of oral lichen planus with thyroid disease in a Finnish population: a retrospective case-control study, *Oral Surg Oral Med Oral Pathol Oral Radiol Endod* 110:319-324, 2010.

17

Pregnancy and Breast Feeding

A pregnant patient, although not considered medically compromised, poses a unique set of management considerations for the dentist. Dental care must be rendered to the mother without adversely affecting the developing fetus, and although routine dental care generally is safe for the pregnant patient, the delivery of such care involves some potentially harmful elements, including the use of ionizing radiation and certain drugs. Thus, the prudent practitioner must balance the beneficial aspects of dentistry with potentially harmful procedures by minimizing or avoiding exposure of the patient (and the developing fetus).

Additional considerations arise during the postpartum period if the mother elects to breast feed her infant. Although most drugs are only minimally transmitted from maternal serum to breast milk, and the infant's exposure is not significant, the dentist should avoid using any drug that is known to be harmful to the infant.

OVERVIEW OF PREGNANCY

Physiology and Complications

To define rational management guidelines, a review of the normal processes of pregnancy and fetal development is provided here.

Endocrine changes are the most significant basic alterations that occur with pregnancy. They result from the increased production of maternal and placental hormones and from modified activity of target end organs.

Fatigue is a common physiologic finding during the first trimester that may have a psychologic impact. A tendency toward syncope and postural hypotension also has been noted. During the second trimester, patients typically have a sense of well-being and relatively few symptoms. During the third trimester, increasing fatigue and discomfort and mild depression may be reported. Several cardiovascular changes occur as well. Blood volume increases by 40% to 50%, cardiac output by 30% to 50%, but red blood cell volume increases by only about 15% to 20%, resulting in a fall in the maternal hematocrit.[1] Despite the increase in cardiac output, blood pressure falls (usually to 100/70 mm Hg or lower) during the second trimester, and a modest increase is noted in the last month of pregnancy. This increase in blood volume is associated with high flow–low resistance circulation, tachycardia, and heart murmurs, and it may unmask glomerulopathies, peripartum cardiomyopathy, arterial aneurysms, or arteriovenous malformations. A benign systolic ejection murmur is a rather common finding occurring in more than 90% of pregnant women, which disappears shortly after delivery.[1] A murmur of this type is considered physiologic or functional. However, a murmur that preceded pregnancy or persisted after delivery would require further evaluation for determination of its significance.

During late pregnancy, a phenomenon known as *supine hypotensive syndrome* may occur that manifests as an abrupt fall in blood pressure, bradycardia, sweating, nausea, weakness, and air hunger when the patient is in a supine position.[1,2] Symptoms and signs are caused by impaired venous return to the heart resulting from compression of the inferior vena cava by the gravid uterus. This leads to decreased blood pressure, reduced cardiac output, and impairment or loss of consciousness. The remedy for the problem is for the patient to roll over onto her left side, which lifts the uterus off the vena cava. Blood pressure should rapidly return to normal.

Blood changes in pregnancy include anemia and a decreased hematocrit value. Anemia occurs because blood volume increases more rapidly than red blood cell mass. As a result, a fall in hemoglobin and a marked need for additional folate and iron occur. A majority of pregnant women have insufficient iron stores—a problem that is exaggerated by significant blood loss. However, there is disagreement over whether or not to routinely provide iron supplementation.[1] Although changes in platelets are usually clinically insignificant, most studies show a mild decrease in platelets during pregnancy.[3] Several blood clotting factors, especially fibrinogen and factors VII, VIII, IX, and X, are increased. As a result of the increase in many of the coagulation factors, combined with venous stasis, pregnancy is associated with a hypercoagulable state. Interestingly, however, the prothrombin time, activated partial thromboplastin time, and thrombin time all fall slightly but remain within the limits of normal nonpregnant values.[1] The overall risk of thromboembolism in pregnancy is estimated to be 1 in 1500 and accounts for 25% of maternal deaths in the United States.[4]

Several white blood cell (WBC) and immunologic changes occur. The WBC count increases progressively throughout pregnancy, primarily because of an increase in neutrophils, and is nearly doubled by term. The reason for the increase is unclear but may involve elevated estrogen and cortisol levels.[5] This increase in neutrophils may complicate the interpretation of the complete blood count during infection. Also, during pregnancy, the immune system shifts from helper T cell type 1 (T_H1) dominance to T_H2 dominance. This shift leads to immune suppression. Clinically, the decrease in cellular immunity leads to increased susceptibility to intracellular pathogens such as cytomegalovirus virus, herpes simplex virus, varicella virus, and the agent of malaria.[1] The decrease in cellular immunity may explain why rheumatoid arthritis frequently improves during gestation, since it is a cell-mediated immunopathologic disease.[6] During the postpartum period, rebound and heightened inflammatory activity occurs.

Changes in respiratory function during pregnancy include elevation of the diaphragm which decreases the volume of the lungs in the resting state, thereby reducing total lung capacity by 5% and the functional residual capacity (FRC), the volume of air in the lungs at the end of quiet exhalation, by 20%.[7] Of interest, the respiratory rate and vital capacity remain unchanged. These ventilatory changes produce an increased rate of respiration (tachypnea) and dyspnea that is worsened by the supine position. Thus, it is not surprising that sleep during pregnancy is impaired, especially during the third trimester.[8]

Pregnancy predisposes the expectant mother to an increased appetite and often a craving for unusual foods. As a result, the diet may be unbalanced, high in sugars, or nonnutritious. This can adversely affect the mother's dentition and also contribute to significant weight gain. Taste alterations and an increased gag response are common as well. The pH and production of saliva are probably unchanged.[9] No evidence exists that pregnancy causes or accelerates the course of dental caries. Nausea and vomiting, or "morning sickness," may complicate up to 70% of pregnancies. Typical onset is between 4 and 8 weeks of gestation, with improvement before 16 weeks; however, 10% to 25% of women still experience symptoms at 20 to 22 weeks of gestation, and some women experience this throughout the pregnancy.[10] The cause is not well understood. Some patients may experience extreme nausea and frequent vomiting, which can be a cause of dental erosion.

The general pattern of fetal development should be understood when dental management plans are being formulated. Normal pregnancy lasts approximately 40 weeks. During the first trimester, organs and systems are formed (organogenesis). Thus, the fetus is most susceptible to malformation during this period. After the first trimester, the major aspects of formation are complete, and the remainder of fetal development is devoted primarily to growth and maturation. Thus, the chances of malformation are markedly diminished after the first trimester. A notable exception to this relative protection is the fetal dentition, which is susceptible to malformation from toxins or radiation, and to tooth discoloration caused by administration of tetracycline.

Complications of pregnancy are infrequent when appropriate prenatal care is provided and the mother is healthy. Unfortunately, complications occur more often in expectant mothers who harbor pathogens (oral and extraoral) and smoke, and in nonwhites than in whites in the United States.[11] Common complications include infection, enhanced inflammatory response, glucose abnormalities, and hypertension.[12] Each of these entities increases the risks for preterm delivery, perinatal mortality, and congenital anomalies. Insulin resistance is a contributing factor to the development of gestational diabetes mellitus (GDM), which occurs in 2% to 6% of pregnant women. GDM increases the risks for infection and large birth weight babies. Hypertension is of particular interest because it can lead to end organ damage or preeclampsia, a clinical condition of pregnancy that manifests as hypertension, proteinuria, edema, and blurred vision. *Preeclampsia,* defined as hypertension with proteinuria, progresses to *eclampsia* if seizures or coma develop. The cause of eclampsia is unknown but appears to involve sympathetic overactivity associated with insulin resistance, the renin-angiotensin system, lipid peroxidation, and inflammatory mediators.[13] Complications of pregnancy that are unresponsive to diet modification and palliative care ultimately require drugs or hospitalization for adequate control.

Another consideration related to fetal growth is spontaneous abortion (miscarriage). Spontaneous abortion is the natural termination of pregnancy before the 20th week of gestation, and occurs in approximately 15% of all pregnancies.[14] The most common causes of spontaneous abortion are morphologic or chromosomal abnormalities which prevent successful implantation. It is most unlikely that any dental procedure would be implicated in spontaneous abortion, provided fetal hypoxia and exposure of the fetus to teratogens are avoided. Febrile illness and sepsis also can precipitate a miscarriage; therefore, prompt treatment of odontogenic infection and periodontitis is advised.

Because of immature liver and enzyme systems, the fetus has a limited ability to metabolize drugs. Pharmacologic challenge of the fetus is to be avoided when possible.

During the postpartum period, the mother may suffer from lack of sleep and postpartum depression. Also during the postpartum period, risks for the occurrence of autoimmune disease, particularly rheumatoid arthritis, multiple sclerosis, and thyroiditis, are increased.

DENTAL MANAGEMENT

Medical Considerations

Management recommendations during pregnancy should be viewed as general guidelines—not as definitive rules. The dentist should assess the general health of the patient through a thorough medical history. Information to ascertain includes current physician, medications taken, use of tobacco, alcohol, or illicit drugs, history of gestational diabetes, miscarriage, hypertension, and morning sickness. If the need arises, the patient's obstetrician should be consulted. Of interest, in a 1992 survey of obstetricians,[15] 91% of respondents indicated that they preferred not to be contacted in regard to "routine" dental care. However, 88% wanted to be consulted before the dentist prescribed antibiotics, and 54% wanted to participate in a consultation before the dentist prescribed analgesics (Box 17-1).

Pregnancy is a special event in a woman's life; hence, it is an emotionally charged experience. Establishing a good patient-dentist relationship that encourages openness, honesty, and trust is an integral part of successful management. This kind of relationship greatly reduces stress and anxiety for both patient and dentist.

As with all patients, measuring vital signs is important for identifying undiagnosed abnormalities and the need for corrective action. At a minimum, blood pressure and pulse should be measured. Systolic pressure at or above 140 mm Hg and diastolic pressure at or above 90 mm Hg are signs of hypertension (see Chapter 3). Also, clinical concern is appropriate if the patient's blood pressure increases 30 mm Hg or more in systolic or increases 15 mm Hg in diastolic blood pressure over prepregnancy values, because these changes can be a sign of preeclampsia.[16] Confirmed hypertensive values dictate that the patient be referred to a physician to ensure that preeclampsia and other cardiovascular disorders are properly diagnosed and managed.

Preventive Program. An important objective in planning dental treatment for a pregnant patient is to establish a healthy oral environment and an optimum level of

BOX 17-1 Dental Management
Considerations in Patients Who Are Pregnant

P

Patient Evaluation/Risk Assessment (see Box 1-1)
- Evaluate and determine trimester of pregnancy.
- Obtain medical consultation if the patient's condition is poorly controlled, if signs and symptoms point to an undiagnosed condition, or if the diagnosis is uncertain.

Potential Issues/Factors of Concern

A	
Antibiotics	If antibiotics are required, consult with the physician. Use those with FDA classification A or B, unless otherwise approved by the physician.
Analgesics	If analgesics are required, consult with the physician. Acetaminophen is the drug of choice. If other analgesics are required, use with approval of physician.
Anesthesia	The usual local anesthetics with vasoconstrictors are safe to use, provided that care is taken not to exceed the recommended dose.
Allergies	No issues.
Anxiety	Avoid most anxiolytics. Short-term use of nitrous oxide, if needed, is permissible, provided that 50% oxygen is used.
B	
Bleeding	No issues.
Breathing	Patient may have difficulty breathing in the supine position.
Blood pressure	Watch for supine hypotension if patient is in the supine position; most likely in late third trimester.
C	
Chair position	Patient may not be able to tolerate a supine chair position in third trimester.
Cardiovascular	Elevated lood pressure could be a sign of preeclampsia.
D	
Drugs	Avoid all drugs if possible. If drugs are needed, use FDA category A or B, if possible.
Devices	No issues.
E	
Equipment	Make only necessary x-ray exposures; use lead apron and thyroid collar.
Emergencies	Anticipate the possibility of supine hypotension if the pregnancy has reached third trimester.
F	
Follow-up	Follow-up evaluation after delivery is recommended, to ensure resumption of needed dental care, with radiographic assessment, as appropriate.

oral hygiene. This essentially consists of a plaque control program that minimizes the exaggerated inflammatory response of gingival tissues to local irritants that commonly accompany the hormonal changes of pregnancy.[17] Maternal plaque control, however, has implications for caries risk for the infant. Studies conducted over the past few deccades have shown that reduced oral streptococcal levels in the pregnant mother reduce the risk that the infant will become infected and develop caries.[18-20]

Acceptable oral hygiene techniques should be taught, reinforced, and monitored. Diet counseling, with emphasis on limiting the intake of refined carbohydrates and carbonated soft drinks, should be provided. Coronal scaling and polishing or root curettage may be performed whenever necessary. Preventive plaque control measures should be provided and emphasized throughout pregnancy, including the first trimester, for benefit to the pregnant mother and the developing baby.[21] Chlorhexidine 0.12% mouth rinse is classified in U.S. Food and Drug Admnistration (FDA) pregnancy risk category B for drugs (discussed later under "Drug Aministration") and thus may be used safely during pregnancy, if needed.

The benefits of prenatal fluoride are controversial. Early studies by Glenn and associates[22-24] concluded that a daily 2.2-mg tablet of sodium fluoride administered to mothers during the second and third trimesters in combination with fluoridated water resulted in 97% of the offspring being caries-free for up to 10 years. Not only were medical or dental defects, including fluorosis, absent in these children, but an association with decreased premature delivery and increased birth weight was seen in the fluoride treatment group. However, in a later randomized, controlled trial of 798 children followed for 5 years after birth, no significant benefit was found with prenatal fluoride compared with placebo.[25] Furthermore, another study failed to find any significant increase in fluoride content of enamel in children who received prenatal fluoride versus placebo.[26] In 2001, the Centers for Disease Control and Prevention (CDC) reported that evidence was insufficient to support a recommendation for the use of prenatal fluoride.[27]

Treatment Timing

Other than as part of a good plaque control program, elective dental care is best avoided during the first trimester because of the potential vulnerability of the fetus (Table 17-1). The second trimester is the safest period during which to provide routine dental care. Emphasis should be placed on controlling active disease and eliminating potential problems that could occur later in pregnancy or during the immediate postpartum period, because providing dental care during these periods often is difficult. Extensive reconstruction or significant surgical procedures are best postponed until after delivery.

The early part of the third trimester is still a good time to provide routine dental care. After the middle of the third trimester, however, elective dental care is best postponed. This is because of the increasing feeling of discomfort that many expectant mothers may experience. Prolonged time in the dental chair should be avoided, to prevent the complication of supine hypotension. If supine hypotension develops, rolling the patient onto her left side affords return of circulation to the heart. Scheduling short appointments, allowing the patient to assume a semireclining position, and encouraging frequent changes of position can help to minimize problems.

TABLE 17-1 Treatment Timing During Pregnancy*

First Trimester	Second Trimester	Third Trimester
Plaque control Oral hygiene instruction Scaling, polishing, curettage Avoid elective treatment; urgent care only	Plaque control Oral hygiene instruction Scaling, polishing, curettage Routine dental care	Plaque control Oral hygiene instruction Scaling, polishing, curettage Routine dental care

*Limit radiographic exposures to only those required for diagnosis and treatment.

Dental Radiographs

Dental radiography is one of the more controversial areas in the management of a pregnant patient. Pregnant patients who require radiographs often have anxiety about the adverse effects of x-rays on their baby. In some instances, their obstetrician or primary care physician may reinforce these fears. In almost all cases involving dental radiography, these fears are unfounded. The safety of dental radiography has been well established, provided that features such as fast exposure techniques (e.g., high-speed film or digital imaging), filtration, collimation, lead aprons, and thyroid collars are used. Of all aids, the most important for the pregnant patient are the protective lead apron and the thyroid collar. In addition, the use of digital radiography markedly reduces radiation exposure to no more than that with the use of F-speed film.[28]

In spite of the safety of dental radiography, ionizing radiation should be avoided, if possible, during pregnancy, especially during the first trimester, because the developing fetus is particularly susceptible to radiation damage.[29] However, should dental treatment become necessary, radiographs may be required for accurate diagnosis and treatment. The American Academy of Pediatrics and the American College of Obstetricians and Gynecologists have published guidelines stating: "Diagnostic radiologic procedures should not be performed during pregnancy unless the information to be obtained from them is necessary for the care of the patient and cannot be obtained by other means."[30,31] Therefore, the dentist should understand the risks of ionizing radiation and know how to proceed as safely as possible in the event that radiographs are needed. In 2004, the American Dental Association (ADA) and the FDA (www.fda.gov) jointly published guidelines for prescribing and taking radiographs, including taking radiographs during pregnancy. These guidelines were updated by the ADA in 2006.[32]

The teratogenicity of ionizing radiation is dose-dependent, so an understanding of the units of measurement is particularly important for use of dental radiography in the pregnant patient.[28] The absorbed dose is a measure of the energy absorbed by any type of ionizing radiation per unit of mass of any type of matter. The traditional unit of the absorbed dose is the rad (radiation absorbed dose). In recent years, however, there has been a move to use the metric-based Système International (SI), and its unit of measurement for absorbed dose is the gray (Gy): 1 Gy equals 100 rads. Thus, 1 centigray (cGy) equals 1 rad. An additional unit, the sievert (Sv), is used as a measure of equivalent dose to compare the biologic effects of different types of radiation on a tissue or organ. For diagnostic x-ray examinations, 1 Sv equals 1 Gy

Increased risk of adverse outcomes has not been detected among animals with continuous low-dose exposure less than 5 rad (5 cGy) throughout pregnancy.[33] Available animal and human data support the conclusion that no increase in gross congenital anomalies or interauterine growth retardation occurs as a result of exposures during pregnancy totaling less than 5 cGy (5 rad)[29,34-37] Table 17-2 provides a comparison of ionizing radiation exposures expressed in cGy. It is obvious that exposures from typical dental radiographs are less than natural daily background radiation. Of note, however, maternal thyroid exposure to diagnostic radiation in excess of 0.4 mGy has been associated with a slight decrease in infant birth weight.[38] This finding reinforces the importance of using a thyroid collar on pregnant patients.

Teratogenicity also is dependent on the gestational age of the fetus at the time of exposure. During the organogenesis period (from the end of the 2nd to the 8th week after conception), the fetus is extremely sensitive to the teratogenic effect of ionizing radiation and particularly the central nervous system (CNS), even though its main formation period is between weeks 8 and 15 of pregnancy, a period in which it is very radiosensitive.[39] From weeks 16 to 25, there is a reduction in the radiosensitivity of the CNS and in many of the other organs. After week 25, the central nervous system becomes relatively radioresistent, and major fetal malformations and functional anomalies are highly improbable.[36,37]

*When risks of dental radiography are further assessed during pregnancy, three reports should be kept in mind. The first states that the maximum risk attributable to 1 cGy (which is more than 1000 full-mouth series with E-speed film and rectangular collimation or 10% to 20% of the threshold dose) of in utero radiation exposure is estimated[35] to be approximately 0.1%. This is a figure thousands of times less than the normal anticipated risks of spontaneous abortion, malformation, or genetic disease. The second report calculates the risk for a first-generation fetal defect from a dental radiographic examination to be 9 in 1 billion.[40] The third report found that the gonadal dose to women, after full mouth radiography, is less than 0.01 μSv, which is at least 1000-fold below the threshold shown to cause congenital damage to newborns.[41] These data indicate that with use of the lead apron, rectangular collimation, and E-speed film or faster techniques, one or two intraoral films are truly of minute significance in terms of radiation effects on the developing fetus. In terms that can be explained to a patient, the following example can be used: The gonadal/fetal dose incurred with two periapical dental films (when a lead apron is used) is 700 times less than that for 1 day of average exposure to natural background radiation in the United States.[42,43]

Despite the negligible risks of dental radiography, the dentist should not be cavalier regarding its use during pregnancy (or at any other time, for that matter). Radiographs should be obtained selectively and only when necessary and appropriate to aid in diagnosis and treatment. Bitewing, panoramic, or selected periapical films are recommended for minimizing patient dose. To further reduce the radiation dose, the following measures should be employed: rectangular collimation, E-speed or F-speed film or faster techniques (digital imaging reduces radiographic exposure by at least 50% in comparison with

TABLE 17-2 Comparative Radiation Exposures to Fetal or Embryonic Tissues

Source of Radiation	Absorbed Exposure (cGy)
Upper gastrointestinal series	0.330
Chest radiograph	0.008
Skull radiograph	0.004
Daily (cosmic) background radiation	0.0004
Full-mouth dental series (18 intraoral radiographs, D film, lead apron)	0.00001

Data from National Council on Radiation Protection and Measurements (NCRP): Medical radiation exposure of pregnant and potentially pregnant women, *NCRP Report No 54, Washington, DC, NCRP Publications, 1977; and DiSaia PJ: Radiation Therapy. In Scott JR, et al, editors:* Danforth's obstetrics and gynecology, *ed 6, Philadelphia, 1990, JB Lippincott.*

*1 cGy (0.01 Gy) = 1 rad (roentgen, R) (e.g., 1 R = 0.01 Gy = 0.01 Sievert [Sv] = 10 mSv). For diagnostic radiology, 1 Sv = 1 Gy)

E-speed exposures), lead shielding (abdominal and thyroid collar), high-kilovoltage (kV) or constant beams, and an ongoing quality assurance program for equipment and technique.

An additional consideration is potential fetal exposure in the pregnant dental auxiliary or dentist. The maximum permissible radiation dose for whole body exposure of the pregnant dental care worker is 0.005 Gy or 5 mSv per year. This dose is equivalent to the maximum permissible radiation dose for the nonoccupationally exposed public and 10-fold less than the level for occupationally exposed nonpregnant workers (50 mSv).[44] The National Council on Radiation Protection and Measurements reports that induction of congenital defects is negligible from fetal exposures of 50 mSv.[44,45] To further ensure safety, the pregnant operator should wear a film badge, stand more than 6 feet from the tube head, and position herself at between 90 and 130 degrees of the beam, preferably behind a protective wall (Figure 17-1). When these guidelines are followed, no clinical contraindication to operation of the x-ray machine by pregnant women arises. However, dentists should familiarize themselves with federal (Code of Federal Regulations, Code 10, Part 20, Section 20.201) and state regulations that would supersede these guidelines.

Drug Administration

During Pregnancy. Another controversial area in the treatment of the pregnant dental patient is drug administration. The principal concern is that a drug may cross the placenta, with the potential for toxic or teratogenic effects on the fetus. Additionally, any drug that is a respiratory depressant may cause maternal hypoxia, resulting in fetal hypoxia, injury, or death.

Ideally, no drug should be administered during pregnancy, especially during the first trimester. Strict adherence to this rule, however, is sometimes impossible. Fortunately, most of the commonly used drugs in dental practice can be given during pregnancy with relative safety, although a few exceptions are notable. Table 17-3 presents a suggested approach to drug usage for pregnant patients.

Before prescribing or administering a drug to a pregnant patient, the dentist should be familiar with the FDA categorization of prescription drugs for pregnancy based on their potential risk of fetal injury.[46] These pregnancy risk classification categories, although not without limitations, are meant to aid clinicians and patients in making decisions about drug therapy. Counseling should be provided to ensure that women who are pregnant clearly

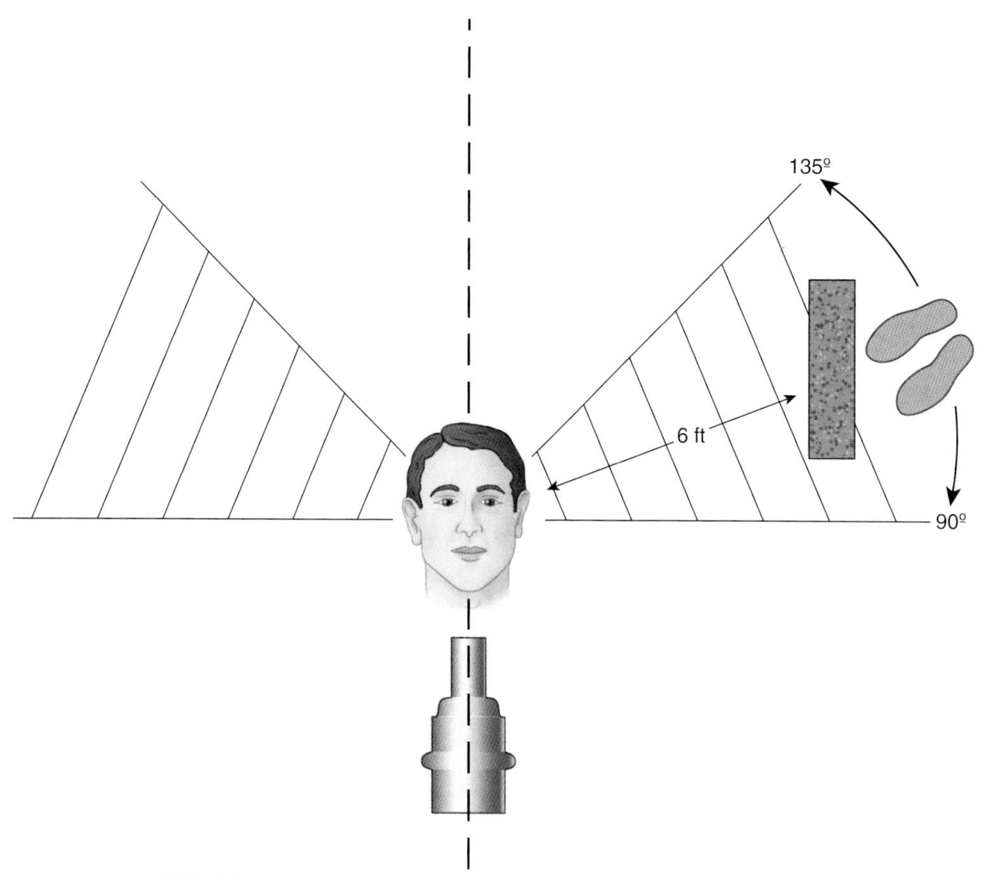

FIGURE 17-1 Proper operator position during exposure of x-ray films.

TABLE 17-3 Drug Administration During Pregnancy and Breast Feeding

Drug	FDA Pregnancy Risk Category	Use During Pregnancy	Risk	Use During Breast Feeding
Local Anesthetics				
Articaine	C	Use with caution; consult physician		Unknown
Bupivacaine	C	Use with caution; consult physician	Fetal bradycardia	Yes
Etidocaine	B	Yes		Yes
Lidocaine	B	Yes		Yes
Mepivacaine	C	Use with caution; consult physician	Fetal bradycardia	Yes
Prilocaine	B	Yes		Yes
Analgesics—Non-Narcotic				
Acetaminophen	B	Yes		Yes
Aspirin	C/D[3]	Caution; avoid in third trimester	Postpartum hemorrhage Constriction ductus arteriosus	Avoid
Cyclooxygenase (COX)-2 inhibitor	C	Avoid in third trimester	May lead to constriction, ductus arteriosus	Yes
Diflunisal, etodolac, mefenamic acid	C/D[3]	Use with caution; avoid in third trimester; consult physician	Delayed labor	No
Ibuprofen, flurbiprofen	B/D[3]	Caution; avoid in third trimester	Delayed labor	Yes
Naproxen	B/D[3]	Caution; avoid in third trimester	Delayed labor	Yes
Analgesics—Narcotic				
Codeine	C/D*	Use with caution (low dose, short duration); consult physician	Neonatal respiratory depression	Yes
Hydrocodone	C/D[3]	Use with caution (low dose, short duration); consult physician	Neonatal respiratory depression	—
Oxycodone	C/D[3]	Use with caution (low dose, short duration); consult physician	Neonatal respiratory depression	Yes
Pentazocine	C	Use with caution (low dose, short duration); consult physician	Neonatal respiratory depression	Yes
Propoxyphene	C	Use with caution (low dose, short duration); consult physician	Neonatal respiratory depression	Yes
Antibiotics				
Cephalosporins	B	Yes		Yes
Clindamycin	B	Yes		Yes
Fluoroquinolones (norfloxacin, ciprofloxacin, ofloxacin, and enoxacin)	C	Use with caution; consult physician	Arthropathy	Caution
Macrolides				
Erythromycin	B	Yes; avoid estolate form		Yes
Azithromycin	B	Yes		Yes
Clarithromycin	C	Use with caution; consult physician		Yes
Metronidazole	B	Yes		Yes
Penicillins	B	Yes		Yes
Tetracycline	D	Avoid	Tooth discoloration, inhibits bone formation	Avoid
Tetracycline—periodontal dosages	C	Avoid	Tooth discoloration, inhibits bone formation	Avoid
Antivirals				
Acyclovir	C	Yes		Yes
Famciclovir	B	Yes		Yes
Valacyclovir	B	Yes		Yes
Antifungals				
Fluconazole	C	Yes		Yes
Nystatin	B/C	Yes		Yes
Corticosteroid				
Prednisone	B	Yes		Yes

Continued

TABLE 17-3 Drug Administration During Pregnancy and Breast Feeding—cont'd

Drug	FDA Pregnancy Risk Category	Use During Pregnancy	Risk	Use During Breast Feeding
Sedative-Hypnotics				
Barbiturates	D	Avoid	Neonatal respiratory depression	Avoid
Benzodiazepines (diazepam, lorazepam)	D	Avoid	Possible risk for oral clefts with prolonged exposure	Avoid
Triazolam	X			
Nitrous oxide	Not assigned	Best used in second and third trimesters and for <30 minutes; consult physician		Yes
Sialagogues				
Cevimeline	C	No information		No information
Pilocarpine	C	Yes		Avoid

*D**, Risk category D if used for prolonged period or at high dose; D^3, risk category D if administered during the third trimester.
Data from Moore PA: Selecting drugs for the pregnant dental patient, J Am Dent Assoc *129:1281-1286, 1998;* Drug information for the health care professional, *ed 2, Rockville, Maryland, 2000, United States Pharmacopeial Convention; and Briggs GG, Freeman RK, Yaffe SJ:* Drugs in pregnancy and lactation: a reference guide to fetal and neonatal risk, *ed 5, Baltimore, 1998, Williams & Wilkins.*

understand the nature and magnitude of the risk associated with a drug. In 2008, the FDA announced that it was eliminating the current pregnancy risk classification system owing to inadequacies; however, at this time the original system is still in place.

The current five pregnancy labeling categories are as follows:

Category A: Controlled studies in humans have failed to demonstrate a risk to the fetus, and the possibility of fetal harm appears remote.

Category B: Animal studies have not indicated fetal risk, and human studies have not been conducted, *or* animal studies have shown a risk, but controlled human studies have not.

Category C: Animal studies have shown a risk, but controlled human studies have not been conducted, *or* studies are not available in humans or animals.

Category D: Positive evidence of human fetal risk exists, but in certain situations, the drug may be used despite its risk.

Category X: Evidence of fetal abnormalities and fetal risk exists based on human experience, and the risk outweighs any possible benefit of use during pregnancy.

Drugs in categories A and B are preferable for prescribing during pregnancy. However, many commonly prescribed drugs used in dentistry fall into category C, so the safety of their use often is uncertain. Drugs in category C present the greatest difficulty for the dentist and the physician in terms of therapeutic and medicolegal decisions; therefore, consultation with the patient's physician may be needed.

Physicians may advise against the use of some of the approved drugs or, conversely, may suggest the use of an uncertain or a questionable drug. The FDA categories are general guidelines and may be incomplete, so differences in practice are not unusual. An example of the occasional use of a questionable drug is be a category C narcotic analgesic for a pregnant patient who is in severe pain.

Local Anesthetics. Local anesthetics administered with epinephrine generally are considered safe for use during pregnancy and are assigned to pregnancy risk classification categories B and C. Although both the local anesthetic and the vasoconstrictor cross the placenta, subtoxic threshold doses have not been shown to cause fetal abnormalities. Because of adverse effects associated with high levels of local anesthetics, it is important not to exceed the manufacturer's recommended maximum dose.

Analgesics. The analgesic of choice during pregnancy is acetaminophen (category B). Aspirin and nonsteroidal antiinflammatory drugs convey risks for constriction of the ductus arteriosus, as well as for postpartum hemorrhage and delayed labor (see Table 17-3).[47,48] The risk of these adverse events increases when agents are administered during the third trimester. Risk also is more closely associated with prolonged administration, high dosage, and selectively potent antiinflammatory drugs, such as indomethacin. Codeine and propoxyphene are associated with multiple congenital defects and should be used cautiously and only if needed.[47,49] The safety of hydrocodone and oxycodone is unclear.

Antibiotics. Penicillins (including amoxicillin), erythromycin (except in estolate form), cephalosporins, metronidazole, and clindamycin are generally considered to be safe for the expectant mother and the developing child.[48] The use of tetracycline, including doxycycline

(FDA category D), is contraindicated during pregnancy. Tetracyclines bind to hydroxyapatite, causing brown discoloration of teeth, hypoplastic enamel, inhibition of bone growth, and other skeletal abnormalities.[47]

Antibiotics and Oral Contraceptives. The concern for potential interactions between antibiotics and oral contraceptives requires mention in this chapter. This concern arises from the ability of select antibiotics such as rifampin, an antituberculosis drug, to reduce plasma levels of circulating oral contraceptives. It has been speculated that this interaction also may be seen with other antibiotics, however, studies to date regarding other antibiotics have been less convincing. To address this concern, the ADA Council on Scientific Affairs[50] issued the following recommendations for prescribing antibiotics to a female patient who takes oral contraceptives:

> The dentist should (1) advise the patient of the potential risk of the antibiotic's reducing the effectiveness of the oral contraceptive, (2) recommend that the patient discuss with her physician the use of an additional nonhormonal means of contraception, [and] (3) advise the patient to maintain compliance with oral contraceptives when concurrently using antibiotics.[50]

The application of these recommendations appears to be prudent until the findings of larger studies become available.

Anxiolytics. Few anxiolytics are considered safe to use during pregnancy. However, a single, short-term exposure to nitrous oxide–oxygen (N_2O-O_2) for less than 35 minutes is not thought to be associated with any human fetal anomalies, including low birth rate.[51,52] By contrast, however, chronic occupational exposure to N_2O-O_2 has been associated with spontaneous abortion and reduced fertility in humans.[53,54] Nitrous oxide may cause inactivation of methionine synthetase and vitamin B_{12}, resulting in altered DNA metabolism, which in turn can lead to cellular abnormalities in animals and birth defects. Accordingly, the following guidelines are recommended if N_2O-O_2 is used during pregnancy[55]:

- Use of N_2O-O_2 inhalation should be minimized to 30 minutes.
- At least 50% oxygen should be delivered to ensure adequate oxygenation at all times.
- Appropriate oxygenation should be provided to avoid diffusion hypoxia at the termination of administration.
- Repeated and prolonged exposures to nitrous oxide are to be avoided.
- The second and third trimesters are safer periods for treatment because organogenesis occurs during the first trimester.

An additional consideration involves the female dentist or dental auxiliary who is pregnant. These women should not be exposed to persistent trace levels of nitrous oxide in the operatory. The use of appropriate scavenging equipment can help alleviate this problem. Female dental health care workers who are chronically exposed to nitrous oxide for more than 3 hours per week, when scavenging equipment is not used, have decreased fertility and increased rates of spontaneous abortion.[47,56] Implementation of National Institute for Occupational Safety and Health (NIOSH) recommendations can reduce occupational exposure to nitrous oxide (Box 17-2).[57,58]

BOX 17-2 Control of Nitrous Oxide in the Dental Office During Pregnancy

1. Inspect nitrous oxide equipment, and replace defective tubing and parts.
2. Check pressure connections for leaks, and fix leaks.
3. Ensure that mask fits well and is secure. Check that the reservoir bag is not overinflated or underinflated.
4. Provide operatory ventilation of 10 or more room air exchanges per hour.
5. Use a scavenging system and appropriate mask sizes. Vacuum should provide outward flow of up to 45 L/minute.
6. Connect and turn on the vacuum pump of the scavenging system before providing nitrous oxide.
7. Regularly conduct air sampling. Maintain low exposure limits (e.g., 25 ppm*) when pregnant dental health care workers are involved.

*This limit is an NIOSH recommendation. By contrast, a time-weighted average (TWA) lower limit of 100 parts per million (ppm) for an 8-hour workday has been suggested (Yagiela JA: Health hazards and nitrous oxide: a time for reappraisal, *Anesth Prog* 38:1-11, 1991).

Adapted from McGlothlin JD, Crouch KG, Mickelsen RL: Control of nitrous oxide in dental operatories, *Cincinnati, Ohio, National Institute for Occupational Safety and Health, 1994, U.S. Department of Health and Human Services (NIOSH) publication 94-129.*

During Breast Feeding. A potential problem arises when a nursing mother requires the administration of a drug in the course of dental treatment. The concern is that the administered drug may enter the breast milk and be transferred to the nursing infant, in whom exposure may result in adverse effects.

Data on which to draw definitive conclusions about drug dosages and effects from breast milk consumption are limited. However, retrospective clinical studies and empirical observations, coupled with known pharmacologic pathways, allow recommendations to be made. The American Academy of Pediatrics concludes that "most drugs likely to be prescribed to the nursing mother should have no effect on milk supply or on infant well-being."[59] A significant fact is that the amount of drug excreted in the breast milk usually is not more than about 1% to 2% of the maternal dose. Therefore, most drugs are of little pharmacologic significance for the infant.[60]

Agreement exists that a few drugs, or categories of drugs, are definitely contraindicated for nursing mothers. These include lithium, anticancer drugs, radioactive pharmaceuticals, and phenindione.[59,60] Table 17-3 presents recommendations adapted from the American Academy of Pediatrics regarding the administration of commonly used dental drugs during breast feeding. As with drug use during pregnancy, individual practitioners may wish to modify these recommendations, which should be viewed only as general guidelines for treatment.

In addition to careful drug selection, nursing mothers may take the drug just after breast feeding and avoid nursing for 4 hours or longer if possible. This timing should result in even further reduced drug concentrations in the breast milk.

Treatment Planning Modifications

No technical modifications are required for the pregnant patient. However, full-mouth radiographs, reconstruction, crown and bridge procedures, and significant surgery are best delayed until after pregnancy. A prominent gag reflex also may dictate a delay in certain dental procedures. Some patients have a concern about mercury exposure from amalgam fillings. In 2009,[61] the FDA investigators concluded that "although data are limited, existing data do not suggest that fetuses are at risk for adverse health effects due to maternal exposure to mercury vapors from dental amalgam." These investigators do note, however, that "maternal exposures are likely to increase temporarily when new dental amalgams are inserted or existing dental amalgams are removed." They furthermore concluded that "existing data support a finding that infants are not at risk for adverse health effects from the breast milk of women exposed to mercury vapors from dental amalgams." Practitioners should be aware, however, that several European countries and Canada have national recommendations advising dentists to limit or avoid the placement and replacement of amalgams during pregnancy.

Regarding the risk to dental personnel from exposure to dental amalgam, the FDA concludes that "existing data indicate that dental professionals generally are not at risk for mercury toxicity except when dental amalgams are improperly used, stored, triturated, or handled."

Oral Complications and Manifestations

The most common oral complication of pregnancy is pregnancy gingivitis (Figure 17-2). This condition results from an exaggerated inflammatory response to local irritants and less-than-meticulous oral hygiene during periods of increased secretion of estrogen and progesterone and altered fibrinolysis.[17,62] Pregnancy gingivitis begins at the marginal and interdental gingiva, usually in the second month of pregnancy. Progression of this condition leads to development of fiery red and edematous interproximal papillae that are tender to palpation. In approximately 1% of gravid women, the hyperplastic response may exacerbate in a localized area, resulting in a pyogenic granuloma or "pregnancy tumor" (Figure 17-3). The most common location for a pyogenic granuloma is the labial aspect of the interdental papilla. The lesion generally is asymptomatic; however, toothbrushing may traumatize the lesion and cause bleeding.

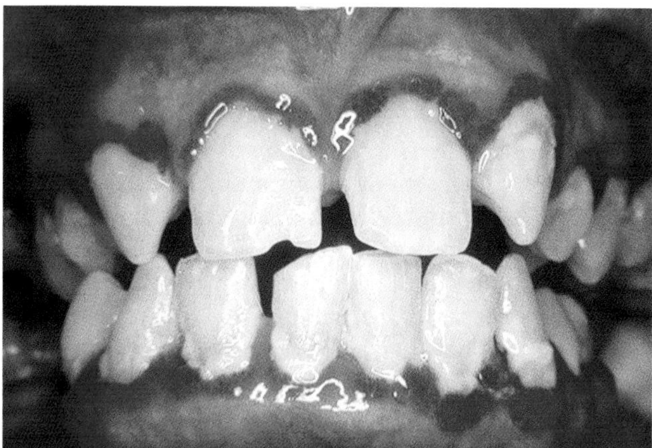

FIGURE 17-2 Generalized gingivitis—"pregnancy gingivitis"—in a woman in her sixth month of pregnancy.

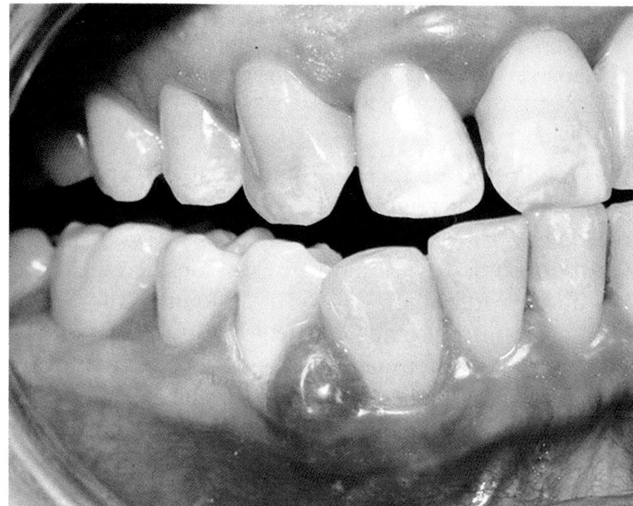

FIGURE 17-3 Pyogenic granuloma—"pregnancy tumor"—occurring during pregnancy.

Hyperplastic gingival changes become apparent around the second month and persist until after parturition, at which time the gingival tissues usually regress and return to normal, provided that proper oral hygiene measures are implemented and any calculus present is removed.[17] Surgical or laser excision occasionally is required as dictated by symptoms, bleeding, or interference with mastication. Pregnancy does not cause periodontal disease but may modify and worsen what is already present. Gestational diabetes mellitus, however, may be associated with an increased risk for periodontal disease.[63] It has been speculated that periodontal disease is a risk factor for preeclampsia and contributes to the frequency of preterm birth and low birth weight in the infant; however, recent reviews do not support this contention.[64-66]

A relationship between dental caries and the physiologic processes of pregnancy has not been demonstrated. Caries activity is attributed to the presence of cariogenic bacteria in the mouth, a diet containing fermentable carbohydrates, and poor oral hygiene. Control of the carious process through use of fluoride and chlorhexidine is important, because maternal saliva is the primary vehicle for transfer of cariogenic streptococci to the infant.[67]

Many women are convinced that pregnancy causes tooth loss (i.e., "a tooth for every pregnancy"), or that calcium is withdrawn from the maternal dentition to supply fetal requirements (i.e., "soft teeth"). Calcium is present in the teeth in a stable crystalline form and hence is not available to the systemic circulation to supply a calcium demand. However, calcium is readily mobilized from bone to supply these demands. Therefore, although calcium supplementation for the purpose of preventing tooth loss or soft teeth is unwarranted, the physician may prescribe calcium to fulfill the general nutritional requirements of mother and fetus.

Tooth mobility, localized or generalized, is an uncommon finding during pregnancy. Mobility is a sign of gingival disease, disturbance of the attachment apparatus, and mineral changes in the lamina dura. Because vitamin deficiencies may contribute to this and other congenital problems (e.g., folate deficiency, spina bifida), the dentist, when discussing oral hygiene, should take this opportunity to educate the patient about the benefits of the use of multivitamins. Daily removal of local irritants, adequate levels of vitamin C, and delivery of the newborn should result in reversal of tooth mobility.

Pregnant women often have a hypersensitive gag reflex. This, in combination with morning sickness, may contribute to episodes of regurgitation, potentially leading to halitosis and enamel erosion. The dentist should advise the patient to rinse after regurgitation with a solution that neutralizes the acid (e.g., baking soda, water).

REFERENCES

1. Gordon MC: Maternal physiology. In Gabbe SG, Niebyl JR, Simpson JL, editors: *Obstetrics: normal and problem pregnancies*, Philadelphia, 2007, Churchill Livingstone.
2. Turner M, Aziz SR: Management of the pregnant oral and maxillofacial surgery patient, *J Oral Maxillofac Surg* 60:1479-1488, 2002.
3. Boehlen F, et al: Platelet count at term pregnancy: a reappraisal of the threshold, *Obstet Gynecol* 95:29, 2000.
4. Johnson RL: Thromboembolic disease complicating pregnancy. In Foley MR, Strong TH, editors: *Obstetric intensive care: a practical manual*, Philadelphia, 1997, WB Saunders.
5. Naccasha N, et al: Phenotypic and metabolic characteristics of monocytes and granulocytes in normal pregnancy and maternal infection, *Am J Obstet Gynecol* 185:1124, 2001.
6. Stirrat G: Pregnancy and immunity: changes occur but pregnancy does not result in immunodeficiency, *BMJ* 308:1385, 1994.
7. Crapo R: Normal cardiopulmonary physiology during pregnancy, *Clin Obstet Gynecol* 39:33, 1996.
8. Santiago J, Nolledo M, Kinzler W: Sleep and sleep disorders in pregnancy, *Ann Intern Med* 134:396, 2001.
9. Kallender D, Sonesson B: Studies on saliva in menstruating, pregnant and postmenopausal women, *Acta Endocrinol (Copenh)* 48, 1965.
10. Furneaux EC, Langley-Evans AJ, Langley-Evans SC: Nausea and vomiting of pregnancy: endocrine basis and contribution to pregnancy outcome, *Obstet Gynecol Surv* 56:775-782, 2001.
11. Martin JA, et al: Births: final data for 2007, *Natl Vital Stat Rep* 58:1-85, 2010.
12. Kaaja RJ, Greer IA: Manifestations of chronic disease during pregnancy, *JAMA*, 294:2751-2757, 2005.
13. Sibai BM: Hypertension. In Gabbe SG, Niebyl JR, Simpson JL, editors: *Obstetrics: normal and problem pregnancies*, Philadelphia, 2007, Churchill Livingstone.
14. Simpson JL, Jauniaux ERM: Pregnancy loss. In Gabbe SG, Niebyl JR, Simpson JL, editors: *Obstetrics: normal and problem pregnancies*, Philadelphia, 2007, Churchill Livingstone.
15. Shrout MK, et al: Treating the pregnant dental patient: four basic rules addressed, *J Am Dent Assoc* 123:75-80, 1992.
16. Solomon CG, Seely EW: Brief review: hypertension in pregnancy: a manifestation of the insulin resistance syndrome? *Hypertension* 37(2):232-239, 2001.
17. Loe H, Silness J: Periodontal disease in pregnancy. I. Prevalence and severity, *Acta Odontol Scand* 21:533-551, 1963.
18. Kohler B, Bratthall D, Krasse B: Preventive measures in mothers influence the establishment of the bacterium *Streptococcus mutans* in their infants, *Arch Oral Biol* 28:225-231, 1983.
19. Kohler B, Andreen I: Influence of caries-preventive measures in mothers on cariogenic bacteria and caries experience in their children, *Arch Oral Biol* 39:907-911, 1994.
20. Brambilla, E., et al: Caries prevention during pregnancy: results of a 30-month study, *J Am Dent Assoc* 129: 871-877, 1998.
21. Fitzsimons D, et al: Nutrition and oral health guidelines for pregnant women, infants, and children, *J Am Diet Assoc* 98:182-186, 189, 1998.
22. Glenn FB: Immunity conveyed by a fluoride supplement during pregnancy, *ASDC J Dent Child* 44:391-395, 1977.
23. Glenn FB: Immunity conveyed by sodium-fluoride supplement during pregnancy: part II, *ASDC J Dent Child* 46:17-24, 1979.
24. Glenn FB, Glenn WD 3rd, Duncan RC: Fluoride tablet supplementation during pregnancy for caries immunity: a study of the offspring produced, *Am J Obstet Gynecol* 143:560-564, 1982.
25. Leverett DH, et al: Randomized clinical trial of the effect of prenatal fluoride supplements in preventing dental caries, *Caries Res* 31:174-179, 1997.
26. Sa Roriz Fonteles C, et al: Fluoride concentrations in enamel and dentin of primary teeth after pre- and postnatal fluoride exposure, *Caries Res* 39:505-508, 2005.
27. Horowitz HS: The 2001 CDC recommendations for using fluoride to prevent and control dental caries in the United States, *J Public Health Dent* 63:3-8, 2003.
28. White SC, Pharoah MJ: *Oral radiology. Principles and interpretation*, ed 6, St. Louis, 2009, Mosby.
29. De Santis M, et al: Ionizing radiations in pregnancy and teratogenesis: a review of literature, *Reprod Toxicol* 20:323-329, 2005.

30. American Academy of Pediatrics and American College of Obstetricians and Gynecologists: *Guidelines for perinatal care*, ed 3, Elk Grove Village, Ill, 1992, American Acdemy of Pediatrics.
31. American College of Obstetricians and Gynecologists: *Guidelines for diagnostic imaging during pregnancy*, ACOG Committee Opinion no. 158, Washington, DC, 1995, ACOG.
32. The use of dental radiographs: update and recommendations, *J Am Dent Assoc* 137:1304-1312, 2006.
33. Brent RL: The effects of embryonic and fetal exposure to x-ray, microwaves, and ultrasound, *Clin Perinatol* 13:615-648, 1986.
34. Lowe SA: Diagnostic radiography in pregnancy: risks and reality, *Aust N Z J Obstet Gynaecol* 44:191-196, 2004
35. Brent RL: The effects of ionizing radiation, microwaves, and ultrasound on the developing embryo: clinical interpretations and applications of the data, *Curr Probl Pediatr* 14:1-87, 1984.
36. Timins JK: Radiation during pregnancy, *N Engl J Med* 98:29-33, 2001.
37. Streffer C, et al: Biological effects after prenatal irradiation (embryo and fetus). A report of the International Commission on Radiological Protection, *Ann ICRP* 33:5-206, 2003.
38. Hujoel PP, et al: Antepartum dental radiography and infant low birth weight, *JAMA* 291:1987-1993, 2004.
39. Mole RH: Detriment in humans after irradiation in utero, *Int J Radiat Biol* 60:561-564, 1991.
40. Danforth RA,Gibbs SJ: Diagnostic radiation: what is the risk? *J Calif Dent Assoc* 8:28-35, 1980.
41. White SC: 1992 assessment of radiation risk from dental radiography, *Dentomaxillofac Radiol* 21:118-126, 1992.
42. *Gonad doses and genetically significant dose from diagnostic radiology: United States, 1964 and 1970*, DHEW Publication (FDA) 76-8034, Rockville, Md, 1976, U.S. Food and Drug Administration.
43. Freeman JP, Brand JW: Radiation doses of commonly used dental radiographic surveys, *Oral Surg Oral Med Oral Pathol* 77:285-289, 1994.
44. National Council on Radiation Protection & Measurements (NCRP): *Recommendations on limits for exposure to ionizing radiation*, Report No. 91, Bethesda, Md, 1987, NCRP.
45. National Council on Radiation Protection & Measurements (NCRP): *Ionizing radiation exposure of the population of the United States*, Report No. 93, Bethesda, Md, 1987, NCRP.
46. Boothby LA, Doering PL: FDA labeling system for drugs in pregnancy, *Ann Pharmacother* 35:1485-1489, 2001.
47. Moore PA: Selecting drugs for the pregnant dental patient, *J Am Dent Assoc* 129:1281-1286, 1998.
48. Rayburn WF, Amanze AC: Prescribing medications safely during pregnancy, *Med Clin North Am* 92:1227-1237, xii, 2008.
49. Heinonen, OP, Sloan D, Shapiro S: *Birth defects and drugs in pregnancy*, Littleton, Miss, 1977, Publishing Sciences Group.
50. Antibiotic interference with oral contraceptives, *J Am Dent Assoc* 133:880, 2002.
51. Crawford JS, Lewis M: Nitrous oxide in early human pregnancy, *Anaesthesia* 41:900-905, 1986.
52. Czeizel AE, Pataki T, Rockenbauer M: Reproductive outcome after exposure to surgery under anesthesia during pregnancy, *Arch Gynecol Obstet* 261:193-199, 1998.
53. Rowland AS, et al: Reduced fertility among women employed as dental assistants exposed to high levels of nitrous oxide, *N Engl J Med* 327:993-997, 1992.
54. Cohen EN, et al: Occupational disease in dentistry and chronic exposure to trace anesthetic gases, *J Am Dent Assoc* 101:21-31, 1980.
55. Suresh L, Radfar L: Pregnancy and lactation, *Oral Surg Oral Med Oral Pathol Oral Radiol Endod* 97:672-682, 2004.
56. Rowland AS, et al: Nitrous oxide and spontaneous abortion in female dental assistants, *Am J Epidemiol* 141:531-538, 1995.
57. Nitrous oxide in the dental office. ADA Council on Scientific Affairs; ADA Council on Dental Practice, *J Am Dent Assoc* 128:364-365, 1997.
58. Control of nitrous oxide in dental operatories. National Institute for Occupational Safety and Health, *Appl Occup Environ Hyg* 14:218-220, 1999.
59. Transfer of drugs and other chemicals into human milk, *Pediatrics* 108:776-789, 2001.
60. Ito S, Lee A: Drug excretion into breast milk—overview, *Adv Drug Deliv Rev* 55:617-627, 2003.
61. Dental devices: classification of dental amalgam, reclassification of dental mercury, designation of special controls for dental amalgam, mercury, and amalgam alloy. Final rule, *Fed Regist* 74:38685-38714, 2009.
62. Silness J, Loe H: Periodontal disease in pregnancy. II. Correlation between oral hygiene and periodontal condition, *Acta Odontol Scand* 22:121-135, 1964.
63. Novak KF, et al: Periodontitis and gestational diabetes mellitus: exploring the link in NHANES III, *J Public Health Dent* 66:163-168, 2006.
64. Uppal A, et al: The effectiveness of periodontal disease treatment during pregnancy in reducing the risk of experiencing preterm birth and low birth weight: a meta-analysis, *J Am Dent Assoc* 141:1423-1434, 2010.
65. Polyzos NP, et al: Obstetric outcomes after treatment of periodontal disease during pregnancy: systematic review and meta-analysis, *BMJ* 341:c7017, 2010.
66. Michalowicz BS, et al: Treatment of periodontal disease and the risk of preterm birth *N Engl J Med* 355:1885-1894, 2006.
67. Caufield PW: Dental caries—a transmissible and infectious disease revisited: a position paper, *Pediatr Dent* 19:491-498, 1997.

PART VII

Immunologic Disease

18

AIDS, HIV Infection, and Related Conditions

On June 5, 1981, when the Centers for Disease Control (CDC) reported five cases of *Pneumocystis carinii* (now *jiroveci*) pneumonia in young homosexual men in Los Angeles, few suspected that it heralded a pandemic of acquired immunodeficiency syndrome (AIDS). In 1983, a retrovirus (later named the human immunodeficiency virus [HIV]) was isolated from a patient with AIDS. Since that first report, more than 70 million persons have been infected with HIV, and more than 30 million have died of AIDS.[1] The total number of deaths has exceeded those caused by the Black Death of 14th-century Europe and the influenza pandemic of 1918 and 1919. About 95% of HIV-infected persons live in low- to middle-income regions, countries, and in sub-Saharan Africa. More than 40% of new infections (excluding those in infants) occur in young people 15 to 24 years of age.[2,3]

AIDS is an infectious disease that is transmitted predominantly through intimate sexual contact and by parenteral means. In view of the nature of this bloodborne pathogen, HIV infection and AIDS have important implications for dental practitioners. Although HIV has rarely been transmitted from patients to health care workers, this may occur, and the patient with HIV infection or AIDS may be medically compromised and may need special dental management considerations. On the basis of current statistics, the average dental practice is predicted to encounter at least two patients infected with HIV per year.

DEFINITION

The definition of AIDS provided by the CDC has been revised several times over the years, and in 2008 it was revised to be *laboratory-confirmed evidence of HIV infection in a person who has stage 3 HIV infection* (i.e., a CD4+ lymphocyte count less than 200 cells/μL).[4] This definition also includes HIV-infected persons whose CD4+ count may be above 200 but have an AIDS-defining condition, as shown in Box 18-1. Of note, because of the provision of antiretroviral drug regimens, not all patients progress to AIDS or develop life-threatening opportunistic infections.[5,6]

Incidence and Prevalence

An estimated 2.7 million people across the globe are newly infected with HIV annually. At the end of 2009, there were an estimated 33.4 million persons globally and an estimated 1.1 million persons in the United States who were infected and living with HIV infection/AIDS.[1] Worldwide, these rates represent a 3-fold higher prevalence since 1990, but a decline since the peak prevalence that occurred in 1999. In the United States, approximately 24% are undiagnosed and unaware of their infection, 42% are HIV-positive but not yet progressed to AIDS, and 34% have AIDS.[7]

The CDC estimated that approximately 56,300 persons were newly infected with HIV in 2006 and 42,000 were newly infected in 2009.[7,8] A majority of those infected are between the ages of 20 and 45, male, and disproportionately black. Recent estimates for cases of HIV infection diagnosed in the United States by age, race, and transmission category are shown in Table 18-1.[9] The overall prevalence (among persons older than 13 years of age) is 70.8 for black men who have sex with men (MSM) and 14.6 for white MSM per 100,000,[10] and the number of cases of HIV infection due to heterosexual transmission remains greater than 15,000 per year.[11]

The estimated number of AIDS diagnoses in the United States for 2009 was approximately 34,000. Adult and adolescent AIDS accounted for about 99% of the cases, 75% of which occurred in males and 25% in females. The cumulative estimated number of AIDS diagnoses through 2009 in the United States was 1.1 million.[7,11]

Since the introduction of protease inhibitors in 1996 and the advent of highly active antiretroviral therapy (HAART), the epidemic of AIDS in the United States has slowed and stabilized. Still, the CDC reports approximately 2250 new cases per month. As of the end of 2006, 565,927 deaths have been reported in the United States due to AIDS, and 14,627 deaths occurred in 2006 alone. Most deaths occur in adults, with few deaths reported in children younger than age 13 in 2006.[12] In the United States, AIDS is the leading cause of death in men 25 to 44 years of age. Worldwide, there are 2 million deaths per year, and more than 30 million persons have died of

BOX 18-1 AIDS-Defining Conditions

- Bacterial infections, multiple or recurrent*
- Candidiasis of bronchi, trachea, or lungs
- Candidiasis of esophagus†
- Cervical cancer, invasive§
- Coccidioidomycosis, disseminated or extrapulmonary
- Cryptococcosis, extrapulmonary
- Cryptosporidiosis, chronic intestinal (longer than 1 month in duration)
- Cytomegalovirus disease (other than liver, spleen, or nodes), onset at age >1 month
- Cytomegalovirus retinitis (with loss of vision)†
- Encephalopathy, HIV-related
- Herpes simplex: chronic ulcers (>1 month's duration) or bronchitis, pneumonitis, or esophagitis (onset at age >1 month)
- Histoplasmosis, disseminated or extrapulmonary
- Isosporiasis, chronic intestinal (>1 month's duration)
- Kaposi sarcoma†
- Lymphoid interstitial pneumonia or pulmonary lymphoid hyperplasia complex*†
- Lymphoma, Burkitt (or equivalent term)
- Lymphoma, immunoblastic (or equivalent term)
- Lymphoma, primary, of brain
- *Mycobacterium avium* complex or *Mycobacterium kansasii* infection, disseminated or extrapulmonary†
- *Mycobacterium tuberculosis* infection of any site, pulmonary,†§ disseminated,† or extrapulmonary†
- *Mycobacterium* infection, other species or unidentified species, disseminated† or extrapulmonary†
- *Pneumocystis jiroveci* pneumonia†
- Pneumonia, recurrent†§
- Progressive multifocal leukoencephalopathy
- *Salmonella* septicemia, recurrent
- Toxoplasmosis of brain, onset at age >1 month†
- Wasting syndrome attributed to HIV

*Only among children younger than 13 years of age. (Data from Centers for Disease Control and Prevention [CDC]: 1994 revised classification system for human immunodeficiency virus infection in children less than 13 years of age, *MMWR Recomm Rep* 43:1, 1994; Centers for Disease Control and Prevention [CDC]: 2008 revised surveillance case definitions for HIV infection among adults, adolescents, and children aged <18 months and for HIV infection and AIDS among children aged 18 months to <13 years—United States, *MMWR Recomm Rep* 57:9, 2008.)
†Condition that might be diagnosed presumptively.
§Only among adults and adolescents 13 years of age and older. (Data from Centers for Disease Control and Prevention [CDC]: 1993 Revised classification system for HIV infection and expanded surveillance case definition for AIDS among adolescents and adults, *MMWR Recomm Rep* 41: 1, 1993.)
AIDS, Acquired immunodeficiency syndrome.

AIDS.[13] AIDS is the world's leading cause of death in women and men aged 15 to 59 years.[2,13]

Several trends in the epidemiology of AIDS have emerged over the decades. In the United States, peak incidence was in 1993 and peak incidence of death was 50,877 in 1995. The past 2 decades witnessed a decline in the number of cases of AIDS associated with blood and blood products in transfusion and hemophiliac patient groups, specifically attributable to improved testing (starting in 1985) of donor blood for HIV antibodies and the heating of factor VIII replacement preparations. Also, an increase in the ratio of infected women to men occurred a decade ago; this ratio has remained stable in about 25% of women but is particularly higher in the 30- to 40-year age group of black women.[11]

At present there is no effective vaccine to prevent HIV infection, although large research efforts have and continue to be made in this arena. Also, a nonpandemic relating strain of HIV, known as HIV-2, occurs less commonly throughout the world. Most cases of HIV-2 infection have occurred in West Africa, with a limited number of cases occurring in Canada and the United States. Most persons infected with HIV-2 are long-term nonprogressors because viral loads generally are low, and the immunosuppression is not as severe.[14,15]

Etiology

AIDS is caused by HIV, a nontransforming retrovirus of the lentivirus family. There are two HIV subtypes, HIV-1 and HIV-2, and many strains of each. HIV-1 was first identified in 1983 by Francoise Barre-Sinoussi in the lab of Luc Montaignier of the Pasteur Institute. They first called it *lymphadenopathy-associated virus.* Within a year of this discovery, a team led by Robert Gallo from the National Institutes of Health isolated a retrovirus identified as the human T lymphotropic virus III (HTLV-III) and labeled it as the etiologic agent for AIDS. In 1984, Jay Levy's team in San Francisco also isolated a retrovirus, AIDS-related virus (ARV), and designated it as the causative agent for AIDS. All three viruses were similar retroviruses, but minor differences were observed in their amino acid sequences. Variation in disease patterns are attributed to the slight sequence differences among HIV strains, which also makes difficult the production of a vaccine. The three groups essentially were describing the same retrovirus, which can change its antigenicity. Until 1986, most workers in the field referred to the virus as HTLV-III and considered it to be the causative agent for AIDS. In 1986, the World Health Organization (WHO) recommended that the AIDS virus be called the *human immunodeficiency virus*[16-18] (Figure 18-1). Subsequent analysis of frozen tissue and serum samples from select patients who died of uncertain causes in the 1950s and 1960s demonstrated that HIV had infected these patients, indicating its presence in humans for more than 60 years.[19]

HIV is an enveloped RNA retrovirus about 100 nM in diameter. Glycoproteins (gp41 and gp120) stud the surface of the envelope and serve to bind to human cells (Figure 18-2). Internal to the envelope is a protein capsid (p24) that surrounds essential viral enzymes (protease, integrase, reverse transcriptase) and an RNA inner core. It infects most human cells. However, the cells most commonly infected are those with CD4+ receptors, including T helper lymphocytes (CD4+ cells) and macrophages.

TABLE 18-1 Select Patient Characteristics in HIV Infection and AIDS*

Patient Characteristic	Estimated No. of Cases		
	HIV Infection	**AIDS**	**AIDS: Cumulative Data**
Age (Years)			
Under 13	166	13	9448
13-19	2057	542	8535
20-29	12,188	5571	172,559
30-39	10,252	8936	448,724
40-49	10,384	11,155	319,617
50-59	5327	6174	111,352
60 and older	1636	1056	38,376
Race or Ethnicity			
American Indian/Alaska Native	189	155	3700
Asian	470	429	8324
Black	21,652	16,741	466,351
Hispanic/Latino	7347	6719	190,263
Native Hawaiian/other Pacific Islander	34	50	839
White	11,803	9467	426,102
Multiple races	516	686	12,726
Transmission Category			
Male-to-male sexual contact	23,846	17,005	529,908
Injection drug use	3932	4942	273,444
Male-to-male sexual contact and injection drug use	1131	1580	77,213
Heterosexual contact	12,860	10,393	198,820
Perinatal	131	12	8640
Other*	111	313	20,583

*U.S. 2009 data, including cases of hemophilia, blood transfusion, and risk not reported or not identified (adults, adolescents, and infants).
Data from Centers for Disease Control and Prevention: HIV/AIDS statistics and surveillance/basic statistics *(article online), http://www.cdc.gov/hiv/topics/surveillance/basic.htm?source=govdelivery#international; accessed on March 5, 2010.*

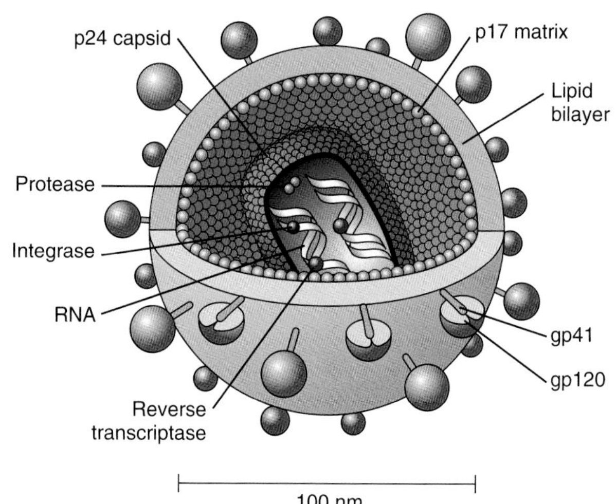

FIGURE 18-1 The structure of human immunodeficiency virus, showing the p24 capsid protein surrounding two strands of viral RNA. *(From Copstead LC, Banasik JL:* Pathophysiology, *ed 4, St. Louis, 2010, Saunders.)*

Accordingly, these cells are most deeply involved in HIV infection. Additional coreceptors that allow HIV to infect human cells include CCR5, CXCR4 (fusin), and CCR2.[20]

HIV-1 infection is divided into stages: *entry, reverse transcription* of RNA to DNA, export of the viral DNA from the cytoplasm to the nucleus and *integration* into the host chromosome, *transcription, translation* and cleavage of the polyproteins produced, *assembly* of virions, and *budding* of virions. The process is largely regulated by the proteins tat, rev, and nef, which are necessary for viral replication. Virulence has been mapped to the carboxyl-terminal half of the gp120, which has been referred to as the V_3 loop.[20] (For additional information see Chapter 182 in Fauci AS, et al., (editors): *Harrison's Principles of Internal Medicine*, ed 17, New York, 2008, McGraw Medical.)

Pathophysiology and Complications

Transmission of HIV is by exchange of infected bodily fluids from sexual contact and through blood and blood products. The most common method of sexual

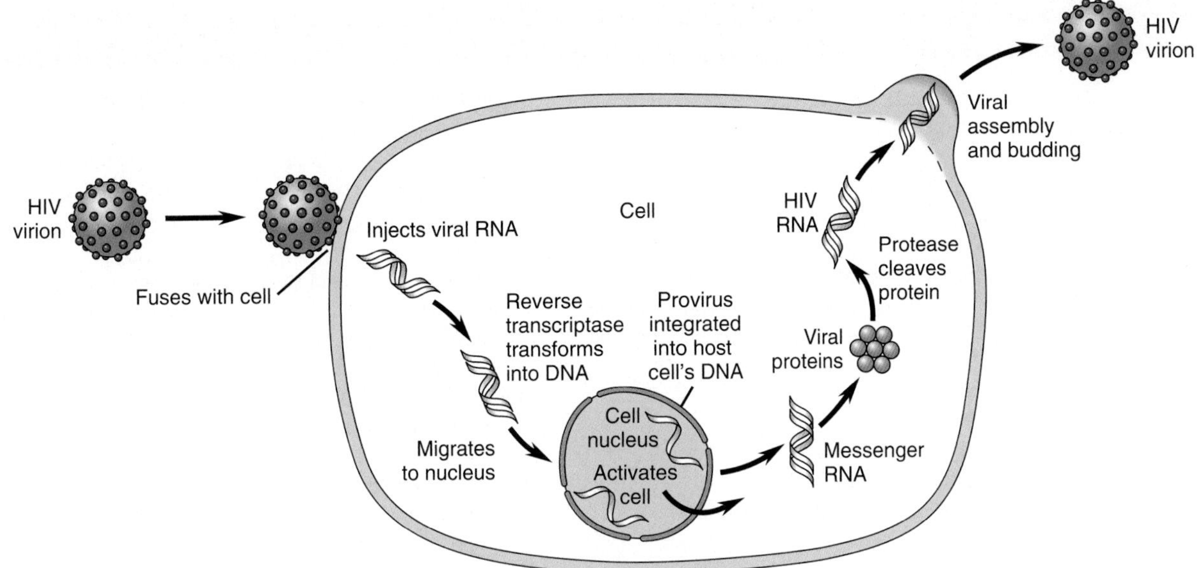

FIGURE 18-2 Life Cycle of the Human Immunodeficiency Virus. *(From Copstead LC, Banasik JL:* Pathophysiology, *ed 4, St. Louis, 2010, Saunders.)*

transmission in the United States is anal intercourse in MSM, in whom the risk of HIV infection is 40 times higher than in other men and in women.[21] Heterosexual transmission (male to female or female to male) is the second most common form of transmission in the United States but accounts for 80% of the world's HIV infections. Heterosexual transmission of HIV can occur through sexual contact of carriers who are heterosexual injection drug users, bisexual men, or blood recipients of either gender. Transmission from injection drug use is the third largest group to be affected in the United States.[22]

The virus is found in blood, seminal fluid, vaginal secretions, tears, breast milk, cerebrospinal fluid, amniotic fluid, and urine. Blood, semen, breast milk, and vaginal secretions are the main fluids that have been shown to be associated with transmission of the virus.

Vertical transmission to infants born of infected mothers can occur at birth or transplacentally. HIV has been found in saliva, and transmission by transfer of saliva possibly contaminated with blood has been reported from providing premasticated food from HIV-infected parents to infants.[23] Casual contact has not been demonstrated as a means of transmission. Inflammation and breaks in the skin or mucosa (e.g., presence of other sexually transmitted diseases) and high concentrations of HIV in bodily fluids increase the risk of transmission.[24-26] Oral sex is an inefficient but documented mode of transmission.[27] The risk of transmission from a blood transfusion is estimated to be less than 1 in 1 million because of current screening measures. Occupational exposure also is a source of transmission and health care provider to patient transmission has occurred (see later under "Dental Management").

Once HIV has gained access to the bloodstream, the virus selectively seeks out T lymphocytes (specifically T4 or T helper lymphocytes) (see Figure 18-2). The virus binds to the CD4+ lymphocyte cell surface specifically through the highly glycosylated outer surface envelope (gp120) proteins. Upon infection, reverse transcriptase catalyzes the synthesis of a haploid, double-stranded DNA provirus, which becomes incorporated into the chromosomal DNA of the host cell. Thus integrated, the provirus genetic material may remain latent in an unexpressed form until events occur that activate it, at which time DNA transcription rapidly occurs and new virions are produced. The virus is lymphotropic; hence, the cells it selects for replication are soon destroyed. Once the virus takes hold, it causes a reduction in the total number of T helper cells, and a marked shift in the ratio of CD4+ to CD8+ lymphocytes occurs. The normal ratio of T helper to T suppressor lymphocytes is about 2:1 (60% T helper, 30% T suppressor). In AIDS, the T4/T8 ratio is reversed. This marked reduction in T helper lymphocytes, to a great degree, explains the lack of an effective immune response seen in patients with AIDS and contributes to the increase in malignant disease that has been found to be associated with AIDS, including Kaposi sarcoma, lymphoma, carcinoma of the cervix, and carcinoma of the rectum.[20]

Table 18-2 presents the clinical stages of HIV infection through frank AIDS. More than 50% of persons exposed to the virus develop an acute and brief viremia (seroconversion sickness) within 2 to 6 weeks of HIV exposure and then develop antibodies (anti-gag, anti-gp120, anti-p24) between weeks 6 and 12. A few may take 6 months or longer to achieve seroconversion. A concomitant, transient fall in CD4+ cells occurs

TABLE 18-2 Features of HIV Infection and Disease Progression

Status	Signs/Symptoms	Laboratory Findings	Comments
Recent infection	No signs or symptoms	HIV nucleic acid: positive p24 antigen; positive DNA PCR assay; ELISA and Western blot may or may not be positive.	Patient is unaware of his or her HIV infection. Can transmit the infection by blood or sexual activity.
Stage 1 *Acute seroconversion syndrome*	Symptoms occur within about 1-3 weeks after infection in about 70% of infected patients: Fever, weakness, diarrhea, nausea, vomiting, myalgia, headache Weight loss Pharyngitis Skin rashes (roseola-like or urticarial) Lymphadenopathy Symptoms clear in about 1 to 2 wk	HIV antibody–negative at start of syndrome. Seroconversion occurs near end of the syndrome. CD4+ and CD8+ lymphocytes reduced in numbers, but >500 cells/μL After acute symptoms, they tend to return toward normal levels. ELISA and Western blot are positive.	The severity of the acute syndrome varies among infected persons. The period for seroconversion of 30% of patients without acute symptoms varies and can be 1-6 months or longer.
Stage 2 *Latent period (asymptomatic stage)*	Median time from initial infection to onset of clinical symptoms: 8-10 years About 50-70% of patients develop persistent generalized lymphadenopathy (PGL).	ELISA and Western blot are positive. A slow but usually steady increase in viral load. Usually, a steady decline in CD4+ cell count; CD4+/CD8+ ratio begins to approach 1.	Viral replication is ongoing and progressive. A steady decline in CD4+ cell counts occurs, except in the less than 1% who are nonprogressors (also have low viral load).
Stage 2 *(Early symptomatic stage)*	Without treatment, lasts for 1 to 3 years. Any of the following: PGL Fungal infections Vaginal yeast and trichomonal infections Oral hairy leukoplakia Herpes zoster Herpes simplex HIV retinopathy Constitutional symptoms: fever, night sweats, fatigue diarrhea, weight loss, weakness	ELISA and Western blot are positive. HIV antigen, RNA, and DNA tests are positive. Signs and symptoms increase as CD4+ cell count declines and approaches 200/μL; often between 200 and 300/μL. Viral load continues to increase. Platelet count may decrease in about 10% of patients.	The spectrum of disease changes as CD4+ cell count declines.
Stage 3 *(AIDS)*	Opportunistic infection(s): *Pneumocystis jiroveci* pneumonia Cryptococcosis Tuberculosis Toxoplasmosis Histoplasmosis Others Malignancies: Kaposi sarcoma Burkitt's lymphoma Non-Hodgkin's lymphoma Primary CNS lymphoma Invasive cervical cancer, carcinoma of rectum Slim (wasting) disease	High viral load. CD4+ cell count below 200/ μL. CD4+ cell count below 50/μL at high risk for lymphoma and death. Platelet count may be low. Neutrophil count may be low. ELISA and Western blot are positive. HIV antigen, RNA, and DNA tests are positive.	Death usually occurs because of wasting, opportunistic infection, or malignancies. The use of combination antiretroviral agents has slowed the death rate, but long-term outlook must depend on vaccines for prevention and treatment because the virus promotes resistance to these agents.

AIDS, Acquired immunodeficiency syndrome; *CNS,* Central nervous system; *ELISA,* Enzyme-linked immunosorbent assay; *HIV,* Human immunodeficiency virus; *PCR,* Polymerase chain reaction.

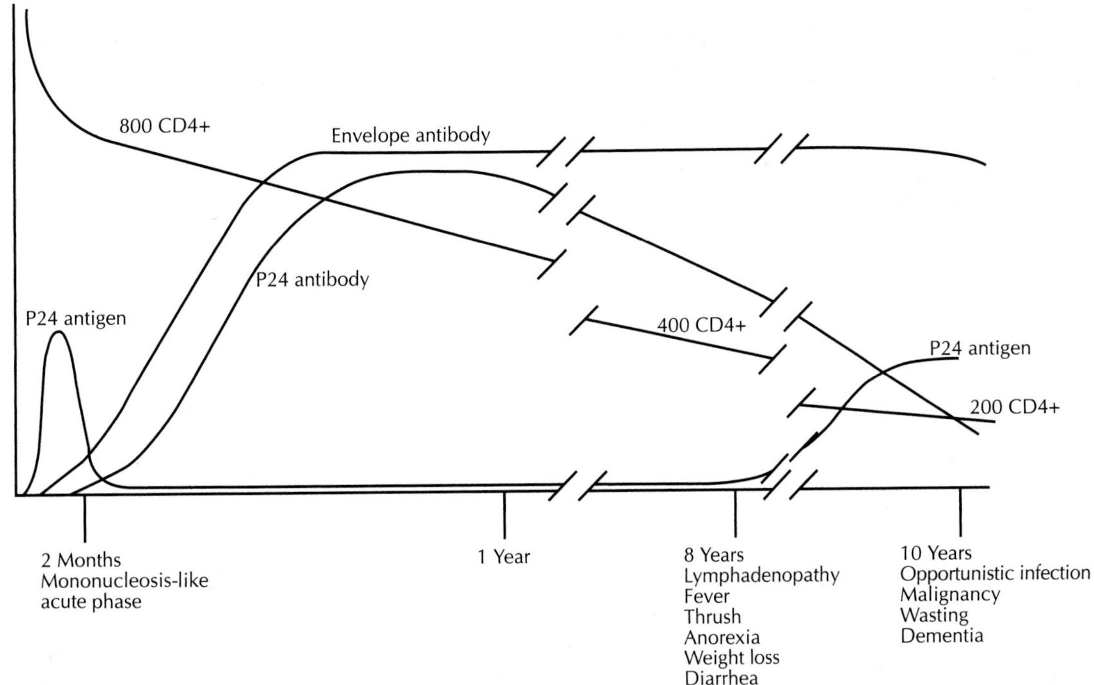

FIGURE 18-3 The natural history of human immunodeficiency virus infection. *(From Brookmeyer R, Gail MH: AIDS epidemiology: a quantitative approach, New York, 1994, Oxford University Press.)*

(lymphopenia, along with high titers of plasma HIV), but patients do not develop evidence of immunosuppression. Various flulike symptoms occur during this acute infection, which usually lasts about 2 to 4 weeks. Only an estimated 20% of affected persons seek medical attention. During primary infection, HIV disseminates throughout the lymphoid tissue, incubates and replicates. These events allow HIV to establish a chronic infection and reservoirs of latently infected cells.

As time progresses, a steady-state viremia develops, and several thousand copies of HIV are present in the blood (Figure 18-3). This clinical latency period is characterized by evolution of the virus within its host to generate closely related, yet distinct mutant viruses that serve to evade the surveying immune response and circulating antibodies. Although the infection is clinically latent, there is a progressive decline in immune function evident as progressive depletion of CD4+ lymphocytes with ultimate pancytopenia, impaired lymphocyte proliferation, and cytokine responses to mitogens and antigens; impaired cytotoxic lymphocyte function and natural killer cell activity; anergy to skin testing; and diminished antibody responses to new antigens.[20]

In untreated persons and in persons in whom therapy is ineffective, the CD4+ count continues to decline while HIV proliferates. As the CD4+ count drops and approaches 200 cells/µL, persons can exhibit weight loss, diarrhea, and night sweats (see Figure 18-3). When the CD4+ count drops to below 200 cells/µL, the person has AIDS and is susceptible to opportunistic infections, including *Pneumocystis* pneumonia, toxoplasmosis, cryptococcosis, influenza, histoplasmosis, tuberculosis, cytomegalovirus (CMV) infection, mucocutaneous diseases such as candidiasis, and neoplasms previously discussed. Neurologic disease is common and includes secondary opportunistic infections as well as primary HIV infection of macrophages, neurons, and microglial cells in the CNS that leads to rapidly progressive dementia.

Evidence suggests that persons most susceptible to developing AIDS are those with repeated exposure to the virus who also have an immune system that has been challenged by repeated exposure to various antigens (semen, hepatitis B, or blood products).[20] The median time from primary infection to the development of AIDS in untreated patients is about 10 years. About 30% of patients with AIDS can be expected to live approximately 2 to 3 years, with most others living 10 years or longer. Long-term survival with HIV infection (beyond 15 years) occurs and is associated with less virulent HIV strains, lower-level viremia, HAART, and robust immune responses.[28]

CLINICAL PRESENTATION

Signs and Symptoms

During the first 2 to 6 weeks after initial infection with HIV, more than 50% of patients develop an acute flulike syndrome marked by viremia that may last 10 to 14 days. Others may not manifest this symptom complex.

BOX 18-2 CDC Staging of HIV Infection in Adults and Adolescents

Stage 1: Laboratory confirmation of HIV infection, no AIDS-defining conditions *and* CD4+ T lymphocyte count of ≥500 cells/μL or CD4+ T lymphocyte percentage of total lymphocytes of ≥29.

Stage 2: Laboratory confirmation of HIV infection, no AIDS-defining condition, and laboratory confirmation of HIV infection *and* CD4+ T lymphocyte count of 200-499 cells/μL *or* CD4+ T lymphocyte percentage of total lymphocytes of 14-28.

Stage 3 (AIDS): Laboratory confirmation of HIV infection *and* CD4+ T lymphocyte count is <200 cells/μL or CD4+ T lymphocyte percentage of total lymphocytes is <14 or documentation of an AIDS-defining condition (see Box 18-1). Documentation of an AIDS-defining condition supersedes a CD4+ T lymphocyte count of ≥200 cells/μL and a CD4+ T lymphocyte percentage of total lymphocytes of ≥14.

CDC, Centers for Disease Control and Prevention; *HIV,* Human immunodeficiency virus; *AIDS,* Acquired immunodeficiency syndrome.

Symptomatic persons often develop lymphadenopathy, fever, pharyngitis and a skin rash but generally do not display circulation antibodies until the 6th week to 6th month. The severity of the initial acute infection with HIV (i.e., level of viremia) is predictive of the course the infection will follow. In one study, 78% of persons with a long-lasting acute illness developed AIDS within 3 years; by contrast, only 10% of those patients with no acute illness at seroconversion developed AIDS within 3 years.[29]

The CDC defines three stages of HIV infection.[4] Box 18-2 illustrates the definitions for each stage. Briefly, stage 1 generally begins immediately after HIV exposure and may last for years. Affected persons are HIV antibody–positive but are asymptomatic and show no other laboratory abnormalities. Stage 2 is characterized by progressive immunosuppression and symptomatic disease. Patients who demonstrate various laboratory changes (i.e., lymphopenia: T helper/T suppressor ratio usually less than 1) in addition to HIV antibody positivity also may show clinical signs or symptoms, such as enlarged lymph nodes, night sweats, weight loss, oral candidiasis, fever, malaise, and diarrhea. Persons in stage 3 have AIDS and can demonstrate a variety of immunesuppression-related diseases. Opportunistic infections predominate as the CD4+ T count approximates 200 cells/μL; then malignancies, wasting syndrome, and a progressive form of dementia can develop. Patients may become confused and disoriented or may experience short-term memory deficits. Others develop severe depression or paranoia and show suicidal tendencies. Figure 18-3 depicts the natural history of HIV, and Table 18-2 lists the diseases associated with the progression of HIV infection through frank AIDS.

Laboratory Findings

Most patients exposed to the virus, with or without clinical evidence of disease, show antibodies to the virus by the 6th month of infection. Patients with advanced HIV infection or AIDS have an altered ratio of CD4+/CD8+ lymphocytes, a decrease in total number of lymphocytes, thrombocytopenia, anemia, a slight alteration in the humoral antibody system, and a decreased ability to show delayed allergic reactions to skin testing (cutaneous anergy).[20] CD4+ and CD8+ cell counts should be performed at the time of HIV diagnosis and then every 3 to 4 months.[2]

The enzyme-linked immunosorbent assay (ELISA) is the screening test for identification of antibodies to HIV. It is 90% sensitive but has a high rate of false-positive results. Current practice is to screen first with ELISA. If the results are positive, a second ELISA is performed. All positive results are then confirmed with Western blot analysis. This combination of tests is accurate more than 99% of the time. Positive ELISA and Western blot test results indicate only that the individual has been exposed to the AIDS virus. If results of the Western blot are indeterminate, HIV infection is rarely, if ever, present. These tests, however, do not indicate the status of the HIV infection or whether AIDS is present. However, patients with positive results on the ELISA and Western blot test are considered potentially infectious. ELISA testing for HIV in saliva is an alternative approach that is 98% sensitive in detecting antibodies to HIV.[30] More recently, Abbott has developed a combination assay, the ARCHITECT HIV Ag/Ab Combo assay (Abbott Laboratories, Abbott Park, Illinois), that can simultaneously detect the combined presence of HIV antigens (the p24 antigen produced by HIV) and antibodies to HIV. This recently FDA approved test is expected to be important for diagnosing HIV infection in the acute phase of the disease when antibodies are not yet present and for ongoing monitoring of patients.[31]

Nucleic acid amplification using polymerase chain reaction (PCR)-based assays of the viral RNA is performed to determine the viral load in the blood (i.e., degree of viremia) and monitor response to therapy. Detection ranges are from 40 copies/mL to more than 750,000 copies/mL. The greatest viral load is found during the first 3 months after initial infection and during late stages of the disease. Direct detection of HIV by PCR assay is superior to testing for HIV antigen in serum, but more expensive.[32] Antiviral resistance testing is recommended when treatment is failing.[33]

MEDICAL MANAGEMENT

Medical management of the HIV-infected patient has four main treatment goals: (1) to reduce HIV-associated morbidity and prolong the duration and quality of survival, (2) to restore and preserve immunologic function, (3) to maximally and durably suppress plasma HIV viral load, and (4) to prevent HIV transmission.[33] The physician managing these patients should be an expert in infectious disease and in the use of antiretroviral drugs. Antiretroviral therapy (ART) should be used in a manner that will achieve viral suppression and immune reconstitution while at the same time preventing emergence of resistance and limiting drug toxicity. Long-term goals are to delay disease progression, prolong life, and improve quality of life. Treatment often is organized into three major areas: (1) ART, (2) prophylaxis for opportunistic infections, and (3) treatment of HIV-related complications. Monitoring response to therapy is a long-term requirement, as more than 70% of HIV infected persons survive beyond 10 years from the time of diagnosis in the United States, especially if treatment is not delayed.[12,34]

ART and HAART

Over the past decade, much progress has been made in the treatment of AIDS because of ART and HAART. Both ART and HAART involve use of combinations of antiretroviral drugs; however strictly speaking, HAART is defined as the use of at least three active antiretroviral medications. Today the terms *ART* and *HAART* are essentially equivalent.

The benefits of ART are now well known. ART increases survival, reduces systemic complications, and improves the quality of life in patients infected with HIV.[2] The major goal of ART is to inhibit HIV replication completely such that the viral load is below the detection limit of the assay at 4 to 6 months. However, there are no conclusive studies that show when therapy should be initiated. Experts recommend starting treatment in all patients with symptoms ascribed to HIV infection, all pregnant mothers infected with HIV, and all HIV-infected infants. ART currently is recommended when the CD4+ count is less than 350 cells/μL and in those with plasma HIV RNA levels greater than 55,000 copies/mL.[33] Treatment is generally initiated for asymptomatic patients who have a rapid drop in CD4+ T cell count or high viral loads. Asymptomatic patients with stable CD4+ T cell counts and low viral loads are generally followed without treatment. ART is strongly recommended for patients with CD4+ T cell counts lower than 200/μL and for those with AIDS.[20,33]

Antiretroviral drugs are used to restore immune dysfunction by inhibiting viral replication. More than 20 antiretroviral drugs are currently available for the management of HIV infection/AIDS (Table 18-3). The antiretroviral agents available are classified into five categories: protease inhibitors (PIs), nucleoside reverse transcriptase inhibitors (NRTIs), non-nucleoside reverse transcriptase inhibitors (NNRTIs), nucleotides, and entry inhibitors. These agents usually are used in combinations known as ART or HAART and should be given long-term.

The drug regimen that is initiated should be individualized to be potent enough to suppress the viral load to below the level of assay detection for a prolonged period, while reducing the virus mutation rates that can lead to drug resistance. Currently, preferred regimens for the ART-naive patient consist of either efavirenz + tenofovir + emtricitabine or ritonavir-boosted atazanavir/darunavir plus tenofovir/emtricitabine, or raltegravir + tenofovir + emtricitabine. Several alternative drug regimens also appear in recent Department of Health and Human Services guidelines; however, no regimen has proved superior to efavirenz-based regimens with respect to virologic responses.[33] Patients who respond to therapy generally show an increase in CD4+ count in the range of 50 to 150 cells/μL per year and viral loads of less than 75 copies/mL.[33] Virologic suppression is defined as less than 48 copies/mL, and virologic failure is defined as a confirmed viral load of greater than 200 copies/mL in the presence of ART.[33]

Patients who are on ART medications must be closely monitored for drug effectiveness (which often wanes over time), development of antiviral resistance, drug toxicity, and drug interactions. Some important toxicities include hyperlactemia, mitochondrial dysfunction, peripheral neuropathy, hepatotoxicity, and lipodystrophy. Compliance also is a major challenge for patients in view of recognized drug toxicities, costs, and inconvenience.[35] To this end, several drugs are now formulated as combination agents to simplify and improve treatment of the disease. *Atripla, Epzicom,* and *Trizivir* are combinations of three antiretrovirals, and *Combivir, Epzicom, Trizivir,* and *Truvada* are combinations of two nucleoside–nucleotide reverse transcriptase inhibitors. Only a decade ago, when cocktails of AIDS drugs began to be used, patients sometimes had to take two dozen or more pills a day. Currently, immune modulators also are being tested in conjunction with ART.

In about 25% of patients, particularly those with a very low CD4+ T cell count, weeks after initiation of ART, an exacerbation of preexisting opportunistic infections occurs.[36] This condition, known as *immune reconstitution inflammatory syndrome* (IRIS), probably results from elicitation of an inflammatory response in association with the antiviral drugs, leading to focal lymphadenitis and reactivation of a viral disease (e.g., shingles) or granulomatous infection.[20]

Chemoprophylaxis. Chemoprophylaxis regimens are recommended when CD4+ lymphocyte counts drop to specific levels to prevent initial episode of a disease or to suppress a developing opportunistic infection. These regimens exist for the prevention of *Pneumocystis* pneumonia, tuberculosis, toxoplasmosis, and other opportunistic diseases. Also, select vaccines are recommended for the HIV-infected adult before the CD4+ T cell count drops to below 200/μL. Standard resources such as the

TABLE 18-3 Antiretroviral Drugs Used to Treat HIV Infection

Drug	Toxicity	Interactions	Comments
Protease Inhibitors (PIs)			
Amprenavir	Nausea, vomiting	Amiodarone	PIs act at the end of the virus replication cycle, blocking the catalytic center of the protease enzyme, resulting in viral particles that are ineffective and immature.
Atazanavir	Nausea, vomiting, liver, tingling arms/legs	Midazolam, triazolam	
Darunavir	Nausea, diarrhea, lipodystrophy	Midazolam, triazolam, quinidine	
Fosamprenavir	Nausea, vomiting	Midazolam, triazolam	
Indinavir	Diarrhea	Quinidine	
Lopinavir*	Abdominal discomfort	Rifampin	
Nelfinavir	Paresthesias	Ergotamine	
Ritonavir*	Fatigue	St. John's wort	
Saquinavir	Anemia, leukopenia	Midazolam	
	Thrombocytopenia	Triazolam	
	Altered taste		
	Hypercholesterolemia		
	Hypertriglyceridemia		
	Xerostomia		
Tipranavir	Nausea, vomiting, diarrhea, liver damage	Midazolam, triazolam, quinidine	
Nucleoside Reverse Transcriptase Inhibitors (NRTIs)			
Abacavir**	Headache	Avoid mixing zidovudine and stavudine, ribavirin, or doxorubicin.	Drug adverse effects often are dose-related and can be minimized with lower doses. Use of zalcitabine is restricted because of the small therapeutic window. Stavudine is the most frequently used drug in the group.
Emtricitabine	Insomnia	Ganciclovir and interferon-α must be avoided.	
Didanosine	Fatigue		
Lamivudine**	Anemia, neutropenia		
Stavudine	Nausea		
Zalcitabine	Diarrhea		
Zidovudine**	Neuropathy		
	Pancreatitis		
	Myopathy		
	Xerostomia		
Non-Nucleoside Reverse Transcriptase Inhibitors (NNRTIs)			
Delavirdine	Dizziness, insomnia, dyslipidemia	Midazolam	The most important negative adverse effects are neuropsychiatric events, skin reactions, GI alterations, and liver alterations.
Efavirenz	Confusion, agitation	Triazolam	
Etravirine	Rash, nausea	Clarithromycin	
Nevirapine	Hallucinations	Clarithromycin (rash, <drug concentration)	
	Depression, mania		
	Skin rashes	Sertraline (<drug concentration)	
	Nausea, vomiting		
	Diarrhea	Warfarin (>drug effect)	
	Stevens-Johnson syndrome	Ketoconazole (<drug concentration)	
	Xerostomia, taste alteration		
Nucleotides			
Adefovir	Dizziness	NSAIDs, acyclovir, and ganciclovir affect the metabolism of tenofovir.	Adefovir is not used often because of GI and renal toxicity. Tenofovir is used in patients on multiple-drug therapy who are not responding. Tenofovir usually is well tolerated.
Tenofovir	Nausea, diarrhea	Vancomycin, NSAIDs, and cyclosporine increase risk for kidney disease.	
	Weakness		
	Depression, anxiety		
	Skin rash—allergy		
	Neuropathy		
	Liver, kidney failure		
	Lactic acidosis (rapid breathing, drowsiness, muscle aches)		

TABLE 18-3 Antiretroviral Drugs Used to Treat HIV Infection—cont'd

Drug	Toxicity	Interactions	Comments
Entry Inhibitors			
Enfuvirtide	Bacterial pneumonia Rash, fever Nausea, vomiting Glomerulonephritis Guillain-Barré syndrome Taste disturbance Hyperglycemia Myalgia Xerostomia Anorexia	No significant drug interactions	Inhibits fusion of HIV-1 and CD4+ T cells. Only one fusion inhibitor has been approved (enfuvirtide), and it has to be injected. Three other entry inhibitors are available.
Maraviroc	Liver	None	
Immune-Based Therapies§			
Chloroquinine, hydroxychloroquine	Stomach upset, muscle weakness, retinopathy	Gold salts	These drugs reduce cellular activation thus reducing HIV replication and boost the immune response. Several others are in testing.
Interleukin-2	Fever, chills, nausea, vomiting	Pain medications, steroids	
Interleukin-7	Transient elevations of liver function tests	None yet reported.	

Agents are grouped by drug class.
*Available in combination as Kaletra.
**Available in combination as Combivir, Epzicom, Trizivir, and Truvada.
ART, Antiretroviral therapy; *GI,* Gastrointestinal; *HIV,* Human immunodeficiency virus; *NSAIDs,* Nonsteroidal antiinflammatory drugs; *VL,* Viral load.
§Although not ART drugs, immune-based therapies also are being used in the management of HIV infection.
ART is associated with many drug interactions, only a few are listed. For more detailed recommendations, see guidelines at http://aidsinfo.nih.gov/guidelines.

National Institutes of Health AIDS information Web site (http://www.aids.info.nih.gov) are available for more information on this topic.

Hope exists for improving outcomes with HIV infection. Vaccine development is ongoing,[37] and stem cell transplantation with CCR5-deficient cells has led to reduction of the HIV viral reservoir in one patient and may prove effective in eradicating HIV in the clinical setting.[38]

DENTAL MANAGEMENT

Health history, head and neck examination, intraoral soft tissue examination, and complete periodontal and dental examinations should be performed on all new patients. History and clinical findings may indicate that the patient has HIV infection/AIDS. Of note, however, patients who know they are seropositive and those at high risk for these conditions may not answer questions honestly, on account of the stigma or concern for privacy. Accordingly, the patient history should be obtained whenever possible with this understanding, verbal communication in a quiet, private location, and the sharing of knowledge and facts in an atmosphere of honesty and openness.

Patients who, on the basis of history or clinical findings, are found to be at high risk for AIDS or related conditions should be referred for HIV testing, and medical evaluation. The dentist can undertake diagnostic laboratory screening using saliva (Oraquick Advance; OraSure Technologies, Inc., Bethlehem, Pennsylvania),[39] or serum testing can be done with a referral to a medical facility. Discussions with the patient should emphasize importance of testing and should ascertain risk factors including sexual habits, intravenous drug use, and so forth. Patients with high-risk factors should be strongly encouraged to seek diagnostic testing.

Patients at high risk for AIDS and those in whom AIDS or HIV has been diagnosed should be treated in a manner identical to that for any other patient—that is, with standard precautions. Several guidelines have emerged regarding the rights of dentists and patients with AIDS, including the following:

- Dental treatment may not be withheld if the patient refuses to undergo testing for HIV exposure. The dentist may then assume that the patient is a potential carrier of HIV and should treat the person using standard precautions, just as for any other patient.
- A patient with AIDS who needs emergency dental treatment may not be refused care simply because the dentist does not want to treat patients with AIDS.
- No medical or scientific reason exists to justify why patients with AIDS who seek routine dental care may

be declined treatment by the dentist, regardless of the practitioner's personal reason. However, if the dentist and the patient agree, the dentist may refer this patient to another provider who is more willing or better suited (in keeping with the patient's oral health status) to provide treatment.

- A patient who has been under the care of a dentist and then develops AIDS or a related condition must be treated by that dentist or receive a referral that is satisfactory for and agreed to by the patient.
- The CDC and the American Dental Association recommend that infected dentists inform the patient of their HIV serostatus and should receive consent or refrain from performing invasive procedures.[40]

Treatment Planning Considerations

A major consideration in dental treatment of the patient with HIV infection/AIDS involves determining the current CD4+ lymphocyte count and level of immunosuppression of the patient. Another point of emphasis in dental treatment planning is the level of viral load, which may be related to susceptibility to opportunistic infections and rate of progression of AIDS. The dentist should be knowledgeable about the presence and status of opportunistic infections and the medications that the patient may be taking for therapy or prophylaxis for such conditions. Patients who have been exposed to the AIDS virus and are HIV-seropositive but asymptomatic may receive all indicated dental treatment. Generally, this is true for patients with a CD4+ cell count of more than 350/μL. Patients who are symptomatic for the early stages of AIDS (i.e., CD4+ cell count lower than 200) have increased susceptibility to opportunistic infection and may be medicated with prophylactic drugs.[33]

The patient with AIDS can receive almost any dental care needed and desired once the possibility of significant immunosuppression, neutropenia, or thrombocytopenia has been ruled out. Complex treatment plans should not be undertaken before an honest and open discussion about the long-term prognosis of the patient's medical condition has occurred.

Dental treatment of the HIV-infected patient without symptoms is no different from that provided for any other patient in the practice.[41] Standard precautions must be used for *all* patients. Any oral lesions found should be diagnosed, then managed by appropriate local and systemic treatment or referred for diagnosis and treatment. Patients with lesions suggestive of HIV infection must be evaluated for possible HIV.

In planning invasive dental procedures, attention must be paid to the prevention of infection and excessive bleeding in patients with severe immunosuppression, neutropenia, and thrombocytopenia. This may involve the use of prophylactic antibiotics in patients with CD4+ cell counts below 200/μL and/or severe neutropenia (neutrophil count lower than 500/μL).[42] White blood cell and differential counts, as well as a platelet count, should be ordered before any surgical procedure is undertaken. Patients with severe thrombocytopenia may require special measures (platelet replacement) before surgical procedures (including scaling and curettage) are performed. Medical consultation should precede any dental treatment for patients with these abnormalities.

Patients may be medicated with drugs that are prophylactic for *Pneumocystis* pneumonia, candidiasis, herpes simplex virus (HSV) or CMV infection, or other opportunistic disease, and these medications must be carefully considered in dental treatment planning. Care in prescribing other medications must be exercised with these, or any, medications after which the patient may experience adverse drug effects, including allergic reactions, toxic drug reactions, hepatotoxicity, immunosuppression, anemia, serious drug interactions, and other potential problems. Most often, consultation with the patient's physician is beneficial.[42] For example, acetaminophen should be used with caution in patients treated with zidovudine (Retrovir) because studies have suggested that granulocytopenia and anemia, associated with zidovudine, may be intensified; also, aspirin should not be given to patients with thrombocytopenia. Meperidine should be avoided in patients taking ritonavir, because ritonavir increases the metabolism of meperidine to normeperidine which is associated with adverse effects such as lethargy, agitation, and seizures. Propoxyphene levels may be increased by ritonavir which may potentially lead to toxic effects such as drowsiness, slurred speech, or incoordination. Antacids, phenytoin, cimetidine, and rifampin should not be given to patients who are being treated with ketoconazole, because of the possibility of altered absorption and metabolism. Also, midazolam and triazolam should be avoided in patients taking select protease inhibitors, because benzodiazepine metabolism may be inhibited, leading to excessive sedation and/or respiratory depression.[42]

Medical consultation is necessary for symptomatic HIV-infected patients before surgical procedures are performed. Current platelet count and white blood cell count should be available. Patients with abnormal test results may require special management. All these matters must be discussed in detail with the patient's physician. Any source of oral or dental infection should be eliminated in HIV-infected patients, who often require more frequent recall appointments for maintenance of periodontal health. Daily use of chlorhexidine mouth rinse may be helpful.[43]

In patients with periodontal disease whose general health status is not clear, periodontal scaling for several teeth can be provided to allow assessment of tissue response and bleeding. If no problems are noted, the rest of the mouth can be treated.[43] Adjunctive antibacterial measures may be required if the patient's CD4+ cell count is below 200/μL or if tissues remain unresponsive to routine therapy. Root canal therapy has good success in patients with HIV infection, and no modifications are required.[44] Infection can be treated through local and systemic measures.

Occupational Exposure to HIV

The risk of HIV transmission from infected patients to health care workers is very low, reportedly about 3 of every 1000 cases (0.3%) in which a needlestick or other sharp instrument transmitted blood from a patient to a health care worker.[35] In comparison, the risk of infection from a needlestick is 3% for hepatitis C and is 30% for hepatitis B.

After a needlestick, the rate of transmission of HIV can be reduced by postexposure prophylaxis (PEP).[45] The CDC recommends PEP as soon as possible after exposure to HIV-infected blood.[45] The number of PEP drugs recommended is based on the severity of the exposure as well as the HIV status of the source-patient.[46] A *less severe exposure* (solid needle or superficial injury) from a source-patient who is asymptomatic or has a low viral load (<1500 viral copies/mL) has a two-drug PEP. Use of at least a three-drug PEP regimen is recommended for *more severe exposure* (large-bore hollow needle, deep puncture, visible blood on device or needle used in patient's artery or vein) or when the patient is symptomatic, has AIDS, or a high viral load. The recommended *basic* regimen for HIV PEP is tenofovir plus emtricitabine or zidovudine plus lamivudine. The *expanded* regimen includes a standard two-drug regimen plus a protease inhibitor such as ritonavir-boosted (/r) lopinavir, darunavir/r, atazanavir/r, or raltegravir. PEP should be continued for 4 weeks, during which time the exposed clinician should be provided expert consultation, and follow-up monitoring for compliance, adverse events, and possible seroconversion. Tests for seroconversion should be performed at 3, 6, and 12 months. To date, there have been six reports of occupational HIV seroconversion despite combination PEP.[45]

If the exposed dental health care worker is pregnant, risk of infection versus unknown yet possible risks of PEP to the fetus, should be discussed.

Risk of Transmission From Health Care Personnel

In 1990, an HIV-infected Florida dentist transmitted, in some undetermined way, HIV infection to six of his patients. All of these patients are now deceased.[47] The only other report of HIV transmission involving dentistry came from Bucaramanga, Colombia, in 1997, where 14 cases of HIV infection occurred among hemodialysis patients at a university hospital. Transmission of the virus appeared to occur through contaminated dental instruments.[48] The risk of transmission in the dental setting is minimized by adherence to standard infection control procedures.[49]

Oral Complications and Manifestations

Oral lesions can be one of the early signs of HIV infection and risk for progression to AIDS. For these reasons, the clinician should be cognizant of the oral manifestations of HIV infection. Common oral manifestations include candidiasis of the oral mucosa (Figures 18-4 to 18-7), bluish purple or red lesion(s) that on biopsy are identified as Kaposi sarcoma (Figures 18-8 to 18-11), and hairy leukoplakia of the lateral borders of the tongue (Figure 18-12). Other oral conditions that occur in association with HIV infection are HSV, herpes zoster, recurrent aphthous ulcerations, linear gingival erythema (Figure 18-13), necrotizing ulcerative periodontitis (Figure 18-14), and necrotizing stomatitis, oral warts (Figure 18-15), facial

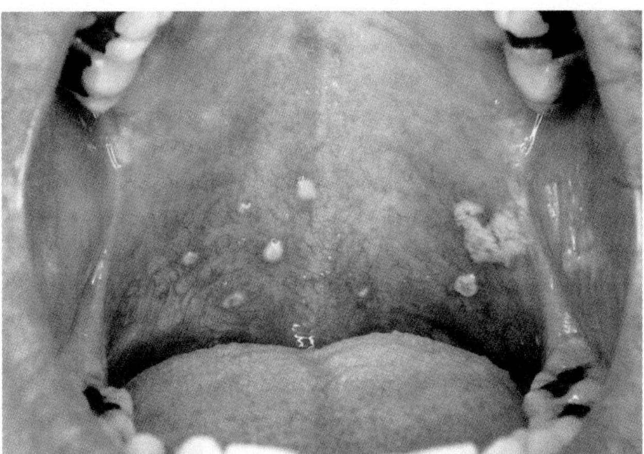

FIGURE 18-4 White lesions on the palate in a patient with AIDS. The lesions could be scraped off with a tongue blade. The underlying mucosa was erythematous. Clinical and cytologic findings supported the diagnosis of pseudomembranous candidiasis. *(From Silverman S Jr: Color atlas of oral manifestations of AIDS, ed 2, St. Louis, 1996, Mosby.)*

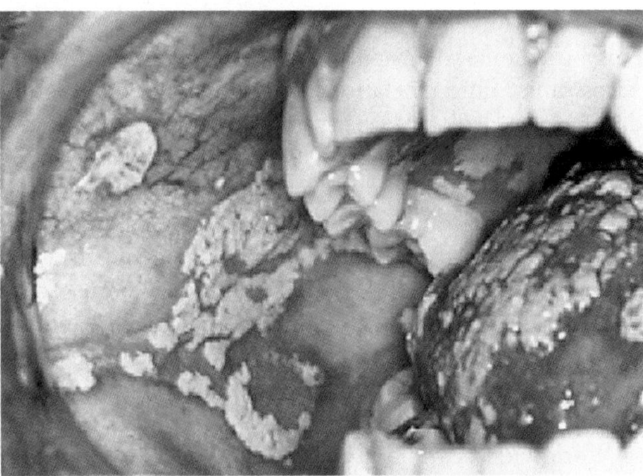

FIGURE 18-5 Note the white lesions on the oral mucosa. The diagnosis of pseudomembranous candidiasis was established. *(Courtesy Eric Haus, Chicago, Illinois.)*

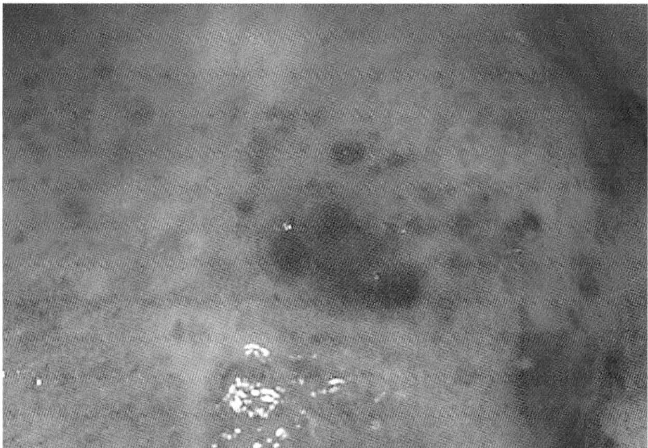

FIGURE 18-6 Erythematous palatal lesion in a human immunodeficiency virus antibody–positive patient. Smears taken from the lesion showed hyphae and spores consistent with *Candida*. The lesion healed after a 2-week course of antifungal medications. A diagnosis of erythematous candidiasis was made on the basis of clinical laboratory findings. *(Courtesy Eric Haus, Chicago, Illinois.)*

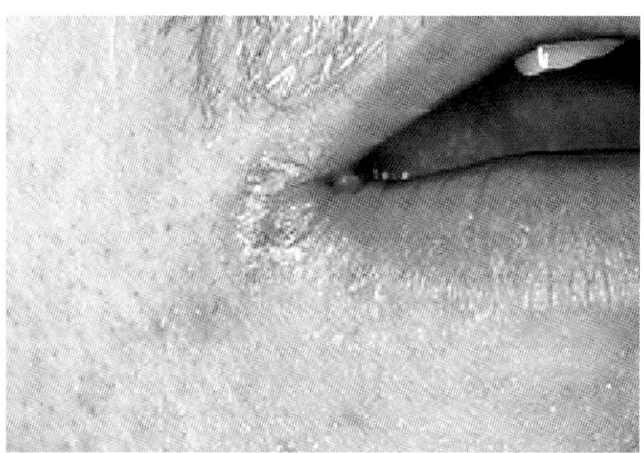

FIGURE 18-7 Angular cheilitis in a patient with AIDS. The lesion responded to antifungal medication. *(Courtesy Eric Haus, Chicago, Illinois.)*

palsy, trigeminal neuropathy, salivary gland enlargement, xerostomia, and melanotic pigmentation.[50,51] Candidiasis, hairy leukoplakia, specific forms of periodontal disease (i.e., linear gingival erythema and necrotizing ulcerative periodontitis), Kaposi sarcoma, and non-Hodgkin's lymphoma are reported to be strongly associated with HIV infection. Features and management of the oral manifestations of HIV infection are discussed in Tables 18-4 and 18-5. In addition, clinicians should be aware that oral lesions can be a feature of the stage of the disease or a sign of treatment failure or disease progression[52,53] (Table 18-6).

Worldwide, candidiasis is the most common oral manifestation of HIV infection. Oral candidiasis diagnosed in HIV-infected patients with persistent generalized lymphadenopathy may be of predictive value for the

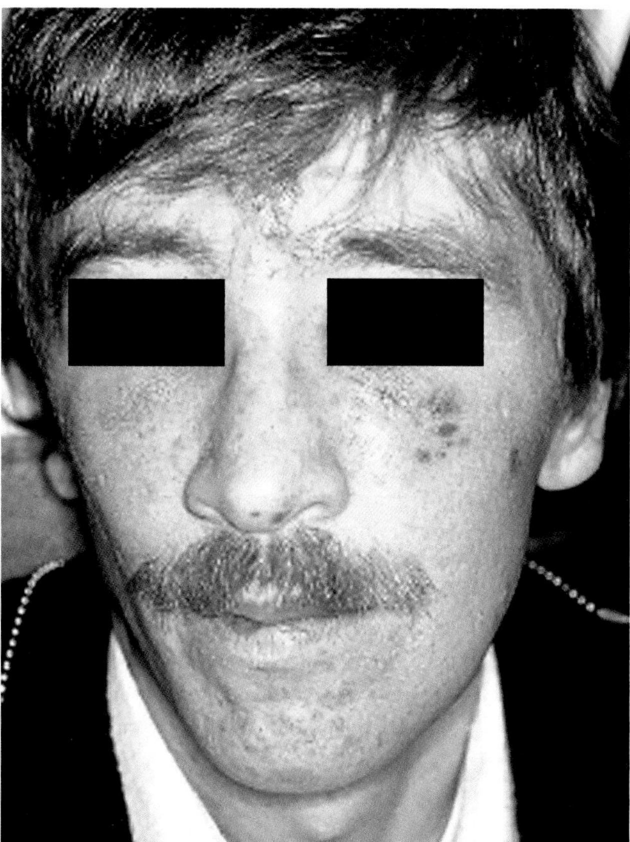

FIGURE 18-8 Multiple erythematous lesions on the face of a patient with AIDS. With the use of biopsy, lesions were established as Kaposi sarcoma. *(Courtesy Sol Silverman, San Francisco, California.)*

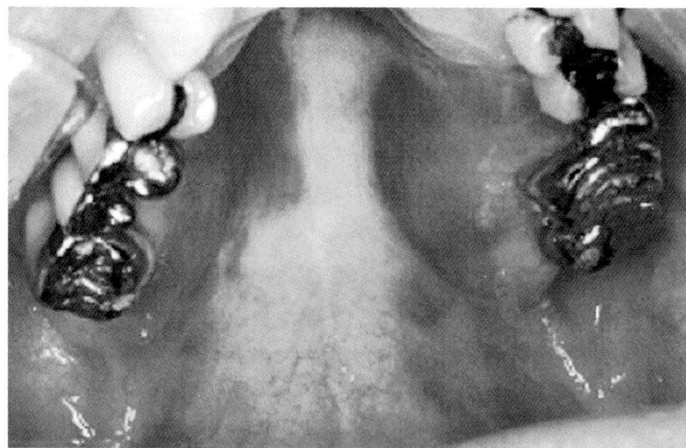

FIGURE 18-9 Multiple large, flat, erythematous lesions involving the palatal mucosa. Biopsy revealed the lesions to be Kaposi sarcoma, and the patient was eventually given a diagnosis of AIDS. *(Courtesy Sol Silverman, San Francisco, California.)*

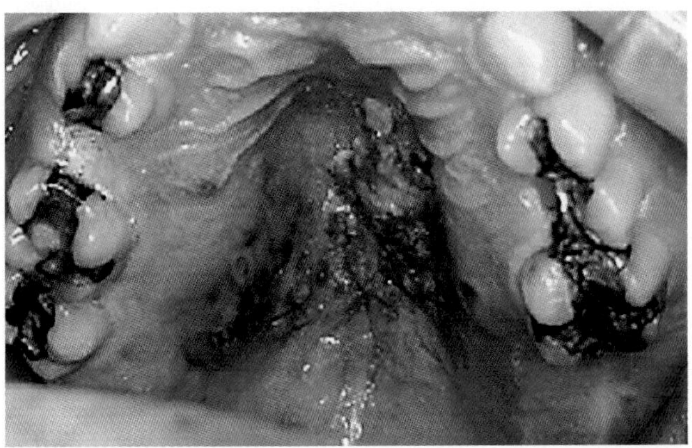

FIGURE 18-10 Palatal lesion in a patient with AIDS. Biopsy revealed Kaposi sarcoma. *(Courtesy Sol Silverman, San Francisco, California.)*

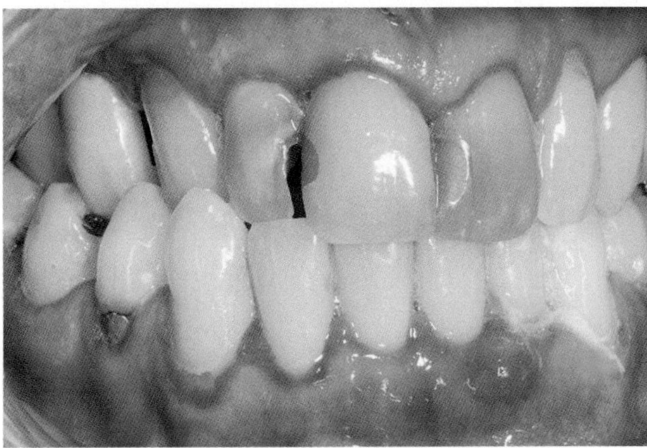

FIGURE 18-13 Band of linear gingival erythema involving the free gingival margin of a human immunodeficiency virus–infected patient. *(From Neville B, et al: Oral and maxillofacial pathology, ed 3,St. Louis, 2009, Saunders.)*

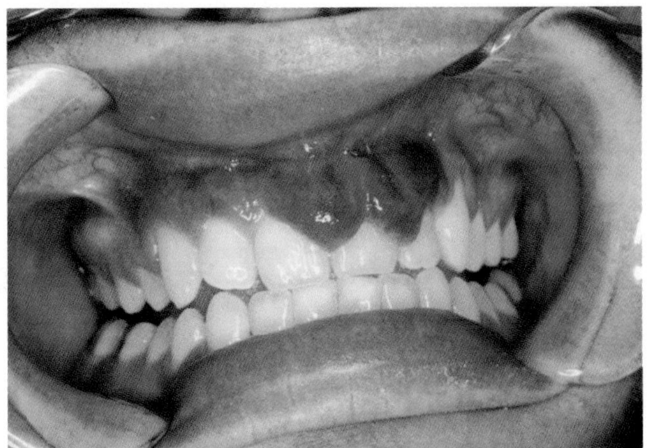

FIGURE 18-11 Kaposi sarcoma of the gingiva. *(From Silverman S Jr: Color atlas of oral manifestations of AIDS, ed 2, St. Louis, 1996, Mosby.)*

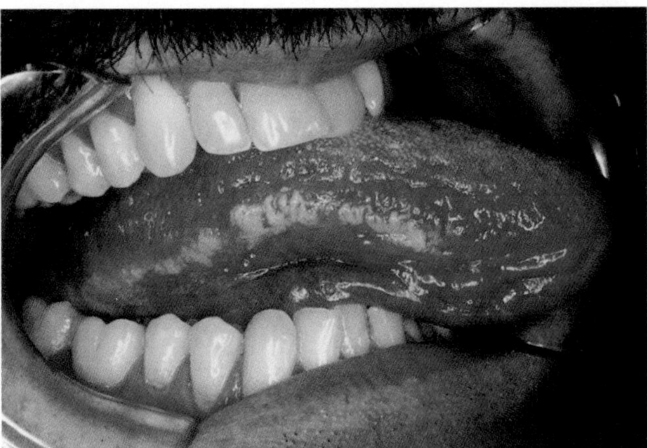

FIGURE 18-12 Diffuse white lesion involving the tongue. Biopsy supported the diagnosis of hairy leukoplakia. *(From Silverman S Jr: Color atlas of oral manifestations of AIDS, ed 2, St. Louis, 1996, Mosby.)*

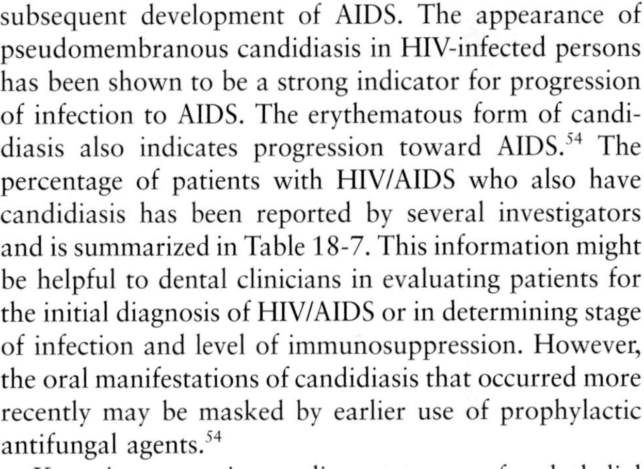

subsequent development of AIDS. The appearance of pseudomembranous candidiasis in HIV-infected persons has been shown to be a strong indicator for progression of infection to AIDS. The erythematous form of candidiasis also indicates progression toward AIDS.[54] The percentage of patients with HIV/AIDS who also have candidiasis has been reported by several investigators and is summarized in Table 18-7. This information might be helpful to dental clinicians in evaluating patients for the initial diagnosis of HIV/AIDS or in determining stage of infection and level of immunosuppression. However, the oral manifestations of candidiasis that occurred more recently may be masked by earlier use of prophylactic antifungal agents.[54]

Kaposi sarcoma is a malignant tumor of endothelial cells caused by human herpesvirus type 8 (HHV-8). MSM who are HIV-infected are more commonly affected. In these patients, Kaposi's sarcoma most often is disseminated throughout the body and runs a fulminant clinical course. Before 1996, the survival rate was 35% at 2 years. However, survival rates have improved to 81% since the introduction of protease inhibitors into the ART regimen.[55]

Hairy leukoplakia is an asymptomatic, corrugated white lesion of the lateral borders of the tongue due to reactivation and replication of Epstein-Barr virus (EBV). This lesion can appear in any patient who is immunosuppressed, irregardless of HIV status. The diagnosis can be made on cell scrapings or from a biopsy. Histologic features include koilocytosis and hyperkeratotic, hairlike surface projections from the lesion. Treatment is with antiviral agents.

Lymphadenopathy at cervical and submandibular locations often is an early finding in patients infected with HIV. This condition is persistent and may be found in the absence of any current infection or medications

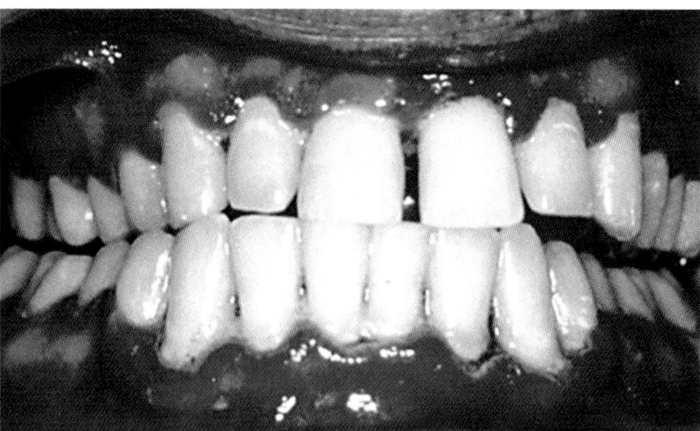

FIGURE 18-14 Necrotizing ulcerative periodontitis in a human immunodeficiency virus–infected patient. The diagnosis was established after the patient was referred for medical evaluation. *(Courtesy Sol Silverman, San Francisco, California.)*

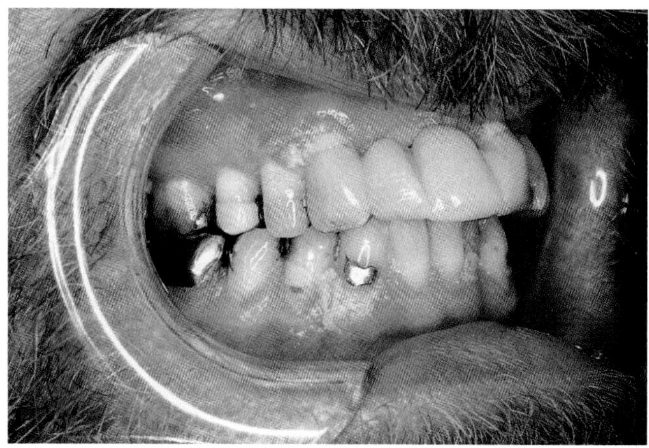

FIGURE 18-15 Multiple areas of condylomata acuminata on the gingivae of a human immunodeficiency virus–positive patient. *(From Silverman S Jr: Color atlas of oral manifestations of AIDS, ed 2, St. Louis, 1996, Mosby.)*

TABLE 18-4 Head, Neck, and Oral Lesions Commonly Associated with HIV Infection and AIDS

Oral Condition	Comment	Treatment
Persistent generalized lymphadenopathy	An early sign of HIV infection, found in about 70% of infected patients during the latent stage of infection. Must be present longer than 3 months and in two or more extrainguinal locations. Anterior and posterior cervical, submandibular, occipital, and axillary nodes are most frequently involved.	Usually not treated directly, may need biopsy to rule out lymphoma or other conditions.
Oral candidiasis Pseudomembranous Erythematous Hyperplastic Angular cheilitis	Most common intraoral manifestation of HIV infection. First found during the early symptomatic stage of infection. This indicates that AIDS will develop within 2 years in untreated patients. About 90% of patients with AIDS will develop oral candidiasis at some time during their disease course.	Nystatin often is ineffective. Topical clotrimazole is effective but has high rate of recurrence. Systemic fluconazole and itraconazole are effective but have a number of drug interactions and may result in drug-resistant candidiasis. If azoles fail, then intravenous amphotericin B can be administered.
HIV-associated periodontal disease		
Linear gingival erythema (LGE)	LGE does not respond to improved plaque control procedures. Condition is associated with candidiasis.	LGE usually responds to plaque removal, improved oral hygiene, and chlorhexidine rinses. Persistent cases usually respond to local measures plus systemic antifungal medications. Therapy for NUG, NUP, and NS involves debridement (removal of necrotic tissue and povidone-iodine irrigation), chlorhexidine rinses, metronidazole, follow-up care, and long-term maintenance.
Necrotizing ulcerative gingivitis (NUG)[16]	NUG relates to ulceration and necrosis of one or more interdental papillae with no loss of periodontal attachment.	
Necrotizing ulcerative periodontitis (NUP)	NUP consists of gingival ulceration and necrosis with attachment loss and does not respond to conventional periodontal therapy.	
Necrotizing stomatitis (NS)	May be seen as an extension of NUP or may involve oral mucosa separate from the gingiva.	

TABLE 18-4 Head, Neck, and Oral Lesions Commonly Associated with HIV Infection and AIDS—cont'd

Oral Condition	Comment	Treatment
Herpes simplex virus (HSV) infection	Immunocompetent persons and HIV-infected patients experience about the same rate of recurrent HSV infection (10-15%), but in HIV-infected patients, the lesions are more widespread, occur in an atypical pattern, and may persist for months.	Systemic acyclovir, valacyclovir, or famciclovir for at least 5 days can be effective. Higher doses may be needed during severe immunosuppression. An elixir or syrup of diphenhydramine (Benadryl) of 12.5 mg/5 mL can be used for pain control.
Varicella-zoster virus (VZV) infection	Recurrent VZV infection is common in HIV-infected patients, but the course is more severe. Intraoral lesions are often severe and can lead to bone involvement with loss of teeth.	Valacyclovir 1 g PO tid; famciclovir 500 mg PO tid; acyclovir 800 mg PO 5 times per day. Intravenous acyclovir may be needed for severe herpes zoster in patients with immunosuppression.
Oral hairy leukoplakia (OHL)	White lesion most often found on the lateral border of the tongue. OHL on rare occasions has been found on the buccal mucosa, soft palate, and pharynx. Associated with Epstein-Barr virus infection. In an untreated patient with HIV symptomatic infection, the finding of OHL indicates that AIDS will develop in the near future.	Treatment often is not needed. Acyclovir or desiclovir can result in rapid resolution, but recurrence is likely. Retinoids or podophyllum resin therapy can lead to temporary remission. HIV therapy with ART can result in significant regression.
Kaposi sarcoma (KS)	Human herpes virus type 8 (HHV-8) involved in KS development. About 50% of patients with KS have oral lesions, and the oral cavity is the initial site of involvement in 20% to 25% of cases. The most common sites are the hard palate, gingival, and tongue. KS that occurs in an HIV-infected patient is diagnostic of AIDS.	Often regresses with HAART. Treatment involves irradiation, local and systemic chemotherapy. Focal symptomatic lesions can be excised, or injected with vinblastine or a sclerosing agent (sodium tetradecyl sulfate). Other options for dealing with these types of lesions are cryotherapy, laser ablation, and electrosurgery, but care must be taken to protect operating personnel from aerosolization of viral particles when the laser or electrosurgery unit is used.

AIDS, Acquired immunodeficiency syndrome; *HIV,* Human immunodeficiency virus.

TABLE 18-5 Less Common Oral Conditions Associated with HIV Infection

Oral Condition	Comment	Treatment
Aphthous stomatitis Minor Major Herpetiform	About 66% of lesions are of the more uncommon forms—major and herpetiform. With more severe reduction of CD4+ cell count, major lesions become more prevalent. Lesions that are chronic or atypical, or that do not respond to treatment, should be biopsied.	Treatment of major lesions that persist involves potent topical or intralesional corticosteroids. Systemic steroids generally are avoided, to prevent further immunosuppression. Thalidomide treatment has yielded good response but should be used for only a short time, because the drug can enhance HIV replication. Granulocyte colony-stimulating factor has produced significant improvement in a limited number of patients.
Human papillomavirus (HPV) Verruca vulgaris (wart) Oral squamous papilloma	The usual HPV types are found in oral lesions, but some uncommon variants such as HPV-7 and HPV-32 also are found. Lesions usually are multiple and may be found on any oral mucosal site.	Treatment of choice is surgical removal of the lesion(s). Other treatment modalities include topical podophyllin, interferon, and cryosurgery. Laser ablation and electrocoagulation have been used, but care must be taken because the plume may contain infectious HPV.

Continued

TABLE 18-5 Less Common Oral Conditions Associated with HIV Infection—cont'd

Oral Condition	Comment	Treatment
Histoplasmosis	Histoplasmosis is the most common endemic respiratory fungal infection in the United States and usually is subclinical and self-limiting. Dissemination of infection occurs in about 5% of patients with AIDS who live in areas in the United States where the fungus is endemic.	The treatment of choice for disseminated histoplasmosis is intravenous amphotericin B. Oral itraconazole also has been found to be effective and has fewer adverse effects, with better patient compliance.
Molluscum contagiosum	Molluscum contagiosum is caused by a poxvirus. The lesions are small papules with a central depressed crater. In immunocompetent persons, the lesions are self-limiting and are found on the genitals and trunk. In patients with AIDS, multiple lesions (hundreds) are found that do not regress (5% to 10% of patients with lesions have lesions of the facial skin).	Curettage, cryosurgery, and cautery have been used to treat these lesions, but they are painful and recurrences are common. Resolution of multiple lesions has been reported with HAART.
Thrombocytopenia	Thrombocytopenia is found in about 10% of HIV-infected patients. It may occur during any stage of the disease. Skin manifestations are most common, but petechiae, ecchymosis, and spontaneous gingival bleeding can occur in the oral cavity.	Platelet counts below 50,000/mm^3 may result in significant bleeding with minor surgical procedures. Platelet replacement may be indicated for these patients.
HIV-associated salivary gland disease	Found in 5% of HIV-infected patients and can occur any time during the infection. Bilateral swelling of the parotid is most common. In some patients, CD8+ lymphocytes infiltrate the gland and are associated with lymphadenopathy. Xerostomia may occur. Patients are at increased risk for B cell lymphoma.	Risk is increased for cysts of the parotid and lymphoma. Treatment involves antiretroviral therapy ± immune modulators. Associated xerostomia can be managed with sialogogues and saliva substitutes.
Hyperpigmentation	Melanin pigmentation has been reported to occur in HIV-infected patients. Several of the medications (ketoconazole, clofazimine, and zidovudine) used to treat these patients may cause melanin pigmentation. Addison-like pigmentation also may occur because of destruction of the adrenal gland. HIV infection itself may cause melanin pigmentation.	Usually, no treatment is indicated. Single lesions may have to be biopsied so that melanoma can be ruled out. Patients with Addison disease may require corticosteroids.
Lymphoma	Found in about 3% of patients with AIDS. Most are found in extranodal locations. Most lesions are non-Hodgkin B cell lymphoma and are related to the EBV. The CNS is the most common site, but oral lesions occur in the palate and gingiva and in other locations.	Treatment usually involves a combination of chemotherapy and radiation and is used for local control of disease. Prognosis is very poor, with death occurring within months of the diagnosis. HAART has reduced the prevalence of opportunistic infections and Kaposi sarcoma in HIV-infected patients but has not affected the prevalence of lymphoma.
Oral squamous cell carcinoma	Can be found in the oral cavity, pharynx, and larynx in HIV-infected persons. The same risk factors apply as for the general population, but the cancer occurs at a younger age (it appears that HIV infection accelerates onset of carcinoma).	Treatment of oral squamous cell carcinoma is the same as for non–HIV-infected patients: surgery, irradiation, chemotherapy, or combination therapy.

AIDS, Acquired immunodeficiency virus; *CNS,* Central nervous system; *EBV,* Epstein-Barr virus; *HAART,* Highly active antiretroviral therapy; *HIV,* Human immunodeficiency virus.

TABLE 18-6 Specific Oral Lesions Related to Stage of HIV Infection: Percentage of Patients with Lesions

Lesion	Seronegative + High Risk (%)	Seropositive, But Data Not Separated Into Clinical Stages (%)	Asymptomatic + PGL (%)	ARC (%)	AIDS (%)
Hairy leukoplakia	0.3-3	19	8-21	9-44	4-23
Candidiasis	0.8-10	11-31	5-17	11-85	29-87
Kaposi's sarcoma	0	0.3-3	1-2	0	35-38
Herpes simplex	0-0.5	0-1	0-5	11-29	0-9
Aphthous	0-2	0-1	2-8	11-14	2-7
Venereal warts	0-0.7	0-1	0-1	0	0-1
NUG	0-0.2	1-5	0-1	0	51
HIV periodontitis	0	0	0-2	0-21	19

AIDS, Acquired immunodeficiency syndrome; *NUG,* Necrotizing ulcerative gingivitis; *ARC,* AIDS-related complex; *HIV,* Human immunodeficiency virus; *PGL,* Persistent generalized lymphadenopathy.

Data from Barone R, et al: Oral Surg *69:169-173, 1990; Barr C, et al;* IADR *1443:289, 1990; Feigal DW, et al:* IADR *65:190, 1989; Little JW, Melnick SL, Rhame FS:* Gen Dent *42:446-450, 1994; Melnick SL, et al:* Oral Surg *68:37-43, 1989; Roberts MW, Brahim JS, Rinne NF:* J Am Dent Assoc *116:863-866, 1988; Silverman S Jr, et al:* J Am Dent Assoc *112:187-192, 1986.*

TABLE 18-7 Summary of Statistics Related to Oral Candidiasis in HIV-Infected Persons*

		Prevalence Frequencies		
Disease State	Published Studies	Range[†]	Weighted Mean (%)	Mean
Oral candidiasis	17	11-96	30.0	45.2
Erythematous	7	10-96	40.5	33.0
Pseudomembranous	6	6-69	22.2	25.6
Hyperplastic	6	2-20	3.8	3.8
Angular cheilitis	4	1-23	12.5	16.0

*Data from 17 published reports in the United States.
[†]Weighted by overall number of patients with oral candidiasis in each study.
HIV, Human immunodeficiency virus.
From Samaranayake LP, Holmstrup P: Oral candidiasis and human immunodeficiency virus infection, J Oral Pathol Med *18:554-564, 1989.*

known to cause lymph node enlargement. The nodes tend to be larger than 1 cm in diameter, and multiple sites of enlargement may be found.

The overall general dental management of the patient with AIDS is summarized in Box 18-3. The dentist should perform head and neck and intraoral soft tissue examinations on all patients. White lesions in the mouth must be identified, and appropriate steps taken to establish a diagnosis. This may involve cell study, culture, and biopsy by the dentist or referral to an oral surgeon. If red or purple lesions are found that cannot be explained by history (e.g., trauma, burn, chemical, physical) or proved by clinical observation (healing within 7 to 10 days), biopsy is indicated. Persistent lymphadenopathy must be investigated by referral for medical evaluation, diagnosis, and treatment.

BOX 18-3 Dental Management
Considerations in the Patient with HIV Infection or AIDS

P

Patient Evaluation/Risk Assessment (see Box 1-1)
- Evaluate and determine whether HIV infection exists.
- Obtain medical consultation if poorly controlled or undiagnosed problem, or if uncertain.

Potential Issues/Factors of Concern

A	
Analgesics	Aspirin and other NSAID use can worsen bleeding in a patient who has thrombocytopenia. Avoid during thrombocytopenic episodes. Check drug interactions before use.
Antibiotics	Prophylactic use not required unless severe immune neutropenia (<500 cells/μL) is present. Manage postoperative infections with usual antibiotic use. Check for drug interactions before use of antibiotics.
Anesthesia	No issues.
Anxiety	No issues.
Allergy	No issues.
B	
Bleeding	Excessive bleeding may occur in the patient with untreated or poorly controlled disease as a result of thrombocytopenia, which fortunately is not a common finding.
Breathing	Ensure that patient does not have a pulmonary infection. Delay treatment until pulmonary infections are resolved.
Blood pressure	No issues.
C	
Chair position	No issues.
Cardiovascular	Confirm cardiovascular status. Some ART drugs can increase risk of cardiovascular disease.
D	
Devices	No issues.
Drugs	There are many drug interactions and drug toxicities associated with ART. Clinicians are advised to check drug reference resources before prescribing medications to patients on ART, to minimize drug interactions. Also, some ART drugs can cause mucosal eruptions (see Table 18-3).
E	
Equipment	No issues.
Emergencies/urgencies	No issues.
F	
Follow-up	Routine and periodic follow-up evaluation is advised for patients in stage 1. Patients in stage 2 or 3 may require more frequent follow-up or additional prophylactic agents and may require hospital-like environment for care. Inspect for oral lesions to monitor for disease progression or ART treatment failure.

REFERENCES

1. Global HIV and AIDS estimates, end of 2009 (article online), http://www.avert.org/worldstats.htm; accessed on March 31, 2011.
2. Piot P: Human immunodeficiency virus infection and acquired immunodeficiency syndrome: a global overview. In Goldman L, Ausiello D, editors: *Cecil textbook of medicine*, ed 23, St. Louis, 2008, Saunders, pp 2553-2554.
3. Merson MH: The HIV-AIDS pandemic at 25—the global response, *N Engl J Med* 354:2414-2417, 2006.
4. Schneider E, et al: Revised surveillance case definitions for HIV infection among adults, adolescents, and children aged <18 months and for HIV infection and AIDS among children aged 18 months to <13 years—United States, 2008, *MMWR Recomm Rep* 57:1-12, 2008.
5. The HIV/AIDS epidemic: the first 10 years, *MMWR Morb Mortal Wkly Rep* 40:357, 1991.
6. World Health Organization (WHO): *WHO case definitions of HIV for surveillance and revised clinical staging and immunological classification of HIV-related disease in adults and children*, Geneva, 2007, WHO Press, available at http://www.who.int/hiv/pub/guidelines/hivstaging/en/index.html; accessed on March 31, 2011.
7. HIV prevalence estimates—United States, 2006, *MMWR Morb Mortal Wkly Rep* 57:1073-1076, 2008.
8. Hall HI, et al: Estimation of HIV incidence in the United States, *JAMA* 300:520-529, 2008.
9. Centers for Disease Control and Prevention: HIV/AIDS statistics and surveillance. Basic statistics (article online), http://www.cdc.gov/hiv/topics/surveillance/basic.htm?source=govdelivery; accessed on March 31, 2011.
10. Hall HI, et al: Racial/ethnic and age disparities in HIV prevalence and disease progression among men who have sex with men in the United States, *Am J Public Health* 97:1060-1066, 2007.
11. Lansky A, et al: Epidemiology of HIV in the United States, *J Acquir Immune Defic Syndr* 55(Suppl 2):S64-S68, 2010.
12. Centers for Disease Control and Prevention: Deaths among persons with AIDS through December 2006. HIV/AIDS Surveillance Supplemental Report, vol 14, no. 3 (publication online), http://www.cdc.gov/hiv/surveillance/resources/reports/2009supp_vol14no3/pdf/table6.pdf; accessed on March 31, 2011.
13. AIDS epidemic update, Geneva, WHO/UNAIDS, 2009; available at http://www.unaids.org/en/media/unaids/contentassets/dataimport/pub/report/2009/jc1700_epi_update_2009_en.pdf; accessed on March 31, 2011.
14. Campbell-Yesufu OT, Gandhi RT: Update on human immunodeficiency virus (HIV)-2 infection, *Clin Infect Dis* 52:780-787, 2011.
15. Update: HIV-2 infection among blood and plasma donors—United States, June 1992-June 1995, *MMWR Morb Mortal Wkly Rep* 44:603-606, 1995.
16. Barre-Sinoussi F, et al: Isolation of a T-lymphotropic retrovirus from a patient at risk for acquired immune deficiency syndrome (AIDS), *Science* 220:868-871, 1983.
17. Gallo RC, et al: Frequent detection and isolation of cytopathic retroviruses (HTLV-III) from patients with AIDS and at risk for AIDS, *Science* 224:500-503, 1984.

18. Levy JA, et al: Isolation of lymphocytopathic retroviruses from San Francisco patients with AIDS, *Science* 225:840-842, 1984.
19. Hillis DM: AIDS. Origins of HIV, *Science* 288:1757-1759, 2000.
20. Fauci AS, Lane HC: HIV disease: AIDS and related disorders. In Fauci AS, et al, editors: *Harrison's principles of internal medicine*, ed 17, New York, 2008, McGraw-Hill, pp 1772-1776.
21. Centers for Disease Control and Prevention: HIV among gay, bisexual and other men who have sex with men (MSM) (article online), http://www.cdc.gov/hiv/topics/msm/index.htm; accessed on March 31, 2011.
22. Centers for Disease Control and Prevention: HIV in the United States (article online), http://www.cdc.gov/hiv/resources/factsheets/us.htm; accessed on March 31, 2011.
23. Gaur AH, et al: Practice of feeding premasticated food to infants: a potential risk factor for HIV transmission, *Pediatrics* 124:658-666, 2009.
24. Abu-Raddad LJ, et al: Genital herpes has played a more important role than any other sexually transmitted infection in driving HIV prevalence in Africa, *PLoS One* 3:e2230, 2008.
25. Gwanzura L, et al: Association between human immunodeficiency virus and herpes simplex virus type 2 seropositivity among male factory workers in Zimbabwe, *J Infect Dis* 177:481-484, 1998.
26. Workowski KA, Berman S: Sexually transmitted diseases treatment guidelines, 2010, *MMWR Recomm Rep* 59:1-110, 2010.
27. Campo J, et al: Oral transmission of HIV, reality or fiction? An update, *Oral Dis* 12:219-228, 2006.
28. Jevtovic DO, et al: Long-term survival of HIV-infected patients treated with highly active antiretroviral therapy in Serbia and Montenegro, *HIV Med* 8:75-79, 2007.
29. Pedersen C, et al: Clinical course of primary HIV infection: consequences for subsequent course of infection, *BMJ* 299:154-157, 1989.
30. Vazquez E: FDA approves two new approaches to HIV testing. Food and Drug Administration, *Posit Aware* 7:8, 1996.
31. Eshleman SH, et al: Detection of individuals with acute HIV-1 infection using the ARCHITECT HIV Ag/Ab Combo assay, *J Acquir Immune Defic Syndr* 52:121-124, 2009.
32. Stekler JD, et al: HIV testing in a high-incidence population: is antibody testing alone good enough? *Clin Infect Dis* 49:444-453, 2009.
33. Guidelines for the use of antiretroviral agents in HIV-1-infected adults and adolescents, January 20, 2011. Developed by the DHHS Panel on Antiretroviral Guidelines for Adults and Adolescents—A Working Group of the Office of AIDS Research Advisory Council (OARAC) (publication online), http://www.aidsinfo.nih.gov/ContentFiles/AdultandAdolescentGL.pdf; accessed on March 31, 2011.
34. Perez-Molina JA, et al: Late initiation of HAART among HIV-infected patients in Spain is frequent and related to a higher rate of virological failure but not to immigrant status, *HIV Clin Trials* 12:1-8, 2011.
35. Masur H, Healey L, Hadigan C: Treatment of human immunodeficiency virus infection and acquired immunodeficiency syndrome. In Goldman L, Ausiello D, editors: *Cecil textbook of medicine*, ed 23, St. Louis, 2008, Saunders, pp 2571-2582.
36. Muller M, et al: Immune reconstitution inflammatory syndrome in patients starting antiretroviral therapy for HIV infection: a systematic review and meta-analysis, *Lancet Infect Dis* 10:251-261, 2010.
37. Kim JH, et al: HIV vaccines: lessons learned and the way forward, *Curr Opin HIV AIDS* 5:428-434, 2010.
38. Allers K, et al: Evidence for the cure of HIV infection by CCR5{delta}32/{delta}32 stem cell transplantation, *Blood* 117:2791-2799, 2011.
39. Vernillo AT, Caplan AL: Routine HIV testing in dental practice: can we cross the Rubicon? *J Dent Educ* 71:1534-1539, 2007.
40. Oral Health Topics: HIV (serial online), http://www.ada.org/5166.aspx?currentTab=1; accessed on March 31, 2011.
41. Campo J, et al: Oral complication risks after invasive and non-invasive dental procedures in HIV-positive patients, *Oral Dis* 13:110-116, 2007.
42. Moswin AH, Epstein JB: Essential medical issues related to HIV in dentistry, *J Can Dent Assoc* 73:945-948, 2007.
43. Reddy J: Control of HIV/AIDS and AIDS-related conditions in Africa with special reference to periodontal diseases, *J Int Acad Periodontol* 9:2-12, 2007.
44. Alley BS, Buchanan TH, Eleazer PD: Comparison of the success of root canal therapy in HIV/AIDS patients and non-infected controls, *Gen Dent* 56:155-157, 2008.
45. Panlilio AL, et al: Updated U.S. Public Health Service guidelines for the management of occupational exposures to HIV and recommendations for postexposure prophylaxis, *MMWR Recomm Rep* 54:1-17, 2005.
46. Occupational postexposure prophylaxis for HIV: The PEPline perspective, *Top HIV Med* 18:174-177, 2010.
47. Update: transmission of HIV infection during invasive dental procedures—Florida, *MMWR Morb Mortal Wkly Rep* 40:377-381, 1991.
48. Bautista LE, Orostegui M: Dental care associated with an outbreak of HIV infection among dialysis patients, *Rev Panam Salud Publica* 2:194-202, 1997.
49. Kohn WG, et al: Guidelines for infection control in dental health-care settings—2003, *MMWR Recomm Rep* 52:1-61, 2003.
50. Leao JC, et al: Oral complications of HIV disease, *Clinics (Sao Paulo)* 64:459-470, 2009.
51. Hodgson TA, Greenspan D, Greenspan JS: Oral lesions of HIV disease and HAART in industrialized countries, *Adv Dent Res* 19:57-62, 2006.
52. Patton LL, Shugars DC: Immunologic and viral markers of HIV-1 disease progression: implications for dentistry, *J Am Dent Assoc* 130:1313-1322, 1999.
53. Glick M, Muzyka BC, Lurie D, Salkin LM: Oral manifestations associated with HIV-related disease as markers for immune suppression and AIDS, *Oral Surg Oral Med Oral Pathol* 77:344-349, 1994.
54. Challacombe SJ, Coogan MM, Williams DM: Overview of the Fourth International Workshop on the Oral Manifestations of HIV Infection, *Oral Dis* 8(Suppl 2):9-14, 2002.
55. Lodi S, et al: Kaposi sarcoma incidence and survival among HIV-infected homosexual men after HIV seroconversion, *J Natl Cancer Inst* 102:784-792, 2010.

CHAPTER

19

Allergy

Allergic diseases are increasing in prevalence and are contributing significantly to health care costs. For example, the number of children with allergies has recently doubled.[1]

One of the most common medical emergencies that can occur in the dental office is that of an acute allergic reaction. Accordingly, a requirement for every dental practitioner is a basic understanding of the pathophysiology of such reactions, as well as risk factors and clinical manifestations. In this context, such knowledge will permit meeting the following goals of safe and effective dental treatment:

- To identify patients with a true allergic history, so acute medical emergencies that might occur in the dental office because of an allergic reaction can be prevented
- To recognize head, neck, and oral tissue changes that might be caused by an allergic reaction
- To identify and plan appropriate dental care for patients who have severe alterations of the immune system secondary to irradiation or drug therapy or related to an immune deficiency disorder
- To recognize signs and symptoms of acute allergic reactions and to manage these problems appropriately

An overview of the significant principles of allergic disease, including the various types of reactions that may be encountered in the dental office, is presented.

DEFINITION

Epidemiology: Incidence and Prevalence

Allergy is an abnormal or hypersensitive response of the immune system to a substance introduced into the body. It is estimated that 15% to 25% of all Americans demonstrate an allergy to some substance, including about 4.5% who have asthma, 4% who are allergic to insect stings, and 5% who are allergic to one or more drugs. Allergic reactions account for about 6% to 10% of all adverse drug reactions. Of these, 46% consist of erythema and rash, 23% urticaria, 10% fixed drug reactions, 5% erythema multiforme, and 1% anaphylaxis. About a 1% to 3% risk for an allergic reaction is associated with administration of any drug. Fatal drug reactions occur in about 0.01% of surgical inpatients and 0.1% of medical inpatients.[1-4]

Drugs are the most common cause of urticarial reaction in adults, and food and infection are the most common causes of these lesions in children. Urticaria occurs in 15% to 20% of young adults. In approximately 70% of patients with chronic urticaria, no etiologic agent can be identified.[1-3,5]

Use of iodinated organic compounds as radiographic contrast media results in about 1 death for every 1400 to 60,000 diagnostic procedures. Animal insulin used to treat patients with type 1 diabetes causes an allergic reaction in about 10% to 56% of these persons, and reports have stated that some 25% of patients with diabetes who are allergic to insulin react to penicillin.[1-3]

About 5% to 10% of people who are given penicillin develop an allergic reaction, and 0.04% to 0.2% of these experience an anaphylactic reaction to the drug. Death occurs in about 1% to 10% of those persons who experience an anaphylactic reaction. Usually, in anaphylactic reactions to penicillin, death occurs within 15 minutes after administration of the drug; 50% of the time, the allergic reaction starts immediately after drug administration. About 70% of affected patients report that they have taken penicillin previously (Box 19-1). The most common causes of anaphylactic death are penicillin, bee stings, and wasp stings; people with an atopic history are more susceptible to anaphylactic death than are patients with no history of allergy. Causes of anaphylaxis of significance in clinical practice are listed in Box 19-2.[1-4]

In rare cases, antihistamines have been reported to cause urticaria through an allergic response to the colored coating material of the capsule. In addition, azo and nonazo dyes used in toothpaste have been reported to cause anaphylactic-like reactions. Aniline dyes used to coat certain steroid tablets have caused serious allergic reactions as well.[1-3]

Parabens (used as preservatives in local anesthetics) have caused anaphylactoid reactions. Sulfites (sodium metabisulfite or acetone sodium bisulfite) used in local anesthetic solutions to prevent oxidation of the

BOX 19-1 Summary of 151 Cases of Penicillin-Related Anaphylactic Deaths

- 21 (14%) of the patients had a history of allergies.
- 106 (70%) of the patients had received penicillin before; of these, 25% experienced a sudden allergic reaction.
- 128 (85%) of patients died within 15 minutes of administration.
- 75 (50%) of the patients experienced symptoms right after first administration of the drug.
- 3 (2%) of the cases were related to oral penicillin.

Data from Idsoe O, et al: Nature and extent of penicillin side-reactions, with particular reference to fatalities from anaphylactic shock, Bull World Health Organ 38:159-188, 1968.

vasoconstrictors can cause serious allergic reactions. The group most susceptible to allergic reactions caused by sulfites includes the 9 to 11 million persons in the United States in whom asthma has been diagnosed.[1-3] Allergy to latex occurs in between 1% and 6% of the general population, and much more commonly in persons who have spina bifida.[4]

Etiology

Allergic diseases result from an immunologic reaction to a noninfectious foreign substance (antigen). They comprise a series of repeat reactions to a foreign substance. These reactions involve different types of immunologic hypersensitivity (Box 19-3) and elements of the nonspecific and specific branches of the immune system (Box 19-4). The three branches of the immune system are the humoral, cellular, and nonspecific branches. Functions of the humoral and cellular branches of the immune system are shown in Table 19-1.[1-3,5]

Foreign substances that trigger hypersensitivity reactions are called *allergens* or *antigens*. Box 19-5 shows some of the characteristics of antigens. Two types of lymphocytes play central roles in the two branches of the specific immune system: B lymphocytes in the humoral branch, and T lymphocytes in the cellular branch. The three branches of the immune system do not operate independently. T lymphocytes play an important role in the regulation of B lymphocytes. The initial function of the humoral and cellular branches of the immune system involves the recognition of antigens; however, cells and chemicals from the nonspecific branch of the immune system are needed to eradicate antigens.[1-3]

Under some circumstances, repeated contact with or exposure to an antigen may cause an inappropriate response (hypersensitivity) that can be harmful or destructive to host tissues; thus, hypersensitivity reactions can involve cellular or humoral components of the immune system.[1-4] Reactions that involve the humoral system most often occur soon after contact with the antigen; three types of hypersensitivity reaction (types I, II, and III) involve elements of the humoral immune system. Type IV hypersensitivity reactions involve the cellular immune system. Allergic reactions that involve the cellular immune system often have delayed onset. Examples include contact dermatitis, graft rejection,

BOX 19-2 Causes of Human Anaphylactic Reactions of Importance in Health Care

Causative Agents

Antibiotics

- Penicillins
- Sulfonamides
- Vancomycin
- Amphotericin B
- Cephalosporins
- Nitrofurantoin
- Ciprofloxacin
- Tetracyclines
- Streptomycin
- Chloramphenicol

Miscellaneous Drugs/Therapeutic Agents

- Acetylsalicylic acid
- Succinylcholine
- *d*-Tubocurarine
- Antitoxins
- Progesterone
- Thiopental
- Vaccines
- Protamine sulfate
- Nonsteroidal antiinflammatory drugs (NSAIDs)
- Opiates
- Mechlorethamine

Diagnostic Agents

- Sodium dehydrocholate
- Radiographic contrast media
- Sulfobromophthalein
- Benzylpenicilloyl polylysine (Pre-Pen)

Hormones

- Insulin
- Parathormone
- Corticotropin
- Synthetic adrenocorticotropic hormone (ACTH)

Enzymes

- Streptokinase
- Penicillinase
- Chymotrypsin
- Asparaginase
- Trypsin
- Chymopapain

Blood Products

- Whole blood
- Plasma
- Gamma globulin
- Cryoprecipitate
- Immunoglobulin A (IgA)

Latex

Data from Grammer LC, Greenberger PA (editors): Patterson's allergic diseases, *ed 7, Phildadelphia, 2009, Lippincott, Williams and Wilkins.*

BOX 19-3 Coombs and Gell Classification of Immunologic Hypersensitivity Reactions

- *Type I*—anaphylactic or IgE-mediated
- *Type II*—cytotoxic
- *Type III*—immune complex–mediated
- *Type IV*—cell-mediated or delayed

IgE, Immunoglobulin E.

BOX 19-4 The Immune System

1. Nonspecific
   a. Mechanical reflexes
      (1) Coughing, sneezing
      (2) Action of cilia
      (3) Sphincter control of bladder
   b. Secretion of bactericidal substances
      (1) Stomach acid
      (2) Earwax (cerumen)
      (3) Enzymes in tears or saliva
   c. Phagocytic cells
      (1) Neutrophils
      (2) Monocytes
      (3) Macrophages
   d. Circulating chemicals
      (1) Complement
      (2) Interferon
2. Specific
   a. Humoral immunity
      (1) Protection against bacterial infection
      (2) Clones of B lymphocytes
      (3) Recognition of chemical configuration
      (4) Production of antibodies by plasma cells
      (5) Eradication of antigen
   b. Cellular immunity
      (1) Protection against viral infection, tuberculosis, leprosy
      (2) Transplant rejection
      (3) Production of cytokines by T lymphocytes
      (4) Eradication of antigen

Adapted from Thomson NC, et al, editors: Handbook of clinical allergy, *Oxford, Blackwell Scientific, 1990, pp 1-36.*

graft-versus-host disease, some drug reactions, and some types of autoimmune disease.[1-3,5]

Pathophysiology and Complications

Humoral Immune System. B lymphocytes recognize specific foreign chemical configurations via receptors on their cell membranes. For the antigen to be recognized by specific B lymphocytes, it must first be processed by T lymphocytes and macrophages. Each clone (family) of B lymphocytes recognizes its own specific chemical structure. Once recognition has taken place, B lymphocytes differentiate and multiply, forming plasma cells and memory B lymphocytes. Memory B lymphocytes remain inactive until contact is made with the same type of antigen. This contact transforms the memory cell into a plasma cell that produces immunoglobulins (antibodies)

BOX 19-5 Antigens

- Materials considered foreign by the body
- Large molecular size
- Certain degree of molecular complexity
- Cell-mediated immune response rarely induced by polysaccharides (T-independent antigens)
- Multiple antigenic determinants or antibody-binding sites (epitopes)
- Various reactions in humans

Adapted from Thomson NC, et al, editors: Handbook of clinical allergy, *Oxford, Blackwell Scientific, 1990, pp 1-36.*

TABLE 19-1 Functions of the Immune System

Function	Humoral	Cellular
Processing of antigen	T helper cells and macrophages	Macrophages plus antigens of major histocompatibility complex (MHC)
Cellular recognition of antigen	Receptors on B lymphocytes are sensitive to specific chemical configurations	T lymphocytes with receptors to specific subsets of MHC antigens
Cellular response to presentation of antigen	Specific clones of B lymphocytes multiply and produce plasma cells and memory cells	Specific clones of T lymphocytes multiply and produce effector T cells and memory T cells
Cellular action against antigen	Plasma cells produce specific immunoglobulins (antibodies); memory cells become plasma cells, with later antigen contact	Effector T cells produce cytokines; Memory T cells become effector T cells, with later antigen contact
Eradication of antigen	Reaction with specific antibody is facilitated by nonspecific branch of the immune system; antigen is removed by cells of a nonspecific branch	Destruction of antigen by cytokines and elements of a nonspecific branch of the immune system

Adapted from Thomson NC, et al, editors: Handbook of clinical allergy, *Oxford, Blackwell Scientific, 1990, pp 1-36.*

BOX 19-6 Functions of Immunoglobulins

1. Immunoglobulin (Ig)G
   a. Most abundant immunoglobulin
   b. Small size allows diffusion into tissue spaces
   c. Can cross the placenta
   d. Opsonizing antibody—facilitates phagocytosis of microorganisms by neutrophils
   e. Four subclasses: IgG1, IgG2, IgG3, IgG4 (IgG can bind to mast cells)
2. IgA
   a. Two types
      (1) Secretory (dimer, secretory components)—found in saliva, tears, and nasal mucus; secretory component protects from proteolysis
      (2) Serum (monomer)
   b. Does not cross the placenta
   c. Last immunoglobulin to appear in childhood
3. IgM
   a. Large molecule
   b. Confined to intravascular space
   c. First immunoglobulin produced
   d. Activates complement
   e. Good agglutinating antibody
4. IgE
   a. Very low concentration in serum (0.004%)
   b. Increased in parasitic and atopic diseases
   c. Binds to mast cells and basophils
   d. Key antibody in pathogenesis of type I hypersensitivity reactions
5. IgD
   a. Low concentration in serum
   b. Little importance

Adapted from Thomson NC, et al, editors: Handbook of clinical allergy, *Oxford, 1990, Blackwell Scientific, pp 1-36.*

specific for the antigen involved. Box 19-6 lists the functions of the five classes of immunoglobulins. Note that immunoglobulin E is the key antibody involved in the pathogenesis of type I hypersensitivity reactions. Normal functions of the humoral immune system are shown in Box 19-7.[1-3,5]

Type I, type II, and type III hypersensitivity reactions involve elements of the humoral immune system. Type I hypersensitivity is summarized in Box 19-8. This is an IgE-mediated reaction that leads to the release of chemical mediators from mast cells and basophils in various target tissues. The role of IgE is clear in such reactions, but that of the other sensitizing antibody, IgG4, is not well understood.[1-3,5]

Type I Hypersensitivity Reactions. Type I hypersensitivity reactions commonly are caused by food substances (e.g., shellfish, nuts, eggs, milk), antibiotics, and insect bites (e.g., bee stings). They are related to the humoral immune system and usually occur soon after second contact with an antigen; however, many people have repeated contacts with a specific drug or material before they become allergic to it (Figure 19-1). The different types of type I hypersensitivity reactions are discussed next.

BOX 19-7 Functions of the Humoral Immune System

1. First encounter with antigen (primary response)
   a. Latent period
      (1) Antigen is processed
      (2) B lymphocyte clone is selected
      (3) Differentiation and proliferation
      (4) Plasma cells produce specific immunoglobulins
   b. Specific immunoglobulin (Ig)M level increases first in serum followed by IgG
   c. IgM levels later fall to zero
   d. IgG levels fall; however, some stay the same
2. Second encounter with antigen (secondary response)
   a. Latent period is shorter
      (1) Antigen is processed
      (2) Memory cells are selected; become plasma cells
      (3) Plasma cells produce specific immunoglobulins
   b. IgM levels increase first
   c. IgG levels increase to 50 times the level found in the primary response
   d. IgM levels fall later
   e. IgG levels fall later, but a significant serum level is usually maintained

Adapted from Thomson NC, et al, editors: Handbook of clinical allergy, *Oxford, 1990, Blackwell Scientific, pp 1-36.*

BOX 19-8 Type I Hypersensitivity

1. Immunoglobulin (Ig)E antibody–mediated
2. Immediate response
3. Usual allergens (antigens)
   a. Dust
   b. Mites
   c. Pollens
   d. Animal danders
   e. Food
   f. Drugs (haptens)
4. Symptoms
   a. Anaphylaxis
   b. Hay fever
   c. Asthma
   d. Urticaria, angioedema
   e. Symptoms on occasion
5. Frequency: affects about 10% of the population
6. Inherited tendency

Anaphylaxis is an acute reaction involving the smooth muscle of the bronchi in which antigen–IgE antibody complexes form on the surface of mast cells which causes sudden histamine release from these cells. The release of histamine, as well as other vasoactive mediators, leads

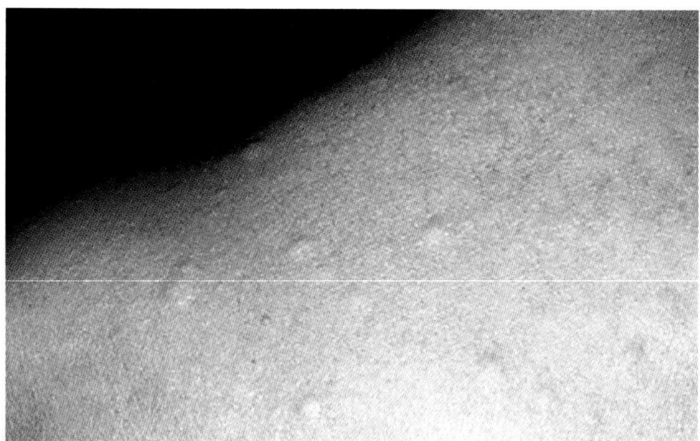

FIGURE 19-1 This generalized urticarial reaction occurred after injection of penicillin for treatment of an acute oral infection. The patient had previously taken penicillin a number of times without any problem.

to smooth muscle contraction and increased vascular permeability. The potential end result is acute respiratory compromise and cardiovascular collapse.

Atopy is a hypersensitivity state that is influenced by hereditary factors. Hay fever, asthma, urticaria, and angioedema are examples of atopic reactions. Lesions most commonly associated with atopic reactions include *urticaria,* which is a superficial lesion of the skin, and *angioedema,* which is a lesion that occurs in the deep dermis or subcutaneous tissues and often involves diffuse enlargement of the lips, infraorbital tissues, larynx, or tongue. In true allergic reactions, these lesions result from the effects of antigens and their antibodies on mast cells in various locations in the body. As is typical for type I hypersensitivity, the antigen–antibody complex causes the release of mediators (histamine) from mast cells. These mediators then produce an increase in the permeability of adjacent vascular structures, resulting in loss of intravascular fluid into surrounding tissue spaces—seen clinically as urticaria, angioedema, and secretions associated with hay fever.[1-3,5]

Of note, there are many types of angioedema. Three types of interest to dentistry are acquired (allergic-based), drug-induced, and hereditary angioedema. Drug-induced angioedema results from impaired bradykinin degradation after administration of certain drugs, such as angiotensin converting enzyme inhibitors. The hereditary form is due to a deficiency or dysfunction of complement C1 inhibitor, which can be triggered by trauma, thus leading to activation of the complement cascade and Hageman factor (factor XII) and overproduction of bradykinin.[5]

Type II Hypersensitivity Reactions. The key elements involved in type II hypersensitivity are shown in Box 19-9. These reactions are IgG- or IgM-mediated. The classic example of type II (cytotoxic) hypersensitivity is transfusion reaction caused by mismatched blood.[1-3,5]

BOX 19-9 Type II Hypersensitivity

1. Antibody-mediated
2. Cytotoxic hypersensitivity
   a. Antibodies combine with host cells recognized as foreign.
   b. Foreign antigens bind to host cell membranes during induced hemolytic anemia or thrombocytopenia.
3. Common examples
   a. Transfusion reactions from mismatched bloods
   b. Rhesus incompatibility
   c. Goodpasture's syndrome

Type III Hypersensitivity Reactions. Type III hypersensitivity is summarized in Box 19-10. These reactions take place in blood vessels and involve soluble immune complexes. They constitute what is referred to as *immune complex–mediated hypersensitivity.* Their key feature is vasculitis. Clinical examples include systemic lupus erythematosus and streptococcal glomerulonephritis.[1-3,5]

BOX 19-10 Type III Hypersensitivity

1. Antibody-mediated through immune complex formation
2. Also known as immune complex–mediated hypersensitivity
3. Local form is Arthus reaction
4. Immune complex formation
   a. Hypersensitivity state: complexes persist and lodge in blood vessel walls, initiating inflammatory reaction.
   b. Large complexes
   c. Removed by neutrophils and macrophages
   d. Soluble complexes (more antigen than antibody)
      (1) Most harmful
      (2) Penetrate vessel wall
      (3) Lodge in the basement membrane
   e. Complement is activated
      (1) Vascular permeability increased
      (2) Neutrophils attracted
      (3) Neutrophils release enzymes
      (4) Vasculitis results
5. Sensitive sites
   a. Renal glomeruli
   b. Synovial membranes
6. Examples
   a. Systemic lupus erythematosus
   b. Poststreptococcal glomerulonephritis

Cellular Immune System. In the cellular or delayed immune system, T lymphocytes play the central role. The primary function of this system is to recognize and eradicate antigens that are fixed in tissues or within cells. This system is involved in protection against viruses, tuberculosis, and leprosy. Antibodies are not operative in the cell-mediated immune system. Effector T lymphocytes produce various cytokines that serve as active agents of this system.[1-3,5]

Type IV Hypersensitivity Reactions. Type IV hypersensitivity reactions, which involve the cellular immune system, include infectious contact dermatitis, transplant rejection, and graft-versus-host disease (Box 19-11). Events in type IV hypersensitivity (contact dermatitis),

BOX 19-11 Type IV Hypersensitivity

Signs and Symptoms Suggestive of an Allergic Reaction

1. Mediated by T lymphocytes
2. Does not involve antibodies
3. Also called delayed-type hypersensitivity (response not seen until about 2 days after antigenic exposure)
4. Examples include the following:
   a. Contact dermatitis
   b. Graft rejection
   c. Graft-versus-host reaction
   d. Some type of drug hypersensitivity
   e. Some types of autoimmune disease

TABLE 19-2 Examples of Newer Antihistamines

Drug	Trade Name(s)	OTC?*
Acrivastine	Semprex, Benadryl Allergy Relief capsules	No
Cetirizine	Zirtec, Zyrtec	Yes
Desloratadine	Neoclarityn	No
Fexofenadine	Telfast 120, Telfast 180, Allegra	No
Levocetrizine	Xyzal	No
Loratadine	Clarityn, Clarityne, Boots Antihistamine Tablets, Claritin	Yes
Mizolastine	Mizollen, Mistamine (superseded by fexofenadine)	No

*Over the counter. Some of these medicines can be purchased without a doctor's prescription in the United States.

which may involve dendritic cells and Langerhans cells, present the antigen to undifferentiated T lymphocytes. Some of the more common antigens that cause contact dermatitis include metal jewelry, perfumes, rubber products, chemicals such as formaldehyde, and medicines such as topical anesthetics. Type IV hypersensitivity reactions usually are delayed and appear about 48 to 72 hours after contact has been made with the antigen.[1-3,5]

Infectious-type allergic reactions are exemplified by the tuberculin skin test, in which a person who has previously been exposed to *Mycobacterium tuberculosis* develops a delayed response, usually within 48 to 72 hours after a second exposure to components of the bacteria. This response is characterized by induration, erythema, swelling, and sometimes ulceration at the site of injection.

Contact allergy occurs when a substance of low molecular weight that is not antigenic by itself comes in contact with a tissue component (primarily a protein) and forms an antigenic complex. This small molecule is called a *hapten* (or one half of an antigen), and the resulting complex causes sensitization of T lymphocytes. Poison ivy is an example of a contact allergy wherein the reaction is delayed (with response occurring 48 to 72 hours after contact is made with the allergen).

Graft rejection occurs when organs or tissues from one body are transplanted into another body. Cellular rejection of transplanted tissue occurs, unless the donor and recipient are genetically identical or the host immune response has been suppressed.

Graft-versus-host reaction is an unusual phenomenon that occurs in bone marrow transplant recipients whose cellular immune system has been rendered deficient by whole body irradiation. Lymphocytes transferred to the host attempt to destroy host tissues.[1-3,5]

Nonallergic Reactions. Other agents may cause mast cells to release their mediators without inciting a true allergic reaction; this occurs in cases of chronic urticaria caused by certain drugs, temperature changes, and emotional states and in some reactions to drugs. Most so-called anaphylactic reactions to local anesthetics do not involve an antigen–antibody reaction but result from damage to the mast cells caused by other mechanisms. These reactions are referred to as anaphylactoid or *anaphylaxis-like*.[1-3,5]

From the clinical standpoint, approaches to management of anaphylactic and anaphylactoid reactions are similar; therefore, these types of drug reactions are viewed as true allergic reactions. Some cases of urticaria and angioedema have a similar pathogenesis and are not considered true allergic reactions.

Nonallergic cases of urticaria, angioedema, and anaphylactoid reactions are caused by the nonspecific release of vasoactive amines from mast cells or by the activation of other forms of nonspecific immunologic effectors involving the complement system and Hageman factor–dependent pathway. One example is hereditary angioedema, in which tissue swelling is triggered by trauma because of an underlying absence or dysfunction of C1 inhibitor, a protein that regulates the complement cascade pathway and the production of bradykinin. More in-depth discussion of the origin of these reactions can be found in standard texts on allergic diseases.[1-3,5]

MEDICAL MANAGEMENT

Patients with atopy may be given injections to gradually desensitize them so that they are no longer allergic to the antigen. Some patients with severe asthma may be forced to move to an area of the country that does not contain the antigen (e.g., in the case of allergy to pollen). Patients with asthma (see Chapter 7), immune complex injury, or cytotoxic immune reactions may be treated with systemic steroids, whereas those with hay fever or urticaria are treated with antihistamines.

Newer antihistamines are highly effective and produce fewer adverse effects (e.g., drowsiness) (Table 19-2). These agents differ in a number of ways, such as size of the tablets, duration of effect, efficacy, extent to which they can cause sleepiness (although all are superior to older antihistamines in this context), adverse effects, and drug interactions, as well as price.

A variety of treatments, including topical steroids, have been used for patients with contact dermatitis. From a dental standpoint, the patient who is being treated for allergies has an increased chance of being allergic to another substance. In addition, if the person is taking steroids, the body's reaction to stress may be impaired (see Chapter 15).

DENTAL MANAGEMENT

Medical Considerations

The dentist often is confronted with problems related to allergy. One of the most common concerns is patient-reported allergy to a local anesthetic, antibiotic, or analgesic. In this case, the history must be expanded, with specific efforts made to determine exactly what the offending substance was and exactly how the patient reacted to it. If the adverse reaction was of an allergic nature, one or more of the classic signs or symptoms of allergy should have been present (Box 19-12). If these signs or symptoms were not reported, the patient probably did not experience a true allergic reaction. Common examples of reactions mislabeled as "allergy" are syncope after injection of a local anesthetic and nausea or vomiting after ingestion of codeine. Adverse drug reactions are listed in Box 19-13.

Local Anesthetics. The reaction most often associated with local anesthetics is a toxic reaction, which usually results from inadvertent intravenous injection of the anesthetic solution (Box 19-14). Excessive amounts of an anesthetic also can cause a toxic reaction or a reaction to the vasoconstrictor. Signs and symptoms associated with toxic reactions to a local anesthetic are shown in Box 19-15. Signs and symptoms of a vasoconstrictor reaction include tachycardia, apprehension, sweating, and hyperactivity. Another common reaction to local anesthetics involves an anxious patient who, because of concern about receiving a "shot," experiences tachycardia, sweating, paleness, and syncope (Box 19-16). True allergic reactions to the local anesthetics (amides) most often used in dentistry are rare.[6]

BOX 19-12 Signs and Symptoms Suggestive of an Allergic Reaction

- Urticaria
- Swelling
- Skin rash
- Chest tightness
- Dyspnea, shortness of breath
- Rhinorrhea
- Conjunctivitis

BOX 19-13 Adverse Drug Reactions

Signs and Symptoms of a Toxic Reaction to Local Anesthetic

Predictable
- Dose-related
- No immunologic basis
- Account for about 80% of all adverse reactions to drugs
- Direct toxicity
- Overdose
- Drug interaction
- Adverse effects of drugs

Unpredictable
- Not dose-related
- Unrelated to expected pharmacologic effects
- Allergy
- Pseudoallergy (anaphylactoid reactions)
- Idiosyncrasy
- Intolerance
- Paradoxical reactions (cause histamine release but not IgE-mediated)
- Underlying genetic defect often present

Data from Lichtenstein LM, Busse WW, Geha R, editors: Current therapy in allergy, immunology, and rheumatology, *ed 6, St. Louis, 2004, Mosby.*

BOX 19-14 Adverse Reactions to Local Anesthetics

- Toxicity
- Central nervous system stimulation
- Central nervous system depression
- Vasoconstrictor effects
- Anxiety
- Allergic reaction

Data from Malamed SF: Allergy and toxic reactions to local anesthetics, Dent Today *22:114-116, 118-121, 2003.*

BOX 19-15 Signs and Symptoms of a Toxic Reaction to Local Anesthetic

- Talkativeness
- Slurred speech
- Dizziness
- Nausea
- Depression
- Euphoria
- Excitement
- Convulsions

Data from Malamed SF: Allergy and toxic reactions to local anesthetics, Dent Today *22:114-116, 118-121, 2003.*

BOX 19-16 Signs and Symptoms of a Psychomotor Response to Injection of a Local Anesthetic

- Hyperventilation
- Vasovagal syncope (bradycardia, pallor, sweating)
- Sympathetic stimulation (anxiety, tremor, tachycardia, hypertension)

If the patient's history supports a toxic or vasoconstrictor reaction, the dentist should explain the nature of the previous reaction and should avoid injecting the local anesthetic solution intravenously by aspirating before the injection and limiting the amount of solution to the recommended dose. If the patient's history supports an interpretation of fainting and not a toxic or allergic reaction, the dentist's primary task will be to work with the patient to reduce anxiety during dental visits. If the history supports a true allergic reaction to a local anesthetic, the dentist should try to identify the type of local anesthetic that was used. Once this has been ascertained, a new anesthetic with a different basic chemical structure can be used. The two main groups of local anesthetics in dentistry consist of the following:

1. *Para*-aminobenzoic acid (PABA) esters (procaine [Novocain] and tetracaine [Pontocaine])
2. Amides (articaine [Septocaine], bupivacaine [Marcaine], lidocaine [Xylocaine], mepivacaine [Carbocaine], and prilocaine [Citanest])

Benzoic acid ester anesthetics may cross-react with each other, whereas amide anesthetics usually do not cross-react. Cross-reaction does not occur between ester and amide local anesthetics.[6,7]

Procaine is the local anesthetic associated with the highest incidence of allergic reactions. Currently, it is available only in multidose vials. Its antigenic component appears to be PABA, one of the metabolic breakdown products of procaine. Cross-reactivity has been reported between lidocaine and procaine; however, this was traced to the presence of a germicide, methylparaben, which previously was used in small amounts as a preservative and is chemically similar to PABA. Methylparaben is no longer used as a preservative, so this problem is no longer a concern.[8] Lidocaine or another amide local anesthetic should be used for patients with a history of allergy to procaine.[6,7]

Patients who have been allergic to local anesthetics but who cannot identify the specific agent to which they reacted present more of a diagnostic problem. The nature of the reaction must be established, and if it is consistent with an allergic reaction, the next step should be to attempt to identify the anesthetic used. When the patient is unable to provide this information, the dentist can attempt to contact the previous dentist involved. If this fails, two additional options are available:

- An antihistamine (e.g., diphenhydramine [Benadryl]) can be used as the local anesthetic.
- The patient may be referred to an allergist for provocative dose testing (PDT) (Box 19-17).

The use of diphenhydramine often is the more practical option. A 1% solution of diphenhydramine that contains 1:100,000 epinephrine can be easily compounded by a pharmacist, but it must be confirmed that methylparaben is not used as a preservative. This solution induces anesthesia of about 30 minutes average duration and can be used for infiltration or block injection. When it is used for a mandibular block, 1 to 4 mL of solution is needed. Some patients have reported a burning sensation, swelling, or erythema after a mandibular block with 1% diphenhydramine, but these effects were not serious and cleared within 1 or 2 days. No more than 50 mg of diphenhydramine should be given during a single appointment. Diphenhydramine also can be used in the patient who reports a previous allergic reaction to either an ester or amide local anesthetic.[6,7]

The dentist may elect to refer the patient to an allergist for evaluation and testing, which usually includes both skin testing and PDT. Most investigators agree that skin testing alone for allergy to local anesthetics is of little benefit because false-positive results are common; therefore, the allergist also should perform PDT. Sending samples for specific testing of the clinician's usual anesthetic agents without vasoconstrictors is of great help.

On the basis of patient history, the allergist selects a local anesthetic for testing that is least likely to cause an allergic reaction; this usually is an anesthetic from the amide group because they generally do not cross-react with each other. At 15-minute intervals, 0.1 mL of test solution is injected subcutaneously, with concentrations increasing from 1:10,000 to 1:1000 to 1:100 to 1:10, followed by undiluted solution; next, 0.5 mL of undiluted test solution is tried; and finally, 1 mL of undiluted solution is given. During PDT, the allergist should be prepared to deal with any adverse reaction that might occur and should report to the dentist on the drug selected, the final dose given, and the absence of any adverse reaction. Under these conditions, a local anesthetic that does not cause a reaction can be used in the tested patient, and the risk of an allergic reaction is no greater than in the general population. Malamed has reported that he has not dealt with a single patient for whom a safe local anesthetic could not be found through the PDT procedure.[6]

When administering an alternative anesthetic to a patient with a history of a local anesthetic allergy, the dentist should follow these steps:

BOX 19-17 Dental Management of a Local Anesthetic Allergy

P

Patient Evaluation/Risk Assessment (see Box 1-1)

- Evaluate and determine whether allergy to local anesthetic exists.
- Obtain medical consultation if undiagnosed or if uncertain.

Potential Issues/Factors of Concern

A	
Anesthesia	Establish history of previous reaction after use of local anesthetic.
Anxiety	Distinguish that the reaction is not a vasovagal/syncopal reaction associated with anxiety.
Allergy	Determine the type of anesthetic used that triggers the allergy. A patient experiencing a true allergic reaction will demonstrate one or more of the following: soft tissue swelling, skin rash, rhinitis, difficulty breathing. If the reaction is consistent with allergic reaction, the following should be done: Select anesthetic from a different chemical group: (1) *Para*-aminobenzoic acid (procaine) (2) Amide (lidocaine, mepivacaine, articaine) Aspirate, inject 1 drop of alternate anesthetic, and wait 5 minutes; if no reaction occurs, inject after the rest of the anesthetic needed is aspirated (be prepared to deal with an allergic reaction, should one occur).
B	
Bleeding	No issues.
Breathing	Breathing difficulties can be avoided by avoiding the allergen (local anesthetic) until after allergy testing is completed; thereafter use a local anesthetic to which patient is not allergic.
Blood pressure	Monitor blood pressure during severe allergic reaction.
C	
Chair position	During allergic reaction and with a conscious patient, place in comfortable position. With unconscious patient, place in supine position.
D	
Devices	No issues.
Drugs	In cases of allergic reaction to several local anesthetic agents, or when a previously used anesthetic cannot be identified, consider using diphenhydramine. Have injectable epinephrine (1:1000) and diphenhydramine available.
E	
Equipment	No issues.
Emergencies/urgencies	For severe allergic reaction (e.g., anaphylaxis), inject 0.3 to 0.5 mL of 1:1000 epinephrine through an intramuscular (into the tongue) or subcutaneous route; supplement with intravenous diphenhydramine 50 to 100 mg if needed. Support respiration, if indicated, by mouth-to-mouth breathing or bag and mask.
F	
Follow-up	If history includes allergy to multiple substances, or if type of local anesthetic used previously cannot be identified, refer the patient to an allergist for provocative dose testing (PDT). Follow-up with physician regarding results of tests.

Data from Lichtenstein LM, Busse WW, Geha R, editors: Current therapy in allergy, immunology, and rheumatology, *ed 6, St. Louis, 2004, Mosby.*

1. Inject slowly, aspirating first to make sure that a vessel is not being injected.
2. Place 1 drop of the solution into the tissues.
3. Withdraw the needle, and wait 5 minutes to see what reaction, if any, occurs. If no allergic reaction occurs, as much anesthetic as is needed for the procedure should be deposited. Be sure to aspirate before giving the second injection (see Box 19-17).

Penicillin. Penicillin is used frequently throughout the world and is a common cause of drug allergy. In the United States, about 5% to 10% of the population is allergic to penicillin and penicillin-related drugs. About 0.04% to 0.2% of patients treated with penicillin develop an anaphylactic reaction, which is fatal in about 10% of these patients, accounting for some 400 to 800 deaths per year. Box 19-18 summarizes current data on risk assessment for penicillin reactions.[1,3,9,10] The possibility of sensitizing a patient to penicillin varies with different routes of administration, as follows[2,3,7]: Oral

BOX 19-18 Penicillin Reactions

Anaphylaxis

- In 0.04% to 0.2% of patients
- Fatal reaction occurs in 1 per 100,000 treated persons
- Atopic predisposition not a risk factor for anaphylaxis but is a risk factor for fatal reaction.
- Risk of reaction is dependent on:
    - History of previous reaction
    - Time interval since previous reaction
    - Persistence of specific immunoglobulin E (IgE) antibodies
    - History of multiple drug sensitivities

Risk Assessment

- Most useful parameter to assess risk in patients with a history of penicillin reaction is skin testing with major and minor determinants
    - Negative result—very little risk
    - Positive result—high risk for serious reaction to penicillin; risk for cross reaction with cephalosporin

Data from Lichtenstein LM, Busse WW, Geha R, editors: Current therapy in allergy, immunology, and rheumatology, *ed 6, St. Louis, 2004, Mosby.*

administration results in sensitization of only about 0.1% of patients, intramuscular injection in about 1% to 2%, and topical application in about 5% to 12%. On the basis of these data, the use of penicillin in a topical ointment is contraindicated. Additionally, if the dentist has a choice, the oral route is preferable for administration whenever possible. Parenteral administration of penicillin evokes a more serious reaction than that typically associated with oral administration. Some investigators have suggested that the risk is equally great for a serious allergic reaction with both routes. Antibodies produced against penicillin cross-react with the semisynthetic penicillins and may cause severe reactions in patients who are allergic to penicillin. Nevertheless, the synthetic penicillins seem to cause fewer new sensitizations in patients who are not allergic to penicillin at the time of administration.

Skin testing for allergy to penicillin is much more reliable than is skin testing for allergy to a local anesthetic; however, some risk is involved, and the allergist must be prepared for adverse reactions. Several points should be considered in the use of skin testing for penicillin sensitivity. To be cost-effective, the test should be conducted only on patients with a history of penicillin reaction who need penicillin for a serious infection. An important point is that penicillin reactivity declines with time; hence, a patient may have reacted to the drug years ago but is now no longer sensitive (negative skin test). The length of time for retaining sensitivity is variable and is dependent on IgE levels. Most anaphylactic reactions to penicillin occur in patients who have been treated in the past with penicillin but reported no adverse reactions.[1,3,5,7]

When skin testing for penicillin sensitivity is performed, both metabolic breakdown products of penicillin (the major derivative, penicilloyl polylysine, and the minor derivative mixture) must be tested; 95% of penicillin is metabolized to the major determinant and 5% to the minor determinants. If skin test results are negative for both breakdown products, the patient is considered not allergic to penicillin; however, if positive skin test results are obtained for one or both of the breakdown products, the patient is considered to be allergic to penicillin, and the drug should not be used. When penicillin must be used, the patient with a positive result on skin testing can be desensitized to it. The incidence of anaphylactic reactions is higher in patients who test positive for the minor derivative mixture than do patients who test positive for the major derivative.[1,3,5,7]

In dentistry, a patient who is allergic to penicillin generally is best treated with an alternative antibiotic. For example, patients with a history of penicillin allergy should be given erythromycin or clindamycin for the treatment of oral infection or clindamycin for prophylaxis against infective endocarditis.[1,3,5,7] Additionally, drugs that may cross-react, including ampicillin, carbenicillin, and methicillin, should be avoided in these patients.[5,7]

Cephalosporins are often used as alternatives to penicillins, however cephalosporins cross-react in 5% to 10% of penicillin-sensitive patients. The risk is greatest with first- and second-generation drugs. Cephalosporins are metabolized to their major determinant, cephaloyl, which may cross-react with the major determinant of penicillin. Cephalosporins usually can be used in patients with a history of distant, nonserious reaction to penicillin. However, skin testing is recommended for these patients by some investigators. If the patient's penicillin skin test result is negative, then penicillin or a cephalosporin may be used. If the penicillin skin test result is positive, a skin test for the specific cephalosporin selected should be performed. If this skin test result is negative, the cephalosporin that was tested can be used. Box 19-19 summarizes the use of cephalosporins in patients with a history of penicillin hypersensitivity.[5-7]

Patients with a negative history of allergy to penicillin can be treated with the drug when indicated, and it should be given by the oral route. The patient is observed for 30 minutes after the first dose, if possible, and is advised to seek immediate care if any of the signs or symptoms of an allergic reaction occur after he or she has left the dental office (Box 19-20).

Analgesics. Aspirin may cause gastrointestinal upset, but this problem can be avoided if it is taken with food or a glass of milk. The discomfort may include "heartburn," nausea, vomiting, or gastrointestinal bleeding.

BOX 19-19 Use of Cephalosporins in Patients with a History of Penicillin Hypersensitivity

1. Cephalosporins are metabolized to major determinant, cephaloyl.
2. Cephaloyl can cross-react with major determinant of penicillin (penicilloyl polylysine).
3. Risk of adverse reaction to cephalosporin is controversial.
   a. Greatest with first- or second-generation drugs
      (1) Cephaloridine, 16.5%
      (2) Cephalothin, 5%
      (3) Cephalexin, 5.4%
   b. Anaphylaxis
      (1) Positive history of penicillin reaction, 0.1%
      (2) Negative history of penicillin reaction, 0.4%
   c. Urticaria
      (1) Positive history of penicillin reaction, 1.3%
      (2) Negative history of penicillin reaction, 0.4%
4. Patient with history of penicillin reaction: first skin test for penicillin sensitivity
   a. Negative—use penicillin or a cephalosporin.
   b. Positive
      (1) Avoid penicillin.
      (2) Skin test is specific for cephalosporin; use cephalosporin if result is negative.

Data from Lichtenstein LM, Busse WW, Geha RS: Current therapy in allergy, immunology and rheumatology, *ed 6, London, 2004, Mosby.*

BOX 19-20 Procedures for Prevention of a Penicillin Reaction

1. Have emergency kit for treatment.
2. Take medical history on all patients, including the following:
   a. Previous contact with penicillin
   b. Reactions to penicillin
   c. Allergic reactions to other agents
3. Do not use penicillin in patient with a history of reactions to drugs.
4. Tell patient when you are going to give penicillin.
5. Do not use penicillin in topical preparations.
6. Do not use penicillinase-resistant penicillins unless infection is caused by penicillinase-producing staphylococci.
7. Use oral penicillin whenever possible.
8. Use disposable syringes for injection of penicillin.
9. Have patient wait in office for 30 minutes after first dose of penicillin is given.
10. Inform patient about signs and symptoms of allergic reaction to penicillin, and if these occur, to seek immediate medical assistance.

Aspirin should not be used by patients with an ulcer, gastritis, or a hiatal hernia and should be used with care by patients whose condition predisposes them to nausea, vomiting, dyspepsia, or gastric ulceration. Aspirin also is known to prolong prothrombin time and to inhibit platelet function, which is usually of little clinical importance, except in patients with a hemorrhagic disease or a peptic ulcer. In such instances, aspirin must be avoided. Many people (about 2 in 1000) are allergic to salicylates. Allergic reactions to aspirin can be serious, and deaths have been reported.[1,3,5]

Aspirin provokes a severe reaction in some patients with asthma. They may react in the same way to other nonsteroidal antiinflammatory drugs (NSAIDs) that inhibit cyclooxygenase, which is the key enzyme involved in the generation of prostaglandin from arachidonic acid. The typical reaction consists of acute bronchospasm, rhinorrhea, and urticaria. Most patients with asthma who react to NSAIDs also have nasal polyps and lack IgE-mediated allergy to airborne allergens. The mechanism for this reaction does not appear to be allergic but remains undefined.[11] The dentist should be aware of the many multiple-entity analgesic preparations that include aspirin or other salicylates. These agents must not be given to the patient who may be endangered by an adverse reaction associated with aspirin or other salicylates.[1,5]

Many NSAIDs are now available, and most of these agents can cause some degree of gastrointestinal irritation. NSAIDs also are inhibitors of prostaglandin formation, platelet aggregation, and prothrombin synthesis. Most have the potential for cross-sensitivity in patients who exhibit an asthma-like reaction to aspirin. NSAIDs should not be given to certain patients with asthma, patients with an ulcer or hemorrhagic disease, and those who are pregnant or nursing. The new cyclooxygenase[12] (COX)-2 inhibitors that are now available cause much less gastrointestinal disturbance.[13] However, selective COX-2 inhibitors may cause renal dysfunction and elevated blood pressure, which, in turn, may precipitate heart failure in vulnerable patients. Although NSAID-related cardiotoxicity is relatively rare and is most commonly seen in elderly persons with concomitant disease, the widespread long-term use of these drugs in high-risk groups is potentially hazardous. The use of NSAIDs by high-risk patients is discouraged.

Codeine is a narcotic analgesic that commonly is used in dentistry. Emesis, nausea, and constipation may occur with analgesic doses of codeine. Miosis and adverse renal, hepatic, cardiovascular, and bronchial effects are not likely to occur with therapeutic doses. Most of the reported reactions to codeine consist of nonallergic gastrointestinal manifestations; nevertheless, these may be severe enough to preclude the use of codeine in certain patients. Alternate drug selections may be made after a drug Web site or current pharmacology text, such as *Physicians' Desk Reference* or *Accepted Dental Therapeutics,* is consulted.

Rubber Products. A number of reports have demonstrated that certain health care workers and patients are at risk for hypersensitivity reactions to latex or agents used in the production of rubber gloves or related materials (e.g., rubber dam, blood pressure cuff, catheters). Latex from surgical gloves has been known to cause cardiovascular collapse in surgical patients, anaphylaxis in physicians, hypersensitivity reactions in health care workers, and anaphylaxis in other patients. About 1% to 6% of the general public is latex-sensitive, whereas between 5% and 18% of health care providers are hypersensitive to latex. Although most cases in health providers are type IV reactions, caused by agents used in the production of rubber products, serious type I hypersensitivity reactions may occur in physicians, dentists, other health care workers, and patients as the result of contact with latex products such as gloves, rubber dam or catheters.[14]

Dentists should be aware that latex allergy can manifest as anaphylaxis during dental work when the patient or the dentist has been sensitized to latex. Anaphylaxis may occur in the sensitized person after contact has been made with rubber gloves, rubber dam material, blood pressure cuffs, or any other product containing latex. Studies have shown that latex-allergic persons have IgE antibodies for specific latex proteins. Latex skin tests are a satisfactory means of identifying individuals who may be sensitized to latex.[14,15] Nitrile gloves should be considered for use to minimize these adverse reactions to latex proteins.[16]

Dental Materials and Products. Type I, type III, and type IV hypersensitivity reactions have been reported to result from various dental materials and products. Topical anesthetic agents have been reported to cause type I reactions consisting of urticarial swelling. Mouth rinses and toothpastes containing phenolic compounds, antiseptics, astringents, or flavoring agents have been known to cause type I, type III, and type IV hypersensitivity reactions involving the oral mucosa or lips. Hand soaps used by dental care workers also have been reported as a cause of type IV reactions. Some of the dental agents that can lead to type IV hypersensitivity (contact stomatitis) include dental amalgam, acrylic, composite resin, nickel, palladium, chromium, cobalt, eugenol, rubber products, talcum powder, mouthwashes, and toothpastes.[14,15,17-20]

Hereditary Angioedema. Hereditary angioedema is a condition that can be provoked by dental surgery and trauma and is best managed by implementation of preventive measures. Androgens such as danazol and stanozolol, which increase hepatic production of C1 inhibitor, help to decrease the number and severity of attacks. Newer agents that include C1 inhibitor concentrate (Cinryze or Berinert) show benefit but are expensive.[21] Use of such preventive agents is important, because hereditary angioedema does not respond well to epinephrine or antihistamines.

Other Conditions. Allergic patients who are being treated with steroids should be managed as described in Chapter 15. Patients who have received an organ transplant should be managed as described in Chapter 21. The dental management of patients with asthma is concerned primarily with preventing severe asthma attacks from occurring in the dental office and dealing with an attack if it happens. In addition, certain important drug considerations must be applied in the management of these patients (see Chapter 7).[13]

Treatment Planning Modifications

The dentist should obtain from each patient a history of any allergic reactions. If a patient has a history of allergy to drugs or materials that may be used in dentistry, a clear entry should be made in the dental record, and any further contact with or use of the antigen(s) should be avoided in that patient. Most allergic patients can receive any indicated dental treatment so long as the antigen is avoided and precautions are taken for patients receiving steroids or have angioedema.

Oral Complications and Manifestations

Hypersensitivity

Type I Hypersensitivity. Oral lesions can be produced by type I hypersensitivity reactions. Atopic reactions to various foods, drugs, or anesthetic agents may occur within or around the oral cavity and usually characterized by urticarial swelling or angioedema (Figure 19-2). The reaction generally is rapid, with the lesion developing within a short time after coming into contact with the antigen. This painless, soft tissue swelling produced by transudate from the surrounding vessels may cause itching and burning. The lesion can be present for 1 to 3 days if untreated but will resolve spontaneously. Oral antihistamines should be given; oral diphenhydramine, 50 mg every 4 hours, is the recommended regimen. Treatment is provided for 1 to 3 days. Further contact with the antigen must be avoided (Box 19-21).[6,22]

Type III Hypersensitivity. Foods, drugs, or agents that are placed within the oral cavity can cause white, erythematous, or ulcerative lesions as determined by the presence of type III hypersensitivity or immune complex reactions. These lesions develop rather quickly, usually within a 24-hour period, after contact is made with the offending antigen. Some cases of aphthous stomatitis (Figure 19-3) may be caused by type III hypersensitivity, but most are related to immune dysfunction that has not been fully characterized.[23,24] Figure 19-4

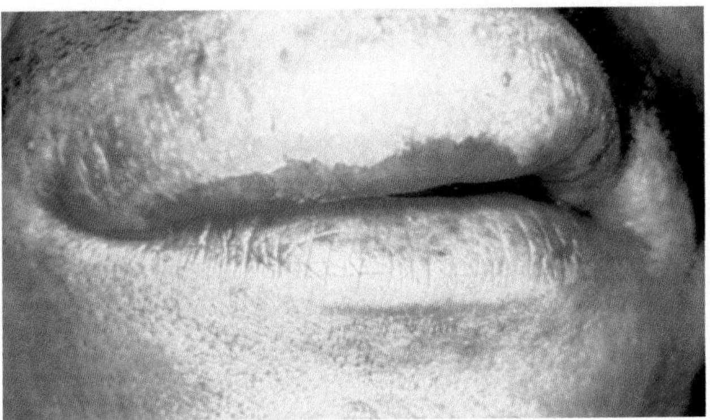

FIGURE 19-2 Angioedema of the upper lip that occurred soon after injection of a local anesthetic.

BOX 19-21 Oral or Paraoral Type I Hypersensitivity Reactions

1. Urticarial swelling (or angioedema)
   a. Reaction occurs soon after contact with antigen.
   b. Reaction consists of painless swelling.
   c. Itching and burning may occur.
   d. Lesion may remain for 1 to 3 days.
2. Treatment
   a. Reaction not involving tongue, pharynx, or larynx and with no respiratory distress noted requires 50 mg of diphenhydramine four times a day until swelling diminishes.
   b. Reaction involving tongue, pharynx, or larynx with respiratory distress noted requires the following:
      (1) 0.5 mL of 1:1000 epinephrine, IM or SC
      (2) Oxygen
      (3) Once immediate danger is over, 50 mg of diphenhydramine should be given four times a day until swelling diminishes.

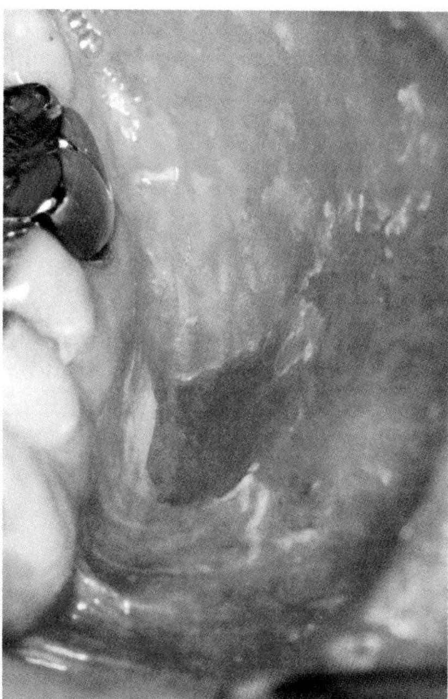

FIGURE 19-3 Stomatitis in a patient who was found to be allergic to the toothpaste he was using. *(From Neville BW, et al:* Oral and maxillofacial pathology, *ed 3, St. Louis, 2009, Saunders.)*

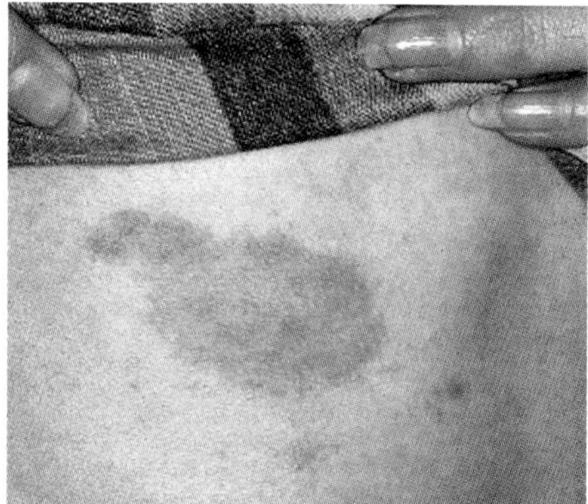

FIGURE 19-4 Allergic rash on the abdomen of a patient in whom orthodontic brackets and archwires were just placed. The patient was tested and was found to be allergic to the nickel in the wires.

shows an allergic dermatitis that occurred after orthodontic brackets and archwires (containing nickel) were placed. Hypersensitivity reactions to orthodontic appliances are rare and seldom occur unless the patient has nickel hypersensitivity and a history of previous cutaneous/skin piercing.[25]

Erythema multiforme represents an immune complex reaction that appears as polymorphous eruption of macules, erosions, and characteristic "target" lesions that are symmetrically distributed on the skin and/or mucosa. In about half of patients in whom erythema multiforme is diagnosed (Figure 19-5) a predisposing factor such as a drug allergy or a herpes simplex infection has been involved in the onset of their disease.[26] Sulfa antibiotics most commonly are associated with the onset of erythema multiforme. Sulfonyl urea hypoglycemic agents (e.g., tolbutamide, tolazamide, glyburide, glipizide), which are used to treat some patients with diabetes, have been found to be associated with the onset of erythema multiforme as well. Many patients with erythema multiforme can be treated with symptomatic therapy, including a bland mouth rinse, syrup of diphenhydramine, and triamcinolone acetonide (Kenalog) in Orabase. Patients with more severe involvement may require systemic steroids (see Appendix C for treatment regimens). If a drug appears to be associated with onset of the disease, the drug should be withdrawn and any further contact with it should be avoided. Box 19-22 summarizes oral type III hypersensitivity reactions.[5,14,19]

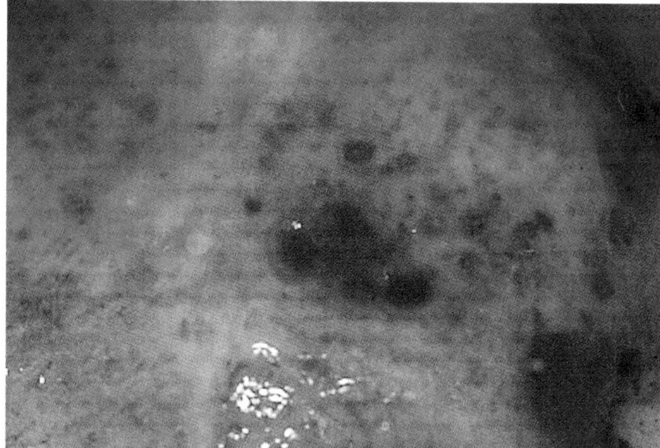

FIGURE 19-5 Erythema multiforme that developed after oral administration of a drug used to treat an oral infection. Ulceration of the palatal mucosa.

BOX 19-22 Type III Hypersensitivity Reactions

1. Usually occur within 24 hours after contact with antigen
2. Consist of:
   a. Erythema
   b. Rash
   c. Ulceration
3. Treatment requires
   a. Topical steroids or systemic steroids (in severe cases)
   b. Identification of antigen
   c. Avoidance/elimination of any further contact with antigen

Type IV Hypersensitivity. Contact stomatitis is a delayed allergic reaction that is associated with the cellular immune response in most cases. Because of the delayed nature of the reaction after contact is made with the allergen, the dentist must inquire about contacts with materials that may have occurred days before the lesions appeared. The antigen may be found in dental materials, toothpaste, mouth rinses, lipsticks, face powders, and so forth. In many cases, no further treatment is necessary once the source of the antigen has been identified and removed from further contact with the patient; however, if the tissue reaction is severe or persistent, topical corticosteroids should be used. A good preparation for topical use is triamcinolone acetonide in Orabase (see Appendix C for treatment regimens).[5,14,19]

Various dental materials have been reported as the cause of allergic reactions in patients. Impression materials containing an aromatic sulfonate catalyst have been reported to cause a delayed allergic reaction in postmenopausal women. The reactive lesion consisted of tissue ulceration and necrosis that became progressively worse with each exposure.[14,19]

Some investigators have reported that oral lesions may be found in close association with amalgam restorations. These (mucosal) lesions have been described as whitish, reddish, ulcerative, or "*lichenoid*" and were thought to be caused by toxic irritation or a hypersensitivity reaction to the silver amalgam restoration. When these restorations were removed, the lesions most often cleared. In some studies, skin testing for mercury sensitivity was performed. Reports have suggested that some of the oral lesions resulted from toxic injury to the mucosa, and others were a result of type IV hypersensitivity reaction to mercury in the amalgam.[27,28]

Several studies performed to date have not correlated symptoms such as depression, fatigue, and headache with the effects of mercury in amalgam restorations. The practice of avoiding the use of amalgam restorations in patients with these nonspecific symptoms has, at present, no scientific basis. However, removal of any amalgam restorations in contact with oral mucosa that shows lesions consistent with a toxic or hypersensitivity reaction to mercury is rational.[27,28]

On rare occasions, dental composite materials have been reported to cause allergic reactions. The acrylic monomer used in denture construction has caused an allergic reaction; however, the vast majority of tissue changes under dentures result from trauma and secondary infection with bacteria or fungi. Gold, nickel, and mercury have been reported to cause allergic reactions that result in tissue erythema and ulceration[19,20,22] (Figure 19-6).

The dentist may wish to test agents that are thought to be possible antigens that cause oral lesions. Oral epimucous testing for contact stomatitis consists of placing the suspected antigen in contact with the oral mucosa and observing for any reaction over a period of several days (e.g., erythema, sloughing, ulceration) that might indicate an allergy to the test material. In most cases, a reaction is not expected to develop for at least 48 to 72 hours. Various techniques have been used to conduct epimucous testing for suspected allergens. One of these involves placing the suspected allergen in a rubber suction cup, placing the cup on the buccal mucosa, and observing at intervals for erythema or ulceration under the cup. Another technique is to place a sample of the suspected antigen in a depression on the palatal aspect of an overlay denture. The denture is inserted and holds the allergen in contact with the palatal mucosa.

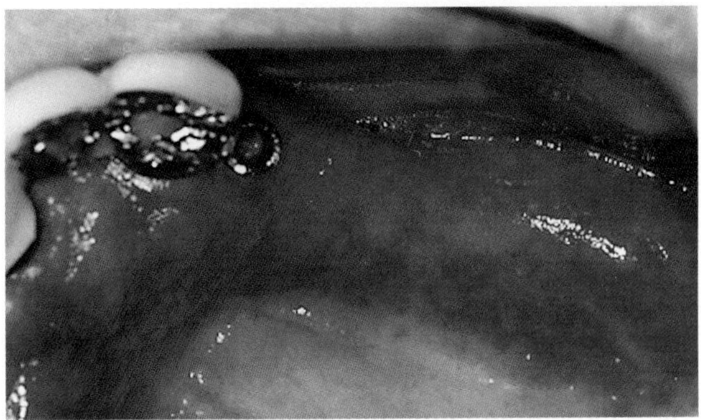

FIGURE 19-6 Allergic reaction to removable partial denture framework. Note the erythematous demarcation.

Another technique consists of incorporating the allergen into Orabase, applying Orabase in the mucobuccal fold, and periodically observing for a reaction. Alternately, the antigen can be incorporated into an oral adhesive spray. Skin testing and oral epimucous testing for potential antigens are not foolproof, by any means; in certain patients, they yield unreliable tissue responses. The response in some cases may be caused by trauma; in others, in which no tissue reaction occurs, the patient may still be allergic to the substance.

Basic management of contact stomatitis requires removal of common sources of antigens known to cause hypersensitivity reactions and assessment for lesion healing. Skin or mucosal testing for sensitivity also can be performed. Once the offending agent or antigen has been identified, the patient should be told to avoid any future contact with the antigen. Again, if the lesions persist, topical steroids can be applied (see Appendix C).

Lichenoid Drug Eruptions. Some patients with skin or oral lesions identical to those of lichen planus will be found to have taken certain drugs before appearance of the lesions. If these drugs are withdrawn, the lesions clear within several days (in most patients) or within a few weeks. The agents most commonly associated with the onset of lichenoid lesions are levamisole (Levantine) and the quinidine drugs. Other agents associated with such lesions are the thiazide drugs, gold, mercury, methyldopa, phenothiazines, quinidine, and certain antibiotics. Biopsy specimens of a lichenoid lesion show a microscopic picture similar to that seen in lichen planus, with the additional finding of eosinophils in the subepithelial infiltrate. These lesions are related to the cellular immune system and therefore could be categorized as a manifestation of contact stomatitis; however, the true nature of the reactions is not clear.

MANAGEMENT OF SEVERE TYPE I HYPERSENSITIVITY REACTIONS

Even when the dentist has taken appropriate precautions, an allergic reaction may occur. Most of these reactions are mild and of a nonemergency nature; however, some may be severe and life-threatening (anaphylactic). The dentist must be ready to deal with either type. In handling the anaphylactic reaction, the dentist should remember that it has an allergic origin. In other words, the reaction should occur soon (within minutes) after the injection, ingestion, or application of a topical anesthetic, medication, drug, local anesthetic, or dental product. The dentist must take the following actions immediately (see Appendix A):

- Place the patient in a head-down or supine position.
- Make certain that the airway is patent.
- Administer oxygen.
- Be prepared to send for help and to support respiration and circulation. The rate and depth of respiration should be noted, as should the patient's other vital signs. Most reactions in dental patients consist of simple fainting, which can be well managed by the preceding actions. In addition, the dentist may administer aromatic spirits of ammonia through inhalation, which encourages breathing through reflex stimulation.
- If these initial steps have not solved the emergency problem, and the cause is highly likely to be allergic, an edematous-type or anaphylactic reaction should be considered.

Angioedema. If an immediate type I hypersensitivity reaction has resulted in edema of the tongue, pharyngeal tissues, or larynx, the dentist must take additional emergency steps to prevent death from respiratory failure. At this point, if the patient has not responded to the initial procedures and is in acute respiratory distress, the dentist should do the following:

- Activate emergency medical service (EMS).
- Inject 0.3 to 0.5 mL of 1:1000 epinephrine by an intramuscular (into the tongue) or subcutaneous route.
- Supplement with intravenous diphenhydramine 50 to 100 mg if needed.
- Support respiration, if indicated, by mouth-to-mouth breathing or bag and mask; the dentist should make sure the chest moves when either of these methods is used.
- Check the carotid or femoral pulse; if a pulse cannot be detected, closed chest cardiac massage should be initiated.
- Confirm emergency medical service is on their way, and transport to medical facility if needed.

Anaphylaxis. An anaphylactic reaction usually takes place within minutes but may take longer. The signs and symptoms associated with anaphylactic reactions are listed in Box 19-23. In contrast with a severe edematous reaction, in which respiratory distress occurs first, both respiratory and circulatory components of depression occur early in the anaphylactic reaction. Anaphylaxis often is fatal unless vigorous, immediate action is taken. Because it occurs often within minutes after contact with the antigen, the dentist should take the following steps (Box 19-24):

BOX 19-23 Signs and Symptoms of Anaphylaxis

- "Itching" of soft palate
- Nausea, vomiting
- Substernal pressure
- Shortness of breath
- Hypotension
- Pruritus
- Urticaria
- Laryngeal edema
- Bronchospasm
- Cardiac arrhythmias

BOX 19-24 Anaphylaxis

Pathophysiologic Basis

1. First contact with antigen results in formation of antibodies by plasma cells.
2. Antibodies circulate in bloodstream (immunoglobulin E [IgE] antibodies).
3. Antibodies attach to target tissues (mast cells near smooth muscle of bronchi).
4. Next contact with antigen may result in combination of antigen with antibody.
5. Antigen-antibody complex causes degranulation of mast cell(s) with release of histamine.
6. Smooth muscle contracts and vessels lose fluid contributing to edema.
7. Acute respiratory distress and cardiovascular collapse may occur within minutes.

Management

1. Call for medical help.
2. Place patient in the supine position.
3. Check for open airway.
4. Administer oxygen.
5. Check pulse, blood pressure, and respiration.
   a. If any of the vital signs is depressed or absent, inject 0.3 to 0.5 mL 1:1000 epinephrine into the tongue.
   b. Provide cardiopulmonary resuscitation if needed.
   c. Repeat intramuscular injection of 0.5 mL 1:1000 epinephrine if no response.

- Have someone in the office call 911 or activate EMS.
- Place the patient in a supine position.
- Assess airway, breathing, circulation, and level of consciousness.
- Establish a patent airway and administer oxygen.
- Inject 0.3 to 0.5 mL of 1:1000 epinephrine by an intramuscular (into the tongue) or subcutaneous route.
- If no pulse is detected, support circulation through closed-chest cardiac massage. Support respiration by mouth-to-mouth breathing.
- Repeat the injection of epinephrine every 5 minutes as needed to control symptoms and blood pressure.

NOTE: Intramuscular injection of epinephrine into the thigh has been reported to provide higher plasma concentrations than those administered into the arm.[29]

REFERENCES

1. Kay AB: Allergy and allergic diseases. First of two parts, *N Engl J Med* 344:30-37, 2001.
2. Austen KF: Allergies, anaphylaxis and systemic mastocytosis. In Fauci AS, et al, editors: *Harrison's principles of internal medicine*, ed 17, New York, 2008, McGraw Medicine, pp 2061-2070.
3. Lichtenstein LM, Busse WW, Geha R, editors: *Current therapy in allergy, immunology, and rheumatology*, ed 6, St. Louis, 2004, Mosby.
4. Neugut AI, Ghatak AT, Miller RL: Anaphylaxis in the United States: an investigation into its epidemiology, *Arch Intern Med* 161:15-21, 2001.
5. Adkinson NF, et al: *Middleton's allergy: principles and practice*, ed 7, St. Louis, 2008, Mosby.
6. Malamed SF: Allergy and toxic reactions to local anesthetics, *Dent Today* 22:114-116, 118-121, 2003.
7. Yagiela JA, et al: *Pharmacology and therapeutics for dentistry*, ed 6, St. Louis, 2011, Mosby.
8. Ivy RS: Anesthetics and methylparaben, *J Am Dent Assoc* 106:302, 1983.
9. Shehab N, et al: Emergency department visits for antibiotic-associated adverse events, *Clin Infect Dis* 47:735-743, 2008.
10. Risk of anaphylaxis in a hospital population in relation to the use of various drugs: an international study, *Pharmacoepidemiol Drug Saf* 12:195-202, 2003.
11. Douglas GC, Karkos PD, Swift AC: Aspirin sensitivity and the nose, *Br J Hosp Med (Lond)* 71:442-445, 2010.
12. Cohen SH, et al: Clinical practice guidelines for *Clostridium difficile* infection in adults: 2010 update by the Society for Healthcare Epidemiology of America (SHEA) and the Infectious Diseases Society of America (IDSA), *Infect Control Hosp Epidemiol* 31:431-455, 2010.
13. Coke JM, Karaki DT: The asthma patient and dental management, *Gen Dent* 50:504-507, 2002.
14. Cullinan P, et al: Latex allergy. A position paper of the British Society of Allergy and Clinical Immunology, *Clin Exp Allergy* 33:1484-1499, 2003.
15. Hamann CP, DePaola LG, Rodgers PA: Occupation-related allergies in dentistry, *J Am Dent Assoc* 136:500-510, 2005.
16. AORN latex guideline, *AORN J* 79:653-672, 2004.
17. Hosoki M, et al: Assessment of allergic hypersensitivity to dental materials, *Biomed Mater Eng* 19:53-61, 2009.
18. Gawkrodger DJ: Investigation of reactions to dental materials, *Br J Dermatol* 153:479-485, 2005.
19. Pretorius E: Allergic reactions caused by dental restorative products, *SADJ* 57:372-375, 2002.
20. Kalimo K, Mattila L, Kautiainen H: Nickel allergy and orthodontic treatment, *J Eur Acad Dermatol Venereol* 18:543-545, 2004.
21. Three new drugs for hereditary angioedema, *Med Lett Drugs Ther* 52:66-67, 2010.
22. Maeda S, et al: Management of oral surgery in patients with hereditary or acquired angioedemas: review and case report, *Oral Surg Oral Med Oral Pathol Oral Radiol Endod* 96:540-543, 2003.
23. Chattopadhyay A, Shetty KV: Recurrent aphthous stomatitis, *Otolaryngol Clin North Am* 44:79-88, v, 2011.
24. Femiano F, et al: Guidelines for diagnosis and management of aphthous stomatitis, *Pediatr Infect Dis J* 26:728-732, 2007.
25. Kolokitha OE, Kaklamanos EG, Papadopoulos MA: Prevalence of nickel hypersensitivity in orthodontic patients: a meta-analysis, *Am J Orthod Dentofacial Orthop* 134:722e1-722e22, 2008.
26. Lamoreux MR, Sternbach MR, Hsu WT: Erythema multiforme, *Am Fam Physician* 74:1883-1888, 2006.
27. Issa Y, et al: Oral lichenoid lesions related to dental restorative materials, *Br Dent J* 198:361-366, 2005.
28. Koch P, Bahmer FA: Oral lesions and symptoms related to metals used in dental restorations: a clinical, allergological, and histologic study, *J Am Acad Dermatol* 41:422-430, 1999.
29. Lieberman P, et al: The diagnosis and management of anaphylaxis practice parameter: 2010 update, *J Allergy Clin Immunol* 126:477-480, e1-e42, 2010.

20

Rheumatologic and Connective Tissue Disorders

Rheumatologic (or rheumatoid) disease is much more than "arthritis" and encompasses a large group of disorders of the rheumatic diseases that affect bones, joints, and muscles.[1] Arthritis is a nonspecific term that means "inflammation of the joints." Often *arthritis* is used interchangeably with *rheumatism* or rheumatoid arthritis to denote aches, pains, and stiffness in the joints and muscles, but these terms are not synonymous. More than 100 rheumatologic (or rheumatoid) diseases affect various parts of the body. Some of the more common types include rheumatoid arthritis (RA), osteoarthritis (OA), systemic lupus erythematosus (SLE), juvenile rheumatoid arthritis (jRA), scleroderma (SD), Sjögren syndrome (SS), gout, ankylosing spondylitis, Lyme disease, giant cell arteritis (or temporal arteritis), fibromyalgia syndrome (FMS), and psoriatic rheumatoid arthritis (pRA).[1]

Rheumatologic (or rheumatoid) diseases have significant personal and economic impact. According to the Arthritis Foundation, more than 40 million Americans suffer from various forms of arthritis, and more than 8 million of them are disabled. In terms of its overall economic impact, arthritis costs the American economy more than $20 billion annually, and nearly 30 million workdays are lost per year.[1]

CATEGORIES OF MUSCULOSKELETAL DISEASES

Musculoskeletal diseases can be classified into nine categories, defined by the predominantly affected tissues, such as joint, synovium, cartilage, or connective tissues (Table 20-1). At each point in the evaluation (history, physical examination, and laboratory testing), it is important to ask what tissues are involved. Recognition of the pattern of predominant tissue involvement can direct attention toward the disease primarily associated with that tissue. Before consideration of clinical approaches to the evaluation of patients with musculoskeletal problems, it is useful to first review the anatomy and pathophysiology of the affected structures.[1]

Anatomy

The structures that are commonly involved in rheumatoid diseases include the joint, the joint cavity, synovial fluid, and periarticular structures. The lining membrane, known as the *synovium,* consists of a thin layer of macrophages (type A cells) and fibroblasts (type B cells) with a sublining of rich, vascular, loose connective tissue. Hyaline cartilage overlies the bony end plates and provides a cushion to joint motion. The cartilage has high water content and obtains its nutrition solely from the synovial fluid, which is derived from the synovium primarily as an ultrafiltrate of plasma. The synovium also secretes specialized molecules into the synovial fluid, such as hyaluronic acid. An intact bony end plate is required to support the cartilage. The joint capsule and ligaments provide further support and blend with the periosteum. Periarticular anatomy is equally important and includes the tendons, bursae, and muscles associated with each joint.[1]

Pathophysiology

The cause of musculoskeletal problems is usually inflammatory, metabolic, degenerative, tumor, or some combination thereof. Synovial inflammatory disorders, such as rheumatoid arthritis, begin in the synovium and secondarily damage the cartilage, joint capsule, and bone. Inflammation at entheses, the insertion sites of tendons or ligaments on bone, is characteristic of the spondyloarthropathies, such as ankylosing spondylitis. Crystal deposition disorders, such as gout or pseudogout, may also cause articular inflammation. Infections primarily involve the joint cavity (septic arthritis) or bone (osteomyelitis). The noninflammatory, degenerative disease osteoarthritis begins in the cartilage and leads to

TABLE 20-1 Classification of Musculoskeletal Diseases

Category	Prototype(s)	Useful Test(s)	Treatment(s)
Synovitis	Rheumatoid arthritis Autoimmune diseases	Rheumatoid factor, ESR Antinuclear antibody test	DMARDs and biologic agents Prednisone and immunosuppressive drugs
Enthesopathy	Ankylosing spondylitis and spondyloarthropathies	Sacroiliac radiographs	NSAIDs, MTX, and biologic agents
Crystal-induced synovitis	Gout CPPD (pseudogout)	Joint fluid crystal examination Radiographic chondrocalcinosis	NSAIDs NSAIDs
Joint space disease	Septic arthritis	Joint fluid culture	Antibiotics
Cartilage degeneration	Osteoarthritis	Radiographs of affected area	NSAIDs, analgesics, and physical therapy
Osteoarticular disease	Osteonecrosis	Radiographs, magnetic resonance imaging	Core decompression or prosthetic joint replacement
Inflammatory myopathy	Polymyositis Dermatomyositis Inclusion body myositis	Muscle enzymes, electromyography, muscle biopsy	Corticosteroids and immunosuppressive drugs
Local and regional conditions	Tendonitis or bursitis	Aspirate bursa if infection is suspected	Local injections
General conditions	Polymyalgia rheumatica Fibromyalgia	Elevated ESR Normal ESR	Corticosteroids Aerobic exercise, stretches, and sleep medications

Biologic agents include anti-tumor necrosis factor (anti-TNF) drugs and others.
CPPD, Calcium pyrophosphate crystal deposition disease; *DMARDs,* Disease-modifying antirheumatic drugs; *ESR,* Erythrocyte sedimentation rate; *MTX,* Methotrexate; *NSAIDs,* Nonsteroidal antiinflammatory drugs.

cartilage loss, subchondral new bone formation, and marginal bony overgrowth. Cartilage loss also may occur secondarily to synovial inflammation or trauma.[1] Osteonecrosis of bone may be associated with secondary cartilage damage after collapse of the bony end plate. Inflammatory diseases of the muscle usually manifest with painless proximal weakness. Periarticular inflammation may involve tendons or bursae, and these structures are common causes of pain and stiffness, often misinterpreted as arising from the joint itself. Finally, the common clinical problem of fibromyalgia (widespread muscle pain) is characterized by soft tissue pain with local tenderness in specific points but without abnormal blood studies.[1]

Although the rheumatologic diseases comprise a group of more than 100 important diseases, this chapter is limited to a discussion of eight: rheumatoid arthritis (RA), osteoarthritis (OA), psoriatic arthritis (PsA), systemic lupus erythematosus (SLE), Lyme disease, fibromyalgia (FMS), temporal arteritis, and Sjögren syndrome (SS), which are among the most common forms encountered, are more dentally related conditions, and can serve as models for the dental management of other forms. Several important items regarding the dental management of patients with rheumatologic and connective tissue disorders, including effects on the temporomandibular joint (TMJ), salivary glands, and oral mucosal tissues, organ and system involvement, and drug therapy, are discussed here.

RHEUMATOID ARTHRITIS

DEFINITION

Incidence and Prevalence

Rheumatoid arthritis (RA) is an autoimmune disease of unknown origin that is characterized by symmetric inflammation of joints, especially of the hands, feet, and knees. Severity of the disease varies widely from patient to patient and from time to time within the same patient. Prevalence is somewhat difficult to determine because of lack of well-defined markers of the disease; however, estimates range from 1% to 2% of the population. Disease onset usually occurs between ages 35 and 50 years. RA is more prevalent in women than in men by a 3:1 ratio.[1]

Etiology

The cause of RA is unknown; however, evidence seems to implicate an interrelationship of infectious agents, genetics, and autoimmunity. One theory suggests that a viral agent alters the immune system in a genetically predisposed person, leading to destruction of synovial tissues. Although the disease can occur within families, suggesting a genetic component, one specific causative gene has not been identified.[2-4] Nevertheless, many people who develop RA have a genetic predisposition that occurs in the form of a tissue marker called HLA-DR4; however, not everyone with this tissue type develops the disease.[2-5]

PATHOPHYSIOLOGY AND COMPLICATIONS

With RA, the fundamental abnormality involves microvascular endothelial cell activation and injury.[2-5] Primary changes occur within the synovium, which is the inner lining of the joint capsule (Figure 20-1). Edema of the synovium occurs, followed by thickening and folding. This excessive tissue, composed of proliferative and invasive granulation tissue, is referred to as *pannus*. In addition, marked infiltration of lymphocytes and plasma cells into the capsule occurs. Eventually, granulation tissue covers the articular surfaces and destroys the cartilage and subchondral bone through enzymatic activity (Figure 20-2). This process also extends to the capsule and ligaments, causing distention and rupture. New bone or fibrous tissue then is deposited, resulting in fusion or loss of mobility.[2-5]

A likely sequence of events begins with a synovitis that stimulates immunoglobulin G (IgG) antibodies. These antibodies form antigenic aggregates in the joint space, leading to the production of rheumatoid factor (autoantibodies). Rheumatoid factor then complexes with IgG complement, a process that produces an inflammatory reaction that injures the joint space.[2-5]

An associated finding in 20% of patients with RA is the presence of subcutaneous nodules, which are commonly found around the elbow and finger joints. These nodules are thought to arise from the same antigen-antibody complex that is found in the joint. Vasculitis confined to small- and medium-sized vessels also may occur and probably is caused by the same complex.[2-5]

RA is a pleomorphic disease with variable expression. The most progressive period of the disease occurs during the earlier years; thereafter, it slows. Onset is gradual in more than 50% of patients, and as many as 20% follow a monocyclic course that abates within 2 years. Another 10% experience relentless crippling that leads to nearly complete disability. The remainder follows a polycyclic or progressive course.[2-5] The long-term prognosis for people with abrupt onset of disease is similar to that for people with gradual disease onset. The course and severity of RA are unpredictable, but the disorder is characterized by remissions and exacerbations. For most patients, however, the disease is a sustained, lifelong problem that can be controlled or modified to allow a normal or nearly normal life.[2-5]

The life expectancy of persons with severe RA is shortened by 10 to 15 years. This increased mortality rate usually is attributed to infection, pulmonary and renal disease, and gastrointestinal bleeding.[2-5]

Many complications may accompany RA. Included among these are digital gangrene, skin ulcers, muscle atrophy, keratoconjunctivitis sicca (Sjögren syndrome), TMJ involvement, pulmonary interstitial fibrosis, pericarditis, amyloidosis, anemia, thrombocytopenia, neutropenia, and splenomegaly (Felty syndrome).[2-5]

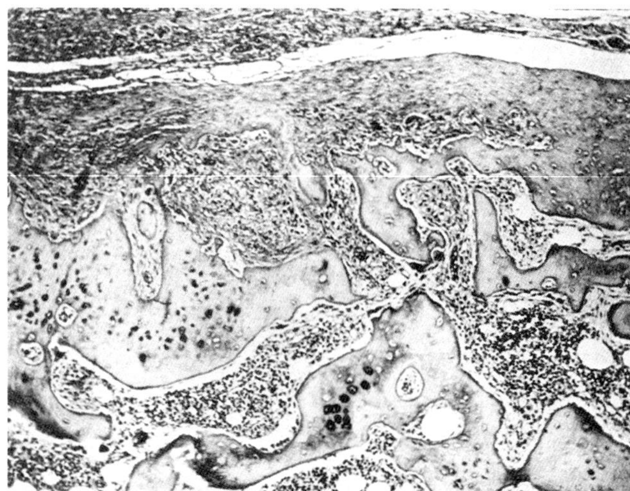

FIGURE 20-1 The joint surface (*top*) has lost its cartilage and consists of granulation tissue with scar tissue. Subchondral bone shows degenerative changes and areas of necrosis. *(Courtesy A. Golden, Lexington, Kentucky.)*

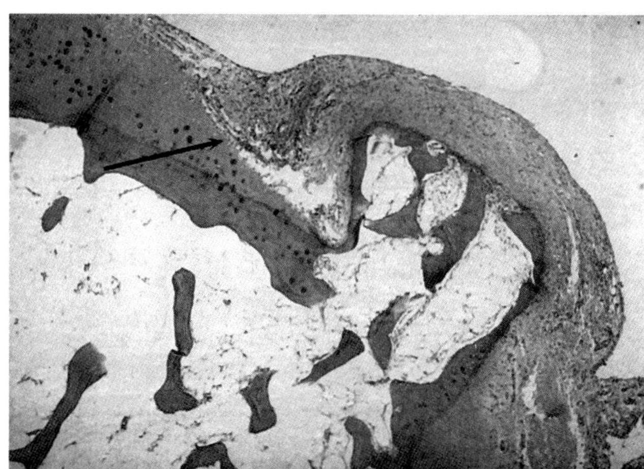

FIGURE 20-2 A micrograph of a pannus resulting from severe synovitis in rheumatoid arthritis. The pannus is eroding articular cartilage and bone (*arrow*). *(Courtesy Richard Estensen, MD, Minneapolis, Minnesota.)*

CLINICAL PRESENTATION

Signs and Symptoms

The usual onset of RA is gradual and subtle (Table 20-2), and the disorder is commonly preceded by a prodromal phase of general fatigue and weakness with joint and muscle aches. Characteristically, these symptoms come and go over varying periods. Then, painful joint swelling, especially of the hands and feet, occurs in several joints and progresses to other joints in a symmetric fashion (Figure 20-3). Joint involvement persists and

TABLE 20-2 Comparison of Rheumatoid Arthritis and Osteoarthritis

Rheumatoid Arthritis	Osteoarthritis
Multiple symmetric joint involvement	Usually one or two joints (or groups) involved
Significant joint inflammation	Joint pain usually without inflammation
Morning joint stiffness lasting longer than 1 hour	Morning joint stiffness lasting less than 15 minutes
Symmetric, spindle-shaped swelling of proximal interphalangeal joints and volar subluxation of metacarpophalangeal joints and Bouchard's nodes of proximal interphalangeal joints	Heberden's nodes of distal interphalangeal joints
Systemic manifestations (fatigue, weakness, malaise)	No systemic involvement

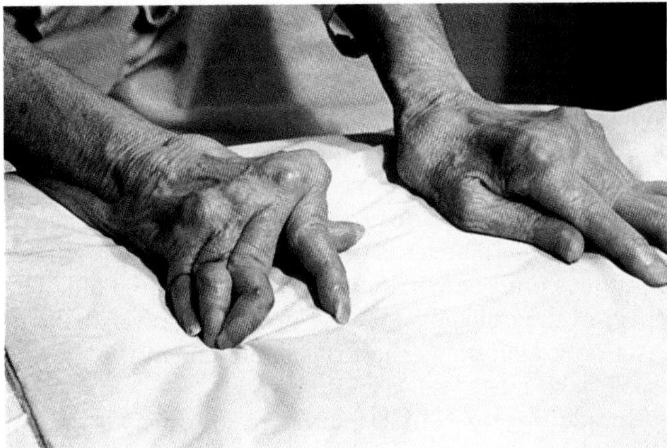

FIGURE 20-3 Hands of a patient with advanced rheumatoid arthritis. *(From Damjanov I:* Pathology for the health professions, *ed 4, St. Louis, 2012, Saunders.)*

gradually progresses to immobility, contractures, subluxation, deviation, and other deformities. Characteristic features include pain in the affected joints aggravated by movement, generalized joint stiffness after inactivity, and morning stiffness that lasts longer than 1 hour. The joints most commonly affected are fingers, wrists, feet, ankles, knees, and elbows. Multiple joint changes noted in the hands include a symmetric spindle-shaped swelling of the proximal interphalangeal (PIP) joints, with dorsal swelling and characteristic volar subluxation of the metacarpophalangeal (MCP) joint (see Figure 20-3). The TMJ is reported to be involved in up to 75% of patients.[2-6] Because of the variable rate of progression and pain intensity, the median period between onset of symptoms of RA and its diagnosis is 36 weeks.[1,7]

Extraarticular manifestations include rheumatoid nodules, vasculitis, skin ulcers, Sjögren syndrome, interstitial lung disease, pericarditis, cervical spine instability,

BOX 20-1 Criteria for the Diagnosis of Rheumatoid Arthritis*

- Morning stiffness
- Arthritis of three or more joint areas
- Arthritis of hand joints
- Symmetric arthritis
- Rheumatoid nodules
- Serum rheumatoid factor
- Radiographic changes

*At least four must be present for a diagnosis of rheumatic arthritis.
Adapted from Arnett FC, et al: The American Rheumatism Association 1987 revised citeria for the classification of rheumatoid arthritis, Arthritis Rheum *31:315-324, 1988.*

entrapment neuropathies, and ischemic neuropathies.[8] The American Rheumatism Association has developed revised criteria for the diagnosis and classification of RA to be used in clinical trials and epidemiologic studies (Box 20-1). These criteria have high specificity (89%) and sensitivity (91% to 94%) compared with control subjects when used to classify patients with RA. For the diagnosis of RA to be made, four of seven criteria must be met.[2-5]

Laboratory Findings

No laboratory tests are pathognomonic or diagnostic of RA, although they are used in conjunction with clinical findings to confirm the diagnosis. Laboratory findings most commonly seen in RA include an increased erythrocyte sedimentation rate (ESR), the presence of C-reactive protein (CRP), a positive result on rheumatoid factor assay in 85% of affected patients, and a hypochromic microcytic anemia. In patients with Felty syndrome (RA with splenomegaly), a marked neutropenia may be present.[2-5]

Antibodies to cyclic citrullinated proteins (CCPs) are autoantibodies, which are important in the diagnosis of RA.[9] Anti-CCP antibodies are highly associated with RA. They occur in 70% to 80% of patients with RA as well as in some other forms of inflammatory arthritis. These antibodies may appear before any signs or symptoms of RA and therefore may prove beneficial as early screening markers for earlier diagnosis and intervention of RA.[9]

Diagnosis

The American College of Rheumatology has established criteria for the diagnosis of RA (see Box 20-1), the classification of severity by radiography, functional classes, and the definition of remission. Although they were not designed for managing individual patients, these criteria are useful as a frame of reference and for describing clinical phenomena.[1,10]

By definition, the diagnosis of RA cannot be made until the disease has been present for at least several weeks. Many extraarticular features of RA, the characteristic symmetry of inflammation, and the typical serologic findings may not be evident during the first month or two after disease onset. Therefore, the diagnosis of RA usually is presumptive early in its course.

Although extraarticular manifestations may dominate in some patients, documentation of an inflammatory synovitis is essential for a diagnosis. Inflammatory synovitis can be documented by demonstration of synovial fluid leukocytosis, defined as white blood cell (WBC) counts greater than 2000/μL, histologic evidence of synovitis, or radiographic evidence of characteristic erosions.[5-7,9,10]

MEDICAL MANAGEMENT

The treatment approach to RA is, by necessity, palliative because no cure as yet exists for the disease. The ultimate aim of management is to achieve disease remission for the patient. Remission is elusive, however, so more practical treatment goals are to reduce joint inflammation and swelling, relieve pain and stiffness, and facilitate and encourage normal function.[8] These goals are accomplished through a basic treatment program that consists of patient education, rest, exercise, physical therapy, and aspirin or other nonsteroidal antiinflammatory drugs (NSAIDs).[2-5]

When an understanding of the determinants of disease outcome is acquired, a treatment strategy that will be useful and acceptable to the individual patient can be devised. These determinants include presence of rheumatoid factor, early onset of severe synovitis with functional limitation, joint erosions, persistent elevation of ESR or CRP, presence of extraarticular manifestations, and a family history of severe RA.[11,12]

The major goals of therapy are to relieve pain, swelling, and fatigue; improve joint function; stop joint damage; and prevent disability and disease-related morbidity. These goals are constant throughout the disease course, although emphasis may shift to address specific patient needs. For example, some patients with advanced joint damage experience minimal swelling or constitutional symptoms and benefit most from physical therapy, joint reconstruction, and pain control. Most patients, however, require continued efforts to control the inflammatory process through disease-modifying therapy.[1,12]

Drugs for the management of RA have been traditionally, but imperfectly, divided into two groups: those used primarily for the control of joint pain and swelling, and those intended to limit joint damage and improve long-term outcome (Table 20-3). Symptoms of pain and swelling in RA are mediated, at least in part, by intense cytokine activity. NSAIDs inhibit proinflammatory prostaglandins and are effective treatments for pain, swelling, and stiffness, but they have no effect on the disease course or on risk of joint damage. On the other hand, antiinflammatory properties have been noted for several disease-modifying antirheumatic drugs (DMARDs), which are used principally to control disease and to limit joint damage.[2-5] These drugs include methotrexate and biologic response modifiers with actions targeted against specific cytokines, such as tumor necrosis factor-α (TNF-α). Corticosteroids are powerful, nonspecific inhibitors of cytokines and, in some studies that compared them with placebo, are reported to effectively delay joint erosion.[1-7]

NSAIDs, especially aspirin, constitute the cornerstone of treatment. Aspirin may be prescribed in large doses on an individual basis. A common approach is to start a patient on three 5-grain tablets four times a day, then to adjust the dosage on the basis of patient response. The most common sign of aspirin toxicity is tinnitus. Should this occur, dosage is decreased. In addition to aspirin, many NSAIDs are available for use (see Table 20-3). Some of the more common NSAIDs include cyclooxygenase (COX)-2 inhibitors, namely, celecoxib (Celebrex); ibuprofen (Motrin, Advil, Rufen, Nuprin); naproxen (Naprosyn, Aleve); sulindac (Clinoril); tolmetin (Tolectin); fenoprofen (Nalfon); piroxicam (Feldene); diclofenac (Voltaren); flurbiprofen (Ansaid); diflunisal (Dolobid); etodolac (Lodine), and nabumetone (Relafen).[1-7]

All NSAIDs can cause a qualitative platelet defect that may result in prolonged bleeding, especially when given in high doses. The effects of aspirin are irreversible for the life of the platelet (10 to 12 days); thus, this effect continues until new platelets have replaced the old. The effect of the other NSAIDs on platelets is reversible and lasts only as long as the drug is present in the plasma (see Chapter 24).[1-7]

In addition to NSAIDs, a variety of other drugs can be used to treat patients with RA (see Table 20-3). Many of these drugs cause blood dyscrasias that may lead to more frequent infection, delayed healing, and prolonged bleeding.[1-7]

DMARDs, which commonly are employed in the treatment of patients with RA, are classified in various groups, each of which consists of multiple drugs (e.g., antimalarial agents, penicillamine, gold compounds) (see Table 20-3).[1-7] Conventional DMARDs include methotrexate, sulfasalazine, hydroxychloroquine, leflunomide, and gold injections. These drugs can be helpful in slowing down the damaging component of the disease process; however, the precise modes of action are still subject to research. The optimal sequencing of DMARDs remains a source of debate, and whether patients should be started on combinations of therapies or a single DMARD is also contentious.[8]

Gold compounds may be effective in decreasing inflammation and retarding the progress of the disease, but the incidence of associated toxicity is high, and dermatitis with mucosal ulceration, proteinuria, neutropenia, and thrombocytopenia may result. Antimalarial drugs (e.g., chloroquine, hydroxychloroquine) are also used to treat

TABLE 20-3 Drugs Used in the Management of Rheumatoid Disorders and Systemic Lupus Erythematosus

Drug(s) (Trade Name)	Dental and Oral Considerations
Salicylates	
Aspirin, Ascriptin, Bufferin, Anacin, Ecotrin, Empirin	Prolonged bleeding but not usually clinically significant
Nonsteroidal Antiinflammatory Drugs (NSAIDs)	
Ibuprofen (Motrin), fenoprofen (Nalfon), indomethacin (Indocin), naproxen (Naprosyn), meclofenamate (Meclomen), piroxicam (Feldene), sulindac (Sulindac), tolmetin (Tolectin), diclofenac (Voltaren), flurbiprofen (Ansaid), diflunisal (Dolobid), etodolac (Lodine), nabumetone (Relafen), oxaprozin, ketorolac	Prolonged bleeding but not usually clinically significant; oral ulceration, stomatitis
Cyclooxygenase (COX)-2 Inhibitors	
Celecoxib Rofecoxib	None
Tumor Necrosis Factor-α Inhibitors	
Etanercept Infliximab	None
Injectable Glucocorticoids	
Triamcinolone hexacetonide Triamcinolone acetonide Prednisolone tebutate Methylprednisolone acetate Dexamethasone acetate Hydrocortisone acetate Triamcinolone diacetate Betamethasone sodium phosphate and acetate Dexamethasone sodium phosphate Prednisolone sodium phosphate	Adrenal suppression, masking of oral infection, impaired healing
Systemic Glucocorticoids	
Hydrocortisone, cortisone, prednisone, prednisolone, dexamethasone, methylprednisolone (Deltasone, Meticorten, Orasone, Articulose-50, Delta-Cortef, Medrol)	Adrenal suppression, masking of oral infection, impaired healing
Disease-Modifying Antirheumatic Drugs (DMARDs)	
Antimalarial Agents	
Hydroxychloroquine, quinine, chloroquine (Plaquenil)	None
Penicillamine	
Cuprimine, Depen	None
Gold Compounds	
Gold sodium thiomalate (Auranofin), aurothioglucose (Myochrysine Ridaura, Solganal)	Increased infections, delayed healing, prolonged bleeding, oral ulcerations
Aralen	Increased infections, delayed healing, prolonged bleeding, glossitis, stomatitis
Sulfasalazine	
Azulfidine	Increased infections, delayed healing, prolonged bleeding, intraoral pigmentation
Immunosuppressives	
Azathioprine, cyclophosphamide	Increased infections, delayed healing, prolonged bleeding
Methotrexate, cyclosporine, chlorambucil (Imuran, Cytoxan, Rheumatrex)	Increased infections, delayed healing, prolonged bleeding, stomatitis

patients with RA; they are usually given in combination with aspirin or corticosteroids.[1-7] Adverse effects include severe eye damage and blue-black intraoral pigmentation. Penicillamine also is used in the treatment of patients with RA. Both the antimalarials and penicillamine, however, are associated with significant toxicity—a fact that limits their use. Corticosteroids (e.g., prednisone, prednisolone) frequently are useful in controlling acute symptoms; however, because of multiple adverse effects, long-term usage is avoided if possible. One of the more potentially significant associated adverse effects is secondary adrenal suppression (see Chapter 15).[1,3,7]

In cases of refractory disease, immunosuppressive therapy has been used successfully and may include methotrexate, cyclophosphamide, or azathioprine. These drugs may produce significant adverse effects, including severe oral ulceration. Methotrexate also may cause hepatic toxicity. COX-2 inhibitors and TNF-α inhibitors have recently proved effective in relieving the symptoms of RA (see Table 20-3). Although COX-2 inhibitors (e.g., celecoxib [Celebrex][1,13]) have shown considerable efficacy in relieving inflammatory pain associated with RA, problems have been reported with these agents, and myocardial infarction has occurred in patients who have used these treatments over the long term.[1-7] Celebrex carries with it warnings regarding potential heart problems that are provided to long-term users. Standard NSAIDs inhibit both cyclooxygenases (COX-1 and COX-2)—the enzymes involved in production of prostaglandins. Whereas COX-2 is active on demand, COX-1 is critical for normal cellular function.[1] A complication that may result from the use of NSAIDs for arthritis (and other conditions) is the adverse effect of gastrointestinal distress. Because COX-2 inhibitors are selective for this enzyme, they produce fewer gastrointestinal adverse effects.[1-7] As treatment options for RA become more effective and more complex, greater attention will be paid to the costs of drug treatments and associated adverse effects with respect to disease control and remission. Drugs that improve the long-term outcomes of disease will be prescribed more frequently, and efforts will be made to limit the use of NSAIDs in persons who are coping with joint pain and swelling.[1-7]

A group of drugs have been developed, labeled "biologic," because they consist of monoclonal antibodies and soluble receptors that specifically modify the disease process by blocking key protein messenger molecules (such as cytokines) or cells (such as B lymphocytes). The development of biologic drugs has been based on an increasing understanding of the disease process. The key drivers of RA include cytokines such as TNF-α, interleukin 1 (IL-1), and interleukin 6 (IL-6). An IL-1 receptor antagonist called anakinra had been appraised by the National Institute for Health and Clinical Excellence (NICE) and rejected for use in the National Health Service as not being cost-effective.[8]

The newer biologic agents etanercept and infliximab (and other TNF-α inhibitors) have been shown to be highly effective in the treatment of patients with early rheumatoid arthritis relative to the "gold standard" agent, methotrexate.[1-7] Although costly and difficult to administer (requiring an injectable route), etanercept (e.g., Enbrel, Immunex) has been shown to significantly reduce symptoms of RA and to more effectively slow joint damage when compared with methotrexate. Likewise, infliximab (Remicade), which also is costly and requires administration by the intravenous route, when used with methotrexate significantly reduced RA symptoms and slowed joint damage to a greater extent than that achieved with methotrexate therapy alone. Although these biologic agents are novel and show great promise, they have had limited widespread use in RA therapy.[1-7]

Combination Therapies

In people with moderate to severe disease activity, methotrexate often is used in combination with other agents.[1-7] In patients who have acute and severe disease, initial therapy often consists of a combination of DMARDs, corticosteroids, and NSAIDs. Combinations of DMARDs also are used to improve disease control; approximately 50% of people with RA who are treated by rheumatologists are prescribed combination therapies with two or three DMARDs. The combination of methotrexate, hydroxychloroquine, and sulfasalazine is among the most popular regimens, although study results are not readily duplicated among prescribing physicians.[1-7] Other successful combination therapies include methotrexate used with such agents as cyclosporine, TNF-α antagonists, leflunomide, and azathioprine.[1-7] Surgical management of severely deformed or dysfunctional joints often is necessary and may involve a variety of procedures, including arthroplasty, reconstruction, synovectomy, and total joint replacement.[1-7]

Clinical tools for monitoring the patient's well-being and the efficacy of therapy include self-assessment of the duration of morning stiffness and severity of fatigue, as well as functional, social, emotional, and pain status, as measured by a health assessment questionnaire. A patient-derived global assessment based on a visual analog scale is a simple and effective means of recording patient well-being. The number of tender and swollen joints is a useful measure of disease activity, as is the presence of anemia, thrombocytosis, and elevated ESR or CRP. Serial radiographs of target joints, including the hands, are useful in assessing disease progression.[1,7]

Patient education is essential early in the disease course and on an ongoing basis. Patients are best served by a multidisciplinary approach with early referral to a rheumatologist and other specially trained medical personnel, including nurses, counselors, and occupational and physical therapists who are skilled and knowledgeable about RA. Appropriate medical care of patients with RA encompasses attention to smoking cessation, immunizations, prompt treatment of infections, and management of comorbid conditions such as diabetes, hypertension, and osteoporosis.[1,7]

DENTAL MANAGEMENT

Medical Considerations

Because patients may have multiple joint involvement with varied degrees of pain and immobility, dental appointments should be kept as short as possible, and the patient should be allowed to make frequent position changes as needed (Box 20-2). The patient also may be more comfortable in a sitting or semisupine position, as opposed to a supine one. Physical supports, such as a pillow or a rolled towel, may be used to provide support for deformed limbs, joints, or neck.

The most significant complications associated with RA are drug-related (see Table 20-3). Aspirin and other NSAIDs can interfere with platelet function and cause prolonged bleeding; however, this effect generally is not found to be of clinical significance. A patient who is taking both aspirin and a corticosteroid may be at greater risk for bleeding. The risk is not great, however, and patients usually can be treated, so long as curettage or surgery is performed conservatively in small segments, with attention to good techniques (see Chapter 24).[14-16]

Patients who are taking gold salts, penicillamine, sulfasalazine, or immunosuppressive agents are susceptible to bone marrow suppression, which can result in anemia, agranulocytosis, and thrombocytopenia. As a rule, these patients should be followed closely by their physician for detection of this problem. If a patient has not undergone recent laboratory testing, a complete blood cell count with a differential white blood cell count should be ordered. Abnormal results should be discussed with the physician. If corticosteroids are used for prolonged periods, the potential for adrenal suppression exists. Management of this problem is discussed in Chapter 15. Corticosteroids may induce a number of adverse effects, which are presented in Table 20-3.

Prosthetic Joints. A potential long-term complication of chronic rheumatoid arthritis (also osteoarthritis[14] and other types, including fractures that do not heal and avascular necrosis) is the ultimate destruction of particular joint structures to the degree that the joint must be replaced with synthetic materials. Patients with prosthetic joints (most commonly, hip and knee replacement, followed by shoulder, elbow, wrist, and ankle) often are encountered in dental practice; when this occurs, a question arises concerning the need for antibiotic prophylaxis to prevent infection of the prosthesis. This is a legitimate

BOX 20-2 Dental Management
Considerations in Patients with Rheumatoid Disorders

P

Patient Evaluation/Risk Assessment (see Box 1-1)
- Evaluate and determine whether rheumatoid or joint disorder exists.
- Obtain medical consultation if disease is poorly controlled or undiagnosed, or if the diagnosis is uncertain.

Potential Issues/Factors of Concern

A	
Analgesics	If patient is taking aspirin or another NSAID or acetaminophen, be aware of dosing and the possibility that pain may be refractory to some analgesics; dosing and/or analgesic choices may need to be modified in consultation with the physician.
Antibiotics	Provide antibiotic prophylaxis in accordance with ADA (2003) guidelines (see Boxes 20-3 and 20-4).
Anesthesia	No issues.
Anxiety	No issues.
Allergy	Allergic reactions or lichenoid reactions are possible in patients taking many medications.
B	
Bleeding	Excessive bleeding may occur if major surgery performed on patients who take aspirin or other NSAIDs. Bleeding usually is not clinically significant and can be controlled with local hemostatic measures.
Blood pressure	No issues.
C	
Chair position	Ensure comfortable chair position. Consider shorter appointments and use supports as needed (e.g., pillows, towels).
D	
Devices	Patients who have a prosthetic joint replacement should be managed according to ADA (2003) guidelines (see Boxes 20-3 and 20-4).
Drugs	Obtain blood cell count with differential if surgery is planned for patients taking gold salts, penicillamine, antimalarials, or immunosuppressives. If patient is taking corticosteroids—secondary adrenal suppression is possible (see Chapter 15).
E	
Equipment	No issues.
Emergencies	If surgery is performed, supplemental techniques may be necessary to control bleeding.
F	
Follow-up	Routine follow-up evaluation is appropriate.

ADA, American Dental Association; *NSAIDs,* Nonsteroidal antiinflammatory drug.

concern; however, whether bacteremia resulting from dental procedures can cause prosthetic joint infection (PJI) is the primary issue. This issue has been debated for many years, although scientific data for decision making are lacking. Recommendations to place dental patients on prophylactic antibiotics have been made empirically by orthopedic surgeons, although little evidence suggests that dentally induced bacteremia may cause PJI.[15]

Although reports in the literature weakly associate PJI with dentally induced bacteremia, authors have questioned the validity of these reports. It appears that wound contamination or skin infection is the source of the vast majority of infections.[15] Even the few cases of PJI caused by presumably oral bacteria were more likely to result from physiologically occurring bacteremia or bacteremia caused by acute or chronic infection than from invasive dental procedures.[15]

Unfortunately, however, many orthopedic surgeons have persisted in requesting that patients continue to receive antibiotic prophylaxis for all dental procedures.[16-18]

In an effort to clarify the issue, in 1997 and updated in 2003, an advisory statement made jointly by the American Dental Association (ADA) and the American Academy of Orthopedic Surgeons (AAOS) was published.[19] The 2003 advisory statement concluded that scientific evidence does not support the need for antibiotic prophylaxis for dental procedures to prevent late prosthetic joint infection (LPJI). It further stated that antibiotic prophylaxis is not indicated for dental patients with pins, plates, and screws, nor is it routinely indicated for most patients with total joint replacement. The statement did indicate, however, that antibiotic prophylaxis can be considered for patients whose joint replacement has been in place for less than 2 years and for patients at increased risk for infection who are undergoing invasive dental procedures (see Box 20-3). No evidence suggests that even these patients are at increased risk for infection from dentally induced bacteremia, and in fact, the microbiology of LPJI in these patients is the same in other patients with LPJI.[17]

A more appropriate interpretation is that these patients are at increased risk for LPJI from the usual sources such as wound contamination and acute infection from distant sites. The advisory statement also is clear that the final decision on whether to provide antibiotic prophylaxis lies with the dentist, who must weigh perceived potential benefits against risks. The advisory statement provides suggested antibiotic regimens, should the practitioner elect to provide antibiotic prophylaxis (see Box 20-4).[19]

In 2009 the AAOS published an information statement that added a great deal of confusion to the dental management of patients with joint replacements. Antibiotic prophylaxis was suggested for all patients with joint replacements for dental procedures that produced bacteremia. This statement was made without input from the ADA and appeared to negate the 2003 advisory statement of the ADA and AAOS.[16]

In 2010 the American Academy of Oral Medicine (AAOM) published a position paper in the *Journal of the American Dental Association* (JADA).[20] It strongly recommended that the ADA, AAOS, and the Infectious Disease Society of America (IDSA) meet to develop evidence-based recommendations for the dental management of patients with joint replacements. Until this occurs, the AAOM position paper recommended three options for the dentist when dealing with patients with joint replacements regarding antibiotic prophylaxis:

1. Informed consent
2. Base clinical decisions on the 2003 ADA/AAOS consensus statement
3. Consultation with the patient's orthopedic surgeon to recommend following the 2003 guidelines until a new joint consensus statement is approved. If the orthopedist elects to recommend antibiotic prophylaxis for a patient who would not receive it on the basis of the 2003 guidelines, the orthopedist can write the prescription for the desired antibiotic.[20]

BOX 20-3 High-Risk Patients with Prosthetic Joints

Immunocompromised/Immunosuppressed Patients
- Inflammatory arthropathies: rheumatoid arthritis; systemic lupus erythematosus; disease-, drug-, or radiation-induced immunosuppression

Other Patients
- Insulin-dependent (type 1) diabetes
- First 2 years after joint replacement
- Previous prosthetic joint infections
- Malnourishment
- Hemophilia

BOX 20-4 Suggested Antibiotic Prophylaxis Regimens

Patients Not Allergic to Penicillin: Cephalexin, Cefradine, or Amoxicillin
2 g orally 30 minutes to 1 hour before the dental procedure

Patients Not Allergic to Penicillin and Unable to Take Oral Medications: Cefazolin or Ampicillin
Cefazolin 1 g *or* ampicillin 2 g intramuscularly or intravenously 30 minutes to 1 hour before the dental procedure

Patients Allergic to Penicillin: Clindamycin
600 mg orally 30 minutes to 1 hour before the dental procedure

Patients Allergic to Penicillin and Unable to Take Oral Medications: Clindamycin
600 mg intravenously 30 minutes to 1 hour before the dental procedure

In November 2010 the ADA, AAOS, and IDSA began a series of meetings with the goal of developing an evidence-based recommendation for the dental management of patients with joint replacements. The process was estimated to take about 1 year. Until this recommendation is available, then, the dentist should consider one of the options suggested in the AAOM position paper.

A study that should have a great influence on the future recommendations of the ADA, AAOS, and IDSA was reported from the Mayo Clinic. The investigators concluded that dental procedure bacteremias were not associated with the onset of LPJIs and that antibiotic prophylaxis did not prevent PJIs.[21]

Treatment Planning Modifications

Treatment planning modifications are dictated by the patient's physical disabilities. A patient with marked systemic disability or limited or painful jaw function due to TMJ involvement should not be subjected to prolonged or extensive treatment, such as complicated crown and bridge procedures. If replacement of missing teeth is desired, consideration should be given to fabrication of a removable prosthesis because of the decreased chair time needed for mouth preparation and the ease of cleaning of the appliance. If a fixed prosthesis is desired, the realistic potential to keep it clean must be a significant factor in design. Unpredictable, progressive, or abrupt changes in occlusion are possible because of erosion of the condylar head. Therefore, the dentist and the patient should take these potential occlusal changes into consideration when considering significant reconstructive treatment.

Disabled patients may have significant difficulty cleaning their teeth. Cleaning aids such as floss holders, toothpicks, irrigating devices, and mechanical toothbrushes may be recommended. Manual toothbrushes can be modified by placement of an acrylic or rubber ball on the handle to improve the grip.

RA is a progressive disease that ultimately may lead to severe disability and crippling in some patients, which can make providing dental care difficult. Therefore, the dentist should be aggressive in providing ongoing preventive care and should attempt to identify and treat or eliminate potential problems before the disease progresses.

Oral Complications and Manifestations

The most significant complication of the oral and maxillofacial complex in RA is TMJ involvement, which is found in up to 45% to 75% of patients with RA. This may present as bilateral preauricular pain, tenderness, swelling, stiffness, and decreased mobility of the TMJ, or it may be asymptomatic. Periods of remission and exacerbation may occur, as with other joint involvement. Fibrosis or bony ankylosis can occur. Clinically, patients may present with tenderness over the lateral pole of the condyle, crepitus, limited opening, and radiographic evidence of structural change. Radiographic changes initially may show increased joint space due to inflammation in the joint. Later, these inflammatory changes progress to erosive degenerative changes and changes in size and shape of the joint and can involve both the condyles and the fossa.[5,6,22-24]

A particularly disturbing event is the development of an anterior open bite, caused by destruction of the condylar heads and loss of condylar height (Figure 20-4). This sudden retrognathia and anterior open bite can be severe and has been reported to cause obstructive sleep apnea. Although palliative treatment such as interocclusal splints, physical therapy, and medication may prove to be helpful, surgical intervention often

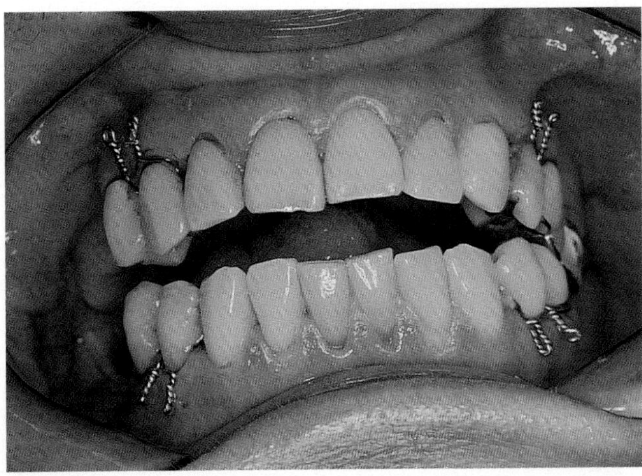

A

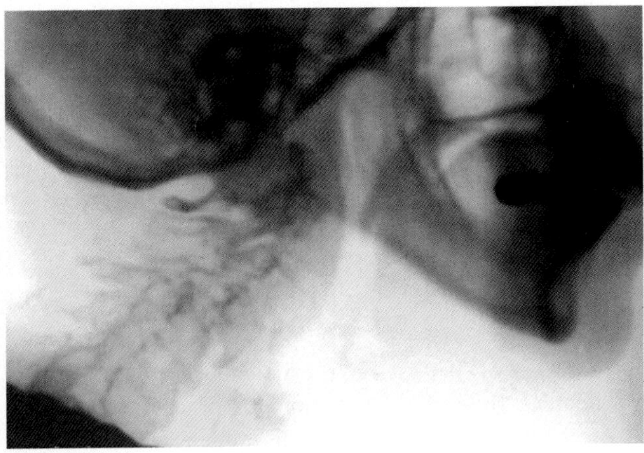

B

FIGURE 20-4 **A,** Anterior open bite resulting from progressive bilateral condylar resorption in a patient with advanced rheumatoid arthritis. **B,** Lateral skull film shows a swan-neck deformity. *(From Quinn PD: Color atlas of temporomandibular joint surgery, St. Louis, 1998, Mosby.)*

becomes necessary to decrease pain, improve appearance, or restore function.[5,6,22-24]

There is some recent evidence that patients with RA have a higher incidence of periodontal disease.[25-30]

An additional complication that may be seen in patients with RA is severe stomatitis that occurs after the administration of drugs such as gold compounds, penicillamine, or immunosuppressive agents.[23,30,31] Stomatitis may be an indication of drug toxicity and should be reported to the physician. Treatment for this problem should include consideration for changing the offending drug, and palliative mouth rinses, diphenhydramine elixir, or a topical emollient such as Orabase (see Appendix C).

OSTEOARTHRITIS

DEFINITION

Another of the rheumatic diseases, osteoarthritis (OA), also called degenerative joint disease, is the most common form of arthritis. Almost everyone older than 60 years of age develops OA to some degree.[32] Most affected persons are minimally symptomatic; however, approximately 17 million people in the United States have OA to the extent that it results in pain. OA is the leading cause of disability within the elderly population.[30]

OA, which is considered a regional disease, usually affects often-used joints such as hips, knees, feet, spine, and hands. The TMJ also is affected. Women are afflicted twice as often as men; however, men are afflicted at an earlier age. It is generally a disease of middle to older age, first appearing after the age of 40. Racial differences have been noted in the prevalence of OA and in the pattern of joint involvement.[33]

Etiology

Although the exact cause of OA is not known, it has been thought to result from normal wear and tear on joints over a long period. However, other factors are now believed to be of significance. Preexisting structural joint abnormalities, intrinsic aging, metabolic factors, genetic predisposition, obesity leading to overloaded joints, and macrotrauma or microtrauma are considered causative or contributory factors in the origin of the disease.[33]

Pathophysiology and Complications

In early stages of the disease, the articular cartilage actually becomes thicker than normal, and water content and the synthesis of proteoglycans are increased. This reflects a repair effort by the chondrocytes and may last for several years. Ultimately, however, the joint surface thins and proteoglycan concentration decreases, leading to softening of the cartilage. Progressive splitting and abrasion of cartilage down to the subchondral bone occur. The exposed bone becomes polished and sclerotic, resembling ivory (eburnation). Some resurfacing with cartilage may occur if the disorder is arrested or stabilized. New bone forms at the margin of the articular cartilage in the non–weight-bearing part of the joint, creating osteophytes (or spurs), often covered by cartilage, that augment the degree of deformity.[33]

In contrast with RA, OA has a more favorable prognosis and less serious complications, depending on the joint or joints involved. The two most important complications associated with OA are pain and disability. Although RA is a more serious disease, OA has a 30-fold greater economic impact, resulting in 68 million lost workdays per year compared with 2 million for RA. Conservative treatment often can retard the progress of the disease; however, surgery may be required to restore function and reduce pain.[33]

CLINICAL PRESENTATION

Signs and Symptoms

The primary symptom of OA is pain localized to one or two joints (see Table 20-2). The pain is described as a dull ache accompanied by stiffness that is typically worse in the morning or after a period of inactivity. The pain and stiffness usually last no longer than 15 minutes. Joint noises or grinding sounds (crepitus) may be detected with movement. Redness and swelling usually are not associated with OA.[32]

The most common sign of OA is appearance of painless bony growths on the medial and lateral aspects of the proximal interphalangeal joints, called Heberden's nodes. When these enlargements occur on the distal interphalangeal joints, they are called Bouchard's nodes (Figure 20-5). On occasion, some pain may be associated with these nodes.[32]

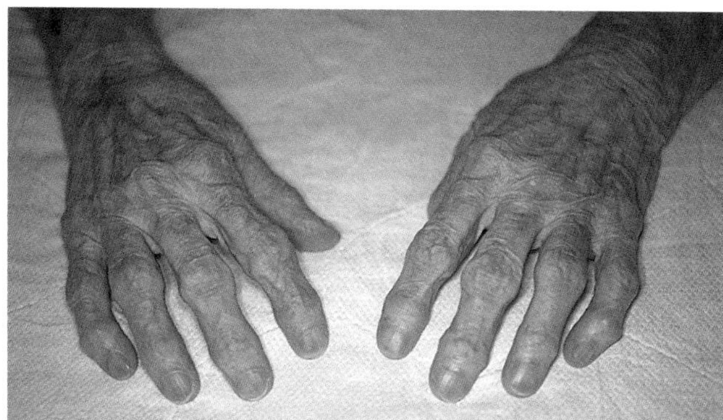

FIGURE 20-5 Heberden's nodes and Bouchard's nodes in osteoarthritis. *(From Swartz MH:* Textbook of physical diagnosis: history and examination, *ed 6, Philadelphia, 2010, Saunders.)*

Depending on which joint or group of joints is involved, patients may experience varying degrees of incapacitation. Hip and knee joints are particularly troublesome and are a common source of disability.

One form of OA, called *primary generalized osteoarthritis,* is characterized by involvement of three or more joints or groups of joints. It occurs most often in women and affects hands, knees, hips, and spine.[32]

Radiographic signs of OA include narrowing of the joint space, articular surface irregularities and remodeling, and osteophytes or spurs. In addition, subchondral sclerosis (eburnation) and ankylosis may be seen. Symptoms often are not well correlated with radiographic signs.[32]

Laboratory Findings

Laboratory findings in OA are essentially unremarkable. The ESR usually is normal, except for a mild elevation in primary generalized cases.[32]

MEDICAL MANAGEMENT

The management of OA is palliative. For the most part, drug therapy is limited to analgesics. Acetaminophen frequently is effective in the management of OA and is recommended as a first-line drug. Aspirin or NSAIDs also are commonly employed when acetaminophen is not effective. Narcotic analgesics are generally used only for acute flares for short periods. Intra-articular steroid injections also may be used for acute flares for short periods. Intra-articular steroid injections may be used intermittently to reduce acute pain and inflammation. Patient education, physical therapy, mild exercise, weight reduction, and joint protection are all important aspects of management. Surgery, including joint replacement, may be required to improve function or relieve pain.[33]

DENTAL MANAGEMENT

Medical Considerations

Depending on which joints are involved, patients may not be comfortable in a supine position in the dental chair. Consideration should be given to providing a more upright chair position, using neck, back, and leg supports, and scheduling short appointments (see Box 20-2). Decreased platelet function caused by large doses of aspirin or other NSAIDs can lead to prolonged bleeding, but this is generally not a clinically significant problem (see Chapter 24).

Adrenal suppression generally is not a concern with occasional intra-articular injections of steroids (see Chapter 15). Patients with OA may also have a joint prosthesis and the same guidelines should apply as with prosthetic joint replacement with RA. These patients usually do not require antibiotic prophylaxis for dental treatment except for the first 2 years or unless a concomitant condition, such as diabetes mellitus, exists, or the patient is otherwise immune suppressed. If antimicrobial prophylaxis is considered, please refer to Box 20-4 for suggested regimens.[20,33]

Treatment Planning Modifications

As with RA, the technical modifications of dental treatment for OA are dictated by the patient's disabilities. For instance, severe disabilities of the hip, knee, or other joint or TMJ involvement may prevent lengthy appointments; therefore, extensive treatment such as reconstruction or a long surgical procedure may not be appropriate. In patients with TMJ OA and restricted range of motion and inflammation, dental providers should not open the mouth too wide or for too long a period of time, as dictated by the patient's level of tolerance. Patients with hand disabilities may have difficulty cleaning their teeth, and aids such as floss holders or electric toothbrushes may be helpful. Modified toothbrush handles also are recommended to facilitate cleaning.

Oral Complications and Manifestations

The TMJ may be affected by OA, and this may constitute a problem for the patient. Figure 20-6 shows osteoarthritic changes in the TMJ.

As would be expected, most people older than 40 years of age show some degree of histologic and radiographic change in the TMJ, but most have no symptoms. Occasional TMJ pain caused by OA has been reported. The usual finding in patients with OA of the TMJ is insidious onset of unilateral preauricular aching and pain with stiffness after a period of inactivity that decreases with mild activity. Severe pain may be elicited on wide

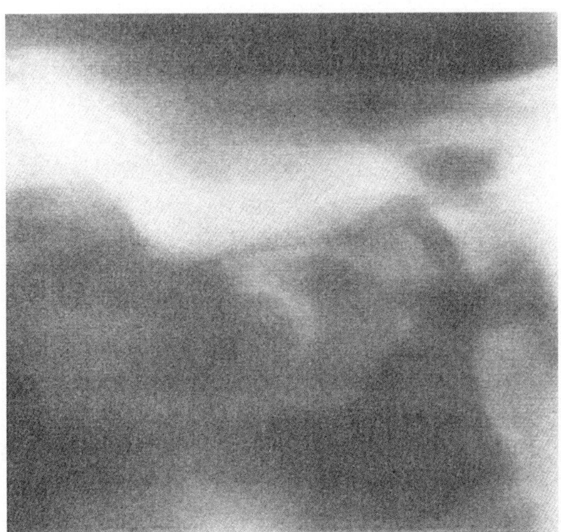

FIGURE 20-6 Osteoarthritic changes in the temporomandibular joint.

opening, and pain occurs with normal function and worsens during the day. Adjacent muscle splinting and spasm may occur. Crepitus is a common finding in the affected joint. In most cases, osteoarthritic pain in the TMJ resolves within 8 months of onset. Radiographic changes include decreased joint space, sclerosis, remodeling, and osteophytes (see Figure 20-6). No correlation exists between TMJ symptoms and radiographic or histologic signs of OA.[7]

In the past, uncertainty was expressed about the relationship between disk displacement and OA. Reports of a 30-year longitudinal study have provided evidence that, for patients with reducing anterior disk displacement, about a 50% chance exists that no progression of the disorder will occur, nor will any significant radiographic changes happen in the TMJ hard or soft tissue structures. For the remaining 50%, progression to nonreducing disk displacement or dislocation (closed lock) is likely. These patients may experience a period of variable pain and dysfunction, but it appears to be self-limiting in most patients. Also, 86% of patients with nonreducing disks demonstrate significant radiographic changes in the condyle and fossa on plain films, along with disk changes on magnetic resonance imaging (MRI). These changes occur rapidly during the first 3 years; then, a stable, persistent, quiescent period is attained. Thus, most patients with disk displacement, whether reducing or nonreducing, can be treated successfully with conservative, reversible therapies.[34]

Treatment of OA of the TMJ consists of acetaminophen, aspirin or NSAIDs, muscle relaxants, approaches to limit jaw function, physical therapy (heat, ice, ultrasound, controlled exercise), and occlusal splints to decrease joint loading. Conservative therapy is successful in controlling symptoms in most cases; however, should pain or dysfunction be severe and persistent, TMJ surgery may be necessary.[34]

PSORIATIC ARTHRITIS

DEFINITION

Epidemiology

Psoriatic arthritis (PsA) develops in 5% to 7% of patients with psoriasis.[35] Although most cases arise in patients with established cutaneous disease, some patients (particularly children) have arthritis that antedates the appearance of the skin lesions. Although the extent of psoriatic skin disease correlates poorly with the development of arthritis, the risk for PsA increases with a family history of rheumatoid arthritis. The age at onset can range from 30 to 55 years, with an equal predilection for women and men. Psoriatic spondylitis has a slight male preponderance.[35]

Pathophysiology

The genetic associations with PsA are complex. Psoriasis itself is associated with HLA-B13, HLA-B16, HLA-B17, and HLA-Cw6. By contrast, HLA-B39 and HLA-B27 have been associated with sacroiliitis and axial involvement.[35,36] No etiologic agent has been proved in PsA, although some investigators have proposed that the disease process represents rheumatoid arthritis in response to cutaneous bacteria. The histopathology of the synovitis of PsA is comparable to that of the other SpAs, with the absence of local production of immunoglobulin and rheumatoid factor being differentiating features from RA. There is the potential for aggressive osteolysis, fibrous ankylosis, and heterotopic new bone formation to occur in PsA. As mentioned earlier, the coexistence of human immunodeficiency virus (HIV) and PsA seems to set the stage for an aggressive course of joint destruction in some patients.[35,36]

Diagnosis

PsA has a variable manifestation and disease course, but several clinical patterns have been identified in prospectively monitored cohorts of patients. The clinical subsets are not mutually exclusive, nor are they static over time. The most common form, in which 30% to 50% of patients are affected, is an asymmetric oligoarthritis that may involve both large and small joints.[35,36] Dactylitis, arising as sausage digits, can be seen in fingers and toes and actually represents an enthesitis. In the second subset there is selective targeting of the distal interphalangeal joints, seen in 10% to 15% of patients. These changes are strongly associated with nail dystrophy, of which the features are onycholysis, subungual keratosis, pitting, and oil drop–like staining (Figure 20-7).[35,36] The third subset (15% to 30% of patients) has a symmetric polyarthritis that mimics RA in many ways except for the

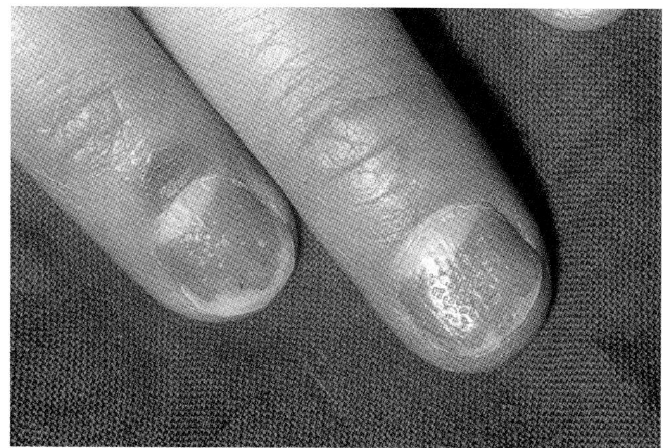

FIGURE 20-7 Nail pitting in a patient with psoriatic arthritis. *(From Goldman L, Ausiello D, editors:* Cecil textbook of medicine, *ed 23, Philadelphia, 2008, Saunders.)*

absence of rheumatoid nodules and rheumatoid factor. The fourth clinical variant is psoriatic spondylitis, which occurs in 20% of patients; 50% of such patients are B27-positive. Finally, arthritis mutilans (5% of patients) is a destructive, erosive arthritis that affects large and small joints. It can be associated with marked deformities and significant disability.[35,36] Figure 20-7 shows nail pitting in psoriasis. The pits are more discrete and regular compared with pits affecting the nail plate in dermatitis.[35,36] Radiographic changes in PsA involve soft tissue swelling (particularly in the case of dactylitis), erosions, and periostitis. Axial involvement may lead to the appearance of asymmetric sacroiliitis with syndesmophytes that are bulky, asymmetric, and nonmarginal. The classic "pencil-in-cup" deformity may be seen in patients with distal interphalangeal joint disease or arthritis mutilans. Acroosteolysis is noted in a minority of patients and reflects an aggressive erosive process.[35,36]

MEDICAL MANAGEMENT

Recently, a new drug for the management for psoriatic arthritis has proved in clinical trials to be an effective treatment. Abatacept selectively inhibits T cell activation via competitive binding to CD80 or CD86 and decreases serum levels of cytokines and inflammatory proteins implicated in the pathogenesis of PsA. Abatacept is an approved treatment for chronic inflammatory conditions such as RA and juvenile idiopathic arthritis, in which T cells are involved in the pathophysiologic progression of the disease. In a phase 3 study of abatacept in patients with psoriasis, clinical improvement was associated with a reduction of the severity in patients with PsA.[37]

DENTAL MANAGEMENT

Dental management for PsA is very similar to that for RA and is reviewed in Box 20-2. The exception may be the skin involvement as well as the choice and/or combination of immunosuppressive drugs. Therefore, the dentist must make a careful assessment of the severity of disease and medical management of the patient's condition.

Depending on which joints are involved, patients may not be comfortable in a supine position in the dental chair. Consideration should be given to providing a more upright chair position, using neck, back, and leg supports, and scheduling short appointments (see Box 20-2). Decreased platelet function caused by large doses of aspirin or other NSAIDs can lead to prolonged bleeding, but this generally is not a clinically significant problem (see Chapter 24).

Adrenal suppression may be a concern with high doses of corticosteroids. Patients with PsA usually do not require antibiotic prophylaxis for dental treatment unless a concomitant condition, such as diabetes mellitus, exists, or the patient is otherwise immune suppressed. If this is the case, consideration of antimicrobial prophylaxis with cephalosporin or clindamycin as the drug of choice is recommended.

TREATMENT PLANNING MODIFICATIONS

As with RA, the technical modifications of dental treatment for PsA are dictated by a patient's disabilities and the immunosuppressive drugs. For instance, severe disabilities of the hip, knee, or other joint or TMJ involvement may prevent lengthy appointments; therefore, extensive treatment such as reconstruction or a long surgical procedure may not be appropriate. Patients with hand disabilities may have difficulty cleaning their teeth, and aids such as floss holders or electric toothbrushes may be helpful. Battery-operated toothbrushes and/or modified toothbrush handles are recommended to facilitate cleaning.

GIANT CELL ARTERITIS

DEFINITION

Giant cell arteritis (GCA) is a systemic vasculitis involving medium-sized and large arteries, most commonly the extracranial branches of the carotid artery. GCA (temporal arteritis) is the most common form of vasculitis. This inflammatory disorder affects women more often than men (as do most autoimmune diseases), almost exclusively after 50 years of age, and the average age is 72 years. Histologically, GCA is represented by a mononulcear cell infiltrate of T cells and macrophages which penetrates through the wall of arteries (typically the temporal artery) (Figure 20-8). Approximately 50% to 60%

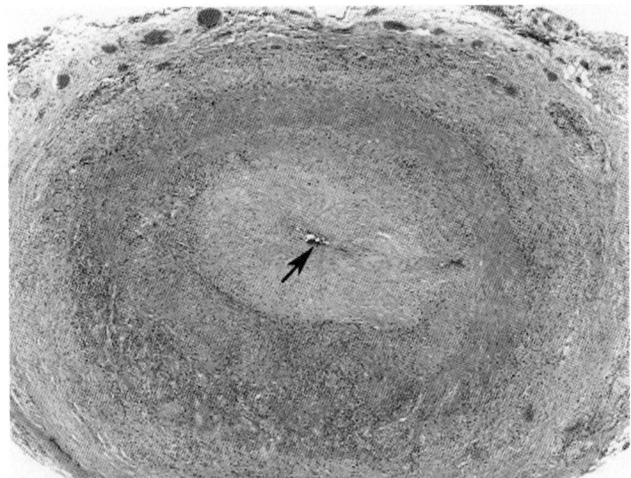

FIGURE 20-8 Histology of giant cell arteritis (GCA). A typical temporal artery affected by GCA shows characteristics such as panmurla mononuclear inflammatory infiltrate, destruction of the internal and external elastic laminae, and concentric intimal hyperplasia. *(From Albert DM, et al:* Albert & Jakobiec's principles & practice of ophthalmology, *ed 3, Edinburgh, 2008, Saunders.)*

of patients with GCA also have polymyalgia rheumatica.[38,39] Because of the occlusive nature of the narrowing of vascular lumen, cranial pain, blindness, transient ischemic attacks (TIAs), and other strokes are common complications in patients with GCA.[39]

Symptoms and signs of GCA (Box 20-5) include excessive sweating, fever, malaise, anorexia, headaches and scalp tenderness, muscle aches (including muscles of mastication), and jaw pain. Obviously, these manifestations are very similar to those of temporomandibular disorders and orofacial pain conditions.[39]

Figure 20-8 illustrates the histologic appearance of GCA. A typical temporal artery affected by GCA shows characteristics such as panmural mononuclear inflammatory infiltrate, destruction of the internal and external elastic laminae, and concentric intimal hyperplasia.[39]

Unfortunately, there are no specific laboratory tests for GCA. Typically, patients will exhibit a high ESR and CRP, but of course, these values are nonspecific. Recently, serum IL-6 has been shown to relate to GCA, but the values also are elevated in other autoimmune diseases as well. Angiography (particularly magnetic resonance angiography [MRA]) is valuable in making the diagnosis.[39]

BOX 20-5 Signs and Symptoms of Giant Cell Arteritis

Commonly Reported Signs and Symptoms

- Excessive sweating
- Fever
- General ill feeling
- Jaw pain, intermittent or when chewing
- Loss of appetite
- Muscle aches
- Throbbing headache on one side of the head or the back of the head
- Scalp sensitivity, tenderness when touching the scalp
- Vision difficulties
  - Blurred vision
  - Double vision
  - Reduced vision (blindness in one eye)
- Weakness, excessive tiredness
- Weight loss (more than 5% of total body weight)

Other, Less Common Signs and Symptoms

- Bleeding gums
- Face pain
- Hearing loss
- Joint stiffness
- Joint pain
- Mouth sores

About 40% of people will have other, nonspecific symptoms such as respiratory complaints (most frequently dry cough) or weakness or pain along many areas. Rarely, paralysis of eye muscles may occur. A persistent fever may be the only symptom.

DIAGNOSIS AND DENTAL IMPLICATIONS

From a dental perspective, GCA is significant for several reasons. Major manifestations are temporal headaches and jaw claudication.[38] Additionally, orofacial manifestations of GCA can lead to misdiagnosis of GCA as temporomandibular disorder. GCA should be included in the differential diagnosis for orofacial pain in elderly persons on the basis of knowledge of related signs and symptoms including masticatory muscle pain, hard "end-feel" limitation of range of motion, and temporal headache.[39]

TREATMENT

The universal treatment for GCA is glucoccortioid therapy. Prednisone (60 mg per day) is the usual initial therapy. Once the immune response has subsided and symptoms diminish, the prednisone may be reduced by 10% per week. However, therapy may need to be resumed when symptoms return. Adjunctive therapy with aspirin also is quite helpful. The primary rationale for aspirin therapy is to reduce ischemic events in the obstructed vessels.[39]

Giant Cell Arteritis Misdiagnosed as Temporomandibular Disorder. The orofacial manifestations of giant cell arteritis frequently may be misdiagnosed as temporomandibular disorder. Early diagnosis and treatment are essential to avoid severe complications. GCA should be included in the differential diagnosis of orofacial pain in the elderly based on the knowledge of related signs and symptoms, mainly jaw claudication, hard end-feel limitation of range of motion, and temporal headache.[38,40]

SYSTEMIC LUPUS ERYTHEMATOSUS

Definition

There are two types of lupus erythematosus (LE): discoid (DLE), which predominantly affects the skin, and a more generalized systemic form (SLE), which affects multiple organ systems. DLE is characterized by chronic, erythematous, scaly plaques on the face, scalp, or ears. Most patients with DLE have very few systemic manifestations, and the course tends to be benign. SLE involves the skin and many other organ systems and is the more serious form.[42] This section focuses only on SLE.

Incidence and Prevalence

SLE is a prototypical autoimmune disease that predominantly affects women of childbearing age, with a female-to-male ratio of 5 : 1; it is more common and more severe among African Americans and Hispanics than among whites.[41,42] A defining feature of SLE is the almost invariable presence in the blood of antibodies directed against one or more components of cell nuclei; certain manifestations of the disease are associated with the presence of one or more of these different antinuclear antibodies.[41,42]

Etiology

The etiology of SLE is unknown, although it is clearly an autoimmune disease. A strong familial aggregation exists, with a much higher frequency noted among first-degree relatives of patients. Studies of patients with SLE suggest that the disease is caused by genetically determined immune abnormalities that can be triggered by exogenous and endogenous factors. Among these triggering factors are infectious agents, stress, diet, toxins, drugs, and sunlight.[41,42]

Pathophysiology and Complications. The production of pathogenic antibodies and immune complexes and their deposition with resultant inflammation and vasculopathy is the basic abnormality that underlies SLE. Antibodies are formed in response to some antigenic stimulus, and the reaction between antigen and circulating antibodies forms antigen-antibody complexes, which are deposited in a wide variety of tissues and organs, including the kidney, skin, blood vessels, muscles and joints, heart, lung, brain, gastrointestinal tract, lymphatics, and eye. Clinical expression of the disease reflects the organs or tissues involved and the extent of that involvement.[41,42]

Despite advances in diagnosis and management, complications attributable to SLE or its treatment continue to cause substantial morbidity. Of reported hospitalizations for SLE, one third occurred because of neurologic or psychiatric involvement; infection, coronary artery disease, and osteonecrosis were other major reasons.[41,42]

Several studies have documented substantial improvement in the survival of patients with SLE, with 5-year survival rates of 90% or greater and 10-year survival rates of more than 80%. The leading causes of death in patients with SLE are infectious complications and clinical manifestations related to lupus itself, such as acute vascular neurologic events, renal failure, and cardiovascular or pulmonary involvement.[41,42]

CLINICAL PRESENTATION

Signs and Symptoms

Because of the widespread systemic involvement of SLE, multiple manifestations are observed in many tissues and organs. Although malaise, overwhelming fatigue, fever, and weight loss are nonspecific manifestations that affect most patients at some time in their disease course, the classic picture of SLE is that of a woman with polyarthritis and a butterfly-shaped rash across the nose and cheeks (Figure 20-9). The presentation of SLE, however, varies widely from mild to severe and depends largely on the extent and selection of organ involvement.[41,42]

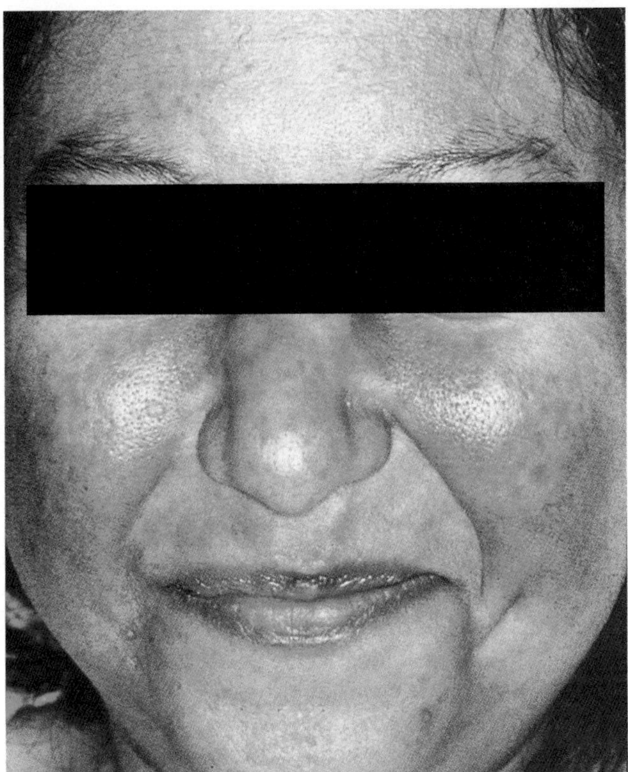

FIGURE 20-9 Female patient with butterfly-shaped rash of systemic lupus erythematosus. *(From Ignatavicius D, Workman ML: Medical-surgical nursing: patient-centered collaborative care, ed 6, St. Louis, 2010, Saunders.)*

Arthritis, the most common manifestation of SLE, is seen in as many as 76% of patients. It affects the small joints and is migratory, and the pain typically is out of proportion to the signs. The classic butterfly rash of the nose and cheeks is found in only about one third of patients with SLE; a rash on the upper trunk or areas of exposed skin is more common. Recurrent noninfectious pharyngitis and oral ulcerations also are common.[41,42]

Serious renal abnormalities occur in less than one third of patients with SLE, although most show some abnormality on renal biopsy. Renal failure, one of the most serious problems, is the best clinical indicator of a poor prognosis.[41,42]

Neuropsychiatric symptoms are common and include organic brain syndrome, psychosis, seizures, stroke, movement disorders, and peripheral neuropathy. Thromboembolism associated with antiphospholipid antibody is an important cause of abnormalities in the central nervous system.[41,42]

Pulmonary manifestations include pleuritis, infection, pulmonary edema, pneumonitis, and pulmonary hypertension. Cardiac involvement is common and consists of pericarditis, myocarditis, endocarditis, and coronary artery disease. Valvular abnormalities can be identified by echocardiography in 25% of patients but rarely result in serious valvular dysfunction. However, Libman-Sacks endocarditis (nonbacterial verrucous endocarditis) is found at autopsy in 50% of patients with SLE. Unfortunately, this is not always demonstrated by echocardiography or by clinical examination findings.[41,42]

A clinically detectable heart murmur found in 18.5% of patients required further investigation for determination of its significance. Approximately 4% of patients had cardiac valve abnormalities that placed them in the moderate risk group for endocarditis.[41,42] However, no cases demonstrated a relationship between endocarditis and SLE. On the basis of 2007 American Heart Association guidelines, none of these patients are recommended for antibiotic prophylaxis for invasive dental procedures (see Chapter 2).

Laboratory Findings

The antinuclear antibody test is the best screening test for SLE because it yields a positive result in 95% of patients.[41,42] A positive result also occurs in patients with other rheumatic diseases. Results of anti-DNA assays—double helix and single helix—also are elevated in 65% to 80% of patients with active untreated SLE.[41,42]

Hematologic abnormalities include hemolytic anemia, leukopenia, lymphopenia, and thrombocytopenia. Leukopenia in SLE usually is not associated with recurrent infection. Autoimmune thrombocytopenia occurs in as many as 25% of patients with SLE and may be severe in 5% of patients. Patients with severe thrombocytopenia are at risk for bleeding spontaneously or after trauma. This event is rare, however, if the platelet count is greater than 50,000/μL.[41,42]

A variety of clotting abnormalities may be seen; the most common of these is the lupus anticoagulant, which is associated with elevated partial thromboplastin time (PTT). This can indicate the presence of antiphospholipid antibodies. These antibodies may be useful in the diagnosis of SLE but are not 100% accurate and can result in false-positive results. This can result in thromboembolic events rather than increased bleeding, and invasive surgery may be performed without correction of this laboratory abnormality. The ESR often is elevated, but this does not reflect disease activity. With active nephritis, proteinuria is present, as are hematuria and cellular or granular casts. Other abnormalities include false-positive results on serologic tests for syphilis.[41,42]

MEDICAL MANAGEMENT

No cure for SLE is known; thus, all treatment is of a symptomatic or palliative nature. Patients with SLE are advised to avoid sun exposure because this may trigger onset or exacerbation of the disease. Many of the drugs used to treat patients with RA also are used in the management of SLE (see Table 20-3). These agents include aspirin and NSAIDs for mild disease, antimalarials for dermatologic disease, glucocorticoids for more severe symptoms, and cytotoxic agents for symptoms unresponsive to other therapies or as adjuncts in severe disease. Several experimental approaches to therapy, including plasmapheresis, lymph node irradiation, cyclosporine injection, sex hormone therapy, and immune gamma globulin, are under investigation.[41,42]

A specific set of quality indicators to evaluate the monitoring of SLE patients in routine clinical practice have been developed recently.[43] These quality indicators have been integrated into the recently developed EULAR recommendations for monitoring SLE patients in routine clinical practice and observational studies. Eleven quality indicators (QIs) have been developed referring to the use of validated activity and damage indices in routine clinical practice, general evaluation of drug toxicity, evaluation of comorbid conditions, eye evaluation, laboratory assessment, evaluation of the presence of chronic viral infections, documentation of vaccination, and antibody testing at baseline. A disease-specific set of quality assessment tools should help physicians deliver high quality of care across populations of patients with SLE.[43]

DENTAL MANAGEMENT

Medical Considerations

Because SLE is such a varied disease with so many potential problems caused by the disease or its treatment, pretreatment consultation with the patient's physician is advised (Box 20-6). As in RA, drug considerations and adverse effects in SLE are of major importance. Table 20-3 lists the dental and oral considerations associated with the use of these drugs. The leukopenia that is common in SLE usually is not associated with a significant increase in infection; however, when combined with corticosteroids or cytotoxic drugs, the likelihood of infection is increased. Therefore, in patients who are taking corticosteroids or cytotoxins who also have leukopenia, the use of prophylactic antibiotics for periodontal and oral surgical procedures may be considered. Patients who are taking corticosteroids also may develop significant adrenal suppression and could require supplementation, especially for surgical procedures or in cases of extreme anxiety (see Chapter 15).

Abnormal bleeding due to thrombocytopenia is a potential problem in some patients with SLE. A coagulation profile that especially notes the platelet count and PTT should be obtained. A platelet count greater than 50,000/μL is an indication of adequate platelet activity. Other abnormalities should be discussed with the physician. As was previously mentioned, an elevated PTT associated with the lupus anticoagulant is not a risk factor for increased bleeding.

BOX 20-6 Key Points in Dental Management of the Patient with Systemic Lupus Erythematosus

1. Consultation with physician
   a. Patient status and stability
   b. Extent of systemic manifestations (i.e., kidney, heart)
   c. Hematologic profile: complete blood cell count (CBC) with differential, prothrombin time (PT), partial thromboplastin time (PTT)
   d. Drug profile
2. Drug considerations
   a. Aspirin and nonsteroidal antiinflammatory drugs (NSAIDs)—bleeding may be increased but is not usually clinically significant; if patient is concurrently taking corticosteroids, bleeding is more likely
   b. Gold salts, antimalarials, penicillamine, and cytotoxic drugs may cause leukopenia and thrombocytopenia; also, severe stomatitis—treat symptomatically
   c. Corticosteroids may cause adrenal suppression
3. Hematologic considerations
   a. Leukopenia with corticosteroids or cytotoxic drugs may predispose patient to infection; use of postoperative antibiotics can be considered with surgical procedures
   b. Platelet count <50,000/μL may result in severe bleeding—consultation with physician
   c. Elevated PTT associated with lupus anticoagulant usually does not cause increased bleeding—surgery can be performed
4. Infective endocarditis is a potential problem—antibiotic prophylaxis is not recommended by the American Heart Association.

Cardiac valvular abnormalities are found in 25% to 50% of patients with SLE and often are not clinically detectable, the potential exists for bacterial endocarditis resulting from physiologic bacteremia. The American Heart Association 2007 Guidelines for endocarditis prevention do not recommend antibiotic prophylaxis for patients with valvular disease associated with SLE when receiving invasive dental procedures. Finally, patients with SLE-associated renal failure have the potential for altered drug metabolism, hematologic disorders, and infection (see Chapter 12 for management recommendations).

Treatment Planning Considerations. No specific treatment planning modifications are required. However, consideration should be given to physical disabilities related to arthritis and myalgia. Additionally, systemic complications such as renal impairment and cardiac problems such as arrhythmia and valvular defects may occur. For patients with SLE, the establishment and maintenance of optimal oral health are of paramount importance.

Oral Complications and Manifestations

Oral lesions of the lips and mucous membranes have been reported to occur in up to 5% to 25% of patients with SLE.[44] These lesions are rather nonspecific and may be erythematous with white spots or radiating peripheral lines; they also may occur as painful ulcerations (Figure 20-10). Lesions frequently resemble lichen planus or leukoplakia. When they occur on the lip, a silvery, scaly margin, similar to that seen on the skin, may develop. Skin and lip lesions frequently are noted after exposure to the sun. Treatment of these lesions is symptomatic, and future sun exposure is avoided (see Appendix C). Other oral manifestations of SLE may include xerostomia and hyposalivation, dysgeusia, and glossodynia. The dentist should always remain alert to oral eruptions and lesions associated with any of a variety of medications used to treat patients with SLE; they may be a sign of toxicity. Similarly, some medications (hydralazine) have been associated with lupus-like eruptions.[44]

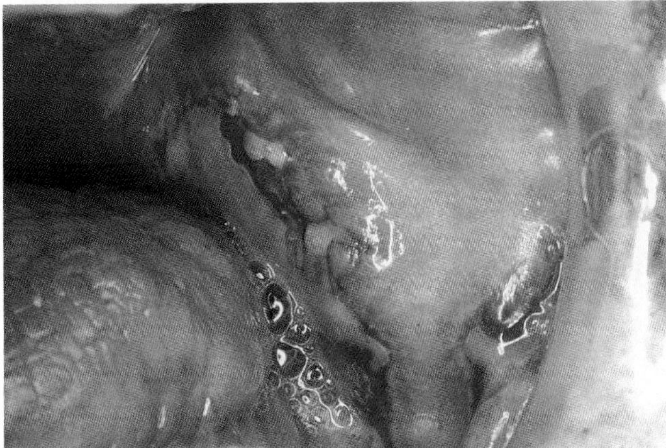

FIGURE 20-10 Systemic lupus erythematosus ulcerations of the buccal mucosa. *(From Neville BW, et al:* Oral and maxillofacial pathology, *ed 3, St. Louis, 2009, Saunders.)*

FIBROMYALGIA

Fibromyalgia (FM) is the most common cause of chronic pain in the United States. FM affects up to 4% of the population, primarily women. The diagnosis of FM is typically difficult and lengthy because there are so many other potential causes for the widespread pain. Chronic (several years) diffuse (muscle) pain accompanied by fatigue, sleep disturbance, and neuropathies (or other neurologic symptoms) are all cardinal symptoms of FM. As with most rheumatologic conditions, there is considerable overlap with FM and other autoimmune conditions. Up to 25% of patients with FM may also be diagnosed with SLE, Sjögren syndrome, and RA, as well as several other conditions.[1,45,46]

In 1990 the American College of Rheumatology adopted diagnostic classification criteria for FM, which are summarized in Figure 20-11. The red dots indicate specific "tender points." To meet the diagnostic criteria, there must be chronic (present for more than 3 months) widespread pain in all four quadrants of the body, and

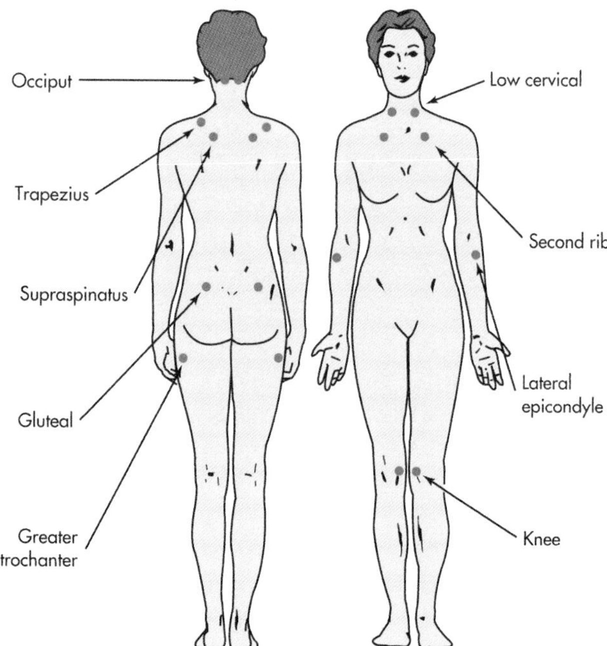

FIGURE 20-11 The American College of Rheumatology defines fibromyalgia as consistent tender points in 11 of these 18 anatomic locations. *(Redrawn from Freundlich B, Leventhal L: The fibromyalgia syndrome. In Schumacher HR Jr, et al, editors:* Primer on the rheumatic diseases, *ed 11, Atlanta, 1997, Arthritis Foundation. Reprinted with permission from The Arthritis Foundation, 1330 W. Peachtree St., Atlanta, GA 30309.)*

11 of the 18 points must be painful on application of only 4 kg pressure.[1,45,46] Symptoms and signs of FM are listed in Box 20-7.[2,46,47]

MEDICAL MANAGEMENT

Successful management of FM requires a thorough analysis of the patient's biopsychosocial issues, including fatigue, sleep, pain, psychological distress, and so on. Management of central sensitization is beneficial using heterocyclic antidepressant agents (HCA) such as amitriptyline, trazadone, or nortriptyline. Highly selective serotonin reuptake inhibitors (SSRIs) such as fluoxetine exhibit a modest pain benefit in patients with FM. Anticonvulsant medications such as gabapentin, topiramate, or pregabalin are effective and are being utilized more frequently in the treatment of FM. Opioids also are commonly used in FM, but long-term trials are lacking and they should not be the first choice of therapy.[46]

DENTAL MANAGEMENT

Medical Considerations

The major discomfort with FM is muscle pain.[1,45,46] Depending on which muscles are involved, patients may not be comfortable in a supine position in the dental chair. Consideration should be given to providing a more upright chair position, using neck, back, and leg supports, and scheduling short appointments (see Box 20-2). Decreased platelet function caused by large doses of aspirin or other NSAIDs can lead to prolonged bleeding, but this is generally not a clinically significant problem (see Chapter 24).[1,45,46]

Often patients with FM are treated with anxiolytic drugs (benzodiazepines) or antidepressants (tricyclics). Although, the American College of Rheumatology has established specific criteria for the diagnosis and classification of FM, there is a strong central psychological component. Patients are often very focused on their chronic symptoms and may become centrally sensitized. They very often require behavioral intervention.[1,45,46]

BOX 20-7 Symptoms of Fibromyalgia

- Body aches
- Chronic facial muscle pain or aching
- Fatigue
- Irritable bowel syndrome
- Memory difficulties and cognitive difficulties
- Multiple tender areas (muscle and joint pain) on the back of the neck, shoulders, sternum, lower back, hips, shins, elbows, knees
- Numbness and tingling
- Palpitations
- Reduced exercise tolerance
- Sleep disturbances
- Tension or migraine headaches

Treatment Planning Modifications

As with the other rheumatic conditions, the technical modifications of dental treatment for FM are dictated by a patient's disabilities and drug therapy. For instance, patients with severe symptoms and/or TMJ involvement may not be capable of enduring lengthy appointments; therefore, extensive treatment such as reconstruction or a long surgical procedure may not be appropriate. Other dental management considerations for the behavioral component (see Chapter 28) may be necessary.[45]

Oral Complications and Manifestations. The TMJ (and other facial muscular tissues) may be affected in patients with FM, and this may constitute a problem for the patient. As would be expected, most people older than 40 years of age show some degree of histologic and radiographic change in the TMJ, but most have no symptoms. Frequently, TMJ pain has been reported in patients with FM. Severe pain may be elicited on wide opening, and pain occurs with normal function and worsens during the day. Adjacent muscle splinting and spasm may occur. Crepitus is a common finding in the affected joint. In most cases, osteoarthritic pain in the TMJ resolves within 8 months of onset.[41,42]

The regional pain found with myofascial pain syndrome (MFP) needs to be distinguished from the widespread muscular pain associated with FM. In both cases, the pain is often described as a "chronic dull aching pain" and is central to the diagnosis of both disorders. These two disorders have many similar characteristics and may represent two ends of a continuous spectrum. The pain in FM is relatively stable and consistent in contrast to MFP, which can vary in intensity and location depending on which muscles are involved. Patients with FM most often have pain in the low back, neck, shoulders, and hips, although these areas are frequently affected by MFP, reflecting the overlap between the two disorders. These studies have also shown that the pain in FM is considerably more severe over a larger body area than pain in patients with other nonlocalized rheumatic disease syndromes.[42,43,46] It should be further noted that when the muscle pain is primarily due to the FM, it may not respond as well as the jaw pain from MFP because FM is a systemic and not a local condition and muscle pain is a typical presentation in FM.

LYME DISEASE

DEFINITION

Lyme disease is a multisystemic inflammatory disease caused by the tickborne spirochete *Borrelia burgdorferi*. The disease was first identified in the United States in 1975 during an outbreak around Lyme, Connecticut, of an inflammatory condition presumed to be juvenile rheumatoid arthritis. The classical pattern of Lyme disease is a characteristic macular skin rash (erythema migrans) that appears within a month after the tick (*Ixodes dammini*) bite. Several different manifestations, including neurologic, articular, and cardiac manifestations, may follow.[47]

Incidence and Prevalence

Lyme disease has been reported in North America, Europe, and Asia. In the United States, more than 90% of all cases of Lyme disease have been reported in only eight states (New York, Connecticut, Pennsylvania, Massachusetts, Rhode Island, New Jersey, Wisconsin, and Minnesota). Differences in the organism and in the immunogenetics of the affected population may explain the differences in clinical presentation of Lyme disease.[47]

Pathophysiology and Complications

Precisely how *B. burgdorferi* causes Lyme disease is not clear. The organism does not make toxins or cause tissue damage. It may activate proteolytic enzymes and induce spirochetemia. Local inflammation results from host response mechanisms. Vasculitis has been implicated in some cases of peripheral neuropathy, and a vascular lesion resembling endarteritis obliterans has been identified in the meninges and synovium of patients with Lyme disease.[47]

The clinical manifestations of Lyme disease can be divided into three phases: early localized, early disseminated, and late disease. Patients with a diagnosis of Lyme disease may not be identified until later stages of the disease. Early localized disease includes erythema migrans and associated findings. Erythema migrans occurs in 50% to 80% of infected patients within 1 month of the tick bite. Only about 30% of patients can recall an associated tick bite. Erythema migrans presents as a "target" or "bull's eye" lesion that typically appears in or near the axilla or belt line, because ticks like warm, moist areas of the human body (Figure 20-12).[47] Most often, the lesion is asymptomatic, although it may itch, burn, or hurt. The lesion typically expands and enlarges over the course of a few days. Some sources have reported that 50% of patients have multiple lesions of erythema migrans because of spirochetemia. Patients also may have an acute viremia-like syndrome with fever, malaise, nausea, myalgia, fatigue, headache, and arthralgias.[47]

The next phase of clinical presentation is early disseminated disease, which may occur within a few days to a few months after the tick bite, possibly without preceding erythema migrans. The primary clinical manifestations of this phase are cardiac and neurologic problems.[47] In the absence of treatment, about 8% of patients infected with Lyme disease manifest some cardiac problems, including heart block and myopericarditis. In most cases, the carditis begins to resolve, even without antibiotic therapy. Neurologic damage occurs in approximately 10% of untreated patients with Lyme disease. Primary manifestations include lymphocytic meningitis, cranial nerve palsy (especially of the facial nerve), and radiculoneuritis. In the late disease stage, which may

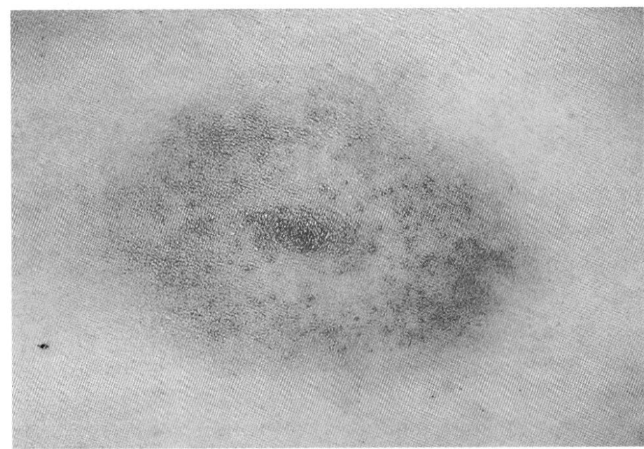

FIGURE 20-12 Classic erythema migrans lesion of Lyme disease. *(From Swartz M: Textbook of physical diagnosis, ed 6, St. Louis, 2010, Saunders.)*

occur months to years after the infection and may not be preceded by the earlier manifestations, musculoskeletal problems are the primary manifestation. Intermittent, migratory episodes of polyarthritis that mimic the "juvenile arthritis" originally described in cases of Lyme disease occur in approximately 50% of patients. Chronic arthritis of the knee is common, along with erosion of bone and cartilage. Chronic inflammatory joint disease may last for 5 to 8 years.[43]

Late neurologic manifestations of Lyme disease, called *tertiary neuroborreliosis,* consist of encephalopathy, neurocognitive dysfunction, and peripheral neuropathy. Symptoms may be subtle and may be reported as headache and fatigue, in addition to cognitive, mood, and sleep disturbances. Neuropsychological testing may be useful in confirming the diagnosis. Fibromyalgia is common in patients with Lyme disease.[41,43]

Laboratory Findings

Although the diagnosis of Lyme disease is based on clinical findings, serologic testing may prove useful. Current practice is to confirm all enzyme-linked immunosorbent assay (ELISA) results with Western blot analysis.[47] Many other conditions (e.g., Epstein-Barr virus [EBV] infections, SLE, infective endocarditis) may mimic Lyme disease; therefore, laboratory testing should be performed for a more precise, definitive diagnosis. Serologic testing has not been standardized between various laboratories; this may be problematic. Antibody responses may be undetectable in infections of less than 6 weeks' duration, and early antibiotic therapy based on symptoms may render the infected patient seronegative. Most patients with late disease manifestations are strongly seropositive.[43]

MEDICAL MANAGEMENT

Antibiotic therapy is effective for the treatment of patients with *B. burgdorferi* infection. Prompt antibiotic therapy when early symptoms are reported usually prevents progression to later stages of Lyme disease. Oral doses of 100 mg of doxycycline given twice daily for 3 to 4 weeks provide first-line treatment for early infection.[47] Alternatively, tetracycline or amoxicillin (250 to 500 mg four times daily) may be given for the same duration. In the late disseminated stages of Lyme disease, intravenous antibiotics may be necessary. Third-generation cephalosporins (ceftriaxone 2 g four times daily, or cefotaxime 3 g twice daily), penicillin G (20 million units in six divided doses), or chloramphenicol (50 mg/kg/day in four divided doses) may be used. Some physicians treat all pregnant women only through the intravenous (IV) route. Some patients with arthritis are refractory to antibiotic therapy. These patients may benefit from intra-articular corticosteroid injections or hydroxychloroquine. Adequate therapy for neurologic damage is elusive, and recovery may be very slow.[43]

DENTAL MANAGEMENT

Medical Considerations

The major dental consideration in Lyme disease is the identification of unusual symptoms in the absence of a clear medical condition. Symptoms of fatigue, malaise, arthralgia, neuritis, or neuralgia, including facial palsy, may indicate the possibility of Lyme disease and the need for referral for proper medical diagnosis. Numerous reports have described facial nerve palsy that closely resembles Bell's palsy caused by Lyme disease.[47] The presentation of this facial palsy may be combined with other neurologic deficits or may stand alone. Involvement of the parotid glands (acute parotitis) has been reported. Along with facial nerve palsy, facial and dental neuralgia and temporomandibular joint symptoms have been reported to occur with Lyme disease.[43]

SJÖGREN SYNDROME

DEFINITION

Sjögren syndrome (SS) is an autoimmune disease complex classified among the many rheumatic diseases that causes exocrinopathy and affects the salivary and lacrimal glands. SS is characterized by a triad of clinical conditions that consists of keratoconjunctivitis sicca, xerostomia, and a connective tissue disease (usually RA).[13] SS manifests in two different forms: primary SS and secondary SS. Primary SS (SS-1) manifests clinically with the primary ocular complication of keratoconjunctivitis sicca; in the oral cavity, it is associated with various levels of salivary gland dysfunction (xerostomia). Secondary SS (SS-2) manifests as the presence of keratoconjunctivitis sicca or xerostomia in the presence of a diagnosed systemic connective tissue disease. The connective tissue disorder from which SS develops most commonly is RA; SLE, primary biliary cirrhosis, fibromyalgia, mixed connective tissue disease, polymyositis, Raynaud's syndrome, and several others are among the associated inflammatory conditions.[45,46]

Incidence and Prevalence

According to the World Health Organization (WHO), the prevalence of SS is unknown. It has been estimated that its prevalence in the adult population is around 2.7%.[48] Today, the prevalence of SS in the United States is estimated at more than 2.5 million. SS has now become the second most common rheumatoid disorder.[49] Originally named for an ophthalmologist from Sweden, SS has been reported in nearly every major country, and the geographic distribution of cases, although accurate data are lacking, appears to be relatively uniform. SS is primarily a disease of women—more than 90% of all patients with SS are female.[48,50,51]

SS typically manifests during the fourth or fifth decade of life, although the condition usually progresses insidiously over several years, often remaining unrecognized. Therefore, some affected persons may exhibit clinical SS at a much earlier age than when it is actually diagnosed. Isolated cases of SS have been reported in children.[48,50,51]

Etiology

The precise cause of SS, as of many of the autoimmune rheumatic disorders, is unknown, although several contributing factors have been identified. One theory is that the disease results from complications of viral infection with EBV.[52,53] Exposure to or reactivation of EBV elicits expression of the HLA (human lymphocyte antigen) complex; this is recognized by the T cell (CD4+) lymphocytes and results in the release of cytokines (tumor necrosis factor [TNF], interleukin 2 [IL-2], interferon-γ [IFN-γ], and others).[52] Chronic inflammation, infiltration of lymphocytes, and ultimate destruction of exocrine gland tissue follow.[46-52]

Pathophysiology and Complications

SS is a chronic, progressive autoimmune disorder that is characterized by exocrinopathy and generalized lymphoproliferation that primarily affect the salivary and lacrimal glands. It can affect the pancreas, biliary tract, and lungs. A genetic marker, HLA-DR4, has been identified as specific for SS.[52,53] Activation of the interferon pathway is important in SS.

Labial salivary gland histopathologic examination has been accepted almost universally as the prima facie diagnostic indicator for definitive diagnosis of SS.[52,53] The classic histopathologic feature of the minor salivary glands in SS is seen as lymphocytic infiltration that includes benign lymphosialadenopathy (focal lymphocytic sialadenitis or benign lymphoepithelial lesion in the major salivary glands). This benign lymphosialadenopathy may manifest as parotid hypertrophy, particularly in patients with primary SS. Small clusters of intralobular ducts enlarge to replace the acinar epithelial parenchyma. The lesion comprises primarily CD4+ T cell lymphocytes, along with polyclonal B cells and plasma cells that are acquired late. Among the lymphocytic foci, approximately 75% are T cells and 5% to 10% are B cells. As the inflammatory process progresses, fibrosis and atrophy of the salivary glands occur, and hyposalivation progresses. Progression to lymphoma is a possibility in SS and is discussed in the patient management section.[54,55]

CLINICAL PRESENTATION

Signs and Symptoms

SS is characterized by eye dryness, hyposalivation, and enlargement of the parotid glands. Secondary outcomes of persistent oral dryness are angular cheilosis, dysgeusia (taste dysfunction), secondary infection, and a significantly increased caries rate (Table 20-4).[46]

Salivary Gland Dysfunction and Hyposalivation

Saliva in normal quantity and composition is rich in constituents that have potent antimicrobial, antacid, lubricative, and homeostatic properties. Saliva contains approximately 60 important protective constituents, including immunoglobulins, electrolytes, buffers, antimicrobial enzymes, digestive enzymes, and many others, all of which almost universally serve to make saliva an essential contributor to the health and homeostasis of the oral cavity. Obviously, when saliva is diminished in quantity or altered in composition, as in SS, deterioration of oral soft and mineralized tissues may occur.[13]

Patients with SS also demonstrate increased levels of dysphagia in comparison with control subjects. Studies have shown that patients with SS have difficulty tasting, tolerating, and swallowing certain foods. Consequently, dietary intake of certain nutrients may be inadequate in these patients.[12]

Among its many beneficial constituents, saliva has been shown to be rich in proteins that have potent antifungal properties; thus, it plays an important role in host defense and protection from yeasts such as *Candida* spp.

TABLE 20-4 Clinical Manifestations of Sjögren Syndrome*

Clinical Manifestation	Prevalence (% of Affected Patients)
Orcheilosis/angular cheilitis	75
Glossitis	60
Mucositis	30
Glossodynia	45
Dysgeusia	75
Dysphagia	45
Candidiasis	75
Dental caries	100
Periodontitis	60-100

*From 62 consecutive patients with Sjögren syndrome who presented to the University of Minnesota Xerostomia Clinic.

Data from Rhodus NL: Xerostomia and glossodynia in patients with autoimmune disorders, Ear Nose Throat J *68:791-794, 1989; and Rhodus NL, et al: Quantitative assessment of dysphagia in patients with primary and secondary Sjögren's syndrome,* Oral Surg Oral Med Oral Pathol Oral Radiol Endod *79:305-310, 1995.*

Therefore, with reduced salivary flow in SS, *Candida* infections are very common.[12] Studies also have shown that patients with SS more frequently exhibit periodontal disease, especially loss of clinical attachment.[12]

Diagnosis

Precise diagnostic criteria for SS remain controversial, although specific laboratory tests are available for the major diagnostic categories of salivary and tear production, histopathologic changes, and serologic inflammatory markers. Five sets of published criteria are available for the diagnosis of SS; several common characteristics and some variations and modifications are summarized in Box 20-8.[50,51,53-61]

Laboratory Findings

On serologic testing, hypergammaglobulinemia is the most frequent laboratory finding (80%) among patients with SS. Hyperactivity of B lymphocytes results in increased rheumatoid factor antibodies, antinuclear antibodies (ANA), and antibodies against organ-specific antigens, such as salivary duct epithelia or thyroid tissue. ANA make up the SS-A (Ro), which is present in approximately 70% of patients with SS-1 and 15% to 90% with SS-1 and SS-B (La) antibodies, which are present in approximately 50% of patients with SS-1 and 5% to 30% with SS-2.[51,52,54-62] These ANA also may be found in other autoimmune disorders. Elevated ESR, mild anemia (approximately 25%), and leukopenia (approximately 10%) also are found in patients with SS. The laboratory tests used to diagnose SS are summarized in Box 20-8).[50,51,53-61]

BOX 20-8 Diagnostic Criteria for Sjögren Syndrome*

Subjects must meet four of six criteria; labial biopsy or serologic studies must be performed.

Ocular Symptoms (1:3)	**Ocular Signs (1:2)**
Daily dry eyes >3 months	+ Shirmer test (<5 mm/5 min)
Sand or gravel sensitivity	Rose Bengal score (>4 vBs)
Use of tear substitutes (>3 times daily)	
Oral Symptoms (1:3)	**Oral Signs: Salivary Function (1:3)**
Daily dry mouth >3 months	+ Scintigraphy
Swollen salivary glands	+ Sialography
Need fluids to swallow food	WUSF < 1.5 mL/15 min (0.1 mL/min)
Labial SG histology	**Autoantibodies (1:2)**
Focus scope biopsy > ¼ mm	anti–SS-Ro
>50 mononuclear cells per field	anti–SS-La

*Modified European-American Criteria, used at the University of Minnesota. *vBs*, von Blisterberg score for eyes; *WUSF*, Whole unstimulated saliva flow.

Sialometry. Sialometry is useful as an initial screening tool for hyposalivation associated with SS and as an assessment for the level of severity of SS. To be valuable as a diagnostic technique, salivary flow collection must be performed precisely according to the type of gland and over a period of at least 5 minutes (often up to 15 minutes).[8]

Imaging. Radiographic findings may appear in advanced stages of fibrosis of the salivary glands. Sialograms are performed with injection of a radiocontrast dye into the salivary ductal system before conventional radiography. Sialograms may reveal punctate radiopaque calcifications or, if more advanced, larger, lobular calcifications. Sialectasis may occur in portions of the ductal system, or these portions may appear dilated or to have areas of absent acinar parenchyma. MRI sialography has been shown to be much more accurate in demonstrating levels of salivary gland destruction in SS. Salivary scintigraphy with technetium-99 m pertechnetate (sodium pertechnetate, a radioisotope of technetium) can be performed to assess the function of the salivary glands through measurement of the rate and density of technetium uptake.[8]

DENTAL MANAGEMENT

Medical Considerations. Patient management for SS traditionally has been palliative and preventive, as there is no known cure. Relief of the primary symptoms of dryness (oral and ocular) and the secondary burning and discomfort is the main goal. Restoration and maintenance of a normal homeostatic oral environment is a secondary goal.[8,61]

Therapy for the oral component of SS may be classified into three major categories:

1. Provision of moisture and lubrication by stimulation or simulation
2. Treatment of secondary mucosal conditions (such as mucositis or candidiasis)
3. Prevention of oral disease, provision of maintenance and general support (such as nutrition)

These therapeutic strategies are outlined in Table 20-5.

Moisture and Lubrication

Patients with SS are quite thirsty and should be counseled to drink plenty of water (8 to 10 glasses per day) and to avoid diuretics such as caffeine, tobacco, and alcoholic beverages. Obviously, certain medications (more than 400) may contribute to and compound the xerostomia, so some may need to be modified or avoided, if possible. Any changes in the patient's medication must be coordinated with the patient's physician. Although salivary substitutes, oral moisturizers, and artificial salivas may provide some relief for the xerostomia

TABLE 20-5 Management of Salivary Dysfunction*

General Measures	Specific Agents/Measures*
Moisture and Lubrication (continuous, as needed)	
Drink (sip water, liquids)	Oasis, Salivart (or other artificial saliva), or moisturizers (especially at night)
Use sugarless candy or gum	Pilocarpine hydrochloride, 2% (5 mg, 3 times daily)
Avoid ethanol	*or*
Avoid tobacco	Cevimeline hydrochloride (Evoxac), 30-mg caps, 3 times daily)
Avoid coffee, tea, and other caffeinated beverages	Sodium carboxymethylcellulose, 0.5% solution
Soft Tissue Lesions and Soreness (treatment and maintenance)	
Oasis, Salivart (or other artificial saliva) or moisturizers (especially at night)	Benadryl + Maalox + nystatin elixir†
	(Carafate, optional)
	(Lidocaine 2%, optional, for acute lesions)
	Decadron, 0.5 mg/5 mL elixir‡ (for acute lesions)
	Triamcinolone 0.1% (in Orabase) (for acute lesions)
	Orabase-HCA (for acute lesions)
	Mycelex 60-mg troches (for candidiasis)
	Mycolog II ointment (lips and tongue)
Prevention of Caries and Periodontal Disease (continuous)	
Meticulous perioral hygiene	Biotene toothpaste (neutral sodium fluoride, 1.0%, trays)
Avoid acids	Prevident, 5000 ppm§
Regular hygiene and prophylaxis recalls	Peridex (chlorhexidine gluconate) (optional)
Sodium bicarbonate rinses (optional)	Waterpik

Manufacturers: Oral Balance, Laclede Pharmaceuticals; Salagen, MGI Pharmaceuticals; Mouthkote, Parnell Pharmaceuticals; Optimoist, Colgate-Hoyt; Salivart, Gebauer; Biotene, Laclede Pharmaceuticals; Benadryl, Parke-Davis; Maalox, Novartis Pharmaceuticals; Carafate, Hoechst, Marion, Roussel Pharmaceuticals; Decadron, Merck & Co. Pharmaceuticals; Orabase, Colgate-Palmolive; Mycelex, ALZA Prevident, Colgate-Hoyte; Peridex, Procter & Gamble; Waterpik, Teledyne.
*Specific treatments are dependent on the diagnosis.
†Benadryl, 25 mg/10 mL + Maalox, 64 mL + nystatin, 100,000 IU/mL = 16 mL.
‡Decadron elixir, 0.5%/5 mL. Dispense 100 mL; to be swished and expectorated, 5 mL 3 times daily.
§Prevident neutral sodium fluoride, 1.0%, to be applied in trays 2 times daily.
Adapted from Rhodus NL: Diagnosis and treatment of Sjögren's syndrome, Quintessence Int *30:689-699, 1999.*

experienced by patients with SS, by and large, they are inadequate. Most are compounds of carboxymethylcellulose or hydroxymethylcellulose are too viscous or not viscous enough for most patients. The retentivity or longevity of their effect is very short-lived, and they provide little more relief than water. To date, these simulated salivas appear to provide little benefit to the patient with SS. Some artificial salivas from Europe (including Saliva Orthana) seem to be effective. On the other hand, pharmacologic stimulation of the salivary glands can be quite successful. Recently, the U.S. Food and Drug Administration (FDA) approved the use of pilocarpine HCl (Salagen) and cevimeline HCl (Evoxac) for the treatment of patients with SS with signs and symptoms of hyposalivation.[8]

Systemic administration of pilocarpine or cevimeline effectively stimulates only the salivary acinar tissue, which remains functional. Therefore, patients with SS who have lost most of the salivary acinar tissue capable of fluid production benefit little from this drug. Conversely, those patients with functional tissue remaining experience an increase in salivary secretion after the administration of pilocarpine relative to the ability of the tissue to become stimulated. The dosage of pilocarpine ranges from 2.5 to 15 mg administered from two to six times daily. The dosage of cevimeline is 30 mg given two to four times daily.[8]

Other pharmacologic sialagogues, such as bethanechol chloride, bromhexine, and anethole trithione, have been shown to stimulate salivary flow, but none has withstood extensive clinical evaluation of safety and efficacy in the United States, and none has been approved by the FDA as of the time of this writing. Very recently, clinical trials have been undertaken to study the safety and efficacy of human interferon (IFN-α) for the treatment of patients with SS. This NSAID appears to have significant promise as a new therapy for SS.[8]

Oral Complications and Manifestations

Among the oral symptoms most commonly associated with SS, aside from xerostomia, is glossodynia (burning tongue). The tongue often becomes depapillated and fissured and develops a scrotal appearance (Figure 20-13). The dorsal epithelium often is atrophic or eroded, erythematous, and potentially secondarily infected. Pain and burning may be spontaneous or may be elicited with acidic or spicy foods, such as those containing ascorbic or acetic acid. The tongue is commonly infected (in as many as 83%) with *C. albicans* in patients with

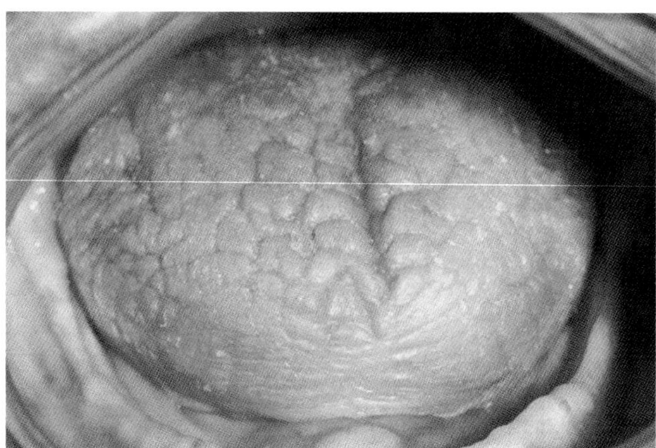

FIGURE 20-13 Dry and fissured tongue in a patient with Sjögren's syndrome. *(From Neville BW, et al: Oral and maxillofacial pathology, ed 3, St. Louis, 2009, Saunders. Courtesy Dr. David Schaffner.)*

SS.[13] Not only must the acute candidal infection be treated, but some type of maintenance therapy must be provided to prevent recurrence of the fungal infection. As long as the oral environment is adversely affected by hyposalivation, susceptibility to recurrence of the oral infection and continued deterioration occur. Atrophy of the epithelium in the dry environment may render the tissue susceptible to painful excoriation and ulceration. Therefore, clinical follow-up evaluation and some phased maintenance therapy may be necessary. Generally, these oral mucosal conditions are treated as if they occurred independently (i.e., with antifungal agents, topical antiinflammatory agents including corticosteroids, analgesics, or anesthetics as indicated) (see Table 20-5).[14]

Prevention and Maintenance

The patient with SS may have less than 5% of the normal quantity of saliva to protect the oral cavity. The risk for caries as well as enamel erosion then is extremely high. Of particular risk is the cervical-cementoenamel junction portion of the tooth. Meticulous oral hygiene with minimally abrasive fluoridated dentifrices and irrigation devices is paramount. In the xerostomic environment, abrasion of the tooth surface should be minimized as much as possible. Shorter professional hygiene recall intervals also are extremely important.

Frequent application of concentrated fluorides delivered as a direct brush-on treatment or with custom-made trays is imperative to prevent the rapid progression of caries. Over-the-counter fluoride rinses are inadequate; 5000 ppm sodium fluoride is preferred because of the unpleasant metallic taste of stannous fluoride, which also may cause some burning symptoms in the xerostomic patient and staining of the enamel. Special dentifrices have been found to be well accepted by patients with SS (see Table 20-5).[12,13,55-63]

Lymphoma

Lymphomas occur in SS-1 patients at a rate higher than in the general population. The prevalence is approximately 5%. It has been estimated that the predicted relative risk in patients with SS is 44 times normal and even higher (67 times) in those patients with SS-1 with chronic parotid enlargement; whether patients had other cancers or had undergone radiation therapy or chemotherapy (then the relative risk may be as high as 100 times greater) was considered.[12,59-63] Progression to lymphoma in patients with SS is thought to be related to chronic inflammatory challenge, as in the case of *Helicobacter pylori* in gastric cancer. In the presence of continued and chronic inflammation (mediated first by type 1 cytokines—TNF-α, IL-2, IFN-γ—and then, later, by type 2 cytokines—IL-4, IL-6, and IL-10), B cells undergo oligoclonality and sometimes, eventually, monoclonality.[52] Patients with SS may then manifest non-Hodgkin's lymphoma. B cell monoclonality seems to be predictive of the occurrence of lymphoma outside the salivary glands.[12,59-63]

Clinical findings associated with lymphoma include anemia, cryoglobulinemia, lymphopenia, cutaneous vasculitis, and peripheral neuropathy. Lymphadenopathy is common (86%) and is associated with enlarged cervical and axillary nodes. Evidence suggests that initial transformation to lymphoma occurs in the salivary glands, and that the presence of B cell monoclonality in labial minor salivary gland (LMSG) tissue is associated with progression to malignancy.[12,55-63]

The most common type of lymphoma in patients with SS involves mucosa-associated lymphoid tissue (MALT); 70% of cases are low-grade, nonaggressive lymphomas, and 15% are the high-grade lymphoblastic type. IL-6 and TNF-α are associated with lesions that undergo transformation to lymphoma.[12,55-63]

ACKNOWLEDGMENT

The authors would like to thank Dr. James Fricton for his suggestions on fibromyalgia and giant cell arteritis.

REFERENCES

1. Kippel JH: Rheumatoid arthritis. In Klippel JH, et al, editors: *Primer on the rheumatic diseases*, New York, 2008, Springer, pp 389-402.
2. Zhao B, et al: Characterization of synovial cell clones isolated from rheumatoid arthritis patients: possible involvement of TNF-alpha in reduction of osteoprotegerin in synovium, *Cytokine* 41:61-70, 2008.
3. Marston B, Palanichamy A, Anolik JH: B cells in the pathogenesis and treatment of rheumatoid arthritis, *Curr Opin Rheumatol* 22:307-315, 2010.
4. Azevedo PM, et al: Interleukin-1 receptor antagonist gene (IL1RN) polymorphism possibly associated to severity of

rheumatic carditis in a Brazilian cohort, *Cytokine* 49:109-113, 2010.

5. Arvidsson LZ, Flato B, Larheim TA: Radiographic TMJ abnormalities in patients with juvenile idiopathic arthritis followed for 27 years, *Oral Surg Oral Med Oral Pathol Oral Radiol Endod* 108:114-123, 2009.
6. Sasaguri K, et al: The temporomandibular joint in a rheumatoid arthritis patient after orthodontic treatment, *Angle Orthod* 79:804-811, 2009.
7. Huntjens E, et al: Condylar asymmetry in children with juvenile idiopathic arthritis assessed by cone-beam computed tomography, *Eur J Orthod* 30:545-551, 2008.
8. Royal College of Physicians: *Rheumatoid arthritis: national clinical guideline for management and treatment in adults*, London, 2009, Lavenham Press.
9. Pistesky D: Laboratory testing in the rheumatic diseases. In Ausiello DA, Goldman L, editors: *Cecil textbook of medicine*, ed 23, Philadelphia, 2008, Saunders.
10. Kelsey JL, Lamster IB: Influence of musculoskeletal conditions on oral health among older adults, *Am J Publ Health* 98:1177-1183, 2008.
11. Ardic F, et al: The comprehensive evaluation of temporomandibular disorders seen in rheumatoid arthritis, *Aust Dent J* 51:23-28, 2006.
12. Lipsky P: Rheumatoid arthritis. In Fauci A, et al, editors: *Harrison's principles of internal medicine*, ed 17, New York, 2008, McGraw-Hill.
13. Rhodus NL: Sjogren's syndrome. *Quintessence Int* 30:689-699, 1999.
14. Figueroa FE, et al: [Presence of bacterial DNA in valvular tissue of patients with chronic rheumatic heart disease], *Rev Med Chil* 135:959-966, 2007.
15. Little J: Patients with prosthetic joints: are they at risk when undergoing dental procedures, *Spec Care Dent* 17:153-160, 1997.
16. American Academy of Orthopedic Surgeons: Antibiotic prophylaxis of bacteremia in patients with joint replacements, 2009, available at http://www.aaos.org(1033).
17. Cutando-Soriano A, Galindo-Moreno P: Antibiotic prophylaxis in dental patients with body prostheses, *Med Oral* 7:348-359, 2002.
18. Bauer T, et al: [Dental care and joint prostheses], *Rev Chir Orthop Reparatrice Appar Mot* 93:607-618, 2007.
19. ADA/AAOS: Antibiotic prophylaxis for dental patients with prosthetic joints, *J Am Dental Assoc* 134:895-897, 2003.
20. Little JW, et al: The dental treatment of patients with joint replacements, *J Am Dental Assoc* 141:667-671, 2010.
21. Barberi EF, et al: Dental procedures as risk factors for prosthetic hip or knee infection: a hospital-based prospective case-control study, *Clin Infect Dis* 50:8-19, 2010.
22. Bracco P, et al: Evaluation of the stomatognathic system in patients with rheumatoid arthritis according to the research diagnostic criteria for temporomandibular disorders, *Cranio* 28:181-186, 2010.
23. Griffin SO, et al: Oral health needs among adults in the United States with chronic diseases, *JADA* 140:1266-1274, 2009.
24. Kristensen KD, et al: Quantitative histological changes of repeated antigen-induced arthritis in the temporomandibular joints of rabbits treated with intra-articular corticosteroid, *J Oral Pathol Med* 37:437-444, 2008.
25. Pischon N, et al: Association among rheumatoid arthritis, oral hygiene, and periodontitis, *J Periodontol* 79:979-986, 2008.
26. Ishi Ede P, et al: Periodontal condition in patients with rheumatoid arthritis, *Braz Oral Res* 22:72-77, 2008.
27. Pers JO, et al: Anti-TNF-alpha immunotherapy is associated with increased gingival inflammation without clinical attachment loss in subjects with rheumatoid arthritis, *J Periodontol* 79:1645-1651, 2008.
28. Biyikoglu B, et al: Gingival crevicular fluid MMP-8 and -13 and TIMP-1 levels in patients with rheumatoid arthritis and inflammatory periodontal disease, *J Periodontol* 80:1307-1314, 2009.
29. Ortiz P, et al: Periodontal therapy reduces the severity of active rheumatoid arthritis in patients treated with or without tumor necrosis factor inhibitors, *J Periodontol* 80:535-540, 2009.
30. Pizzo G, et al: Dentistry and internal medicine: from the focal infection theory to the periodontal medicine concept, *Eur J Intern Med* 21:496-502, 2010.
31. Aramaki T, et al: A significantly impaired natural killer cell activity due to a low activity on a per-cell basis in rheumatoid arthritis, *Mod Rheumatol* 19:245-252, 2009.
32. Lane NE, Schnitzer TJ: Osteoarthritis. In Ausiello DA, Goldman L, editors: *Cecil textbook of medicine*, ed 23, Philadelphia, 2007, Saunders.
33. Lockhart PB, et al: The evidence base for the efficacy of antibiotic prophylaxis in dental practice, *JADA* 138:458-474, 2007.
34. de Leeuw R, et al: Radiographic signs of TMJ osteoarthritis, *Oral Surg Oral Med Oral Pathol* 79:382-392, 1995.
35. Inman R: Psoriatic arthritis. In Ausiello DA, Goldman L, editors: *Cecil textbook of medicine*, ed 23, Philadelphia, 2007, Saunders.
36. Ritchlin C: Psoriatic disease—from skin to bone, *Nat Clin Pract Rheumatol* 3:698-706, 2007.
37. Mease P, et al: Abatacept in the treatment of patients with psoriatic arthritis: results of a six-month, multicenter, randomized, double-blind, placebo-controlled, phase II trial, *Arthritis Rheum* 63:939-948, 2011.
38. Reiter S, et al: Giant cell arteritis misdiagnosed as temporomandibular disorder: a case report and review of the literature, *J Orofac Pain* 23:360-365, 2009.
39. Weyland CM, Goronzy JJ: Giant cell arteritis. In Klippel JH, et al, editors: *Primer on the rheumatic diseases*, New York, 2008, Springer, pp 398-424.
40. Reiter S, et al: Giant cell arteritis misdiagnosed as temporomandibular disorder: a case report and review of the literature, *J Orofac Pain* 23:360-365, 2009.
41. Powers DB: Systemic lupus erythematosus and discoid lupus erythematosus, *Oral Maxillofac Surg Clin North Am* 20:651-662, 2008.
42. Albilia JB, et al: Systemic lupus erythematosus: a review for dentists, *J Can Dent Assoc* 73:823-828, 2007.
43. Mosca M, et al: Development of quality indicators to evaluate the monitoring of SLE patients in routine clinical practice, *Autoimmun Rev* 69:1269-1274, 2011.
44. Rhodus NL, Johnson DK: The prevalence of oral manifestations of systemic lupus erythematosus, *Quintessence Int* 21:461-465, 1990.
45. Rhodus NL, et al: Oral symptoms associated with fibromyalgia syndrome, *J Rheumatol* 30:1841-1845, 2003.
46. Bennett RM: Fibromyalgia and chronic fatigue syndrome. In Ausiello DA, Goldman L, editors: *Cecil a textbook of medicine*, ed 23, Philadelphia, 2007, Saunders.
47. Rhodus NL, Falace DA: Oral concerns in Lyme disease, *Northwest Dent* 81:17-18, 2002.
48. Westhoff G, Zink A: [Epidemiology of primary Sjogren's syndrome], *Z Rheumatol* 69:41-49, 2010.
49. Youinou P, Pers JO: The international symposium on Sjogren's syndrome in Brest: the "top of the tops" at the "tip of the tips," *Autoimmun Rev* 9:589-590, 2010.
50. Witte T: [Pathogenesis and diagnosis of Sjogren's syndrome], *Z Rheumatol* 69:50-56, 2010.
51. Witte T: Diagnostic markers of Sjogren's syndrome. *Dev Ophthalmol* 45:123-128, 2010.
52. Emamian ES, et al: Peripheral blood gene expression profiling in Sjogren's syndrome. *Genes Immun* 10:285-296, 2009.

53. Daniels TE, et al: An early view of the international Sjogren's syndrome registry. *Arthritis Rheum* 61:711-714, 2009.
54. Singh M, Palmer C, Papas AS: Sjogren's syndrome: dental considerations, *Dent Today* 29:64, 66-67, 2010.
55. Shapira Y, Agmon-Levin N, Shoenfeld Y: Geoepidemiology of autoimmune rheumatic diseases, *Nat Rev Rheumatol* 6:468-476, 2010.
56. Seror R, et al: EULAR Sjogren's syndrome disease activity index: development of a consensus systemic disease activity index for primary Sjogren's syndrome, *Ann Rheum Dis* 69:1103-1109, 2010.
57. Seror R, et al: Accurate detection of changes in disease activity in primary Sjogren's syndrome by the European League Against Rheumatism Sjogren's Syndrome Disease Activity Index. *Arthritis Care Res* 62:551-558, 2010.
58. Scully C: Aspects of human disease. Human disease. 56. Sjogren's syndrome, *Dent Update* 37:413, 2010.
59. Schmidt RE, Witte T, Dorner T: [Sjogren's syndrome], *Z Rheumatol* 69:9-10, 2010.
60. Moutsopoulos HM: Sjogren's syndrome. In Fauci AS, et al, editors: *Harrison's principles of internal medicine*, ed 17, New York, 2008, McGraw-Hill, pp 2117-2121.
61. Daniels T: Sjogren's syndrome. In Klippel JH, et al, editors: *Primer on the rheumatic diseases*, New York, 2008, Springer, pp 389-402.
62. Vissink A: [Theses 25 years after date 23. Developments in the prevention and treatment of xerostomia], *Ned Tijdschr Tandheelkd* 117:453-459, 2010.
63. Segal BA, et al: Genetics and genomics of Sjogren's syndrome: research provides clues to pathogenesis and novel therapies, *Oral Surg Oral Med Oral Pathol Oral Radiol Endod* 111:673-680, 2011.

21

Organ and Bone Marrow Transplantation

On average, over the past 10 years there have been more than 26,000 solid organ transplant procedures in the United States annually, with nearly 95,000 persons on the Organ Procurement and Sharing Network (OPTN) waiting list for transplant organs.[1,2] The total number of transplanted organs has now exceeded half a million.[3] During the past 10 years the number of living donors increased by about 3%, for a total of 108,400, while the number of deceased donors grew by 11%, totalling 391,000, according to the OPTN.[1,4] Some of this increase can likely be attributed to efforts that focus on increasing the supply of organs for transplantation.[2,4] Although in 2010 the number of donors actually decreased by about 6000, overall this figure will continue to increase.[5]

Key outcomes after transplantation include (1) survival of transplant recipients and (2) the function of transplanted grafts. Reported 1-year patient survival rates are highest for kidney and pancreas recipients, ranging from about 95% to 98%; the median survival rate with renal transplantation from living donors has increased from 17 years in 1988 to nearly 38 years at 2010. Corresponding survival rates at 1 year for liver, intestine, and heart transplant recipients were approximately 86% to 88%, about 83% for lung, and lowest for the small number of heart-lung recipients at around 58%.[4,6] The survival rates for solid organ transplant procedures are summarized in Table 21-1.

Because more organ and bone marrow transplant procedures are being performed successfully and technologic proficiency will continue to increase, so that more post-transplantation patients are surviving longer, more of these patients will be seeking dental care. Although there are no precise guidelines drawn from evidence-based clinical trials for the dental management of organ transplant patients, a number of principles have been identified that apply in the care of the dental patient before, during, and after the solid organ transplant process. This chapter reviews the epidemiology, pathophysiology, process, complications, and dental management recommendations for these patients.[7]

DEFINITION

Organ transplant procedures are common today and may be performed in several organ systems, depending on the mix of recipients and donors. Heart, liver, kidney, pancreas, heart-lung, bone marrow, and other transplants may be available for the appropriate recipient. The ideal combination involves the transplantation of an organ from an identical twin to the other twin (syngeneic). The next best match for organ survival is transplantation of an organ from one living relative to another (allogeneic), followed by transplantation of an organ between living nonrelated people (xenograft). Each of these combinations, however, is limited by the fact that unless at least two organs are present, the donor cannot survive. Thus, these types of matches are basically limited to kidney and bone marrow donors. Nevertheless, recent studies have shown success with transplantation of a portion of a liver or pancreas from living donors. The largest organ pool for transplantation is cadaver organs, but the match also is poorest.[8-12]

Incidence and Prevalence

Dr. Joseph E. Murray, a Nobel laureate, performed the first successful human organ transplant procedure in Boston in 1954, using a kidney donated by the patient's identical twin brother. Then Murray performed the first successful kidney allograft transplant procedure in 1959, applying total body irradiation for immunosuppression, and the first successful human kidney cadaver transplant procedure in 1962, introducing Imuran (azathioprine), an immunosuppressive drug. Before these early transplant procedures, patients with renal failure, hypertension, and azotemia were undergoing renal dialysis, which was not nearly as successful in addressing the deficits in kidney function. Since those early days, more than one-half million kidney transplant procedures have been performed in the United States.[9]

Since 1987, all organ transplant procedures performed in the United States have been reported to the OPTN.

TABLE 21-1 Patient Survival Rates After Organ Transplant Procedures*

Organ With No. of Transplants	Patient Survival Rate	
	Deceased Donor	Living Donor
Kidney: 16,067†		
1-year survival	95.0%	98.2%
5-year survival	81.0%	90.6%
Pancreas alone: 122†		
1-year survival	97.9%	
5-year survival	88.7%	
Pancreas after kidney: 214†		
1-year survival	97.3%	
5-year survival	93.9%	
Kidney-pancreas: 825†		
1-year survival	95.1%	
5-year survival	86.6%	
Liver: 5817†		
1-year survival	87.1%	87.9%
5-year survival	73.3%	77.3%
Intestine: 69†		
1-year survival	81.4%	
5-year survival	56.2%	
Heart: 2085†		
1-year survival	87.6%	
5-year survival	73.9%	
Lung: 1473†		
1-year survival	83.6%	
5-year survival	53.4%	
Heart-lung: 26†		
1-year survival	73.8%	
5-year survival	46.5%	

*Total of 27,281 solid organ transplants in 2008.
†Numbers based on 2008 statistics.
Data from OPTN/STTR Annual Report, 2008.

Since that time, renal transplants have averaged over 10,000 per year nationwide.[13-15] Nearly 600 medical centers perform kidney transplantations in the United States. Improvements in preparation of the patient before the transplant procedure, with better immunosuppressive techniques, have increased the success of the procedure and extended the longevity of the transplant recipient. The 1-year survival rate among renal transplant recipients is more than 97%, and the 5-year survival rate is more than 90% (see Table 21-1).[4]

The first human heart transplantation was performed in 1967 and at that time the 1-year survival rate was only about 20%. At present, more than 70,000 heart transplantations have been performed at the rate of approximately 3400 per year at more than 250 U.S. hospitals. The 1-year survival rate is more than 87%, with the 5-year survival rate over 70% (see Table 21-1).[4]

The first orthotopic liver transplantation was performed in 1963. However, the first transplant resulting in an extended survival of 13 months was not achieved until 1967. By 1980, only 300 liver transplants had been performed, with a 1-year survival rate of only 28%. At present, more than 6000 liver transplant procedures are performed each year, with about the same number on the waiting list for a liver transplant. More than 100,000 liver transplantations have been performed in the United States. Survival rates for patients receiving transplants in 1988 were 75.5% at 1 year and 68.6% at 2 years after the operation. Currently, the survival rates have increased to approximately 80% for 1 year and 70% for 5 years[2,12,16,17] (see Table 21-1).

The first pancreas transplant procedure, which also included a duodenum and a kidney, was performed in 1966, by Kelly and Lillehei at the University of Minnesota, in a patient with diabetic nephropathy. Now more than 1000 pancreas transplantations are performed each year. The 5-year survival rate is nearly 90%. Recently, pancreatic islet cell transplant procedures also have shown considerable success.[16]

In 1990 only five lung transplant procedures had been performed. Since that time, more than 10,000 lungs have been transplanted at 119 centers, most within the last 5 years. The first heart-lung combination transplant procedure was performed in 1981. Since that time, more than 1000 have been performed, with a 1-year survival rate of almost 60%.[16]

To date, only a few small bowel transplant procedures have been performed (some combined with liver transplantation) at only a few transplant centers (in Cambridge, England, and London, Ontario, and in Pittsburgh and Omaha). However, much progress is being made in this area for the treatment of end-stage intestinal failure, with a current 1-year survival rate of approximately 70%.[16]

The modern era of bone marrow transplantation (BMT) was ushered in by the seminal experiments of Jacobsen (1950) and Lorenz (1951) and their colleagues, who demonstrated that mice could be protected from the lethal irradiation that was used to treat severe aplastic anemia or leukemia by shielding the spleen or with intravenous infusion of bone marrow. By 1956, several laboratories had demonstrated that the protective effects against otherwise lethal doses of total body irradiation were caused by the colonization of the recipient bone marrow by the infused donor cells.

In 1957, E. Donnell Thomas described the clinical technique of large quantities of marrow infused intravenously into patients with leukemia with safety and efficacy and demonstrated a transient bone marrow transplant in humans. In 1958, BMT was performed in six victims of a radiation accident.[10]

Most early BMTs were performed in only terminally ill patients, and the grafts could not be evaluated because the patient did not live long enough. The few successful allogeneic grafts were followed by lethal immunologic reaction of graft-versus-host disease (GVHD). Many years of research, first in rodents and then in dogs and monkeys, paved the way for the ultimate success of BMT in humans. Recent advances in knowledge of histocompatability typing and in the prevention of GVHD, as well as more supportive measures for the patient, have resulted in greater success and more frequent BMTs.[10]

The first attempts at transplantation in the 1950s and 1960s all were followed by increased activity in transplantation that resulted in very poor survival rates. A period followed during which few transplants were attempted. Increased research activity in the 1960s led to development of techniques that dealt with the major limiting factor in organ transplantation rejection of the organ by the host immune system.[18-20]

With the development of effective immunosuppressive agents, improved surgical techniques (including percutaneous biopsy of solid transplanted organs to monitor rejection), and the acceptance of the concept of "brain death" as a definition for determining the death of potential donors, major advances in organ transplantation have occurred.[18-20]

Transplantation of the heart, liver, and kidney is no longer considered an experimental procedure and is available as a treatment option for selected patients with end-organ disease. Transplantation of the pancreas also is considered a major treatment option for uremic diabetic patients who are receiving a kidney transplant.

The International Bone Marrow Transplant Registry reported that more than 20,000 patients had received allogeneic bone marrow transplants between 1955 and 1987. More than 50% of these were performed during the 3 years between 1985 and 1987. By 1991, that figure had doubled, and through 1999 nearly 90,000 BMTs had been performed. BMT is the treatment of choice for patients with myelogenous leukemia and for those with other blood dyscrasias (see Table 21-1), those in whom conventional therapy for acute leukemia fails to confer benefit, and patients with a variety of immune deficiency disorders.[9,11,12]

For many patients in whom a remission from leukemia cannot be achieved or the disease has not responded to chemotherapy, stem cell transplantation is an option. Currently, more than 15% of patients with end-stage disease will survive after stem cell transplantation.[15] Ideally, use of stem cells from an HLA-identical sibling donor offers the best outcome, and if transplantation is performed earlier in the disease process, the survival rate may reach as high as 30%. Because toxicity associated with stem cell transplantation increases with age, most centers limit use of such procedures to patients younger than 55 years of age. Autologous stem cell transplantation offers an alternative for patients without HLA-matched sibling donors, and in clinical trials, use of this technique after consolidation chemotherapy significantly prolonged the duration of disease-free survival in patients with acute myelogenous leukemia.[15,21]

Etiology

The most common indications for heart transplantation are cardiomyopathy and severe coronary artery disease.[13,22] The most common diseases in adults for which liver transplantation is indicated are primary biliary cirrhosis, chronic hepatitis, sclerosing cholangitis, fulminant hepatic failure, and metabolic disorders.[23-25] In children, most liver transplant procedures are performed for extrahepatic biliary atresia or metabolic disorders.[26,27] Common indications for kidney transplantation are bilateral chronic disease or end-stage renal disease. Glomerulonephritis, pyelonephritis, diabetic nephropathy, and congenital kidney disorders are the most frequent conditions leading to end-stage renal disease.[26,27] The most common indication for pancreas transplantation is severe diabetes leading to end-stage renal disease. Diabetic patients who are going to receive a kidney transplant also are good candidates for pancreas transplantation. The most common indications for bone marrow transplantation are acute and chronic myelogenous leukemia, acute lymphoblastic leukemia, aplastic anemia, and immune deficiency syndromes.[11,12]

Pathophysiology and Complications

All candidates for heart, liver, and bone marrow transplantation have severe end-stage organ disease and would die without transplantation. Patients with end-stage renal disease can be kept alive by hemodialysis. However, the quality of life for such patients can be greatly improved by renal transplantation. Patients with severe diabetes also can be kept alive with daily insulin injections, but their lives also may be greatly improved by pancreas transplantation.[11,12]

CLINICAL PRESENTATION

Signs and Symptoms

Signs and symptoms for the diseases necessitating transplantation are discussed in the chapters indicated:

- Advanced cardiac disease (Chapters 4, 5, and 6)
- Advanced liver disease (Chapter 10)
- End-stage renal disease (Chapter 12)
- Advanced diabetes mellitus (Chapter 14)
- Red blood cell disorders and white blood cell disorders (Chapters 22 and 23)

Laboratory Findings

Laboratory findings of particular importance in the care of dental patients who are scheduled for a transplant procedure include bleeding time, platelet count, white blood cell (WBC) count with differential, prothrombin time, hematocrit, partial thromboplastin time, blood urea nitrogen, aspartate aminotransaminase, serum creatinine, specific gravity of urine, serum bilirubin, alkaline phosphatase, and urinary levels of albumin and other proteins. Elevation of aspartate aminotransaminase, alkaline phosphatase, prothrombin time, and serum bilirubin would suggest advanced liver disease. Increased bleeding time, low platelet count, decreased WBC count, and decreased hematocrit are associated with many of the blood dyscrasias. Elevation of serum creatinine and blood urea nitrogen and increased specific gravity of urine and proteinuria are associated with advanced renal disease. In addition, a low hematocrit, prolonged partial thromboplastin time, and decreased WBC count can be found in patients with advanced renal disease. These patients may be potential bleeders, are prone to infection, and will experience buildup of toxic levels of drugs that are metabolized by the liver or kidney, depending on the organ involved (Table 21-2).[9,10,28]

TABLE 21-2 Screening Laboratory Tests Used to Evaluate Status of Kidney, Liver, Pancreas, and Bone Marrow Function*

Test	Normal Range	Abnormal Result	Organ Affected
Complete Blood Count			
White blood cell count	4400-11,000/mL	Decreased	Bone marrow
Hematocrit—male	41.5-50.4%		
Hematocrit—female	35.9-44.6%		
Hemoglobin—male	13.5-17.5 g/dL		
Hemoglobin—female	12.3-15.3 g/dL		
Platelet count	150,000-450,000/μL		
Differential Blood Count			
Neutrophils	43-47%	Decreased	Bone marrow
Lymphocytes	17-47%		
Monocytes	0-9%		
Platelet count	150,000-450,000/μL	<80,000/μL	
Hemostasis			
PFA-100	Closure <175 seconds	Prolonged	Bone marrow, kidney
Prothrombin time (PT)	10-13 seconds		
Activated partial thromboplastin time (aPTT)	25-35 seconds		
Thrombin time (TT)	9-13 seconds		
Serum Chemistry			
Glucose (fasting)	70-110 mg/dL	>126 mg/dL	Pancreas
Glucose	<180 mg/dL	>200 mg/dL	Pancreas
Blood urea nitrogen (BUN)	8-23 mg/dL	Elevated	Kidney
Creatinine	0.6-1.2 mg/dL	Elevated	Kidney
Serum Electrolytes			
Sodium	136-142 mEq/L	Elevated	Kidney
Potassium	3.9-5.0 mEq/L		
Chloride	95-103 mEq/L		
Serum Enzymes			
Alkaline phosphatase	20-130 IU/L	Elevated	Liver
Alanine aminotransferase	4-36 μ/L	Elevated	Liver
Aspartate aminotransferase	8-33 μ/L	Elevated	Liver
Amylase	16-120 Somogyi units/dL	Elevated	Pancreas
Urinalysis			
Specific gravity	1.0003-1.03	Elevated	Kidney
pH	4.8-7.5	Decreased	
Protein	None	Present	
Blood	None	Present	

*Normal values may vary depending on the techniques used.
PFA-100, Platelet function analyzer 100.
Data from McPherson RA, Pincus MR, editors: Henry's clinical diagnosis and management by laboratory methods, *ed 22, Philadelphia, 2012, Saunders.*

TABLE 21-3 Current Immunosuppressive Agents for Use in Early Posttransplantation Period

Agent	Class	Mechanism of Action
Prednisone	Corticosteroid	Blocks cytokine gene transcription
Cyclosporine	Calcineurin inhibitor	Inhibits IL-2 gene transcription Reduces activation of T cells
Tacrolimus	Calcineurin inhibitor	Inhibits IL-2 gene transcription Reduces activation of T cells
Azathioprine	Nucleoside inhibitor	Impairs DNA synthesis Inhibits B cell proliferation
Mycophenolate mofetil	Nucleoside inhibitor	Impairs DNA synthesis Inhibits B cell proliferation
Rapamycin (sirolimus)	TOR inhibitor	Inhibits tyrosine kinase
Everolimus (RAD)	TOR inhibitor	Inhibits tyrosine kinase

IL, Interleukin; *TOR,* Transplanted organ rejection.
Data from Little, JW, Rhodus, NL: Dental treatment of the liver transplant patient. *Oral Surg Oral Med Oral Pathol, 73(4):419-426, 1992.*

MEDICAL AND SURGICAL MANAGEMENT

Immunosuppression

The immunosuppressive agents now used for most heart, liver, kidney, and pancreas transplantations are cyclosporine, azathioprine, prednisone, and an antilymphocyte agent (Table 21-3). Since the 1980s, cyclosporine has been the standard immunosuppressive drug used to prevent organ graft rejection. Antilymphocyte agents include the Minnesota antilymphocyte globulin, equine antithymocyte globulin, rabbit antithymocyte globulin, and Orthoclone monoclonal antibody. The best clinical results are obtained with triple-drug immunosuppressive therapy—cyclosporine, prednisone, and azathioprine or mycophenolate mofetil (MMF). Antilymphocyte agents are used at the time of induction of immunosuppression and for acute rejection episodes. More recently, the immunosuppressive agent tacrolimus (FK 506) is being used with organ transplantation.[29] Tacrolimus is a xenobiotic immunosuppressive drug that was discovered in Japan in 1984 and has been proved effective in the prevention of graft rejection. It is now used in organ transplant recipients as a primary immunosuppressive drug or as a rescue drug in cases of therapy-resistant acute rejection. It seems to produce fewer or less severe adverse side effects than those typical for other forms of immunosuppressive therapy. The immunosuppression regimens vary from center to center in terms of dosage, timing, and duration of use of the various agents. After transplantation, doses of the immunosuppression agents are reduced as much as possible to prevent rejection of the graft[6,11,12,28] (see Table 21-3).

Anti-interleukin-2 receptor antibodies (IL-2Rα), daclizumab (humanized anti-IL-2Rα) and basiliximab (chimeric anti-IL-2Rα) have proved quite successful in furthering the immunosupression. Another important new drug is sirolimus, which is a macrocyclic lactone and blocks IL-2 receptors. Organ rejection and the need for antilymphocyte globulin have been reduced by sirolimus.[6]

Total body irradiation (1000 cGy) has been the most effective means of conditioning the bone marrow graft recipient. Cyclophosphamide usually is given in the immunosuppressive phase before (4 to 5 days) transplantation. Busulfan also has been used for conditioning the graft recipient. Cyclosporine, prednisone, and methotrexate are used after marrow transplantation to prevent or ameliorate GVHD.[10]

Surgical Procedure

Heart Transplantation. Heart transplantation involves the surgical removal of the heart from the donor by one surgical team and the removal of the recipient's diseased heart and the attachment of the donor's heart to the major vessels of the recipient's heart by a second surgical team (Figure 21-1). In addition to the immunosuppressive agents given to the recipient, other medications are given at the time of transplantation. These drugs include such agents as dipyridamole (for platelet suppression), trimethoprim-sulfamethoxazole (to prevent infection), and nystatin (Mycostatin) (*Candida* prophylaxis). Surveillance right ventricular endomyocardial biopsy specimens are obtained after transplantation to check for signs of acute or chronic rejection. Starting 1 year after transplantation, coronary angiography often is performed to look for evidence of coronary artery disease.[11]

Heart-Lung Transplantation. In addition to the surgical protocol for cardiac transplantation, the lungs are generally combined in patients with primary pulmonary hypertension, pulmonary fibrosis, cystic fibrosis, certain congenital heart conditions, and primary cardiac disease accompanied by secondary pulmonary hypertension. Heart-lung transplantation also involves the surgical removal of the heart and lungs from the donor by one surgical team and the removal of the recipient's diseased heart and lungs and the attachment of the donor's heart and lungs with anastomotic sites at the trachea, the right atrium, and the aorta by the second surgical team (Figure 21-2). The typical immunosuppressive agents are used as in heart transplantation.[11,30]

An additional complication, however, that may be seen with heart-lung combination transplantation is the implantation response. The incidence of this particular complication is highest between 4 and 21 days after transplantation. It is a reversible condition characterized by fever, tachypnea, diffuse pulmonary infiltrates on the chest radiograph, decreased partial pressure of oxygen in arterial blood (PaO_2) and increased partial pressure of

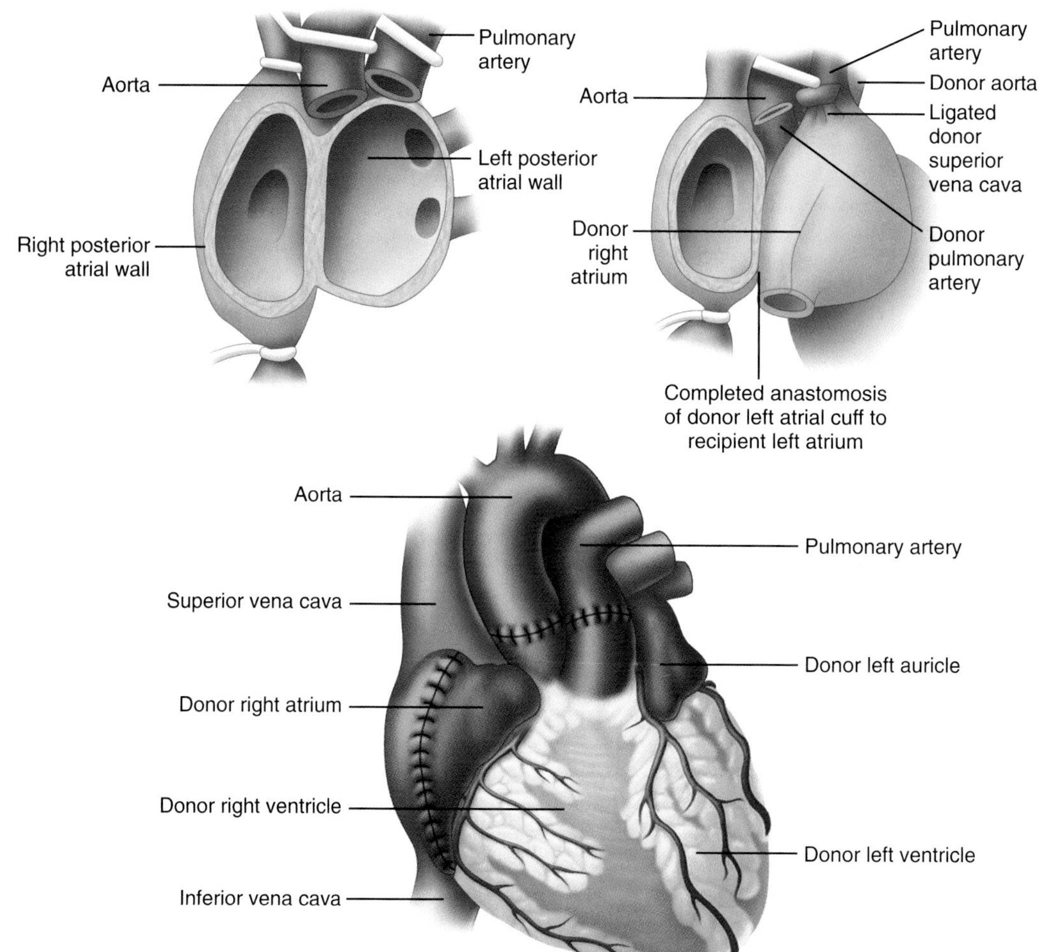

FIGURE 21-1 Orthotopic heart transplant. In this procedure, a patient's atria and ventricles are completely replaced. *(Redrawn from Lamb J: Cardiac transplantation.* Am J Nurs *80:1786, 1980.)*

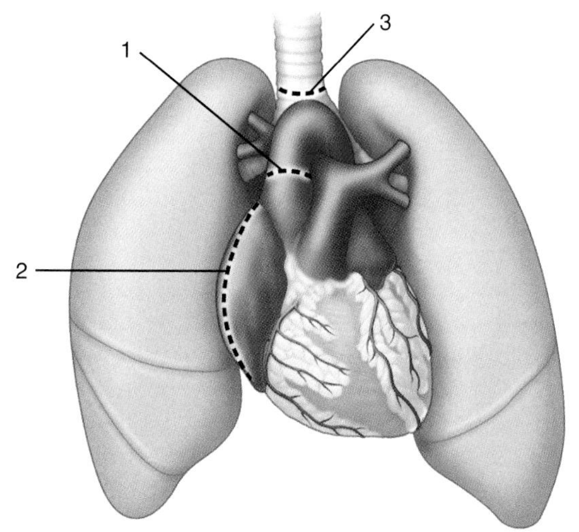

FIGURE 21-2 Anastomotic sites in a completed combination heart-lung transplant: *1,* aorta; *2,* right atrium; *3,* trachea.

carbon dioxide in arterial blood ($PaCO_2$). The cause is multifactorial, involving lymphatic interruption, ischemia, denervation, and surgical trauma. The patient may need short-term mechanical ventilation. Acute rejection of the transplanted organs also is a major complication and constitutes the most common cause of death within the first year.[11,30]

Liver Transplantation. Liver transplantation involves the excision of the diseased recipient's liver with reconstruction of the vena cava, portal vein, and biliary tree (Figures 21-3 and 21-4). The transplant procedure[12] commonly is divided into three phases: (1) dissection, during which the recipient's liver is dissected free of surrounding structures; (2) anhepatic, when blood flow through the vena cava, portal vein, and hepatic artery is interrupted (during this time, the recipient's liver is resected and the donor liver is revascularized); and (3) reperfusion, in which the implanted donor's liver is filled with blood. The final step is biliary anastomosis.[19,30]

Liver transplant procedures have been performed in patients with hemophilia, and their factor VIII deficiency

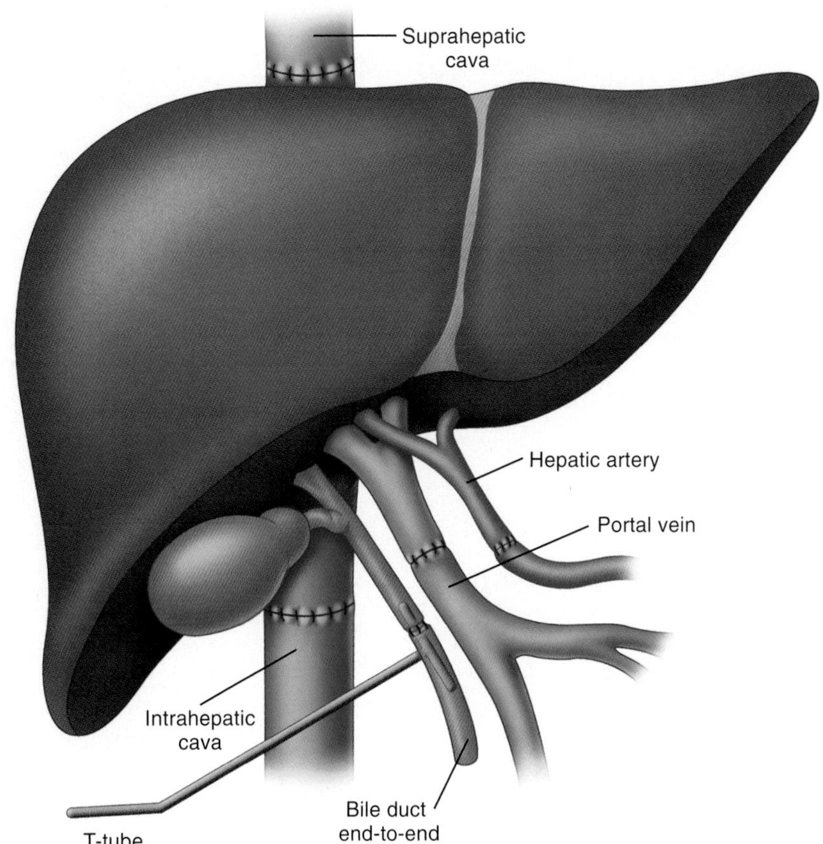

FIGURE 21-3 Completed liver transplant procedure. Vascular anastomoses include the suprahepatic vena cava, infrahepatic vena cava, portal vein, and hepatic artery. A choledochocholedochostomy biliary reconstruction is depicted. *(Redrawn from Kaplowitz N, editor:* Liver and biliary diseases, *Baltimore, 1992, Williams & Wilkins.)*

subsequently was corrected. Obviously, then, factor VIII is produced by the liver and not endothelial cells.[31]

Small Bowel Transplantation. Few small bowel transplantations (SBTs) have been performed. Because of its quasi-experimental nature, use of SBT currently is restricted to patients with end-stage intestinal failure in whom conventional treatments were of no benefit. Intestinal failure is characterized by the inability to maintain nutrition and intestinal fluid and electrolyte balance. Several causes of this condition are recognized, the most common being massive small bowel resection with consequent *short gut syndrome,* which results in rapid intestinal transit without proper absorption of nutrients.[32] Nearly 2 million patients with intestinal failure are diagnosed per year in the United States. SBT commonly is performed in conjunction with liver transplantation. The small bowel is unique among solid organ transplant grafts in the large amount of lymphoid tissue contained in the mesenteric lymph nodes, Peyer's patches, and lamina propria, and in the heavy colonization with microorganisms and large quantities of antigens on the surface of the intestinal epithelium. These factors contribute to a high rate of GVHD, graft rejection, and sepsis.

The surgical technique for SBT is shown in Figure 21-5. The transplanted small bowel has anastomotic sites at the superior end of the native gastrointestinal tract at the jejunum, and at its distal end a stoma is created exteriorly. The superior mesenteric artery is attached to the native aorta below the renal arteries.[33]

Kidney Transplantation. Patients who have a living related donor available for kidney transplantation usually are admitted to the hospital 2 days before transplantation. When a kidney recipient is to receive a cadaver kidney, the patient is admitted to the hospital on an urgent basis. Current preservation techniques allow kidney storage for up to 72 hours.[34]

The indications for renal transplantation generally include chronic renal disease or end-stage renal disease (ESRD). ESRD is a progressive, bilateral deterioration of kidney nephrons that results in uremia and, ultimately, death. ESRD is associated with glomerulonephritis, nephrosclerosis, pyelonephritis, diabetic nephropathy, congenital renal disorders, drug-induced nephropathy, obstructive uropathy, and hypertension.[35]

Accompanying hypertension, diabetes, congestive heart failure, infections, volume depletion, urinary tract obstruction, hypercalcemia, and hyperuricemia must be constantly managed. After conservative care (i.e., drug therapy, dietary restrictions, management of underlying disease), to control waste products, fluid balance, and electrolyte levels becomes inadequate, renal dialysis is

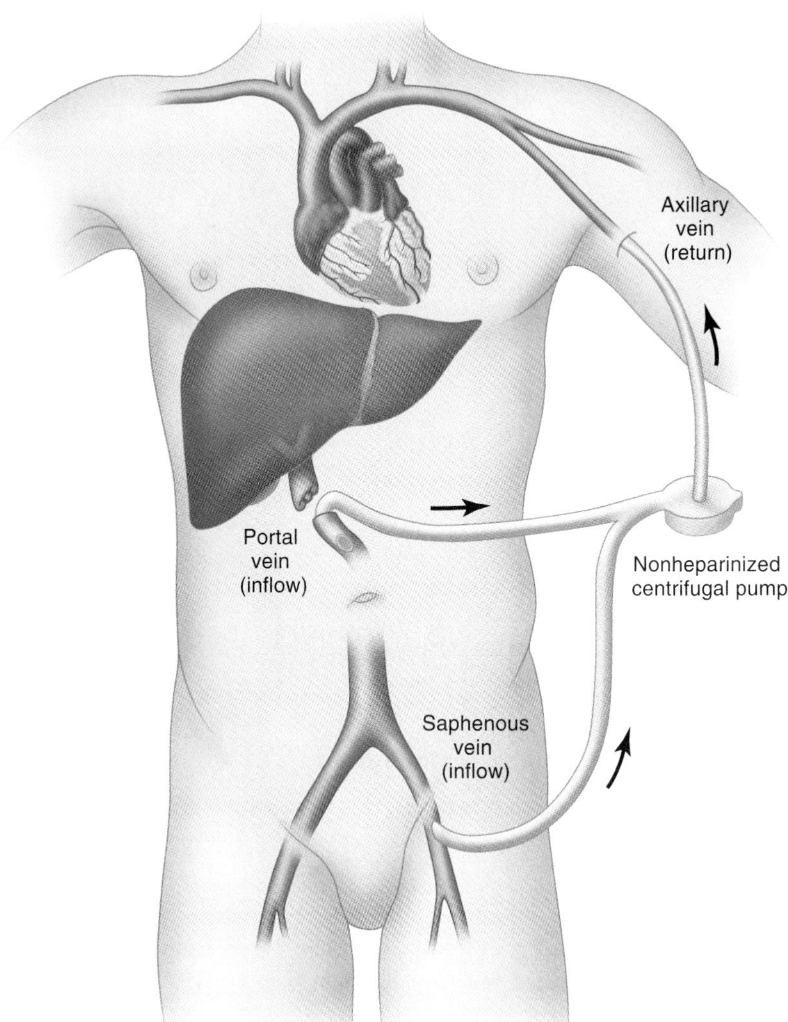

FIGURE 21-4 Venovenous bypass. The portal vein is divided, and devascularization of the liver is completed. Then the portal vein is cannulated and a second cannula is placed in the iliac vein via the saphenous vein. The blood is pumped by a centrifugal pump through a nonheparinized system and returned to the patient by way of a cannula placed in the axillary vein. Flows of 2 to 5 L/min are commonly attained. Flow must be maintained above 700 to 1000 mL/min to prevent thrombosis. *(Redrawn Kaplowitz N, editor:* Liver and biliary diseases, *Baltimore, 1992, Williams & Wilkins.)*

the next step. As renal disease progresses, and more nephrons are destroyed, azotemia cannot be controlled, and the patient must have the blood artificially filtered. Therefore, the therapy of peritoneal dialysis or hemodialysis begins.[9,35]

More than 80,000 patients are currently being maintained on hemodialysis in the United States. Hemodialysis treatment must be performed every 2 to 3 days, and each such treatment requires 4 to 5 hours. The cost in terms of time, money, patient inconvenience, and so on is enormous, and this management mode is extremely confining (see Chapter 12). An alternative to dialysis is transplantation of a kidney from either a living donor or a cadaver. The transplant frees the patient from not only the burden of dialysis but also almost all of the chronic consequences of ESRD. Renal transplantation has become a standard surgical procedure in most major hospitals today.[9,35]

The recipients of a kidney transplant require immunosuppressive preparation so that they will not reject the graft. As with all major transplant procedures, the major problem in renal transplantation is rejection of the graft. The type of preparation depends on the nature of the underlying renal disease. Intensive chemotherapy commonly is used. Chemotherapy with cytotoxic agents (azathioprine) or steroids (prednisone) and administration of antilymphocyte globulin (ALG) are effective. However, greater success has been attained with cyclosporine instead of prednisone or azathioprine.[9,35]

With the immunosuppression, the patient is rendered susceptible to infection and poor wound healing. Sepsis is a major complication in renal transplant recipients. Adrenal function may be suppressed and, likewise, endogenous cortisol production (Box 21-1) (see Chapter 15).

In addition to being given immunosuppressive medications, the patient receives a bladder injection of antibiotic solution through a Foley catheter and a second-generation cephalosporin. In children, the donor renal artery usually is anastomosed to the aorta, and the renal

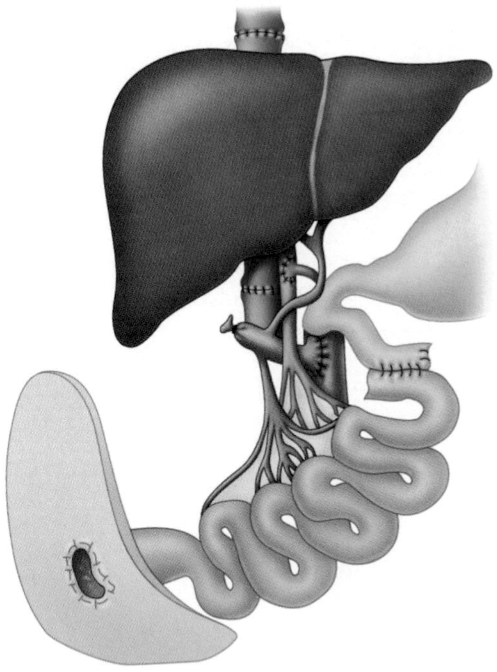

FIGURE 21-5 Small bowel transplantation. Anastomoses are at the superior end of the small intestine at the jejunum, and the terminus is exteriorized in a stoma. Here the liver also has been transplanted. *(Redrawn from Asfar S, Zhong R, Grant D: Small bowel transplantation,* Surg Clin North Am *74:1197-1207, 1994.)*

BOX 21-1 Signs of Overimmunosuppression in Posttransplant Patients

- Viral infections (HSV, CMV, HBV, HIV)
- Bacterial infections (respiratory, wound,)
- Fungal infections (candidiasis, pulmonary)
- Delayed healing
- Excessive bleeding
- Hypertension
- Cushingoid reaction (edema, ascites)
- Addison's reaction (adverse reaction to stress, other factors)
- Diabetes mellitus
- Anemia
- Osteoporosis
- Tumors

CMV, Cytomegalovirus; *HBV,* Hepatitis B virus; *HIV,* Human immunodeficiency virus; *HSV,* Herpes simplex virus.

vein to the vena cava. In adults, the renal artery is anastomosed to either the internal or the external iliac artery. After the kidneys are reperfused, urethral implantation is done. The antibiotics that were started just before surgery are stopped 3 days after surgery, and the patient is given trimethoprim-sulfamethoxazole (Bactrim) daily for as long as the graft is functioning. Acyclovir and nystatin usually are given for the first 3 months to prevent herpes simplex virus (HSV), cytomegalovirus (CMV), and *Candida* infections.[9,35]

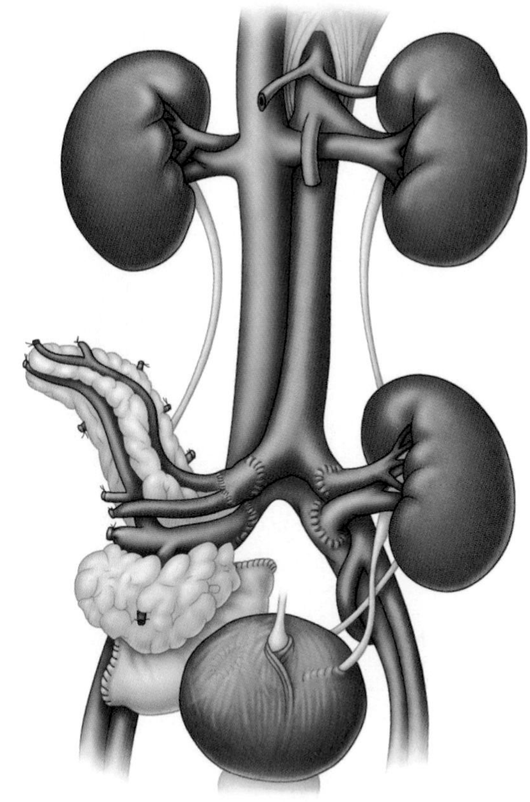

FIGURE 21-6 Pancreaticoduodenocystostomy. Combined kidney and pancreas transplants. *(Redrawn from Groshek M, Smith VL: In Norris MK, House MA, editors:* Organ and tissue transplantation, *Philadelphia, 1991, FA Davis.)*

Pancreas Transplantation. Pancreas transplantation can be done (1) simultaneously with kidney transplantation (Figure 21-6), (2) after kidney transplantation, or (3) as a separate procedure (Figures 21-7 and 21-8). Living related donor grafts usually are used for recipients of pancreas transplants alone or a pancreas transplant after a previous kidney transplant. However, cadaver grafts can be transplanted to all recipient categories. Cadaver donor pancreas grafts can be preserved by cold storage in a silica gel–filtered plasma solution for about 10 to 24 hours. In most grafts, the pancreatic duct is drained into the bladder. Urine amylase levels (25% reduction) are used in patients with bladder-drained pancreas transplants to monitor for rejection. Decreased urinary amylase activity precedes hyperglycemia as a manifestation of rejection. In patients who have simultaneous kidney and pancreas transplants, an increase in serum creatinine indicates the possible onset of rejection before changes in urinary amylase are detected.[36]

A relatively new, revolutionary technique that may have far-reaching implications for the management of diabetes is transplantation of islet cells from a donor's pancreas into the liver of the recipient. The response to the transplanted beta cells has helped in many cases of diabetes. One impediment to the success of this

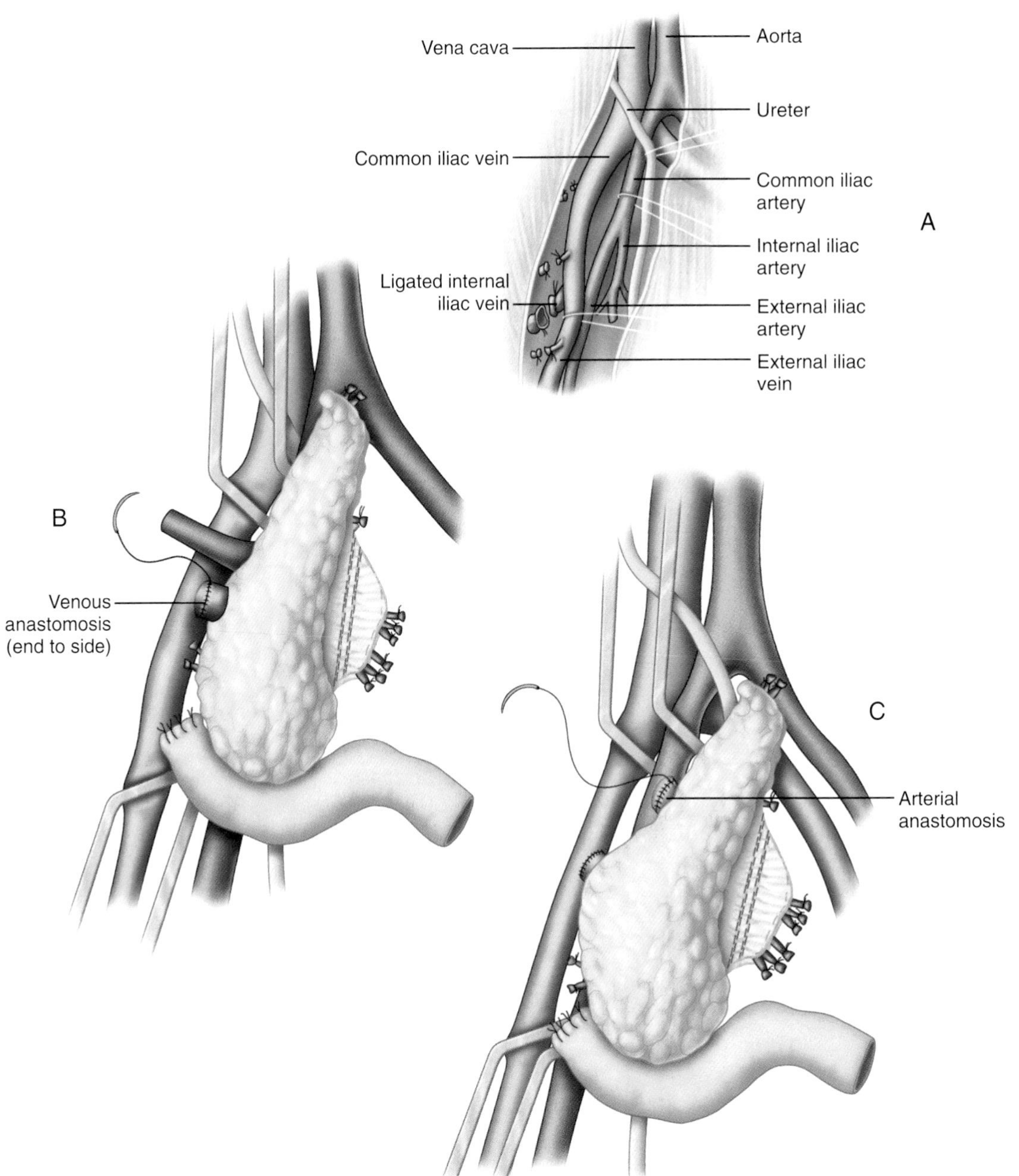

FIGURE 21-7 Transplantation of the pancreaticoduodenal allografts. **A,** Preparation of the recipient vessels. Note that all deep branches of the common and external iliac veins are ligated and divided. The vein is brought lateral to the artery. The ureter is mobilized and brought medial to the artery. **B,** The venous anastomosis is performed end-to-side, with the portal vein of the pancreas graft anastomosed to the proximal external or distal common iliac vein. **C,** The arterial anastomosis is performed after the venous anastomosis and placed superior to the venous anastomosis. The common iliac artery of the recipient is used as the site for the arterial anastomosis. *(Redrawn from In Cameron JL, Cameron AM, editors:* Current surgical therapy, *ed 10, St. Louis, 2011, Mosby.)*

technique has been the need to avoid immune attacks from the recipient on the transplanted donor cells. However, this technique certainly holds much promise for the future.[37]

Bone Marrow Transplantation. Patients who are going to receive a bone marrow transplant are prepared using different preoperative regimens, depending on the patient's disease. The greatest chance of success from BMT is in patients with chronic myelogenous leukemia. Commonly, patients with aplastic anemia, lymphoma, Hodgkin disease, neuroblastoma, or genetic diseases (i.e., immunodeficiency, Hurler syndrome) undergo BMT as well. Chronic myelogenous leukemia is 100% fatal without BMT, but with BMT, the cure rate is approximately 60% to 70%. Acute myelogenous leukemia is 40% to 60% curable, and acute lymphoblastic leukemia has a 20% to 25% cure rate. Cyclophosphamide and total body irradiation or busulfan may be used for

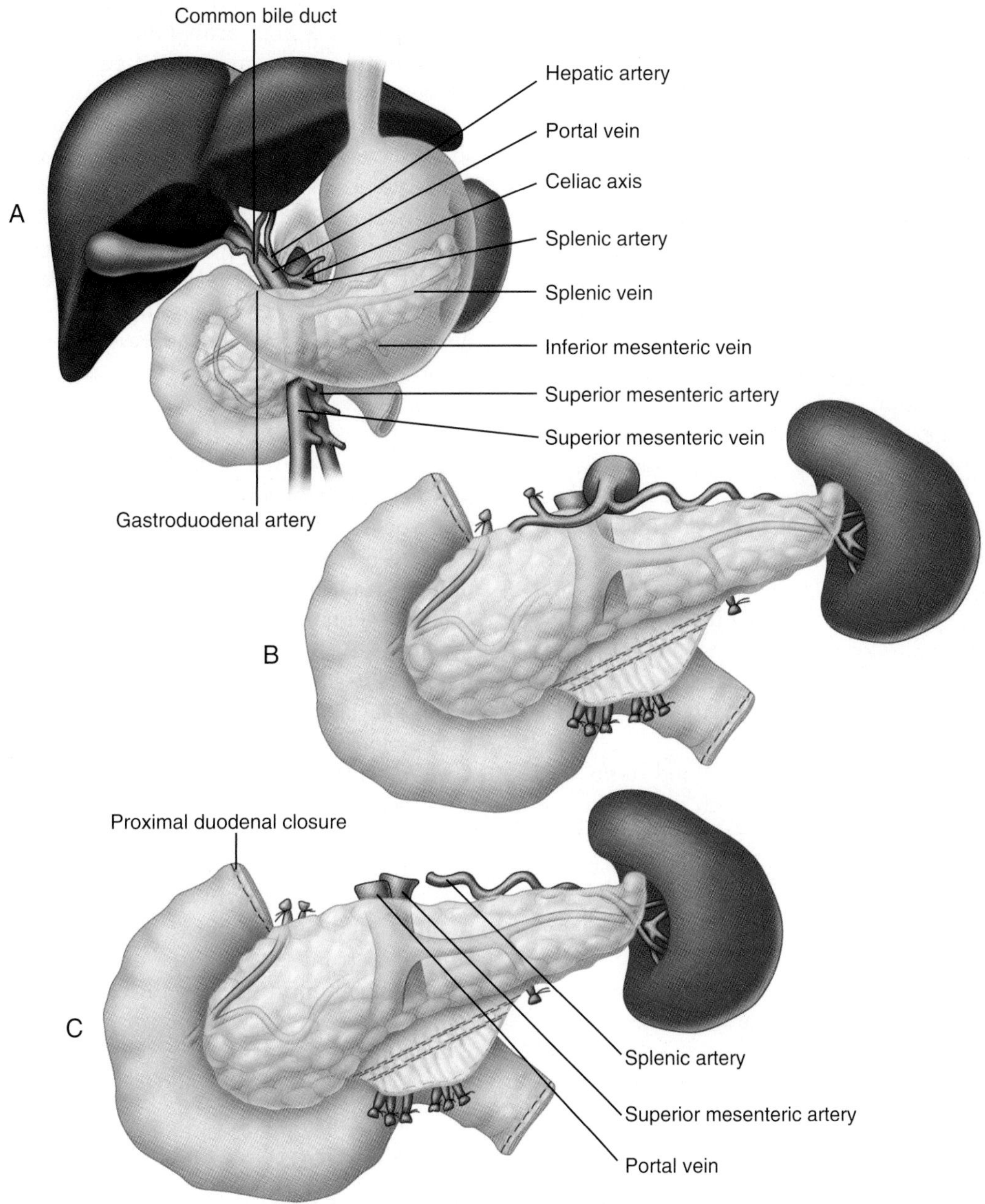

FIGURE 21-8 Procurement of the pancreaticoduodenal allograft. **A,** Vascular anatomy of the liver and pancreas. Note the gastroduodenal artery, which is divided during simultaneous procurement of the liver and the pancreas but not during procurement of the pancreas alone. **B,** Pancreaticoduodenal allograft after procurement (from a nonliver donor). Note that the proximal duodenum has been divided with the gastrointestinal anastomosis (GIA) stapler. The mesentery of the small intestine inferior to the pancreas also has been ligated and divided after placement of two parallel rows of TA 90 staples. **C,** Pancreaticoduodenal allograft after procurement from a donor whose liver also was procured. Note the splenic and superior mesenteric arteries, which require ex vivo reconstruction. *(Redrawn from Cameron JL, Cameron AM, editors:* Current surgical therapy, *ed 10, St. Louis, 2011, Mosby.)*

patients with leukemia. Patients with a lymphoma may be given cyclophosphamide and total body irradiation, busulfan and cyclophosphamide, or busulfan alone. Patients with aplastic anemia may be given cyclophosphamide alone.

The preoperative regimens start 7 to 10 days before transplantation. At transplantation, the donor's marrow is infused into the recipient. The recipient of a syngeneic marrow graft (from an identical twin) requires no immunosuppressive preparation. Similarly, the patient with severe immunologic deficiency requires no immunosuppressive preparation because of the very nature of the disease. All other recipients of BMT, however, must undergo some form of immunosuppressive therapy so that they will not reject the graft. The type of preparation depends on the nature of the underlying disease. BMT is not the cure for the cancer. The intensive chemotherapy or total body irradiation kills the cancer. However, these treatments also may kill the patient, so BMT is used as a "rescue" modality allowing the patient to combat the lethal effects of the chemoradiation therapy.

The marrow is harvested from the donor's iliac bones by numerous needle aspirations performed with use of spinal anesthesia in an operating room environment. The typical quantity of marrow obtained per needle aspiration is 1 to 3 mL (400 to 800 mL is required).[32] Generally, the procedure is well tolerated and involves few complications. In nonmalignant conditions (i.e., aplastic anemia), the preparation of the recipient can be directed solely toward the problem of immunosuppression without worrying about destroying cancerous cells. In malignant disorders, however, specifically, acute myelogenous leukemia, the preparation of the recipient must not only accomplish immunosuppression but likewise kill all or nearly all of the malignant leukemic cells. Total body irradiation (1000 cGy) has been the most effective means of such conditioning in a bone marrow graft recipient. Cyclophosphamide (50 mg/kg) is used in the immunosuppressive phase before (4 to 5 days) the transplantation.[32]

Histocompatibility. Matching of blood type and human lymphocyte antigens (HLAs) with tissue compatibility tests usually results in longer graft and patient survival. The best matching occurs in identical twins; however, with appropriate screening tests, acceptable matches can be found for other potential organ recipients and living or cadaver donors.[9]

With *syngeneic* or isogeneic human marrow transplantation, both donor and recipient carry the same tissue antigens, as in identical twins. Consequently, no immunologic barrier exists to transplantation. An *autologous* marrow graft refers to the transplantation of the patient's own marrow, which was harvested earlier and set aside before the intense chemotherapy or total body irradiation used in preparation for the transplantation. An *allogeneic* marrow graft involves a donor and a recipient of different genetic origins within the same species (usually 50% to 70% of transplant procedures). Siblings provide grafts with the best chance of survival, which are a partial match (haploidentical), or parents may donate the marrow (providing usually 30% to 50% of bone marrow transplants). *Allogeneic* grafts also may involve unrelated donors (usually 10% to 15%). These transplants involve moderate to severe histoincompatibility, with a bidirectional immunologic barrier to transplantation. The recipient may react adversely to the donated marrow and reject it, or the infused marrow cells from the donor transplant, containing immunologically competent cells, may react against the host to produce GVHD.[32,38]

In humans, the major histocompatibility complex (H-2) involves two closely associated serologically detected loci, the first "LA" locus and the second "4" locus (HLA-A4). Marrow grafts between unrelated humans carry a high probability of major histocompatibility problems because of the complex polymorphism of the histocompatibility complex. With transplantation between members of the same family, however, the situation is simplified considerably, because only four haplotypes can be involved. HLA typing of the family can therefore identify the most ideal donor.[10,32,38]

Before the grafting procedure begins, almost all patients scheduled for BMT experience a period of no marrow function as a consequence of their underlying disease and the immunosuppressive preparation. After the transplant procedure, 10 to 20 days are required before the transplanted marrow begins to function. Naturally, this is a critical period for the patient's recovery and for success of the BMT. The posttransplantation period consists of three phases of recovery: the pancytopenic phase (absolute neutrophil count greater than 500 for 4 to 6 weeks), the immune recovery phase (3 to 12 months), and the long-term immunocompetent phase (1 to 3 years). Most patients are given cyclosporine, methotrexate, or steroids after transplantation. Patients who test positive for HSV are given prophylactic intravenous acyclovir. Patients usually are given an antifungal medication such as intravenous miconazole to prevent *Candida* infection. These medications are continued after BMT throughout the critical period needed for the transplanted marrow to begin functioning. As noted, this critical period may last up to 20 days or more. Once the transplanted marrow starts to function, the risk of infection decreases. However, long-term therapy using broad-spectrum antibiotics such as the combination agent trimethoprim-sulfamethoxazole (Bactrim, Septra) is needed to reduce the risk of infection. Patients who develop evidence of GVHD are treated with methotrexate.[10,32,38]

Complications

Complications associated with organ transplantation generally consist of technical problems involving the surgical procedure, problems related to immunosuppression, and special problems specific to the organ transplanted. A discussion of surgical complications is beyond the scope of this book and would seldom apply to dental management of such patients (Box 21-2).

Immunosuppression

Excessive immunosuppression increases the risk for infection and must be avoided. Invasive (biopsy) and noninvasive techniques are used to evaluate patients for signs of excessive immunosuppression. Clinical evidence of such immunosuppression includes occurrence of opportunistic infections and development of tumors known to be related to these agents (see Box 21-1).

BOX 21-2 Major Medical Complications Associated with Transplantation

- Excessive immunosuppression
- Infection
- Tumors
- Delayed healing
- Rejection of allograft
- Graft failure—heart, kidney, liver, pancreas
- Increased risk for excessive bleeding—liver, kidney, bone marrow transplants
- Overdosage—if drugs metabolized or excreted by kidney or liver are administered in normal amounts
- Death or retransplantation—heart, liver, bone marrow transplants
- Insulin, hemodialysis, or retransplantation—kidney, pancreas transplants
- Side effects caused by immunosuppressant agents
- Hypertension
- Diabetes mellitus
- Infection
- Excessive bleeding
- Anemia
- Osteoporosis
- Adrenal crisis (significant stress from surgery, trauma)
- Special organ complications:
    - Heart transplants—accelerated coronary artery atherosclerosis
    - Bone marrow transplants—graft-versus-host disease

When evidence of excessive immunosuppression is found, the dosage of the immunosuppressant drugs must be reduced.

Of course, signs of overimmunosuppression can exist in all types of transplant patients. These signs include infections, delayed healing, hypertension, diabetes, Addison's disease–type reactions, cushingoid features (e.g., edema, ascites, buffalo hump, moon facies), increased susceptibility to infection, weakness, and fatigue (see Box 21-1).[10,32,38]

Rejection

Rejection of the transplanted organ is evidenced by the appearance of signs and symptoms of organ failure. Organ biopsy is used to confirm the rejection reaction (Figure 21-9). When evidence of acute rejection is found, the dosage of the immunosuppressive agents usually is increased.

Chronic rejection occurs insidiously and is progressive. It cannot be reversed with intensified therapy. Chronic rejection of the organ graft is associated with signs and symptoms of organ failure. Classic evidence of chronic rejection is found by biopsy.[10,32,38]

Drug Side Effects

The agents used for immunosuppression have several important side effects. A major side effect of azathioprine is bone marrow suppression with resulting

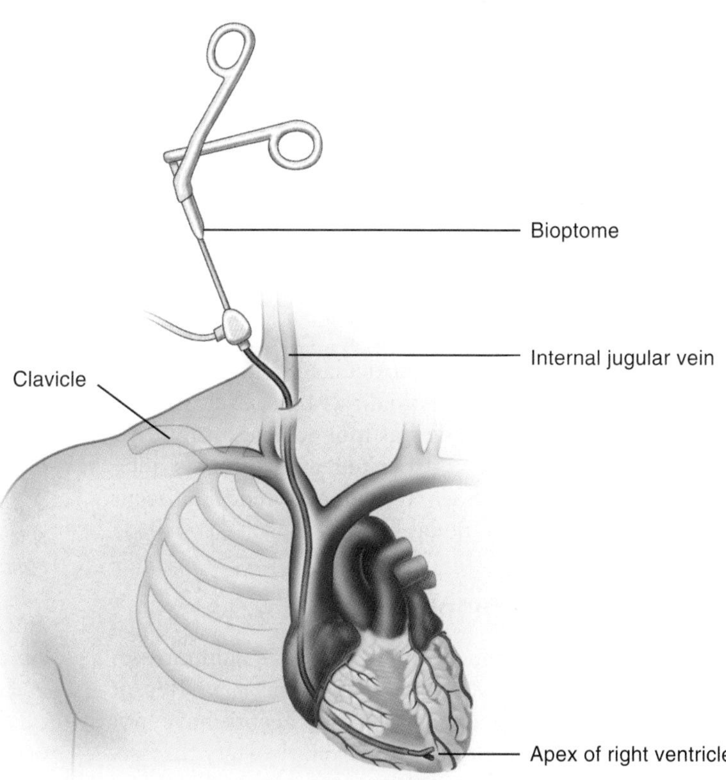

FIGURE 21-9 Endomyocardial biopsy technique, with the bioptome in place in the right ventricle. *(Redrawn from Copeland JG, Stinson EB: Human heart transplantation,* Curr Probl Cardiol *4:1-5, 1979.)*

leukopenia, thrombocytopenia, and anemia. These changes place the patient at greater risk for infection and excessive bleeding. Cyclosporine has replaced azathioprine as the key agent for immunosuppression in transplant patients because it does not suppress the bone marrow. However, cyclosporine does have important side effects: It may cause severe kidney and liver changes, which can lead to hypertension, bleeding problems, and anemia, and it may potentiate renal injury caused by other agents. Cyclosporine also is associated with an increased incidence of gingival hyperplasia, hirsutism, gynecomastia, and cancers of the skin and cervix. Antithymocyte globulin (ATG) and ALG both act as lymphocyte-selective immunosuppressants. Important side effects associated with these agents include fever, hemolysis, leukopenia, thrombocytopenia, tumor development, and increased risk for infection.[9-12,28]

Prednisone has important side effects including hypertension, diabetes mellitus, osteoporosis, impaired healing, mental depression, psychoses, and increased risk for infection (see Chapter 15). In addition to these side effects, prednisone therapy may cause adrenal gland suppression. If adrenal suppression occurs, the patient is unable to produce and release increased amounts of steroids needed to deal with the stress of infection, trauma, surgery, or extreme anxiety.[32]

Immunosuppressed patients exhibit an increased incidence of certain cancers. Overall, approximately 6% of these patients develop various forms of cancer. Cancers commonly seen in the general population (carcinomas of lung, breast, prostate, and colon) show no change in occurrence in immunosuppressed patients. However, two types of cancer found commonly in the general population are found with increased frequency in immunosuppressed patients: squamous cell carcinoma of the skin and in situ carcinomas of the uterine cervix. Cancers that are uncommon in the general population but that occur with increased frequency in immunosuppressed patients are lymphomas, lip carcinomas, Kaposi sarcoma, carcinomas of the kidney, and carcinomas of the vulva and perineum (Table 21-4). Cancer is a complication of intense immunosuppression per se, rather than being related to the use of any particular agent. However, certain agents may play a more direct role. Cyclosporine is one of these agents, as well as monoclonal antibodies. Both of these agents are associated with a higher incidence of lymphoma. Such lymphomas tend to occur earlier and show more nodal involvement.[32,39]

TABLE 21-4 Cancer Development in the General Population and in Transplant Recipients

Tumor	Frequency (%) General Population	Frequency (%) Transplant Recipients
Lymphoma	<5.3	20
Lip carcinoma	<0.3	28
Kaposi sarcoma	<0.1	26
Carcinoma of kidney	2.1	25
Carcinoma of vulva and perineum	<0.6	2

From Najarian JS, Sutherland DER: Pancreas transplantation—1991. Transplant Proc *24:1293-1296, 1992.*

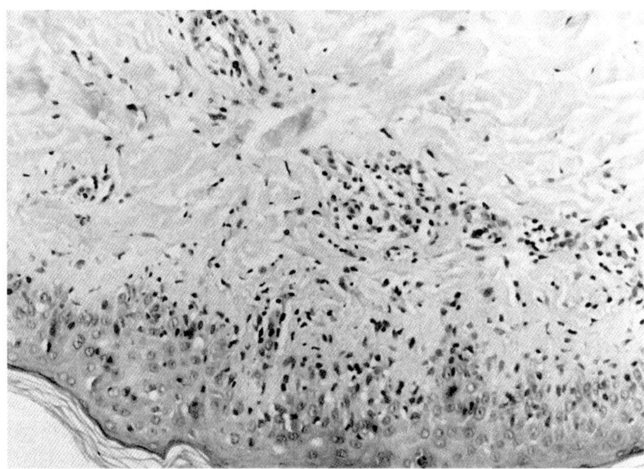

FIGURE 21-10 Photomicrograph of histologic changes of graft-versus-host disease (GVHD) in a patient after bone marrow transplantation.

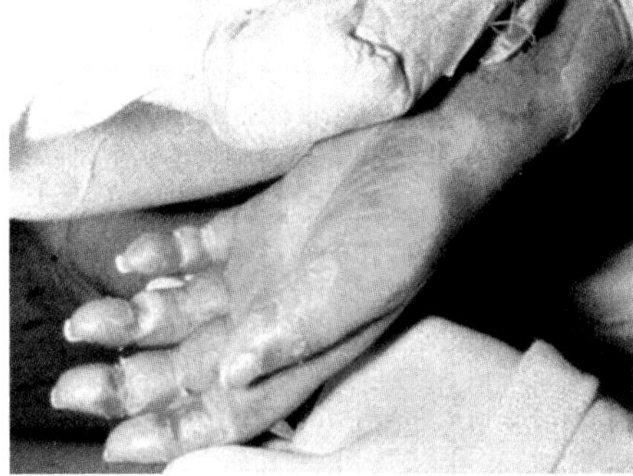

FIGURE 21-11 Other changes of graft-versus-host disease in a bone marrow transplant recipient. Note areas of necrosis. *(Courtesy Norma Ramsay MD, University of Minnesota Hospital, Minneapolis, Minnesota.)*

Special Organ Complications

The major specific organ complications of immunosuppression involve the heart and bone marrow. Recent improvements in immunosuppressant agents have not altered the development of graft coronary artery disease. In one study, the incidence of coronary artery disease in transplanted patients was 10% at 1 year, 25% at 3 years, and 36% at 5 years. Coronary artery disease was responsible for 60% of late deaths.[9-12]

GVHD is an important and often lethal complication of allogenic bone marrow transplantation. Acute GVHD occurs within the first 3 months after transplantation and is characterized by mucosal, skin, liver, and gastrointestinal tract involvement (Figures 21-10 to 21-12).

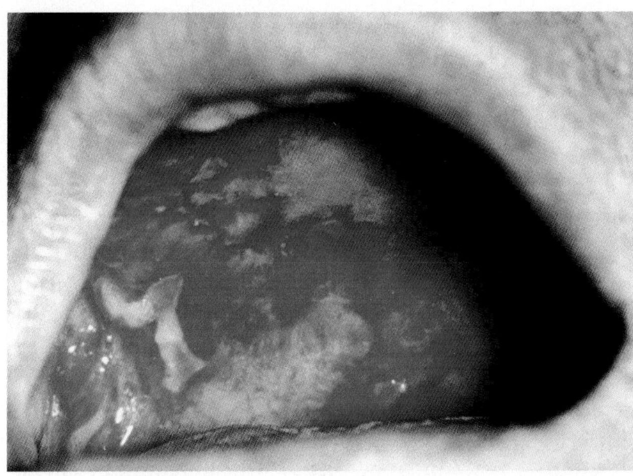

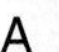

A

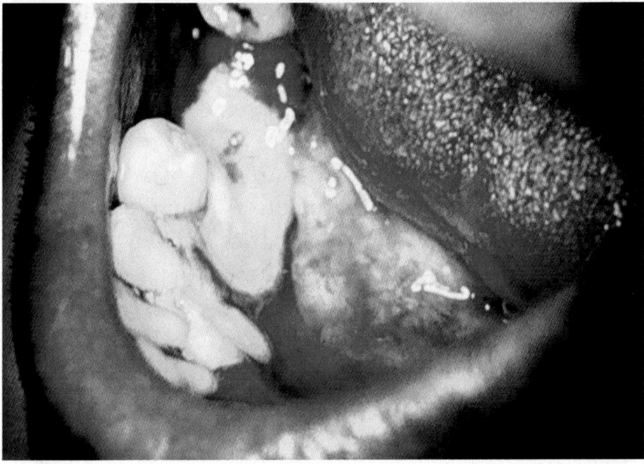

B

FIGURE 21-12 Oral mucositis/candidiasis after bone marrow transplantation: **A,** hard and soft palate; **B,** gingiva and floor of mouth. *(Courtesy Norma Ramsay, MD, University of Minnesota Hospital, Minneapolis, Minnesota.)*

Intraorally there are nonspecific mucosal ulcers and palatal mucoceles. Chronic GVHD occurs later (often after day 100) and is characterized by skin changes similar to those in scleroderma, sicca syndrome, malabsorption, and features of autoimmunity. Cyclosporine appears to be more effective than methotrexate in preventing GVHD in HLA-identical siblings who have received a bone marrow transplant for severe aplastic anemia. Methotrexate appears to be more effective for acute leukemia.[9-12]

DENTAL MANAGEMENT

Pretransplant Medical Considerations

A number of significant medical problems must be considered during the dental management of patients being prepared for transplantation. First, the patient will have significant end-organ disease from the organ system for which a transplant is necessary. The problems associated with advanced coronary artery disease, significant cardiac arrhythmias, and congestive heart failure are discussed in Chapters 4, 5, and 6. The medical considerations that affect the dental treatment of patients with end-stage liver disease and renal failure are discussed in Chapters 10 and 12. The medical considerations affecting dental treatment for severely diabetic patients being considered for kidney and pancreas transplantation are covered in Chapters 12 and 14. Therefore, the dentist must manage the pretransplantation patient as indicated for severe medical complications from the particular organ system.[9-12]

Second, a thorough dental evaluation will be necessary and is required by most transplant centers to diagnose and treat any existing dental disease, particularly any infection or any oral condition that could result either in an infection or the need for oral surgery during the immediate posttransplantation phase, when the patient will be immunocompromised and very susceptible to infection.

Immediately after the transplant procedure and for several weeks thereafter, the patient will be extremely immunosuppressed from induction immunosuppression, which will be directed to prevent graft rejection. Therefore, the likelihood of associated morbidity is extremely high, with potentially devastating consequences.[28]

Obviously, a consultation with the transplant surgeon and team will be important to determine precisely the patient's physical status as well as the details of the procedure as well as the likelihood of posttransplantation complications including infections. Infections are a very serious concern in the transplant patient, and any potential source of infection in the posttransplant period must be identified and prevented. Therefore, antibiotics may be needed (Table 21-5). Because protocols vary from transplant center to center, no standard regimen has emerged. In many instances, transplant physicians and medical insurance request the dental evaluation to be performed as a medically necessary, inpatient service.

Furthermore, it is best to avoid any dental treatment for about 6 months after transplantation, owing to many associated potential complications aside from infections, such as fatigue, medication interactions and side effects, and inadvertent saliva aspiration leading to aspiration pneumonia.[28]

The patient who is a candidate for a bone marrow transplant generally is very ill and prone to infection, bleeding, and delayed healing secondary to thrombocytopenia and leukopenia (see Chapters 22 and 23).

The transplantation preparation may be a very difficult process, because the patient typically may have been unable to maintain good dental health previously. The ideal treatment plan should restore the patient to optimal oral health before the surgery and therefore may necessarily need to be expeditious, because the transplant surgery may be imminent (less than 1 week). Past dental

TABLE 21-5 Recommended Standard Prophylactic Regimen for Dental/Oral Procedures in the Posttransplant Patient*

Medication	Regimen
Amoxicillin	2 g orally 1 hour before the procedure
plus metronidazole	500 mg orally 1 hour before procedure
If amoxicillin-penicillin allergy[†]: Vancomycin	1 g IV Infused slowly over 1 hour preoperatively
or	
Imipenem	1 g IV Infused slowly over 1 hour preoperatively
Unable to take oral medication	
Ampicillin	2 g IV 1 hour before procedure
plus metronidazole	500 mg IV 1 hour before procedure

*Only when prophylactic antibiotics are indicated.
[†]For the prevention of spontaneous bacterial peritonitis.
NOTE: Clindamycin should not be used in most organ transplant recipients because of the potential for acute liver toxicity.

history as well as prognosis and attitudes toward maintenance of oral health may strongly influence the scenario of aggressive treatment before the transplant. Other factors that may affect the treatment plan include financial concerns, ability to tolerate dental procedures and to access dental care after transplantation, general medical stability, and the constraints of the organ donor. Priority must be given to the patient's overall medical status and the ultimate success of the transplant procedure.[29,40-44]

Posttransplantation Medical Considerations

Medical considerations of clinical importance in the dental management of the patient who has received an organ transplant can be divided into three stages: (1) immediate posttransplantation period, (2) stable posttransplantation period, and (3) chronic rejection period.[9-12]

During the immediate posttransplantation period, which generally encompasses the first 3 months after the transplant procedure, the patient will be started on immunosuppressive therapy to prevent cytotoxic T cells from destroying the graft. During this period, the patient is at the greatest risk for technical complications, acute rejection, and infection. The duration of this period will vary, depending on a number of factors. Cyclosporine, prednisone, and other immunosuppressive agents (azothioprine, antilymphocyte globulin) have great benefit in increasing the survival and preventing rejection in posttransplant patients (see Table 21-3). However, these agents also have significant major side effects and are associated with substantial risk for infection. Also, many drugs exist that may adversely interact with cyclosporine and other immunosuppressive agents, in the transplant patient including several drugs that dentists may use (i.e., erythromycin, ketoconazole, carbamazepine, phenytoin, and others) (Table 21-6). The dentist needs to consult with the patient's physician to confirm current health status, ascertain the level and severity of immunosuppression, and identify potential drug interactions and to determine whether the patient has progressed beyond this critical stage.

Medical complications are relatively common during the immediate posttransplant period. The patient may have acute respiratory distress syndrome; viral, bacterial, and fungal infections of varying types and severity; bleeding problems; hypertension; acute renal and/or hepatic failure; acute pancreatitis; and other problems. For these reasons, during the first 3 months after an organ transplant procedure, the patient should receive only emergency dental treatment, as required, and elective procedures should be postponed. Even the emergency dental treatment must be provided in close association with the patient's physician(s). Although there is no overall recommendation for antibiotic prophylaxis for transplant patients, antibiotics should be used during this time because of the immunosuppression and increased risk for infections. The type of agents and regimen for this antibiotic prophylaxis are specific for transplant patients and is presented in Table 21-5.[9-12]

The next stage is the period during which the graft is stable and functional. In most cases, this is approximately 3 months after transplantation. The patient has undergone graft healing and the new organ should be functioning nearly normally. In most cases, the coagulation factors and susceptibility to bleeding and the blood chemistry profiles will have returned to normal limits, although this should be confirmed by the patient's physician. The medical considerations during this stage relate to the effects of immunosuppressive agents. The patient will still be susceptible to infections (Table 21-7), but at this time the major concern is overimmunosuppression, which increases the risk for infection, and underimmunosuppression, which increases the risk for acute rejection. If rejection of the graft occurs, the organ begins to fail, and the problems associated with end-stage heart, liver, kidney, and pancreas failure will have to be considered and managed when present.

The side effects of the immunosuppressive agents may present significant medical problems during any of the stages after transplantation. However, those occurring during the stable graft stage are of greatest clinical concern for the dental practitioner. These side effects may increase the risk for infection; excessive bleeding; bone fractures; circulatory collapse after significant

TABLE 21-6 Drug Adjustments in Chronic Renal Disease

Drug	Route of Elimination and Metabolism	Removed by Dialysis	Dosage Adjustment for Renal Failure: Method	GFR (mL/min): 30->50	GFR (mL/min): <50 >10 (between 10 and 50) 2950	GFR (mL/min): <10	Supplement Dose After Hemodialysis
Analgesic							
Aspirin	Liver[50] (kidney)	Yes	I	100%, q4h	100%, q6h	Avoid	Yes
Acetaminophen	Liver	Yes (HD); no (PD)	I	100%, q4h	100%, q6h	q8h	No
Ibuprofen (Motrin)	Liver	?	—	100%	100%	100%	No
Propoxyphene* (Darvon)	Liver[50] (kidney)	No	DR	100%	100%	Avoid	No
Codeine	Liver	?	DR	100%, 75%	100%	50%	No
Meperidine† (Demerol)	Liver	?	DR	100%, 75%	75%	50%	No
Anesthetic							
Lidocaine (Xylocaine)	Liver[50] (kidney)	No	—	100%	100%	100%	N/A
Antimicrobial							
Acyclovir (Zovirax)	Kidney	Yes	I, DR	q8h, 100%	100%, q12-24h	50%, q24-48h	Yes
Amoxicillin, Penicillin V	Kidney[51]	No	I	q8h	q8-12h	q24h	Yes
Cephalexin (Keflex)	Kidney	Yes	I	q6-8h	q8-12h	q12-24h	Yes; 50% of usual dose after HD
Clindamycin (Cleocin)	Liver	No	D	100%	100%	100%	No
Erythromycin	Liver	No	DR	100%	100%	50-100%	No
Ketoconazole (Nizoral)	Liver	No	—	100%	100%		No
Metronidazole (Flagyl)	Liver[50] (kidney)	Yes	DR	100%	100%	100%	Yes (HD); no (PD)
Tetracycline* (Doxycycline)	Kidney[51]	No	I	q8-12h	q12-24h	q24h	No
Benzodiazepine							
Diazepam (Valium)†; Triazolam (Halcion)	Liver	?	D	100%	100%	100%	No
Corticosteroid							
Dexamethasone	Local site and liver		—		100%		No

*Tetracyclines and aminoglycosides are nephrotoxic and should be avoided in patients with chronic kidney disease. Toxic metabolites can build up in severe end-stage renal disease. Nafcillin, clindamycin, and ceftriaxone do not need dosage adjustment in patients with chronic kidney disease. NOTE: NSAIDs can aggravate sodium retention and edema, and full-dose aspirin can aggravate coagulaopathy.

†Active metabolites can accumulate in renal failure, so reduce dose if drug is given longer than a few days

DR, Dosage reduction; *GFR,* Glomerular filtration rate; *HD,* Hemodialysis; *I,* Increased interval extension between doses; *NSAIDs,* Nonsteroidal antiinflammatory drugs; *PD,* Peritoneal dialysis.

NOTE: 100% means no dosage adjustment required.

Adapted from Bennett WM, et al: Drug prescribing in renal failure: dosing guidelines for adults and children, *ed 5, Philadelphia, 2007, American College of Physicians.*

TABLE 21-7 Potential Posttransplantation Infections

Infection	Time to Onset After Surgery	Susceptibility Period
Viral infections		
Hepatitis B	Immediate	4 to 5 weeks
Hepatitis C	3 to 4 weeks	Continuous
HIV infection	3 to 4 weeks	Continuous
HSV infection	3 to 4 weeks	8 to 10 weeks
CMV infection	4 to 5 weeks	Continuous
Bacterial infections		
Staphylococcal wound infection	Immediate	4 to 5 weeks
Staphylococcal pneumonia	Immediate	4 to 5 weeks*
Urinary tract infection (bacteremia/pyelonephritis)	Immediate	4 to 5 weeks
Tuberculosis, *Pneumocystis jiroveci* pneumonia, toxoplasmosis	4 to 5 weeks	25 to 30 weeks
Fungal infections	4 to 5 weeks	Continuous

*Community-acquired pneumonia may occur/recur after approximately 6 months.

CMV, Cytomegalovirus; *HIV,* Human immunodeficiency virus; *HSV,* Herpes simplex virus.

Adapted from Rubin RH, et al: Infection in the renal transplant recipient, Am J Med *70:405-411, 1981.*

BOX 21-3 Dental Management of the Patient Being Prepared for Transplantation

Consultation with physician(s)
Complete dental evaluation:

- Poor dental status—consider extractions and dentures
- Good dental status—maintain dentition
- Other—decide on individual patient basis

Patients Maintaining Their Dentition

1. Extract all nonrestorable teeth.
2. Extract all teeth with severe periodontal disease (clinical attachment loss of 5 mm or greater).
3. Perform endodontic treatment or extraction of nonvital teeth.
4. Perform denture adjustments (if needed).
5. Perform dental prophylaxis.
6. Provide elective dental treatment as time and necessity permit.
7. Initiate an active, effective, oral hygiene program:
   a. Toothbrushing, flossing
   b. Diet modification if indicated
   c. Topical fluorides
   d. Plaque control, calculus removal
   e. Chlorhexidine or Listerine mouthwash (daily)

Patients Receiving Dental Treatment Including Dental Prophylaxis

1. Medical consultation
   a. Degree of organ failure
   b. Current status of patient
   c. Need for antibiotic prophylaxis (WBC count depressed)
   d. Need to modify drug selection or dosage (kidney or liver failure)
   e. Need to take special precautions to avoid excessive bleeding
   f. Other special management procedures that may be required
2. Laboratory tests (surgical procedures planned)
   a. Access to current PT, aPTT, bleeding time, platelet count
   b. Access to WBC count and differential

aPTT, Activated partial thromboplastin time; *PT,* Prothrombin time; *WBC,* White blood cell.

emotional, physical, or surgical stress; hypertension; diabetes mellitus; and anemia.[9-12,28]

Posttransplant patients also are particularly susceptible to fungal infections, especially with *Candida albicans* (see Table 21-7). Therefore, prevention and aggressive management with antifungal agents should be a consideration. Special organ complications found in heart and bone marrow transplantation recipients must be considered during the stable graft period. Symptomatic coronary artery disease develops in many of the heart transplantation patients. However, one important clinical feature of coronary insufficiency or myocardial infarction is missing in these patients: The transplanted heart has no nerve supply, so pain is not associated with angina or infarction.[10,32,38]

In some cases following heart transplantation, valvular degeneration will occur, in those cases antibiotic prophylaxis according to the American Heart Association guidelines should be used prior to dental treatment. Bone marrow transplantation recipients may develop GVHD after transplantation. Acute GVHD occurs during the immediate posttransplantation period, whereas the chronic form of the disease may appear in the stable period. The patient is particularly susceptible to community-based infections such as influenza and pneumonia, so appropriate precautionary measures such as vaccination are important.

The chronic rejection period begins with signs and symptoms usually associated with organ failure along with histologic findings on biopsy indicating chronic rejection of the graft. This reaction is not reversible and will necessitate retransplantation or lead to death in heart and liver transplant recipients. Kidney transplant recipients will require dialysis or retransplantation. Pancreas transplant recipients will require insulin or retransplantation.[9-12,28]

TREATMENT PLANNING CONSIDERATIONS

Pretransplantation Patients

Patients being prepared for transplantation (Box 21-3) should be referred for an evaluation of their dental status. Whenever possible, patients found to have active dental disease should receive indicated dental care before the transplant operation. Patients with advanced periodontal disease may best be advised to have their teeth extracted and dentures constructed. The same consideration would be involved for patients who have extensive caries and have demonstrated little interest in or ability necessary for improving the level of oral hygiene or to modify the diet.[10,32,38,43]

Patients who enjoy a very good level of dental health should be encouraged to keep their teeth, but they must be advised of the risks and problems involved if significant dental disease were to develop after transplantation. The need for effective preventive dental procedures and more frequent recall visits to the dentist after transplantation must be pointed out to the patient (see Box 21-3).

Recommendations concerning retention of teeth for patients who have a dental status that falls between the extremes of poor and very good are more difficult to make. The risks involved regarding infection, the steps needed to prevent these complications, and the costs involved must be discussed with the patient and the transplant surgeon. Patients with poor oral hygiene who have failed to become motivated to improve their level of home care should be encouraged to consider the extraction of teeth and the construction of dentures.[9-12,28,43]

Before transplantation, all nonrestorable teeth and teeth with advanced periodontal disease should be extracted in those patients deciding to retain their dentition. Nonvital teeth should be endodontically treated or extracted, and all active carious lesions should be restored in these patients. Preventive dentistry techniques including toothbrushing and flossing, diet modification, and the use of topical fluorides should be initiated, reviewed, and implemented. The importance of using effective hygiene procedures, including antiseptic mouth rinses such as chlorhexidine or Listerine, and the need for maintenance of good oral hygiene must be emphasized (see Box 21-3).[28]

Before invasive dental procedures are performed on the patient and before transplantation, the dentist must consult with the patient's physician to establish the degree of organ dysfunction, need for prophylactic antibiotics to prevent local or distant infection, the ability of the patient to tolerate dental treatment, and the need to obtain other management suggestions. In most cases, the earlier that most dental treatment should be performed before the transplant, the better.[9-12,28]

No data exist to show that prophylactic antibiotics are indicated in the dental management of patients with advanced heart, liver, kidney, and pancreatic disease unless patients are subject to endocarditis or endarteritis.[43] In patients with a depressed WBC count, a case can be made for using prophylactic antibiotics. The presence of infection in the operative field might be used as an additional indication for the use of antibiotics. Patients being prepared for bone marrow transplantation may require antibiotic prophylaxis. The need for prophylactic antibiotic treatment for invasive dental procedures in patients with advanced heart, liver, kidney, or bone marrow disease should be discussed with the patient's physician before treatment.[43] The possibility exists for spontaneous bacterial peritonitis after transplantation, so antibiotic prophylaxis may be indicated.[45] If the decision is made to use prophylactic antibiotics for certain patients, no general agreement on antibiotic, dosage, or duration of administration has emerged. The current American Heart Association standard regimen used for prevention of endocarditis appears to be adequate for this need (see Table 21-5). Patients facing BMT may require a more aggressive prophylactic regimen than do those with advanced heart, liver, and kidney disease.[9-12,28]

Results of selective screening tests shown in Table 21-2 should be reviewed. If they are not available through medical consultation, they should be ordered before any invasive dental procedure is performed. If the screening tests reveal significant alterations in bleeding time or coagulation status (prothrombin time [PT], thrombin time [TT], and activated partial thromboplastin time [aPTT]), the dentist should consider using antifibrinolytic agents, fresh frozen plasma, vitamin K, and platelet replacement. The approach selected should be based on consultation with the patient's physician. The physician also should be consulted regarding drug selection and dosage modification.[9-12,28]

In patients with end-stage liver or kidney disease, the dentist should not use drugs that are metabolized by these organs, or should prescribe such drugs in a reduced dosage to prevent increased or unexpected effects (see Table 21-6). Patients with severe diabetes mellitus must be managed as described in Chapter 14. If infection is present, an increase in insulin dosage may be required. Again, the dentist should consult with the patient's physician to confirm the patient's current status and specific management needs (see Box 21-3).

Posttransplant Patients

The dental management of the patient after transplantation can be divided in three phases: (1) immediate posttransplant period, (2) stable graft period, (3) chronic rejection period (Box 21-4), or, in bone marrow transplants, the onset of significant GVHD.

Immediate Posttransplantation Period. During this phase, when operative complications and acute rejection of the graft are the major medical concerns, no routine dentistry is indicated. Only emergency dental care should be provided, as confirmed by medical consultation, and it should be as noninvasive as possible[9-12,28,43] (see Box 21-4).

Stable Posttransplantation Period. Once the graft has healed and the acute rejection reaction has been controlled, the patient is considered to be in the stable phase.

BOX 21-4 Dental Management of Patients with Transplanted Organs

Immediate Posttransplantation Period (up to 6 months)

Consultation with physician(s)

1. Avoid routine dental treatment.
2. Continue oral hygiene procedures.
3. Provide emergency dental care as needed (eliminate infections).
   a. Medical consultation
   b. Conservative selection of treatment

Stable Graft Period

Consultation with physician(s)

1. Maintain effective oral hygiene procedures.
2. Initiate active *recall* program with appointments every 3 to 6 months.
3. Schedule *medical consultation* regarding patient status and management.
4. Treat all new *dental disease.*
5. Use *standard precautions* in controlling infection.
6. Have staff *vaccinated* against HBV infection.
7. Avoid infection.
   a. Medical consultation—need for antibiotic prophylaxis (no evidence that it is needed)
   b. Screening tests—WBC count, differential, CD4+ and CD8+ counts
   c. American Heart Association (AHA) standard regimen as option
8. Avoid excessive bleeding.
   a. Screening tests—INR (PT), aPTT, platelet count
   b. Special precautions
9. Alter *drug selection* or reduce dosage.
   a. Liver or kidney failure
   b. Avoid drugs toxic to liver or kidney (i.e., NSAIDs)
10. Establish need for *steroid supplementation* and be able to identify and deal with acute adrenal crisis if it should occur.
11. Examine for oral signs and symptoms of *overimmunosuppression* or *graft rejection.*
12. Monitor blood pressure in patients taking cyclosporine or prednisone; if blood pressure increases above established baseline, refer for medical evaluation.

Chronic Rejection Period

Consultation with physician(s)

1. Render immediate or emergency dental treatment (especially infections).
2. Follow recommendations for patients with stable grafts if dental treatment is needed.

aPTT, Activated partial thromboplastin time; *HBV,* Hepatitis B virus; *INR,* International normalized ratio; *NSAIDs,* Nonsteroidal antiinflammatory drugs; *PT,* Prothrombin time.

This period should be confirmed by medical consultation with the transplant surgeon. Usually any indicated dental treatment can be performed during this period if the procedures shown in Box 21-4 are adhered to completely. Many of the dental management problems in the stable posttransplantation period are similar regardless of the organ that was transplanted. However, some problems are unique to patients with specific transplanted organs.[9-12,28]

Risk of Infection. Many posttransplantation infections may occur (see Table 21-7). The health care professional must be aware of the clinical appearance, signs, and symptoms of these various infections. In some cases, specific prophylaxis may be indicated.

The increased risk for infection in the immunosuppressed transplant patient makes the case for use of prophylactic antibiotics stronger. Many transplant centers recommend prophylactic coverage for all dental procedures that can produce transient bacteremias in these patients. The rationale for this practice is based on the increased risk for local and systemic infection resulting from suppression of the immune system. Again, no data indicate if this practice is effective or necessary for all immunosuppressed transplant patients. To further complicate the situation, the oral flora in these patients is altered by the immunosuppressive therapy, making the selection of the best antibiotics for prophylaxis difficult. In addition, repeated antibiotic prophylaxis itself may alter the oral flora. Patients who have shown evidence of rejection and are receiving an increased dose of immunosuppressive agents are considered to be at greater risk for infection. A stronger case for the use of prophylactic antibiotics could be made for these patients.[9-12,28]

Because of the lack of scientific information indicating any benefit from antibiotic prophylaxis in the prevention of local or systemic infection in organ transplant patients receiving invasive dental procedures, antibiotic use should be determined on an individual patient basis. Thus, the decision to use antibiotic prophylaxis and the regimen to follow should be made in consultation with the patient's transplant physician. Patients in excellent to good dental health, whose grafts are stable, and who are not undergoing extensive dental procedures may not require prophylaxis. By contrast, patients needing increased dosage of immunosuppressants, or those with active dental infection (chronic periodontitis), may best be managed using antibiotic prophylaxis for invasive dental procedures (see Table 21-5).[43]

The recommendations for antibiotic prophylaxis in posttransplant patients are somewhat different from those for prevention of infective endocarditis. Part of the rationale for this is the susceptibility of posttransplant patients to subacute bacterial peritonitis.[45,46] The basic prophylactic regimen is with amoxicillin 2 g 1 hour before the dental procedure plus metronidazole 500 mg 1 hour before the dental procedure. In patients allergic to amoxicillin, vancomycin, or imipenem 1 g infused slowly over 1 hour before the dental procedure should be used. Clindamycin may be toxic to the liver and kidneys and therefore should not be used in most posttransplant patients. In patients who cannot take a drug by the oral route, intravenous ampicillin 1 g with metronidazole 500 mg 1 hour before the dental procedure should be used (see Table 21-5).[9-12,28]

The immunosuppressive agents used in the transplant recipient may mask the early signs and symptoms of oral infection, making the diagnosis of the problem more difficult. When acute infection does occur, it often is more advanced and severe than that found in normal patients. The dentist should examine carefully for any evidence of acute infection in all transplant patients. The overimmunosuppressed patient can be more prone to oral infection, as can be the patient with bone marrow suppression caused by the side effects of azathioprine, ALG, or ATG.[47,48]

Viral Infections. Posttransplant patients may be especially susceptible to viral infections. The agents include: herpes simplex viruses (HSV), Epstein-Barr virus (EBV), cytomegalovirus (CMV), hepatitis B and hepatitis C virus (HBV, HCV), and human immunodeficiency virus (HIV). The most common infection in these patients is CMV. Effective infection control procedures must be used when transplant patients receive dental treatment. Patients who receive a transplant because of chronic hepatitis complications may still be infected with HBV or HCV. In addition, during transplant surgery, additional blood is used, increasing the risk of infection with HBV or HCV. A few transplant patients also become HIV infected (see Table 21-7). Excessively immunosuppressed patients may be infected with HSV, CMV, EBV, or other microorganisms that potentially may be transmitted to dental staff or other patients. Patients also are at increased risk for infection transmitted to them in the dental operatory. The use of barrier techniques and the practice of standard precautions (recommended for all patients being treated in the dental office) are considered adequate to manage posttransplant patients with stable grafts. In addition, hepatitis B vaccine should be administered to all members of the dental staff to protect against infection from HBV.[47,48]

Excessive Bleeding. Liver transplant patients may be taking anticoagulants to prevent recurrence of hepatic vein thrombosis. Heart transplant patients may be taking anticoagulants to prevent thrombosis of the coronary vessels. Transplant patients taking anticoagulants may need to have the dosage reduced by their physician before any dental surgical procedures. If the level of anticoagulation is greater than that for an international normalized ratio (INR) of 3.5, the dosage of the medication may need to be reduced by the patient's physician (see Chapter 24). At least 3 to 4 days are required for the effect of the reduced dosage to lower the PT. When the patient's INR has been appropriately reduced, the surgery can be performed. If the INR is greater than 3.5, the surgery may need to be delayed. After surgery, the dentist must be prepared to deal with excessive bleeding, by use of splints, thrombin, hemostatic agents, or antifibrinolytic agents.

Liver, kidney, and bone marrow transplant patients who are not taking anticoagulants still could be potential bleeders if rejection of the graft or GVHD and significant organ dysfunction occur. Therefore, before any dental surgical procedure, the patient's physician should be consulted to determine the patient's current bleeding status. If necessary, selected screening tests should be ordered (aPTT, PT, TT, platelet count).[9-12,28]

Adverse Reaction to Stress. Transplant patients who are receiving steroids may not be able to adjust to the stress of various dental surgical procedures because of adrenal suppression and may require additional steroids before and after these surgical procedures to protect against an acute adrenal crisis (see Chapter 15). The need for supplemental steroids should be established by medical consultation. If steroid supplementation is recommended, the dosage and timing in relation to the dental procedure should be confirmed with the patient's physician. Dental treatment such as surgery or extended appointments may require supplementation. If postoperative pain or complications are anticipated, the need for supplementation is increased. Patients taking a very large daily dose of prednisone usually will not require supplementation (see Chapter 15). Also, many routine dental procedures, such as examinations, orthodontics, prophylaxis, simple restorations, and even minor oral surgery, may not need supplementation.

Even with adequate precautions and management of the patient with appropriate increase in steroid dosage, the dentist should remain alert to the possibility of an acute adrenal crisis. Signs and symptoms of acute adrenal insufficiency include hypotension, weakness, nausea, vomiting, headache, and frequently, fever. Immediate treatment of this complication is required and consists of 100 mg of hydrocortisone (SoluCortef), given intravenously or intramuscularly, and emergency transportation to a medical facility (see Chapter 15).[9-12,28]

Hypertension. An important side effect of cyclosporine is renal damage with associated hypertension (see Chapter 3). Prednisone also can cause hypertension, as well as other adverse effects (see Chapter 15). The dentist must determine, by medical consultation once the graft is stable, what the "baseline" blood pressure is for each patient treated with cyclosporine or prednisone. As a part of each visit to the dentist, the patient's blood pressure should be measured; if it becomes elevated above the patient's baseline level, the patient's physician should be consulted immediately.[28,49]

Chronic Rejection Period. The third posttransplantation period begins with the appearance of significant signs and symptoms of chronic rejection of the graft or GVHD. Onset of this phase should be established by medical consultation. In general, only emergency or immediate dental needs should be treated during this period.[50,51]

Oral Complications and Manifestations

Oral complications associated with advanced heart, liver, and kidney diseases are discussed in Chapters 4, 5,

6, 10, and 12. Oral complications seen in patients with blood dyscrasias are covered in Chapters 22 and 23. Oral complications seen in patients with organ transplants usually are caused by (1) rejection, (2) overimmunosuppression, (3) side effects of the immunosuppressive agents, and (4) in bone marrow transplants (e.g., GVHD).

Oral findings associated with graft rejection are the same as those in patients with organ failure before transplantation. If lesions are found by the dentist that could be associated with organ failure, the patient should immediately be referred to the transplant physician for evaluation for possible organ rejection. Management of ulcerative or infectious lesions associated with organ transplantation is described in Appendix C.[9-12,28]

Oral findings that may indicate overimmunosuppression include mucositis, herpes simplex infections, herpes zoster, CMV infection, candidiasis, large and slow-to-heal aphthous ulcers and other ulcerations, unusual alveolar bone loss, and on occasion, lymphoma, Kaposi sarcoma, squamous cell carcinoma of the lip, and hairy leukoplakia.[9-12,28]

In addition, the potential is present for progressive gingival and periodontal disease. The presence of any of these lesions may indicate that the transplant patient is overimmunosuppressed.

Oral complications associated with the side effects of the immunosuppressive agents include infection, bleeding, poor healing, and tumor formation. Azathioprine may cause bone marrow suppression, which may be accompanied by the appearance of oral ulcerations, petechiae, and bleeding. ATG and ALG may cause bone marrow suppression, thereby increasing the risk for bleeding and infection. Cyclosporine may cause poor healing, increase the risk for infection, and produce gingival hyperplasia. The increased incidence of lymphoma in transplant patients is related to immunosuppression in general but also is related to the side effects of cyclosporine and antilymphocyte monoclonal antibodies. Oral ulcerations developing after liver transplantation were found to decrease once the dosage of the immunosuppressive agent (tacrolimus) was decreased. After proper investigation, the transplant physician may need to reduce the dosage of the immunosuppressant agents.[9-12,28]

Oral manifestations of GVHD include nonspecific mucosal ulcerations, salivary gland hypofunction, and palatal mucoceles.

REFERENCES

1. United Network for Organ Sharing (UNOS) data for organ allocation, available at http://www.unos.org/donation/index.php?topic=organ_allocation, 2010.
2. U.S. Department of Health and Human Services: *2006 annual report of the U.S. Organ Procurement and Transplantation Network and the Scientific Registry for Transplant Recipients: transplant data 2002-2005*, Washington, DC, 2006, U.S. Department of Health and Human Services.
3. U.S. Department of Health and Human Services: 2010 annual report of the U.S. Organ Procurement and Transplantation Network and the Scientific Registry for Transplant Recipients: transplant data (article online), http://optn.transplant.hrsa.gov/latestData/rptData.asp, 2010; accessed on March 5, 2010.
4. U.S. Department of Health and Human Services: *2006 annual report of the U.S. Organ Procurement and Transplantation Network and the Scientific Registry for Transplant Recipients: Transplant data 2002-2005*, Washington, DC, 2006, Department of Health and Human Services.
5. Neumann ME: UNOS data shows largest drop in organ donations in 20 years, *Nephrol News Issues* 24:30, 2010.
6. Terasaki PI: *Clinical transplants*, Los Angeles, 1999, UCLA Immunogenetics Center.
7. Henderson W, editor: *Complications of immunosuppression in organ transplants: transplant surgery*, New York, 1988, Elsevier.
8. Cecka JM, Terasaki PI: *Clinical transplants*, Los Angeles, 1999, UCLA Immunogenetics Center.
9. Rhodus NL, Little JW: Dental management of the renal transplant patient, *Compendium* 14:518-524, 1993.
10. Rhodus NL, Little JW: Dental management of the bone marrow transplant patient, *Compendium* 13:1040, 1042-1050, 1992.
11. Little JW, Rhodus NL: Dental management of the heart transplant patient, *Gen Dent* 40:126-131, 1992.
12. Little JW, Rhodus NL: Dental treatment of the liver transplant patient, *Oral Surg Oral Med Oral Pathol* 73:419-426, 1992.
13. Weiss ES, et al: Outcomes in bicaval versus biatrial techniques in heart transplantation: an analysis of the UNOS database, *J Heart Lung Transplant* 27:178-183, 2008.
14. Lin YT, Yang FT: Gingival enlargement in the cyclosporine-administered liver transplant children, *J Periodontol* 81:1250-1255, 2010.
15. Appelbaum FL: The leukemias. In Goldman L, Ausiello DA, editors: *Cecil textbook of medicine*, ed 23, Philadelphia, 2008, Saunders Elsevier.
16. Hornick D, Rose ML: *Transplantation immunology: methods and protocols*, Clifton, NJ, 2006, Humana Press, p 429.
17. Kashyap R, et al: Living donor and deceased donor liver transplantation for autoimmune and cholestatic liver diseases—an analysis of the UNOS database, *J Gastrointest Surg* 14:1362-1369, 2010.
18. Frazier D: Heart transplants in horizons in organ transplantation, *Surg Clin North Am* 74:1169-1189, 1994.
19. Ozaki S: Liver transplants in horizons in organ transplantation, *Surg Clin North Am* 74:1197-1209, 1994.
20. Hornick D: *Transplantation Immunology: methods and protocols*, Clifton, NJ, 2006, Humana Press, p 429.
21. Tallman M, Gilliland DG, Row JM: Drug therapy for acute myeloid leukemia, *Blood* 106:1154-1163, 2006.
22. Weiss ES, et al: Outcomes in patients older than 60 years of age undergoing orthotopic heart transplantation: an analysis of the UNOS database, *J Heart Lung Transplant* 27:184-191, 2008.
23. Rodriguez JA, et al: Long-term outcomes following liver transplantation for hepatic hemangioendothelioma: the UNOS experience from 1987 to 2005, *J Gastrointest Surg* 12:110-116, 2008.
24. Goh A: An analysis of liver transplant survival rates from the UNOS registry, *Clin Transpl* 19-34, 2008.
25. Waki K: UNOS Liver registry: ten year survivals, *Clin Transpl* 29-39, 2006.
26. Kaneku HK, Terasaki PI: Thirty year trend in kidney transplants: UCLA and UNOS renal transplant registry, *Clin Transpl* 1-27, 2006.

27. Bajwa M, et al: Donor biopsy and kidney transplant outcomes: an analysis using the organ procurement and transplantation network/united network for organ sharing (OPTN/UNOS) database, *Transplantation* 84:1399-1405, 2007.
28. Guggenheimer J, Eghtesad B, Stock DJ: Dental management of the (solid) organ transplant patient, *Oral Surg Oral Med Oral Pathol Oral Radiol Endod* 95:383-389, 2003.
29. Shiboski CH, et al: Gingival enlargement in pediatric organ transplant recipients in relation to tacrolimus-based immunosuppressive regimens, *Pediatr Dent* 31:38-46, 2009.
30. Frazier D: Heart transplants in horizons in organ transplantation, *Surg Clin North Am* 74:1169-1181, 1994.
31. Maio R, et al: Erythropoietin preserves the integrity and quality of organs for transplantation after cardiac death, *Shock* 35:126-133, 2011.
32. Kahan BC: Immunosuppressive drugs in horizons in organ transplantation, *Surg Clin North Am* 74:1015-1027, 1994.
33. Asfar A: Small bowel transplants in horizons in organ transplantation, *Surg Clin North Am* 74:1197-1207, 1994.
34. O'Connor KJ, Delmonico FL: Increasing the supply of kidneys for transplantation, *Semin Dial* 18:460-462, 2005.
35. Browne R: Renal transplants in horizons in organ transplantation, *Surg Clin North Am* 74:1097-1111, 1994.
36. Sollinger T: Pancreas transplants in horizons in organ transplantation, *Surg Clin North Am* 74:1183-1193, 1994.
37. Lacy P: Treating diabetes with transplanted islet cells, *Sci Am* 89:50-55, 1995.
38. Heimdahl A, et al: The oral cavity as a portal of entry for early infections in patients treated with bone marrow transplantation, *Oral Surg* 68:711-716, 1989.
39. King GN: Increased prevalence of dysplastic and malignant oral lesions in renal transplant recipitents, *N Engl J Med* 332:677-681, 1995.
40. Ojha J, et al: Post-transplant lymphoproliferative disorders of oral cavity, *Oral Surg Oral Med Oral Pathol Oral Radiol Endod* 105:589-596, 2008.
41. Vasanthan A, Dallal N: Periodontal treatment considerations for cell transplant and organ transplant patients, *J Periodontol 2000* 44:82-102, 2007.
42. Shiboski CH, et al: Oral disease burden and utilization of dental care patterns among pediatric solid organ transplant recipients, *J Public Health Dent* 69:48-55, 2009.
43. Scully C, Kumar N, Diz Dios P: Hot topics in special care dentistry. 5. Transplant patients, *Dent Update* 36:445, 2009.
44. Schander K, et al: Oral infections and their influence on medical rehabilitation in kidney transplant patients, *Swed Dent J* 33:97-103, 2009.
45. Cai J: Double- and single-lung transplantation: an analysis of twenty years of OPTN/UNOS registry data, *Clin Transpl* 1-8, 2007.
46. Correia-Silva JF, et al: Saliva as a source of HCMV DNA in allogeneic stem cell transplantation patients. *Oral Dis* 16:210-216, 2010.
47. Morimoto Y, et al: Dental management prior to hematopoietic stem cell transplantation, *Spec Care Dentist* 24:287-292, 2004.
48. Cawley MM, Benson LM: Current trends in managing oral mucositis, *Clin J Oncol Nurs* 9:584-592, 2005.
49. Golla K, Epstein JB, Cabay RJ: Liver disease: current perspectives on medical and dental management, *Oral Surg Oral Med Oral Pathol Oral Radiol Endod* 98:516-521, 2004.
50. National Kidney Foundation: KDOQI Clinical Practice Guidelines for Bone Metabolism and Disease in Chronic Kidney Disease 2010 (article online), available at http://www.kidney.org/PROFESSIONALS/kdoqi/guidelines_bone/; accessed December 21, 2010.
51. Oliver R, et al: Antibiotics for the prophylaxis of bacterial endocarditis in dentistry, *Cochrane Database Syst Rev* 4:CD003813, 2008.

PART VIII

Hematologic and Oncologic Disease

CHAPTER

22

Disorders of Red Blood Cells

Disorders of the red blood cells (RBCs), which in large part consist of the anemias, are of clinical importance in dental practice for several reasons. First, the dentist serves an important role in detecting patients with anemia through history, clinical examination, and results of screening laboratory tests. These screening procedures should lead to early referral to a physician and the establishment of the diagnosis. Clinical recognition of anemia can significantly affect morbidity and mortality risks, because anemia often occurs as an underlying condition that requires attention and medical treatment. Also of note, anemia is an independent risk factor for adverse cardiovascular outcomes (i.e., acute myocardial infarction and death) in a variety of patient populations (as defined by chronic kidney disease, acute coronary syndrome, or old age, for example).[1-4] Accordingly, implementation of measures to prevent or relieve anxiety should be considered in the performance of stressful dental procedures in patients diagnosed with anemia.

ANEMIA

DEFINITION

Anemia, which is defined as a reduction in the oxygen-carrying capacity of the blood, usually is associated with a decreased number of circulating RBCs or an abnormality in the Hb contained within the RBCs. Anemia is not a disease but rather a symptom complex that may result from one of three underlying causes: (1) decreased production of RBCs (iron deficiency, pernicious anemia, folate deficiency), (2) blood loss, or (3) increased rate of destruction of circulating RBCs (hypersplenism, autoimmune destruction).

Erythropoiesis

About 1% of the circulating erythrocyte mass is generated by the bone marrow each day. Precursors of RBCs are reticulocytes, which account for 1% of the total RBC count. The normal RBC is about 33% hemoglobin by volume. Hemoglobin (Hb), the oxygen-carrying molecule of erythrocytes, consists of two pairs of globin chains (i.e., α plus β, δ, or γ) that form a shell around four oxygen-binding heme groups. Healthy adults have about 95% HbA ($\alpha2\beta2$) and small amounts of HbA2 ($\alpha2\delta2$) and HbF ($\alpha2\gamma2$). Genes on chromosome 16 encode α globin chains; β chains are encoded on chromosome 11.[5] Oxygen demand (hypoxia) serves as the stimulus for erythropoiesis. The kidney serves as the primary sensor for determining the level of oxygenation. If the level is low, the kidney releases erythropoietin, a hormone that stimulates the bone marrow to release RBCs. About 95% of erythropoietin is produced by cortical cells in the kidney. The other 5% is produced by the liver.[6,7]

EPIDEMIOLOGY

It is estimated that about 3.4 million Americans have anemia.[8] Approximately 4% of men and 8% of women in the United States have anemia, defined as Hb values below 13 g/dL for men and below 12 g/dL for women.[8,9] In the United States, iron deficiency anemia is the most common type.[10] Of the approximately 2000 patients treated in the average dental practice, about 12 men and 24 women will be anemic. In most of these patients, the condition may be undiagnosed.

Etiology

Anemia has numerous causes (Table 22-1). A partial list includes genetic disorders that produce aberrant RBCs that result in RBC destruction (hemolysis), nutritional disorders that limit the production of RBCs, immune-mediated disorders that result in attacks on RBCs, bleeding disorders that cause loss of RBCs, chronic diseases (rheumatoid arthritis), infections, and diseases of bone marrow. Figure 22-1 shows the most common causes of anemia found in general medical practice.[8] This chapter discusses select examples relevant to the practice of dentistry, to demonstrate the clinical problems involved in the management of patients with anemia.

TABLE 22-1 Types of Anemia

Classification by RBC Size and Shape	Cause
Microcytic (MCV ≤ 80 fL*)	
Iron deficiency anemia	Decreased production of RBCs
Thalassemias	Defective hemoglobin synthesis
Lead poisoning	Inhibition of hemoglobin synthesis
Normocytic (MCV 80-100 fL*)	
Hemolytic anemia	Increased destruction of RBCs
Sickle cell anemia	
Glucose-6-phosphate dehydrogenase deficiency	
Aplastic anemia	Decreased production of RBCs
Renal failure	Decreased production of RBCs
Anemia of chronic disease	Decreased production of RBCs
Macrocytic (MCV > 100 fL*)	
Pernicious anemia	Decreased production of RBCs
Folate deficiency	Decreased production of RBCs
Hypothyroidism	Decreased production of RBCs

*Also expressed in μm^3 units.
fL, Femtoliter; *MCV*, Mean corpuscular volume; *RBC*, Red blood cell.

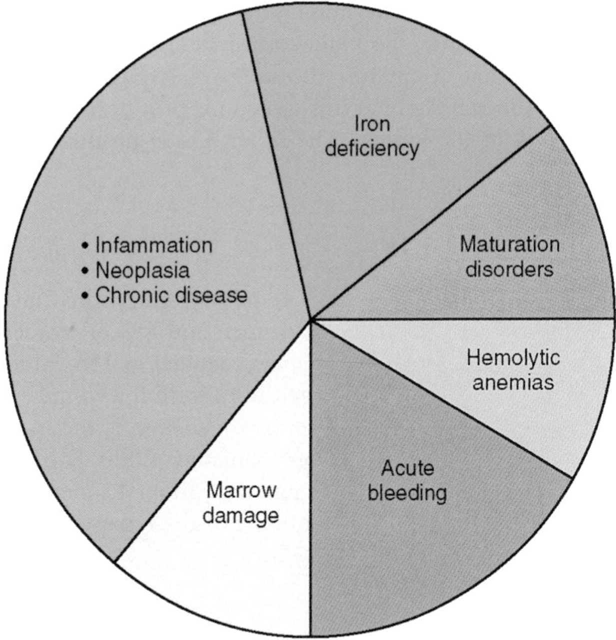

FIGURE 22-1 Relative frequencies of anemia in clinical practice. *(Redrawn from Hillman RS, Finch CA, editors:* Red cell manual, *ed 7, Philadelphia, 1996, FA Davis.)*

TYPES OF ANEMIA

Iron Deficiency Anemia

Iron deficiency anemia is a microcytic anemia (Figure 22-2) that can be caused by excessive blood loss, poor iron intake, poor iron absorption, or increased demand for iron. Blood loss may occur with menstruation or be caused by bleeding from the gastrointestinal tract. Poor intake is more common in children who live in developing countries, where cereals and formula fortified with iron are not readily available. Malabsorption of iron can result from gastrectomy or intestinal disease that reduces absorption of iron from the duodenum and the jejunum. Increased demand is associated with chronic inflammation (autoimmune disease).

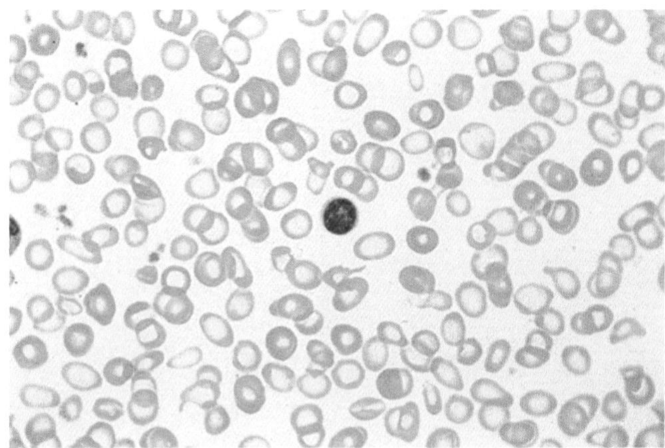

FIGURE 22-2 Microcytic anemia associated with iron deficiency. Peripheral blood smear shows red blood cells (RBCs) that are small and have marked hypochromic central pallor.

In women, menstruation and pregnancy contribute to the development of iron deficiency anemia. The repeated loss of blood associated with menses can lead to depletion of iron, resulting in a mild state of anemia. During pregnancy, the expectant mother experiences an increased demand for additional iron and vitamins to support the growth of her fetus, and unless sufficient amounts of these nutrients have been provided in some form, she may become anemic. Approximately 20% of pregnant women have iron deficiency anemia.[11] Also, 30% to 60% of persons with rheumatoid arthritis (who more commonly are women) have this type of anemia.[12]

By contrast, mild anemia in men usually indicates the presence of a serious underlying medical problem (e.g., gastrointestinal bleeding, malignancy). Under normal physiologic conditions, men lose little iron, and because iron can be stored for months, iron deficiency anemia is rare in men. Therefore, any man who is found to be anemic should be promptly referred for medical evaluation.

Folate Deficiency Anemia and Pernicious Anemia

Vitamin B_{12} (cobalamin) and folic acid are needed for RBC formation and growth within bone marrow. Vitamin B_{12} is a cofactor in methionine-associated enzymatic reactions required of protein synthesis and thus in the maturation of RBCs. Folate is needed for enzymatic reactions required for the synthesis of purines and pyrimidines of deoxyribonucleic acid (DNA) and ribonucleic acid (RNA) and thus for the synthesis of proteins. A deficiency in daily intake (as in chronic alcoholism) or absorption (due to celiac disease or tropical sprue) of these vitamins can result in anemia.

Folate is found in fruits and leafy vegetables. It is not stored in the body in large amounts, so a continual dietary supply is needed. Its absorption and metabolism are interfered with by alcohol consumption and certain drugs (methotrexate, phenytoin [Dilantin]). Risk factors for folate deficiency include poor diet (seen frequently in the poor, elderly persons, and people who do not eat fresh fruits or vegetables), alcoholism, history of malabsorption disorders, and pregnancy (especially the third trimester). Folate deficiency anemia occurs in about 4 of 100,000 people.

Pernicious anemia is caused by a deficiency of intrinsic factor, a substance secreted by the stomach parietal cells that is necessary for absorption of vitamin B_{12} (cobalamin). Because vitamin B_{12} may be stored for several years, this form of nutritional deficiency is rare and usually does not develop until late adulthood. Most often, it occurs in 40- to 70-year-old northern Europeans of fair complexion, with one notable exception. Early onset in black American women, 21% of whom were younger than 40 years of age, has been observed.[13,14] Most patients with pernicious anemia have chronic atrophic gastritis with decreased intrinsic factor and hydrochloric acid secretion. Antibodies against parietal cells and intrinsic factor also are present in the sera of most patients.[14] This finding strongly suggests that the disease involves an autoimmune process.

Long–standing pernicious anemia is associated with increased risk for development of gastric carcinoma. In addition, an association with myxedema, rheumatoid arthritis, and neuropsychiatric and neuromuscular abnormalities (due to a defect in myelin synthesis) has been reported.[13,14]

Hemolytic Anemia

Hemolytic anemias are caused by immune attack, extrinsic factors (infection, splenomegaly, drugs, eclampsia), disorders of the RBC membrane (spherocytosis), enzymopathies (glucose-6-phosphate dehydrogenase [G-6-PD] deficiency), and hemoglobinopathies (sickle cell anemia, thalassemia). G-6-PD deficiency and sickle cell anemia are discussed here to illustrate the problems presented by the hemolytic anemias.[15,16]

Hemolytic Anemia: Glucose-6-Phosphate Dehydrogenase Deficiency

The search during World War II for a substitute quinine led to the use of newer antimalarial drugs and the discovery of deficiency of glucose-6-phosphate dehydrogenase (G-6-PD), an enzyme that helps the RBC to turn carbohydrates into energy. This discovery occurred after several persons who were given primaquine developed hemolytic anemia because they lacked G-6-PD, an enzyme needed for the hexose monophosphate shunt pathway.[13]

Glucose enters the RBC through a carrier mechanism, independent of insulin. About 90% of glucose is metabolized by the glycolytic pathway. The remaining glucose is metabolized by the hexose monophosphate shunt pathway. The byproduct of the glycolytic pathway is adenosine triphosphate, which provides energy for the cell. The byproduct of the hexose monophosphate shunt pathway is nicotinamide adenine dinucleotide phosphate (NADPH), which is used to reduce various cellular oxidants.[15,16] Blockade of the hexose monophosphate shunt pathway in persons with G-6-PD deficiency allows accumulation of harmful oxidants within RBCs. These substances, which produce methemoglobin and denatured Hb, precipitate to form Heinz bodies, which attach to cell membranes. These alterations in cell membranes lead to hemolysis of the cell (hemolytic anemia).[15,16]

G-6-PD is the most common enzymopathy of humans.[15] At present, more than 350 G-6-PD variants have been identified. They are grouped into five classes designated I to V, with class I being severely deficient, on the basis of level of enzyme deficiency.[15] The G-6-PD gene is located on the X chromosome; thus, disease inheritance is gender linked. G-6-PD A, the variant most commonly associated with hemolysis, is found in 11% of African Americans. G-6-PD MED, the second most common variant associated with hemolysis, occurs in ethnic groups from the Mediterranean, the Middle East, and Asia and is associated with sickle cell anemia.[15]

Clinical features of G-6-PD deficiency involve acute intravascular hemolysis, which may be severe. Jaundice, palpitations, dyspnea, and dizziness may result. Infection is the event that most commonly triggers hemolysis in G-6-PD A deficiency. Drugs are the most common trigger for hemolysis in G-6-PD MED deficiency. Of more than 40 drugs that can induce hemolysis, those of significance in dental practice include acetylsalicylic acid, acetophenetidin (phenacetin), dapsone, ascorbic acid, and vitamin K. Fava bean ingestion is the most common dietary cause of hemolytic anemia in persons with G-6-PD deficiency.[15]

Sickle Cell Anemia

Sickle cell hemoglobin (HbS) was the first Hb variant of the more than 600 inherited human Hb variants (hemoglobinopathies) to be recognized. Of these, more than 90% have single amino acid substitutions in the Hb chain. HbS is the result of substitution of a single amino acid—valine for glutamic acid—at the sixth residue of the β chain. In contrast, the thalassemias, another type of hemoglobinopathy, are caused by deletions or mutations of the α or β globin gene that result in a defect in globin synthesis (reduced or absent synthesis of one or more globin chains).[17] The hemoglobinopathies are more commonly found in regions of malarial endemicity and in populations who have migrated from these regions, because the mutated gene(s) confer advantages against infection by *Plasmodium falciparum* (the agent of malaria). Hemoglobinopathies such as sickle cell anemia are inherited as autosomal recessive traits.[17,18]

Sickle cell disorders are distinguished by the number of globin genes affected. The two most common types are sickle cell trait and sickle cell (disease) anemia. *Sickle cell trait* is the heterozygous state in which the affected person carries one gene for HbS. Approximately 8% to 10% of African Americans carry the trait. In western Africa, 25% to 30% of the population may be carriers. *Sickle cell anemia* is the homozygous state. A gene from each parent contributes to formation of the HbS molecule responsible for the disease. The RBC in sickle cell anemia becomes sickle-shaped when blood experiences lowered oxygen tension or decreased pH, or when the patient becomes dehydrated.[18,19] Approximately 50,000 African Americans (about 0.003% to 0.15%), or 1 in 600, have sickle cell anemia.[20,21]

Distortion of the RBC into a sickled shape results from deoxygenation or decreased blood pH, causing partial crystallization of HbS, polymerization, and realignment of the defective Hb molecule (Figure 22-3). Cellular rigidity and membrane damage occur, and irreversible sickling is the final result. The net effects of these changes are erythrostasis, increased blood viscosity, reduced blood flow, hypoxia, increased adhesion of RBCs, vascular occlusion, and further sickling.[18,19] Sickling crises are rare in persons with the sickle cell trait.[18,19]

In patients with sickle cell anemia, more than 80% of the Hb is HbS. Clinical signs and symptoms of sickle cell anemia are the result of chronic anemia and small blood vessel occlusion. These manifestations include jaundice, pallor, dactylitis (hand and foot warmth and tenderness), leg ulcers, organomegaly, cardiac failure, stroke, attacks of abdominal and bone pain (aseptic necrosis), and delays in growth and development (Figure 22-4). Aplastic crisis, an acute illness wherein production of RBCs stops and severe anemia occurs, may develop from

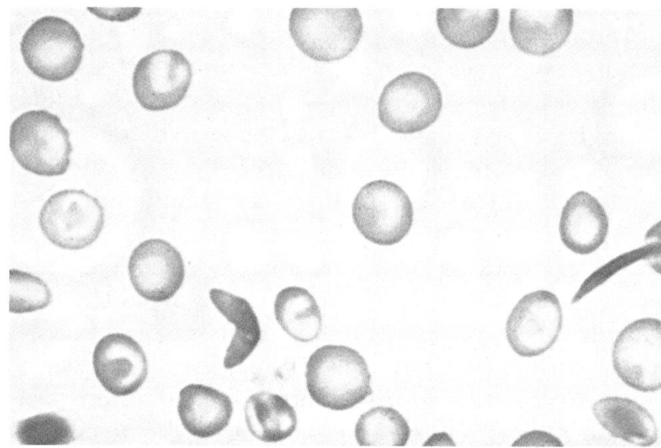

FIGURE 22-3 Sickle cell anemia. Peripheral blood smear shows characteristic abnormal sickle-shaped red blood cells (RBCs).

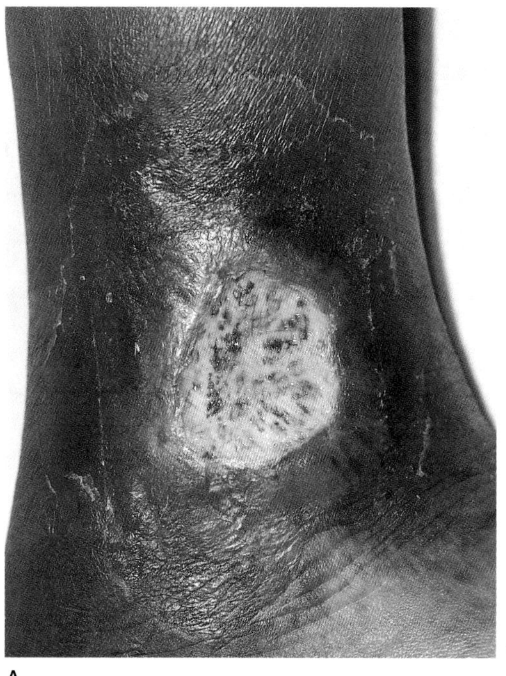

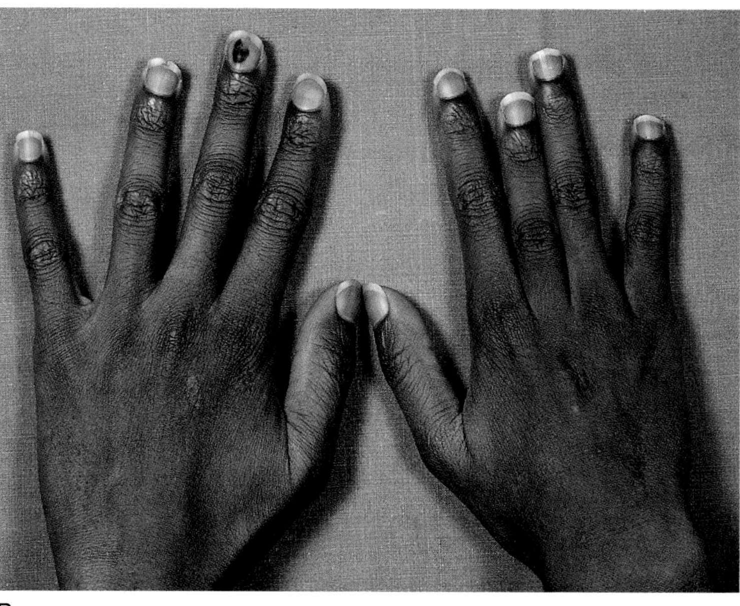

A B

FIGURE 22-4 Sickle cell anemia may cause various complications. **A,** Leg ulcer secondary to a vasoocclusive attack. **B,** Growth deformation of the middle finger from dactylitis of the growth plate. *(From Hoffbrand AV, Pettit JE:* Color atlas of clinical hematology, *ed 4, London, 2010, Mosby.)*

infection, hypersensitivity reactions, hypoxia, systemic disease, acidosis, dehydration, or trauma. Diagnosis requires use of RBC indices and tests in which deoxygenating agents are used (Sickledex). Confirmatory tests use electrophoresis or high-performance liquid chromatography.[18,19,22]

Complications of sickle cell anemia can occur at any age, but patients in the following age groups are more likely to manifest certain complications:

1. *Birth to 20 years of age:* painful events, stroke, acute chest syndrome (fever, chest pain, wheezing, cough, and hypoxia), acute anemia and infection
2. *From 20 to 40 years of age:* osteonecrosis of hip and shoulder joints, leg ulcers, priapism, liver disease, and gallstones
3. *Older than 40 years of age:* pulmonary hypertension, nephropathy, proliferative retinopathy, and cardiac enlargement, heart murmurs, and sudden death due to arrhythmias[19]

People with the sickle cell trait generally have no symptoms unless they encounter situations in which abnormally low concentrations of oxygen are present (e.g., in an unpressurized airplane, through the injudicious administration of general anesthesia). Patients with sickle cell trait are much more resistant to sickling stimuli, because only 20% to 45% of their Hb is HbS. Patients with sickle cell trait are not at risk for adverse events during dental treatment unless severe hypoxia, severe infection, or dehydration also is present.[19-21]

Aplastic Anemia

Aplastic anemia occurs when the bone marrow is unable to produce adequate numbers of RBCs, white blood cells, and platelets. The hematopoietic stem cells are unable to proliferate, differentiate, or give rise to mature blood cells.[23] The incidence in the United States is about 2 cases per 1 million persons per year. The incidence is about two times higher in Asia. Aplastic anemia is most common in young adults (15 to 30 years of age) and in persons older than 60 years of age.[23-25]

Some cases of aplastic anemia are caused by drugs, viruses, organic compounds, and radiation. A few, such as Fanconi's anemia, are inherited. A majority of cases, however, are idiopathic (50% to 65%).[23-25] Anticonvulsants, antibacterials, antidiabetic drugs, diuretics, sulfonamides, and synthetic antithyroid drugs are the drugs most commonly associated with aplastic anemia. Benzene and insecticides also have been shown to cause aplastic anemia. The most common viral infection associated with aplastic anemia is viral hepatitis. A few cases of aplastic anemia have been associated with pregnancy.[23-25]

The most common initial signs and symptoms of aplastic anemia are caused by anemia and thrombocytopenia: weakness, fatigue, headaches, dyspnea with exertion, petechiae, ecchymoses, epistaxis, metrorrhagia (bleeding between expected menstrual periods), and gingival bleeding. Infection is rare as an initial presentation, even in cases of severe neutropenia.[23-25]

Aplastic anemia is described as moderate, severe, or very severe based on the degree of pancytopenia. Moderate aplastic anemia is defined as more than 500 neutrophils/μL, more than 20,000 platelets/μL, and more than 20,000 reticulocytes/μL. Severe aplastic anemia is defined as (two or more) neutrophils less than 500/μL, platelets less than 20,000/μL, and reticulocytes less than 20,000/μL. The values for platelets and reticulocytes are the same in the very severe form of aplastic anemia as in the severe form, but the neutrophil count is less than 200/μL. The prognosis is poorest for patients with the very severe form of the disease.[23-25]

If a specific cause is suspected, the drug should be discontinued. In cases associated with pregnancy delivery or therapeutic abortion is indicated. Aplastic anemia associated with hepatitis B may resolve after antiviral therapy.[23]

Renal Disease

The kidney produces the hormone erythropoietin, which stimulates RBC production by the bone marrow. If significant renal damage occurs, lack of production of this hormone results in anemia. Patients who have chronic renal failure and are on dialysis often have anemia and low erythropoietin levels. Erythropoietic drug therapy is offered to these patients.

Organ Transplantation

Patients who undergo organ (kidney, liver, bone marrow) transplantation and acquire immunosuppression develop anemia as a result of bone marrow suppression.

CLINICAL PRESENTATION

Signs and Symptoms

Symptoms of anemia occur in proportion to the rate of development of anemia; rapidly developing anemia has more profound features than slowly developing anemia. Because in most affected patients anemia develops slowly, most experience few symptoms until the condition worsens. Usual symptoms include fatigue, lethargy, palpitations, shortness of breath, abdominal pain, bone pain, tinnitus, irritability, dizziness, tingling of fingers and toes, and muscular weakness.[7,26] Specific to iron deficiency anemia are impaired immunity and resistance to infection and diminished exercise tolerance and work performance.[26]

Signs of anemia may include jaundice, pallor, cracking, splitting and spooning of the fingernails, increased size of the liver and spleen, lymphadenopathy, and blood

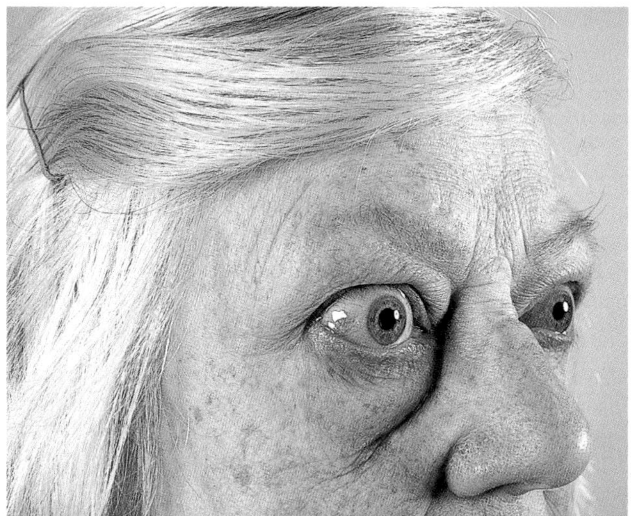

FIGURE 22-5 Pernicious anemia. This 38-year-old woman has blue eyes and vitiligo and shows premature graying of the hair—three features that are more common in patients with pernicious anemia than in control subjects. *(From Hoffbrand AV, Pettit JE:* Color atlas of clinical hematology, *ed 4, London, 2010, Mosby.)*

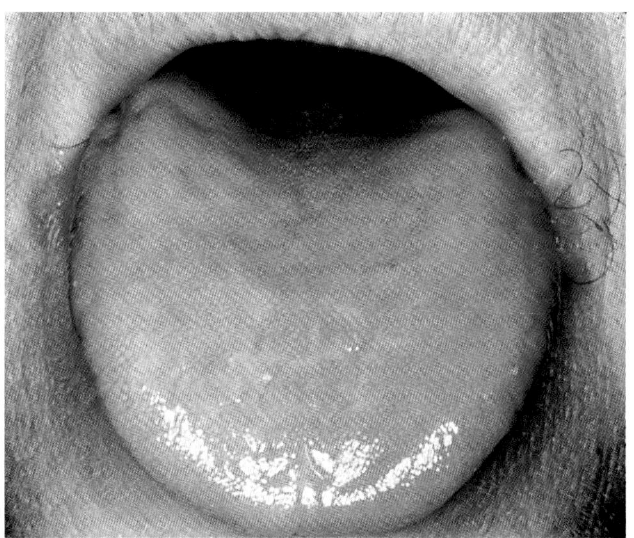

FIGURE 22-6 Smooth red tongue and angular cheilitis in a patient found to have iron deficiency anemia.

in the stool. Premature graying of hair and yellowing of the skin (due to jaundice) have been reported with pernicious anemia (Figure 22-5).[7,27] Patients with anemia also may describe a sore or painful tongue (glossitis), a smooth tongue, or redness of the tongue or cheilosis (Figure 22-6). Some patients may complain of loss of taste sensation.

Screening Laboratory Tests

If the dentist identifies a patient with signs or symptoms suggestive of anemia, this patient should be sent to a commercial laboratory for a complete blood count and differential, or referred to a physician for evaluation. Hb

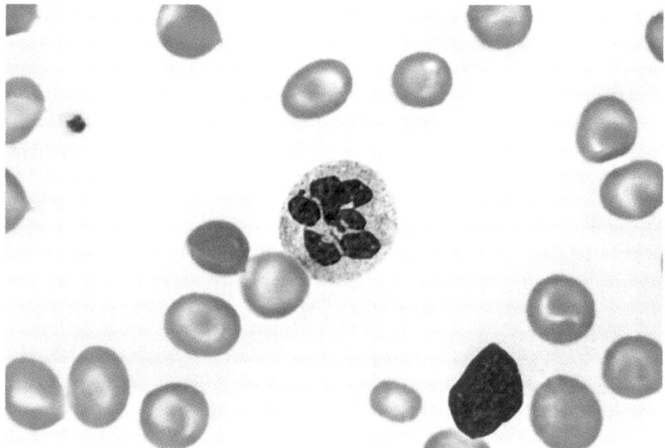

FIGURE 22-7 Megaloblastic anemia. Peripheral blood smear shows a hypersegmented neutrophil with a six-lobed nucleus. *(From Kumar V, Abbas A, Fausto N:* Robbins & Cotran pathologic basis of disease, *ed 8, Philadelphia, Saunders, 2010. Courtesy Dr. Robert W. McKenna, Department of Pathology, University of Texas Southwestern Medical School, Dallas, Texas.)*

level, hematocrit, and RBC indices (mean corpuscular volume [MCV], mean corpuscular hemoglobin [MCH], red blood cell distribution width [RDW], and mean corpuscular hemoglobin concentration [MCHC]) are tests that are used to screen the patient. In addition, total white blood cell (WBC) count and platelet count should be obtained to determine whether a generalized bone marrow defect has occurred and to inspect for hypersegmented neutrophils (see Chapter 1).

Anemia generally is defined as Hb level less than 12 g/dL for women and less than 13 g/dL for men.[8,22] In accordance with the size of RBCs, anemia is classified as microcytic (MCV less than 80 fL [or μm^3]), macrocytic (MCV greater than 100 fL), or normocytic (MCV of 80 to 100 fL).[28] A reticulocyte count (based on percentage of RBCs) of less than 0.5% indicates inadequate RBC production in the bone marrow, whereas a value greater than 1.5% indicates increased production in response to bleeding or destruction. Based on the absolute reticulocyte count in the presence of anemia, a value below 75,000/μL indicates hypoproliferative anemias, and a value greater 100,000/μL indicates hemolysis or an appropriate erythropoietic response.[28] To further distinguish between the various types of anemias, key laboratory tests, as shown in Table 22-2, are performed.

Deficiencies in iron would reveal a microcytic anemia, low serum ferritin, low serum iron, and a high total iron-binding capacity (TIBC).

Deficiencies of vitamin B_{12} and folic acid are associated with macrocytic anemia and the presence of hypersegmented polymorphonuclear leukocytes in the peripheral blood smear (Figure 22-7). Measures of serum methylmalonic acid and homocysteine levels and serologic testing for parietal cell and intrinsic factor antibodies are used to further screen for the deficiency.[12-14]

TABLE 22-2 Laboratory Assessments to Aid in the Diagnosis of Anemia*

Type	Etiology	Tests to Discriminate Types of Anemia
Microcytic anemia	Iron deficiency	Serum iron, ferritin, total iron-binding capacity (TIBC), transferrin saturation, bone marrow aspirate; also, stool examination for occult blood
Macrocytic anemia	Folate deficiency	CBC, serum folate level
Macrocytic anemia	Pernicious anemia	CBC, serum vitamin B_{12} (cobalamin) assay levels, Schilling test, serum antiparietal cell, and intrinsic factor antibodies
Normocytic anemia	G-6-PD	Staining peripheral blood smear with methyl or crystal violet, cyanide-ascorbate assay, qualitative (fluorescent spot) test and quantitative test for G-6-PD, reticulocyte count, indirect bilirubin levels
Normocytic anemia	Sickle cell anemia	Sickledex, high-performance liquid chromatography, hemoglobin electrophoresis, reticulocyte count, indirect bilirubin levels
Normocytic anemia	Aplastic anemia	Erythropoietin levels, bone marrow aspirate

**MCV,* Mean corpuscular volume; *MCH,* Mean corpuscular hemoglobin; *MCHC,* Mean corpuscular hemoglobin concentration have been assessed, and values indicate that anemia is present. These tests are ordered after the initial CBC and differential, including red blood cell indices.
CBC, Complete blood count; *G-6-PD,* glucose-6-phosphate dehydrogenase.

Use of the serum cobalamin assay followed by the Schilling test helps to establish the diagnosis of pernicious anemia.[11,13,14,22] For the Schilling test, the fasting patient receives a small oral dose of radioactive vitamin B_{12} and then a larger dose of nonradioactive vitamin B_{12} as a parenteral flush. At 24 hours, the amount of radioactive cyanocobalamin in the urine is measured. About 7% of the radioactive vitamin B_{12} dose is excreted during the first 24 hours; however, persons with pernicious anemia excrete less than 3%.[14,22]

Screening tests for Heinz bodies (hemoglobin precipitates) (Figure 22-8) or NADPH may be used to detect G-6-PD deficiency. More sensitive tests use direct fluorescent measures of NADPH. Other tests used to detect this deficiency include the cyanide-ascorbate assay, the quantitative assay of G-6-PD, and G-6-PD-tetrazolium cytochemical test.[15,22]

All African American patients should be questioned about the presence of sickle cell disease in their family histories. If the patient or family members have not been screened, the dentist should arrange for the patient to be tested. This can be done in the dental office with the Sickledex test (Streck, Inc., Omaha, Nebraska), in a commercial clinical laboratory, or by a physician. The Sickledex test uses deoxygenating agents which will cause RBCs to sickle in shape. Confirmatory tests use electrophoresis or high-performance liquid chromatography.[18,19,22]

The diagnosis of *aplastic anemia* is based on the presence of anemia (normochromic, normocytic), thrombocytopenia (normal sized platelets), neutropenia, and no abnormal cells in the leukocyte differential. The diagnosis is confirmed by findings on bone marrow biopsy and examination consisting of numerous bone spicules with empty fatty spaces and few hematopoietic cells. Lymphocytes, plasma cells, and mast cells are increased in numbers and represent more than 65% of the cells found in the samples.[23-25]

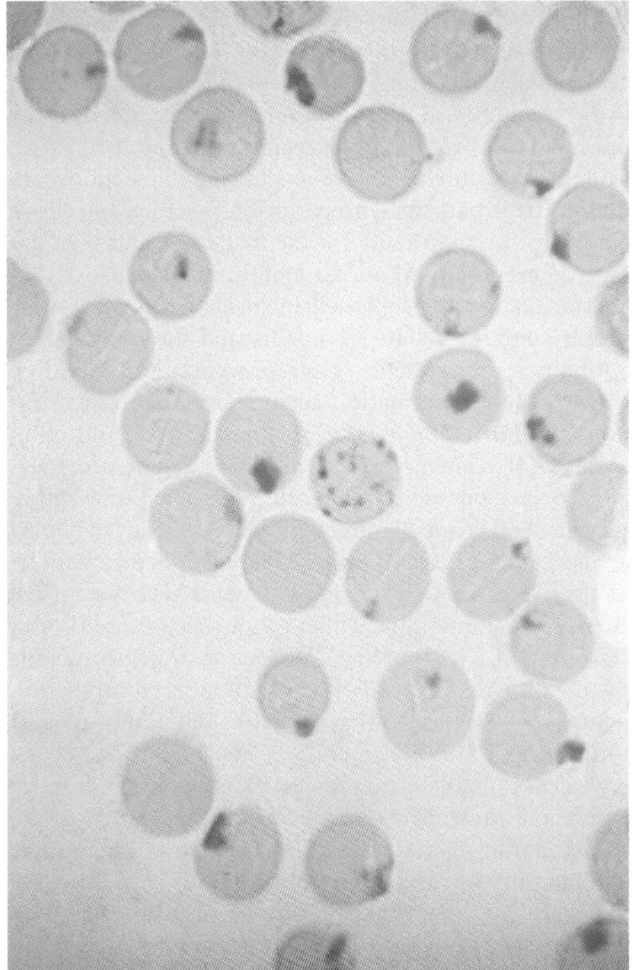

FIGURE 22-8 Deficiency of glucose 6-phosphate dehydrogenase: Peripheral blood film shows Heinz bodies in red blood cells and a single reticulocyte. (Supravital new methylene blue stain.) *(From Hoffbrand AV, Pettit JE:* Color atlas of clinical hematology, *ed 4, London, 2010, Mosby.)*

MEDICAL MANAGEMENT

The goal of treatment is to eliminate the underlying cause. Presented in this section are management protocols for several types of anemia.

In microcytic anemia (iron deficiency), the physician should look for a source of bleeding. Iron deficiency associated with pregnancy often resolves after childbirth. In children, iron supplements (ferrous sulfate, 2 to 6 mg/kg/day) are recommended to arrest motor and cognitive impairment brought on by iron deficiency.[10,29] In patients who have undergone a gastrectomy, iron supplements (ferrous sulfate, ferrous fumarate or ferrous gluconate) are provided on a long-term basis. The preferred route of iron administration is oral. In cases in which blood loss is uncontrollable, iron cannot be absorbed, or iron is not tolerated, parenteral iron is given by either intravenous or intramuscular injection.[10] In men, management often involves treatment of the underlying cause (e.g., peptic ulcer disease, gastrointestinal malignancy).

Folate deficiency is managed by administering folic acid supplements and by increasing the intake of green, leafy vegetables and citrus fruits. In the case of poor intestinal absorption, replacement therapy with folic acid may be lifelong. Cyanocobalamin injections are used to treat patients with pernicious anemia. Injections generally are given daily for the first week and then are tapered eventually to once a month, as needed.

Management of sickle cell anemia is based on routine prophylactic penicillin for infants and the early use of antibiotics to prevent severe infection.[18,19] Children should receive vaccination against *Streptococcus pneumoniae, Haemophilus influenzae,* hepatitis B, and influenza.[18,19] If contemporary health care is not provided, 50% of persons with sickle cell anemia will die before the age of 30 years. Because folic acid deficiency may play a role in the causes of crises, folic acid dietary supplements are given daily to most patients with sickle cell anemia. In addition, penicillin prophylaxis is used for at least the first 5 years of life. Therapeutic strategies include the use of hydroxyurea (with or without erythropoietin), which induces production of HbF and thus prevents formation of HbS polymers.[18,19,30] Once a crisis occurs, high doses of folic acid, analgesics for pain, hydration, and blood transfusions are used to treat the patient.[18,19,30] Stem cell transplantation with bone marrow as the source in a majority of cases from sibling donors carries a 10% mortality rate, with a 90% overall survival rate, with a mean follow-up of 54 months.[18] Patients older than 16 years of age are much less likely to have successful grafts.[19] Only about 1% of the patients with sickle cell anemia meet the criteria for stem cell transplantation.[31]

Once the diagnosis of aplastic anemia is established, family human leukocyte antigen (HLA) typing is recommended for patients 50 years of age or younger for possible stem cell transplantation from a histocompatible sibling. Transplantation is curative but is associated with an early-mortality rate of 10% in children and young adults and more than 20% in older patients.[23-25] Immunosuppression with antithymocyte globulin (ATG) alone or with cyclosporine is the most common therapy for aplastic anemia. About 60% to 80% of patients respond to immunosuppression therapy with about 20% to 30% having a complete recovery. The other 50% to 70% achieve a partial response and become transfusion-independent. The patients who do not respond to immunosuppression can benefit from a second course of immunosuppression (about 75% of these patients respond to the second treatment).[23-25]

HLA-matched related bone marrow transplantation is curative for 80% to 90% of patients.[23-25] In long-term survivors, however, the development of chronic graft-versus-host disease (GVHD) is not uncommon (see Chapter 21).[24,25] GVHD occurs in about 20% of the patients younger than 20 years of age and in about 40% of those older than 40.[25] Immunosuppressive therapy is associated with fewer early adverse effects and results in partial remission in 60% to 80% of patients but is not curative.[23]

Treatment of patients with chronic renal failure often requires dialysis and long-term use of recombinant erythropoietin (see Chapter 12). Erythropoietic growth factors may be used when Hb levels are less than 9.5 g/dL, or 9.5 to 11.0 g/dL in the setting of symptomatic anemia.[32] Long-term use of erythropoietin is associated with hypertension and prothrombotic and inflammatory states.[33]

Anemic patients may require hospitalization if the hematocrit value is less than 20%. Transfusion with RBCs is reserved for patients who are actively bleeding and for those with severe and symptomatic anemia who have underlying disease.

DENTAL MANAGEMENT

Medical Considerations

The dentist should obtain a careful history to identify conditions associated with anemia. This assessment should include questions concerning dietary intake, malnutrition, alcohol or drug use, use of nonsteroidal anti-inflammatory drugs, menstrual blood loss, pregnancies, hypothyroidism, jaundice, gallstones, splenectomy, bleeding disorders and abnormal Hb, and organ transplantation. Historical information concerning family members also is important for identifying hereditary risk for hemolytic anemias.

In children, the history should identify patterns of growth. When the patient is a woman, questions that reveal the onset, nature, and regularity of the menstrual cycle may be important. Women with a history of regular periods but with heavy flow may be anemic and should be referred for appropriate medical advice and treatment. Patients who report a change in the pattern, onset, duration, or rate of menstrual flow should be encouraged to seek medical evaluation. Patients who stopped having periods long before expected should be referred for medical evaluation, as should those who have experienced bleeding between regular periods. In addition, in women who are pregnant or who recently experienced childbirth, the history should establish whether the patient had excessive bleeding during pregnancy, and whether the patient has other children and when they were born, because the closer together the pregnancies were, the greater is the risk for development of iron deficiency anemia. Once the baby is born, the mother may lose additional iron during delivery and breastfeeding.

The dentist should be keen to identify signs and symptoms of anemia in patients who are seen for dental treatment (Figure 22-9). A patient with classic signs or symptoms of anemia should be referred directly to a physician and screened by appropriate laboratory tests (see Table 22-2). Screening tests should include complete and differential blood counts, a smear for cell morphologic study, determination of Hb or hematocrit, a Sickledex test (for African American patients), and platelet count. If screening tests are ordered by the dentist and results of one or more are abnormal, the patient should be referred for medical evaluation and treatment.

Patients with anemia, particularly men, may have a serious underlying disease such as peptic ulcer or carcinoma, for which early detection may be lifesaving. Patients with sickle cell anemia may be in grave danger if the disease is not detected before dental treatment is started. Thus, it is important for the dentist to attempt to identify these patients through history and clinical examination before starting any treatment.

Assessment of the severity of a patient's anemia is important for preventing complications. First and foremost, the dentist should ensure that the patient's underlying condition is under good medical control before proceeding with routine dental treatment. In many cases, anemia is associated with chronic illness; thus, treatment may be provided in the presence of anemia. To minimize the risk of medical complications, Hb levels should be above 11 g/dL, and the patient should be free from symptoms. Patients who are short of breath and in whom Hb levels are less than 11 g/dL, an abnormal heart rate, or oxygen saturation less than 91% (as determined by pulse oximetry) are considered medically unstable, and routine treatment should be deferred until their health status improves.

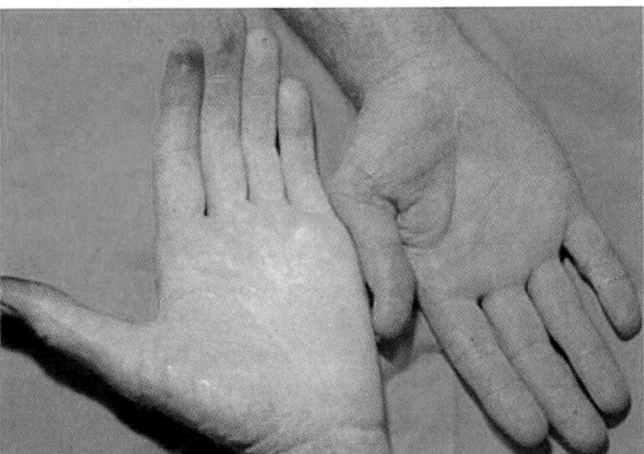

FIGURE 22-9 Pallor of the hand in anemia is obvious in this patient, especially when compared with the physician's hand on the right. The patient's hemoglobin was 7 g/dL. The patient's hand also shows that he was a heavy smoker. The cause of the anemia was chronic blood loss from carcinoma of the esophagus. *(From Forbes CD, Jackson WF: Color atlas and text of clinical medicine, ed 3, Edinburgh, 2003, Mosby.)*

Patients with G-6-PD deficiency exhibit an increased incidence of drug sensitivity, with sulfonamides (sulfamethoxazole), aspirin, and chloramphenicol being the prime offenders. Penicillin, streptomycin, and isoniazid also have been linked to hemolysis in these patients.[15,34] Dental infection may accelerate the rate of hemolysis in patients with this type of anemia.[21,35] Thus, dental infections should be avoided, and if they occur, they must be dealt with effectively. The astute clinician will recognize that febrile illness and elevated bilirubin are features of this condition. The drugs listed previously should not be used in these patients.

African Americans with sickle cell anemia can receive routine dental care during noncrisis periods; however, long and complicated procedures should be avoided. Good dental repair and preventive dental care are important, because oral infection can precipitate a crisis. If infection occurs, it must be treated expeditiously using local and systemic measures such as incision and drainage, heat, high doses of appropriate antibiotics, pulpectomy, and extraction. If cellulitis develops, the patient's physician must be consulted and hospitalization considered.[21] Adequate fluid intake is important for avoiding dehydration. Dental management considerations for the patient with sickle cell anemia are summarized in Box 22-1.

For routine dental care, appointments should be short (to reduce stress) for patients with sickle cell anemia. The use of a local anesthetic is acceptable (avoid prilocaine and general anesthesia); however, inclusion of small amounts of epinephrine in the local anesthetic is controversial in that some authors believe it may impair circulation and cause vascular occlusion.[36] The benefits of a vasoconstrictor probably outweigh the risk of local impairment of circulation.[36] Thus, the use of a local anesthetic with epinephrine 1:100,000 to attain hemostasis and profound anesthesia is warranted. Stronger concentrations of epinephrine must be avoided. If required, nitrous oxide–oxygen (N_2O-O_2) should be used for short periods, with at least 50% oxygen concentration provided.[36]

Intravenous sedation must be used with extreme caution in patients who have a history of sickle cell anemia. Barbiturates and narcotics should be avoided

BOX 22-1 Dental Management
Considerations in the Patient with Sickle Cell Anemia

P

Patient Evaluation/Risk Assessment (see Box 1-1)

- Screening tests include white blood cell count with differential, hemoglobin or hematocrit determination, blood smear, and Sickledex test.
- Confirm with patient's physician that condition is stable.

Potential Issues/Factors of Concern

A	
Antibiotics	Antibiotic prophylaxis is recommended for major surgical procedures.
Analgesics	Avoid strong narcotics and high doses of salicylates. Use acetaminophen with or without small doses of codeine
Anesthesia	Consider using local anesthetic without epinephrine for routine dental care. For surgical procedures, use 1:100,000 epinephrine in local anesthetic. Avoid general anesthesia, particularly if the hemoglobin level is below 10 g/dL.
Allergies	No issues.
Anxiety	No issues.
B	
Bleeding	No issues.
Breathing	No issues.
Blood pressure	No issues.
C	
Chair position	No issues.
Cardiovascular	No issues.
Consultation	Consult with patient's physician before surgical procedures are performed.
D	
Drugs	Avoid barbiturates and strong narcotics; sedation may be obtained with midazolam (Versed). When using nitrous oxide, provide oxygen at greater than 50% with high flow rate and good ventilation.
Devices	No issues.
E	
Equipment	Use pulse oximeter and maintain oxygen saturation above 95%.
Emergencies	Treat acute infection with incision and drainage if indicated; local heat and high doses of appropriate antibiotics will help avoid a crisis. Dehydration should be avoided. If sickling crisis occurs, hospitalization is indicated.
F	
Follow-up	Follow-up consultation with patient's physician is advised.

because suppression of the respiratory center by these agents leads to hypoxia and acidosis, which may precipitate an acute crisis. Light sedation can be provided with midazolam (Versed) or nalbuphine hydrochloride.[36,37] Additional oxygen provided by nasal cannula and liberal use of intravenous fluids during sedation are advised.[30] General anesthesia is not recommended when the Hb level falls below 10 g/dL. High doses of salicylates should be avoided, because the "acid" effect can precipitate a crisis. Pain control may be attempted with use of acetaminophen and small doses of codeine.[38,39]

Although there is no evidence supporting their use, prophylactic antibiotics are often recommended for sickle cell anemia when major surgical procedures are performed to prevent wound infection or osteomyelitis. Penicillin is the drug of choice in nonallergic patients. Intramuscular or intravenous antibiotics should be considered for use in sickle cell anemic patients who have an acute dental infection. Dehydration must be avoided during surgery and the postoperative period. Consultation with the patient's physician is a must before any surgical procedure. The dentist must establish the patient's current status, and, if blood transfusion is indicated, must correct severe anemia or its complications before surgery.[39]

Persons with aplastic anemia are susceptible to infection and bleeding, so clinical recognition of such patients before invasive dental procedures are performed is important. Patients with signs and symptoms of anemia, petechiae, ecchymoses, and gingival bleeding should be referred to a physician for evaluation, diagnosis, and treatment as indicated. The dental management of the patient treated by immunosuppression or bone marrow transplantation is covered in Chapter 21.

Treatment Planning Modifications

Delays in dental treatment may be required for patients who have anemia due to severe underlying conditions. Treatment planning modifications are directed primarily toward patients who have severe anemia or sickle cell anemia. Elective surgical procedures are best avoided in patients with sickle cell anemia. Routine dental care can be rendered for patients with sickle cell trait and for those in whom the disease is in a noncrisis state. Special emphasis should be placed on oral hygiene procedures to avoid development of dental caries, gingival inflammation, and infection, which can lead to osteomyelitis. Adequate oxygenation should be provided during nitrous oxide inhalation procedures. Pulse oximetry monitoring is prudent during dental treatment of all patients with anemia.

Oral Complications and Manifestations

Oral findings in patients with anemia usually relate to the underlying cause of the anemia. The oral mucosa often appears pale. Patients with nutritional causes of anemia (e.g., vitamin B_{12} or iron deficiency) may show loss of papillae from the tongue and atrophic changes in the oral mucosa (see Figure 22-6). Angular cheilitis and aphthae may be found. Patients also may report a burning or sore tongue. Some patients with iron deficiency anemia develop Plummer-Vinson syndrome (Figure 22-10), which is characterized by a sore mouth, dysphagia (resulting from muscular degeneration in the esophagus with esophageal stenosis or "webbing"), and an increased frequency of carcinoma of the oral cavity and pharynx. Patients with this syndrome should be monitored closely for any oral or pharyngeal tissue changes that might be early indicators of carcinoma.[21,40,41]

Patients with hemolytic anemia (e.g., sickle cell anemia) may show pallor and oral evidence of jaundice caused by hyperbilirubinemia caused by excessive erythrocyte destruction. The trabecular pattern of the bone on dental radiographs may be affected because of hyperplasia of marrow elements in response to increased destruction of RBCs. Therefore, dental radiographs may show enlarged bone marrow (medullary) spaces associated with bone marrow hyperplasia, increased widening and decreased numbers of trabeculations, and generalized osteoporosis (thinning of the inferior border of the mandible). Because of compensatory marrow expansion, the bone appears more radiolucent, with prominent lamellar striations.[21,41] Specifically, the trabeculae between teeth may appear as horizontal rows or in a "stepladder" configuration (Figure 22-11). This can also manifest as frontal bossing or "hair on end" appearance in the cortical regions of a skull film (Figure 22-12).

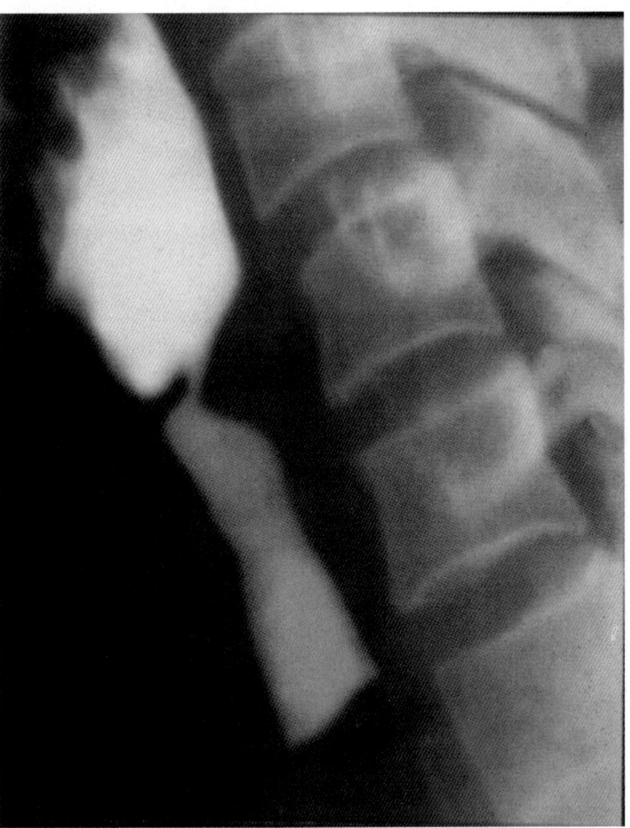

FIGURE 22-10 Feature of Plummer-Vinson syndrome. Barium contrast radiograph demonstrates esophageal webbing. *(From Bricker SL, Langlais RP, Miller CS:* Oral diagnosis, oral medicine, and treatment planning, *ed 2, Hamilton, Ontario, 2002, BC Decker. Courtesy Dr. Thomas J. Vaughan.)*

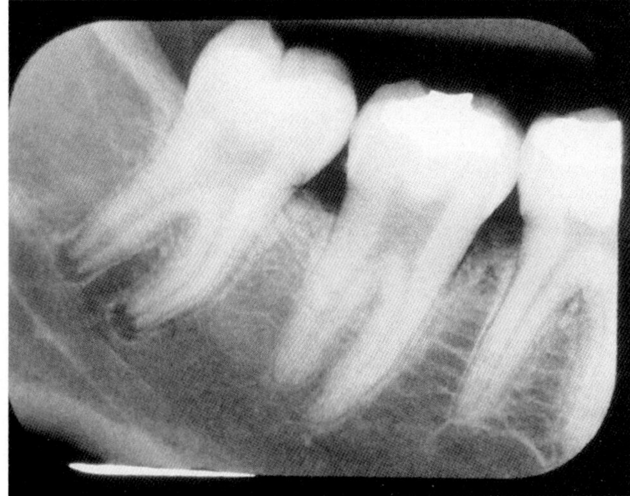

FIGURE 22-11 Periapical radiograph of the mandible in a patient with sickle cell anemia. Note the prominent horizontal trabeculations and the dense lamina dura.

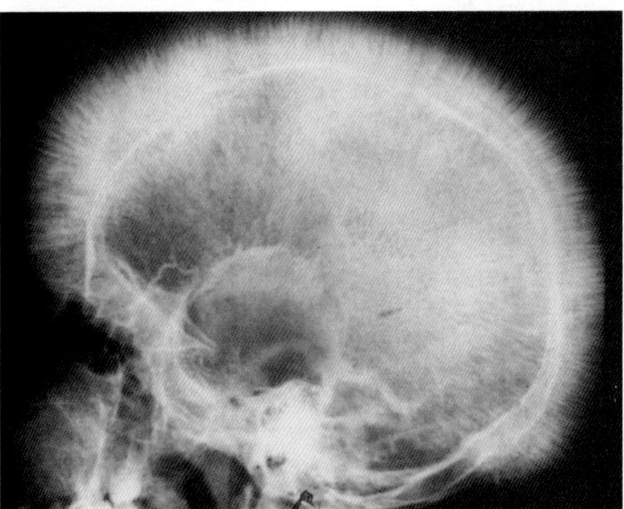

FIGURE 22-12 Skull film in a patient with hemolytic anemia shows new bone formation on the outer table, producing perpendicular radiations or "hair on end" appearance. *(From Kumar V, Abbas A, Fausto N:* Robbins & Cotran pathologic basis of disease, *ed 8, Philadelphia, 2010, Saunders. Courtesy Dr. Jack Reynolds, Department of Radiology, University of Texas Southwestern Medical School, Dallas, Texas.)*

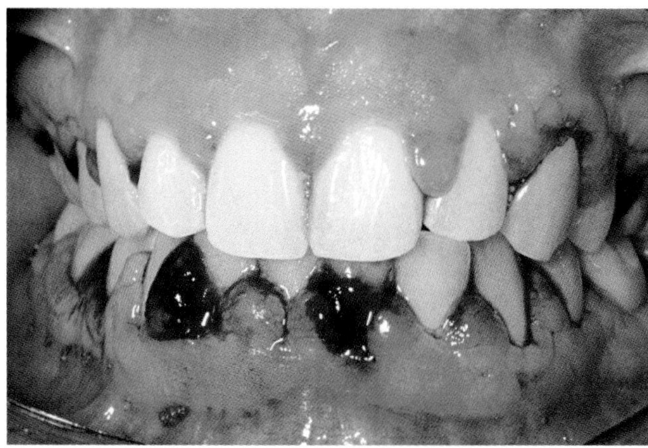

FIGURE 22-13 Aplastic anemia. Diffuse gingival hyperplasia with sulcal hemorrhage. *(From Neville BW, et al, editors:* Oral and maxillofacial pathology, *ed 3, St. Louis, 2009, Saunders.)*

Vasoocclusive events can promote asymptomatic pulpal necrosis, osteomyelitis, ischemic necrosis within the mandible, and peripheral neuropathy. Patients with sickle cell anemia often have delayed eruption of teeth and dental hypoplasia.[21,31]

The oral findings associated with aplastic anemia include petechiae, ecchymoses, mucosal pallor, ulceration (infection), gingival bleeding, and gingival hyperplasia.[31] Figure 22-13 shows an example of diffuse gingival hyperplasia with sulcal bleeding. Another oral finding of aplastic anemia is necrotizing gingivostomatitis.[42] Chapter 21 describes oral complications of immunosuppression and bone marrow transplantation and their management.

REFERENCES

1. Cavusoglu E: Usefulness of anemia in men as an independent predictor of two-year cardiovascular outcome in patients presenting with acute coronary syndrome, *Am J Cardiol* 98:580-584, 2006.
2. Penninx BW: Anemia in old age is associated with increased mortality and hospitalization, *J Gerontol A Biol Sci Med Sci* 61(5):474-479, 2006.
3. Swaak A: Anemia of chronic disease in patients with rheumatoid arthritis: aspects of prevalence, outcome, diagnosis, and the effect of treatment on disease activity, *J Rheumatol* 33:1467-1468, 2006.
4. Walker AM: Anemia as a predictor of cardiovascular events in patients with elevated serum creatinine, *J Am Soc Nephrol* 17:2293-2298, 2006.
5. Rodgers GP: Hemoglobinopathies: the thalassemias. In Goldman L, Ausiello D, editors: *Cecil medicine*, ed 23, Philadelphia, 2008, Saunders, pp 1212-1216.
6. Adamson JW: Iron deficiency and other hypoproliferative anemias. In Fauci AS, et al, editors: *Harrison's principles of internal medicine*, ed 17, New York, 2008, McGraw-Hill, pp 628-634.
7. Zuckerman KS: Approach to the anemias. In Goldman L, Ausiello D, editors: *Cecil medicine*, ed 23, Philadelphia, 2008, Saunders, pp 1179-1188.
8. Silver BJ: Anemia. In Carey WD, et al, editors: *Current clinical medicine 2009, Cleveland Clinic*, Philadelphia, 2009, Saunders, pp 615-620.
9. Frith-Terhune AL: Iron deficiency anemia: higher prevalence in Mexican American than in non-Hispanic white females in the Third National Health and Nutrition Examination Survey, 1988-1994, *Am J Clin Nutr* 72:963-968, 2000.
10. Ginder GD: Microcytic and hypochromic anemias. In Goldman L, Ausiello D, editors: *Cecil medicine*, ed 23, Philadelphia, 2008, Saunders, pp 1187-1193.
11. Suresh L, Radfar L: Pregnancy and lactation, *Oral Surg Oral Med Oral Pathol Oral Radiol Endod* 97:672-682, 2004.
12. Wilson A: Prevalence and outcomes of anemia in rheumatoid arthritis: a systematic review of the literature, *Am J Med Suppl* 7A:50S-57S, 2004.
13. Babior BM: Folate, colbalamin and megaloblastic anemias. In Lichtman MA, et al, editors: *Williams hematology*, New York, 2006, McGraw-Hill.
14. Antony AC: Megaloblastic anemias. In Hoffman R, et al, editors: *Hematology: basic principles and practice*, ed 5, Philadelphia, Churchill Livingstone, 2009, pp 491-524.
15. Golan DE: Hemolytic anemias: red cell membrane and metabolic defects. In Goldman L, Ausiello D, editors: *Cecil medicine*, ed 23, Philadelphia, 2008, Saunders, pp 1203-1211.
16. Gallagher PG, Jarolim P: Red blood cell membrane disorders. In Hoffman R, et al, editors: *Hematology: basic principles and practice*, ed 5, Philadelphia, 2009, Churchill Livingstone, pp 623-643.
17. Giardia PJ, Forget BG: Thalassemia syndromes. In Hoffman R, et al, editors: *Hematology: basic principles and practice*, ed 5, Philadelphia, 2009, Churchill Livingstone, pp 535-564.
18. Saunthararajah Y, Vichinsky EP: Sickle cell disease. Clinical features and management. In Hoffman R, et al, editors: *Hematology: basic principles and practice*, ed 5, Philadelphia, 2009, Churchill Livingstone, pp 577-602.
19. Steinberg MH: Sickle cell disease and associated hemoglobinopathies. In Goldman L, Ausiello D, editors: *Cecil medicine*, ed 23, Philadelphia, 2008, Saunders, pp 1217-1225.
20. Bsoul SA: Sickle cell disease. *Quintessence Int* 34:76-77, 2003.
21. DeRossi SS, Garfunkel A, Greenberg MS: Hematologic diseases. In Lynch MA, editor: *Burket's oral medicine: diagnosis and treatment*, ed 10, Hamilton, Ontario, 2003, BCDecker.
22. Elghetany MT, Banki K: Erythrocytic disorders. In McPherson RA, Pincus MR, editors: *Henry's clinical diagnosis and management by laboratory methods*, ed 21, Philadelphia, 2007, Saunders.
23. Castro-Malaspina H, O'Reilly RJ: Aplastic anemia and related disorders. In Goldman L, Ausiello D, editors: *Cecil medicine*, ed 23, Philadelphia, 2008, Saunders, pp 1241-1247.
24. Young NS: Aplastic anemia, myelodysplasia and related bone marrow failure. In Fauci AS, et al, editors: *Harrison's principles of internal medicine*, ed 17, New York, 2008, McGraw-Hill, pp 663-670.
25. Young NS, Maciejewski JP: Aplastic anemia. In Hoffman R, et al, editors: *Hematology: basic principles and practice*, ed 5, Philadelphia, 2009, Churchill Livingstone, pp 359-384.
26. Brittenham GM: Disorders of iron metabolism: iron deficiency and iron overload. In Hoffman R, et al, editors: *Hematology: basic principles and practice*, ed 5, Philadelphia, 2009, Churchill Livingstone, pp 453-468.
27. Forbes CD, Jackson WF: *Color atlas and text of clinical medicine*, ed 3, St. Louis, 2003, Mosby.
28. Marks PW, Gladere B: Approach to anemia in the adult and child. In Hoffman R, et al, editors: *Hematology: basic principles and practice*, ed 5, Philadelphia, 2009, Churchill Livingstone, pp 439-446.

29. Centers for Disease Control and Prevention: Recommendation to prevent and control iron deficiency in the United States, *MMWR Recomm Rep* 47:1-29, 1998.
30. Davies SC, Gilmore A: The role of hydroxyurea in the management of sickle cell disease, *Blood Rev* 17:99-109, 2003.
31. Neville BW: Hematologic disorders. In Neville BW, et al, editors: *Oral and maxillofacial pathology*, ed 3, St. Louis, 2009, Saunders, pp 571-612.
32. Dubois RW: Identification, diagnosis, and management of anemia in adult ambulatory patients treated by primary care physicians: evidence-based and consensus recommendations, *Curr Med Res Opin* 22:385-395, 2006.
33. Agarwal R: Overcoming barriers that inhibit proper treatment of anemia. *Kidney Int* 101:S9-S12, 2006.
34. Gregg XT, Prchal JT: Red blood cell enzymopathies. In Hoffman R, et al, editors: *Hematology: basic principles and practice*, ed 5, Philadelphia, 2009, Churchill Livingstone, pp 611-622.
35. Micromedex: *Drug information for the health care professional*, Taunton, Mass, 2006, Thomson Micromedex.
36. Lockhart PB: *Dental care of the medically complex patient*, ed 5, St. Louis, 2004, Wright Elsevier.
37. Ruwende C, Hill A: Glucose-6 phosphate dehydrogenase deficiency and malaria, *J Mol Med* 76:581-588, 1998.
38. Sansevere JJ, Milles M: Management of the oral and maxillofacial surgery patient with sickle cell disease and related hemoglobinopathies, *J Oral Maxillofac Surg* 51:912-916, 1993.
39. Smith HB, McDonald DK, Miller RI: Dental management of patients with sickle cell disorders, *J Am Dent Assoc* 114:85-87, 1987.
40. Neville BW, et al: *Oral and maxillofacial pathology*, ed 2, Philadelphia, 2002, WB Saunders.
41. Shafer WG, Hine MK, Levy BM: *A textbook of oral pathology*, ed 4, Philadelphia, 1983, WB Saunders.
42. Tewari S, et al: Necrotizing stomatitis: a possible periodontal manifestation of deferiprone-induced agranulocytosis, *Oral Surg Oral Med Oral Pathol Oral Radiol Endod* 108(4):e13-e19, 2009.

CHAPTER

23

Disorders of White Blood Cells

Disorders of white blood cells (WBCs) in the dental patient can greatly influence clinical decision making as well as the specifics of care, because WBCs provide the primary defense against microbial infections and are critical for mounting an immune response (Box 23-1). Defects in WBCs can manifest as delayed healing, infection, or mucosal ulceration and, in some cases, may be fatal. To ensure the health of the patient, the dentist should be able to detect WBC abnormalities through history, clinical examination, and screening laboratory tests and should provide prompt referral to a physician for diagnosis and treatment before invasive dental procedures are performed. Patients with known life-threatening disorders who are under medical care should not receive dental care until after the dentist has consulted with the patient's physician.

Three groups of WBCs are found in the peripheral circulation: granulocytes, lymphocytes, and monocytes. Of the granulocyte population, 90% is composed of neutrophils; the remainder consists of eosinophils and basophils. Circulating lymphocytes are of three types: T lymphocytes (thymus mediated), B lymphocytes (bursa-derived), and natural killer (NK) cells. Lymphocytes are subdivided by the surface markers they exhibit and by the cytokines they produce.[1,2]

The primary function of neutrophils is to defend the body against certain infectious agents (primarily bacteria) through phagocytosis and enzymatic destruction. Eosinophils and basophils are involved in inflammatory allergic reactions and mediate these reactions through release of their cytoplasmic granules. Eosinophils also combat infection by parasites. T lymphocytes (T cells) are involved with the delayed, or cellular, immune reaction, whereas B lymphocytes (B cells) play an important role in the immediate, or humoral, immune system involving the production of plasma cells and immunoglobulins (IgA, IgD, IgE, IgG, and IgM). Monocytes have diverse functions that include phagocytosis, intracellular killing (especially of mycobacteria, fungi, and protozoa), and mediating of the immune and inflammatory response through the production of more than 100 substances, such as cytokines and growth factors, that increase the activity of lymphocytes. In addition, monocytes serve as antigen-presenting cells and migrate into tissues. In tissue, these antigen-presenting cells are known as dendritic cells (in lymph nodes) or Langerhans cells (in skin and mucosa). Monocytes in tissue that phagocytose microbes are known as macrophages.[1,2]

Most WBCs are produced primarily in the bone marrow (granulocytes and monocytes), and these cells form several "pools" in the marrow: (1) the mitotic pool, which consists of immature precursor cells; (2) a maturing pool, which consists of cells undergoing maturation; and (3) a storage pool of functional cells, which can be released as needed.

WBCs released by the bone marrow that circulate in the peripheral blood account for only 5% of the total WBC mass and form two pools of cells: a marginal one and a circulating one. Cells in the marginal pool adhere to vessel walls and are readily available. When infection threatens the body, the storage and marginal pools can be called on to help fight the invading organisms.

Growth-promoting substances called *colony-stimulating factors* (CSFs) are responsible for the growth of committed granulocyte-monocyte stem cells. The major function of CSFs is to amplify leukopoiesis rather than recruit new stem cells into the granulocyte-monocyte differentiation pathway. Thus, through the local release of CSFs, the bone marrow can increase the production of granulocytes and monocytes. This process occurs in response to infection.[3]

Lymphocytes localize primarily in three regions: lymph nodes, the spleen, and the mucosa-associated lymphoid tissue (MALT) lining the respiratory and gastrointestinal tracts. At these sites, microbial antigens are trapped and presented to B or T lymphocytes (cells). Antigens bind B cells through cell surface immunoglobulins, whereupon B cells are activated, proliferate, and produce large amounts of immunoglobulin to aid in opsonization. Antigens are presented to CD4+ (helper) T cells by major histocompatibility complex (MHC) class I molecules, and to CD8+ T cells by MHC class II molecules. CD4+ T cells activate B cells and macrophages by producing cytokines and through direct contact. CD8+ T cells kill virus-infected cells.

BOX 23-1 Classification and Features of White Blood Cell (WBC) Dyscrasias

Leukocytosis—increased number of circulating WBCs
Leukopenia—decreased number of circulating WBCs
Myeloproliferative disorders
1. Acute myeloid leukemia—immature neoplastic malignancy of myeloid cells
2. Chronic myeloid leukemia—mature neoplastic malignancy of myeloid cells

Lymphoproliferative disorders
1. Acute lymphoblastic leukemia—immature neoplastic malignancy of lymphoid cells
2. Chronic lymphocytic leukemia—mature neoplastic malignancy of lymphoid cells
3. Lymphomas
   a. Hodgkin lymphoma—malignant growth of B lymphocytes, primarily in lymph nodes
   b. Non-Hodgkin lymphoma—B or T cell malignant neoplasms, many types and locations; most are of B cell lineage
      (1) Burkitt lymphoma—non-Hodgkin B cell lymphoma involving bone and lymph nodes
4. Multiple myeloma—Overproduction of malignant plasma cells involving bone

LEUKOCYTOSIS AND LEUKOPENIA

The number of circulating WBCs normally ranges from 4400 to 11,000/μL in adults.[4] The differential WBC count is an estimation of the percentage of each cell type per microliter of blood. A normal differential count consists of neutrophils, 50% to 60%; eosinophils, 1% to 3%; basophils, less than 1%; lymphocytes, 20% to 34%; and monocytes, 3% to 7%. The term *leukocytosis* is defined as an increase in the number of circulating WBCs (lymphocytes or granulocytes) to more than 11,000/μL, and *leukopenia* as a reduction in the number of circulating WBCs (usually to less than 4400/μL).

Many causes of leukocytosis are known. Exercise, pregnancy, and emotional stress can lead to increased numbers of WBCs in the peripheral circulation. Leukocytosis resulting from these causes is called *physiologic leukocytosis*. Pathologic leukocytosis can be caused by infection, neoplasia, or necrosis. Pyogenic infections induce a type of leukocytosis that is characterized by an increased number of neutrophils. If excessive numbers of immature neutrophils (stab cells) are released into the circulation in response to a bacterial infection, a shift to the left is said to have occurred. Tuberculosis, syphilis, and viral infections produce a type of leukocytosis that is characterized by increased numbers of lymphocytes. Protozoal infections often produce a type of leukocytosis that increases the numbers of monocytes. Allergies and parasitic infections caused by certain helminths increase the numbers of circulating eosinophils. Cellular necrosis increases the numbers of circulating neutrophils. Leukemia (cancer of the WBCs) is characterized by a great increase in the numbers of circulating immature leukocytes. Carcinoma of glandular tissues may cause an increase in the number of circulating neutrophils. Acute bleeding also can result in leukocytosis.[2,4]

Many causes of deficient numbers of leukocytes (less than 4400/μL) in the blood are evident. Leukopenia may occur in the early phase of leukemia and lymphoma as a result of bone marrow replacement through excessive proliferation of WBCs. Leukopenia also occurs during agranulocytosis (reduction of granulocytes) and pancytopenia (decreased WBCs and RBCs) that result from toxic effects of drugs and chemicals. Leukopenia is a common complication that results from the use of chemotherapeutic (anticancer) drugs.[2,4]

Cyclic Neutropenia

An important form of leukopenia involving the cyclic depression of circulating neutrophils is a disorder called *cyclic neutropenia*. It is associated with mutations located near the junction of exons 4 and 5 of the neutrophil elastase gene (*ELA2*).[2] The estimated frequency of cyclic neutropenia is about 1 in 1 million.[5] In this condition, patients have a periodic decrease (at least a 40% drop) in the number of neutrophils (about every 21 to 28 days). During the period in which few circulating neutrophils are present, the patient is susceptible to infection and oral manifestations (see under "Oral Complications and Manifestations" later on).[2,6] Up to 10% of patients die from pneumonia, cellulitis, or peritonitis.[2]

Patients with leukocytosis or leukopenia may have bone marrow abnormalities that can cause thrombocytopenia. Examination of the patient's bone marrow aspirate is important for making the final diagnosis. Infectious diseases that can cause leukocytosis and leukopenia are discussed in Chapters 7, 13, and 18.

LEUKEMIA AND LYMPHOMA

The remainder of this chapter focuses on leukemia and malignancies of lymphoid cells (lymphoma and multiple myeloma). Leukemia and lymphoma account for about 8% of all new malignancies each year in the United States, which amounts to approximately 117,080 cases per year.[7,8] These patients become gravely ill if they are not properly identified and do not receive appropriate medical care. In addition, patients are usually immunosuppressed as a result of the disease itself or because of the treatment used to control it. Hence, they are prone to develop serious infection and often bleed easily because of thrombocytopenia. A dental practice that manages 2000 patients is predicted to have 1 to 3 patients with leukemia or a malignancy of lymphoid cells.

Leukemia

Leukemia is cancer of the WBCs that affects the bone marrow and circulating blood. It involves exponential proliferation of a clonal myeloid or lymphoid cell and occurs in both acute and chronic forms. Acute leukemia is a rapidly progressive disease that results from accumulation of immature, functionless WBCs in the marrow and blood. Chronic leukemias have a slower onset, which allows production of larger numbers of more mature (terminally differentiated), functional cells. This section focuses on four types of leukemia: (1) acute lymphocytic leukemia (ALL), (2) acute myelogenous leukemia (AML), (3) chronic lymphocytic leukemia (CLL), and (4) chronic myelogenous leukemia (CML).

Leukemia occurs in all races, at any age, at an incidence of 12.3 per 100,000.[8] Approximately 43,050 new cases were diagnosed in 2010 in the United States.[7,8] The incidence of leukemia has remained somewhat stable in the United States since about 1956.[9] In general, the likelihood of dying from most types of leukemia, lymphoma, or myeloma decreased from 1998 to 2007.[8] All types of leukemia are somewhat more common in men. In 2010 the incidence of acute leukemia was 9740 cases in men and 7920 cases in women and the incidence of chronic leukemia was 11,670 in men and 8190 in women.[7,8] In 2010, more cases of chronic leukemia (19,860) were reported than acute leukemia (17,860).[7]

Leukemia is much more common in adults than in children, with more than half of all cases occurring after age 65 years. The most common types of leukemia in adults are acute myelogenous leukemia, with an estimated 12,330 new cases in 2010, and chronic lymphocytic leukemia, with some 14,990 new cases in 2010.[7] Chronic myelogenous leukemia is estimated to affect about 4870 persons in 2010.[7] The most common form of leukemia among people younger than 19 years of age is acute lymphocytic leukemia. It accounted for about 5330 cases in 2010.[7] Other unclassified forms of leukemia account for the remaining 5530 cases.[7]

The cause of leukemia remains unknown. Increased risk is associated with large doses of ionizing radiation, certain chemicals (benzene), and infection with specific viruses (e.g., Epstein-Barr virus [EBV], human lymphotropic virus [HTLV]-1). Cigarette smoking and exposure to electromagnetic fields also have been proposed to be causative.[8-11]

ACUTE MYELOGENOUS LEUKEMIA

DEFINITION

AML is a neoplasm of myeloid (immature) WBCs, which demonstrate uncontrolled proliferation in the bone marrow space and subsequently appear in the peripheral blood.

Epidemiology

In 2010, AMLs accounted for 28.6% of all leukemias.[7] AML is a disease of adults.[11] Incidence increases with age and rises rapidly after the age of 50 years,[11] reaching 22 per 100,000 by age 80. The mean age of persons with AML in the United States is 65 years.[11]

Etiology

AML arises de novo in younger adults or secondarily in elderly persons as a consequence of myelodysplasia. Environmental factors such as tobacco smoke, benzene-containing products, chemotherapies for cancer, and radiation exposure appear to be risk factors.[11] It is estimated that 10% to 20% of all cases of AML are now therapy-related.[11] Genetic factors (e.g., translocation and rearrangement of chromosomes) may cause cytogenetic abnormalities that affect transcriptional cascades of myeloid precursor cells and uncontrolled proliferation of these cells. Certain genetic disorders increase the risk for AML including Down syndrome, Klinefelter's syndrome, Fanconi's anemia, and von Recklinghausen disease.[11]

Pathophysiology and Complications

AML has a sudden onset and leads to death in 1 to 3 months if left untreated.[12] It involves increased numbers of immature myeloid WBCs in the bone marrow space and peripheral circulation (Figure 23-1). As a result, patients are susceptible to excessive bleeding, anemia, poor healing, and infection after surgical procedures.[12] Hemorrhage and infection, frequent complications of chemotherapy, are the chief causes of death.

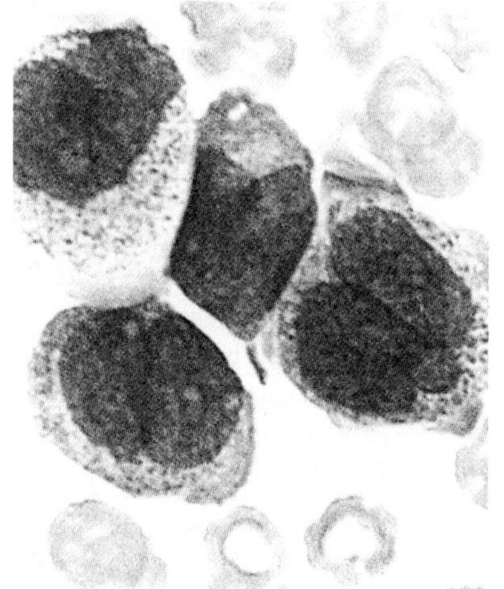

FIGURE 23-1 Acute myeloid leukemia. Peripheral blood smear shows many myeloid cells with large nuclei and azurophilic granules. *(From Hoffbrand AV, Pettit JE:* Color atlas of clinical hematology, *ed 4, London, 2010, Mosby. Courtesy Prof. J.M. Chessells.)*

CLINICAL PRESENTATION

Signs and Symptoms

AML produces a leukemic infiltration of marrow and organs that causes cytopenia and diverse nonspecific signs and symptoms, including fatigue, easy bruising, and bone pain. Many patients complain of flulike symptoms for 4 to 6 weeks before the diagnosis. Anemia and thrombocytopenia usually manifest as malaise, pallor, dyspnea on exertion, and bleeding and small hemorrhage (petechiae, ecchymoses) in the skin and mucous membranes (Figure 23-2, *A*).[10,11] Because of granulocytopenia, at least one third of patients have recurrent infections (nonhealing wounds), oral ulcerations, and fever. Enlargement of the tonsils, lymph nodes, spleen, and gingiva (see Figure 23-2, *B*) occurs as a result of leukemic infiltration of these tissues.[11] Infiltration of the central nervous system (CNS) occurs in about 35% of the cases of AML with increased eosinophils (the M4Eo variant).[11] Most of these patients are asymptomatic, but some will present with meningeal signs and symptoms and symptoms associated with increased intracranial pressure.[11] Skin lesions consisting of collections of leukemic cells termed leukemic cutis, granulocytic sarcomas, and chloromas may occur.[10]

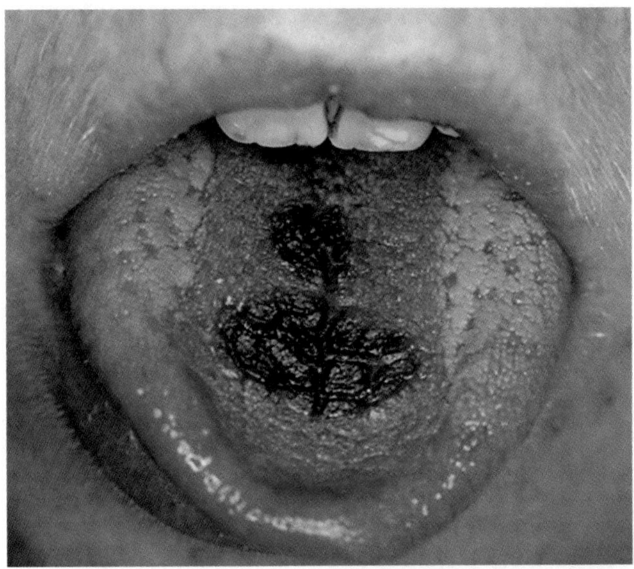
A

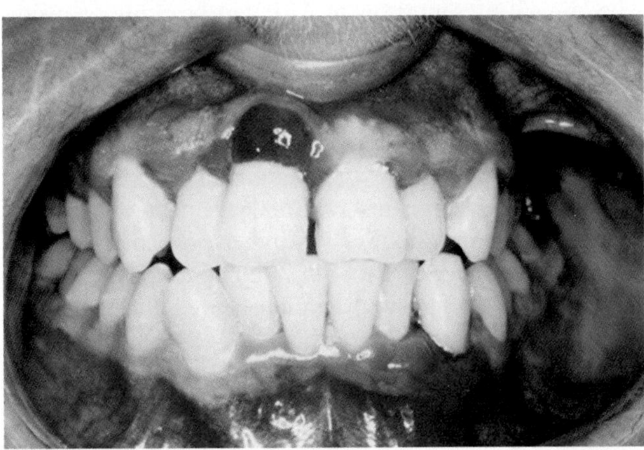
B

FIGURE 23-2 **A,** Acute myeloid leukemia presenting as bleeding and ecchymosis of the tongue in a 14-year-old. **B,** Gingival leukemia infiltrate in a patient with acute myeloid leukemia.

Laboratory Findings

The diagnosis of leukemia is made through examination of peripheral blood and bone marrow stained with Wright-Giemsa. Cytochemical staining, immunophenotyping, and cytogenetic analyses are used to characterize the type and subtype, to allow for specific treatment approaches, and to detect residual disease after therapy is provided. Granulocytopenia and thrombocytopenia are common.

The diagnosis of AML is made when myeloblasts are found in the bone marrow or peripheral blood at a rate of at least 20%. Myeloblasts stain positive for myeloperoxidase and are immunotype-positive for several of the following markers: CD13, CD33, CD34, CD65, and CD117.[13] The French-American-British (FAB) classification categorizes AML into eight subtypes (Table 23-1). The WHO classification describes four subtypes that differ in terms of genetic abnormalities, evolution, and response to therapy.[10,11]

ACUTE LYMPHOID LEUKEMIA

DEFINITION

ALL is the result of uncontrolled monoclonal proliferation of immature lymphoid cells in the bone marrow and peripheral blood. These neoplastic cells may also expand in the lymph nodes, liver, spleen, or CNS.

EPIDEMIOLOGY

In 2010 there were 5330 cases of ALL reported in the United States.[7] It occurs at an incidence of 1.6 in 100,000 and typically occurs in children.[14] ALL accounts for about 25% of all neoplasms in children and 80% of leukemias in children.[15] A remarkable peak of incidence occurs in children who are 2 to 3 years old, with 75% of cases reported in this age group.[16] Boys are affected slightly more often than girls. In adults the greatest number of cases occur in those older than 65 years.[16]

Etiology

Although environmental, infectious, and genetic factors are considered likely causes of the disease, causal links for ALL have not been established. The disease is

TABLE 23-1 Classification of Acute Leukemias and Associated Clinical,* Cytologic, and Immunologic Abnormalities

FAB Subtype	Common Name (% of Cases)	Cell Surface Markers	Chromosomal Abnormality(ies)
M0	Acute undifferentiated leukemia (3-5%)	Anti-CD13, CD14, CD33, CD34	Various
M1	Acute myeloblastic leukemia with minimal differentiation (15-20%)	Anti-CD13, CD33, CD33, CD34	Various
M2	Acute myeloid leukemia with differentiation (25-30%)	Anti-CD14, CD15, CD33, CD34	Various, including t(8;21)
M3	Acute promyelocytic leukemia (10-15%)	Anti-CD13, CD15, CD33, CD65	t(15;17)
M4	Acute myelomonocyticleukemia (20-30%)	Anti-CD13, CD15, CD33, CD34	Various including inv/del (16)
M5a and M5b Type a: 80% monoblasts Type b: >20% promonocytes	Acute monocytic leukemia (5a 2-9%) (5b 2-5%)	HLADR, Anti-CD13, CD15, CD33, CD34	Various including abnormalities of 11q23
M6	Acute erythroleukemia (3-5%)	Antiglycopherin antispectrin	
M7	Acute megakaryocytic leukemia (3-5%)	CD41,CD61	
L1, childhood variant	Acute lymphoid leukemia Small, uniform blasts, nucleoli indistinct	About 65% react with anti-CD10; 20% with T cell phenotype: anti-CD1, 2, 3, 5, or 7	t(9;22), t(4;11), and t(1;9)
L2, adult variant	Acute lymphoid leukemia Larger, more irregular nucleoli present		
L3, Burkitt-like	Acute lymphoid leukemia Large, with strong basophilic cytoplasm and vacuoles	Anti-CD19, 20	t(8;14)

*Clinical signs of leukemia: pallor, lymphadenopathy, petechiae, ecchymoses, gingival enlargement, oral ulcerations, loose teeth, pulpal abscess, enlarged tonsils, gingival bleeding, and recurrent infections.

NOTE: The WHO classifies AML into four major categories: acute myeloid leukemia with recurrent genetic abnormalities (four subtypes), acute myeloid leukemia with multilineage dysplasia (two subtypes), acute myeloid leukemia and myelodysplastic syndromes (two subtypes), acute myeloid leukemia, and not otherwise categorized (11 subtypes).

Adapted from Appelbaum FR: Acute myeloid leukemia in adults. In Goldman L, Ausiello D, editors: Cecil medicine, *ed 23, Philadelphia, 2008, Saunders, pp 1390-1396.*

18- to 20-fold more common in patients with Down syndrome (trisomy 21). Cytogenetic studies frequently display the Philadelphia chromosome [t(9;22)], a shortened chromosome 22, as a result of translocation of genes between the long arms of chromosomes 9 and 22. About 5% of children and 25% of adults with ALL have cytogenetics showing the Philadelphia chromosome. Patients with the Philadelphia chromosome have slightly lower complete remission rates and greatly reduced remission durations. Other chromosomal anomalies are also common.[9,14]

Pathophysiology and Complications

Similar to AML, ALL results in suppression of normal hematopoiesis, leaving patients susceptible to excessive bleeding, anemia, poor healing, and infection after surgical procedures have been performed.[9,14] Treatment of children results in remission rates that exceed 90% and cure rates above 70%. In adults, long-term survival from ALL occurs at rates of only about 50% to 60%.[9,14]

CLINICAL PRESENTATION

Signs and Symptoms

The clinical presentation of ALL can be acute or insidious. Presenting signs and symptoms relate to anemia, thrombocytopenia, fever, and neutropenia. Frequently, bone and joint pain have effects on walking. In one large study one third of the patients presented with infection or fever and one third with hemorrhagic episodes, and over half of the patients with enlargement of the liver, spleen, and lymph nodes.[14] A higher propensity toward CNS disease occurs with ALL compared with AML. Patients may present with cranial nerve deficiencies.[14]

Laboratory Findings

ALL is diagnosed when massive replacement of the bone marrow space with leukemic blast cells is observed. Figure 23-3 shows a peripheral blood smear of ALL. A correspondingly high number of lymphoblasts are detected in the peripheral blood smear and levels of Hb,

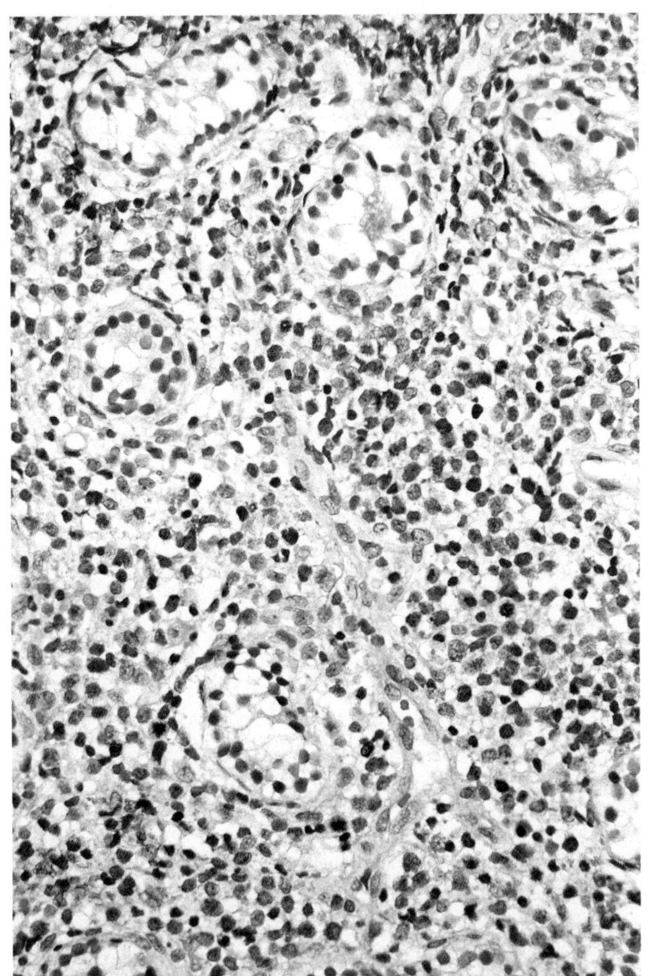

FIGURE 23-3 Peripheral blood smear of acute lymphoblastic leukemia. *(From Hoffbrand AV, Pettit JE:* Color atlas of clinical hematology, *ed 4, London, 2010, Mosby.)*

hematocrit, and platelets are depressed, reflecting large replacement of marrow by lymphoblasts. Immunotyping and flow cytometry is the preferred method of lineage assignment and assessment of cell maturation. Detection of a nuclear enzyme, terminal deoxynucleotidyl transferase (Tdt), along with (B cell) antigen (CD10, originally designated CALLA) and CD19, CD22, and HLA-DR, allows histologic classification of ALL.[9,14]

According to the French-American-British Cooperative Group, three distinct subtypes are based on type and size of neoplastic lymphocytes: L1 (cells small and homogeneous), L2 (cells pleomorphic and often large), and L3 (cells homogeneous and of medium size with dispersed chromatin).[9,14]

MEDICAL MANAGEMENT OF ACUTE LEUKEMIA

The ability to cure a patient of acute leukemia is related to tumor burden and the rapid elimination of malignant WBCs. Normal bone marrow consists of 0.3% to 5% blast cells. Patients with acute leukemia have 100-fold more (about a trillion) blast cells. Once effective chemotherapy has been given, the number of blast cells is reduced from trillions to billions, leukemic cells can no longer be detected, and the patient is said to be in remission. With a 5-day generation time for the remaining undetectable leukemic cell mass, 10 doublings in 50 days could restore the leukemic cell mass to a trillion cells, and the patient would again show signs and symptoms of leukemia. This would constitute a short remission with relapse.[17]

Chemotherapy for acute leukemia consists of three phases. The purpose of the first phase (induction) is to hit hard and induce a state of remission by killing tumor cells with cytotoxic agents. Agents used to treat the acute leukemias are shown in Table 23-2. The second phase (consolidation or intensification) focuses on consolidating the kill of remaining leukemic cells. During the third phase (complete remission), maintenance therapy is provided to prevent expansion of any remaining leukemic cell mass. The criteria for complete remission include the following: platelet count higher than 100,000/μL, neutrophil count greater than 1000/μL, and bone marrow specimen with less than 5% blasts.[18] During induction and consolidation, myeloid growth factors (granulocyte colony-stimulating factor [G-CSF] and granulocyte-monocyte colony-stimulating factor [GM-CSF]) are administered at some institutes to shorten the duration of neutropenia and reduce the incidence of severe infection.

Patients are cured of leukemia when no leukemic cells remain. Long-term survival occurs when the leukemic cell mass is greatly reduced and is kept from increasing over a long period. In general, once a patient relapses, a second remission is more difficult to induce, and if it occurs, it will be of a shorter duration. Bone marrow transplantation (BMT) generally is reserved for patients younger than 45 years of age and for children and young adults who relapse when a suitable sibling match is available (allogeneic).[9,14] The marrow transplant or, more recently, the peripheral blood stem cell transplant procedure is preceded by high-dose chemotherapy (including busulfan) and radiation therapy.

Treatment of patients with AML is shown in Table 23-3. In 1966 the median survival of adults with AML was 40 days.[10] Today patients younger than 60 years have complete remission rates of 70% to 80% after induction therapy but overall survival rate is only 50% for those who go into complete remission and 30% overall.[10] The prognosis of AML in adults who are 60 years or older is poorer. The remission rate for older patients is 52% for patients 60 to 69 years and only 26% for patients 70 years or older with long-term survival rates of only 5% to 10% (Table 23-4).[9,10]

Treatment for ALL is shown in Table 23-3. The prognosis for children with ALL is very good, with cure now being attained in more than 70% of cases. The prognosis

TABLE 23-2 Classes of Drugs Used to Treat Leukemia

Drug Class	Chemotherapeutic Agents	Mechanism of Action
Alkylating agents	Busulfan, carmustine, cyclophosphamide, dacarbazine, lomustine nitrogen mustard *Derivative*: chlorambucil	Produce alkyl radicals, causing cross-linking of DNA and inhibition of DNA synthesis in rapidly replicating tumor cells
Antibiotics	Bleomycin, daunorubicin, doxorubicin, idarubicin, mitomycin C	Disrupt cellular functions, such as RNA synthesis, or inhibit mitosis
Antimetabolites	Folic acid analogues: methotrexate Purine analogues: cladribine, fludarabine, fluorouracil 6-mercaptopurine, thioguanine Pyrimidine nucleoside analogues: arabinosyl cytosine (Ara-C, cytarabine)	Disrupt enzymatic processes or nucleic acid synthesis
Biologicals	Interferon alfa	Causes a direct antiproliferative effect on CML progenitor cells
	Rituximab	Monoclonal antibody to CD20
	Alemtuzumab	Monoclonal antibody to CD52
	All-*trans* retinoic acid (ATRA) [tretinoin]	Binds antigen target on malignant lymphocyte Induces differentiation and apoptosis of malignant promyelocytes in APML
Enzymes	Asparaginase	Inhibits synthesis of asparagines, which is required for protein synthesis in leukemic lymphoblasts
Mitotic inhibitors	Vincristine, vinblastine	Act as mitotic spindle inhibitors causing metaphase arrest
	Etoposide	Topoisomerase II inhibitor
Steroid	Prednisone	Hormone that has antiinflammatory and antilymphocytic properties
Newer agents	Arsenic trioxide	Inorganic compound
	Gemtuzumab ozogamicin	Monoclonal antibody to CD33
	Decitabine	Inhibits DNA methyltransferase
	Colofrabine	Purine nucleoside antimetabolite
	Imatinib mesylate	Tyrosine kinase inhibitor (inhibits signal transduction in cancer cells)
Agents in clinical trials	Farnesyltransferase inhibitors	Signal transduction inhibitor
	Flavopiridol	Kinase inhibitor
	Lenalidomide	Immunomodulatory
	Ofatumumab	Monoclonal antibody to CD20
	Lumiliximab	Monoclonal antibody to CD23

APML, Acute promyelocytic leukemia; *CML*, Chronic myelogenous leukemia.

is worse in persons older than 30 years of age, with a blast count greater than 50,000/μL, with mature B cell ALL phenotype, multiorgan involvement, and chromosomal translocations t(9;22) and t(4;11). In these patients, remission can be achieved with chemotherapy; however, the duration of remission is short. The overall long-term survival (cure) rate for adults is less than 20%.[19] Relapse can result in second remission in 75%, but less than 30% of these patients are cured.

Another concern related to treatment of patients with acute leukemia is that leukemic cells can migrate to areas in the body where chemotherapeutic agents cannot reach them. These areas are called *sanctuaries*, and they require special treatment. The most important sanctuary in patients with ALL is the CNS. Thus, patients with ALL are treated with systemic chemotherapy plus high-dose methotrexate intravenously and cytarabine or intrathecal methotrexate and radiation to the cranium plus high-dose systemic chemotherapy. Another important sanctuary (in males) is the testes.[9,14,19]

Oral Manifestations of Acute Leukemia

Leukemic patients are prone to develop gingival enlargement, ulceration, and oral infection. Localized or generalized gingival enlargement is caused by inflammation and infiltration of atypical and immature WBCs (see Figure 23-2). It occurs in up to 36% of those with acute leukemia (most frequently with the acute myelomonocytic types) and in about 10% of those with chronic leukemia.[20] The gingiva is boggy and bleeds easily, and multiple tooth sites are typically affected. Generalized gingival enlargement is more common and is particularly prevalent when oral hygiene is poor and in patients who have AML (particularly the monocytic type [M5]; see Table 23-1). The combination of poor oral hygiene and gingival

TABLE 23-3 Medical Treatment for Leukemia and Lymphoma

Condition	Induction Chemotherapy	Consolidation Chemotherapy	Maintenance Chemotherapy	Other
AML	Daunomycin Idarubicin Cytarabine	Daunomycin Cytarabine	High-dose cytarabine	*Older patients:* gemtuzumab ozogamicin
APML	All-*trans*-retinoic acid (ATRA) Daunomycin Cytarabine	ATRA Daunomycin	ATRA	
ALL	L-Asparaginase Doxorubicin Vincristine Prednisone	Methotrexate Cytarabine	6-Mercaptopurine Methotrexate	*Ph chromosome–positive cases:* add imatinib mesylate Stem cell transplantation
CML	Imatinib mesylate	Imatinib mesylate	Imatinib mesylate	Stem cell transplantation Nilotinib (for cases resistant to imatinib mesylate)
CLL	Chlorambucil Fludarabine monophosphate COP regimen (cyclophosphamide, vincristine, and prednisone) Rituximab combined with fludarabine		COP adjusted to dosage that obtains desired effect or until thrombocytopenia or neutropenia develops	Radiation therapy as a palliative treatment to shrink large nodal masses or enlarged spleen Stem cell transplantation has no proven benefit
Non-Hodgkin lymphoma	CHOP-R (cyclophosphamide, doxorubicin, vincristine, prednisone, rituximab) CVP-R (cyclophosphamide, vincristine, prednisone, rituximab) FCR (fludarabine, cyclophosphamide, rituximab)			Surgery for localized MALT lymphomas Splenectomy to improve cytopenias Radiation therapy
Hodgkin lymphoma	*Limited-stage:* ABVD (Adriamycin [doxorubicin], bleomycin, vinblastine, dacarbazine) *Advanced-stage:* ABVD or Stanford V regimen (doxorubicin, vinblastine, mechlorethamine, etoposide, vincristine, bleomycin, prednisone)			*Limited-stage:* also involved-field irradiation *Advanced-stage:* post chemotherapy irradiation to sites of initial or residual tumor bulk Stem cell transplantation for patients not cured by chemotherapy

ALL, Acute lymphocytic leukemia; *AML,* Acute myelogenous leukemia; *APML,* Acute promyelocytic leukemia; *CLL,* Chronic lymphocytic leukemia; *CML,* Chronic myelogenous leukemia; *MALT,* Mucosa-associated lymphoid tissue.

TABLE 23-4 Clinical Factors in Acute and Chronic Leukemias

	Type of Leukemia			
Factor	**ALL**	**AML**	**CLL**	**CML**
Age	Children (75%)	Adults (85%)	Over 40 years	30-50 years
Prognosis	Very good	Poor	Good	Poor
Survival, mean	—	2 years	Stage I (19 months)	3-4 years
			Stage IV (12 years)	—
Remissions	90%	60-80%	—	—
Duration	Usually long term	9-24 months	—	—
Cures	50-70%	10-30%	—	
	ALL	**AML**	**CLL**	**CML**
Age	Adults (25%)	Children (15%)	Children (rare)	Children (rare)
Prognosis	Poor	Poor	—	—
Survival, mean	26 months	—	—	—
Remissions	50-70%	56-66%	—	—
Duration	10-19 months	8-12 months	—	—
Cures	20%	20-40%	—	

ALL, Acute lymphocytic leukemia; *AML,* Acute myelogenous leukemia; *CLL,* Chronic lymphocytic leukemia; *CML,* Chronic myelogenous leukemia.
Data from Wetzler M, Byrd JC, Bloomfield CD: Acute and chronic myeloid leukemia. In Kasper DL, et al, editors: Harrison's principles of internal medicine, *ed 16, New York, 2005, McGraw-Hill; and Armitage JO, Longo DL: Malignancies of lymphoid cells. In Kasper DL, et al, editors:* Harrison's principles of internal medicine, *ed 16, New York, 2005, McGraw-Hill.*

enlargement contributes to gingival bleeding and fetor oris. Gingival bleeding is exacerbated by the presence of thrombocytopenia. Plaque control measures, chlorhexidine, and chemotherapy promote resolution of the condition.

A localized mass of leukemic cells (in the gingiva or other sites) is specifically known as a *granulocytic sarcoma* or *chloroma*. These extramedullary tumors have been observed in the maxilla and the palate.[5]

CHRONIC MYELOGENOUS LEUKEMIA

DEFINITION

Chronic myelogenous leukemia (CML) is a neoplasm of mature myeloid WBCs.

EPIDEMIOLOGY

CML has an incidence of 1 to 1.5 cases per 100,000 population, with 4870 cases reported for 2010 in the United States.[7,21] It accounts for 15% to 20% of all leukemias and is much less common than CLL in the United States.[21] The median age at diagnosis is 67 years, and the incidence increases with age. CML occurs slightly more common in men than in women. CML causes 3% of childhood leukemias.[21]

Etiology

The etiology is unknown, but radiation exposure increases risk for the disease. The genetic defect consists of translocation of the cellular oncogene *ABL* (Abelson leukemia virus gene) from chromosome 9 to the *BCR* (breakpoint cluster region) gene of chromosome 22 and a reciprocal translocation of part of *BCR* from chromosome 22 to the *ABL* gene in chromosome 9. A shortened chromosome 22, the Philadelphia (Ph) chromosome, results from the translocations and is evident in more than 90% of cases of CML.[21] The Philadelphia chromosome also is present in ALL. Translocation contributes to increased tyrosine kinase activity and myeloid proliferation.[21]

Pathophysiology and Complications

CML progresses slowly through a chronic phase for 3 to 5 years and then moves on to an accelerated phase, followed by a blast phase (or crisis). More than 90% of the patients when first diagnosed are in the chronic phase of the disease. During the chronic phase of CML, leukemic cells are functional; thus, infection is not a major problem. However, once transformation to the blastic stage has occurred, the leukemic cells are immature and nonfunctional. As a result, anemia, thrombocytopenia, and infection become problems. In about 25% of patients with CML per year exhibit progression to the blast phase of the disease 6 to 12 months after diagnosis. The blast phase is characterized by 30% or more leukemic blast cells in the peripheral blood or marrow.[21,22] More than 85% of patients with CML die in the blast phase, and patients without the Philadelphia chromosome have a worse prognosis. The overall prognosis for CML was poor, and survival from the time of diagnosis was about 3.5 years before tyrosine kinase inhibitor treatment with imatinib mesylate therapy was initiated.[21,22] Patients treated in the chronic phase with imatinib obtain complete remission, and about 70% of the patients remain in remission after 5 years. Allogeneic transplantation is associated with 10-year survival rates of 70% or better for younger patients in the early chronic phase of the disease. Patients treated in the accelerated or blast phase of the disease have a much poorer prognosis.[21,22]

CLINICAL PRESENTATION

Signs and Symptoms

In nearly 90% of patients, CML is diagnosed during the chronic phase. Up to half of these patients are asymptomatic, and diagnosis is based on their complete blood cell count. Common symptoms are fatigue, weakness, abdominal (upper left quadrant) pain, abdominal fullness, weight loss, night sweats due to anemia, an enlarged and painful spleen (splenomegaly), and altered hematopoiesis. Hyperviscosity of the blood may cause a stroke.[21,22]

Laboratory Findings

Patients are identified by marked elevation of their WBC count during routine examination (Figure 23-4). WBC count usually is above 50,000/μL at the time of diagnosis, and basophilia and eosinophilia are present. Cytogenetic analysis, a part of the standard diagnostic workup, reveals the Philadelphia chromosome in more than 90% of cases. Serum chemistry reveals elevated levels of lactate dehydrogenase (LDH) and low levels of leukocyte alkaline phosphatase. The bone marrow is markedly hypercellular.[21,22]

MEDICAL MANAGEMENT

Patients with CML were historically treated during the chronic phase with hydroxyurea or busulfan; this approach resulted in good symptom and blood count control, along with significant toxicity. Interferon-α or imatinib mesylate (Gleevec), an inhibitor of tyrosine kinase, is widely used today.[21,22] Two second-generation tyrosine kinase inhibitors, dasatinib and nilotinib, are being used to overcome imatinib resistance (see Table 23-3).[21,23] Stem cell transplantation has resulted in remission in more than 70% of patients at 10 years when treatment is provided before the accelerated or blastic

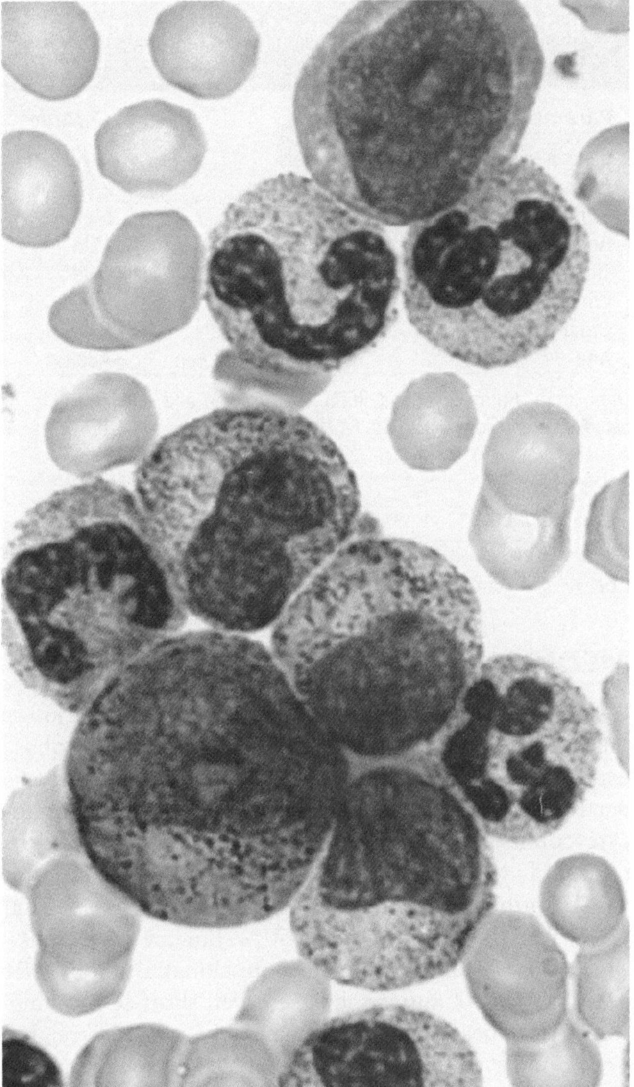

FIGURE 23-4 Chronic myeloid leukemia. Peripheral blood smear shows myeloblasts, promyelocytes, and segmented neutrophils. *(From Hoffbrand AV, Pettit JE:* Color atlas of clinical hematology, *ed 3, London, 2000, Mosby.)*

phase.[24] Stem cell transplants generally are recommended for younger patients who have an adequate human leukocyte antigen (HLA) match.

Oral Manifestations

Chronic forms of leukemia are less likely to demonstrate oral manifestations than are acute forms of leukemia. Generalized lymphadenopathy, pallor of the oral mucosa, and soft tissue infection may be present.

CHRONIC LYMPHOCYTIC LEUKEMIA

DEFINITION

Chronic lymphocytic leukemia (CLL) is a neoplasm of mature clonal CD5+ B lymphocytes.

EPIDEMIOLOGY

CLL is the most common type of leukemia in adults. In 2010 there were 14,990 cases of CLL reported in the United States. The incidence rate is 4 to 5.3 cases per 100,000.[25,26] The median age at diagnosis is about 72 years. CLL is very uncommon before the age of 45 and infrequent in patients under 65 years of age. The 5-year survival rate is 75.9%, with more than 95,123 patients living with CLL.[26] It is more common in men than in women; however, 5-year and 10-year survival rates are higher for women. It is more common in Jewish people from Russian or Eastern European ancestry. This disease is rare in Asia and in children throughout the world.[26]

Etiology

The etiology of CLL is unknown, and risk factors are more related to familial inheritance than to exposure to harmful environmental agents. Neoplastic B cells have various genetic aberrations, most commonly gene deletions (e.g., on chromosome 11, 12, or 17) that lead to loss of cell cycle control.[22,26] The specific genetic defect dictates the course of the disease. Cytogenetic analysis shows the following abnormalities: 13q deletion (40-50%), 11q deletion (15-20%), trisomy 12 (15-20%), and 17p deletion (5-10%). In most cases, low levels of expression of monoclonal immunoglobulin are demonstrated on the cell surface, which includes CD19, CD20, CD21, CD23, CD24, and CD38.[22,26,27] Genetic mutations in p53 and ATM plus serum markers thymidine kinase and β_2-microglobulin also are helpful in predicting the clinical course of CLL.[27]

Pathophysiology and Complications

The pathophysiology of CLL relates directly to the slow lymphocytic infiltration of the bone marrow. This eventually results in marrow failure and anemia, hepatosplenomegaly, hypogammaglobulinemia, which contributes to poor wound healing, and risk for infection. Although the course of the disease is variable, median survival is 4 to 6 years.[6] A possible link of CLL to Merkel cell carcinoma of the skin has been suggested through members of the polyomavirus family.[28]

CLINICAL PRESENTATION

Signs and Symptoms

Most patients with CLL are asymptomatic at presentation. When symptoms occur, fatigue, anorexia, and weight loss are the most common complaints. Patients have an enlarged spleen, lymphadenopathy (Figure 23-5), and decreased serum immunoglobulin levels (hypogammaglobulinemia) that contribute to susceptibility to

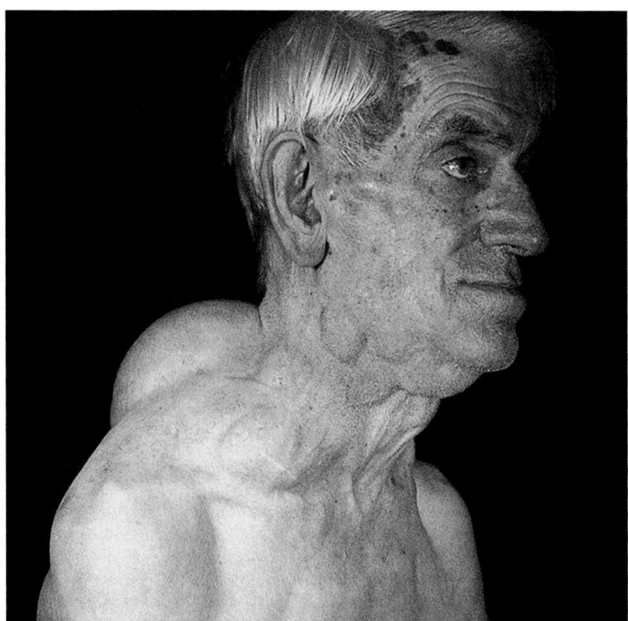

FIGURE 23-5 Chronic lymphocytic leukemia in a 65-year-old man with bilateral cervical lymphadenopathy. *(From Hoffbrand AV, Pettit JE:* Color atlas of clinical hematology, *ed 3, London, 2000, Mosby.)*

infection. Less frequently, patients with CLL develop autoantibodies against red blood cells (RBCs) or platelets that produce hemolytic anemia or thrombocytopenia. In about 15% of patients, CLL evolves into a more aggressive malignancy with increasing lymphadenopathy, hepatosplenomegaly, fever, abdominal pain, weight loss, progressive anemia, and thrombocytopenia. Second malignancies occur because of immune defects associated with the disease. Survival after this transformation lasts less than 1 year.[29] The clinical factors and prognosis in acute and chronic leukemia are summarized in Table 23-4.

Laboratory Findings

CLL requires the presence of more than 5000 mature lymphocytes per microliter in the peripheral blood smear. Also evident in the smear are numerous small, round lymphocytes with scant cytoplasm. Immunotyping reveals the neoplastic cells to be B lymphocytes that are positive for CD3, CD19, CD20, CD21, CD23, and CD24.[22,26]

CLL is classified with the use of an international staging system (BINET). Three stages are identified: stage A (two or fewer lymph node groups, no anemia or thrombocytopenia); stage B (three or more lymph node groups, no anemia or thrombocytopenia); and stage C (anemia and thrombocytopenia, any number of lymph node groups). Lymph node groups include cervical, axillary, inguinal, liver, and spleen. Mean survival time for patients with stage A disease is longer than 10 years (about one third will never require treatment); with stage B, about 5 years; and with stage C, only about 2 years.[22,26]

TABLE 23-5 Comparison of Acute and Chronic Leukemias

Parameter	Acute	Chronic
Clinical onset	Sudden	Insidious
Course (untreated)	<6 months	2-6 years
Leukemic cells	Immature	Mature
Anemia	Mild to severe	Mild
Thrombocytopenia	Mild to severe	Mild
White blood cell count	Variable	Increased
Organomegaly	Mild	Prominent
Age	Adults and children	Adults

Data from Harming DM: Clinical hematology and fundamentals of hemostasis, *Philadelphia, 2009, FA Davis.*

MEDICAL MANAGEMENT

CLL is not a curable disease, and treatment has little effect on survival times. Patients in the asymptomatic phase usually are not treated. Only moderate effectiveness has been reported for some treatments in reducing lymphocyte counts and alleviating symptoms. Agents used to treat CLL are shown in Table 23-3. Rituximab, a monoclonal antibody targeting the CD20 antigen, is associated with a remission rate of about 50%. But complete remission is rare. Alemtuzumab, a monoclonal antibody that binds the CD52 antigen, has achieved short-term remissions.[22,26] These agents are used when disease-related symptoms (e.g., fevers, chills, anemia, thrombocytopenia, hepatosplenomegaly) affect the patient's quality of life. Prednisone is used to treat autoimmune complications. Ofatumumab (an anti-CD20 monoclonal antibody) and lenalidomide (an immunomodulatory agent) are being investigated for use in patients with fludarabine resistance.[30] Stem cell transplantation has no proven benefit in terms of survival or long-term disease control. Radiation therapy is used to shrink unsightly or painful enlarged nodes or an enlarged spleen.[22,26] Drugs that are being tested in clinical trials for the treatment of CLL include ofatumumab (CD20 monoclonal antibody), lumiliximab (CD23 monoclonal antibody), lenalidomide (an immunomodulatory drug), and flavopiridol (a chlorophenyl flavone that stimulates apoptosis that is p53-dependent.[26] Table 23-5 presents a comparison of acute and chronic leukemia.

Oral Manifestations

Generalized lymphadenopathy and pallor of the oral mucosa are features of CLL. Oral soft tissue infection may become evident as the patient develops hypoglobulinemia.

LYMPHOMAS

Lymphoma is cancer of the lymphoid organs and tissues that presents as discrete tissue masses. Lymphomas represent the seventh most common malignancy worldwide and in 2010 affected 74,030 Americans.[7,31] Lymphomas are classified by cell type (B cell, T cell, MALT, plasma cell), appearance (small or large cell, cleaved or non-cleaved nucleus), and clinical behavior (of low, intermediate, and high grade); higher grades have been noted to be more aggressive. Of more than 20 types, 3 common lymphomas—Hodgkin lymphoma, non-Hodgkin lymphoma, and Burkitt's lymphoma—and a plasma cell malignancy—multiple myeloma (MM)—are considered here. These diseases are of importance in dental management because initial signs often occur in the mouth (e.g., Waldeyer's ring) and in the head and neck region, and precautions must be taken before any dental treatment is provided.

HODGKIN LYMPHOMA

DEFINITION

Hodgkin lymphoma (HL) is a neoplasm (exhibiting uncontrolled growth) of B lymphocytes that was named for Thomas Hodgkin, the British pathologist who first described it. This neoplasm contains a characteristic tumor cell called the *Reed-Sternberg cell* that represents usually less than 1% of the cellular infiltrate in affected tissues.[32] For a long time HL was referred to as Hodgkin's disease and NHL as non-Hodgkin's lymphoma. References cited in this book use both sets of identification.

EPIDEMIOLOGY

In 2010, 8490 cases of HL were reported.[7] It is the most common lymphoma in young adults. HL has two peaks of incidence—one in early adulthood and the other around the fifth decade of life.[33] Men are at slightly higher risk for developing the disease (1.4 : 1 male-female ratio).[33] In developing countries, HL is found primarily in children, and the incidence decreases with age, in contrast with industrialized countries, where it is uncommon in children.[33]

Etiology

The cause of HL is unknown, but EBV frequently is present (50% of cases in the Western world) in malignant lymphocytes.[33] This virus can immortalize B cells in vitro and encodes a protein known as latent membrane protein 1 that has oncogenic potential.[34] Increased risk is associated with presence of the disease in first-degree relatives and with human immunodeficiency virus (HIV)-seropositive status.[32,33]

Pathophysiology and Complications

Enlarging tumorous nodes may cause lung or vascular obstruction, and enlarging mediastinal nodes can cause cough, shortness of breath, or dysphagia. The disease spreads predictably over weeks to months, first to other lymphoid sites (other lymph nodes and spleen) and then hematogenously to extranodal sites, including bone marrow, liver, and lung. Without treatment, death occurs as a result of complications from bone marrow failure or infection.

CLINICAL PRESENTATION

Signs and Symptoms

HL presents most commonly as a painless mass or a group of firm, nontender, enlarged lymph nodes, often (i.e., in more than 50% of cases) affecting the mediastinal nodes or the neck nodes (Figure 23-6, *A*).[32,33] Enlarged lymph nodes in the underarm or groin are also common presentations. Fever, weight loss, and night sweats occur

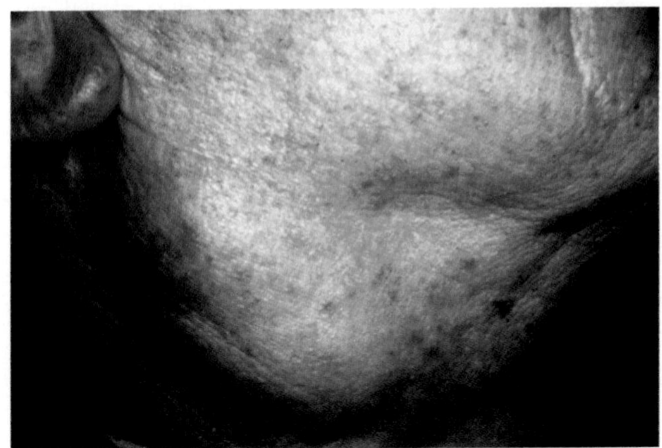

A

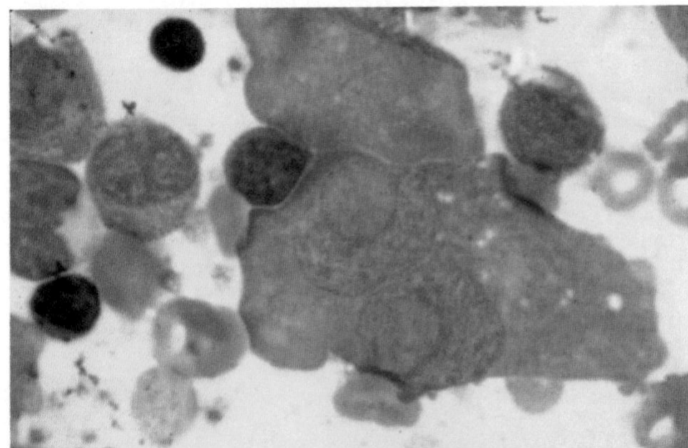

B

FIGURE 23-6 Hodgkin lymphoma. **A,** Cervical lymphadenopathy due to tumor infiltrate. **B,** Large Reed-Sternberg cells are seen in this bone marrow specimen.

in about one third of patients.[32,33] Pruritus and fatigue develop and may precede the appearance of enlarging lymph nodes. Palpation of the lymph nodes reveals a rubbery consistency.

Laboratory Findings

The diagnosis of lymphoma is made on the basis of nodal biopsy or bone marrow aspirate. Microscopically, tumorous tissue typically shows large, multinucleated Reed-Sternberg reticulum (monoclonal B) cells (Figure 23-6, *B*). Four pathologic variants of classic HL have been described: nodular sclerosing (65%), mixed cellularity (12%), lymphocyte-depleted type (2%), and lymphocyte-predominant type (3%). Two other variants of HL are nodular lymphocyte-predominant HL (6%) and HL not otherwise classifiable.[32]

MEDICAL MANAGEMENT

Effective management requires accurate staging of the disease. Staging is performed on the basis of biopsies, medical history, physical examination findings, laboratory evaluation of the abdominal organs, and computed tomography (CT) and gallium scans that reveal the extent of disease (Figure 23-7). Positron emission tomography (PET) is more sensitive and specific than CT or gallium scanning both for staging and for assessment of residual masses after treatment. However, it has not been proved that by adding it to the standard staging imaging tests for HL it will improve outcome. Thus, its primary use is in the assessment of residual masses after treatment.[32] Poorer survival rates are associated with mixed cellularity and lymphocyte-depleted types, male sex, presence of B symptoms (more than 10% of baseline weight loss, night sweats, and persistent fever), a large number of involved nodal sites, and bulky disease.[32,33]

The current cure rate for HL is about 90%.[32,33] Historically, radiation (therapeutic dose greater than 3.5 gray [Gy]) to involved sites was the primary mode of therapy. Contemporary strategies use a lower dose (less than 3.0 Gy) and more precise targeting of radiation to involved sites after disease volume has been reduced by chemotherapy.[33] Table 23-3 summarizes the treatment regimen for patients with limited and advanced-stage HL (stages IIIA, IIIB, IVA, and IVB).[32]

Relapses, if they occur, generally occur within 2 years of therapy and seldom appear after 5 years. To prevent relapse, those who have received radiation therapy alone are provided subsequent ABVD (Adriamycin [doxorubicin], bleomycin, vinblastine, dacarbazine) chemotherapy (known as salvage therapy). If relapse occurs after standard radiation regimens or chemotherapy, autologous peripheral stem cell transplantation is recommended.[32,33]

Long-term complications of chemotherapy and radiation therapy used to manage patients with HL can occur in the lungs, heart, thyroid, breasts, and gonads. Radiation pneumonitis occurs in 5% to 10% of irradiated patients with mediastinal lymphadenopathy. Myocarditis, myocardial necrosis, arrhythmias, myocardial infarction, and pericarditis occur in 2% to 4% of patients

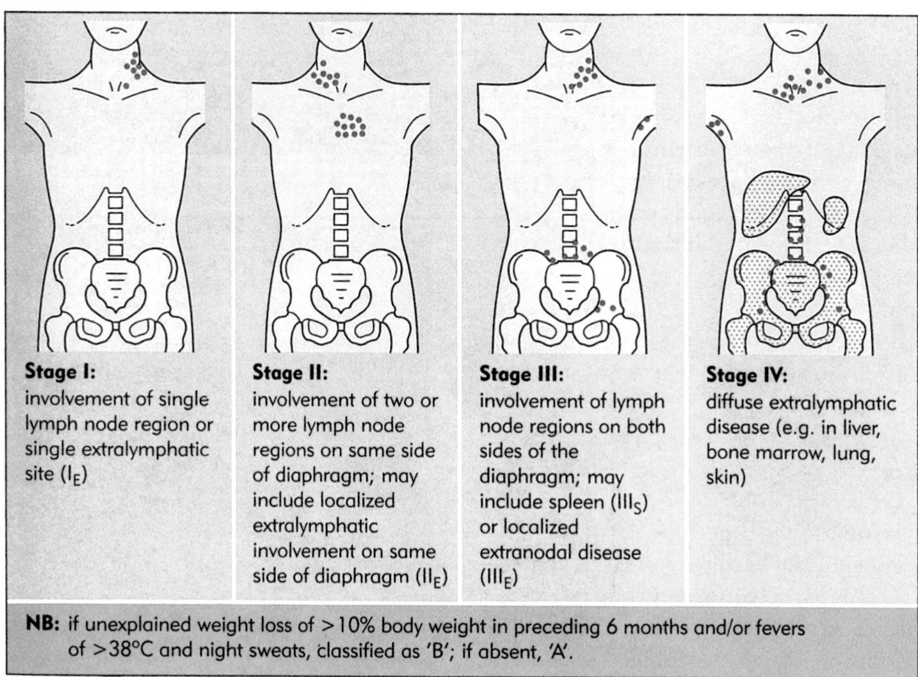

FIGURE 23-7 Ann Arbor staging system for Hodgkin lymphoma. *(From Hoffbrand AV, Pettit JE:* Color atlas of clinical hematology, *ed 4, London, 2010, Mosby. Originally modified from Hoffbrand AV, Pettit JE:* Essential haematology, *ed 3, Oxford, 1993, Blackwell Science Publications.)*

receiving chemotherapy and radiation treatment. Valvular heart disease and coronary artery disease have been reported as late complications of radiation therapy to the chest area. Secondary neoplasia is a complication of treatment of HL include acute leukemia, lung cancer, breast cancer, and thyroid cancer.[33]

NON-HODGKIN LYMPHOMA

DEFINITION

Non-Hodgkin lymphoma (NHL) comprises a large group of lymphoproliferative disorders classified as of B cell or T cell origin. More than 80% of these neoplasms are of B cell origin.[6] The World Health Organization (WHO) classification system uses immunophenotype, cytogenetics, and epidemiologic/etiologic factors to distinguish the many types of NHL. Four major categories of NHL are described: precursor (immature) B cell neoplasms, peripheral (mature) B cell neoplasms, precursor (immature) T cell neoplasms, and peripheral (mature) T cell and natural killer (NK) cell neoplasms.[6,35] Subcategories are based on pattern of distribution (diffuse or nodular), cell type (lymphocytic, histiocytic, mixed), and degree of differentiation of cells (good, moderate, poor). Of the more than 20 types of NHL that have been identified, diffuse large B cell and follicular lymphomas account for about 60% of cases.[36]

EPIDEMIOLOGY

In 2010, 65,540 cases of NHL were reported in the United States.[7] The incidence rates increased dramatically from 1950 to 1970 and then doubled since the early 1970s to 2000.[37,38] Since the late 1990s the incidence of NHL has declined slightly.[37,38] All races and age groups are affected. NHL is the sixth most common cancer in men and the fifth most common cancer in women in the United States.[15] NHL results in about 21,000 deaths per year and is the seventh leading cause of death in the United States.[7,31,38] Median age at the time of diagnosis is 67 years.[39]

Etiology

The cause of NHL is unknown, but genetic factors, infectious agents, herbicides, radiation, and some forms of chemotherapy are increasingly recognized as causative agents. At the molecular level, malignant lymphocytes have chromosomal translocations or mutations in genes that regulate lymphocyte growth (*BCL6*) or survival (*BCL2*). Persistent inflammation from *Helicobacter pylori* infection of the stomach contributes to gastric lymphoma. Oncogenic viruses such as EBV, Kaposi sarcoma herpesvirus (KSHV), and retroviruses are associated with several types of NHL. Patients with autoimmune disease (Sjögren syndrome) or immunodeficiency states (acquired immunodeficiency syndrome [AIDS], after chemotherapy) are at increased risk for the disease.[36]

Pathophysiology and Complications

The course of NHL varies from highly proliferative and rapidly fatal disorders (aggressive) to slowly progressing (indolent) malignancies that are tolerated for 10 to 20 years.[38,40] Tumorous cells behave in similar fashion to that for the cell of origin: Tumorous B cells home to follicular regions of lymph nodes, and T cells have a propensity for paracortical T cell zones. These neoplasms cause tumorous enlargements and abnormalities of the immune system. Tumors often are widespread at the time of diagnosis and more variable in location (involving various organs such as liver and spleen) than in Hodgkin disease. Anemic and leukemic manifestations are common.

CLINICAL PRESENTATION

Signs and Symptoms

NHLs may occur at any age and often are marked by enlarged lymph nodes, fever, and weight loss. In contrast with Hodgkin disease, which often begins with a single focus of tumor, NHL usually is multifocal when first detected.[37,38,40] About 20% to 40% of lymphomas develop outside of lymph nodes and are termed extranodal lymphomas.[5] The most prominent sign of NHL is a painless lymph node(s) swelling of longer than 2 weeks' duration. Additional signs and symptoms include persistent fever of unknown cause, weight loss, malaise, sweating, tender lymphadenopathy, abdominal or chest pain, and on occasion, extranodal tumors.[31,38,40] *B symptoms,* defined as fever, drenching night sweats, and weight loss of more than 10%, indicate a more aggressive clinical course.[38,40]

Laboratory Findings

The diagnosis of NHL is based on findings on excisional biopsy of the involved lymph node. Tumorous cells are classified first by lineage (B, T, or NK cell) and second by level of differentiation. Immunologic and molecular genetic assays are performed to facilitate diagnosis. Proper staging of disease requires complete blood cell count, chemistry screen, chest radiographs, CT scans, and bone marrow biopsy.

MEDICAL MANAGEMENT

Medical treatment of patients with the two most common NHLs (follicular and diffuse large B cell lymphoma) is reviewed in this section. Follicular lymphoma is radiosensitive, and the typical total dose is 35 Gy. Asymptomatic patients, elderly persons, and those with other medical illnesses can be managed by a "watch and wait" approach. However, most patients with follicular lymphoma will require treatment, with 30% to 50% of the neoplasms undergoing histologic transformation to diffuse large B cell lymphoma. Once the patient becomes symptomatic, selective therapy can be started.

About 5% to 15% of patients with follicular lymphoma have localized disease, which usually is treated with involved-field irradiation, with overall survival rates of 60% to 70%. Most patients with follicular lymphoma present with extensive disease at diagnosis. The median survival time for these patients is 8 to 10 years. Treatment protocols are shown in Table 23-3.[37,38,40] In addition, radiation therapy is used for patients with a localized site of symptomatic disease.

About 30% of patients with diffuse large B cell lymphoma have stage I or minimal stage II disease. Although some of these patients my occasionally be cured with radiation therapy alone, the more effective treatment is chemotherapy followed by radiation therapy (see Table 23-3).

Stem cell transplantation and monoclonal antibodies against antigens expressed by malignant lymphocytes (in addition to rituximab, ^{131}I-tositumobab and ^{90}Y-ibritumomab are FDA approved for treatment of NHL), combined with chemotherapy (cispatin, etoposide, caroplatin, and ifosfamide), help patients who respond poorly to traditional therapies (see Table 23-3). Extranodal lymphomas in the oral/pharyngeal region have a poor prognosis. Table 23-6 compares the findings of Hodgkin disease and NHL and emphasizes that disease-free survival with NHL is not very good.

TABLE 23-6 Comparison of Non-Hodgkin and Hodgkin Lymphomas

Parameter	Non-Hodgkin	Hodgkin
Cellular derivation site	>80% B cell, 10-19% T cell or NK cell	B cell
Localized	Uncommon	Common
Waldeyer's ring	Commonly involved	Rarely involved
Extranodal	Common	Uncommon
Abdominal (mesenteric nodes)	Common	Uncommon
Mediastinal	Uncommon	Common
Bone marrow	Common	Uncommon
"B" symptoms (fever, night sweats, weight loss)	Uncommon	Common
Curability	<25%	>75%

NK, Natural killer.
Data from Armitage JO, Longo DL: Malignancies of lymphoid cells. In Kasper DL, et al, editors: *Harrison's principles of internal medicine,* ed 16, New York, 2005, McGraw-Hill.

Oral Complications and Manifestations

Patients with HL or NHL may present with cervical lymphadenopathy and extranodal or intraoral tumors (Figure 23-8). Lymphoma in the oral cavity usually appears as extranodal disease.[5] This situation is of particular concern in immunosuppressed patients and in those with Sjögren syndrome, who are at increased risk for the development of lymphoma. Patients should be periodically monitored for the development of orofacial neoplasia.[5]

Intraoral lymphoma most commonly involves Waldeyer's ring (soft palate and oropharynx)[41]; less often, the salivary glands and mandible are affected. Intraoral lymphomas appear as rapidly expanding (or chronic), unexplained swellings of the head and neck lymph nodes, palate, gingiva, buccal sulcus, or floor of the mouth. Enlargements may be painless or painful. Infrequent findings include deep "crateriform" oral ulcers and fever.[42] The presence of these orofacial abnormalities requires prompt evaluation by biopsy using needle, incisional, or excisional techniques.

Patients with lymphoma who have received medical treatment for their disease sometimes report burning mouth symptoms, similar to those noted by patients with

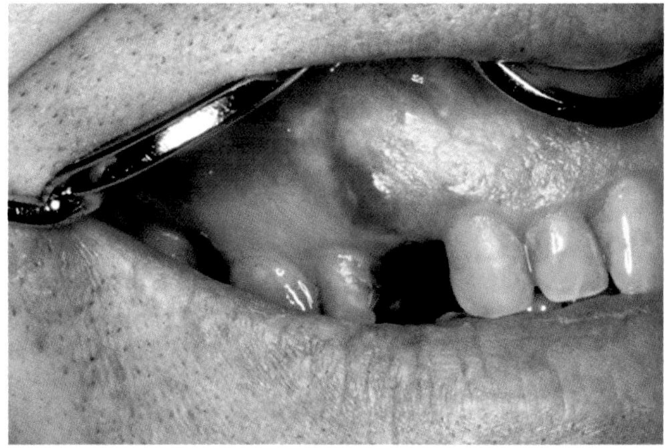

A

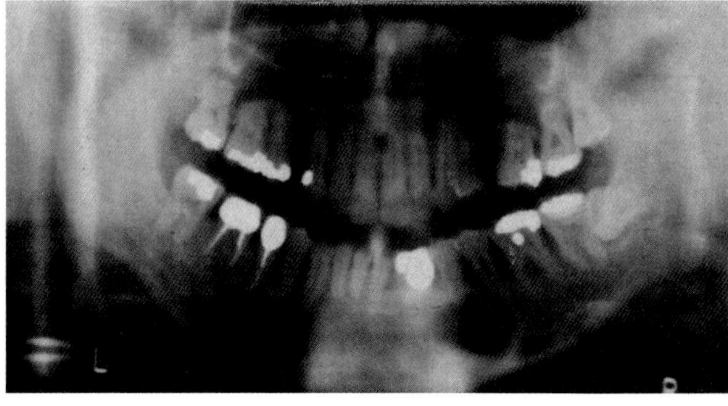

B

FIGURE 23-8 Non-Hodgkin lymphoma manifesting as a gingival enlargement that also involved the underlying alveolar bone (**A**) and an osteolytic lesion of the mandible (**B**).

leukemia, which may be related to drug toxicity, xerostomia, candidiasis, or anemia (see Appendix C for management regimens). Patients who have been given more than 25 Gy are susceptible to xerostomia and would benefit from salivary substitutes or pilocarpine.[41] Radiation also can damage taste buds, cause trismus of the masticatory muscles, and stunt craniomandibular growth and development. Osteoradionecrosis is a long-term risk associated with radiation doses to the jaws in excess of 50 Gy. The usual dose of irradiation to patients with lymphoma seldom puts them at risk for osteoradionecrosis, but they may develop xerostomia.[41] Protocols to reduce the risk of osteoradionecrosis have included the use of prophylactic antibiotics and hyperbaric oxygen, as well as antibiotics during the week of healing (see Chapter 26).

Head, neck, and intraabdominal manifestations occur fairly often. Less frequently, an oral presentation (e.g., as a firm swelling arising from the posterior hard palate) may be seen.[41]

BURKITT LYMPHOMA

DEFINITION

Burkitt lymphoma is an aggressive B cell (non-Hodgkin) lymphoma that originally was described by Denis Burkitt.[43] The tumors are composed of mature B cells that express surface IgM.

EPIDEMIOLOGY

Burkitt lymphoma is the most common lymphoma of childhood. It affects children and young adults at a rate of 0.05 cases per 100,000.[17,36] Two types are commonly described. Burkitt lymphoma that is found most often in Central Africa is known as endemic Burkitt lymphoma and affects children with a peak prevalence of about 7 years of age.[5] Over 50% to 70% of endemic cases present in the jaws (90% in 3-year-old patients and 25% in patients older than age 15).[5] Sporadic (nonendemic) Burkitt lymphoma is more common in Western societies and affects slightly older children and adults in their 30s. A third aggressive type that occurs in HIV-infected people is also described. Burkitt lymphoma is more common among men.[5,6]

Etiology

Burkitt's lymphoma is a mature B cell lymphoma expressing surface immunoglobulin, usually IgM. All Burkitt's lymphomas are associated with translocation of the *c-myc* gene (a gene involved in cellular proliferation) onto chromosome 8. In most cases, the immunoglobulin gene is translocated to chromosome 14 [t(8;14)], but it may also be translocated to chromosome 2 [t(2;8)] or 22 [t(8;22)].[44] These regions regulate immunoglobulin class (isotype) switching. Recent studies have suggested that mutation of the *TP53* gene may play a role in the development of Burkitt lymphoma.[44] Over 90% of endemic tumors contain latent EBV. EBV is present in about 15% to 20% of sporadic lymphomas and in about 25% of HIV-associated tumors.[5,44]

Pathophysiology and Complications

This malignancy is very aggressive and grows very rapidly. Tumors can double in size every 3 days; thus, obstruction of the airway, alimentary canal, and vasculature is possible. The tumor also has a propensity for spread to the central nervous system (CNS).

CLINICAL PRESENTATION

Signs and Symptoms

Most Burkitt's lymphomas arise at extranodal sites. The endemic form shows a predilection for tumors of the jaw and for involvement of select abdominal organs, particularly the kidneys, ovaries, and adrenal glands. Jaw involvement is more common in patients younger than 5 years of age than among those older than age 10 (Figure 23-9). Nonendemic Burkitt lymphoma often presents as an abdominal mass that involves the lymph nodes of the intestine and peritoneum, with jaw lesions being less common. Tumors that enlarge as abdominal masses are accompanied by fluid buildup, pain, and possibly vomiting. The bone marrow is infrequently involved.

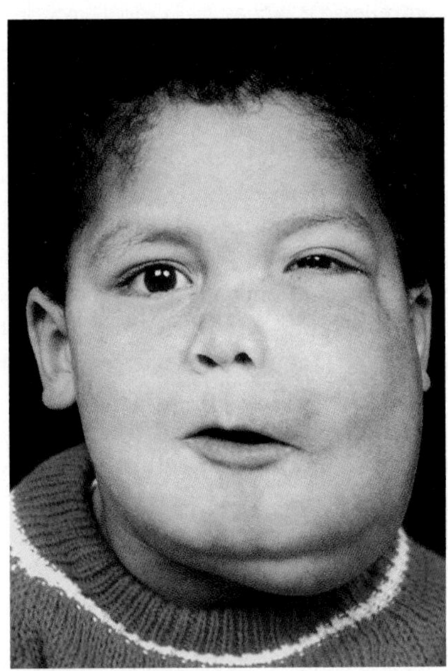

FIGURE 23-9 Burkitt lymphoma showing characteristic facial swelling caused by extensive tumor involvement of the mandible and surrounding soft tissues. *(From Hoffbrand AV, Pettit JE: Color atlas of clinical hematology, ed 4, London, 2010, Mosby. Courtesy Prof. J.M. Chessells.)*

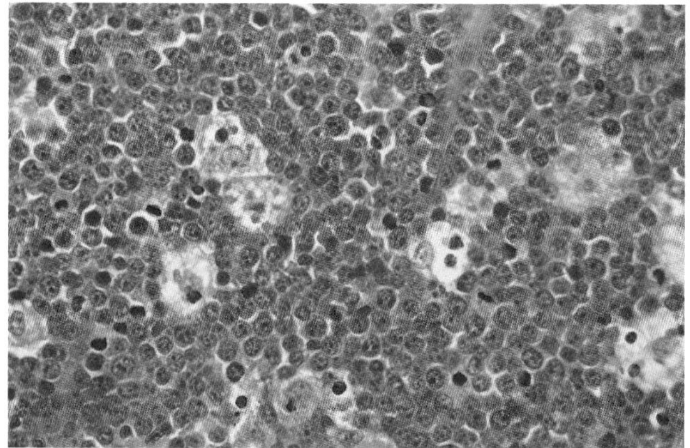

A

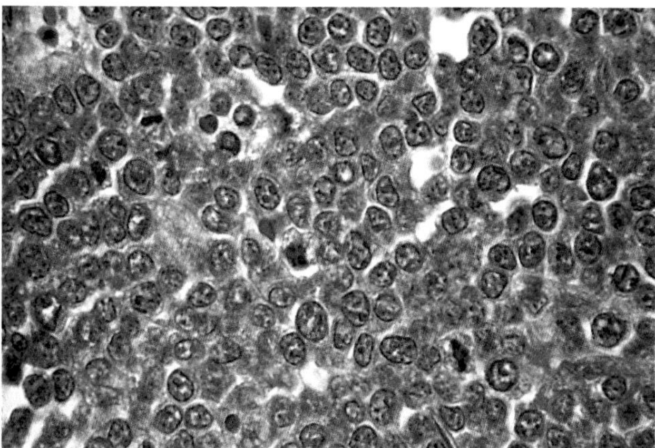

B

FIGURE 23-10 Burkitt lymphoma. **A,** At low power, numerous pale macrophages are evident, interspersed among the tumor cells, producing a "starry sky" appearance. **B,** At high power, tumor cells are seen to have multiple small nucleoli and a high mitotic index. (*A and B from Kumar V, Abbas A, Fausto N, editors:* Robbins & Cotran pathologic basis of disease, *ed 7, Philadelphia, 2005, Saunders. B courtesy Dr. Jose Hernandez, Department of Pathology, University of Texas Southwestern Medical School, Dallas, Texas.*)

Laboratory Findings

The diagnosis is based on radiographic features and a histologic pattern of numerous small, noncleaved atypical B (CD10) lymphocytes interspersed with lightly stained histiocytes ("starry sky" pattern) (Figure 23-10). Histologically, tumor cells are darkly stained and have small prominent nucleoli and a high mitotic index (feature of malignancy).[6] Intraoral radiographs of tumors of the endemic type reveal osteolytic jaw lesions with ill-defined margins and tooth displacement (floating teeth). Usually these develop distal to the last mandibular molar.

MEDICAL MANAGEMENT

The disease responds well to high-dose chemotherapy. Tumors are particularly sensitive to cyclophosphamide. Combination chemotherapy with vincristine, doxorubicin, methotrexate, or cytarabine has achieved remission in more than 90% of patients. Those who live beyond 2 years often enjoy long-term remission.[45]

Oral Complications and Manifestations

Endemic Burkitt lymphoma often presents as a rapidly expanding tumorous mass in the posterior region of the maxilla or mandible with about 50% to 70% of the cases with jaw lesions.[5] Rapid growth pushes adjacent teeth, causing the teeth to become mobile and abnormally positioned. Pain and paresthesia accompany the condition. Radiographically, the tumor produces an osteolytic lesion with poorly demarcated margins, erosion of the cortical plate, and soft tissue involvement.

MULTIPLE MYELOMA

DEFINITION

Multiple myeloma (MM) is a lymphoproliferative disorder that results from overproduction of cloned malignant plasma cells that results in multiple tumorous masses scattered throughout the skeletal system. Malignant plasma cells secrete monoclonal immunoglobulins and various cytokines. Monoclonal gammopathy of undetermined significance (MGUS), consisting of increased numbers of plasma cells with no other clinical manifestations, may precede MM. Another condition preceding full-blown MM is smoldering myeloma, which is an early form of MM not associated with overt clinical signs and symptoms.[7]

EPIDEMIOLOGY

About 20,180 new cases of MM occur each year; these account for more than 14% of hematologic malignancies.[7,46] In 2010 there were over 66,500 people living with MM or in remission in the United States.[46] Men are affected slightly more often than women (with a male-to-female ratio of 1.5 : 1), and most cases are diagnosed after the age of 65 years.[47] The lifetime risk for MM is 1 : 159 (0.68%).[7] The median age at diagnosis of MM for men is 69 years and for women, 71 years.[48] The disease is diagnosed in fewer than 5% of patients younger than 40 years of age.[48]

Etiology

The etiology of MM is unknown but involves uncontrolled division of a clonal cell that produces daughter cells of the same genetic makeup. Chromosomal translocations that frequently involve the immunoglobulin heavy chain locus (IgH), at 14q32, are common. The translocated gene is placed under transcriptional control of potent IgH enhancers, resulting in their overexpression.[48,49] Deletions in chromosome 13 (accounting for

30% of cases) and chromosome 17 have been reported. Malignant plasma cells express certain cluster differentiation glycoproteins on the surface: CD38, CD56, CD138, and CD20 in 20% of cases. Abnormalities of the following oncogenes has been reported: c-Myc (early), N-ras and K-ras (late), and p53.[7] Various cytokines (interleukin [IL] 1α and RANKL [receptor activator for nuclear factor-κB ligand]) are also overproduced. Production of IL-6 by neoplastic plasma cells and normal stromal cells aids in the proliferation of tumor cells. Additional cytokines act as osteoclast-activating factors that stimulate osteoclasts to resorb bone.[7,48-50]

Pathophysiology and Complications

The disease consists of plasma and myeloma cell proliferation, immunoglobulin production, bone resorption at tumor sites, and bone marrow replacement. Resorption of bone leads to release of calcium and serum hypercalcemia. Bone marrow replacement leads to anemia, leukopenia, thrombocytopenia, and eventually a decrease in plasma immunoglobulins. During the early to middle stages of disease, increased plasma viscosity contributes to altered platelet function, excessive bleeding, renal impairment, and neuropathy. Renal failure results from tubular damage caused by excretion of light chains (of immunoglobulin) or by glomerular deposition of amyloid, hyperuricemia, recurrent pyelonephritis, or local infiltration of tumor cells. Infections are common because of diffuse hypogammaglobulinemia (an immune deficiency state) that is caused by decreased production of normal antibodies. Infection is a primary cause of death in MM. Renal failure is the second most common cause of death.[7,48-50]

CLINICAL PRESENTATION

Signs and Symptoms

The most prominent feature of MM is observed radiographically. This disease produces multiple "punched-out" lesions or mottled areas, which represent areas of tumor that appear in the spine, ribs, and cortical regions of the skull (Figure 23-11). Osteolytic lesions of the jaw occur in up to 30% of patients. Amyloid deposition is seen in various soft tissues (heart, liver, nervous system). Because of the hypogammaglobulinemia, pneumonia and pyelonephritis commonly develop.

The most prominent symptom is persistent bone pain. The sites most commonly affected are along the spine, ribs, and sternum. As bone marrow is replaced, anemia develops, along with associated features of weakness, weight loss, and recurrent infection. Headache and peripheral neuropathy are associated with hypercalcemia. Tumor destruction of bone may cause pathologic fracture.

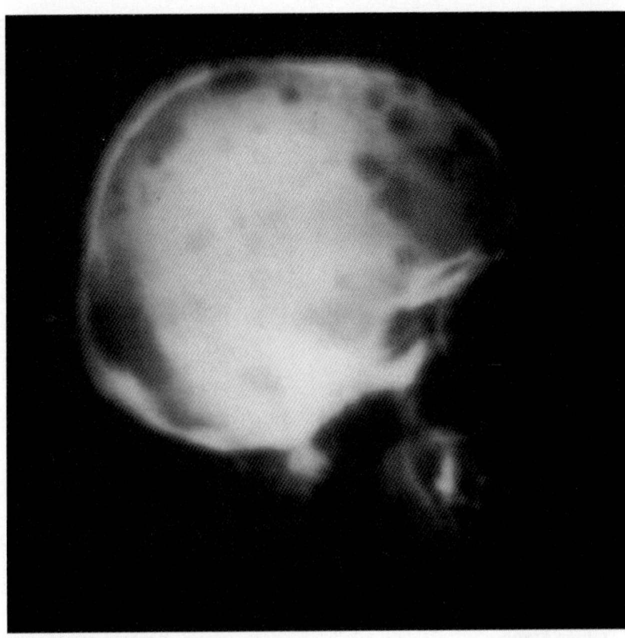

FIGURE 23-11 Multiple myeloma. Punched-out lytic lesions in the skull containing malignant plasma cells.

Laboratory Findings

Osteolytic bone lesions, elevated serum calcium, increased immunoglobulins in the blood, abnormal immunoglobulin light chains (Bence-Jones proteins) in the urine, and anemia (normocytic and normochromic), neutropenia, and thrombocytopenia are features of MM. The diagnosis is typically confirmed by protein electrophoresis of serum or urine that shows the presence of the myeloma or monoclonal (M) protein band. The immunoglobulin most commonly detected is IgG, followed by IgA and IgM. Tumor biopsy reveals sheets of plasmacytoid cells. Bone marrow aspirates show monoclonal plasma cells that constitute more than 30% of the marrow cellularity. Elevated blood urea nitrogen and serum creatinine indicate renal involvement. Low serum albumin level and increasing levels of β_2-microglobulin indicate a poorer prognosis.[7,48,49]

MEDICAL MANAGEMENT

Treatment of patients with MM is shown in Table 23-7. Thalidomide and proteasome inhibitors (Bortezomib) are also used. Thalidomide is a potent inhibitor of angiogenesis and immune response (it inhibits secretion of tumor necrosis factor-α and IL-6). Proteasome inhibitors block proteases required for the accumulation of regulatory proteins important in cell cycle control. Radiation therapy is used as palliative treatment (see Table 23-7).

Interventions are provided to manage anemia, to prevent infection, and to treat or prevent bone disease. Usually, anemia is controlled with recombinant erythropoietin. Intravenous immunoglobulins and antibiotics are given selectively to prevent infection.

TABLE 23-7 Treatment of Multiple Myeloma

Type of Therapy	Agent(s)/Technique(s)	Complications
Traditional chemotherapy	Melphalan Vincristine Cyclophosphamide Carmustine Doxorubicin	Hair loss Mouth sores (ulceration) Loss of appetite Nausea and vomiting Low blood counts Increased risk of infection Bleeding and bruising Tiredness
Corticosteroids	Dexamethasone Prednisone	Increase blood sugar Increased appetite Problems sleeping Infection (weakened immune system)
Immunomodulating agents	Thalidomide Lenalidomide	Sleepiness Tiredness Nerve damage Infection (decrease in WBCs) Bleeding (decrease in platelets)
Other drugs	Bortezomib (proteasome inhibitor)	Nausea and vomiting Tiredness Diarrhea or constipation Bleeding and bruising Decreased appetite Fever Peripheral neuropathy
Bisphosphonates (*slow the rate of bone resorption*)	Intravenous pamidronate Intravenous zoledronic acid	Osteonecrosis of the jaws
Radiation therapy (*for bone lesions that do not respond to drugs for pain relief*)		
Surgery (*relieve spinal cord compression, placement of rods for long bone support*)		
Biologic therapy	Interferon (prolong remissions) Erythropoietin (increase red blood cell numbers)	Tiredness Flu-like symptoms
Stem cell transplantation		
Autologous	Tandem transplant	Infection
Allogeneic	Use of graft-versus-tumor effect	Graft-versus-host disease
Nonmyeloablastive (mini-transplant)	Marrow not completely killed	
Plasmapheresis	Used to reduce hyerviscosity of blood in advanced cases of multiple myeloma	

WBCs, White blood cells.

Bisphosphonates are used to maintain bone strength and to reduce bone pain in early-stage and advanced disease.[7,48-50]

According to the International Staging System, median survival can be predicted on the basis of serum β_2-microglobulin and serum albumin levels (Table 23-8). Patients with low levels of β_2-microglobulin (less than 3.5 mg/L) and high albumin levels (less than 3.5 mg/dL) have an estimated survival of 62 months from the time of diagnosis, whereas patients with high β_2-microglobulin levels (greater than 5.5 mg/L) have a median survival of 29 months.[7,48,50] Reported 5-year survival rates for MM, based on data up to 2006, range from 28% to 41%.[51]

Oral Complications and Manifestations

Patients with MM may have jaw lesions, soft tissue lesions, and soft tissue deposits of amyloid. Bone and soft tissue lesions often are painful.[41] Dental radiographs may show "punched-out" lesions or mottled areas that represent areas of tumor. These osteolytic lesions are more common in the posterior body of the mandible and may be associated with cortical plate expansion. Extramedullary plasma cell tumors can occur in the oral pharynx. An amyloid-like protein is found sometimes in oral soft tissues (e.g., tongue) as a result of MM, and these areas may be swollen and painful. Biopsy and special amyloid stains can be used for diagnosis.[41]

TABLE 23-8 Staging and Prognostic Factors in Multiple Myeloma

Staging and Prognostic Factors	Median Survival
I. International Staging System (serum β_2-microglobulin and albumin)	
Stage I (serum β_2-microglobulin <3.5 mg/L and serum albumin >3.5 g/dL)	62 months
Stage II (neither stage I or III)	44 months
Stage III (serum β_2-microglobulin >5.5 mg/L)	29 months
II. Risk Stratification	
High-risk myeloma—any of the following:	24-36 months
Karyotyping: deletion 13 or hypodiploidy	
Molecular genetics: t4;14, t14;16, deletion 17p	
Plasma cell labeling index >3%	
III. Other Adverse Prognostic Factors	
Elevated lactate dehydrogenase level	
Poor performance status	
Increased circulating plasma cells	
Plasmablastic morphology	
High C-reactive protein level	

From Goldman L, Ausiello D, editors: Cecil medicine, *ed 23, Philadelphia, 2008, Saunders.*

DENTAL MANAGEMENT

Recognition of Disorders of White Blood Cells and Medical Considerations

A diligent search for evidence of WBC disorders is essential in all patients who present for dental treatment. Clinical recognition of such disorders is critical, because patients with leukemia or lymphoma may be at risk for catastrophic outcomes if the disease is not detected before dental treatment is started. Leukemic patients whose disease has not been diagnosed may experience serious bleeding problems after any surgical procedure, may have problems with healing of surgical wounds, and are prone to postsurgical infection. Thus, it is important for the dentist to attempt to identify these patients through history and clinical examination before starting any treatment.

Physical evaluation requires a consistent approach by which important medical, historical, and clinical information is attained from the patient. Specific questions regarding blood disorders and cancer in family members, weight loss, fever, swollen or enlarged lymph nodes, and bleeding tendencies should be asked. In addition, the dentist should emphasize the importance of routine annual physical examinations that will provide screening of the patient's blood for potential abnormalities.

After the history is complete, clinical examination is mandatory. Examination of the head, neck, and mouth should include a thorough inspection of the oropharynx, head, and cervical and supraclavicular lymph nodes. The dentist should be cognizant that an enlarged supraclavicular node is highly suggestive of malignancy. Cranial nerve examination is important for identifying abnormalities suggestive of invasive neoplasms. Panoramic films also will provide insight into potential osteolytic lesions associated with WBC disorders (see Figure 23-8).

A patient who displays the classic signs or symptoms of leukemia, lymphoma, or MM (see Table 23-5) should be referred directly to a physician. Patients with signs and symptoms suggestive of these disorders should be screened by appropriate laboratory tests or biopsy of soft tissue and osseous lesions. Referral to a surgeon for excisional biopsy of a lymph node may be required. Screening laboratory tests can be conducted at a commercial clinical laboratory or in a physician's office. Screening tests should include total and differential WBC counts, a smear for cell morphologic study, Hb or hematocrit, and platelet count. If screening tests are ordered by the dentist and one or more are abnormal, the patient should be referred for medical evaluation and treatment. Biopsy specimens that contain WBCs should be immunophenotyped with the use of a panel of monoclonal antibodies. Immunophenotyping allows determination of the cell of origin (B or T cell or nonlymphoid). Accurate diagnosis also requires culturing of WBCs for analyses of the chromosomes through cytogenetic methods.

Treatment Planning Modifications

Dental management of patients in whom a WBC disorder is diagnosed requires consideration of the three phases of medical therapy. Planning involves (1) pretreatment assessment and preparation of the patient, (2) oral health care during medical therapy, and (3) posttreatment management, including long-term considerations and possible remission.

Pretreatment Evaluation and Considerations. The dentist must be cognizant of the specific diagnosis and the severity of the disorder, the type of treatment selected for the patient, and whether the WBC disorder can be controlled through consultation with the physician. Full knowledge of this information is required for effective decision making regarding dental treatment. For example, a patient who is receiving only palliative treatment is not a good candidate for extensive restorative or prosthodontic procedures that require months for completion.

For the patient in whom leukemia or lymphoma has been recently diagnosed, the dentist should become involved early—during the treatment planning stages of cancer therapy. Guidance regarding the health of the oral cavity and jaws can help prevent severe oral infection. Accordingly, pretreatment assessment should include a thorough extraoral and intraoral examination, panoramic film, and review of blood laboratory findings, with the overall goal of minimizing or eliminating oral disease before the start of chemotherapy. Inspection of radiographs for undiagnosed or latent disease, retained root tips, impacted teeth, and latent osseous disease is important for clearing the oral cavity of disease.

Pretreatment care should include oral hygiene instructions that emphasize the importance of meticulous plaque removal. Caries and infection should be eliminated, if possible, before chemotherapy is begun, and treatment should be directed first toward acute needs (e.g., periapical disease, large lesions treated before small carious lesions). If pulpal disease is present, the dentist may recommend root canal therapy or extraction of teeth before chemotherapy. Dental attention is given to oral hygiene procedures, including using fluoride gels, encouraging a noncariogenic diet, eliminating mucosal and periodontal disease, eliminating sources of mucosal injury, and protecting salivary glands (with lead-lined stents or drugs) if head and neck irradiation is planned. Extraction should be considered if periodontal pocket depths are greater than 5 mm, periapical inflammation is present, the tooth is nonfunctional or partially erupted (as with third molars), or the patient is noncompliant with oral hygiene measures and routine dental care.[52]

Guidelines for extraction in patients before chemotherapy include scheduling a minimum of 10 to 14 days (3 weeks preferable) between the time of extraction and initiation of chemotherapy or radiotherapy, attaining primary closure, avoiding invasive procedures if the platelet count is less than 50,000/μL, and transfusing if the platelet count is less than 40,000/μL. It is important to note that chemotherapy is initiated in many cases of acute leukemia within a few days of diagnosis, so dental treatment may have to be provided promptly before the patient becomes neutropenic as a result of chemotherapy.

Patients who are neutropenic should not undergo invasive dental procedures without special preparation and precautions. The patient's physician may select to use recombinant human granulocyte colony-stimulating factor to promote growth and differentiation of neutrophils before surgical procedures. After necessary treatment is cleared with the patient's physician, the use of prophylactic antibiotics is dictated by WBC and neutrophil counts. Prophylactic antibiotics often are recommended if the WBC count is less than 2000, or the neutrophil count is less than 500 (or 1000 at some institutions). Antibiotic regimens are empirical. Penicillin VK 2 g given 1 hour before the procedure and 500 mg given four times daily for 1 week is a reasonable selection, when needed. There is no evidence that antibiotic prophylaxis is effective under these circumstances, but it often is recommended.

Oral Health Care and Oral Complications During Medical Therapy. Patients who are undergoing chemotherapy or radiotherapy are susceptible to many oral complications, including mucositis, neutropenia, infection, excessive bleeding, graft-versus-host disease, and alterations in growth and development. Fortunately, improved therapy protocols have resulted in a decline in the incidence (to about 30% of cases) of oral complications.

Mucositis. Mucosae of the mouth and gastrointestinal tract grow rapidly and are likely to be affected by cancer therapy. Thus, these patients often develop mucositis, which usually begins 7 to 10 days after initiation of chemotherapy and resolves after cessation of chemotherapy. Cytotoxic agent treatments affect epithelial cells that have high replication rates. Thus, younger persons have a greater prevalence of mucositis of nonkeratinized sites (ventral tongue, labial and buccal mucosae, floor of mouth) and are more severely affected.[53] Affected mucosa becomes red, raw, and tender. Breakdown of the epithelial barrier produces oral ulcerations that may become secondarily infected and can serve as a source of systemic infection. Oral hygiene should be maintained to minimize infection complications. A bland mouth rinse can be used to clean the surface of the ulcer (commercial mouth rinses are not recommended because they contain alcohol and tend to irritate ulcerated tissues). After the bland mouth rinse, use of a topical anesthetic and systemic analgesics makes the mouth more comfortable. Various solutions of antihistamines (benzydamine) that have local anesthetic properties are effective, and a thin layer of Orabase is useful in protecting ulcers from surface irritation. (See Appendix C for suggested regimens.)[54] This protocol can be repeated four to six times a day. In addition, removal of sharp edges of teeth and restorations is palliative. Antiseptic and antimicrobial rinses (e.g., chlorhexidine) are recommended to promote healing of oral ulcerations and to prevent oral infection.[55] Additional novel cytoprotective agents (e.g., amifostine, keratinocyte growth factor [Palifermin]) can be considered for patients not responding to other agents.[53]

Neutropenia and Infection. Patients may present with neutropenia alone, neutropenia combined with leukemia or lymphoma, or neutropenia that results from medical treatment (chemotherapy- or drug-induced) (Figure 23-12). Patients who have neutropenia are unable to provide a protective response against oral microbes. Accordingly, these patients develop acute gingival inflammation and mucosal ulcerations. Chronic neutropenia contributes to severe destruction of the periodontium with loss of attachment when oral hygiene is less than optimal. Periodontal therapy that includes instruction on oral hygiene, frequent scaling, and antimicrobial therapy can reduce the adverse effects associated with this disorder.[20]

Oral infection is less of a problem in patients with chronic leukemia than in those with acute leukemia because the cells are more mature and functional in chronic leukemia. However, in the later stages of both CML and CLL, infection can become a serious complication. Splenectomy due to massive splenomegaly may also increase the risk of infection.

Because of neutropenia, signs of infection are often masked in patients with leukemia. The swelling and

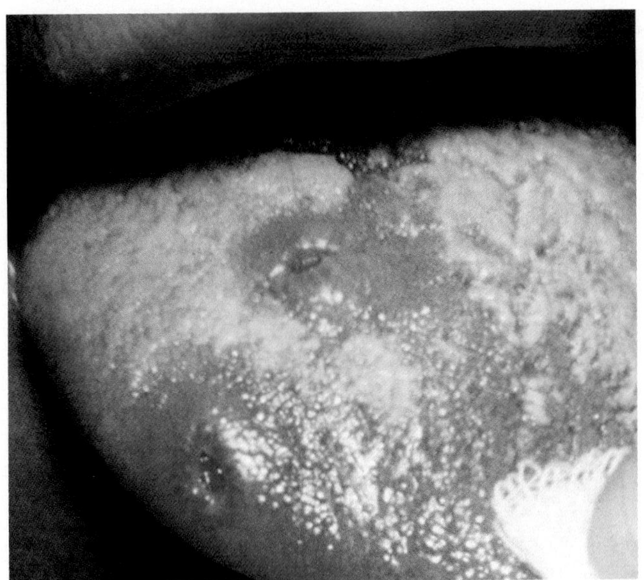

FIGURE 23-12 Oral ulcers due to neutropenia.

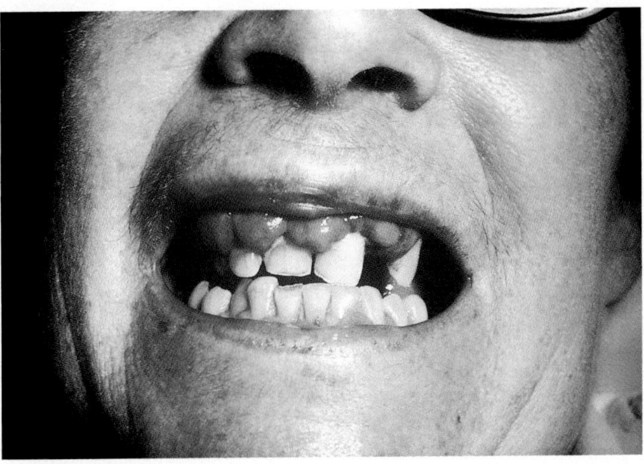

FIGURE 23-13 Leukemic gingival enlargement in a patient who has acute myeloid leukemia. Enlargement is due to leukemic infiltrations in the gingival tissue. *(From Hoffbrand AV, Pettit JE:* Color atlas of clinical hematology, *ed 4, London, 2010, Mosby.)*

erythema usually associated with oral infection are often less marked. In these patients, severe infection can occur with minimal clinical signs, which can make clinical diagnosis more difficult. Infections often develop in the presence of neutropenia as the result of invasion by unusual oral pathogens (i.e., bacteria that do not cause oral infection in most patients seen by the dentist). Unusual infections may be caused by *Pseudomonas, Klebsiella, Proteus, Escherichia coli,* or *Enterobacter.* Often, these infections present as oral ulcerations. When oral infection develops in such patients, a specimen of exudate should be sent for culture, diagnosis, and antibiotic sensitivity testing. If a bacterial infection is suspected, penicillin therapy should be started (if the patient is not allergic to penicillin). If the clinical course shows little or no improvement in several days, laboratory data should be used to select a more appropriate antimicrobial agent, and referral to a physician should be considered.

Opportunistic infections (bacterial, fungal, and viral) are common in leukemic patients because (1) malignant leukocytes are immature, (2) chemotherapy induces an immunocompromised state, and (3) use of broad-spectrum antibiotics produces selective antimicrobial killing. A common opportunistic infection is acute pseudomembranous candidiasis. When this complication occurs, the patient should be treated with one of the antifungal medications listed in Appendix C. Infrequently, unusual oral fungal infections (torulopsis, aspergillosis, and mucormycosis) occur, or fungal septicemia may originate from the oral cavity. These patients require potent systemic antifungal agents such as fluconazole or amphotericin B.

Another common infection in patients receiving chemotherapy is recurrent HSV infection. Herpetic lesions tend to be larger and take longer to heal than herpetic lesions found in nonleukemic patients. Generally, to prevent recurrence, antiviral agents (acyclovir, valacyclovir, famciclovir) are prescribed to HSV antibody–positive patients who are undergoing chemotherapy. In patients in whom HSV infection develops, diagnosis can be made rapidly using an enzyme-linked immunoassay.[56] Immunocompromised leukemic patients also are susceptible to varicella-zoster and cytomegalovirus infections. Lesions in the oral cavity have been reported.[57]

Bleeding. Small or large areas of submucosal hemorrhage may be found in the leukemic patient (see Figure 23-2, *A*). These lesions result from minor trauma (e.g., tongue biting) and are related to thrombocytopenia. Leukemic patients also may report spontaneous and severe gingival bleeding that is aggravated by poor oral hygiene. Enlarged and boggy gingiva (Figure 23-13) bleeds easily, especially if significant thrombocytopenia is present. The dentist should make efforts to improve oral hygiene and should use local measures to control bleeding. A gelatin sponge with thrombin or microfibrillar collagen can be placed over the area, or an oral antifibrinolytic rinse may be used. If local measures fail, medical help will be needed and may involve platelet transfusion.[58] Platelet counts should be at least 50,000/μL before performance of invasive dental procedures.

Graft-versus-Host Disease. Graft-versus-host disease (GVHD) is a common sequela of patients who undergo BMT or stem cell transplantation. It occurs when immunologically active donor T cells react against histocompatibility antigens of the host. The acute stage develops within the first 100 days (median, 2 to 3 weeks) and is marked by rash, mucosal ulcerations, elevated liver enzymes, and diarrhea. The chronic stage occurs at between 3 and 12 months and produces features that mimic Sjögren syndrome and scleroderma, including thickening and lichenoid changes of the skin and mucosa, arthritis, xerostomia, xerophthalmia, mucositis, and dysphagia. Damage to the liver, esophagus (stricture), and immune system may result in recurrent and

BOX 23-2 Dental Management of Patients with Leukemia and Lymphoma

P

Patient Evaluation/Risk Assessment (see Box 1-1)

- Evaluate and determine whether leukemia or lymphoma exists.
- Obtain medical consultation if undiagnosed, poorly controlled, or if uncertain.

Potential Issues/Factors of Concern

A

Analgesics	No issues.
Antimicrobials	Patient with white blood cell (WBC) count less than 2000 µL or a neutrophil count less than 500 µL are candidates for antibiotic prophylaxis when invasive dental procedures are performed. Although there is no standard antibiotic regimen, penicillin VK is used most often. Antibiotic sensitivity testing should be done for oral infections; infections should be treated in a conservative manner with heat, indicated antibiotic, and strong analgesics for pain. Chlorhexidine rinse may be helpful to promote healing of mucositis. Provide antifungal medications for oral candidiasis.
Anesthesia	Mucositis is painful and requires management with bland mouth rinses, antihistamine solutions, and topical anesthetic gel such as Orabase.
Anxiety	No issues.
Allergies	No issues.

B

Bleeding	If the platelet count is less than 50,000/µL, platelet transfusion may be needed before certain invasive and surgical procedures. Confirm by medical consultation.
Breathing	No issues.
Blood pressure	No issues.

C

Chair position	No issues.
Cardiovascular	Radiation and chemotherapeutic agents can cause cardiac damage to the myocardium, valves, and coronary arteries. They also can be associated with serious cardiac arrhythmias. Consult with patient's physician to determine if there is cardiac damage, and take appropriate action to avoid complications.

D

Drugs	A few patients on chemotherapy may complain of paresthesias; those receiving cyclosporine (for bone marrow transplantation) may develop gingival hyperplasia.
Devices	No issues.

E

Equipment	No issues.
Emergencies	No issues.

F

Follow-up	Follow-up evaluation during hospitalization to ensure oral health and minimize the discomfort of mucositis is recommended. After hospitalization, routine follow-up is recommended.

life-threatening infections. To prevent this complication, patients who are preparing for BMT typically undergo T cell depletion of the graft and prophylactic treatment with immunosuppressive agents, such as corticosteroids, cyclosporine, methotrexate, or tacrolimus.

Adverse Drug Effects. A small number of leukemic patients describe paresthesias that result from leukemic infiltration of the peripheral nerves or as adverse effects of chemotherapy (vincristine). An adverse effect of cyclosporine use in BMT patients is gingival overgrowth.

Growth and Development. Chemotherapy during childhood can affect growth and development of the teeth and facial bones. This effect is not observed in adults. Restricted growth of the jaws leads to micrognathia, retrognathia, or malocclusion. Damage to the teeth that occurs at the time of chemotherapy can manifest as shortened or blunted roots, dilacerations, calcification abnormalities, pulp enlargement, microdontia, and hypodontia.

Posttreatment Management. Patients who have WBC disorders and are in a state of remission can receive most indicated dental treatment (Box 23-2). Patients who have advanced disease and a limited prognosis, as occurs in many cases of leukemia and MM, should receive emergency care only. Complex restorative procedures, extensive dental restorations, and other procedures usually are not indicated.

If invasive (scaling) or surgical procedures are planned for a patient who has a WBC disorder that is under good medical control, platelet count should be obtained on the day of the procedure. This is done to ensure that an adequate number of platelets are present. The number of platelets can be depressed in these patients by the leukemic process or by agents used to treat the patient. If the platelet count is low the procedure should be delayed until the patient's physician is consulted. In patients whose disease is under good control but who are still thrombocytopenic, platelet replacement by the physician can be instituted if a dental procedure must be done. Dental management of the patient receiving radiation or chemotherapy is discussed further in Chapter 26.

In HL, the spleen may be involved and surgically removed. Subsequently, the patient is at risk for bacterial infection. Risk for such infection is greatest during the first 6 months after splenectomy.[56] McKenna[56] suggests that antibiotic prophylaxis should be provided for invasive procedures during the first 6 months after splenectomy. The need for prophylaxis after 6 months has not been defined.[56,59] The benefit of antibiotic prophylaxis for invasive dental procedures in these patients has not been established. The dentist should consult with the patient's physician concerning the need for prophylaxis. If prophylaxis is selected the antibiotic regimen is empirical. Penicillin VK 2 g given 1 hour before the procedure and 500 mg given four times daily for 1 week is a reasonable selection.

Up to 80% of patients in whom MM is newly diagnosed present with osteopenia, osteolysis, and pathologic fractures. Patients often are treated with bisphosphonates—drugs that inhibit osteoclast activity. An infrequent adverse effect of bisphosphonates is osteonecrosis of the jaws (BONJ).[52,60-62] Greatest risk for this complication is associated with use of intravenous bisphosphonates (pamidronate and zoledronic acid) for at least 1 year and orally administered nitrogen-containing bisphosphonate (alendronate therapy [Fosamax], risedronate [Actonel], ibandronate [Boniva]) administered for 5 years or longer.[52,63,64] The condition often is triggered by the extraction of a painful tooth or teeth, most commonly a mandibular posterior tooth. In a study of 2408 patients with BONJ, 43% were associated with MM, 67% followed tooth extractions, and only 35% were cured.[60] The typical presenting lesion is a severely painful and unexpected nonhealing extraction socket or exposed area of bone. However, the necrotic bone may be asymptomatic for weeks and may be noticed only on routine examination. Treatment is directed toward controlling and limiting progression by means of local débridement (bone and wound irrigation with antiseptics), together with long-term or intermittent courses of penicillin-type antibiotics (clindamycin or azithromycin if penicillin allergic).[63,64] To minimize the likelihood that osteonecrosis will develop in these patients, the following recommendations should be followed: (1) treat infections (periapical pathoses, sinus tracts, purulent periodontal pockets, severe periodontitis, and active abscesses) early; (2) nonsurgical approaches are preferable to surgical approaches; (3) if surgery or extractions are required, conservative surgical techniques should be used (limit the procedure to as few teeth as possible and to one sextant); (4) wait 2 months before performing surgery/extraction in a different sextant; (5) provide antibiotic coverage during the extraction and healing period and consider alveolectomy;[65] and (6) be aware of and discuss the risks of osteonecrosis (including implant bone preparation) with the patient who is considering undergoing surgery.[63] Chapter 26 presents more in-depth information regarding the management of BONJ.

REFERENCES

1. Roit I, Brostoff J, Male D: *Immunology*, ed 5, Edinburgh, 2001, Mosby.
2. Bagby GCJ: Leukopenia and leukocytosis. In Goldman L, Ausiello D, editors: *Cecil medicine*, ed 23, Philadelphia, 2008, Saunders, pp 1252-1263.
3. Quesenberry PJ: Hematopoiesis and hematopoietic growth factors. In Goldman L, Ausiello D, editors: *Cecil medicine*, ed 23, Philadelphia, 2008, Saunders, pp 1165-1172.
4. Viswanatha DS, Larson RS: Molecular diagnosis of hematopoietic neoplasms. In McPherson RA, Pincus MR, editors: *Henry's clinical diagnosis and management by laboratory methods*, ed 21, Philadelphia, 2007, Saunders.
5. Neville BW: Hematologic disorders. In Neville BW, et al, editors: *Oral and maxillofacial pathology*, ed 3, St. Louis, 2009, Saunders, pp 571-612.
6. Aster JC: Diseases of white blood cells, lymph nodes, spleen and thymus. In Kumar VK, Abbas AK, Fausto N, editors: *Robbins and Cotran pathologic basis of disease*, ed 7, Philadelphia, 2005, Elsevier Saunders.
7. American Cancer Society: *Cancer facts and figures 2010: leukemia, lymphoma and myeloma*, Atlanta, 2010, American Cancer Society.
8. Leukemia and Lymphoma Society: *Leukemia*, White Plains, NY, 2010, Leukemia and Lymphoma Society.
9. Appelbaum FR: The acute leukemias. In Goldman L, Ausiello D, editors: *Cecil medicine*, ed 23, Philadelphia, 2008, Saunders, pp 1390-1396.
10. Fanning SR, et al: Acute myelogenous leukemia. In Carey WD, et al, editors: *Current clinical medicine 2009—Cleveland Clinic*, Philadelphia, 2009, Saunders, pp 610-614.
11. Miller KB, Pihan G: Clinical manifestations of acute myeloid leukemia. In Hoffman R, et al, editors: *Hematology: basic principles and practice*, ed 5, Philadelphia, 2009, Churchill Livingstone, pp 933-964.
12. Wetzler M, Byrd JC, Bloomfield CD. Acute and chronic myeloid leukemia. In Kasper DL, et al, editors: *Harrison's principles of internal medicine*, ed 16, New York, 2005, McGraw-Hill.
13. Appelbaum FR: Acute myeloid leukemia in adults. In Abeloff MD, et al, editors: *Clinical oncology*, ed 3, Philadelphia, 2004, Saunders.
14. Hoeizer D, Gokbuget N: Acute lymphocytic leukemia in adults. In Hoffman R, et al, editors: *Hematology: basic principles and practice*, ed 5, Philadelphia, 2009, Churchill Livingstone, pp 1033-1050.
15. Dechartres A, et al: Inclusion of patients with acute leukemia in clinical trials: a prospective multicenter survey of 1066 cases. *Ann Oncol* 22:224-233, 2011.
16. Rabin KR, et al: Clinical manifestations of acute lymphoblastic leukemia. In Hoffman R, et al, editors: *Hematology: basic principles and practice*, ed 5, Philadelphia, 2009, Churchill Livingstone, pp 1019-1026.
17. O'Mura GA: The leukemias. In Rose LF, Kaye D, editors: *Internal medicine for dentistry*, ed 2, St. Louis, 1990, Mosby.
18. Rowe JM, Avivi I: Therapy for acute myeloid leukemia. In Hoffman R, et al, editors: *Hematology: basic principles and practice*, ed 5, Philadelphia, 2009, Churchill Livingstone, pp 965-989.
19. Wang ES, Berliner N: Clonal disorders of the hematopoietic stem cell. In Andreoli TE, et al, editors: *Cecil essentials of medicine*, ed 6, Philadelphia, 2004, Saunders.
20. Kinane D: Blood and lymphoreticular disorders, *Periodontology* 21:84-93, 2000.
21. Bhatia R, Radich JP: Chronic myeloid leukemia. In Hoffman R, et al, editors: *Hematology: basic principles and practice*, ed 5, Philadelphia, 2009, Churchill Livingstone, pp 1109-1124.

22. Kantarjian H, O'Brien S: The chronic leukemias. In Goldman L, Ausiello DA, editors: *Cecil medicine*, ed 23, Philadelphia, 2008, Saunders, pp 1397-1407.
23. Traer E, Deininger MW: How much and how long: tyrosine kinase inhibitor therapy in chronic myeloid leukemia, *Clin Lymphoma Myeloma Leuk* 10(Suppl 1):S20-S26, 2010.
24. Kantarjian H, et al: Dasatinib versus imatinib in newly diagnosed chronic-phase chronic myeloid leukemia, *N Engl J Med* 362:2260-2270, 2010.
25. Chesan BD: Chronic lymphoid leukemias. In Abeloff MD, et al, editors: *Clinical oncology*, ed 3, Philadelphia, 2004, Saunders.
26. Lin TS, et al: Chronic lymphocytic leukemia. In Hoffman R, et al, editors: *Hematology: basic principles and practice*, ed 5, Philadelphia, 2009, Churchill Livingstone, pp 1327-1348.
27. Zenz T, et al: Moving from prognostic to predictive factors in chronic lymphocytic leukaemia (CLL), *Best Pract Res Clin Haematol* 23:71-84, 2010.
28. Tadmor T, Aviv A, Polliack A: Merkel cell carcinoma, chronic lymphocytic leukemia and other lymphoproliferative disorders: an old bond with possible new viral ties, *Ann Oncol* 22:250-256, 2011.
29. Yee KW, O'Brien SW: Chronic lymphocytic leukemia: diagnosis and treatment, *Mayo Clin Proc* 81:1105-1129, 2006.
30. Tsimberidou AM, Keating MJ: Treatment of patients with fludarabine-refractory chronic lymphocytic leukemia: need for new treatment options, *Leuk Lymphoma* 51:1188-1199, 2010.
31. Leukemia and Lymphoma Society: *Lymphoma*, White Plains, NY, 2010, Leukemia and Lymphoma Society.
32. Connors JM: Hodgkin's lymphoma. In Goldman L, Ausiello D, editors: *Cecil medicine*, ed 23, Philadelphia, 2008, Saunders, pp 1420-1425.
33. Diehl V, et al: Hodgkin lymphoma: clinical manifestations, staging and therapy. In Hoffman R, et al, editors: *Hematology: basic principles and practice*, ed 5, Philadelphia, 2009, Churchill Livingstone, pp 1239-1264.
34. Knecht H, et al: The role of Epstein-Barr virus in neoplastic transformation, *Oncology* 60:289-302, 2001.
35. Keating MJ: Chronic leukemias. In Goldman L, Bennett JC, editors: *Cecil textbook of medicine*, ed 21, Philadelphia, 2000, WB Saunders.
36. Lister TA, Coiffier B, Armitage JO: Non-Hodgkin's lymphoma. In Abeloff MD, Armitage JO, Niederhuber JE, editors: *Clinical oncology*, ed 3, Philadelphia, 2004, Saunders.
37. Bierman PJ, et al: Non-Hodgkin's lymphomas. In Goldman L, Ausiello D, editors: *Cecil medicine*, ed 23, Philadelphia, 2008, Saunders, pp 1408-1419.
38. Gribben JG: Clinical manifestations, staging, and treatment of indolent non-Hodgkin lymphoma. In Hoffman R, et al, editors: *Hematology: basic principles and practice*, ed 5, Philadelphia, 2009, Churchill Livingstone, pp 1281-1292.
39. Institute USNC. Cancer statistics fact sheets, 2006.
40. Dunleavy K, Wilson WH: Diagnosis and treatment of non-Hodgkin lymphoma (aggressive). In Hoffman R, et al, editors: *Hematology: basic principles and practice*, ed 5, Philadelphia, 2009, Churchill Livingstone, pp 1293-1302.
41. Silverman SJ: *Oral cancer*, ed 5, Hamilton, Ontario, 2003, BC Decker.
42. Raut A, et al: Unusual gingival presentation of post-transplantation lymphoproliferative disorder: a case report and review of the literature, *Oral Surg Oral Med Oral Pathol Oral Radiol Endod* 90:436-441, 2000.
43. Burkitt DP: The discovery of Burkitt's lymphoma, *Cancer* 51:1177-1286, 1983.
44. Sandlund JTJ, Link MP: Malignant lymphomas in childhood. In Hoffman R, et al, editors: *Hematology: basic principles and practice*, ed 5, Philadelphia, 2009, Churchill Livingstone, pp 1303-1314.
45. Kasamon YL, Swinnen LJ: Treatment advances in adult Burkitt lymphoma and leukemia, *Curr Opin Oncol* 16:429-435, 2004.
46. Leukemia and Lymphoma Society: *Myeloma*, White Plains, NY, 2010, Leukemia and Lymphoma Society.
47. Dispenzieri A, Kyle RA: Multiple myeloma: clinical features and indications for therapy, *Best Pract Res Clin Haematol* 18:553-568, 2005.
48. Tricot G: Multiple myeloma. In Hoffman R, et al, editors: *Hematology: basic principles and practice*, ed 5, Philadelphia, 2009, Churchill Livingstone, pp 1387-1412.
49. Baz R, Bolwell B: Multiple myeloma. In Carey WD, et al, editors: *Current clinical medicine 2009—Cleveland Clinic*, Philadelphia, 2009, Saunders, pp 647-654.
50. Rajkumar SV, Kyle RA: Plasma cell disorders. In Goldman L, Ausiello D, editors: *Cecil medicine*, ed 23, Philadelphia, 2008, Saunders Elsevier, pp 1426-1436.
51. Storm HH, et al: Trends in the survival of patients diagnosed with malignant neoplasms of lymphoid, haematopoietic, and related tissue in the Nordic countries 1964-2003 followed up to the end of 2006, *Acta Oncol* 49:694-712, 2010.
52. Migliorati CA, Siegel MA, Elting LS: Bisphosphonate-associated osteonecrosis: a long-term complication of bisphosphonate treatment, *Lancet Oncol* 7:508-514, 2006.
53. Scully C, Sonis S, Diz PD: Oral mucositis, *Oral Dis* 12:229-241, 2006.
54. McGuire DB, et al: The role of basic oral care and good clinical practice principles in the management of oral mucositis, *Support Care Cancer* 14:541-547, 2006.
55. DeRossie SS, et al: Hematologic diseases. In Greenberg MS, Glick M, editors: *Burket's oral medicine: diagnosis and treatment*, ed 10, Hamilton, Ontario, 2003, BC Decker.
56. McKenna SJ: Immunocompromised host and infection. In Topazian RG, Goldberg MH, Hupp JR, editors: *Oral and maxillofacial infections*, ed 4, Philadelphia, 2002, Saunders.
57. Sonis S: Oral complications of cancer chemotherapy. In Peterson D, Sonis S, editors: *Epidemiology, frequency, distribution, mechanisms and histopathology*, The Hague, 1983, Martinus Nijhoff.
58. Barosi G, et al: Management of multiple myeloma and related disorders: guidelines from the Italian Society of Hematology (SIE), Italian Society of Experimental Hematology (SIES) and Italian Group for Bone Marrow Transplantation (GITMO), *Haematologica* 89:717-741, 2004.
59. Scully C, Cawson RA: Immunodeficiencies other than HIV/AIDS. In Scully C, Cawson RA, editors: *Medical problems in dentistry*, ed 5, Edinburgh, 2005, Elsevier.
60. Filleul O, Crompot E, Saussez S: Bisphosphonate-induced osteonecrosis of the jaw: a review of 2,400 patient cases, *J Cancer Res Clin Oncol* 136:1117-1124, 2010.
61. Lipton A: Bone continuum of cancer, *Am J Clin Oncol* 33(3 Suppl):S1-S7, 2010.
62. Walter C, et al: Prevalence of bisphosphonate associated osteonecrosis of the jaws in multiple myeloma patients, *Head Face Med* 6:11, 2010.
63. American Dental Association Council on Scientific Affairs: Dental management of patients receiving oral bisphosphonate therapy: expert panel recommendations, *J Am Dent Assoc* 137:1144-1150, 2006.
64. Marx RE: Pamidronate (Aredia) and zoledronate (Zometa) induced avascular necrosis of the jaws: a growing epidemic, *J Oral Maxillofac Surg* 61:1115-1117, 2003.
65. Ferlito S, Puzzo S, Liardo C: Preventive protocol for tooth extractions in patients treated with zoledronate: a case series, *J Oral Maxillofac Surg* 69:e1-4, 2011.

CHAPTER

24

Acquired Bleeding and Hypercoagulable Disorders

A number of procedures that are performed in dentistry may cause bleeding. Under normal circumstances, these procedures can be performed with little clinical risk; however, in the patient whose ability to control bleeding has been altered by drugs or disease such procedures may be associated with potentially catastrophic outcomes unless the dental practitioner identifies the problem before initiation of treatment. In most instances, once the patient with a bleeding problem due to drugs or disease has been identified, appropriate dental management will greatly reduce the associated risks. This chapter presents an overview of the physiologic mechanisms involved in the control of bleeding and the pathophysiology of acquired bleeding disorders and hypercoagulable states. Congenital bleeding disorders and genetic hypercoagulable conditions are covered in Chapter 25.

DEFINITION

Bleeding disorders are conditions that alter the ability of blood vessels, platelets, and coagulation factors to maintain hemostasis. Acquired bleeding disorders may occur as the result of diseases, drugs, radiation, or chemotherapy for cancer in which vascular wall integrity, platelet production or function, or coagulation factors are impaired.

Most bleeding disorders are iatrogenic. Every patient who receives coumarin to prevent recurrent thrombosis has a potential bleeding problem. Most of these patients are receiving anticoagulant medication because they have had a recent myocardial infarction, a cerebrovascular accident, or thrombophlebitis. Patients who have atrial fibrillation; who have had open heart surgery to correct a congenital defect, replace diseased arteries, or repair or replace damaged heart valves; or who have had recent total hip or knee replacement also may be receiving long-term anticoagulation therapy. Patients treated with antiplatelet medications to prevent cardiovascular complications also may have a potential bleeding problem. Some people treated with aspirin for chronic illnesses, such as rheumatoid arthritis, may have potential bleeding problems.

In a dental practice of 2000 adults, about 100 to 150 patients may have a possible bleeding problem. This is a rough estimate, however, and the number could be higher.

Epidemiology: Incidence and Prevalence

Patients on low-intensity warfarin therapy (with an international normalized ratio [INR] goal of 2.0 to 3.0) for prophylaxis of venous thromboembolism have a risk of major bleeding of less than 1% and about an 8% risk for minor bleeding. Patients on high-intensity warfarin therapy (with an INR goal of 2.5 to 3.5) have up to a five-fold greater risk for bleeding.[1-4]

Patients with acute or chronic leukemia may have clinical bleeding tendencies because of thrombocytopenia, which may result from overgrowth of malignant cells in the bone marrow that leaves no room for red blood cells or platelet precursors. In addition, leukemic patients may develop thrombocytopenia from the toxic effects of the various chemotherapeutic agents used to treat the disease. The etiology and incidence of leukemia are reviewed in Chapter 23.

It is difficult to obtain accurate information about the incidence of other systemic conditions, such as liver disease, renal failure, thrombocytopenia, and drug-induced vascular wall defects, that may render the patient susceptible to prolonged bleeding after injury or surgery. However, when the prevalence of drug-influenced or disease-produced defects in the normal control of blood loss is considered, a busy dental practice will contain a large number of patients who may be potential "bleeders."

ETIOLOGY

A pathologic alteration of blood vessel walls, a significant reduction in the number of platelets, defective platelets or platelet function, a deficiency of one or more coagulation factors, the administration of anticoagulant or antiplatelet drugs, a disorder of platelet release, or the inability to destroy free plasmin can result in significant

BOX 24-1 Classification of Acquired Bleeding and Thrombotic Disorders

Nonthrombocytopenic Purpuras

Vascular Wall Alteration

- Scurvy
- Infections
- Chemicals
- Allergy

Disorders of Platelet Function

- Drugs
  - Aspirin, other NSAIDs
  - Other antiplatelet drugs
  - Dipyridamole and aspirin (Aggrenox)
  - Ticlopidine (Ticlid)
  - Clopidogrel (Plavix)
  - Abciximab (ReoPro)
  - Eptifibatide (Integrilin)
  - Tirofiban (Aggrastat)
  - Alcohol
  - Beta-lactam antibiotics
  - Cephalothins
  - Herbal medications
  - Vitamin E Allergy
- Autoimmune disease
- Uremia

Thrombocytopenic Purpuras

Primary

Idiopathic

Secondary

- Chemicals
- Physical agents (radiation)
- Systemic disease (leukemia and others)
- Metastatic cancer to bone
- Splenomegaly
- Drugs
  - Alcohol
  - Thiazide diuretics
  - Estrogens
  - Gold salts
- Vasculitis
- Mechanical prosthetic heart valves
- Viral or bacterial infections

Disorders of Coagulation

- Liver disease
- Vitamin K deficiency
  - Biliary tract obstruction
  - Malabsorption
  - Excessive use of broad-spectrum antibiotics
- Anticoagulation drugs
  - Heparin
  - Low-molecular-weight heparins
    - Enoxaparin (Lovenox)
    - Ardeparin (Normiflo)
    - Dalteparin (Fragmin)
    - Nadroparin (Fraxiparine)
    - Reviparin (Clivarin)
    - Tinzaparin (Innohep)
  - Synthetic heparin
    - Fondaparinux (Arixtra)
    - Idraparinux (completed phase III trials)
  - Coumarin (warfarin), oral
  - Direct thrombin inhibitors
    - Lepirudin (Reflucan)
    - Desirudin (Revasc)
    - Argatroban (Acova)
    - Bivalirudan (Angiox)
    - Dabigatran (Pradaxa), oral
- Disseminated intravascular coagulation
- Primary fibrinogenolysis

Hypercoagulable States

- Old age
- Immobilization
- Obesity
- Infection
- Hospitalization
- Major surgery
- Hormonal therapy
- Atherosclerosis
- Malignancy
- Hyperchomocysteinemia
- Antiphospholipid antibody syndromes
  - Lupus erythematosus
  - Rheumatoid arthritis
  - Sjögren syndrome

abnormal clinical bleeding. This may occur even after minor injuries and may lead to death in some patients if immediate action is not taken.

The classification given in Box 24-1 is based on bleeding problems in patients with normal numbers of platelets (nonthrombocytopenic purpura), decreased numbers of platelets (thrombocytopenic purpura), disorders of coagulation, and hypercoagulable states.

Infections, chemicals, collagen disorders, or certain types of allergy can alter the structure and function of the vascular wall to the point that the patient may have a clinical bleeding problem. A patient may have normal numbers of platelets, but they may be defective or unable to perform their proper function in the control of blood loss from damaged tissues. If the total number of circulating platelets is reduced to below 50,000/μL of blood, the patient may be a bleeder. In some cases, the total platelet count is reduced by unknown mechanisms; this is called *primary* or *idiopathic thrombocytopenia.* Chemicals, radiation, and various systemic diseases (e.g., leukemia) may have a direct effect on the bone marrow, potentially resulting in secondary thrombocytopenia.[5,6]

Acquired coagulation disorders are the most common cause of prolonged bleeding. Liver disease and disseminated intravascular coagulation (DIC) can lead to severe bleeding problems. Many of the other acquired coagulation disorders may become apparent in patients only after trauma or surgical procedures. In contrast with the congenital coagulation disorders, in which only one factor is affected, the acquired coagulation disorders usually have multiple factor deficiencies.[1,7-9]

The liver produces all of the protein coagulation factors; thus, any patient with significant liver disease may have a bleeding problem. In addition to having a possible disorder in coagulation, the patient with liver disease who develops portal hypertension and hypersplenism may be thrombocytopenic as a result of splenic overactivity, which leads to increased sequestration of platelets in the spleen.[10]

Any condition that so disrupts the intestinal flora that vitamin K is not produced in sufficient amounts will result in a decreased plasma level of the vitamin K–dependent coagulation factors. Vitamin K is needed by the liver to produce prothrombin (factor II) and factors VII, IX, and X. Biliary tract obstruction, malabsorption syndrome, and excessive use of broad-spectrum antibiotics all can lead to low levels of prothrombin and factors VII, IX, and X on this basis.[10]

Drugs, such as heparin and coumarin derivatives, can cause a bleeding disorder because they may disrupt the coagulation process. Antiplatelet medications, aspirin, other nonsteroidal antiinflammatory drugs (NSAIDs), penicillin, cephalosporins, and alcohol also may interfere with platelet function.[11]

Many herbal supplements can impair hemostatic function for the control of bleeding. Fish oil or concentrated omega-3 fatty acid supplements may impair platelet activation. Diets naturally rich in omega-3 fatty acids can result in a prolonged bleeding time and abnormal platelet aggregation.[1] Fish oil supplements prolong bleeding time, inhibit platelet aggregation, and decrease thromboxane A_2 (TXA_2) production.[12] Vitamin E appears to inhibit protein kinase C–mediated platelet aggregation and nitric oxide production.[1] The following herbal supplements have potential antiplatelet activity: ginkgo, garlic, bilberry, ginger, dong quai, Asian ginseng, tumeric, meadow sweet, willow, coumarin-containing herbs, chamomile, horse chestnut, red clover, and fenugreek. In patients with unexplained bruising or bleeding, it is prudent to review any new medications or supplements and discontinue those that may be associated with bleeding.[1]

Pathophysiology

The three phases of hemostasis for controlling bleeding are vascular, platelet, and coagulation. The vascular and platelet phases are referred to as primary, and the coagulation phase is secondary. The coagulation phase is followed by the fibrinolytic phase, during which the clot is dissolved (Box 24-2).

Vascular Phase. The vascular phase begins immediately after injury and involves vasoconstriction of arteries and veins in the area of injury, retraction of arteries that have been cut, and buildup of extravascular pressure by blood loss from cut vessels. This pressure aids in collapsing the adjacent capillaries and veins in the area of injury. Vascular wall integrity is important for maintaining the fluidity of blood. The smooth endothelial lining consists of a nonwettable surface that, under normal conditions, does not activate platelet adhesion or coagulation. In fact, the endothelial cells synthesize and secrete three potent antiplatelet agents: prostacyclin, nitric oxide, and certain adenine nucleotides.[8,13-15]

BOX 24-2 Normal Control of Bleeding

1. Vascular phase
   a. Vasoconstriction occurs in area of injury.
   b. Begins immediately after injury.
2. Platelet phase
   a. Platelets and vessel wall become "sticky."
   b. Mechanical plug of platelets seals off openings of cut vessels.
   c. Begins seconds after injury.
3. Coagulation phase
   a. Blood lost into surrounding area coagulates through extrinsic and common pathways.
   b. Blood in vessels in area of injury coagulates through intrinsic and common pathways.
   c. Takes place more slowly than other phases.
4. Fibrinolytic phase
   a. Release of antithrombotic agents
   b. Destruction of antithrombotic agents by spleen and liver

Vascular endothelial cells also are involved in antithrombotic and prothrombotic activities. The major antithrombotic activity consists of secretion of heparin-like glycosaminoglycans (heparin sulfate) that catalyze inactivation of serine proteases such as thrombin and factor Xa by antithrombin III. Endothelial cells also produce thrombomodulin, which combines with thrombin to form a complex that activates protein C. Activated protein C (APC) then binds to endothelially released protein S, causing proteolysis of factor Va and factor VIIIa that inhibits coagulation. Tissue-type plasminogen activator (tPA) is released by injured endothelial cells to initiate fibrinolysis.[8,13-15]

Vessel wall components contribute prothrombotic activities. Exposure of vessel wall subendothelial tissues, collagen, and basement membrane through chemical or traumatic injury serves as a tissue factor (TF)—for which the old term was *tissue thromboplastin*—and initiates coagulation by way of the extrinsic pathway. The extrinsic pathway can be turned off by tissue factor pathway inhibitor (TFPI). An inducible endothelial cell prothrombin activator may directly generate thrombin. Injured endothelial cells release adenosine diphosphate (ADP), which induces platelet adhesion. Vessel wall injury also promotes platelet adhesion and thrombus formation through exposure of subendothelial tissues to von Willebrand factor (vWF). Endothelial cells also contribute to normal homeostasis and vascular integrity through synthesis of type IV collagen, fibronectin, and vWF.[8,13-15]

Platelet Phase. Platelets are cellular fragments from the cytoplasm of megakaryocytes that last 8 to 12 days in the circulation. About 30% of platelets are sequestered in the microvasculature or spleen and serve as a functional reserve. Platelets do not have a nucleus; thus, they are unable to repair inhibited enzyme systems through drugs such as aspirin. Aged or nonviable platelets are removed and destroyed by the spleen and liver.[8,13,16] Functions of platelets include maintenance of vascular integrity, formation of a platelet plug to aid in initial control of bleeding, and stabilization of the platelet plug through involvement in the coagulation process. About 10% of platelets are used to nurture endothelial cells, allowing for endothelial and smooth muscle regeneration.

Subendothelial tissues are exposed at the site of injury and, through contact activation, cause the platelets to become sticky and adhere to subendothelial tissues, platelet membrane glycoprotein Ib (GPIb) binds with vWF, which is attached to the subendothelial tissue, and glycoprotein Ia/IIa (GPIa/IIa) and glycoprotein VI (GPVI) bind to collagen in the injured vessel wall.

ADP released by damaged endothelial cells initiates aggregation of platelets (primary wave), and when platelets release their secretions, a second wave of aggregation results. Platelets bind with fibrinogen by the membrane glycoprotein IIb (GPIIb) the fibrinogen is then converted to fibrin, which stabilizes the platelet plug. The result of the preceding processes is a clot of platelets and fibrin attached to the subendothelial tissue.[8,13,16] Box 24-3 summarizes the functions of platelets.

A product of platelets, thromboxane, is needed to induce platelet aggregation. The enzyme cyclooxygenase is essential in the process for generation of thromboxane. Endothelial cells, through a similar process (also dependent on cyclooxygenase), generate prostacyclin, which inhibits platelet aggregation. Aspirin acts as an inhibitor of cyclooxygenase, and this causes irreversible damage to the platelets. However, endothelial cells can, after a short period, recover and synthesize cyclooxygenase; thus, aspirin has only a short effect on the availability of prostacyclin from these cells. The net result of aspirin therapy is to inhibit platelet aggregation. This effect can last up to 9 days (time needed for all old platelets to be cleared from the blood).[8,13,16]

Coagulation Phase. The process of the fibrin-forming (coagulation) system is shown in Figure 24-1. The overall time involved from injury to a fibrin-stabilized clot is about 9 to 18 minutes. Platelets, blood proteins, lipids, and ions are involved in the process. Thrombin is generated on the surface of the platelets, and bound fibrinogen is converted to fibrin.[8,16] The end product of coagulation is a fibrin clot that can stop further blood loss from injured tissues (Figures 24-2 and 24-3).

BOX 24-3 Platelet Functions and Activation

1. Plasma membrane receptors
   a. Glycoprotein Ib reacts with von Willebrand factor, which attaches to subendothelial tissue.
   b. Glycoprotein Ia/IIa binds to collagen in the injured vessel wall.
   c. Glycoprotein VI binds to collagen in the injured vessel wall.
   d. Glycoproteins IIb and IIIa attach to fibrinogen or fibronectin.
2. Platelets contain three types of secretory granules:
   a. Lysosomes
   b. Alpha granules—contain platelet factor 4, β-thromboglobulin, and several growth factors including platelet-derived growth factor (PDGF), endothelial cell growth factor (PD-ECGF), and transforming growth factor-βa (TGF-β); also several hemostatic proteins: fibrinogen, factor V, and von Willebrand factor
   c. Dense bodies (electron-dense organelles)—contain ATP, ADP, calcium, and serotonin
3. Platelets provide a surface for activation of soluble coagulation factors:
   a. Activated platelets expose specific receptors that bind factors Xa and Va, thus increasing their local concentration, thereby accelerating prothrombin activation.
   b. Factor X also is activated by factors IXa and VIII on the surface of the platelet.
4. Platelets contain a membrane phospholipase C:
   a. When activated, it forms diglyceride.
   b. Diglyceride is converted to arachidonic acid by diglyceride lipase.
   c. Arachidonic acid is a substrate for prostaglandin synthetase (cyclooxygenase).
   d. Cyclooxygenase formation is inhibited by aspirin and nonsteroidal antiinflammatory drugs.
   e. The prostaglandin endoperoxide PGG_2, is required for ADP-induced aggregation and release, as is thromboxane A_2. The formation of both of these agents is dependent on cyclooxygenase.
5. The functions of platelets include:
   a. Nurturing endothelial cells
   b. Endothelial and smooth muscle regeneration
   c. Formation of a platelet plug for initial control of bleeding
   d. Stabilization of the platelet plug

Data from McMillan R: Hemorrhagic disorders: abnormalities of platelet and vascular function. In Goldman L, Ausiello D, editors: Cecil medicine, ed 23, *Philadelphia, 2008, Saunders; and Baz R, Mekhail T: Disorders of platelet function and number. In Carey WD, et al, editors:* Current clinical medicine 2009—Cleveland Clinic, *Philadelphia, 2009, Saunders.*

Coagulation of blood involves the components shown in Table 24-1. Many of the coagulation factors are proenzymes that become activated in a "waterfall" or cascade manner—that is, one factor becomes activated, and it, in turn, activates another, and so on in an ordered sequence.[17] For example, the proenzyme (zymogen) factor XI is activated to the enzyme factor XIa through contact with injury-exposed subendothelial tissues in vivo to start the intrinsic pathway. In vitro, the intrinsic

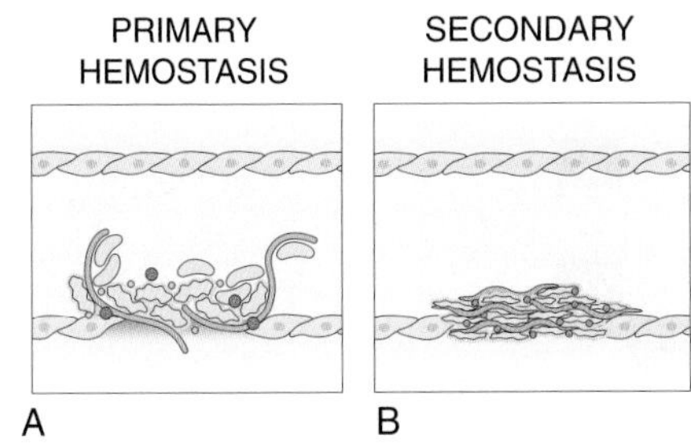

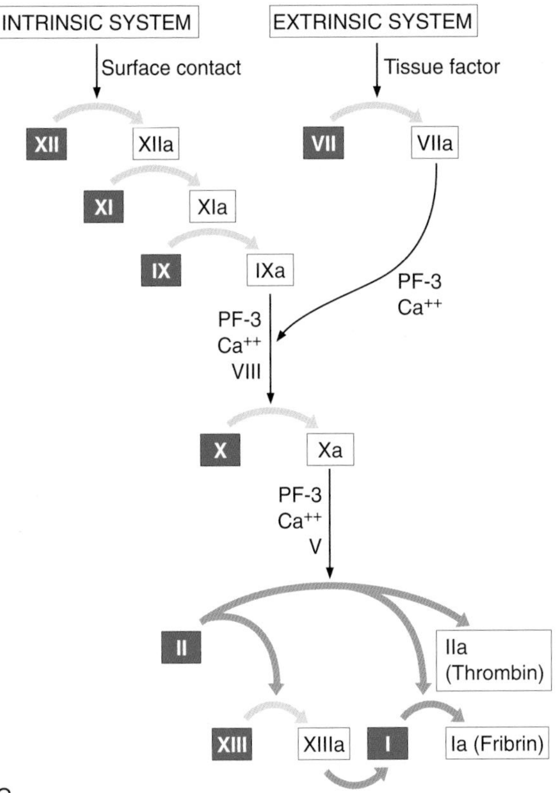

FIGURE 24-1 The primary (vascular/platelet) system (**A**), the secondary (coagulation) system for the control of bleeding (**B**), and the coagulation cascade (**C**). The intrinsic coagulation system is triggered by surface contact; the extrinsic system, by release of tissue factor from injured tissues; and the common pathway, by factor X. *(From Ragni MV: The hemophilias: factor VIII and factor IX deficiencies. In Young NS, Gerson SL, High KA, editors:* Clinical hematology, *St. Louis, 2006, Mosby.)*

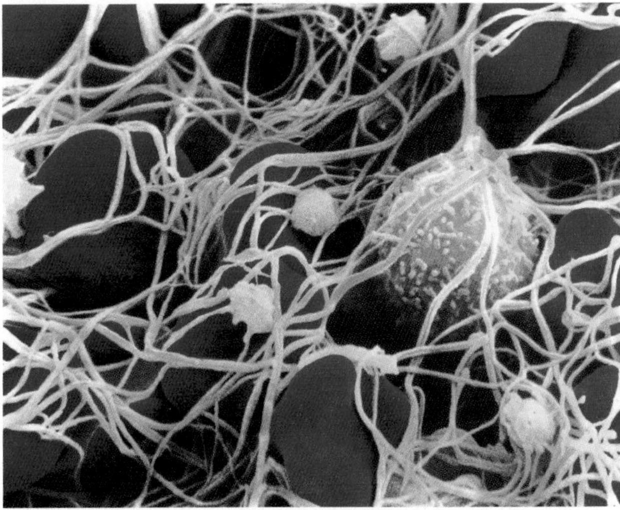

FIGURE 24-2 The end product of the coagulation system, which shows a fibrin clot or thrombus. White threads are fibrin, the structure with yellow on the surface is a white blood cell, platelets are green, and the red structures are red blood cells. *(Reprinted with permission of CNRI/Photo Researchers, Inc.)*

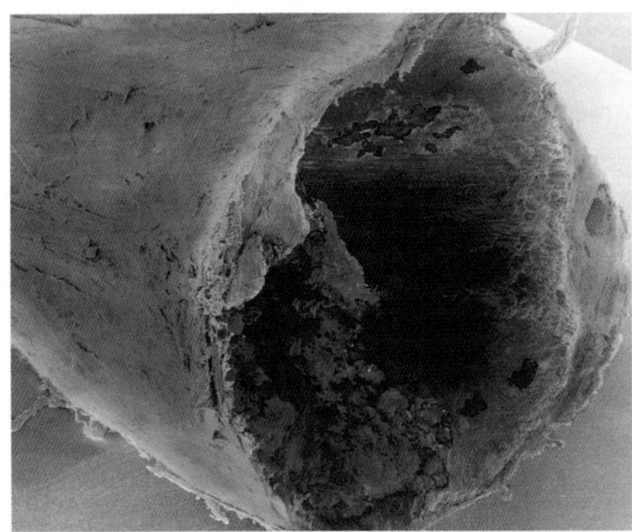

FIGURE 24-3 A colored scanning electron micrograph of a blood clot or thrombus inside the coronary artery of a human heart. *(Reprinted with permission of P. M. Motta, G. Macchiarelli, S. A. Nottola/Photo Researchers, Inc.)*

pathway is initiated by contact activation of factor XII. Coagulation proceeds through two pathways—the intrinsic and the extrinsic. Both use a common pathway to form the end product, fibrin.[8,16] Figure 24-1 shows these coagulation pathways.

The (faster) extrinsic pathway is initiated through tissue factor (an integral membrane protein) and is released or exposed through injury to tissues; this process activates factor VII (VIIa). In the past, the trigger for initiating the extrinsic pathway was referred to as a tissue *thromboplastin.* It has since been shown that the real activator is the tissue factor (TF). The term *extrinsic pathway* continues to be used today, despite the fact that it is somewhat outdated. This is because TF is not always extrinsic to the circulatory system but is expressed on the surface of vascular endothelial cells and leukocytes.[8,16]

Thrombin generated by the faster extrinsic and common pathway is used to accelerate the slower intrinsic and common pathway. Activation of factor XII acts as a common link between the component parts of the homeostatic mechanism: coagulation, fibrinolytic, kinin, and complement systems. As a result, thrombin is generated; in turn, fibrinogen is converted to fibrin, activates

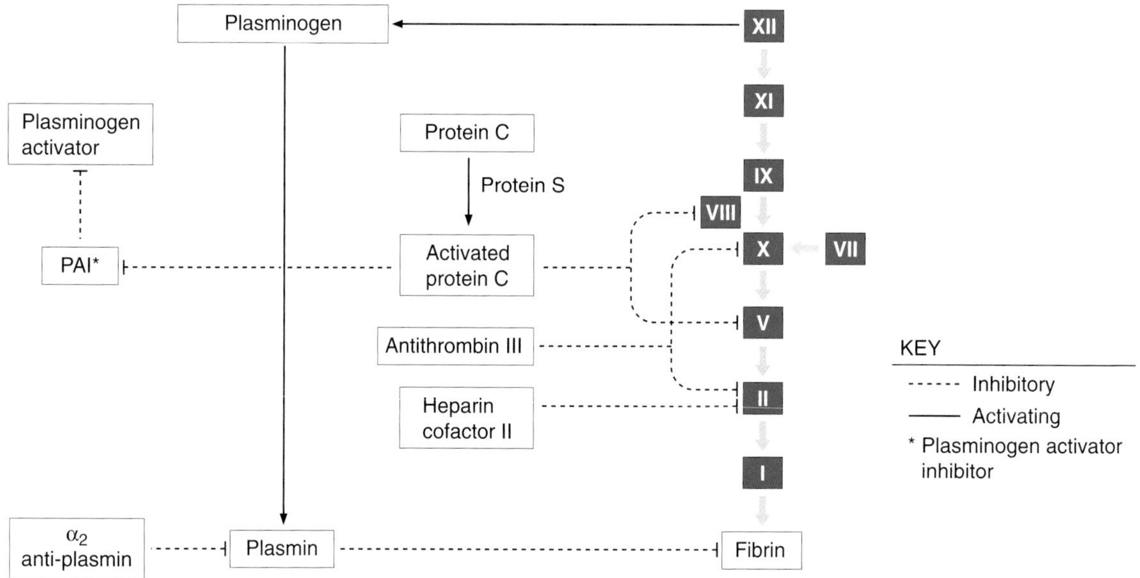

FIGURE 24-4 The coagulation and fibrinolytic pathways with inhibitors. *(From Bontempo FA: Hematologic abnormalities in liver disease. In Young NS, Gerson SL, High KA, editors:* Clinical hematology, *St. Louis, 2006, Mosby.)*

TABLE 24-1 Blood Coagulation Components

Factor	Deficiency	Function
Factor II (prothrombin)	Acquired—common	Protease zymogen
Factor X	Acquired—common	Protease zymogen
Factor IX	Acquired—common	Protease zymogen
Factor VII	Acquired—common	Protease zymogen
Factor VIII	Acquired—rare	Cofactor
Factor V	Acquired—rare	Cofactor
Factor XI	Acquired—common	Protease zymogen
Factor I (fibrinogen)	Acquired—common	Structural
von Willebrand Factor	Acquired—rare	Adhesion

From McVey JH: Coagulation factors. In Young NS, Gerson SL, High KA, editors: Clinical hematology, *St. Louis, 2006, Elsevier.*

factor XIII, enhances factor V and factor VIII activity, and stimulates aggregation of additional platelets.[8,16]

Fibrinolytic Phase. The fibrin-lysing (fibrinolytic) system is needed to prevent coagulation of intravascular blood away from the site of injury and to dissolve the clot, once it has served its function in homeostasis (Figure 24-4). This system involves plasminogen, a proenzyme for the enzyme plasmin, which is produced in the liver, and various plasminogen activators and inhibitors of plasmin. The prime endogenous plasminogen activator is tissue-type plasminogen activator (tPA), which is released by endothelial cells at the site of injury.

The tPA released by injured endothelial cells binds to fibrin as it activates the conversion of fibrin-bound plasminogen to plasmin. Circulating plasminogen (i.e., not fibrin bound) is not activated by tPA. Thus, tPA is efficient in dissolving a clot without causing systemic fibrinolysis.[8,17,18]

The effect of plasmin on fibrin and fibrinogen is to split off large pieces that are broken up into smaller and smaller segments. The final smaller pieces are called *split products*. These split products also are referred to as *fibrin degradation products* (FDPs). FDPs increase vascular permeability and interfere with thrombin-induced fibrin formation; this can provide the basis for clinical bleeding problems.[8,19] Box 24-4 summarizes the fibrinlysing system.

Antiplasmin factors present in circulating blood rapidly destroy free plasmin but are relatively ineffective against plasmin that is bound to fibrin (Box 24-5). Free plasmin is rapidly destroyed and does not interfere with the formation of a clot. Bound plasmin is not inactivated, and it is free to dispose of the fibrin clot after its function in homeostasis has been fulfilled. In a sense, the clot is "programmed" at the time of its formation to self-destruct.[8,19]

Timing of Clinical Bleeding. A significant disorder that may occur in the vascular or platelet phase leads to an immediate clinical bleeding problem after injury or surgery. These phases are concerned with controlling blood loss immediately after an injury and, if defective, will lead to an early problem. However, if the vascular and platelet phases are normal, and the coagulation phase is abnormal, the bleeding problem will not be detected until several hours or longer after the injury or surgical procedure. In the case of small cuts, for example, little bleeding would occur until several hours after the injury, and then a slow trickle of bleeding would start. If the coagulation defect were severe, this slow loss of blood could continue for days. Even with this "trivial"

BOX 24-4 Fibrin-Lysing (Fibrinolytic) System

1. Activation of coagulation also activates fibrinolysis.
2. Active enzyme: plasmin
3. Plasminogen activated to plasmin
   a. Tissue-type plasminogen activator (t-PA)
   b. Prourokinase (scu-PA)
   c. Urokinase (u-PA), streptokinase
4. Tissue plasminogen activator (t-PA)
   a. t-PA is produced by endothelial cells.
   b. It is released by injury.
   c. It activates plasminogen bound to fibrin.
   d. Circulating plasminogen is not activated.
   e. t-PA will dissolve clot, not cause systemic fibrinolysis.
5. Action of plasmin:
   a. Plasmin splits large pieces of alpha and beta polypeptides from fibrin.
   b. It splits small pieces of gamma chains.
   c. First product is X monomer.
   d. Each X monomer splits into one E fragment and two D fragments.
   e. Split products are called fibrin split products (FSPs) and fibrin degradation products (FDPs).
6. Action of fibrin degradation products:
   a. Increase vascular permeability
   b. Interfere with thrombin-induced fibrin formation

Data from Lijnen HR, Collen D: Molecular and cellular basis of fibrinolysis. In Hoffman R, et al, editors: Hematology: basic principles and practice, *Philadelphia, 2009, Churchill Livingstone; and Kessler CM: Hemorrhagic disorders: coagulation factor deficiencies. In Goldman L, Ausiello D, editors:* Cecil textbook of medicine, *ed 23, Philadelphia, 2008, Saunders.*

BOX 24-5 Physiologic Antithrombotic Systems

1. Normal endothelium promotes blood fluidity by inhibiting platelet activation.
2. Endothelium also plays a role in anticoagulation by preventing fibrin formation.
3. Antithrombin III
   a. It is the major protease inhibitor of the coagulation system.
   b. It inactivates thrombin and other activated coagulation factors.
   c. Heparin acts as an anticoagulant by binding to antithrombin and greatly accelerates the ability of antithrombin to inhibit coagulation proteases.
   d. Heparin and heparin sulfate proteoglycans are naturally present on endothelial cells.
4. Activated protein C, with its cofactor protein S, acts as a natural anticoagulant by destroying factors Va and VIIIa.
5. Tissue factor pathway inhibitor (TFPI), a plasma protease inhibitor, inhibits factor VIIa and the extrinsic pathway.
6. The endogenous fibrinolytic system degrades any fibrin produced despite the above-mentioned antithrombotic mechanisms.
7. Inherited deficiencies of antithrombin, protein C, or protein S are associated with a lifelong thrombotic tendency.
8. TFPI deficiency has yet to be related to clinical problems.

Data from Dahlback B, Stenflo J: Regulatory mechanisms in hemostasis: natural anticoagulants. In Hoffman R, et al, editors: Hematology: basic principles and practice, *ed 5, Philadelphia, 2009, Churchill Livingstone.*

rate, a significant loss of blood might occur (0.5 mL/minute or about 3 U/day).[9]

CLINICAL PRESENTATION

Signs and Symptoms

Signs associated with bleeding disorders may appear in the skin or mucous membranes or after trauma or invasive procedures. Jaundice (Figure 24-5), spider angiomas (Figure 24-6), and ecchymoses (Figure 24-7) may be seen in the person with liver disease. A fine tremor of the hands when held out also may be observed in these patients. In about 50% of persons with liver disease, a reduction in platelets occurs because of hypersplenism that results from the effects of portal hypertension; these patients may show petechiae on the skin and mucosa.[8,9,18,20]

The signs seen most commonly in patients with abnormal platelets or thrombocytopenia are petechiae (Figure 24-8) and ecchymoses.[21]

Patients with acute or chronic leukemia may reveal one or more of the following signs: ulceration of the oral mucosa, hyperplasia of the gingivae (Figure 24-9), petechiae of the skin or mucous membranes (Figure 24-10), ecchymoses of skin or mucous membranes, and

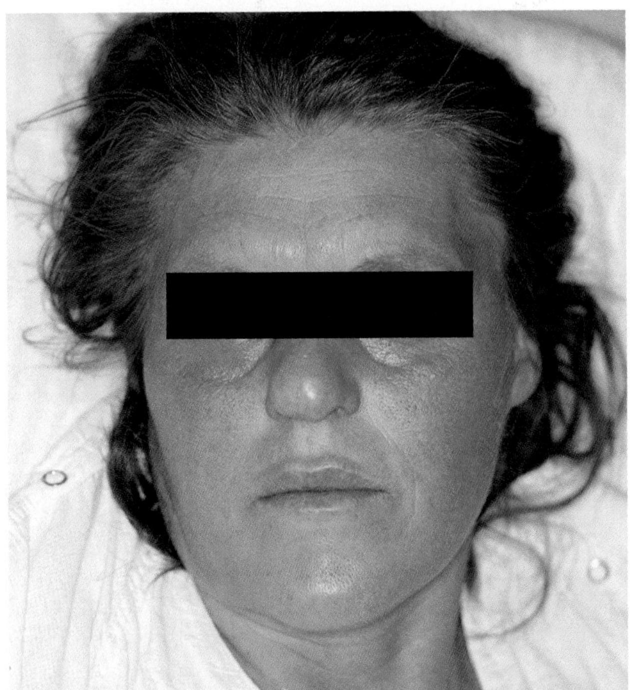

FIGURE 24-5 Jaundice of the skin in a patient with chronic liver disease.

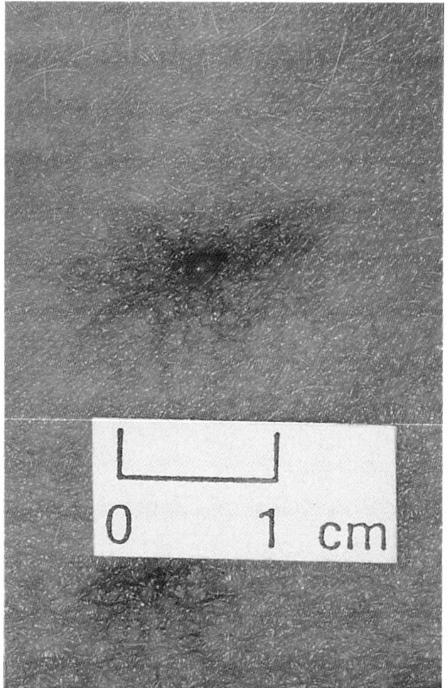

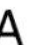
A

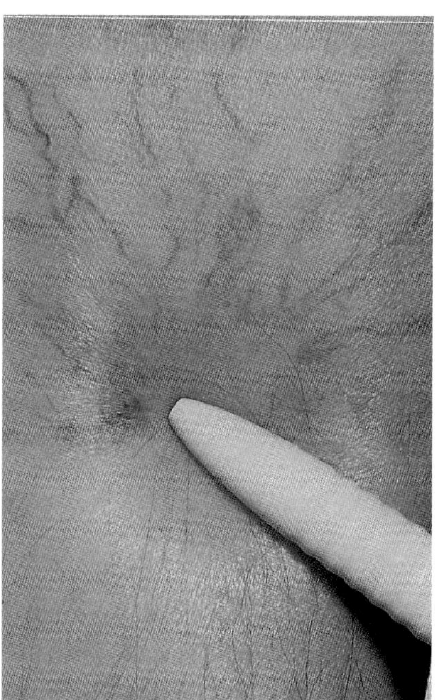
B

FIGURE 24-6 **A**, Spider angioma on the skin of a patient with chronic liver disease **B**, Note how the spider legs of the angioma blanch with pressure on the central arteriole. *(From Forbes CD, Jackson WF:* Color atlas and text of clinical medicine, *ed 3, Edinburgh, 2003, Mosby.)*

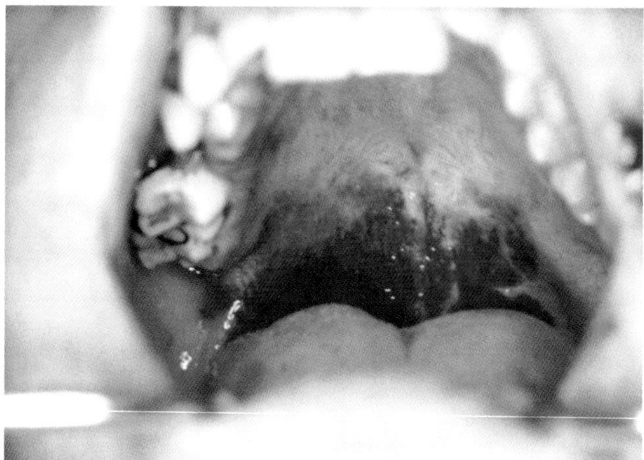

FIGURE 24-7 Ecchymoses on the mucosa of the hard and soft palate in a patient with chronic liver disease.

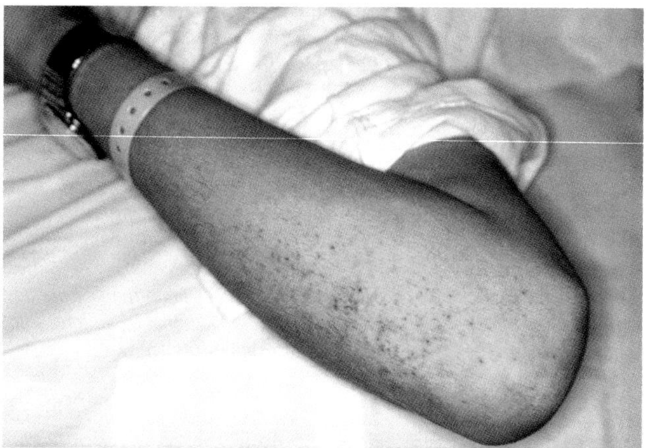

FIGURE 24-8 The arm of a patient with thrombocytopenia shows numerous petechiae.

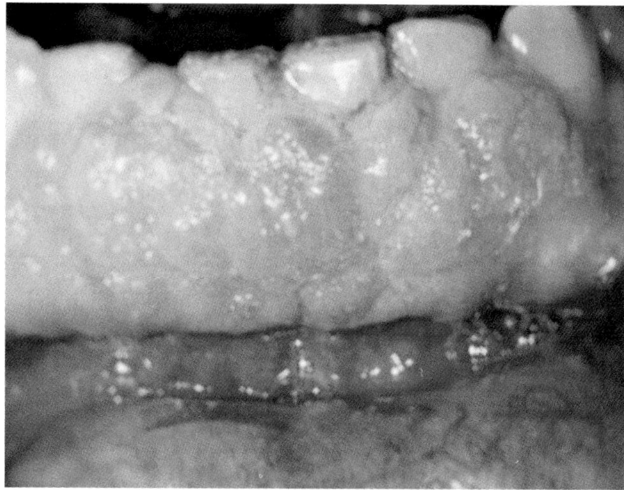

FIGURE 24-9 Hyperplastic gingiva in a patient with leukemia.

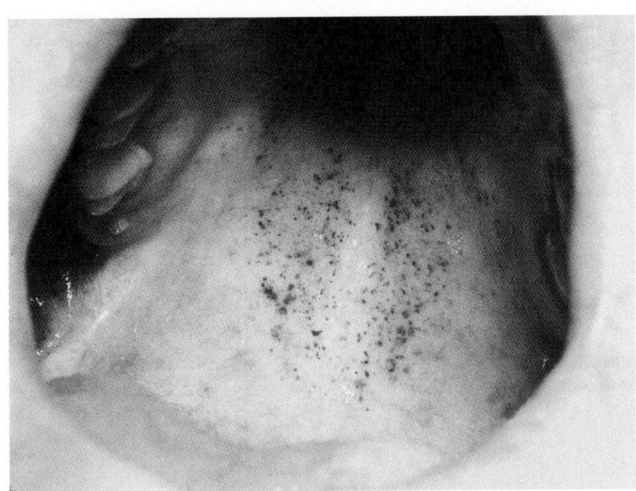

FIGURE 24-10 Palatal petechiae in a patient with leukemia. *(From Hoffbrand AV: Color atlas of clinical hematology, ed 3, St. Louis, 2000, Mosby.)*

lymphadenopathy. Chapter 23 discusses these findings in greater detail.

A number of patients with bleeding disorders may show no objective signs that suggest the underlying problem. Severe or chronic bleeding can lead to anemia with features of pallor, fatigue, and so forth. Anemia is discussed in detail in Chapter 22.

Laboratory Tests

Several tests are available to screen patients for bleeding disorders and to help pinpoint the specific deficiency. In general, screening is done in dentistry when the patient reveals a history of a bleeding problem or a family member with a history of a bleeding problem, or when signs of bleeding disorders are found during the clinical examination. The dentist can order the screening tests, or the patient can be referred to a hematologist for screening. In medicine, routine screening is done for patients before major surgical procedures such as open heart surgery are performed.

The Ivy bleeding time (BT) has been used to screen for disorders of platelet function and thrombocytopenia. It has been found to be unreliable and is no longer used as a screening test. The platelet function analyzer (PFA-100), an instrument that measures platelet-dependent coagulation under flow conditions, is more sensitive and specific for platelet disorders and von Willebrand disease (vWD) than the bleeding time; however, it is not sensitive enough to rule out underlying mild bleeding disorders. Also, it has not been evaluated prospectively to determine its utility in predicting bleeding risk, although such studies are underway. Therefore, the BT and PFA-100 are not recommended as screening tests to be used by the dentist.

Three tests are recommended for use in initial screening for possible bleeding disorders:[1,13,22] activated partial thromboplastin time (aPTT), prothrombin time (PT), and platelet count (Figure 24-11). In the absence of clues to the cause of the bleeding problem, if the dentist is ordering the tests through a commercial laboratory, an additional test can be added to the initial screen: the thrombin time (TT).[1,13,22]

Patients with positive screening tests should be evaluated further so the specific deficiency can be identified and the presence of inhibitors ruled out. A hematologist orders these tests, establishes a diagnosis that is based on the additional testing, and makes recommendations for treatment of the patient who is found to have a significant bleeding problem.

Screening Tests: *Partial Thromboplastin Time.* Partial thromboplastin time (PTT) is used to check the intrinsic system (factors VIII, IX, XI, and XII) and the common pathways (factors V and X, prothrombin, and fibrinogen). It also is the best single screening test for coagulation disorders. A phospholipid platelet substitute is added to the patient's blood to initiate the coagulation process via the intrinsic pathway. When a contact activator, such as kaolin, is added, the test is referred to as *activated PTT* (aPTT). A control sample must be run with the test sample. In general, aPTT ranges from 25 to 35 seconds, and results in excess of 35 seconds are considered abnormal or prolonged. The aPTT is prolonged in cases of mild to severe deficiency of factor VIII or IX. The test result is abnormal when a given factor is 15% to 30% below its normal value.[1,13,22,23]

Prothrombin Time. The prothrombin time (PT) is used to check the extrinsic pathway (factor VII) and the common pathway (factors V and X, prothrombin, and fibrinogen). For this test, tissue thromboplastin is added to the test sample to serve as the activating agent. Again, a control must be run, and results vary from one laboratory to another. In general, the normal range is 11 to 15 seconds. PT is prolonged when the plasma level of any factor is below 10% of its normal value. When the test is used to evaluate the level of anticoagulation with coumarin-like drugs the INR format is recommended. INR, a method that standardizes PT assays, is defined later in this chapter.[1,13,22,23] In this book the term INR will be used only for PT tests from patients on coumarin-like drugs.[24]

Platelet Count. Platelet count is used to screen for possible bleeding problems due to thrombocytopenia. Normal platelet count is 140,000 to 400,000/μL of blood. Patients with a platelet count of between 50,000 and 100,000/μL manifest excessive bleeding only with severe trauma. Patients with counts below 50,000/μL demonstrate skin and mucosal purpura and bleed excessively with minor trauma. Patients with platelet counts below 20,000/μL may experience spontaneous bleeding.[1,13,22,24]

Thrombin Time. In this test, thrombin is added to the patient's blood sample as the activating agent. It converts fibrinogen in the blood to insoluble fibrin,

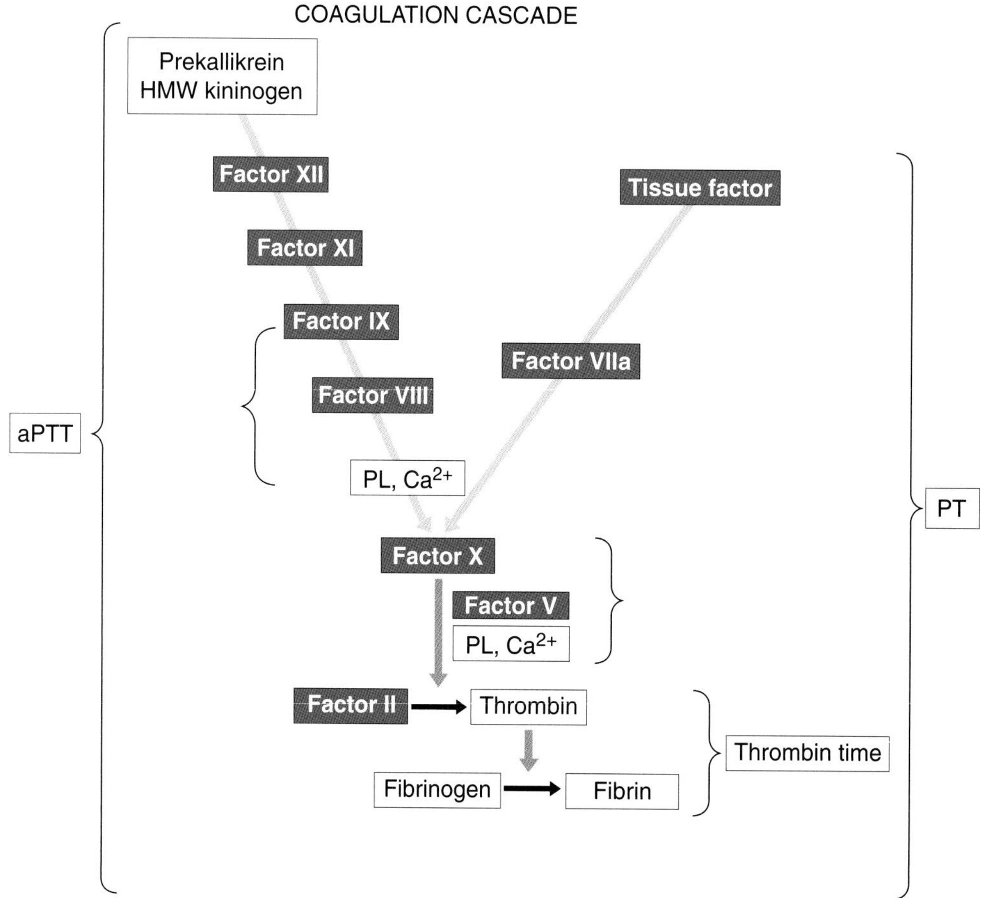

FIGURE 24-11 Coagulation cascade indicating the intrinsic pathway measured by activated partial thromboplastin time (aPTT), the extrinsic pathway measured by prothrombin time (PT), and the conversion of fibrinogen to fibrin, which is measured by thrombin time (TT). Other proteins—prekallikrein and high-molecular-weight (HMW) kininogen—participate in the contact activation phase but are not considered coagulation factors. *Ca^{2+}*, Calcium; *PL*, Phospholipid. *(From Rick ME: Coagulation testing. In Young NS, Gerson SL, High KA, editors:* Clinical hematology, *St. Louis, 2006, Mosby.)*

which makes up the essential portion of a blood clot. Again, a control must be run, and results vary from laboratory to laboratory. This test bypasses the intrinsic, extrinsic, and most of the common pathway. For example, patients with hemophilia A or factor V deficiency have a normal TT. Generally, the normal range for the TT test is 9 to 13 seconds, and results in excess of 16 to 18 seconds are considered abnormal or prolonged.[22,23] Abnormal test results usually are caused by excessive plasmin or fibrin split products.

Diagnostic Tests Performed by the Hematologist. When one or more of the screening tests yield an abnormal result, the hematologist runs additional tests to pinpoint the specific defect of the bleeding disorder.

Platelet Disorders. Platelet count is very effective for identifying patients with thrombocytopenia. It is not effective for identifying patients with disorders of platelet function such as von Willebrand disease, Bernard-Soulier disease, Glanzmann's disease, uremia, and drug-induced platelet release defects. BT may be prolonged in these patients, but test results are inconsistent. Platelet aggregation tests, ristocetin-induced agglutination, platelet release reaction, and other tests may have to be performed for the nature of the clinical bleeding problem to become apparent.[1,13,22,24]

Additional laboratory tests are needed to establish the diagnosis and to identify the type of von Willebrand disease. These consist of ristocetin cofactor activity, ristocetin-induced platelet aggregation, immunoassay of vWF, multimeric analysis of vWF, and specific assays for factor VIII.[1,13,22,24]

Disorders of the Intrinsic Pathway. Screening tests show prolonged aPTT, normal PT, and normal platelet count (except in some cases of von Willebrand disease). The next step is to mix (mixing tests) the patient's blood with a sample of pooled plasma and repeat the aPTT. If this test is normal, then the specific missing factor is identified by specific assays. If the mixing test is abnormal, tests for inhibitor activity (antibodies to the factor) are performed. Some acquired coagulation disorders can produce prolonged aPTT along with normal PT. These include the lupus inhibitor, antibodies to factor VIII, and heparin therapy.[1,13,22,24]

Disorders of the Extrinsic Pathway. A normal aPTT and a prolonged PT suggest a factor VII deficiency, which is very rare, or inhibitors to factor VII. Factor VII deficiency is confirmed by specific assay. Mixing studies are used to rule out factor VII inhibitors.[1,13,22,24]

Disorders of the Common Pathway. A prolonged aPTT and a prolonged PT in a patient with a history of a congenital bleeding disorder indicate a common pathway factor deficiency. Congenital deficiency of factors V and X, prothrombin, or fibrinogen is rare. When both of these tests are prolonged, an acquired common pathway factor deficiency is usually indicated. Often, multiple factors are found to be deficient. Conditions that can cause both tests to be abnormal are vitamin K deficiency, liver disease, and DIC. When both tests are prolonged in a patient with a history suggestive of a congenital bleeding problem, the next step is to exclude or identify an abnormality of fibrinogen in the laboratory. This involves measuring the plasma fibrinogen level and performing tests for D-dimer of FDPs. Once a problem involving fibrinogen has been ruled out, the next step is to perform mixing studies to rule out inhibitor activity. If these studies are negative, then specific assays for deficiency of factor V or X or prothrombin are performed.[1,13,22,23]

Degradation Products of Fibrin or Fibrinogen. In patients with prolonged aPTT, PT, and TT, the defect involves the last stage of the common pathway, which is the activation of fibrinogen to form fibrin to stabilize the clot. The plasma level of fibrinogen is determined, and if it is within normal limits, then tests for fibrinolysis are performed. These tests, which detect the presence of fibrinogen and/or FDPs, consist of staphylococcal clumping assay, agglutination of latex particles coated with antifibrinogen antibody, and euglobulin clot lysis time.[1,13,22,23]

Disorders with Normal Primary Screening Results. Patients with vascular abnormalities that can cause clinical bleeding may not be identified through the use of recommended screening tests. BT is the only finding that might be abnormal in these patients. However, it has clearly been shown that BT is inconsistent in these patients. Thus, this test is not reliable for identifying these patients. In most cases, the diagnosis must be based on history and clinical findings.[1,13,22,23]

Three known defects in the coagulation system do not affect PT, aPTT, or TT. These are rare and include factor XIII deficiency, alpha$_2$ plasmin inhibitor deficiency, and PAI-1 deficiency (major inhibitor of plasminogen activators). Patients with a strong clinical history of bleeding and normal coagulation test results (PT, aPTT, and TT) require additional testing, such as the use of 5M urea.[13,24]

Another small group of patients with a history of significant bleeding problems will have negative test results when screened by means of currently recommended methods. It appears that current methods are unable to reveal whatever disorder these patients may have. A clear-cut history of prolonged bleeding after trauma or surgical procedures is always more significant than negative laboratory data.[13,24]

MEDICAL MANAGEMENT

In this section, conditions that may cause clinical bleeding are considered. The emphasis is on detection of patients with a potential bleeding problem and management of such patients if surgical procedures are needed. Disorders affecting the vascular, platelet, coagulation, and fibrinolytic phases are discussed. DIC, disorders of platelet release, and primary fibrinogenolysis are described to show the nature of acquired bleeding disorders. These diseases reflect the roles of various factors involved in the control of excessive bleeding after injury, and they reveal what happens when these factors are defective. Table 24-2 summarizes the nature of the

TABLE 24-2 Medical Treatment of Acquired Bleeding Disorders

Condition	Defect	Medical Treatment
Primary thrombocytopenia (idiopathic thrombocytopenia)	Platelets destroyed by autoimmune processes	Prednisone Intravenous gamma globulin Platelet transfusion
Secondary thrombocytopenia	Deficiency of platelets due to accelerated destruction or consumption, deficient production, or abnormal pooling	Platelet transfusion
Liver disease	Multiple coagulation factor defects Patients with portal hypertension may be thrombocytopenic.	Vitamin K Replacement therapy only for serious bleeding or before surgical procedures Desmopressin provides some benefit.
Disseminated intravascular coagulation	Multiple coagulation factor defects due to triggered consumption Formation of fibrin and fibrinogen degradation products due to fibrinolysis Thrombocytopenia	Treatment of primary disorder Heparin Cryoprecipitate or fresh frozen plasma for replacement of fibrinogen Platelet transfusion Other blood product replacements lead to mixed results.

defects and the medical treatment available for excessive bleeding in patients with several of the more common acquired disorders covered in this section.

Vascular Defects

Bleeding disorders caused by vascular abnormalities may be caused by structural malformation of vessels, hereditary disorders of connective tissue, and acquired connective tissue disorders.

Acquired connective tissue disorders that may be complicated by bleeding include scurvy, small vessel vasculitis, and skin disorders. In scurvy, deficiency of vitamin C leads to lack of peptidyl hydroxylation of procollagen, resulting in weakened collagen fibers. The abnormal collagen results in defective perivascular supportive tissues, which can lead to capillary fragility and delayed wound healing. In patients on long-term use of steroids, thinning of connective tissues may result in bleeding after minor trauma.[8,25-27]

Small vessel vasculitis may be caused by a variety of conditions that produce inflammation of small vessels, including arterioles, venules, and capillaries. Serum sickness can lead to purpura through immune complex deposits into vessel walls. Drugs such as penicillin, hydralazine, sulfonamides, and thiazide diuretics and hepatitis have been associated with serum sickness–like reactions.[8,26-28]

Platelet Disorders

Disorders of Platelet Function. Platelets participate directly in the clotting cascade by serving as constituents of factor X and prothrombin-converting complexes through the release of platelet factor 3 (PF3). The potency of this release effect is increased by increased participation of platelets in the clotting process. In some cases, platelets may fail to complete the release reaction of PF3. Sometimes, this is caused by defective production of thromboxane, other times by a deficiency in the production of dense-granule ADP.

Defective thromboxane production almost always results from the administration of antiinflammatory drugs. The best-known example is aspirin, which inactivates cyclooxygenase, the first enzyme of the prostaglandin-thromboxane synthetic pathway. Other drugs that interfere with thromboxane formation include NSAIDs (indomethacin, phenylbutazone, ibuprofen, sulfinpyrazone), beta-lactam antibiotics; calcium channel–blocking drugs (verapamil, diltiazem, and nifedipine), phenytoin, nitrates, phenothiazines, and tricyclic antidepressants. All platelet release defects produce about the same clinical picture.[6,16,26]

In otherwise healthy people, the impairment of platelet function that is produced by drugs usually is of no clinical significance. However, in patients with coagulation disorders, uremic or thrombocytopenic patients, and those receiving heparin or coumarin anticoagulants, drug-induced platelet dysfunction can result in serious bleeding. Platelet function studies often show an absence of secondary wave aggregation. Patients can be screened with standard screening tests; if these results are normal, surgical procedures can be performed.[6,25,28]

Uremia may interfere with platelet function. This effect can be severe in patients with grossly abnormal platelet function. Such patients are in danger of bleeding to death if injury occurs or surgery is performed. They respond to dialysis, cryoprecipitate, or kidney transplantation but not to platelet replacement. Although beta-lactam antibiotics (penicillin and cephalothins) may cause platelet dysfunction, usually no treatment is required. In some undetermined way, alcohol may impair platelet function; this effect may be severe enough to contraindicate surgery unless corrective measures are taken.[6,16,26,29]

Coagulation Disorders

Disseminated Intravascular Coagulation. DIC has been reported to occur in about 1 in 1000 hospital admissions. The syndrome is associated with a number of disorders such as infection, obstetric complications, cancer, and snakebites. In fact, worldwide, the most common cause of DIC is snakebite. DIC is a condition that results when the clotting system is activated in all or a major part of the vascular system. Despite widespread fibrin production, the major clinical problem is bleeding, not thrombosis. DIC is caused when large quantities of thromboplastic substances are introduced into the vascular system and "trip" the clotting cascade. Acute DIC may be caused by obstetric complications (abruptio placentae, missed abortion, amniotic fluid embolism), infection, injuries and burns, antigen-antibody complexes, shock, and acidosis.[29-31]

Clinical Findings. Clinical manifestations of acute DIC include severe bleeding from small wounds, purpura, and spontaneous bleeding from the nose, gums, gastrointestinal tract, or urinary tract (Figure 24-12). Traumatic hemolytic anemia may occur when red blood cells are "sliced" by fibrin strands. On rare occasions, bilateral necrosis of the renal cortex has developed. Chronic DIC may occur in association with certain types of cancer. Malignant cells can release thromboplastic material as they die within the tumor mass. Antigen-antibody complexes associated with systemic lupus erythematosus may cause chronic DIC. In the chronic form of the disease, thrombosis is more common than bleeding.[30-32]

Laboratory Diagnosis. The laboratory diagnosis of severe, acute DIC is not usually difficult. Consumption and inhibition of the function of clotting factors cause prolongation of the PT, aPTT, and thrombin time. Consumption of platelets causes thrombocytopenia. Secondary fibrinolysis generates increased titers of FDPs, which can be measured by latex agglutination or D-dimer assays. Chronic or compensated forms of DIC are more

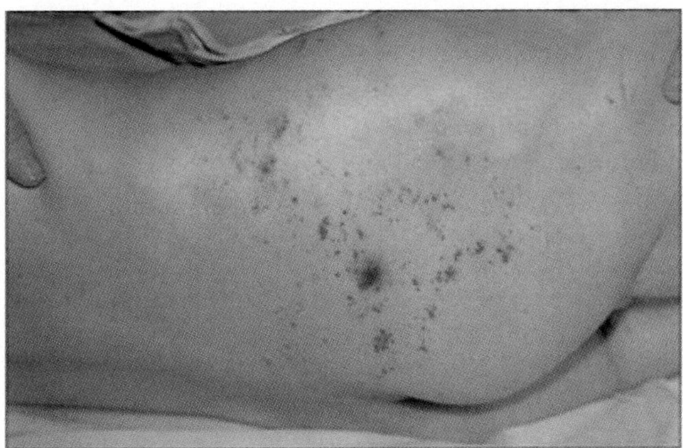

FIGURE 24-12 Disseminated intravascular coagulation resulting from staphylococcal septicemia in a 56-year-old man. Note the characteristic skin hemorrhage, ranging in extent from small purpuric lesions to larger ecchymoses. The patient had non–insulin-dependent (type 2) diabetes, and the septicemia originated with an untreated large boil on his thigh. *(From Forbes CD, Jackson WF:* Color atlas and text of clinical medicine, *ed 3, Edinburgh, 2003, Mosby.)*

difficult to diagnose, with highly variable patterns of abnormalities in "DIC screen" coagulation tests. Increased FDPs and a prolonged PT are generally more sensitive measures than abnormalities of the aPTT and platelet count are. Overcompensated synthesis of consumed clotting factors and platelets in some chronic forms of DIC may actually cause shortening of the PT and aPTT or thrombocytosis (or both), even though elevated levels of FDPs indicate secondary fibrinolysis in such cases. The most difficult differential diagnosis of DIC occurs in patients who have coexisting liver disease.[30] The coagulopathy of liver failure is often indistinguishable from that of DIC, partly because advanced hepatic dysfunction is accompanied by a state of DIC. In liver failure, the combination of decreased synthesis of clotting factors, impaired clearance of activated clotting factors, secondary fibrinolysis, and thrombocytopenia from portal hypertension and hypersplenism may make the coagulopathy practically impossible to differentiate from DIC.[30]

Treatment. Treatment of patients with DIC consists of an attempt to reverse the cause, control of the major symptom (bleeding or thrombosis), and a prophylactic regimen to prevent recurrence in cases of chronic DIC. Consumed coagulation factors need to be replaced, along with missing platelets. Fibrinogen levels must be restored. Cryoprecipitate is used if bleeding is the major problem. Fresh frozen plasma also may be used. If thrombosis is the major problem (early in the process), intravenous heparin is used. Long-term heparin infusion is used for prophylaxis in cases of chronic DIC.[29-31] The use of aminocaproic acid (Amicar), desmopression, and tranexamic acid preparations is not recommended, because increased bleeding may occur.[30]

Fibrinolytic Disorders

Fibrinolysis and Fibrinogenolysis. Primary fibrinogenolysis may develop if active plasmin is generated in the circulation at a time when the clotting cascade is not in operation. It can occur in patients with liver disease, cancer of the lung, cancer of the prostate, or heatstroke. Severe bleeding results from the depletion of fibrinogen (split by plasmin) and the formation of fibrin split products (with their anticoagulant properties) from fibrinogen.[8,19,32,33]

Fibrinogenolysis can be treated with ε-aminocaproic acid or tranexamic acid, which inhibits both plasmin and plasmin activators; however, these drugs may be dangerous if used in DIC, because diffuse thromboses may result. Thus, exclusion of the diagnosis of DIC before antifibrinolytic agents are begun is very important. A specific test such as D-dimer measurement can be used for this purpose.[8,18,33,34]

Thrombosis and Antithrombotic Therapy

Thrombosis is the formation, from components of blood, of an abnormal mass within the vascular system. It involves the interaction of vascular, cellular, and humoral factors within a flowing stream of blood. Thrombosis and the complicating emboli that may result are one of the most important causes of sickness and death in developed countries. Thrombosis is of greater overall clinical importance in terms of morbidity and mortality than are all of the hemorrhagic disorders combined. Excessive activation of coagulation or inhibition of anticoagulant mechanisms may result in hypercoagulability and thrombosis. Injury to the vessel wall, alterations in blood flow, and changes in the composition of blood are major factors leading to thrombosis.[2,4,34,35]

The common causes of acquired venous thrombosis are age, history of thrombosis, immobilization, obesity, infection, hospitalization, major surgery, and pregnancy. Common causes of both venous and arterial thrombosis are malignancy, hormonal therapy, and DIC. The most common cause of arterial thrombosis is atherosclerosis.[1,34]

Patients should be considered for laboratory evaluation for inherited thrombotic disorders if they are younger than 45 years of age and have recurrent thrombosis. In addition, patients who have experienced a single thrombotic event and have a family history of thrombosis should be tested.[2,4,35,36] The inherited thrombotic disorders are covered in Chapter 25.

The pathologic basis for arterial thrombosis involves atherosclerotic vascular disease associated with platelet thrombi. Thrombin is a major mediator in this type of thrombosis. Drug therapy for arterial thrombi involves agents with antithrombin and antiplatelet activity. Venous thrombi usually occur in otherwise normal vessel walls; stasis and hypercoagulability are major predisposing

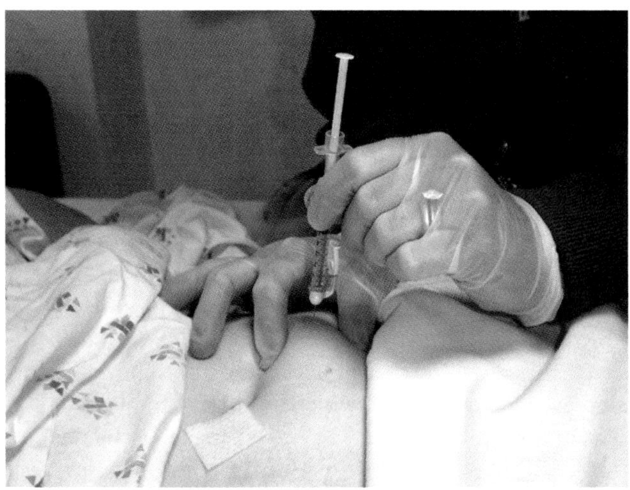

FIGURE 24-13 Subcutaneous heparin is used to reduce the risk of deep vein thrombosis in medical and surgical procedures. *(From Potter PA, Perry AG, Stockert P:* Basci nursing, *ed 7, St. Louis, 2011, Mosby.)*

factors. Drugs that prevent thrombin formation or lyse fibrin clots are the main agents used to treat venous thrombi.[34,37,38] Antidotes are available for overdosing of heparin (protamine) and warfarin (vitamin K); however, none is available for overdosing of the newer anticoagulant drugs.[36,37]

Anticoagulant Drugs

Heparin. Heparin is used in high doses to treat thromboembolism (intravenous bolus of 5000 U followed by infusion over a 5- to 10-day period) and in low-dose form for prophylaxis of thromboembolism. Heparin itself is not an anticoagulant. Plasma antithrombin III (ATIII) is the actual anticoagulant, and heparin serves as a catalyst. Patients older than 40 years of age who are about to undergo major surgery should receive prophylaxis with graded compression elastic stockings, low-dose heparin therapy, or intermittent pneumatic compression. If heparin prophylaxis is used, 5000 U is given subcutaneously 2 hours before surgery and every 8 to 12 hours thereafter until the patient is ambulatory (Figure 24-13). Low-molecular-weight heparin (LMWH) can be used instead of regular heparin and is rapidly becoming the treatment of choice. Patients who are about to undergo total hip or knee replacement should receive postoperative LMWH.[33,36,37]

Standard heparin consists of an unfractionated heterogeneous mixture of polysaccharide chains with a mean molecular weight of 12,000 to 16,000. It inhibits factor Xa and thrombin equally. Treatment with standard heparin usually consists of intravenous infusion in a hospital setting and requires monitoring with aPTT. Standard heparin has a half-life of 1 to 2 hours. LMWH is prepared by depolymerization of unfractionated heparin chains, yielding heparin fragments with a mean molecular weight of 4000 to 6000. LMWH preparations have greater activity against factor Xa than thrombin. LMWHs exhibit less binding to plasma proteins, endothelial cells, and macrophages than is seen with standard heparin. Thus, they have better bioavailability when administered subcutaneously, longer half-lives, and more predictable anticoagulant effects. LMWHs are administered subcutaneously in the abdomen. The dosage is based on body weight, and no laboratory monitoring is needed. The half-life of these preparations is about 2 to 4 hours. Treatment with LMWHs may be provided on an outpatient basis.[33,36,37]

LMWH preparations that are used commonly in North America for the treatment of deep vein thrombi and asymptomatic pulmonary embolism include dalteparin (Fragmin), enoxaparin (Lovenox), and tinzaparin (Innohep). Their mean molecular weight ranges from 4200 for enoxaparin to 6000 for dalteparin. Their anti-Xa–to–thrombin ratio ranges from 1.9 for tinzaparin to 3.8 for enoxaparin.[38,39]

Patients with deep vein thrombosis or pulmonary embolism usually are treated with intravenous heparin in dosages sufficient to prolong the aPTT to a range corresponding to a heparin level of 0.2 to 0.4 u/mL (1.5 to 2.5 times control value). Heparin therapy is continued for 5 days or longer. Oral anticoagulation with warfarin is started early and should overlap heparin treatment for 4 to 5 days. Heparin treatment is stopped after 5 to 10 days, and warfarin treatment is continued for at least 3 months. Complications with heparin treatment include thrombocytopenia and thrombosis. Starting warfarin therapy early after heparin is first started minimizes these complications. Overdosing of heparin can cause significant clinical bleeding.[34,37,38]

Synthetic Heparins. Two synthetic heparin analogues are now available for anticoagulant use. Fondaparinux has been approved for thrombophylaxis in high-risk orthopedic patients; it also appears to provide a useful alternative to heparin or LMWH for the treatment of patients with established venous thromboembolism or pulmonary embolism (5 to 10 mg given once per day with warfarin). It is also given for prophylaxis for major orthopedic surgery at 2.5 mg once per day, starting 6 hours after surgery. The second agent, idraparinux, has a very long half-life (80 hours) and is administered by the subcutaneous route once per week; its efficacy and safety have not been established. Phase III clinical trials of idraparinux have been completed.[33,36,37]

Direct Thrombin Inhibitors. Heparin and LMWH are indirect inhibitors of thrombin because their activity is mediated by antithrombin. Direct thrombin inhibitors that do not require a plasma cofactor are now available for clinical use. Parenteral direct thrombin inhibitors now available include lepirudin, desirudin, argatroban, and bivalirudin. Lepirudin, desirudin, and bivalirudin are hirudins produced by recombinant DNA technology. Desirudin is given subcutaneously to patients who are about to undergo hip replacement. Lepirudin is given intravenously to patients with history of heparin-induced thrombocytopenia (HIT) for treatment of deep venous thrombosis or for hip replacement. Bivalirudin is administered to patients about to undergo percutaneous coronary intervention. Argatroban may also be used in patients with a history of HIT. It is given by continuous infusion.[34,37,38] In 2008, the first orally administered direct thrombin inhibitor, dabigatran (Pradaxa), became available for clinical use in Canada and gained FDA approval in 2010 for use to prevent stroke in patients with atrial fibrillation in the United States.[40,41] Dabigatran has the potential to replace warfarin as the standard anticoagulant with the main advantage that INR monitoring is not needed.

Direct Factor Xa Inhibitors. Several new anticoagulants that act as direct factor Xa inhibitors are under development. One is rivaroxaban (Xaretto), an orally administered anticoagulant that has been approved for use in Europe and was approved in 2011 for use in the United States. Apixaban and betrixaban are in phase III trials.[42-46]

Coumarin. Warfarin (Coumadin), the most widely used coumarin in the United States, is an oral anticoagulant that inhibits the biosynthesis of vitamin K–dependent coagulation proteins (factors VII, IX, and X and prothrombin). Warfarin is named after the patent holder, Wisconsin Alumni Research Foundation. Warfarin is bound to albumin, metabolized through hydroxylation by the liver, and excreted in the urine. PT is used to monitor warfarin therapy because it measures three of the vitamin K–dependent coagulation proteins: factors VII and X and prothrombin. PT is particularly sensitive to factor VII deficiency. Therapeutic anticoagulation with warfarin takes 4 to 5 days.[34,37,38]

PT has been shown to be imprecise and variable. Little comparability has been seen of PT values obtained from different laboratories. These differences are caused by the source of thromboplastin (human brain, rabbit brain), the brand of thromboplastin, and the type of instrumentation used. This has caused problems with bleeding that results from a high degree of anticoagulation based on an artificially low PTT. INR is now used to monitor patients on warfarin therapy. Reliance on the INR (INR = $[PTR]^{ISI}$; PTR = prothrombin time ratio; ISI = international sensitivity index for the thromboplastin used) allows better comparison of PT values among different laboratories and minimizes the risk of bleeding due to artificially low PT values.[33,36,37] The recommended INR goal for a patient on low-intensity warfarin therapy is 2.5, with a range of 2.0 to 3.0. With a patient on high-intensity anticoagulation therapy, the INR goal is 3.0, with a range of 2.5 to 3.5. Table 24-3 shows the conditions for which warfarin therapy is recommended and the recommended INR.[33,36,37] Figure 24-14 shows a patient with deep venous thrombosis, which is one of the conditions for which warfarin treatment is required. Table 24-4 summarizes the anticoagulants now in use and in later stages of clinical trials.

TABLE 24-3 Recommended Therapeutic Range for Warfarin Therapy

INR 2.0 to 3.0 With Target of 2.5
Prophylaxis of venous thrombosis (high-risk surgery)
Treatment of venous thrombosis
Treatment of pulmonary embolism
Prevention of systemic embolism
Tissue heart valves in aortic or mitral position for first 3 months
Tissue heart valves with history of pulmonary embolism
Tissue heart valves with atrial fibrillation
Acute myocardial infarction
Atrial fibrillation
Valvular heart disease
Mitral valve prolapse with history of atrial fibrillation or embolism
INR 2.5 to 3.5 With Target of 3.0
Mechanical prosthetic heart valves
Prevention of recurrent myocardial infarction
Treatment of thrombosis associated with antiphospholipid antibodies

INR, International normalized ratio.

Data from Hirsh J, Schulman S: Antithrombotic therapy. In Goldman L, Ausiello D, editors: Cecil textbook of medicine, *ed 23, Philadelphia, 2008, Saunders; Begelman SM: Venous thromboembolism. In Carey WD, et al, editors:* Current clinical medicine 2009—Cleveland Clinic, *Philadelphia, 2009, Saunders, pp 205-211; and Lim W, et al: Venous thromboembolism. In Hoffman R, et al, editors:* Hematology: basic principles and practice, *ed 5, Philadelphia, 2009, Churchill Livingstone.*

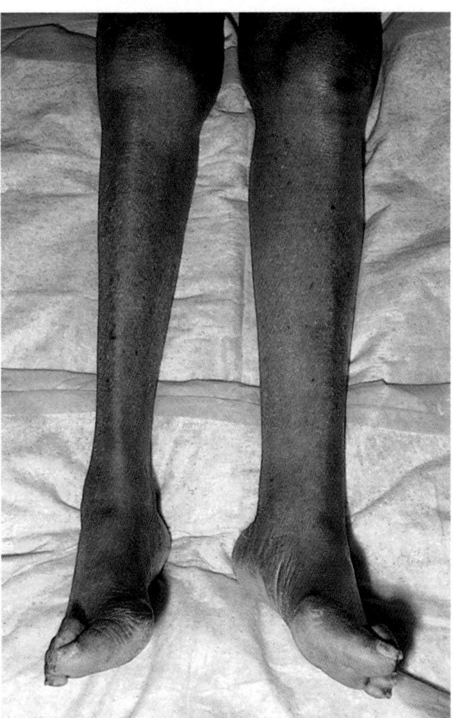

FIGURE 24-14 Deep vein thrombosis manifesting as an acutely swollen left leg. *(From Swartz MH:* Textbook of physical diagnosis: history and examination, *ed 6, Philadelphia, 2010, Saunders.)*

TABLE 24-4 Current Antithrombotic Agents: Anticoagulants

Agent	Indications	Dosage	Monitoring	Complications
Standard heparin, high-dose	Treatment of DVT Treatment of PE Prevention of DVT	IV bolus 5000-10,000 units, IV infusion at rate of 1300 U/hr over 5-10 days	aPTT 1.5-2.5 times the mean laboratory control value	Bleeding Thrombocytopenia
Standard heparin, low-dose	Prevention of DVT	SC; 5000 units 2 hr before surgery and q8-12h until ambulatory	None	Bleeding Thrombocytopenia
Warfarin (Coumadin)	Treatment of DVT, PE Prevention of DVT, or thrombosis in AF:	Oral, 5-7 mg/day for 3 to 6 months	INR: 2.0 to 3.0	Bleeding intolerance Alopecia GI discomfort
	MPHV Prevention of recurrent MI	Oral, 7-10 mg/day, long term	INR: 2.5 to 3.5	Rash, skin necrosis
LMWHs				
Enoxaparin (Lovenox)	Prevention of DVT Prevention of PE Treatment of DVT	*Enoxaparin*: 30 mg SC every 12 hours for up to 14 days (knee or hip) 40 mg SC once daily, with first dose 2 hours before abdominal surgery 1 mg/kg SC q12h up to 5 days	None Oral warfarin started within 72 hr	Bleeding Thrombocytopenia Anemia Fever Peripheral edema
Ardeparin (Normiflo) Dalteparin (Fragmin) Nadroparin (Fraxiparine) Reviparin (Clivarin) Tinzaparin (Innohep)				
Synthetic heparins				
Fondaparinux (Atrixtra)	Prevention and treatment of DVT, PE	Given SC, 2.5 mg to 10 mg per day	None	Bleeding
Idraparinux	Idraparinux in phase III trials			
Direct thrombin inhibitors Lepirudin (Refludan) Desirudin (Revasc) Argatroban (Acova) Bivalirudin (Angiox)	Used in patients with history of HIT; prevention or treatment of DVT	*Lepirudin*: IV 0.4 mg/kg bolus, with IV infusion 0.15 mg/kg	aPTT: 1.5-2.5 times laboratory normal test time	Bleeding Allergy Anaphylaxis
Dabigatran (Pradaxa)	FDA approval for preventing stroke in patients with atrial fibrillation	Given orally, 110 mg or 150 mg twice per day	None	Bleeding Dyspepsia Hypersensitivity Gastritis-like symptoms
Direct factor Xa inhibitors				
Rivaroxaban (Xarelto)	Rivaroxaban gained FDA approval in July of 2011 for prevention of DVT in orthopedic patients, and approval for Apixaban is expected by the end of 2011	Rivaroxaban given orally, 10 mg/day for 13 days for knee replacement surgery and for 35 days for hip replacements	None	Bleeding Nausea, vomiting Anemia Xerostomia Increase in liver transaminases
Apixaban (Eliquis)				

AF, Atrial fibrillation; *DVT*, Deep venous thrombosis; *HIT*, Heparin-induced thrombocytopenia; *IV*, Intravenously; *MI*, Myocardial infarction; *MPHV*, Mechanical prosthetic heart valve; *PE*, Pulmonary embolus; *SC*, Subcutaneously; *TIA*, Transient ischemic attack; *FDA*, Federal Drug Administration.

Antiplatelet Drugs

Platelets are an important contributor to arterial thrombi. Antiplatelet treatment has been reported to reduce overall mortality rate from vascular disease by 15% and to reduce nonfatal vascular complications by 30%. Aspirin, the prototypical antiplatelet drug, exerts its antithrombotic action by irreversibly inhibiting platelet cyclooxygenase, preventing synthesis of thromboxane A_2, and impairing platelet secretion and aggregation. Aspirin is the least expensive, most widely used, and most widely studied antiplatelet drug. NSAIDs such as ibuprofen and indobufen act as reversible inhibitors of cyclooxygenase and are used clinically to some extent. Dipyridamole, which increases cyclic adenosine monophosphate; ticlopidine and clopidogrel, which inhibit

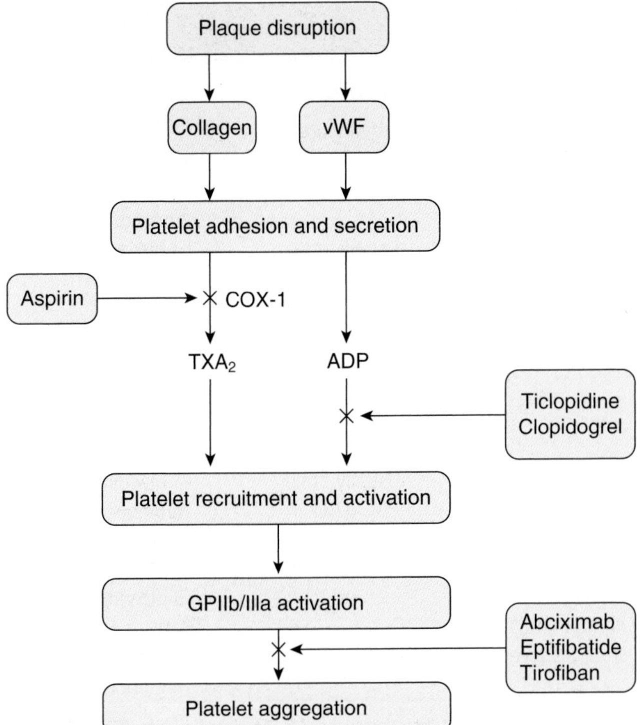

FIGURE 24-15 Site of action of antiplatelet drugs. Aspirin inhibits thromboxane A_2 (TXA_2) synthesis by irreversibly acetylating cyclooxygenase-1 (COX-1). Reduced TXA_2 release attenuates platelet activation and recruitment to the site of vascular injury. Ticlopidine and clopidogrel irreversibly block $P2Y_{12}$, a key adenosine diphosphate (ADP) receptor on the platelet surface. Therefore, these agents also attenuate platelet recruitment. Abciximab, eptifibatide, and tirofiban inhibit the final common pathway of platelet aggregation by blocking fibrinogen binding to activated glycoprotein (GP) IIb/IIIa. *(From Weitz IC: Antithrombotic drugs. In Hoffman R, et al, editors:* Hematology: basic principles and practice, *ed 5, Philadelphia, 2009, Churchill Livingstone.)*

adenosine diphosphate (ADP); and abciximab, a monoclonal antibody; and the small molecule inhibitors, eptifibatide and tirofiban, that block the fibrinogen receptor glycoprotein IIb/IIIa are all used as antiplatelet agents (Figure 24-15). However, dipyridamole alone has been reported to be ineffective and now, when used, is given with aspirin.[33,36,42] The antiplatelet drugs are summarized in Table 24-5.

Clopidogrel is metabolized by the liver resulting in active metabolites. Thus the inhibitory effect of this drug on platelet function is delayed following administration. Clopidogrel is associated with a low risk for development of neutropenia or thrombocytopenia.[35] Aspirin and clopidogrel are used in combination to maintain patency of arterial stents.[35] Abciximab produces an immediate and profound inhibition of platelet activity which lasts for 6 to 12 hours after the last dosage. Eptifibatide and tirofiban have shorter half-lives, and platelet function returns to normal within 4 to 8 hours after the last dosage. Drug-induced thrombocytopenia is more common with abciximab than with the eptifibatide and tirofiban.[35]

PREOPERATIVE EVALUATION OF HEMOSTASIS

Most experts do not recommend routine preoperative screening for potential bleeding disorders in patients with a negative history and clinical findings who are scheduled for minor surgery such as dental extractions and biopsy procedures. It is recommended that patients with a negative history for excessive bleeding who are scheduled for major surgery be screened with use of platelet count and aPTT. Patients with an equivocal bleeding history who are scheduled for major surgery involving hemostatic impairment (heart bypass machine) should be screened with use of PT, aPTT, platelet count, factor XIII assay, and euglobulin clot lysis time. All patients with a positive bleeding history who are scheduled for minor or major surgery should be screened with use of PT, aPTT, platelet count, factor XIII assay, and euglobulin clot lysis time.[8,24] The suggestions for dentistry are based on these recommendations. Patients with a significant history of a bleeding disorder should be referred to a hematologist for all screening and diagnostic testing. Patients with a history suggestive of a possible bleeding disorder may be screened by the dentist at a commercial laboratory or may be referred to a hematologist for screening. If the dentist orders screening tests, aPTT, PT, TT, and platelet count should be used.

DENTAL MANAGEMENT

Patient Identification

The four methods by which the dentist can identify the patient who may have a bleeding problem are listed here. Skills acquired through application of these methods determine how well dentists can protect certain patients from the dangers of excessive bleeding after dental surgical treatment. These four methods consist of the following:

- A thorough history
- Physical examination
- Screening clinical laboratory tests
- Observation of excessive bleeding after a surgical procedure (Box 24-6)

History and Symptoms

The history provides the basis for the search for a potential bleeder in dental practice. To maximize the value of the patient's history in identifying the patient who may be a bleeder, several points must be considered.[9] Some healthy persons have been shown to consider their bleeding and bruising excessive; 23% in one study reported a positive bleeding history.[9] Patients with severe coagulation disorders may have dramatic abnormal bleeding histories but often do not volunteer this information unless asked. Patients with mild to moderate bleeding abnormalities may not have experienced excessive

TABLE 24-5 Current Antithrombotic Agents: Antiplatelet Drugs

Agent	Indication(s)	Dosage	Monitoring	Complications
Aspirin	Prevention: recurrent MI, stroke, coronary thrombosis	Oral; 75-325 mg once daily	Usually none	GI bleeding Tinnitus Urticaria Bronchospasm
Aspirin plus dipyridamole (Aggrenox)	Stroke prevention (history of TIA)	Oral; a*spirin*: 50 mg bid; *dipyridamole*: 200 mg	Usually none	GI bleeding GI ulceration Urticaria Bronchospasm
NSAIDs Ibuprofen (Advil, Motrin)	Prevention: recurrent MI, stroke, coronary thrombosis.	Oral; 400 mg once daily	Usually none	GI bleeding GI ulceration Rash, urticaria Tinnitus
ADP inhibitors Clopidogrel (Plavix) Ticlopidine (Ticlid)	TIA, stroke, and MI prevention	Oral; *clopidogrel*: 75 mg once daily; *ticlopidine*: 250 mg bid	Usually none CBC q2wk	GI bleeding Thrombocytopenia Diarrhea
Fibrinogen receptor inhibitors (GP IIb/IIIa) Tirofiban (Aggrastat) Abciximab (ReoPro) Eptifibatide (Integrilin)	Prevention: recurrent MI, stroke, TIA	*Tirofiban*: IV 0.4 μg/kg/min for 30 minutes, then 0.1 μg/kg/min until steady state achieved	Usually none	GI bleeding GI ulceration Rash Neutropenia Thrombocytopenia

ADP, Adenosine diphosphate; *CBC,* Complete blood count; *GI,* Gastrointestinal; *GP,* Glycoprotein; *IV,* Intravenously; *MI,* Myocardial infarction; *NSAIDs,* Nonsteroidal antiinflammatory drugs; *Rx,* Prescription; *TIA,* Transient ischemic attack.

bleeding symptoms or may be unable to recognize subtle symptoms as abnormal.

In obtaining a good bleeding history, the dentist must go beyond a list of questions that the patient can respond to on a questionnaire. This involves an active process led by the dentist that starts with the patient's initial responses on the questionnaire and continues with expansion and clarification of this information.

The history should include questions on the following topics:

1. Presence of bleeding problems in relatives
2. Excessive bleeding after operations, surgical procedures, and tooth extractions
3. Excessive bleeding after trauma
4. Use of drugs for the prevention of coagulation or chronic pain
5. Past and present illness
6. Occurrence of spontaneous bleeding

Bleeding Problems in Relatives. Presence of bleeding problems in relatives is covered in Chapter 25 on congenital bleeding disorders.

Bleeding Problems After Operations and Tooth Extraction. Each new patient should be questioned about excessive bleeding after major or minor operations. The number of patients who have had an appendectomy, a tonsillectomy, periodontal procedures (surgery or root scaling), or tooth extraction is large. Usually, the extraction of molar teeth is more traumatic than the extraction of incisors. A patient who reports prolonged bleeding after tooth extraction or other dental procedures should be asked whether it was necessary to return to the dentist for packing, suturing, or referral for transfusion of blood products.

Persons who have undergone major operations without a bleeding problem do not have a significant inherited coagulation disorder. Nevertheless, absence of a significant acquired bleeding problem at the time of the operative procedure does not mean that the patient is free of such a problem that may have been acquired since the last surgery.

Establishing the length of prolonged bleeding and the amount of blood that was lost is important. For example, normally, a small amount of blood may ooze from an extraction site for several hours or so. Oozing of blood from an extraction site for several days is abnormal unless a local infection was present. Some blood may be found on a pillow on the day after an extraction, but a pillow soaked with blood would be abnormal. Another area to ask about is the need for blood replacement after surgery; this would be most important if it was required during the postoperative period. Another important question explores whether the patient required hospitalization for the bleeding problem.

The patient should be asked whether the excessive bleeding started soon after minor surgical procedures or whether it was delayed in its onset. When excessive bleeding has been reported after minor surgery, the patient should be asked whether he or she sought medical attention and treatment. If treatment was rendered, the dentist should attempt to establish what type of treatment was

BOX 24-6 Clinical Recognition of the Patient Who Is a "Bleeder"

1. History
   a. Bleeding problems in relatives
   b. Bleeding problems after operations and tooth extractions
   c. Bleeding problems after trauma (e.g., cuts, scrapes)
   d. Medications that may cause bleeding problems
      (1) Aspirin
      (2) Anticoagulants
      (3) Long-term antibiotic therapy
      (4) Certain herbal preparations
   e. Presence of illnesses that may be associated with bleeding problems
      (1) Leukemia
      (2) Liver disease
      (3) Hemophilia
      (4) Congenital heart disease
      (5) Renal disease—uremia
   f. Spontaneous bleeding from nose, mouth, ears
2. Examination findings
   a. Jaundice, pallor
   b. Spider angiomas
   c. Ecchymoses
   d. Petechiae
   e. Oral ulcers
   f. Hyperplastic gingival tissues
   g. Hemarthrosis
3. Screening laboratory tests
   a. PT
   b. aPTT
   c. TT
   d. Platelet count
4. Surgical procedure—excessive bleeding after surgery may be first clue to underlying bleeding problem

aPTT, Activated partial thromboplastin time; *PT,* Prothrombin time; *TT,* Thrombin time.

given. Recall patients should be asked about any surgical procedures that have been performed since the last dental visit, and whether excessive bleeding occurred.

The patient should be asked about visits to other doctors for bleeding problems and any laboratory data that may be available; a history of transfusion of whole blood, packed red blood cells, plasma, platelets, or coagulation factor concentrates; a history of hospitalization for a bleeding problem; and a documented history of anemia or physician-prescribed iron therapy.[9]

Bleeding Problems After Trauma. All new dental patients and recall patients should be asked whether they have experienced any recent trauma and, if so, whether excessive bleeding followed it. The more severe the trauma (knife wounds, automobile accidents), the more likely it is that the presence of an underlying bleeding disorder will be exposed. Small cuts in patients with coagulation disorders may not cause excessive bleeding initially because the vascular and platelet phases may be sufficient to control blood loss, even if a defect in coagulation is found. However, small cuts in patients with platelet or vascular deficiencies usually result in excessive bleeding, and in patients with severe coagulation disorders, this may lead to bleeding several hours after the injury.

The most meaningful data are reported as a recent negative or positive history of excessive bleeding after a major hemostatic challenge. With a negative history, the patient is not a bleeder. By contrast, the patient with a positive history is a bleeder. A negative history of bleeding after minor insults in a patient with a mild bleeding diathesis does not rule out a problem with more severe surgical or traumatic events. Thus, the more recent and severe the surgical or traumatic event, the more accurate it will be in revealing the presence of a bleeding disorder.

Medications That May Cause Bleeding. All new and recall dental patients should be asked whether they are taking an anticoagulant drug such as heparin (by the intravenous toute), LMWH (by the subcutaneous route), or a coumarin derivative. If the patient is receiving one of these drugs, the dentist should contact the patient's physician to find out what degree of anticoagulation is being maintained and the purpose for which the drug is being used. All patients should be asked whether they have been taking aspirin or drugs that contain aspirin or other antiplatelet medications. Patients also should be asked whether they have undergone recent treatment with a broad-spectrum antibiotic and about excessive use of alcohol. Some herbal preparations and vitamin supplements may cause excessive bleeding (see Appendix E), as may some over-the-counter medications. The dentist must inquire about the use of such medications, particularly in the patient with a bleeding history.

Presence of Illness Potentially Associated with Bleeding Problems. The past and current medical status of the patient must be reviewed. This assessment should identify a history of liver disease, biliary tract obstruction, malabsorption problems, infectious diseases, genetic coagulation disorders, chronic inflammatory diseases, chronic renal disease, or leukemia or other types of cancer, and whether they have received radiation therapy or have been exposed to large amounts of radiation. It also must be determined whether patients with cancer are being treated with chemotherapy, because such treatment can cause significant suppression of platelet production.

Spontaneous Bleeding. Each patient should be asked about a history of spontaneous bleeding, including gingival, nasal, urinary, rectal, gastrointestinal, oral, pulmonary, and, in women, vaginal sources of bleeding. If spontaneous bleeding has occurred, the frequency, amount of blood lost, appearance of the blood, and steps that were necessary to stop it should be determined. A history of gingival bleeding is given by as many as 5% of healthy men and 50% of healthy women.[9] This bleeding may be related to periodontal disease or to the use of stiff-bristled toothbrushes. It is important to establish the

BOX 24-7 Screening Laboratory Tests for Detection of a Potential "Bleeder"

1. PT—activated by tissue thromboplastin
   a. Tests extrinsic and common pathways.
   b. Control should be run.
   c. Normal PT is 11 to 15 seconds, depending on laboratory.
   c. Control must be in normal range.
2. aPTT—initiated by phospholipid platelet substitute and activated by addition of contact activator (kaolin)
   a. Tests intrinsic and common pathways.
   b. Control should be run.
   c. Normal aPTT is 25 to 35 seconds, depending on laboratory.
   d. Control must be in normal range
3. TT—activated by thrombin
   a. Tests ability to form initial clot from fibrinogen.
   b. Controls should be run.
   c. Normal TT is 9 to 13 seconds.
4. Platelet count
   a. Tests platelet phase for adequate number of platelets.
   b. Normal count is 140,000 to 400,000/µL.
   c. Clinical bleeding problem can occur if count is less than 50,000//µL.

aPTT, Activated partial thromboplastin time; *PT,* Prothrombin time; *TT,* Thrombin time.

frequency of gingival bleeding and to determine whether the bleeding occurs spontaneously. Excessive gingival bleeding, when it occurs, usually is related to thrombocytopenia, platelet disorders, or von Willebrand disease.

Physical Examination

The dentist should inspect the exposed skin and mucosa of the oral cavity and pharynx of the patient for signs that might indicate a possible bleeding disorder. These include petechiae, ecchymoses (bruises), spider angioma, telangiectasias, jaundice, pallor, and cyanosis. When any of these signs are found by the dentist and cannot be explained by the history or other clinical findings, the patient should be referred for medical evaluation.

Screening Laboratory Tests

The dentist can use four clinical laboratory tests to screen patients for bleeding disorders (Box 24-7): platelet count, aPTT, PT, and TT. The platelet count is ordered to screen for thrombocytopenia. The aPTT test is used to measure the status of the intrinsic and common pathways of coagulation. This test reflects the ability of blood remaining within vessels in the area of injury to coagulate. It will be prolonged in coagulation disorders affecting the intrinsic and common pathways (hemophilia, liver disease) and in cases of excessive fibrinolysis.

The PT test is used to measure the status of the extrinsic and common pathways of coagulation. This test reflects the ability of blood lost from vessels in the area of injury to coagulate. It will be prolonged in cases of factor VII deficiency (which is rare) and in disorders affecting the common pathway and fibrinolysis. This test usually is normal in patients with intrinsic pathway defects (hemophilia).

The TT test uses thrombin as the test-activating agent; hence, it measures only the ability of fibrinogen to form an initial clot. Because FDPs tend to prolong TT, this test becomes reasonably sensitive for fibrinolysis disorders. When performed along with PT and aPTT tests, it allows for the identification of coagulation disorders involving the last "stage" of the sequence—for example, if PT, aPTT, and TT all were prolonged, the problem in the coagulation system would occur at the point of conversion of fibrinogen to the initial clot.

If positive, the results of these screening tests direct the hematologist to the possible source of a bleeding disorder and allow for the selection of more specific tests to identify the nature of the defect.

Surgical Procedures

Prolonged bleeding after a surgical procedure may be the first indication of a bleeding problem in a patient with a negative history and clinical findings. The dentist should use the appropriate local procedures (shown in Table 24-6) in an attempt to control the bleeding. If these measures should fail, consultation with the patient's physician or hematologist is indicated. Screening laboratory tests may be ordered to better identify the source of the problem before the consultation.

Medical Considerations

No surgical procedures should be performed on a patient who is suspected of having a bleeding problem on the basis of history and physical examination findings. Such a patient should be screened by the dentist through appropriate clinical laboratory tests or should be referred to a hematologist for screening. Patients screened by the dentist with abnormal test results should be referred to a hematologist for diagnosis, treatment, and management recommendations. Patients under medical care who may have a bleeding problem should not receive dental treatment until consultation with the patient's physician has taken place, and appropriate preparations have been made to avoid excessive bleeding after dental procedures.

Certain specific clinical situations often present the dentist with the question of whether a given patient has a bleeding problem. Each of these situations is discussed in Box 24-8.

Absence of Clinical or Historical Clues to Cause a Bleeding Problem. A person with a potential bleeding problem may have no subjective or objective findings that suggest the condition. The first indication may be prolonged bleeding after a dental surgical procedure. For

TABLE 24-6 Topical Hemostatic Agents Used to Control Bleeding

Product	Company/Dealer	Description	Indications and Features
Gauze		2×2 inch sterile gauze pads—placed over the wound, with pressure applied by patient (by closing jaws or with fingers)	Bleeding immediately after extractions or minor surgical procedures
Gelfoam	Pharmacia & Upjohn	Absorbable gelatin sponge made from purified gelatin solution—absorbs in 3-5 days	Useful for most patients taking an antithrombotic agent; helpful to place topical thrombin on Gelfoam; for extensive or invasive surgery, can be placed inside a splint
HemCon Dental Dressing	HemCon Medical Technologies	10×12 mm or 1×3 inch dressing—place on wound (best if some blood is present, helps stick dressing to the wound); made of chitosan from shellfish	Can be used on extraction sites, oral wounds; can be used in patients taking anticoagulants
Cellulose			
Surgicel	Johnson & Johnson	Oxidized regenerated cellulose—exerts physical effect rather than physiologic; swells on contact with blood with resulting pressure adding to hemostasis; thrombin ineffective with these agents due to inactivation as a result of pH factors	After 24-48 hours it becomes gelatinous; can be left in place or removed; useful to control bleeding when other agents ineffective
Oxycel	Becton Dickinson		
Collagen			
Instat	Johnson & Johnson	Absorbable collagen made from purified/lyophilized bovine dermal collagen—can be cut or shaped; adheres to bleeding surfaces when wet, but does not stick to instruments, gloves, or gauze sponges	Mild to moderate bleeding usually controlled in 2-5 minutes; more expensive than Gelfoam
Avitene	MedChem Products	Microfibrillar collagen hemostat—dry, sterile, fibrous, water insoluble, HCl acid salt–purified bovine corium collagen; MCH attracts platelets and triggers aggregation in fibrous mass	Thrombin ineffective with these agents due to inactivation as a result of pH factors; moderate to severe bleeding
Helistat	Marion Merrell Dow		
Colla-Cote, Tape, Plug	Zimmer Dental	Absorbable collagen dressings from bovine sources—can be sutured into place, used under stents, dentures, or alone; fully resorbed in 10-14 days	Shaped according to intended use: "cote" $\frac{3}{4} \times 1.5$ inch, tape 1×3 inch;, plug $\frac{3}{8} \times \frac{3}{4}$ inch; all are superior hemostats for moderate-severe bleeding
Thrombin			
Thrombostat	Parke-Davis	Topical thrombin—directly converts fibrinogen to fibrin; derived from bovine sources	One 5000-unit vial dissolved in 5 mL saline can clot equal amount of blood in <1 second; useful in severe bleeding.
Thrombinar	Jones Medical		
Thrombogen	Johnson & Johnson—Merck		
Tranexamic acid		Tranexamic acid—works as a competitive inhibitor of plasminogen activation; used as a mouth wash (5%), taken orally as a tablet or given IV	Useful in short term for preventing hemorrhage after dental extractions
Lysteda (Tablets)	Xanodyne		
Cyklokapron (IV)	Pfizer		
Aminocaproic acid	Wyeth-Ayerest	Aminocaproic acid—works as a competitive inhibitor of plasminogen activation; used as a rinse	Useful in short-term to prevent bleeding
Amicar			
Beriplast	Behringwerke	Fibrin/tissue glue	Not available in U.S. at this time

this, local measures should be taken to control the bleeding; if these fail, a hematologist may have to be consulted. Once the problem has been brought under control, the patient should be screened with the appropriate laboratory tests (PT, aPTT, platelet count, and TT) by the dentist through a commercial clinical laboratory, or by a hematologist.

History or Clinical Findings, or Both, Suggestive of Possible Bleeding Problem in the Absence of Clues to Its Cause. When no clues are evident regarding the cause of a potential bleeding problem in a patient, all four screening laboratory tests should be performed. The stronger the history of excessive bleeding, the more advantageous it is to refer the patient to a hematologist

BOX 24-8 Selection of Screening Laboratory Tests for Clinical Recognition of the Patient with a Potential Bleeding Problem Based on History and Examination Findings

1. No clinical or historical clues to cause of bleeding problem: excessive bleeding occurs after surgery
2. History or clinical findings or both suggest possible bleeding problem but no clues to the cause: PT, aPTT, TT, platelet count
3. Aspirin therapy: PFA-100 if available
4. Warfarin (Coumadin) therapy: INR; low-molecular-weight heparin: aPPT
5. Possible liver disease: platelet count, PT
6. Chronic leukemia: platelet count
7. Malabsorption syndrome or long-term antibiotic therapy: PT
8. Renal dialysis (heparin): aPTT
9. Vascular wall alteration: BT (results often inconsistent)
10. Primary fibrinogenolysis (active plasmin in circulation), cancers (lung, prostate): TT

aPTT, Activated partial thromboplastin time; *BT,* Bleeding time; *INR,* International normalized ratio; *PT,* Prothrombin time; *TT,* Thrombin time.

for screening and diagnosis. In other cases, the patient's physician can order these tests, or the dentist can order them through a clinical laboratory facility (see Box 24-7).

Antiplatelet Therapy. Patients who are receiving *aspirin* therapy may have a bleeding problem because of the drug's effect on platelets. Some of these patients may have been receiving high doses (20 g or more, or 4 or more tablets) of aspirin each day for a prolonged period (longer than a week). Others have been taking 1 tablet a day or 1 tablet every other day to prevent coronary thrombosis. Even this low dosage of aspirin is enough to inhibit platelet thromboxane production and platelet aggregation. Although these effects are nonreversible, they may or may not be clinically significant.[6,34] Although the PFA-100 is not recommended for general patient screening for possible bleeding problems, it can play a role in assessment of the patient on aspirin therapy: If the PFA-100 is moderately prolonged, the patient will not experience excessive bleeding with minor surgery unless some other bleeding disorder is present.

Although aspirin affects platelets and the coagulation process through its effects on platelet release, this effect does not usually lead to a significant bleeding problem and invasive dental procedures can be performed. If major surgery must be performed under emergency conditions, desmopressin (DDAVP) can be used to reduce the risk of excessive bleeding. This should be done in consultation with the patient's physician or hematologist.[6,34,47]

NSAIDs can also inhibit platelet cyclooxygenase, thereby blocking the formation of thromboxane A_2. These drugs produce a systemic bleeding tendency by impairing thromboxane-dependent platelet aggregation. However, they inhibit cyclooxygenase reversibly, and the duration of their action depends on the specific drug dose given, the serum level, and the half-life. Most invasive dental procedures can be performed without adjusting the dosage of the NSAID. If the patient's physician recommends stopping the drug, after three half-lives of the drug have passed, the drug levels will be sufficiently eliminated to allow return of normal platelet function. It should be remembered that the clinical risks of bleeding with aspirin or nonaspirin NSAIDs are enhanced by the use of alcohol or anticoagulants and by associated conditions such as advanced age, liver disease, and other coexisting coagulopathies.[6,33,44]

A common use for the antiplatelet ADP inhibitors, clopidogrel and ticlopidine, is to prevent thrombosis in arterial stents. Clopidogrel is used the most often and is given as a single agent or as a dual agent with aspirin. In 2007, a science advisory from the American Heart Association, American College of Cardiology, Society for Cardiovascular Angiography and Interventions, American College of Surgeons, and American Dental Association, with representation from the American College of Physicians, was published.[45] This advisory stressed the importance of 12 months of dual antiplatelet therapy after placement of a drug-eluting stent and educating patients and health care providers about hazards of premature discontinuation. It also recommends postponing elective surgery for 1 year, and if surgery cannot be deferred, considering the continuation of aspirin during the perioperative period in high-risk patients with drug-eluting stents.[45]

In a recent study involving patients taking single or dual antiplatelet therapy who had invasive dental procedures (extractions, periodontal surgery, subgingival scaling, and root planning) it was found that no episodes of prolonged bleeding occurred.[46] At this time it appears to be safe for patients taking single ticlopidine or clopidogrel therapy or dual therapy with aspirin to be maintained on their medication(s) for invasive dental procedures. For major oral surgical procedures that can't be delayed the thienopyridines may have to be discontinued until after the surgery. Consultation with the patient's physician is recommended.

The *fibrinogen receptor inhibitors* tirofiban, abciximab, and eptifibatide, are injectable (IV) antiplatelet drugs used in emergency coronary situations, usually in a hospital setting. The dentist is very unlikely to be faced with the management of patients on these drugs unless called to the hospital for dental emergency care for a patient with acute coronary syndrome or myocardial infarction. Under these conditions the dentist should consult with the attending physician regarding the management of the patient. In general, the most conservative dental treatment should be selected to deal with the dental problem without any changes in the patient's medications or dosage.

Coumarin Therapy. The major concern in performing surgical or invasive dental procedures on patients who are taking warfarin (Coumadin) is the potential for excessive bleeding. In contrast, if the anticoagulant is discontinued in preparation for the dental procedure, the major medical concern is thrombosis, which could be life-threatening. The literature clearly supports the continuation of warfarin anticoagulation therapy for minor oral surgery and other similarly invasive dental procedures if the INR is 3.5 or less.[37,47-52] It is estimated that for every increase of 1.0 in the INR over 3.5, the risk for bleeding doubles.[39] For major oral surgery, the literature is less clear on management of the warfarin level. If other bleeding problems, such as liver disease and renal disease, are present, or if other drugs (e.g., aspirin, antibiotics, NSAIDs) are being taken, management of the patient will have to be planned on an individual basis. Before performing surgical or invasive dental procedures, the dentist should obtain medical consultation for all patients who are taking warfarin.

If acute infection is present, surgery should be avoided until the infection has been treated. When the patient is free of acute infection and the INR is 3.5 or less, minor surgery can be performed. The procedure should be done with as little trauma as possible.

The American College of Chest Physicians and the American Heart Association/American College of Cardiology also recommend that warfarin therapy should not be interrupted for invasive dental procedures, and that a tranexamic acid (Cyklokapron) or EACA (Amicar) mouthwash should be applied during the first 2 postoperative days to help control excessive bleeding.[51,53] Tranexamic acid rinses are used in other countries and are not readily available in the United States. For stability and sterility reasons, the Amicar solution can be prepared in the dental clinic on the day it is to be used.[54] A 5-g vial for injection (20 mL, contains 5 g of Amicar and 0.9% benzyl alcohol preservative) may be diluted with sterile water to a total volume of 100 mL. The patient is instructed to hold 10 mL of the Amicar solution (1.00 g of Amicar) in the area of the dental or surgical procedure for 2 minutes just before the procedure and every 1 to 2 hours after the procedure until all of the solution is gone. The patient is instructed not to "swish" to avoid dislodging a clot. Activities such as sucking on a straw or candy should be avoided because negative pressure may dislodge the clot.[54]

If excessive postoperative bleeding occurs after an extraction, Gelfoam with thrombin may be placed in the socket to control it. In addition, primary closure over the socket is desirable. Oxycel, Surgicel, or microfibrillar collagen may be used in place of Gelfoam (see Table 24-6). However, thrombin should not be used in combination with these agents because it is inactivated as a result of pH factors, thus representing an additional cost with no real benefits. An inhibitor of fibrinolysis (tranexamic acid or EACA) also can be applied.[55-57]

If excessive bleeding cannot be controlled by the local methods listed earlier, the dentist should consult the patient's physician. Available options include discontinuation of warfarin, which would take several days before an effect on bleeding would occur; administration of vitamin K; and administration of fresh frozen plasma or a prothrombin concentrate. Vitamin K can be given by the intravenous route (rapid response but slight risk of anaphylaxis), subcutaneously (response is unpredictable and sometimes delayed), or orally (predictable response, effective, convenient, safe, and effect seen within 24 hours). Fresh frozen plasma carries a risk of infection, and prothrombin concentrate is associated with a risk of thromboembolic complications. Another option is to administer recombinant factor VIIa.[37,39,58,59]

Box 24-9 summarizes appropriate dental management of the patient who is taking warfarin or Coumadin. If the dosage of anticoagulant must be adjusted, the patient's physician should instruct the patient. It will take 3 to 5 days before the effect of the dose reduction is reflected in the lower INR. On the day of surgery, the INR should be checked again to determine whether the desired reduction has occurred. If no excessive bleeding occurs on the day after the dental procedure is performed, the patient's physician can direct the patient to return to his or her usual warfarin dosage.

Patients who are about to undergo major oral surgery and are receiving warfarin therapy should have input from their physician regarding the INR level that would be indicated. An INR above 3.0 may need to be adjusted by the physician. Again, it will take 3 to 5 days for any effective reduction of the INR to occur.

Another option for these patients is Coumadin Lovenox bridging.[60-62] One approach is to have the patient's physician discontinue warfarin therapy 4 days before major oral surgery and to begin a series of 30-mg subcutaneous enoxaparin (Lovenox and LMWH) injections every 12 hours (at 9 AM and 9 PM) on an outpatient basis, starting 3 days before the surgery is to be performed (referred to as Coumadin Lovenox bridging).[63] Through discontinuation of warfarin, the INR is allowed to normalize, and enoxaparin provides anticoagulation. The last enoxaparin injection is given at 9 PM on the evening before surgery. The INR should be checked on the morning of surgery and, if within normal values (1.0), the surgery can be performed.[63] Enoxaparin injections are started again on the evening after the surgery; oral warfarin therapy is also restarted that evening. After 3 days, the postoperative enoxaparin injections are stopped.[63] A potential problem with this approach is that a temporary hypercoagulable state may occur when warfarin therapy is stopped.

The dentist must be aware that certain drugs will affect the action of warfarin (Coumadin). Drugs the dentist may use that potentiate the anticoagulant action of warfarin include acetaminophen, metronidazole, salicylates, broad-spectrum antibiotics, erythromycin, and the new cyclooxygenase (COX)-2–specific inhibitors (celecoxib and rofecoxib). Other drugs that have the same effect are cimetidine, chloral hydrate, phenytoin, propranolol, and thyroid drugs. Drugs that the dentist

BOX 24-9 Dental Management

Considerations in the Patient Taking Warfarin (Coumadin)

P

Patient Evaluation/Risk Assessment (see Box 1-1)

- Confirm INR level before surgical procedures.

Potential Issues/Factors of Concern

A

Analgesics	Avoid aspirin, aspirin-containing compounds, and other NSAIDs; acetaminophen with or without codeine is suggested for most patients.
Antibiotics	Not indicated unless acute infection is present.
Anesthesia	No issues.
Anxiety	No issues.
Allergy	No issues.

B

Bleeding	The risk for excessive bleeding after invasive dental procedures depends on the level of the patient's INR. If the INR is greater than 3.5, significant bleeding may occur after invasive dental and surgical procedures. These procedures can be performed with little risk of significant bleeding if the INR is between 2.0 and 3.5. If the INR is between 3.0 and 3.5, significant bleeding may occur with major oral surgery and the INR may have to be reduced to 3.0 or lower.
Breathing	No issues.
Blood pressure	No issues.

C

Chair position	No issues.
Cardiovascular	Determine reason for anticoagulation therapy; if for cardiac reason, take appropriate management actions.
Consultation	The dentist should consult with the patient's physician to determine the level of anticoagulation being maintained with warfarin therapy. If invasive procedures or minor oral surgery are planned and the patient's INR is between 2.0 and 3.5 no adjustment in the warfarin dosage is indicated. If the INR is greater than 3.5, the dentist should request that the dosage be reduced to allow the INR to fall in the range of 2.0 to 3.5. Also, if major oral surgery is planned and the patient's INR is between 3.0 and 3.5, the dentist may request that the dosage be reduced to allow the INR to fall in the range of 2.0 to 3.0. If the dosage of warfarin is reduced by the patient's physician it will take 3 to 5 days for the desired reduction to occur. The reduction should be confirmed by INR before the dental or surgical procedure which should be scheduled within 2 days after confirmation of the reduction. Once it has been determined by the dentist that there are no significant complications (bleeding, infection, poor healing), the patient's physician should be contacted to resume the patient's usual warfarin dosage.

D

Devices	No issues.
Drugs	Avoid all drugs that may cause bleeding or potentiate the anticoagulation action of warfarin, such as aspirin or other NSAIDs, metronidazole, broad-spectrum antibiotics, erythromycin, herbal medications, and over-the-counter drugs containing aspirin. Also, drugs such as barbiturates, steroids, and nafcillin that will antagonize the action of warfarin should be avoided.

E

Equipment	No issues.
Emergencies	Excessive bleeding may occur after invasive dental procedures or surgery, and local means may be required to control the bleeding (see Table 24-5).

F

Follow-up	Patients should be contacted or examined within 24 to 48 hours after surgical procedures to determine that excessive bleeding or infection is not occurring.

INR, International normalized ratio [INR = $(PTR)^{ISI}$]; *ISI*, International sensitivity index (based on sensitivity of thromboplastin used in PT); *PT*, Prothrombin time; *PTR*, Prothrombin time ratio.

may use that will antagonize the anticoagulant action of warfarin are barbiturates, steroids, and nafcillin. Other drugs that have the same effect are carbamazepine, cholestyramine, griseofulvin, rifampin, and trazodone.[37]

Postoperative pain control can be attained with the use of minimal doses of acetaminophen with or without codeine. Aspirin and NSAIDs must be avoided. When used at the indicated dosage, COX-2–specific inhibitors (celecoxib and rofecoxib) do not affect platelet count, PT, and PPT and do not inhibit platelet aggregation. However, they can increase PT and INR in patients who are taking warfarin; if used, the dosage should be reduced. With recent concerns over the possible role that COX-2 inhibitors may play in increasing the risk of myocardial infarction, it may be best to avoid these agents, even though they would be used only for a short time.

Heparin Therapy. Most patients treated with standard heparin are hospitalized and will be prescribed warfarin once discharged. Dental emergencies in these patients during hospitalization should be treated as conservatively as possible, with avoidance of invasive procedures, if possible. Patients treated with hemodialysis are given heparin. The half-life of heparin is only 1 to 2 hours; thus, if they wait until the day after dialysis, these patients can receive invasive dental treatment. The dental management of these patients is presented in Chapter 12.

The dentist may see patients who are being treated on an outpatient basis with an LMWH or a synthetic heparin. These agents are used in patients with recent total hip or knee replacement and those being treated on an outpatient basis for deep vein thrombi or asymptomatic pulmonary embolism. Elective surgical procedures can be delayed until the patient is taken off the LMWH or synthetic heparin, which, in most cases, will occur within 3 to 6 months. If an invasive procedure must be performed, the dentist has several options. First, the dentist should consult with the patient's physician regarding the need for and the type of surgery. The half-life of the LMWHs and fondaparinux is less than 1 day. Thus, the physician could suggest that the drug be stopped and the surgery be performed within 1 to 2 days. The other option is to go ahead with the surgery and deal with any bleeding complications on a local basis. It appears that these patients can undergo minor surgical procedures with little risk for any serious bleeding complications.[56,64]

Direct Thrombin Inhibitors. The direct thrombin inhibitors, lepirudin, desirudin, argatroban, and bivalirudin, are injectable drugs used primarily in patients with a history of heparin-induced thrombocytopenia. They all have a very short half-life of only several hours. Again, the dentist is unlikely to have patients on any of these medications as they are used most often in a hospital setting. However, if the dentist has a patient taking one of these drugs many invasive dental procedures can be done without stopping the drug. Most invasive dental procedures can be performed for patients taking the oral direct thrombin inhibitor dabigatran. Consultation with the patient's physician is recommended. Because of the short half-life of these drugs, only a day would be needed without the drug for more invasive procedures.

Possible Liver Disease. A patient with a history of jaundice or heavy alcohol use may have significant liver disease. Most coagulation factors are produced in the liver; therefore, if enough liver damage has occurred, the patient could have a serious bleeding problem because of a defect in the coagulation phase. In addition, about 50% of patients with significant liver disease (with portal hypertension present) will be thrombocytopenic as a result of sequestration of platelets in the spleen. Alcohol also can have a direct effect on homeostasis by interfering with platelet function. The PT test can be used to screen for a defect in the coagulation phase in patients with a history that indicates liver disease (see Chapter 10 for blood tests indicative of alcoholism). A platelet count should be obtained to see if the platelet phase has been affected. The amount of liver damage that has occurred may not be great enough to affect the coagulation phase, but the effect on the platelet phase could be severe enough to lead to a serious bleeding problem. If both the PT and the platelet count are normal, surgery can be performed on these patients with little risk of a postoperative bleeding problem. If results of both tests are abnormal, then the dentist should consult with the patient's physician regarding stabilization of the patient's bleeding status before surgery. Appropriate management may involve vitamin K administration, platelet replacement, or other special physician-directed procedures.

Chronic Leukemia. Chapter 23 describes the dental management of patients with leukemia.

Malabsorption Syndrome or Long-Term Antibiotic Therapy. In patients with malabsorption syndrome and in those receiving long-term antibiotic therapy, bacteria in the intestine that produce vitamin K may be adversely affected. The liver needs vitamin K for the production and function of prothrombin (factor II) and related coagulation factors (factors VII, IX, and X). The PT test can be ordered to screen for a possible bleeding problem; if results are normal, surgery can be performed on these patients without risk of a bleeding problem. The patient's physician should be consulted regarding the patient's health status before surgery, because complicating factors may occur, in addition to the possible bleeding problem that would contraindicate surgery. Parenteral vitamin K may have to be administered in some of these cases.

End-Stage Renal Disease and Renal Dialysis. Management of patients with end-stage renal disease (ESRD) and those on renal dialysis is covered in Chapter 12.

Vascular Wall Alteration. In patients with autoimmune disease, infectious disease, structural malformation of vessels, scurvy, steroid therapy, small vessel vasculitis, or deposits of paraproteins, alterations of the vessel wall can result in excessive bleeding after surgical procedures. No reliable screening tests can detect those patients who will be bleeders. The Ivy BT test can be used in an attempt to identify potential bleeders, but, as stated earlier, this is not a reliable test. The dentist must rely on the medical history (questions related to excessive bleeding problems), clinical findings, and consultation with the patient's physician to identify these patients.

Management of the Patient with a Serious Bleeding Disorder

Thrombocytopenia. Patients found to have severe thrombocytopenia may require hospitalization and special preparation for surgery. A hematologist should be involved with the diagnosis, presurgical assessment, preparation, and postsurgical management of these patients.

Infiltration and block injections of local anesthesia can be provided in patients with platelet counts above 30,000/µL. Also, most routine dental procedures can be performed. If the platelet count is below this level, routine dental treatment involving minor tissue injury should be delayed. For urgent or emergency dental needs, platelet replacement is indicated. If the platelet count is above 50,000/µL, extractions and dentoalveolar surgery can be performed. For more advanced surgery, the platelet count should be 80,000/µL and 100,000/µL or higher. Patients with platelet counts below these levels will need platelet replacement before undergoing the planned procedures.[56,65]

Two types of platelet transfusions are used in the United States. Platelet concentrates are prepared from pooled donor whole blood through centrifugation, or pheresis devices are used to provide continuous centrifugation of blood donated by a single donor, thereby providing apheresis units of concentrated platelets. These products must be used within several days or must be cryopreserved for future use. Platelets from a single donor reduce the risk of infection. Lyophilization of platelets for replacement use is being clinically tested but has not yet been approved for general use.[65]

The need for platelet transfusions can be reduced through the use of local measures (see Table 24-6), along with desmopressin and EACA or tranexamic acid to control bleeding. Also, topical platelet concentrates can be applied.[56]

Patients who fail to respond to platelet replacement therapy have what is called *platelet transfusion refractoriness*. This may occur on an immune or a nonimmune basis. Platelet transfusion refractoriness presents management problems that are beyond the scope of this presentation. The hematologist who is involved with the patient will make recommendations on how to prepare the patient for surgical procedures.[65,66]

Treatment Planning Modifications

With proper preparation, most indicated dental treatment can be provided for patients with various bleeding problems. Patients with bleeding problems related to diseases that may be in the terminal phase should, in general, be offered only conservative dental treatment. Aspirin and other NSAIDs should not be used for pain relief in those who have known bleeding disorders or who are receiving anticoagulant medication. Such medication include the various compounds that contain aspirin, such as Anacin, Synalgos-DC, Fiorinal, Bufferin, Alka-Seltzer, Empirin with Codeine, and Excedrin. Herbal medications that may cause bleeding also should be avoided.

Oral Complications and Manifestations

Patients with bleeding disorders may experience spontaneous gingival bleeding. Oral tissues (e.g., soft palate, tongue, buccal mucosa) may show petechiae, ecchymoses, jaundice, pallor, and ulcers. Spontaneous gingival bleeding and petechiae usually are found in patients with thrombocytopenia. Hemarthrosis of the temporomandibular joint (TMJ) is a rare finding in patients with coagulation disorders and is not found in patients with thrombocytopenia. Enlargement of the parotid glands may be associated with chronic liver disease that is most often seen in alcoholics (see Chapter 10). Patients with leukemia may exhibit generalized hyperplasia of the gingiva (see Chapter 23). Patients with neoplastic disease may show osseous lesions on radiographs, as well as oral ulcers or tumors. These patients also may have drifting and loosening of teeth and may complain of paresthesias (e.g., burning of the tongue, numbness of the lip) (see Chapter 26).

REFERENCES

1. Konkle BA: Bleeding and thrombosis. In Fauci AS, et al, editors: *Harrison's principles of internal medicine*, ed 17, New York, 2008, McGraw-Hill, pp 363-369.
2. Rosendaal FR, Buller HR: Venous thrombosis. In Fauci AS, et al, editors: *Harrison's principles of internal medicine*, ed 17, New York, 2008, McGraw-Hill, pp 731-734.
3. Deitcher SR: Hypercoagulable states. In Carey WD, et al, editors: *Current clinical medicine 2009—Cleveland Clinic*, Philadelphia, 2009, Saunders, pp 639-646.
4. Lim W, et al: Venous thromboembolism. In Hoffman R, et al, editors: *Hematology: basic principles and practice*, ed 5, Philadelphia, 2009, Churchill Livingstone, pp 2043-2054.
5. Bennett JS: Hereditary disorders of platelet function. In Hoffman R, et al, editors: *Hematology: basic principles and practice*, ed 5, Philadelphia, 2009, Churchill Livingstone, pp 2133-2144.
6. Lopez JA, Lockhart E: Acquired disorders of platelet function. In Hoffman R, et al, editors: *Hematology: basic principles and practice*, ed 5, Philadelphia, 2009, Churchill Livingstone, pp 2145-2160.
7. Arruda V, High KA: Coagulation disorders. In Fauci AS, et al, editors: *Harrison's principles of internal medicine*, ed 17, New York, 2008, McGraw-Hill, pp 725-730.
8. Baz R, Mekhail T: Bleeding disorders. In Carey WD, et al, editors: *Current clinical medicine 2009—Cleveland Clinic*, Philadelphia, 2009, Saunders, pp 669-674.

9. Coller BS, Schneiderman PI: Clinical evaluation of hemorrhagic disorders: the bleeding history and differential diagnosis of purpura. In Hoffman R, et al, editors: *Hematology: basic principles and practice*, ed 5, Philadelphia, 2009, Churchill Livingstone, pp 1851-1876.
10. Liebman HA, Weitz IC: Disseminated intravascular coagulation. In Hoffman R, et al, editors: *Hematology basic principles and practices*, ed 4, Philadelphia, 2005, Churchill Livingstone, pp 2169-2183.
11. George JN: Drug-induced thrombocytopenia. In Young NS, Gerson SL, High KA, editors: *Clinical hematology*, St. Louis, 2006, Mosby, pp 791-802.
12. Schauss AG: Fish oils (omega-3 fatty acids, docosahexanoic acid, eicosapentaenoic acid, dietary fish, and fish oils). In Pizzorno JEJ, Murray MT, editors: *Textbook of natural medicine*, St. Louis, 2006, Churchill Livingstone, pp 945-947.
13. Schafer AI: Approach to the patient with bleeding and thrombosis. In Goldman L, Ausiello D, editors: *Cecil medicine*, ed 23, Philadelphia, 2008, Saunders, pp 1286-1288.
14. Brass LF: The molecular basis of platelet activation. In Hoffman R, et al, editors: *Hematology: basic principles and practice*, ed 5, Philadelphia, 2009, Churchill Livingstone, pp 1793-1804.
15. Karsan A, Harlan JM: The blood vessel wall. In Hoffman R, et al, editors: *Hematology: basic principles and practice*, ed 5, Philadelphia, 2009, Churchill Livingstone, pp 1805-1818.
16. Furie B, Furie B: Molecular basis of blood coagulation. In Hoffman R, et al, editors: *Hematology: basic principles and practice*, ed 5, Philadelphia, 2009, Churchill Livingstone, pp 1819-1836.
17. McVey JH: Coagulation factors. In Young NS, Gerson SL, High KA, editors: *Clinical hematology*, St. Louis, 2006, Mosby, pp 103-123.
18. Ragni MV, et al: Clinical aspects and therapy of hemophilia. In Hoffman R, et al, editors: *Hematology: basic principles and practice*, ed 5, Philadelphia, 2009, Churchill Livingstone, pp 1911-1930.
19. Lijnen HR, Collen D: Molecular and cellular basis of fibrinolysis. In Hoffman R, et al, editors: *Hematology: basic principles and practice*, ed 5, Philadelphia, 2009, Churchill Livingstone, pp 1837-1842.
20. White GCI, Sadler JE: von Willebrand disease: clinical aspects and therapy. In Hoffman R, et al, editors: *Hematology: basic principles and practice*, ed 5, Philadelphia, 2009, Churchill Livingstone, pp 1961-1972.
21. Bennett JS: Inherited and acquired disorders of platelet function. In Young NS, Gerson SL, High KA, editors: *Clinical hematology*, St. Louis, 2006, Mosby, pp 767-781.
22. Watzke HH: Evaluation of the acutely bleeding patient. In Young NS, Gerson SL, High KA, editors: *Clinical hematology*, St. Louis, 2006, Mosby, pp 1169-1179.
23. Rand JH, Senzel L: Laboratory evaluation of hemostatic disorders. In Hoffman R, et al, editors: *Hematology: basic principles and practices*, ed 4, Philadelphia, 2005, Churchill Livingstone, pp 2001-2011.
24. Schmaier AH: Laboratory evaluation of hemostatic and thrombotic disorders. In Hoffman R, et al, editors: *Hematology: basic principles and practice*, ed 5, Philadelphia, 2009, Churchill Livingstone, pp 1877-1884.
25. Konkle BA: Disorders of platelets and vessel wall. In Fauci AS, et al, editors: *Harrison's principles of internal medicine*, ed 17, New York, 2008, McGraw-Hill, pp 718-724.
26. Bolognia JL, Braverman IM: Skin manifestations of internal disease. In Fauci AS, et al, editors: *Harrison's principles of internal medicine*, ed 17, New York, 2008, McGraw-Hill, pp 321-335.
27. Grandinetti LM, Tomecki KJ: Dermatologic signs of systemic disease. In Carey WD, et al, editors: *Current clinical medicine 2009—Cleveland Clinic*, Philadelphia, 2009, Saunders, pp 244-256.
28. Baz R, Mekhail T: Disorders of platelet function and number. In Carey WD, et al, editors: *Current clinical medicine 2009—Cleveland Clinic*, Philadelphia, 2009, Saunders, pp 669-674.
29. Toh CH: Disseminated intravascular coagulation. In Young NS, Gerson SL, High KA, editors: *Clinical hematology*, St. Louis, 2006, Elsevier Mosby, pp 1134-1155.
30. Schafer AI: Hemorrhagic disorders: disseminated intravascular coagulation, liver failure, and vitamin K deficiency. In Goldman L, Ausiello D, editors: *Cecil medicine*, ed 23, Philadelphia, 2008, Saunders, pp 1314-1317.
31. Liebman HA, Weitz IC: Disseminated intravascular coagulation. In Hoffman R, et al, editors: *Hematology: basic principles and practice*, ed 5, Philadelphia, 2009, Churchill Livingstone, pp 1999-2009.
32. LoRusso KL, Macik BG: Chronic bruising and bleeding diathesis. In Young NS, Gerson SL, High KA, editors: *Clinical hematology*, St. Louis, 2006, Mosby, pp 1079-1089.
33. Weitz JI: Antiplatelet, anticoagulant, and fibrinolytic drugs. In Fauci AS, editor: *Harrison's principles of internal medicine*, ed 17, New York, 2008, McGraw-Hill, pp 735-748.
34. Schafer AI: Thrombotic disorders: hypercoagulable states. In Goldman L, Ausiello D, editors: *Cecil medicine*, ed 23, Philadelphia, 2008, Saunders, pp 1318-1323.
35. Krakow EF, et al: Arterial thromboembolism. In Hoffman R, et al, editors: *Hematology: basic principles and practice*, ed 5, Philadelphia, 2009, Churchill Livingstone, pp 2055-2066.
36. Hirsh J, Schulman S: Antithrombotic therapy. In Goldman L, Ausiello D, editors: *Cecil medicine*, ed 23, Philadelphia, 2008, Saunders, pp 197-205.
37. Weitz IC: Antithrombotic drugs. In Hoffman R, et al, editors: *Hematology: basic principles and practice*, ed 5, Philadelphia, 2009, Churchill Livingstone, pp 2067-2082.
38. Elliott G: Concise review: low-molecular-weight heparin in the treatment of acute pulmonary embolism. In Fauci AS, et al, editors: *Harrison's principles of internal medicine*, ed 14, New York, 2000, McGraw-Hill, pp 1-4.
39. Warkentin TE, Crowther MA: Anticoagulant and thrombolytic therapy. In Young NS, Gerson SL, High KA, editors: *Clinical hematology*, St. Louis, 2006, Mosby, pp 1114-1134.
40. Nowak G: [New anticoagulants for secondary haemostasis—anti IIa inhibitors.] *Hamostaseologie* 29:256-259, 2009.
41. U.S. Food and Drug Administration: *FDA approves Pradaxa to prevent stroke in people with atrial fibrillation*, Washington, DC, 2010, U.S. Food and Drug Administration.
42. Weitz JI: New oral anticoagulants in development, *Thromb Haemost* 103:62-70, 2009.
43. Coller BS, Schneiderman PI: Clinical evaluation of hemorrhagic disorders: the bleeding history and differential diagnosis of purpura. In Hoffman R, et al, editors: *Hematology: basic principles and practices*, ed 4, Philadelphia, 2005, Churchill Livingstone, pp 1975-2001.
44. Fitzgerald GA: Prostaglandins, aspirin, and related compounds. In Goldman L, Ausiello D, editors: *Cecil medicine*, ed 23, Philadelphia, 2008, Saunders, pp 189-196.
45. Grines CL, et al: Prevention of premature discontinuation of dual antiplatelet therapy in patients with coronary artery stents: a science advisory from the American Heart Association, American College of Cardiology, Society for Cardiovascular Angiography and Interventions, American College of Surgeons, and American Dental Association, with representation from the American College of Physicians, *J Am Dent Assoc* 138:652-655, 2007.
46. Napeñas JJ, et al: The frequency of bleeding complications after invasive dental treatment in patients receiving single and

dual antiplatelet therapy, *J Am Dent Assoc* 140:690-695, 2009.
47. Blinder D, et al: Dental extractions in patients maintained on oral anticoagulant therapy: comparison of INR value with occurrence of postoperative bleeding, *Int J Oral Maxillofac Surg* 30:518-521, 2001.
48. Wahl M: Dental surgery in anticoagulated patients, *Arch Intern Med* 158:1610-1616, 1998.
49. Wahl MJ: Myths of dental surgery in patients receiving anticoagulant therapy, *J Am Dent Assoc* 131:77-81, 2000.
50. Zanon E, et al: Safety of dental extraction among consecutive patients on oral anticoagulant treatment managed using a specific dental management protocol, *Blood Coagul Fibrinolysis* 14:27-30, 2003.
51. Hirsh J, et al: American Heart Association/American College of Cardiology Foundation guide to warfarin therapy, *J Am Coll Cardiol* 41:1633-1652, 2003.
52. Akopov S: Withdrawal of warfarin prior to a surgical procedure: time to follow the guidelines? *Cerebrovasc Dis* 19:337-342, 2005.
53. Ansell J, et al: Managing oral anticoagulant therapy, *Chest* 119(1Suppl):22S-38S, 2001.
54. Bussey HI: Should I stop my patient's warfarin prior to a dental procedure? Available at http://www.clotcare.com., accessed 1/11/2011, 2005.
55. Federici AB, et al: Optimising local therapy during oral surgery in patients with von Willebrand disease: effective results from a retrospective analysis of 63 cases, *Haemophilia* 6:71-77, 2000.
56. Scully C, Cawson RA: *Medical problems in dentistry*, ed 5, Edinburgh, 2005, Elsevier.
57. Zanon E, et al: Proposal of a standard approach to dental extraction in haemophilia patients. A case-control study with good results, *Haemophilia* 6:533-536, 2000.
58. Furie B, Furie BC: Vitamin K: metabolism and disorders. In Hoffman R, et al, editors: *Hematology: basic principles and practices*, ed 4, Philadelphia, 2005, Churchill Livingstone, pp 2136-2143.
59. Roberts HR, Escobar MA: Other clotting factor deficiencies. In Hoffman R, et al, editors: *Hematology: basic principles and practices*, ed 4, Philadelphia, 2005, Churchill Livingstone, pp 2081-2097.
60. Bajkin BV, Popovic SL, Selakovic SD: Randomized, prospective trial comparing bridging therapy using low-molecular-weight heparin with maintenance of oral anticoagulation during extraction of teeth, *J Oral Maxillofac Surg* 67:990-995, 2009.
61. Brejcha M, et al: [Preparation of patients on anticoagulant treatment for invasive surgery.] *Vnitr Lek* 55:272-275, 2009.
62. Ahmed I, et al: Continuing warfarin therapy is superior to interrupting warfarin with or without bridging anticoagulation therapy in patients undergoing pacemaker and defibrillator implantation, *Heart Rhythm* 7:745-749, 2010.
63. Johnson-Leong C, Rada RE: The use of low-molecular-weight heparins in outpatient oral surgery for patients receiving anticoagulation therapy, *J Am Dent Assoc* 133:1083-1087, 2002.
64. Little JW, et al: Antithrombotic agents: implications in dentistry, *Oral Surg Oral Med Oral Path Oral Radiol Endod* 93:544-551, 2002.
65. Kickler TS: Principles of platelet transfusion therapy. In Hoffman R, et al, editors: *Hematology: basic principles and practices*, ed 4, Philadelphia, 2005, Churchill Livingstone, pp 2433-2441.
66. Shuman M: Hemorrhagic disorders: abnormalities of platelet and vascular function. In Goldman L, Ausiello D, editors: *Cecil textbook of medicine*, Philadelphia, 2004, WB Saunders, pp 1060-1069.

CHAPTER

25

Congenital Bleeding and Hypercoagulable Disorders

A number of procedures that are performed in dentistry may cause bleeding. Under normal circumstances, these procedures can be performed with little risk to the patient; however, the patient whose ability to control bleeding has been altered by congenital defects in coagulation factors, platelets, or blood vessels may be in grave danger unless the dentist identifies the problem before performing any dental procedure. In most cases, once the patient with a congenital bleeding problem has been identified, steps can be taken to greatly reduce the risks associated with dental procedures. The following disorders are discussed in this chapter: hereditary hemorrhagic telangiectasia (Osler-Weber-Rendu syndrome), von Willebrand disease, Bernard-Soulier disease, Glanzmann's thrombasthenia, hemophilia A, hemophilia B (Christmas disease), and congenital hypercoagulability disorders.

DEFINITION

Inherited (congenital) bleeding disorders are genetically transmitted. They may involve a deficiency of one of the coagulation factors, abnormal construction of platelets, deficiency of von Willebrand factor, or malformation of vessels (Box 25-1). They are not nearly as prevalent as acquired bleeding disorders. In a typical dental practice of 2000 patients, at the most 10 to 20 patients will have a congenital bleeding disorder. Inherited hypercoagulability disorders increase the risk for thromboembolism due to a genetic deficiency of an antithrombotic factor or increasing a prothrombotic factor. They are more common than the inherited bleeding disorders.

Epidemiology: Incidence and Prevalence

The most common inherited bleeding disorder is von Willebrand disease. It affects about 1% of the U.S. population. The disease usually is inherited as an autosomal dominant trait. Hemophilia A, factor VIII deficiency, is the most common of the inherited coagulation bleeding disorders. It occurs in about 1 of every 5000 male births. More than 20,000 individuals in the United States have hemophilia A.[1,2] Because of its genetic mode of transfer, certain areas of the United States contain higher concentrations of people with hemophilia. Hemophilia B (Christmas disease), a factor IX deficiency, is found in about 1 of every 30,000 male births.[1] About 80% of all genetic coagulation disorders are hemophilia A, 13% are hemophilia B, and 6% are factor XI deficiency.[1] Bernard-Soulier disease and Glanzmann's thrombasthenia are rare inherited platelet disorders.[3] Hereditary hemorrhagic telangiectasia (HHT) is a rare (1:8000 to 1:50,000) vascular disorder.[4] Ehlers-Danlos disease, osteogenesis imperfecta, pseudoxanthoma elasticum, and Marfan syndrome are rare hereditary connective tissue disorders that may be associated with bleeding problems but are not covered in this chapter.[4] An inherited hypercoagulable state has been reported in more than 60% of patients presenting with idiopathic venothromboembolism.[5]

ETIOLOGY

Patients may be born with a deficiency of one of the factors needed for blood coagulation—for example, factor VIII deficiency as in hemophilia A or factor IX deficiency as in hemophilia B or Christmas disease. Congenital deficiencies of the other coagulation factors have been reported but are rare (Table 25-1). When congenital deficiency of a coagulation factor occurs, only a single factor is affected.[1,6]

In von Willebrand disease, the primary problem involves lack of various sizes of von Willebrand factor (vWF), which are needed to attach platelets to damaged vascular wall tissues and to carry factor VIII in circulation.[7] In the most severe form of the disease, bleeding occurs as a consequence of lack of platelet adhesion and deficiency of factor VIII.[7] Bernard-Soulier disease is a disorder of platelet adhesion to vWF due to the lack of glycoprotein Ib on the platelet membrane.[4] These platelets are unable to bind to vWF and thus are unable to adhere to the subendothelium. Glanzmann's thrombasthenia is a disorder of platelet aggregation due to abnormality of the platelet membrane complex glycoprotein

BOX 25-1 Classification of Congenital Bleeding and Thrombotic Disorders

Nonthrombocytopenic Purpuras

Vascular Wall Alterations

Hereditary hemorrhagic telangiectasia

Disorders of Platelet Function

von Willebrand's disease (may have secondary factor VIII deficiency)
Bernard-Soulier disease*
Glanzmann's thrombasthenia
Others

Thrombocytopenic Purpuras (all are very rare)

Gray platelet syndrome
May-Hegglin anomaly
Hereditary thrombocytopenia, deafness, and renal disease
Fechtner syndrome
Alport's syndrome
Sebastian platelet syndrome
Others

Disorders of Coagulation

Hemophilia A (factor VIII deficiency)
Hemophilia B (factor IX deficiency)
Other coagulation factor deficiencies

Hypercoagulable States

Antithrombin III deficiency
Protein C deficiency
Protein S deficiency
Factor V Leiden mutation
Prothrombin G2021A mutation
Hyperchomocysteinemia

*Bernard-Soulier disease also has been classified as a thrombocytopenic disorder.

IIb/IIIa.[4] The platelets can adhere to the subendothelium but cannot bind to fibrinogen.

HHT is a disorder consisting of multiple telangiectatic lesions involving the skin and mucous membranes.[4] Bleeding occurs because of the inherent mechanical fragility of the affected vessels. Problems with the construction of connective tissue components of the vessel wall are the underlying weakness in Ehlers-Danlos disease, osteogenesis imperfecta, pseudoxanthoma elasticum, and Marfan syndrome.[4,8] The reader is referred to other sources for further information on these latter diseases.

Pathophysiology

The three phases of hemostasis for controlling bleeding are vascular, platelet, and coagulation. The vascular and platelet phases are referred to as primary, and the coagulation phase is secondary. The coagulation phase is followed by the fibrinolytic phase, during which the clot is dissolved. These hemostatic mechanisms are discussed in detail in Chapter 24, on acquired bleeding disorders.

TABLE 25-1 Blood Coagulation Components

Factor	Deficiency	Function
Factor II (prothrombin)	Congenital—rare	Protease zymogen
Factor X	Congenital—rare	Protease zymogen
Factor IX	Congenital—rare	Protease zymogen
Factor VII	Congenital—very rare	Protease zymogen
Factor VIII	Congenital—more common	Cofactor
Factor V	Congenital—rare	Cofactor
Factor XI	Congenital—rare	Protease zymogen
Factor XII	Deficiency reported but does not cause bleeding; aPTT will be prolonged	Protease zymogen
Factor I (fibrinogen)	Congenital—rare	Structural
von Willebrand factor	Congenital—most common	Adhesion
Tissue factor	Not applicable	Cofactor initiator
Factor XIII	Congenital—rare; will cause bleeding, but aPTT and PT will be normal	Fibrin stabilization
High-molecular-weight kininogen	Deficiency does not cause bleeding; will prolong aPTT	Coenzyme
Prekallikrein	Deficiency does not cause bleeding; will prolong aPTT	Coenzyme

Data from McVey JH: Coagulation factors. In Young NS, Gerson SL, High KA, editors: Clinical hematology, *St. Louis, 2006, Mosby.*

CLINICAL PRESENTATION

Signs and Symptoms

The most common objective findings in patients with genetic coagulation disorders are ecchymoses, hemarthrosis, and dissecting hematomas (Figures 25-1 and 25-2).[1,6,9] The signs seen most commonly in patients with abnormal platelets or thrombocytopenia are petechiae and ecchymoses (Figure 25-3).[2,10,11] The signs seen most commonly in patients with vascular defects are petechiae and bleeding from the skin or mucous membrane.[4]

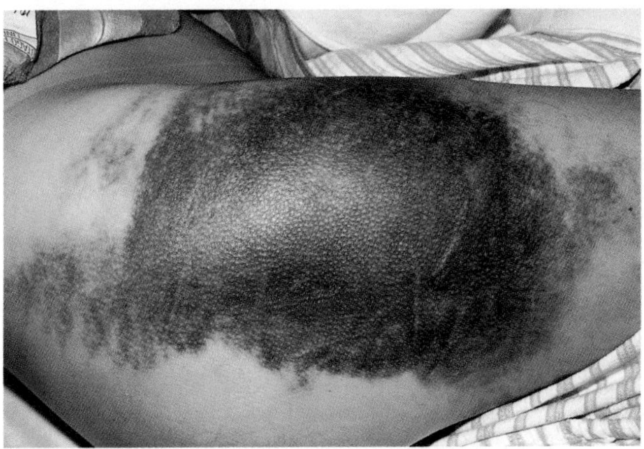

FIGURE 25-1 Large Area of Subcutaneous Ecchymoses Due to Trauma in a Patient with Hemophilia. *(From Hoffbrand AV, Pettit JE:* Color atlas of clinical hematology, *ed 4, London, 2010, Mosby.)*

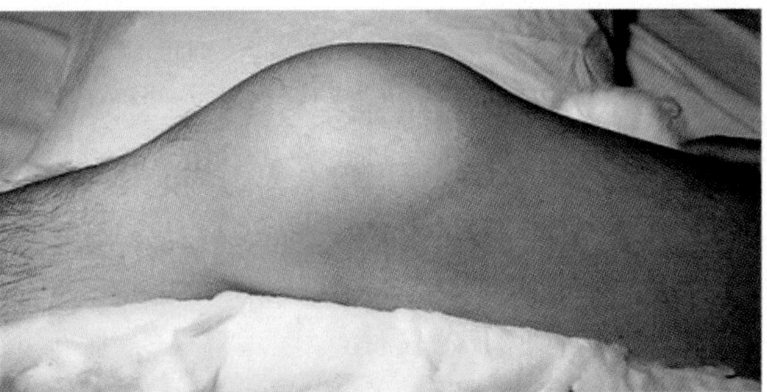

FIGURE 25-2 **Acute Hemarthrosis of the Knee is a Common Complication of Hemophilia.** It may be confused with acute infection unless the patient's coagulation disorder is known, because the knee is hot, red, swollen, and painful. *(From Forbes CD, Jackson WF:* Color atlas and text of clinical medicine, *ed 3, London, 2003, Mosby.)*

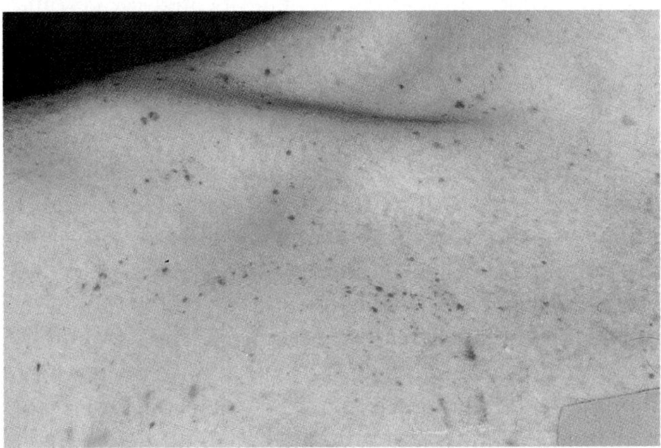

FIGURE 25-3 **Purpura (Petechiae)- in this Case Throbocytopenia Purpura (TP).** The patient was a 15-year-old boy whose antiepileptic treatment regimen had recently been modified to include sodium valproate. This is just one of a number of drugs that may induce TP, but the disorder is almost always reversible if the drug therapy is stopped. *(From Forbes CD, Jackson WF:* Color atlas and text of clinical medicine, *ed 3, London, 2003, Mosby.)*

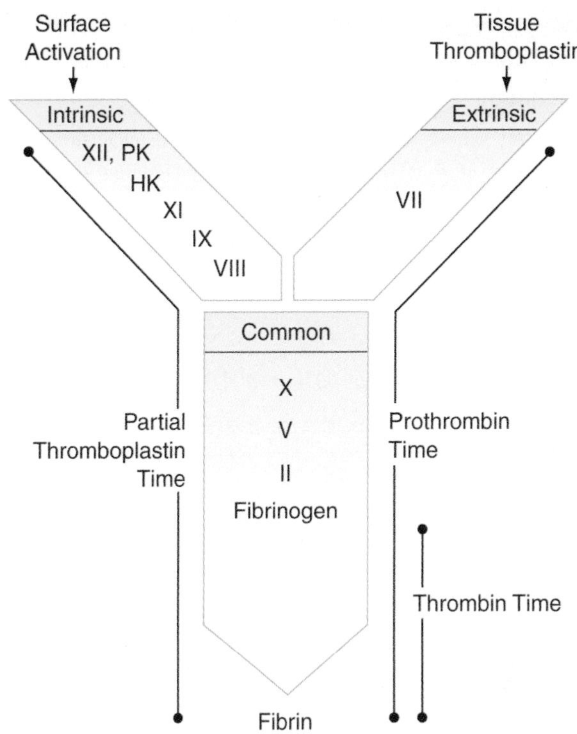

FIGURE 25-4 Organization of the coagulation system based on current screening assays. The intrinsic coagulation system consists of the protein factors XII, XI, IX, and VIII and prekallikrein (PK) and high-molecular-weight kininogen (HK). The extrinsic coagulation system consists of tissue factor and factor VII. The common pathway of the coagulation system consists of factors X, V, and II and fibrinogen (I). The activated partial thromboplastin time requires the presence of every protein except tissue factor and factor VII. The prothrombin time (PT) requires tissue factor; factors VII, X, V, and II; and fibrinogen. The thrombin clotting time only tests the integrity of fibrinogen. *(From McPherson RA, Pincus MR, editors:* Henry's clinical diagnosis and management by laboratory methods, *ed 22, London, 2012, Saunders.)*

Laboratory Tests

Three tests are recommended for use in initial screening for possible bleeding disorders[12-14]: activated partial thromboplastin time (aPTT), prothrombin time (PT), and platelet count (Figure 25-4). If no clues are evident as to the cause of the bleeding problem, and the dentist is ordering the tests through a commercial laboratory, an additional test can be added to the initial screen: thrombin time (TT).[12-14]

Patients with positive results on screening tests should be evaluated further so that the specific deficiency can be identified and the presence of inhibitors ruled out. A hematologist orders these tests, establishes a diagnosis that is based on the additional testing, and makes recommendations for treatment of the patient who is found to have a significant bleeding problem. The screening laboratory tests are discussed in detail in Chapter 24.

In patients with prolonged aPTT, PT, and TT, the defect involves the last stage of the common pathway, which is the activation of fibrinogen to form fibrin to stabilize the clot. The plasma level of fibrinogen is

TABLE 25-2 Medical Treatment of Congenital Bleeding Disorders

Condition	Defect	Medical Management
Hereditary hemorrhagic telangiectasia	Multiple telangiectasias with mechanical fragility of the abnormal vessels	Laser Surgery Estrogen Estrogen plus progesterone Thalidomide
von Willebrand disease	Deficiency or defect in vWF causing poor platelet adhesion and in some cases deficiency of F-VIII	Desmopressin Aminocaproic acid Factor VIII replacement that retains vWF
Hemophilia A	Deficiency or defect in F-VIII	Desmopressin Aminocaproic acid Factor VIII
	Some patients develop antibodies (inhibitors) to F-VIII	Porcine factor VIII, PCC, aPCC, factor VIIa, and/or steroids for patients with inhibitors
Hemophilia B	Deficiency or defect in F-IX	Desmopressin Aminocaproic acid Factor IX
	Development of antibodies (inhibitors) to F-IX is much less common than with hemophilia A	PCC, aPCC, factor VIIa,* and/or steroids for patients with inhibitors
Bernard-Soulier disease	Genetic defect in platelet membrane, absence of glycoprotein Ib (GP-Ib) causes disorder in platelet adhesion	Platelet transfusion Desmopressin Factor VIIa
Glanzmann's thrombasthenia	Genetic defect in platelet membrane, absence of glycoprotein IIb/IIIa (GPIIb/IIIa)	Platelet transfusion Desmopressin Factor VIIa

*Factor VIIa is activated factor VII.
aPCC, Activated prothrombin complex concentrates; *PCC,* Prothrombin complex concentrates; *vWF,* von Willebrand factor.

determined, and if it is within normal limits, then tests for fibrinolysis are performed. These tests, which detect the presence of fibrinogen and/or fibrin-degradation products, consist of staphylococcal clumping assay, agglutination of latex particles coated with antifibrinogen antibody, and euglobulin clot lysis time.[12-14]

MEDICAL MANAGEMENT

In this section, congenital conditions that may cause clinical bleeding are considered. The emphasis is placed on identification of patients with a potential bleeding problem and management of these patients if surgical procedures are needed.

Table 25-2 summarizes the nature of the defects and the medical treatment available for excessive bleeding in patients with the disorders covered in this section. Tables 25-3 and 25-4 list the commercial products that are available to treat bleeding problems in these disorders.

Vascular Defects

HHT, also referred to as Osler-Weber-Rendu syndrome, is a rare autosomal dominant disorder that is characterized by multiple telangiectatic lesions involving the skin, mucous membranes, and viscera. One form of the disorder, characterized by a high frequency of symptomatic pulmonary arteriovenous malformations and cerebral abscesses, has been identified as being due to abnormalities in the endothelial protein endoglin (ENG), encoded by the gene *HHT1,* located on chromosome 9. A second form of the disease has been linked to the activin receptor-like kinase 1 gene located on chromosome 12 (*HHT2*). Other forms of the disease have been linked to loci on chromosome 5q (*HHT3*), 7p14 (*HHT4*), and a region of chromosome 3 encoding the TGF-βII receptor (*HHT5*).[4]

The telangiectasias consist of focal dilation of postcapillary venules with connections to dilated arterioles, initially through capillaries and later directly. Perivascular mononuclear cell infiltrates also are observed. The vessels of HHT show a discontinuous endothelium and an incomplete smooth muscle cell layer. The surrounding stroma lacks elastin. Thus, the bleeding tendencies are thought to be due to mechanical fragility of the abnormal vessels.[4] Lesions usually appear in affected persons by the age of 40, and they increase in number with age.[4,15-18]

Clinical Findings. On clinical examination, venous lakes and papular, punctate, matlike, and linear telangiectasias appear on all areas of the skin and mucous membranes, with a predominance of lesions on and

TABLE 25-3 FDA-Approved Clotting Concentrates for Hemophilia A and B

Preparation with Virucidal Technique(s)	Type/Manufacturer	Specific Activity (IU/mg Protein)
Ultrapure recombinant factor VIII		
Immunoaffinity; ion exchange chromatography	Recombinate (Baxter)	>4000
Ion exchange chromatography, nanofiltration	Refacto (Wyeth)	11,200-15,000
Ion exchange chromatography, ultrafiltration	Kogenate FS (Bayer Inc.)	>4000
No human or animal protein used in culture; immunoaffinity and ion exchange chromatography	Advate (Baxter)	>4000-10,000
Ultrapure human plasma factor VIII		
Chromatography and pasteurization	Monoclate P (ZLB Behring)	>3000
Chromatography and solvent detergent	Hemofil M (Baxter)	>3000
High-purity human plasma factor VIII		
Chromatography, solvent detergent, dry heating	Alphanate SD (Grifols) vWF	50->400
Solvent detergent, dry heating	Koate-DVI (Bayer) vWF	50-100
Pasteurization (heating in solution)	Humate-P (ZLB-Behring) vWF	1-10
Porcine plasma-derived factor VIII		
Solvent detergent viral attenuation	Hyate-C (Ibsen/Biomeasure, Inc.)	>50
Ultrapure recombinant factor IX		
Affinity chromatography and ultrafiltration	BeneFix (Wyeth)	>200
Very highly purified plasma factor IX		
Chromatography and solvent detergent	AlphaNine SD (Grifols, Inc.)	>200
Monoclonal antibody ultrafiltration	Mononine (ZLB-Behring, Inc.)	>160
Low-purity plasma factor IX complex		
Solvent detergent	Profilnine SD (Grifols, Inc.)	<50
Vapor heat	Bebulin VH (Baxter)	<50
Activated plasma factor IX complex concentrate (used primarily for patients with alloantibody and autoantibody factor VIII and IX inhibitor)		
Vapor heat	FEIBA VH (Baxter)	<50
Recombinate factor VIIa (indicated for patients with alloantibody and autoantibody factor VIII and IX inhibitors)		
Affinity chromatography, solvent detergent	NovoSeven (Novo Nordisk, Inc.)	50,000

FDA, U.S. Food and Drug Administration; *vWF*, Von Willebrand factor.
Data from Kessler CM: Hemorrhagic disorders: coagulation factor deficiencies. In Goldman L, Ausiello D, editors: Cecil medicine, *ed 23, Philadelphia, 2008, Saunders.*

under the tongue and on the face, lips, perioral region, nasal mucosa, fingertips, toes, and trunk.[4] Recurrent epistaxis is a common finding in patients with this disorder; symptoms tend to worsen with age. Thus, the severity of the disorder often can be gauged by the age at which the nosebleeds begin, with the most severely affected patients experiencing recurrent epistaxis during childhood. Cutaneous changes usually begin at puberty and progress throughout life. Bleeding can occur in virtually every organ, with gastrointestinal, oral, and urogenital sites most commonly affected (Figure 25-5). In the gastrointestinal tract, the stomach and duodenum are more frequent sites of bleeding than is the colon. Other features may include hepatic and splenic arteriovenous shunts, as well as intracranial, aortic, and splenic aneurysms. Pulmonary arteriovenous fistulas are associated with oxygen desaturation, hemoptysis, hemothorax, brain abscess, and cerebral ischemia due to paradoxical emboli. Cirrhosis of the liver has been reported in some families.[4,15,16]

Laboratory Tests. There are no reliable laboratory tests to determine the tendency for bleeding to occur in affected persons. The Ivy bleeding time is not useful. Clinical findings and a history of bleeding problems are the only effective means to identify patients at risk.

Treatment. Therapy for HHT remains fragmented and problematic, consisting of laser treatment for cutaneous lesions; split-thickness skin grafting, embolization of arteriovenous communications, or hormonal therapy (estrogen or estrogens plus progesterone) for epistaxis; pulmonary resection or embolization for pulmonary arteriovenous malformations; and hormonal therapy and laser coagulation for gastrointestinal lesions.[4] Estrogen or progesterone treatment has been advised, but no benefit has been demonstrated in a placebo-controlled randomized trial.[15] A recent study suggested that treatment with thalidomide reduced the severity and frequency of nosebleeds (epistaxis) in subjects with HHT.[19]

The nasal vasculature pattern may help to predict the response to laser therapy versus septodermaplasty.

TABLE 25-4 FDA-Approved Coagulation Proteins and Replacement Therapies Available in the United States

Deficiency	Inheritance	Prevalence	Minimum Hemostatic Level	Replacement Source(s)
Factor I			50-100 mg	Cryoprecipitate/FFP
Afibrinogenemia	Autosomal R	Rare; <300 families		
Dysfibrogenemia	Autosomal D or R	Rare; >variants		
Factor II (prothrombin)	Autosomal D or R	Rare; 25 kindreds	30% normal	FFP, factor IX complex
Factor V (labile factor)	Autosomal R	1/1 million births	25% normal	FFP
Factor VII	Autosomal R	1/500,000 births	25% normal	Recombinant factor VIIa
Factor VIII (antihemophilic factor)	X-linked R	1/5000 births	25-30% for minor bleeds, 50% for serious bleeds, 80-100% for surgery or life-threatening bleeds	Factor VIII concentrates
von Willebrand disease				
Types 1 and 2	Autosomal D	1% prevalence	>50% vWF	Desmopressin
Type 3	Autosomal R	1/1 million births	>50% vWF	Factor VIII concentrate with vWF
Factor IX (Christmas factor)	X-linked R	1/30,000 births	25-50% normal	Factor IX complex concentrates
Factor X (Stuart-Prower factor)	Autosomal R	1/500,000 births	10-25% normal	FFP or factor IX complex concentrates
Factor XI (hemophilia C)	Autosomal D, severe type R	4% Ashkenazi Jews; 1/1 million in general population	20-40% normal	FFP or factor IX concentrate
Factor XII (Hageman factor)	Autosomal R	Not available	No treatment necessary	
Factor XIII (fibrin-stabilizing factor)	Autosomal R	1/3 million births	5% of normal	FFP, cryoprecipitate or virus-attenuated factor XIII concentrate

D, Dominant; *FDA,* U.S. Food and Drug Administration; *FFP,* Fresh frozen plasma; *R,* Recessive; *vWF,* von Willebrand factor.
From Kessler CM: Hemorrhagic disorders: coagulation factor deficiencies. In Goldman L, Ausiello D, editors: Cecil medicine, *ed 23, Philadelphia, 2008, Saunders.*

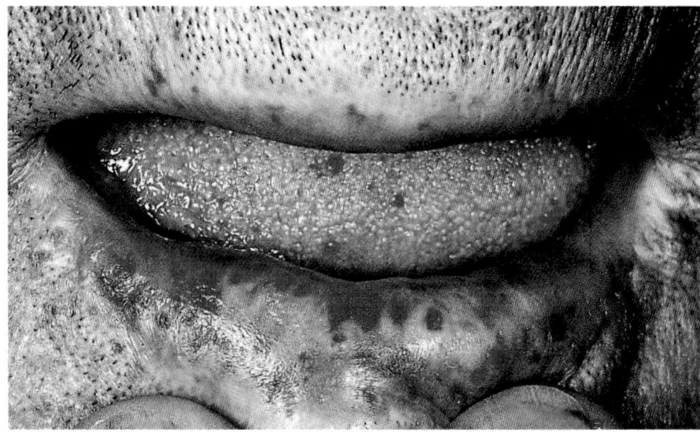

FIGURE 25-5 **Hereditary Haemorrhagic Telangiectasia (HHT).** HHT is a condition in which occult blood loss in the gut may lead to severe iron deficiency anemia. The diagnosis usually is clear from a careful clinical examination, although the telangiectases are not always as obvious, as in this patient with multiple lesions on the face, lip, and tongue. The patient had received multiple blood transfusions over many years because of HHT-associated gastrointestinal blood loss, and he had developed cirrhosis associated with hepatitis B antigen positivity—probably as a result of transmission of hepatitis B in transfused blood. *(From Forbes CD, Jackson WF:* Color atlas and text of clinical medicine, *ed 3, London, 2003, Mosby.)*

Resurfacing the nasomaxillary cavity with radial forearm fasciocutaneous free flaps has been reported to be effective in patients with refractory epistaxis. The antifibrinolytic agents aminocaproic acid and tranexamic acid have been reported to be beneficial in controlling hemorrhage, but negative results with antifibrinolytic therapy also have been reported. Improvement in lesions has been reported in cases using an antagonist to vascular endothelial growth factor and sirolimus and aspirin. Patients with gastrointestinal bleeding should receive supplemental iron and folate; red blood cell transfusions and parenteral iron may be required in some patients.[4,15,16]

Platelet Disorders

von Willebrand Disease. The most common inherited bleeding disorder is von Willebrand disease, which is caused by an inherited defect involving platelet adhesion. The vWF gene and protein and points of mutation are shown in Figure 25-6. The cause of platelet dysfunction in von Willebrand disease is a deficiency or a qualitative defect in vWF, which is made from a group of

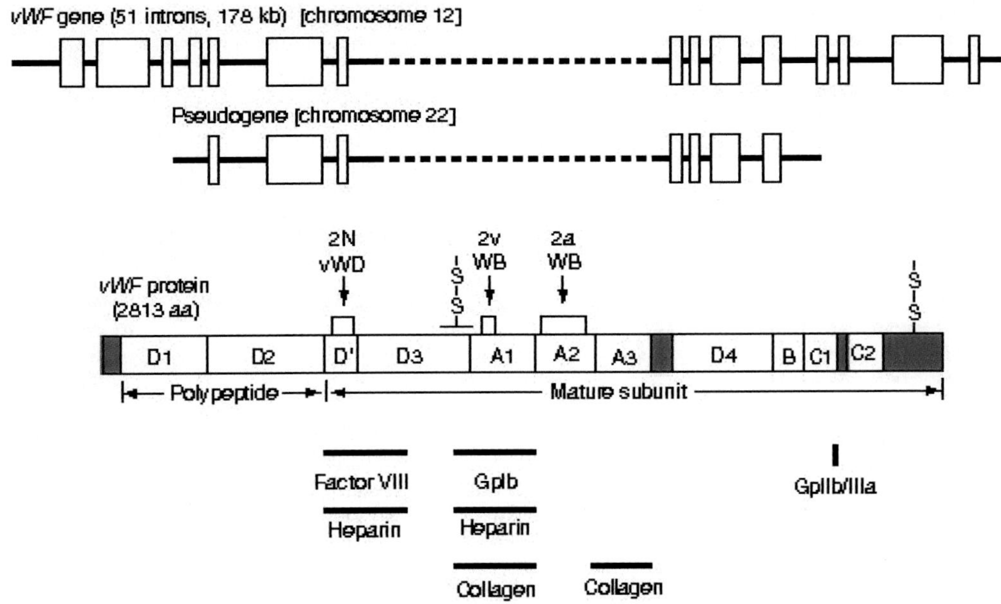

FIGURE 25-6 The structure of the *vWF* gene and protein. The structures of the *vWF* gene and pseudogene are indicated schematically at the top of the figure. The corresponding protein also is depicted, including the homologous repeat domain structure. The localization within *vWF* of point mutations associated with VWD variants also is indicated. *AA*, Amino acids; *vWD*, von Willebrand disease; *vWF*, von Willebrand factor. *(From Hoffman R, et al, editors:* Hematology: basic principles and practice, *ed 5, Philadelphia, 2009, Churchill Livingstone.)*

TABLE 25-5 Multimeric Patterns of von Willebrand Disease and Laboratory Diagnosis by Type

Type	Multimeric Pattern	Ristocetin Cofactor Activity	Factor VIII Activity	High-Molecular-Weight vWF Multimers	Ristocetin-Induced Platelet Aggregation
1 (classic)	Uniform reduced in all	Mildly decreased	Moderately decreased	Normal	Mildly decreased or normal
2A	Reduced in large and intermediate multimers	Moderately decreased	Mildly decreased or normal	Moderately decreased	Mildly decreased
2B	Reduced in large multimers	Moderately decreased	Mildly decreased or normal	Mildly decreased	Increased
2M	Mildly decreased or normal	Mildly decreased	Mildly decreased or normal	Normal	Mildly decreased
2N	Normal	Normal	Moderately decreased	Normal	Normal
3	Absent	Markedly decreased	Markedly decreased	Markedly decreased or absent	Markedly decreased

vWF, von Willebrand factor.
Data from Kessler CM: Hemorrhagic disorders: coagulation factor deficiencies. In Goldman L, Ausiello D, editors: Cecil medicine, *ed 23, Philadelphia, Saunders, 2008, pp 1301-1313; and Baz R, Mekhail T: Disorders of platelet function and number. In Carey WD, et al, editors:* Current clinical medicine 2009—Cleveland Clinic, *Philadelphia, 2009, Saunders.*

glycoproteins produced by megakaryocytes and endothelial cells. They are formed into a single monomer that polymerizes into huge complexes, which are needed to carry (bind) factor VIII and to allow platelets to adhere to surfaces. Unbound factor VIII is destroyed in the circulation.[2,7,10,11]

The disease has several variants, depending on the severity of genetic expression (Table 25-5). Most of the variants are transmitted as autosomal dominant traits (types 1 and 2). These variants of the disease tend to result in mild to moderate clinical bleeding problems. Type 1 is the most common form of von Willebrand disease. It accounts for about 70% to 80% of the cases. The greater the deficiency of vWF in type 1 disease, the more likely it is that signs and symptoms of hemophilia A will be found. Type 2A is responsible for 15% to 20% of cases. The other variants of the disease are uncommon.[6] Type 3, which is rare, is transmitted as an autosomal recessive trait that leads to severe deficiency of vWF and FVIII.[2,7,10,11] Variants of von Willebrand disease with a significant reduction in vWF or with a vWF that is unable to bind factor VIII may show signs and symptoms of hemophilia A, in addition to those associated with defective platelet adhesion. In mild cases, bleeding

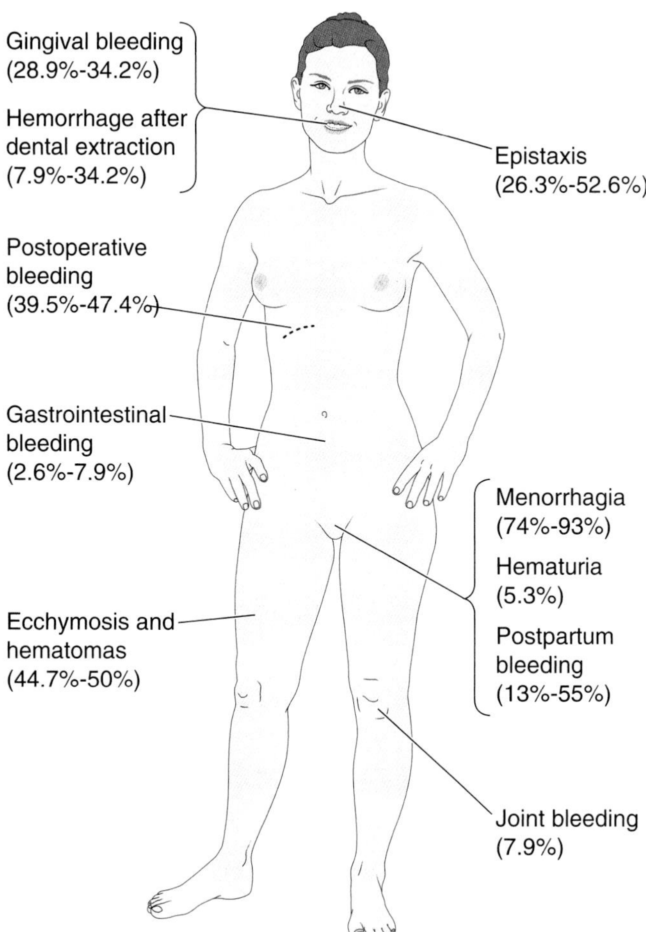

FIGURE 25-7 Clinical bleeding symptoms by type and frequency (%) in patients with type 1 von Willebrand disease. *(From Armstrong E, Konkle BA: von Willebrand disease. In Young NS, Gerson SL, High KA, editors:* Clinical hematology, *St. Louis, 2006, Mosby.)*

occurs only after surgery or trauma. In the more severe cases—type 2N and type 3—spontaneous epistaxis or oral mucosal bleeding may be noted.[2,7,10,11]

Clinical Findings. Mild variants of von Willebrand disease are characterized by a history of cutaneous and mucosal bleeding because platelet adhesion is lacking. In the more severe forms of the disease, in which factor VIII levels are low, hemarthroses and dissecting intramuscular hematomas are part of the clinical picture. Petechiae are rare in these patients. However, gastrointestinal bleeding, epistaxis, and menorrhagia are very common. Figure 25-7 shows the sites and frequency of bleeding in patients with type 1 von Willebrand disease. Serious bleeding can occur in these patients after trauma or surgical procedures. Patients with more severe forms of the disease may describe a family history of bleeding and also may report having had problems with bleeding after injury or surgery. Patients with mild forms of the disease may have a negative history for bleeding problems.

Laboratory Tests. Laboratory investigation is needed to make the diagnosis. Screening laboratory tests may show prolonged aPTT, normal or slightly reduced platelet count, normal PT, and normal TT. Additional laboratory tests are needed to establish the diagnosis and type of von Willebrand disease. These consist of ristocetin cofactor activity, ristocetin-induced platelet aggregation, immunoassay of vWF, multimeric analysis of vWF, and specific assays for factor VIII.[2,7,10,11]

Treatment. Treatment depends on the clinical condition of the patient and the type of von Willebrand disease that is diagnosed. Available treatment options include cryoprecipitate, factor VIII concentrates that retain HMW vWF multimers (Humate-P, Koate HS), and desmopressin (1-deamino-8-D-arginine vasopressin [DDAVP]). Before desmopressin is given, the patient must be tested for response to the agent as some patients are nonresponsive. Desmopressin can be given parenterally or by nasal spray 1 hour before surgery. With parenteral administration, the dose of desmopressin is 0.3 μg/kg of body weight, with a maximum dose of 20 to 24 μg. The nasal spray, Stimate, contains 1.5 mg/mL of desmopressin and is given at a dose of 300 mg/kg. Usually, one dose is sufficient. If a second dose is needed, it is given 8 to 24 hours after the first dose. Desmopressin should be used with caution in older patients with cardiovascular disease because of the potential risk of drug-induced thrombosis.[2,7,10,11]

Patients with type 1 von Willebrand disease are the best candidates for desmopressin therapy. Desmopressin treatment must not be started without previous testing to determine which variant form of von Willebrand disease is involved. It is not effective for type 3 and most variants of type 2 von Willebrand disease. These patients are treated with factor VIII replacement that retains the HMW (high molecular weight) vWF multimers (Humate-P or Koate HS). In patients with type 2 variants with qualitative defects in vWF, Humate-P or Koate HS supplies functional HMW vWF and factor VIII for those with decreased levels. In patients with type 3 von Willebrand disease, these replacement agents supply deficient materials, vWF, and factor VIII. Affected women are often given oral contraceptive agents to suppress menses and avoid excessive physiologic loss of blood.[2,7,10,11]

Other Hereditary Platelet Function Disorders. The two most common hereditary platelet function disorders (HPFDs), Bernard-Soulier syndrome and Glanzmann's thrombasthenia, are discussed in this chapter as examples of platelet function disorders. Other HPFDs include an abnormal alpha granule formation as in the gray platelet syndrome (with marrow myelofibrosis), and of organelle biogenesis in the Hermansky-Pudlak and Chédiak-Higashi syndromes where platelet dense body defects are linked to abnormalities of other lysosome-like organelles including melanosomes. Finally, defects involving surface receptors (P2Y[12], TPα) needed for activating stimuli, of proteins essential for signaling pathways (including Wiskott-Aldrich syndrome), and of platelet-derived procoagulant activity (Scott syndrome) can result in HPFDs.[20,21] The two most common HPFDs, Bernard-Soulier syndrome and Glanzmann's thrombasthenia, are discussed below.

Hereditary thrombocytopenia (HT) is very rare. Several conditions are classified as HT. These include Fechtner syndrome, Alport's syndrome, Sebastian platelet syndrome, and a syndrome consisting of HT, deafness and renal disease.[22-24] Owing to the rarity of these conditions, they are not covered in this book, and the reader is referred to standard hematology textbooks for more information regarding these disorders.

Bernard-Soulier Syndrome. Bernard-Soulier syndrome represents one of the more common hereditary disorders of platelet adhesion; in this disease, the platelets are large and defective and unable to interact with vWF.[25] In some cases the platelet count will be decreased and hence the tendency of some authors to classify the syndrome as an HT disorder.[24] The disease is caused by mutations in genes controlling the expression of the platelet glycoprotein Ib/IX complex.[26] The basic defect is the absence of glycoprotein Ib from the membrane of the platelet. Glycoprotein Ib appears to function as a receptor for vWF.[25,27-29]

Clinical Findings. Classic clinical findings in Bernard-Soulier syndrome include epistaxis, easy bruising, mucous membrane bleeding, perioperative bleeding and menorrhagia. Ecchymosis and gingival and gastrointestinal bleeding may occur. Bleeding may be intermittent and unpredictable.[29,30]

Laboratory Tests. Appropriate laboratory testing for the platelet-type bleeding disorders hinges on an adequate assessment by history and physical examination. Patients with a lifelong history of platelet-type bleeding symptoms and perhaps a positive family history of bleeding are appropriate for testing. For those patients thought to have an inherited disorder, testing for von Willebrand disease should be done initially because approximately 1% of the population has the disorder. The complete von Willebrand disease panel (factor VIII coagulant activity, vWf antigen, ristocetin cofactor activity) should be performed because many patients will have abnormalities of only one particular panel component.[2,3,14] If these studies are normal, platelet aggregation testing should be performed, ensuring that no antiplatelet medications have been ingested at least 1 week before testing.[2,3,14]

Platelet morphology can easily be evaluated to screen for two uncommon qualitative platelet disorders: Bernard-Soulier syndrome (associated with giant platelets) and gray platelet syndrome, a subtype of storage pool disorder in which platelet granulation is morphologically abnormal by light microscopy.[28] The lack of well-standardized test systems continue to make the diagnosis of platelet defects cumbersome for the practicing clinician. Patient history and description of clinical bleeding symptoms are essential.[29] Exclusion of von Willebrand disease, platelet count, and investigation of blood smears may provide a tentative diagnosis. Light transmission aggregometry is still considered the "gold standard" modality for assessing platelet function.[29,31] In summary, laboratory tests show a low platelet count, large platelets, faulty platelet adhesion, and poor aggregation with ristocetin.[3,29,31]

Treatment. Treatment of Bernard-Soulier syndrome generally is supportive, with platelet transfusions when absolutely necessary and avoidance of antiplatelet medications. Recombinant activated factor VII and desmopressin have been used in attempts to shorten bleeding times; however, no definitive studies regarding their effectiveness have been reported.[3,26,30,32]

Glanzmann's Thrombasthenia. Glanzmann's thrombasthenia is a rare autosomal recessive disease of platelet dysfunction. This disease is characterized by a deficiency or defect of the fibrinogen receptor (GPIIb/IIIa) on the platelet surface. The GPIIb/IIIa receptor has an essential function in the adhesion and aggregation of the platelets. The platelets of these patients cannot bind fibrinogen and aggregation does not occur.[33,34] These platelets can adhere to the subendothelium by means of vWF but not to fibrinogen. Bleeding in this condition is very unpredictable.[3,35,36]

Glanzmann's thrombasthenia occurs in high frequency in certain ethnic populations with an increased incidence of consanguinity such as in Indians, Iranians, Iraqi Jews, Palestinian and Jordanian Arabs, and French Gypsies. Carrier detection is important to control the disorder in family members. Carrier detection can be done by both protein analysis and direct gene analysis.[35]

Clinical Findings. The recurrent features of GT are epistaxis, easy bruising, oral and gingival hemorrhage, gastrointestinal bleeding, perioperative bleeding, hemarthrosis, and menorrhagia. Bleeding may be intermittent and unpredictable. Patients complain of bleeding from minor cuts and trauma.[29,35,37,38]

Laboratory Tests. The use of the laboratory in the diagnosis of GT is the same as described for Bernard-Soulier syndrome.

Treatment. Lifestyle advice and patient education programs, local measures, antifibrinolytic agents, hormone treatment, platelet transfusions, and recombinant activated factor VII are used to control bleeding.[34] Activated factor VII at a dose of 80 to 120 μg/kg has been reported to be effective in controlling bleeding after tonsillectomy and severe epistaxis refractory to platelet transfusion.[37,38]

Coagulation Disorders

Hemophilia A. The hemostatic abnormality in hemophilia A is caused by a deficiency or a defect of factor VIII. Factor VIII circulates in plasma bound to vWF. Unbound factor VIII is destroyed. Factor VIII was thought to be produced by endothelial cells and not by the liver, as most coagulation factors are. However, when disease was corrected by transplantation in several liver transplant recipients with hemophilia, it became clear that liver parenchymal cells also produce factor VIII.[39-41]

Hemophilia A is inherited as an X-linked recessive trait. The defective gene is located on the X chromosome (*F8* gene).[9] An affected man will not transmit the disease to his sons; however, all of his daughters will be carriers of the trait because they inherit his X chromosome. A female carrier will transmit the disorder to half of her sons and the carrier state to half of her daughters. Severity of bleeding varies from kindred to kindred. Within a given kindred, the clinical severity of the disorder is constant; for example, relatives of severe hemophiliacs are likely to be affected severely. The mutation rate for the responsible gene is unusually high (up to 30%), which explains why a rare condition such as hemophilia A does not die out after several generations. Because of the high mutation rate of the responsible gene, a negative family history is of limited value in excluding the possibility of hemophilia A.[1,9]

The assay of factor VIII activity can be used to identify female carriers of the trait. About 35% of carriers will show a decrease in factor VIII (about 50% of normal factor VIII levels). Other carriers may have normal levels of factor VIII. Immunoassays for vWF can greatly improve the detection rate among carriers of hemophilia A. Polymorphic DNA probes are now available that are capable of detecting 90% of affected families and 96% or more of carriers.[1,9]

Hemophilia A can manifest in women. This occurs in a mating between an affected male and a female carrier. One half of the daughters of such a mating would inherit two abnormal X chromosomes—one from the affected father and one from the carrier mother. These daughters would have homozygous hemophilia. In addition, hemophilia may occur in a minority of heterozygous carriers. Rare cases of hemophilia in females have been attributed to a newly mutant gene.[1,9]

Normal homeostasis requires at least 30% factor VIII activity. Symptomatic patients usually have factor VIII levels below 5%. Severe forms of the disease occur when the level is less than 1% of normal. Patients with levels between 1% and 5% have moderate disease. Those with factor VIII levels between 5% and 30% have a mild form of the disease. About 60% of cases of hemophilia are severe.[1,9]

Clinical Findings. Patients with severe hemophilia A bleed extensively from trivial injuries. However, the most characteristic bleeding manifestations associated with hemophilia A, such as hemarthrosis, often develop without significant trauma (Figure 25-8). The frequency and severity of bleeding problems in hemophiliac patients are generally related to the blood level of factor VIII. Patients with severe hemophilia (less than 1% of factor VIII) may experience severe, spontaneous bleeding. Hemarthrosis, ecchymoses, and soft tissue hematomas are common (Figures 25-9 and 25-10).

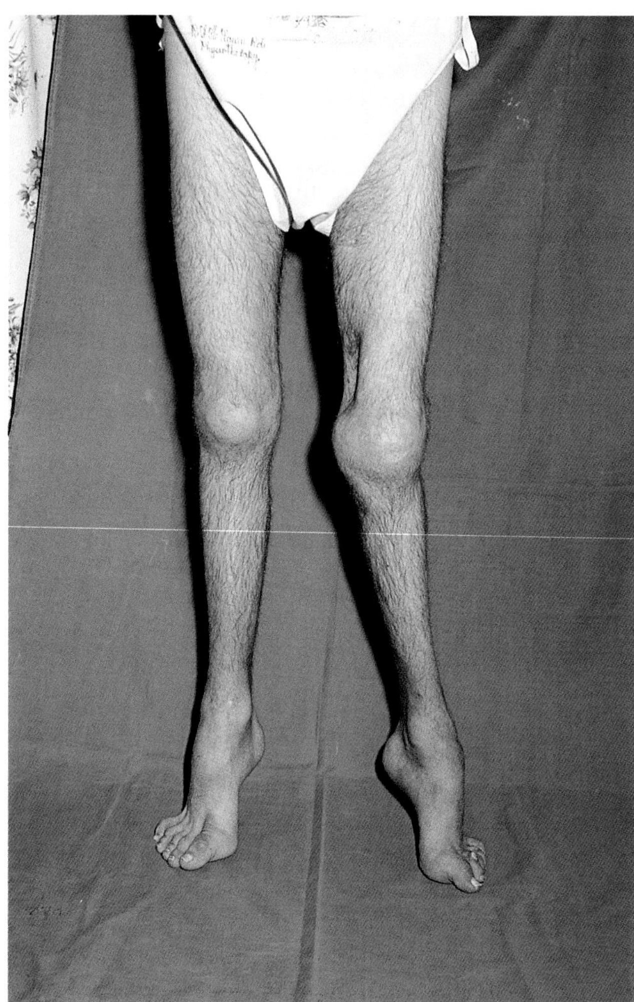

FIGURE 25-8 Hemarthrosis of the right knee in a patient with hemophilia. *(From Hoffbrand AV: Color atlas of clinical hematology, ed 3, St. Louis, 2000, Mosby.)*

Gastrointestinal and genitourinary bleeding also is common in severe hemophilia. Spontaneous bleeding from the mouth, gingivae, lips, tongue, and nose may occur in these patients. Those with moderate hemophilia (1% to 5% of factor VIII) exhibit moderate bleeding with minimal trauma or surgery. Hemarthrosis and soft tissue hematomas occur less often. Persons with mild hemophilia (5% to 30% of factor VIII) may experience mild bleeding after major trauma or surgery. Hemarthrosis and soft tissue hematomas are seldom found in these patients.[1,6,9]

Hemophiliac patients usually do not bleed abnormally from small cuts such as razor nicks. After larger injuries, however, bleeding out of proportion to the extent of injury is common. This bleeding may be massive and life-threatening, or it may persist as a slow, continuous oozing for days, weeks, or months. The onset of excessive bleeding usually is delayed. At the time of surgery or injury, hemostasis appears to be normal. Bleeding of sudden onset and serious proportions may develop several hours or even several days later. Venipuncture, if

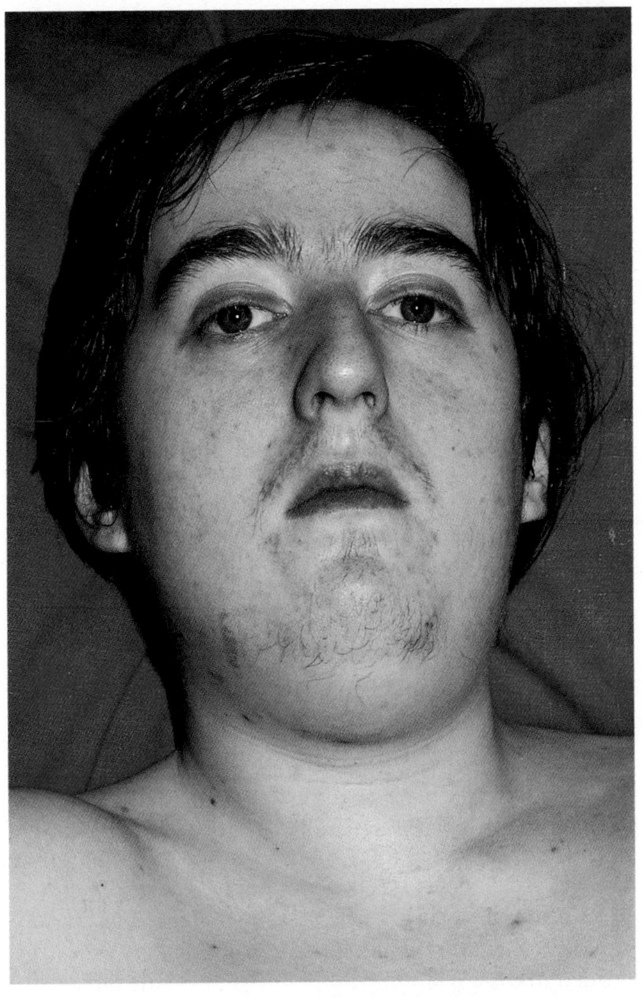

A

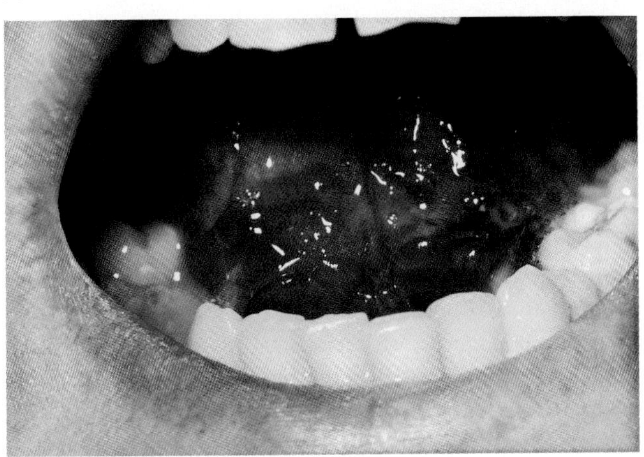

B

FIGURE 25-9 **A,** The swelling in the submandibular region in a patient with hemophilia was caused by bleeding after intraoral trauma. **B,** The floor of the mouth has been elevated because of the bleeding. *(From Hoffbrand AV:* Color atlas of clinical hematology, *ed 3, St. Louis, 2000, Mosby.)*

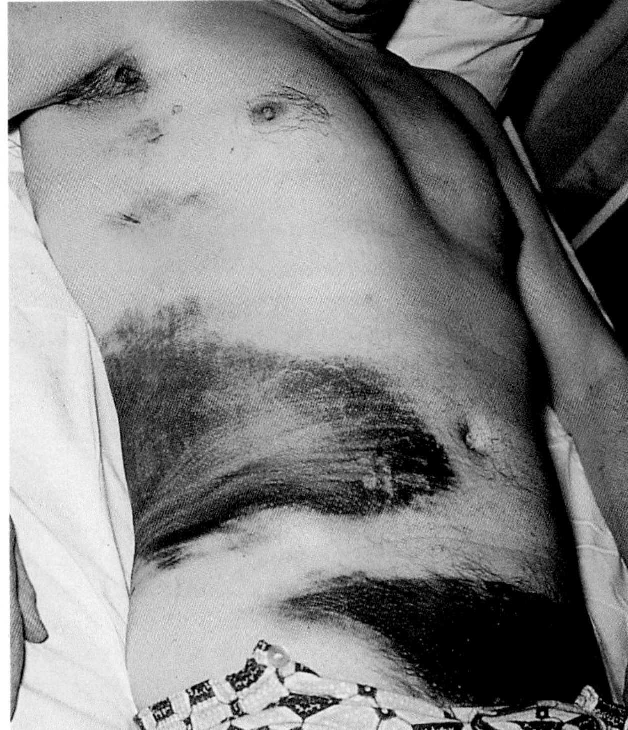

FIGURE 25-10 **Massive Hematomas in a Patient with Hemophilia.** In the absence of major trauma, hematomas of this size always indicate a severe coagulation abnormality. Possible causes include hemophilia, Christmas disease, von Willebrand disease, and uncontrolled anticoagulant therapy. Internal bleeding is a common accompaniment, and patients require urgent investigation and treatment. *(From Forbes CD, Jackson WF:* Color atlas and text of clinical medicine, *ed 3, London, 2003, Mosby.)*

skillfully performed, is of no danger to the hemophiliac patient because of the elasticity of the venous walls.[42]

Laboratory Tests. Screening tests that show prolonged aPTT, normal PT, and normal platelet count (except in some cases of von Willebrand disease) indicate a problem in the intrinsic pathway. The next step is to mix (mixing tests) the patient's blood with a sample of pooled plasma and repeat the aPTT. If this test is normal, then the specific missing factor is identified by specific assays. If the mixing test is abnormal, tests for inhibitor activity (antibodies to the factor) are performed.[1,6,9]

Prognosis. The long-term survival of hemophiliac patients has been greatly affected by contamination of donated blood with human immunodeficiency virus (HIV) and hepatitis C virus (HCV). HIV has tripled the death rate in hemophiliac patients and currently is responsible for more than 55% of all deaths related to hemophilia.[6] By contrast, the lifetime risk of death from intracranial hemorrhage is 2% to 8%. More than 75% of adults with hemophilia A and 45% of adults with hemophilia B are HIV-positive. The anti-HIV protease inhibitors result in prolonged HIV disease survival among this group of patients. With the exception of HIV and HCV infection, life expectancy is related to the severity of hemophilia, and the mortality rate is four to six times higher for severe disease than for mild to moderate disease. The mortality rate among patients with inhibitors is much greater than among those without inhibitors.[6]

Replacement Factors. Factor VIII replacement guidelines for the control of bleeding from trauma or surgical procedures in patients with severe hemophilia are as follows. For minor spontaneous bleeding or minor traumatic bleeding, 25% to 30% replacement of factor VIII is required. For treatment or prevention of severe bleeding during procedures such as major dental surgery or maintenance replacement therapy after major surgery, 50% replacement or greater is needed. Treatment of life-threatening bleeding and limb-threatening bleeding during major surgery requires 80% to 100% replacement of factor VIII.[1,6,9]

The choice of which type of factor concentrate should be used is based on specific findings from the patient's management history and infectious disease exposure (see Table 25-3). The efficacy of replacement preparations, whether recombinant or plasma derived, is the same. Recombinant factor VIII concentrates are recommended for all patients with no history of factor concentrate treatment, for those who have received concentrates but are HCV and HIV seronegative, and after surgery or trauma for those with mild or moderate hemophilia that does not respond sufficiently to desmopressin therapy. Plasma-derived concentrates are recommended for patients who are HCV- and HIV-seropositive. High-purity products are preferred in regimens for immune tolerance induction and prophylaxis.[1,6,9]

Hemophiliacs without Inhibitors. All types of general surgical procedures can now be performed in patients without inducible inhibitors of factor VIII (inhibitors are antibodies to factor VIII that result from previous contact with factor VIII replacement). The expected rate of postoperative bleeding problems is 6% to 23%; with orthopedic surgery on the knee, this rate increases to 40%. Patients with mild deficiency of factor VIII often undergo surgical procedures when desmopressin (1-deamino-8-D-arginine [DDAVP], also called vasopressin) is used alone or in combination with ε-aminocaproic acid (aminocaproic acid). Desmopressin, which transiently increases the factor VIII level, can be given parenterally at a dose of 0.3 mg/kg or at an intranasal dose of 300 mg/kg. A second dose can be given if needed 8 to 24 hours after the first dose.[1,13,43,44]

Aminocaproic acid is a potent antifibrinolytic agent that can inhibit plasminogen activators present in oral secretions and stabilize clot formation in oral tissue. Patients with more severe anti–hemophilic factor (AHF) deficiency require factor VIII replacement. Aminocaproic acid also is given to patients who are receiving factor replacement. Aspirin, aspirin-containing drugs, and other NSAIDs, which impair platelet function and may cause severe bleeding, must not be used. Factor VIIa, a newer recombinant product, is now used in some patients with severe hemophilia A with inducible inhibitors.[1,13,43,44]

Hemophiliac Patients with Inhibitors. A complication that poses great difficulties in the management of patients with hemophilia is the appearance of factor VIII inhibitors. These inhibitors are usually immunoglobulin G (IgG) antibodies to factor VIII. Factor VIII inhibitors (antibodies) develop in patients who have received multiple factor VIII replacement therapy. About 5% to 10% of patients with hemophilia have factor VIII inhibitors. The increasing use of factor VIII concentrates increases the risk for development of factor VIII inhibitors; 20% to 30% of severe hemophiliac patients are affected. Patients who have low inhibitor levels of 5 Bethesda units (BU) or less that do not rise with further use of factor VIII concentrates are identified as *low responders.* About 40% of hemophiliac patients with inhibitors are low responders. Hemophiliac patients whose inhibitor levels rise with additional contact with factor VIII concentrates are called *high responders*; this situation is found in about 60% of hemophiliac patients with inhibitors. The medical management of hemophiliac patients is determined by the absence of inhibitors and low or high responder status. Patients who are most difficult to manage are high responders.[6,45]

Low responders with minor bleeding can be treated with human factor VIII concentrates. The dosage for these patients is larger than for those without inhibitors. Major bleeding in low responders is treated with human factor VIII concentrates but at a higher dosage and given by continuous infusion after an initial large bolus. Activated prothrombin complex concentrates may be used if needed in this group of patients. Also, porcine factor VIII can be used if low levels of cross-reactivity with this agent occur. For surgical or invasive procedures in low responders, any of these treatments may be used.

With the development of recombinant activated factor VIIa (NovoSeven), which was initiated in 1986 by Novo Nordisk (Bagsvaerd, Denmark) and first licensed in Europe in 1996 and the United States in 1999, an effective treatment became available for the management of hemophiliacs who are high responders.[46-48] Bleeding in high responders with a low level of inhibitor titers who are undergoing immune tolerance therapy can be treated with human factor VIII concentrates. Those with high anti–human factor VIII titers, but with low anti–porcine factor VIII titers can be treated with porcine factor VIII. High responders with high titers to both human and porcine factor VIII are treated for bleeding with factor VIIa concentrates. Factor VIIa is also used for surgery or invasive procedures in this group of patients.[6,45]

Hemophilia B. In hemophilia B (Christmas disease), factor IX is deficient or defective. Hemophilia B is inherited as an X-linked recessive trait (*F9* gene).[9] Factor IX levels below 10% have been reported in a few women. Similar to hemophilia A, the disorder manifests primarily in males. Severe disease, in which affected patients have less than 1% of normal amounts of factor IX, is less common than in hemophilia A. Clinical manifestations of the two disorders are identical. Screening laboratory test results are similar for both diseases. Specific factor assays for factor IX establish the diagnosis. Purified factor IX products (see Table 25-3) are recommended for the treatment of minor and major bleeding. Recombinant factor IX is now available for clinical use.[6,45]

Gene Therapy. Hemophilia A and B are model diseases for gene therapy, because they are caused by specific, well-defined gene mutations.[6] A number of gene therapy studies have been initiated in the United States.[49-51] These studies have been designed to prove that patients with hemophilia A or hemophilia B can benefit from this form of treatment.[39,52] Problems with vector safety, vector immune response, and inhibitor antibody formation have not yet been solved, however, and optimal levels of transgene expression have yet to be determined.[1,6]

Other Genetic Clotting Factor Deficiencies. Congenital deficiency of prothrombin occurs rarely. Factor V deficiency also is rare; only about 1 case per 1 million people is reported.[1] Factor VII, which is inherited as an autosomal recessive trait, affects males and females equally; incidence is about 1 in 500,000.[1] Factor X deficiency also is found in about 1 in 500,000 persons.[1] Factor XI deficiency most often occurs in Ashkenazi Jews but also is seen in non-Jewish populations. Subjects with a deficiency of factor XII, prekallikrein, or high-molecular-weight kininogen do not have clinical bleeding problems but do have prolonged aPTT. Another very rare clotting deficiency with significant bleeding problems involves factor XIII; this has been described in just over 100 clinical cases. PT and aPTT test results are normal in these patients.[53]

Another small group of patients with a history of significant bleeding problems will have negative test results when screened by means of currently recommended methods. It appears that current methods are unable to reveal whatever disorder these patients may have. A clear-cut history of prolonged bleeding after trauma or surgical procedures is always more significant than negative laboratory data.[4,6,9,13]

Three known defects in the coagulation system do not affect PT, aPTT, or TT. These are very rare and include factor XIII deficiency, α_2 plasmin inhibitor deficiency, and PAI-1 deficiency (major inhibitor of plasminogen activators). Patients with a strong clinical history of bleeding and normal coagulation test results (PT, aPTT, and TT) require additional testing, such as the use of 5M urea.[1,9,54]

Risk of Infection with Replacement Products

The use of cryoprecipitates, some factor VIII concentrates, and fresh frozen plasma carries several important risks. For example, transmission of hepatitis B virus (HBV), HCV, and HIV may occur.[42]

In the 1980s, more than 90% of multiply-transfused hemophiliac patients became HIV-positive, with the subsequent development of acquired immunodeficiency syndrome (AIDS). Many of these patients have died from the disease. The advent of sterile concentrates, together with rigid donor testing begun in 1985, and the availability of recombinant products have greatly reduced the risk of HIV infection through blood product administration. AIDS cases associated with hemophilia B has been less common, probably because of the rarity of this condition. A look at hemophilia mortality from 1900 to 1990 reveals the terrible impact of HIV infection. Survival increased from 1970, when factor VIII replacement first became available, to 1980, with a median life expectancy of 68 years. From 1980 to 1990, this decreased to 49 years. Most of this effect was caused by infection with HIV from contaminated blood products.[42]

During the 1970s and 1980s, more than 90% of patients treated with plasma-derived clotting factor concentrates became infected with HCV. This exposure rate has been greatly reduced on the basis of donor screening for HCV antibodies since the later 1980s, viral inactivation procedures started in 1985, and the use of ultrapure concentrates. As a result of the earlier contaminated blood pool, however, more than 80% of adult hemophiliac patients are infected with HCV. More than 25% of adult hemophiliac patients have biopsy-demonstrated cirrhosis, and HCV infection is the second leading cause of death in this population. Coinfection with HIV increases the risk for liver failure.[1,39,41]

Transmission of other infectious agents in blood products has occurred in the past. These agents have included various hepatitis viruses (HAV, HBV, HDV, and HGV) and parvovirus B19. Because of screening procedures and viral inactivation procedures, the hepatitis viruses (A, B, D, and G) have not been a major concern since 1985. Many hemophiliac patients who received multiple concentrate replacements before 1985 were infected with HBV. However, the rate of chronic infection was about 5% to 10%, and liver failure occurred late in some of these patients. Evidence of parvovirus B19 infection is found in 1 of every 1000 blood donors. About 80% of adult hemophiliac patients show evidence of infection with parvovirus B19, which occurs even in those who are given viral attenuated products.[1,39,41]

The long-term consequences of parvovirus B19 infection in hemophilia are not established. To date, parvovirus B19, a non–lipid-enveloped virus, has been resistant to inactivation by all available heating and solvent-detergent techniques, used alone or in combination, in the manufacture of concentrates. Adjunctive nanofiltration steps have been implemented for additional viral depletion. Of concern to many physicians who care for patients with hemophilia is the fact that parvovirus B19 is representative of other non–lipid-enveloped viral pathogens (known or unknown) that might contaminate plasma-derived concentrates. These concerns have served as the rationale for administering only recombinant factor VIII or factor IX to parvovirus B19-seronegative patients, previously untreated hemophiliacs, or pregnant carriers.[1]

Screening of blood donors, viral inactivation procedures, preparation of ultrapure concentrates, and the advent of porcine factor VIII have eliminated or greatly reduced the risk of infection in hemophiliac patients with HIV, HCV, HBV, HGV, and other agents.[1,39,41]

Congenital Hypercoagulability

Many patients with venous thromboembolism have an inherited basis for hypercoagulability. The initial episode of venous thromboembolism usually occurs in early adulthood, but onset may be at any time from early childhood to old age. Arterial thrombosis is unusual in patients with inherited hypercoagulable states. Primary hypercoagulable states result from a deficiency of antithrombotic factors (antithrombin III, protein C or protein S) or increased prothrombotic factors (factor Va [activated protein C resistance, factor V Leiden]: prothrombin [prothrombin G20210A mutation]; factors VII, XI, IX, VIII: von Willebrand factor; fibrinogen; and hyperchomocysteinemia) (Figure 25-11).[55,56]

Inherited quantitative or qualitative deficiency of *antithrombin III* leads to increased fibrin accumulation and a lifelong propensity to thrombosis. Antithrombin is the major physiologic inhibitor of thrombin and other activated coagulation factors; therefore, its deficiency leads to unregulated protease activity and fibrin formation. The frequency of asymptomatic heterozygous antithrombin deficiency in the general population may be 1 in 350. Most of the affected persons have clinically silent mutations and never have thrombotic manifestations. The frequency of symptomatic antithrombin deficiency in the general population has been estimated to be between 1 in 2000 and 1 in 5000. Among all patients seen with venous thromboembolism, antithrombin deficiency is detected in only about 1%.[55]

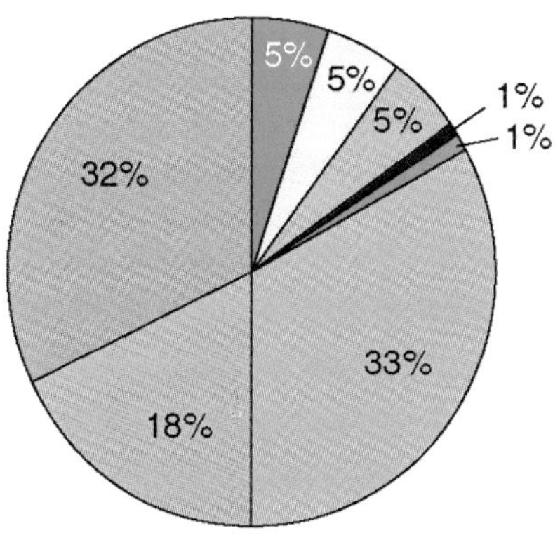

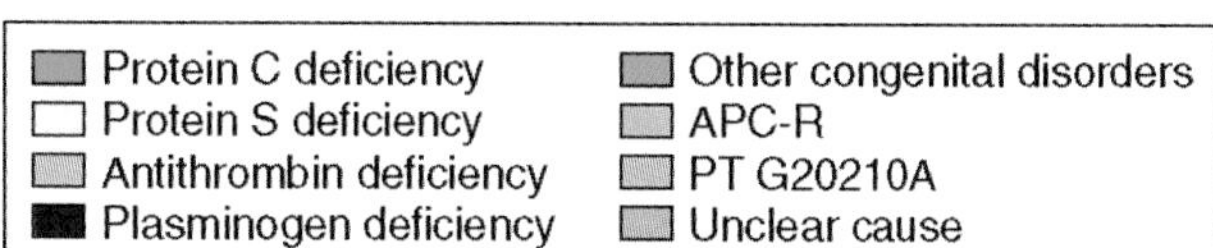

FIGURE 25-11 Results of testing for congenital hypercoagulable states projected for patients who had experienced idiopathic deep venous thrombosis in 2003. *APC-R,* Activated protein C resistance; *PT G20210A,* Prothrombin G20210A mutation. *(From Deitcher SR: Hypercoagulable states. In Carey WD, et al, editors:* Cleveland Clinic's current clinical medicine, *ed 2, Philadelphia, 2010, Saunders.)*

Protein C deficiency leads to unregulated fibrin generation because of impaired inactivation of factors VIIIa and Va, two essential cofactors in the coagulation cascade. The prevalence of heterozygous protein C deficiency in the general population is about 1 per 200 to 500. Protein C deficiency is found in 3% to 4% of all patients with venous thromboembolism.[55]

Protein S is the principal cofactor of activated protein C (APC), and its deficiency mimics that of protein C in causing loss of regulation of fibrin generation by impaired inactivation of factors VIIIa and Va. The prevalence of protein S deficiency in the general population is unknown. Its frequency in all patients evaluated for venous thromboembolism (2% to 3%) is comparable, however, to that of protein C deficiency.[55]

The *factor V Leiden* mutation (activated protein C resistance) is remarkably frequent (3% to 7%) in healthy white populations but is far less prevalent in certain black and Asian populations. In various studies, activated protein C resistance was found in a wide range of frequencies (10% to 64%) among patients with venous thromboembolism.[55,56]

The substitution of G for A at nucleotide 20210 of the prothrombin gene has been associated with elevated plasma levels of prothrombin and an increased risk for venous thrombosis. The allele frequency for this gain-of-function mutation is 1% to 6% in white populations, but it is much less prevalent in other racial groups. The *prothrombin G20210A mutation* is found in 6% to 8% of all patients with venous thromboembolism.[55,56]

The laboratory diagnosis of the primary hypercoagulable states requires testing for each of the disorders individually because no general screening test is available to determine whether a patient may have such a condition. At this time, functional, immunologic, or DNA-based assays are available to test for antithrombin deficiency, protein C deficiency, protein S deficiency, APC resistance (factor V Leiden), and the prothrombin G20210A mutation.[55,56]

More detailed information on the diagnosis and medical management of patients with primary hypercoagulable states is available in standard medicine and hematology textbooks. In general, any needed dental treatment can be provided for these patients.

DENTAL MANAGEMENT

Patient Identification

The four methods by which the dentist can identify the patient who may have a bleeding problem are a good history, careful physical examination, screening laboratory tests, and occurrence of excessive bleeding after a surgical or invasive dental procedure. These are described in detail in Chapter 24.

History and Symptoms

Patients with severe coagulation disorders may have dramatic abnormal bleeding histories but often do not volunteer this information unless asked. A history of spontaneous hemarthroses and muscle hemorrhages is highly suggestive of severe hemophilia. By contrast, epistaxis, gingival bleeding, and menorrhagia are reported found in patients with thrombocytopenia, platelet disorders, or von Willebrand disease.[4] Several hemorrhagic symptoms are more specific for certain disorders—for example, a history of prolonged bleeding after extraction of teeth is more suggestive of von Willebrand disease or platelet disorders than of hemophilia. Patients with a history of bruising and bleeding but with normal results on coagulation tests and normal platelet counts may be afflicted with blood vessel diseases such as HHT, Cushing's disease, scurvy, Ehlers-Danlos syndrome, or other similar conditions.[4] Dermatologic disorders must be considered in patients whose hemorrhagic symptoms are confined to the skin.

The history should include questions on six topics: bleeding problems in relatives; excessive bleeding after operations, surgical procedures, and tooth extractions; excessive bleeding after trauma; use of drugs for prevention of coagulation or chronic pain; past and present illness; and occurrence of spontaneous bleeding. These topics, with the exception of bleeding problems in relatives, are covered in Chapter 24.

Bleeding Problems in Relatives

Male offspring of parents with a family history of hemophilia are at risk for the disease. Hemophilia is very rare in females but can occur when a male with hemophilia marries a female carrier and they have female children, half of whom will have hemophilia. Children of a parent with von Willebrand disease type 1, also are at risk; about 33% of them will inherit the disorder. Children of parents with a hereditary disorder of connective tissue or hereditary hemorrhagic telangiectasia are at risk for a bleeding disorder. In rare cases of a family history of disorders of platelet function, such as Bernard-Soulier syndrome or Glanzmann's thrombasthenia, the bleeding disorder may be passed to offspring.

The most meaningful data are reported as a recent negative or positive history of excessive bleeding after a major hemostatic challenge. With a negative history, the patient is not a bleeder. By contrast, the patient with a positive history is a bleeder. A negative history of bleeding after minor insults in a patient with a mild bleeding diathesis does not rule out a problem with more severe surgical or traumatic events. Thus, the more recent and severe the surgical or traumatic event, the more accurate it will be in revealing the presence of a bleeding disorder.

Physical Examination

The dentist should inspect the exposed skin and mucosa of the oral cavity and pharynx of the patient for signs that might indicate a possible bleeding disorder. These include petechiae, ecchymoses (bruises), spider angioma, telangiectasias, jaundice, pallor, and cyanosis (possible thrombocytopenia). When any of these signs are found by the dentist and cannot be explained by the history or other clinical findings, the patient should be referred for medial evaluation.

Screening Laboratory Tests

The dentist can use four clinical laboratory tests to screen patients for congenital bleeding disorders: platelet count, aPTT, PT, and TT. The platelet count is ordered to screen for thrombocytopenia. The aPTT test is used to measure the status of the intrinsic and common pathways of coagulation. This test reflects the ability of blood remaining within vessels in the area of injury to coagulate. It will be prolonged in coagulation disorders affecting the intrinsic and common pathways (hemophilia, liver disease) and in cases of excessive fibrinolysis.

If positive, the results of these screening tests direct the hematologist to the possible source of a bleeding disorder and allow for the selection of more specific tests to identify the nature of the defect.

Medical Considerations

No surgical procedures should be performed on a patient who is suspected of having a bleeding problem on the basis of history and physical examination findings. Such a patient should be screened by the dentist through appropriate clinical laboratory tests or should be referred to a hematologist for screening. Patients screened by the dentist with abnormal test results should be referred to a hematologist for diagnosis, treatment, and management recommendations. Patients under medical care who may have a bleeding problem should not receive dental treatment until consultation with the patient's physician has taken place, and after appropriate preparations have been made to avoid excessive bleeding after dental procedures.

Management of the Patient with a Serious Bleeding Disorder

Dental treatment of patients with hemophilia A and with von Willebrand disease is used here to show how patients with a serious congential bleeding disorder can be managed to avoid significant bleeding complications.

Before any dental treatment is performed for a patient with a bleeding disorder, the dentist must consult with the patient's physician to determine the severity of the disorder and the need for special preparations for dental treatment. Patients with significant bleeding disorders are at increased risk for spontaneous gingival bleeding or excessive bleeding after minor trauma to the oral tissues. The risk of such problems will be even greater if surgical procedures are performed without special preparations.

Hemophilia. Hemophilia A (factor VIII deficiency) can be used to illustrate some of the management problems involved in dealing with a serious coagulation disorder. When a patient with this medical diagnosis (or with a clinical history suggestive of the disorder) presents for dental treatment, consultation with a hematologist is essential. The hematologist first establishes the diagnosis and determines the degree of factor VIII deficiency, whether any factor VIII inhibitors are present, if the patient is a low or a high responder, and whether hospitalization will be needed. The type of replacement material is selected (Box 25-2; see also Table 25-3), and the hematologist determines the dosage of replacement material that should be used.[1,13]

Patients with severe hemophilia A exhibit signs and symptoms at a very early age. It is important that preventive dentistry practices be initiated early and maintained through adulthood for all hemophiliac patients. Dental caries and periodontal disease should be minimized in these patients. The use of fluorides and fissure sealants and dietary recommendations regarding refined carbohydrate restriction are important for minimizing tooth loss.

BOX 25-2 Dental Management of Patients with Hemophilia

P

Patient Evaluation/Risk Assessment (see Box 1-1)

- Evaluate and determine whether a bleeding disorder (e.g., hemophilia) exists.
- Obtain medical consultation if undiagnosed, poorly controlled, or if uncertain. Screen patients with bleeding history or clinical signs of a bleeding disorder with PT, PTT, TT, and platelet count.

Potential Issues/Factors of Concern

A	
Analgesics	Avoid aspirin, aspirin-containing compounds, and other NSAIDs; acetaminophen with or without codeine is suggested for most patients.
Antibiotics	Not indicated unless acute infection is present.
Anesthesia	Avoid block anesthetic injections in patients not on desmopressin, aminocaproic acid, and/or factor concentrates.
Anxiety	No issues.
Allergy	Patients placed on factor VIII replacement need to be observed for signs and symptoms of allergy.
B	
Bleeding	These patients are at great risk of bleeding from invasive dental procedures. Special precautions must be taken before invasive procedures. Patients with mild to moderate hemophilia can be managed using desmopressin and aminocaproic acid for many dental procedures. Factor VIII replacement is needed for patients with more severe hemophilia. Patients who are low responders for inhibitors (antibody response to factor VIII) will require higher doses of factor VIII. Patients who are high responders are most difficult to manage and will require activated factor VII, porcine factor VIII, steroids, or other special preparations such as prothrombin complex concentrates or activated prothrombin complex concentrations.
Breathing	No issues.
Blood pressure	No issues.
C	
Chair position	No issues.
Cardiovascular	No issues.
Consultation	The patient's hematologist must be consulted before any invasive dental procedures being performed. The severity of the disease must be established. The presence of inhibitors and the level of response to FVIII need to be determined. Determine if the patient can be managed with desmopressin and aminocaproic acid. Establish the type and dosage of factor replacement needed for invasive dental procedures or surgery. Determine if the patient can be managed in the dental office or will require hospitalization.
D	
Devices	Splints may be constructed before multiple extractions or surgical procedures in patients with severe hemophilia.
Drugs	Avoid all drugs that may cause bleeding, such as aspirin and other NSAIDs, certain herbal medications, and over-the-counter drugs containing aspirin.
E	
Equipment	No issues.
Emergencies	Excessive bleeding may occur after invasive dental procedures or surgery. Systemic and local means may be required to control the bleeding (see Tables 25-3 and 25-6). Allergic reactions may occur in patients receiving factor replacement.
F	
Follow-up	Patients should be seen and examined for signs of allergy or bleeding within 24 to 48 hours after surgical procedures

NSAIDs, Nonsteroidal antiinflammatory drugs.

Toothbrushing, flossing, and regular dental visits, including cleaning of the teeth, are important for prevention of caries and periodontal disease, which should be treated when detected. Through maintenance of good oral hygiene and dental repair, the need for dental procedures requiring factor VIII replacement can be minimized.

In general, block anesthesia, lingual infiltrations, or injections into the floor of the mouth, and intramuscular injections must be avoided unless appropriate replacement factors have been used in patients with moderate to severe factor VIII deficiency. Complex restorative procedures usually require replacement therapy.

Infiltration anesthesia and intraligamentary injections usually can be given without replacement therapy. Simple restorative procedures often can be performed without replacement therapy, as can endodontic treatment of nonvital teeth. However, overinstrumentation and overfilling must be avoided. Some experts recommend topical application of 10% cocaine to exposed pulp when a pulpectomy is performed. Intracanal injection of a local anesthetic along with epinephrine will help to control bleeding. Topical application of 1:1000 epinephrine with paper points also will help to control bleeding until the pulp has been removed.[57]

Orthodontic treatment can be provided to hemophiliac patients, but sharp edges on appliances must be avoided. Sharp edges can injure the mucosa, causing significant bleeding in patients with severe to moderate hemophilia.

Periodontal surgery, root planning, extractions, dentoalveolar surgery, soft tissue surgery, and complex oral surgery usually require factor replacement in patients with moderate to severe factor VIII deficiency. When mucoperiosteal flaps are required in the mandibular region, the buccal or labial approach is suggested. Also, the buccal approach is recommended for surgical removal of mandibular third molars. Trauma to mandibular lingual tissues increases the risk of bleeding, which can lead to airway obstruction. Mandibular acrylic splints are not used as often as they were in the past because of problems with tissue trauma and infection.[57] If local bleeding occurs, one or more of the procedures listed in Table 25-6 can be used to control it.

Conservative periodontal procedures, including polishing with a prophy cup and supragingival calculus removal, often can be performed without replacement therapy, so long as injury to the gingival tissues is avoided. In children, primary teeth should be removed soon after they become loose. Patients with mild factor VIII deficiency and no inhibitors often can be managed in the dental office for less invasive procedures such as scaling, soft tissue surgery, and extractions without factor VIII replacement; desmopressin and Aminocaproic acid or tranexamic acid may be used. Patients with moderate factor VIII deficiency without inhibitors may require factor VIII replacement for less invasive dental procedures. Patients with moderate hemophilia and no inhibitors will require factor VIII replacement for major oral surgery. Patients with severe hemophilia will require factor VIII replacement for all invasive dental treatments.[1,13,57] One or more of the local procedures listed in Table 25-6 can be used as adjuncts to aid in the control of bleeding.

Tranexamic acid can be administered orally, IV, or as a mouth wash. Oral Cyklokapron (tablet) was approved for use by the FDA in 1986 and later was discontinued. In 2009 the FDA approved oral tranexamic acid tablets (Lysteda, Ferring Pharmaceuticals, Saint-Prex, Switzerland) for use in patients with heavy menstrual bleeding. An intravenous form of tranexamic acid, Cyklokapron (IV), (Pfizer, New York), has been approved for use in the United States. Tranexamic acid preparations originally were approved for use in hemophilia to reduce or prevent hemorrhage during or after tooth extraction and to control heavy menstrual bleeding. However, tranexamic acid is now used to control bleeding in a number of situations. Care must be taken with use of this drug because of the risk for thrombotic events, particularly in older patients and with long-term use.[2,58]

Cyklokapron (IV), 10 mg/kg, is given just before the surgical procedure and then three times per day as needed. It is supplied in 100-mg vials. Lysteda comes in 500-mg tablets, 25 mg/kg, and is given just before the surgery and then three to four times per day as needed. The dentist can request the pharmacy to prepare a 5% solution of tranexamic acid to be used as a mouth wash. The patient is instructed to take 5 mL of the solution and hold in the mouth for 2 minutes and then spit it out. The first dose should be taken just before the procedure and repeated four times per day as needed.[13,58,59]

Hemophiliac patients with inhibitors who are low responders usually will require factor VIII replacement for any invasive dental procedure. Human, porcine, or ultrapure factor VIII replacements may be used, depending on the clinical situation. Hemophiliac patients who are high responders will require factor VIIa concentrate for all invasive dental procedures.

Hemophiliac patients who have undergone invasive dental procedures should be seen within 24 to 48 hours by the dentist to check on control of bleeding. If bleeding is occurring, the hematologist may have to give additional factor VIII replacement concentrates, and/or the dentist may need to apply one or more of the local procedures listed in Table 25-6. Patients who have received factor VIII replacements also must be examined within 24 to 48 hours after surgery for any evidence of an allergic reaction to the concentrates, and to determine whether the wound is healing without complications.

Before surgery, the dentist can make splints, so that mechanical displacement of the clot in wounds healing by secondary intention is prevented. Care should be taken in the construction of the splints so that pressure is not placed on soft tissues; such pressure could lead to tissue injury, bleeding, and infection. For these reasons,

TABLE 25-6 Topical Hemostatic Agents Used to Control Bleeding

Product	Company/ Dealer	Description	Indications and Features
Gauze		2 × 2 inch sterile gauze pads—placed over the wound, with pressure applied by patient (by closing jaws or with fingers)	Bleeding immediately after extractions or minor surgical procedures
Gelfoam	Pharmacia & Upjohn	Absorbable gelatin sponge made from purified gelatin solution—absorbs in 3-5 days	Useful for most patients taking an antithrombotic agent; helpful to place topical thrombin on Gelfoam; for extensive or invasive surgery, can be placed inside a splint
HemCon Dental Dressing	HemCon Medical Technologies	10 × 12 mm or 1 × 3 inch dressing—place on wound (best if some blood is present, helps stick dressing to the wound); made of chitosan from shellfish	Can be used on extraction sites, oral wounds; can be used in patients taking anticoagulants
Cellulose			
Surgicel Oxycel	Johnson & Johnson Becton Dickinson	Oxidized regenerated cellulose—exerts physical effect rather than physiologic; swells on contact with blood with resulting pressure adding to hemostasis; thrombin ineffective with these agents due to inactivation as a result of pH factors	After 24-48 hours it becomes gelatinous; can be left in place or removed; useful to control bleeding when other agents ineffective
Collagen			
Instat	Johnson & Johnson	Absorbable collagen made from purified/ lyophilized bovine dermal collagen—can be cut or shaped; adheres to bleeding surfaces when wet, but does not stick to instruments, gloves, or gauze sponges	Mild to moderate bleeding usually controlled in 2-5 minutes; more expensive than Gelfoam
Avitene Helistat	MedChem Products Marion Merrell Dow	Microfibrillar collagen hemostat—dry, sterile, fibrous, water insoluble, HCl acid salt–purified bovine corium collagen; MCH attracts platelets and triggers aggregation in fibrous mass	Thrombin ineffective with these agents due to inactivation as a result of pH factors; moderate to severe bleeding
Colla-Cote, Tape, Plug	Zimmer Dental	Absorbable collagen dressings from bovine sources—can be sutured into place, used under stents, dentures, or alone; fully resorbed in 10-14 days	Shaped according to intended use: "cote" $\frac{3}{4}$ × 1.5 inch, tape 1 × 3 inch; plug $\frac{3}{8}$ × $\frac{3}{4}$ inch; all are superior hemostats for moderate-severe bleeding
Thrombin			
Thrombostat Thrombinar Thrombogen	Parke-Davis Jones Medical Johnson & Johnson—Merck	Topical thrombin—directly converts fibrinogen to fibrin; derived from bovine sources	One 5000-unit vial dissolved in 5 mL saline can clot equal amount of blood in <1 second; useful in severe bleeding.
Tranexamic acid Lysteda (Tablets) Cyklokapron (IV)	 Xanodyne Pfizer	Tranexamic acid—works as a competitive inhibitor of plasminogen activation; used as a mouth wash (5%), taken orally as a tablet or given IV	Useful in short term for preventing hemorrhage after dental extractions
Amicar Tablets (500 mg) Syrup (1.25 g/5 mL) IV (250 mg/mL)	Wyeth-Ayerest	ε-Aminocaproic acid—works as a competitive inhibitor of plasminogen activation; Most often used as a mouth wash, can be taken orally or by IV	Useful in short-term to prevent bleeding
Histocryl	B. Braun	Active ingredient is N-Butyl-2 cyanoacrylate, serves as a glue to protect surgical wounds	Useful in the short-term to prevent bleeding
Beriplast	Behringwerke	Fibrin/tissue glue	Not available in U.S. at this time

BOX 25-3 Dental Management *Considerations in Patients with von Willebrand Disease*

P

Patient Evaluation/Risk Assessment (see Box 1-1)

- Evaluate and determine whether bleeding disorder (e.g., von Willebrand) exists.
- Obtain medical consultation if signs and symptoms are suggestive of the disease, if the disease is poorly controlled or if the diagnosis is uncertain. Screen patients with bleeding history or clinical signs of a bleeding disorder with PT, PTT, TT, and platelet count.

Potential Issues/Factors of Concern

A	
Analgesics	Avoid aspirin, aspirin-containing compounds, and other NSAIDs; acetaminophen with or without codeine is suggested for most patients.
Antibiotics	Not indicated unless acute infection is present.
Anesthesia	Avoid infiltration and block anesthetic injections in patients not on desmopressin, aminocaproic acid, and/or factor concentrates.
Anxiety	No issues.
Allergy	Patients placed on factor VIII with vWF replacement need to be observed for signs and symptoms of allergy.
B	
Bleeding	These patients may be at risk for bleeding from invasive dental procedures. Patients with type 2N and type 3 vWD are at greatest risk. Special precautions must be taken before invasive dental procedures and surgery. Most patients can be managed with desmopressin and aminocaproic acid. A few patients will require factor VIII with vWF
Breathing	No issues.
Blood pressure	No issues.
C	
Chair position	No issues.
Cardiovascular	No issues.
Consultation	The patient's hematologist must be consulted before any invasive dental procedures being performed. The diagnosis needs to be confirmed, the type of variant established, and the need for desmopressin factor VIII with vWF, and aminocaproic acid determined. Patients with type 1 vWD, which is by far the most common (70% to 80%), usually can be managed in the dental office using desmopressin; consultation will identify the few patients who may require factor VIII with vWF. Patients with type 2 disease (20% to 30%) usually can be managed with desmopressin; in some cases, factor VIII with vWF also is needed. The patient's physician needs to test for desmopressin response. Type 3 vWD is rare and requires factor VIII with vWF in all cases. Patients with type 3 vWD and some with type 2 vWD may require hospitalization for surgical procedures.
D	
Devices	Splints may be constructed before multiple extractions or surgical procedures in patients with type 3 vWD. Splints should not place excessive pressure on tissue and should be removed once bleeding is controlled so that tissue heals properly. Use local hemostatic agents as needed (see Table 25-6).
Drugs	Avoid all drugs that may cause bleeding such as aspirin and other NSAIDs, herbal medications, and over-the-counter drugs containing aspirin.
E	
Equipment	No issues.
Emergencies	Excessive bleeding may occur after invasive dental procedures or surgery. Systemic and local means may be required to control the bleeding (see Tables 25-3 and 25-6). Allergic reactions may occur in patients receiving factor replacement.
F	
Follow-up	Patients should be seen and examined for signs of bleeding within 24 to 48 hours after surgical procedures.

NSAIDs, Nonsteroidal antiinflammatory drugs; *vWD,* von Willebrand disease; *vWF,* von Willebrand factor.

mandibular acrylic splints may no longer be used. All extraction sites should be packed with microfibrillar collagen, and the wound should be closed with sutures for primary healing whenever possible. Endodontic procedures should be performed, rather than extractions, whenever possible because the risk for serious bleeding is lessened by this approach.

In many instances, the patient must be hospitalized for dental surgical procedures. This decision should be made according to the procedure planned and in consultation with the patient's hematologist. Patients who have a mild to moderate form of hemophilia without inhibitors can be managed on an outpatient basis with the use of desmopressin, aminocaproic acid, or tranexamic acid, or with replacement therapy plus aminocaproic acid. When replacement therapy is used, the dentist and the hematologist must observe the patient for any signs of allergic reaction and must be prepared to take appropriate action. Box 25-2 reviews the roles and functions of the hematologist and the dentist in managing the patient with hemophilia. Postoperative pain control usually can be obtained with the use of acetaminophen with or without codeine (see Box 25-2).

von Willebrand's Disease. Surgical procedures can be performed in patients with mild von Willebrand disease (type 1 and some type 2 variants) with the use of desmopressin and EACA or tranexamic acid. Patients with more severe types of von Willebrand disease will require factor VIII concentrates such as Humate-P that retain vWF multimers to replace the missing vWF and factor VIII. A study by Federici and colleagues[60] reported the results of bleeding complications in 63 consecutive patients with von Willebrand disease. Of these cases, 31 had type 1, 22 had type 2 variants, and 10 had type 3 von Willebrand disease. All patients had undergone extractions or periodontal surgery. In all cases, tranexamic acid was given before and for 7 days after surgery. Fibrin glue (not available in the United States) was used as local therapy in several patients during surgery. Desmopressin or factor VIII concentrates with vWF were given systemically as indicated. Of these patients, 29 were treated with tranexamic acid and local measures and did not experience excessive bleeding. Desmopressin was given to 24 patients, and 6 received factor VIII with vWF. Excessive bleeding after surgery occurred in only two patients. The investigators[60] concluded that tranexamic acid, fibrin glue, and desmopressin can prevent bleeding complications in the vast majority of patients with von Willebrand disease (84%). Box 25-3 reviews the roles and functions of the hematologist and dentist in the management of patients with von Willebrand disease.

Treatment Planning Modifications

With proper preparation, most indicated dental treatment can be provided for patients with various bleeding problems. Patients with congenital coagulation

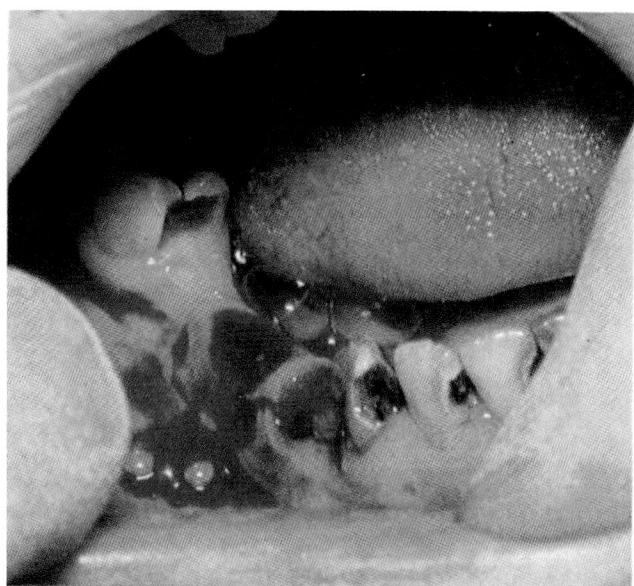

FIGURE 25-12 Severe hemorrhage after dental extraction often is the first clue to more minor degrees of coagulation disorder and is a common presentation in hemophilia, Christmas disease, and von Willebrand disease. *(From Forbes CD, Jackson WF:* Color atlas and text of clinical medicine, *ed 3, London, 2003, Mosby.)*

defects must be encouraged to improve and maintain good oral health, because most dental treatment for these patients at present is complicated by the need for replacement of the missing factor. Dental treatment often requires hospitalization for patients with severe defects. Aspirin and other NSAIDs should not be used for pain relief in patients who have known bleeding disorders or who are receiving anticoagulant medication. Such medication includes the various compounds that contain aspirin, such as Anacin, Synalgos-DC, Fiorinal, Bufferin, Alka-Seltzer, Empirin with Codeine, and Excedrin. Also, herbal medications that may be associated with excessive bleeding are to be avoided (see Appendix E).

Oral Complications and Manifestations

Patients with congenital bleeding disorders may experience spontaneous gingival bleeding. Oral tissues (e.g., soft palate, tongue, buccal mucosa) may show ecchymoses and petechiae. Bleeding occurring after the extraction of teeth may be the first evidence of mild coagulation disorders such as hemophilia A, hemophilia B, or von Willebrand disease variants with factor VIII deficiency (Figure 25-12). Spontaneous gingival bleeding and petechiae usually are found in patients with genetic platelet disorders or HHT. Hemarthrosis of the temporomandibular joint (TMJ) is a rare finding in patients with genetic coagulation disorders.

REFERENCES

1. Ragni MV, et al: Clinical aspects and therapy of hemophilia. In Hoffman R, et al, editors: *Hematology: basic principles and practice*, ed 5, Philadelphia, 2009, Churchill Livingstone, pp 1911-1930.
2. Baz R, Mekhail T: Disorders of platelet function and number. In Carey WD, et al, editors: *Current clinical medicine 2009—Cleveland Clinic*, Philadelphia, 2009, Saunders, pp 669-674.
3. Bennett JS: Hereditary disorders of platelet function. In Hoffman R, et al, editors: *Hematology: basic principles and practice*, ed 5, Philadelphia, 2009, Churchill Livingstone, pp 2133-2144.
4. Coller BS, Schneiderman PI: Clinical evaluation of hemorrhagic disorders: the bleeding history and differential diagnosis of purpura. In Hoffman R, et al, editors: *Hematology: basic principles and practice*, ed 5, Philadelphia, 2009, Churchill Livingstone, pp 1851-1876.
5. Deitcher SR: Hypercoagulable states. In Carey WD, et al, editors: *Current clinical medicine 2009—Cleveland Clinic*, Philadelphia, 2009, Saunders, pp 639-646.
6. Kessler CM: Hemorrhagic disorders: coagulation factor deficiencies. In Goldman L, Ausiello D, editors: *Cecil medicine*, ed 23, Philadelphia, 2008, Saunders, pp 1301-1313.
7. White GCI, Sadler JE: von Willebrand disease: clinical aspects and therapy. In Hoffman R, et al, editors: *Hematology: basic principles and practice*, ed 5, Philadelphia, 2009, Churchill Livingstone, pp 1961-1972.
8. Karsan A, Harlan JM: The blood vessel wall. In Hoffman R, et al, editors: *Hematology: basic principles and practice*, ed 5, Philadelphia, 2009, Churchill Livingstone, pp 1805-1818.
9. Arruda V, High KA. Coagulation disorders. In Fauci AS, et al, editors: *Harrison's principles of internal medicine*, ed 17, New York, 2008, McGraw-Hill, pp 725-730.
10. Konkle BA. Disorders of platelets and vessel wall. In Fauci AS, et al, editors: *Harrison's principles of internal medicine*, ed 17, New York, 2008, McGraw-Hill, pp 718-724.
11. Schafer AI. Approach to the patient with bleeding and thrombosis. In Goldman L, Ausiello D, editors: *Cecil medicine*, ed 23, Philadelphia, 2008, Saunders, pp 1286-1288.
12. Konkle BA. Bleeding and thrombosis. In Fauci AS, et al, editors: *Harrison's principles of internal medicine*, ed 17, New York, 2008, McGraw-Hill, pp 363-369.
13. Baz R, Mekhail T: Bleeding disorders. In Carey WD, et al, editors: *Current Clinical Medicine 2009—Cleveland Clinic*, Philadelphia, 2009, Saunders, pp 669-674.
14. Schmaier AH: Laboratory evaluation of hemostatic and thrombotic disorders. In Hoffman R, et al, editors: *Hematology: basic principles and practice*, ed 5, Philadelphia, 2009, Churchill Livingstone, pp 1877-1884.
15. McMillan R: Hemorrhagic disorders: abnormalities of platelet and vascular function. In Goldman L, Ausiello D, editors: *Cecil medicine*, ed 23, Philadelphia, 2008, Saunders, pp 1289-1300.
16. Grandinetti LM, Tomecki KJ: Dermatologic signs of systemic disease. In Carey WD, et al, editors: *Current clinical medicine 2009—Cleveland Clinic*, Philadelphia, 2009, Saunders, pp 244-256.
17. Rees MM, Rodgers GM: Bleeding disorders caused by vascular abnormalities. In Lee GR, et al, editors: *Wintrobe's clinical hematology*, ed 10, Philadelphia, 1999, Lippincott Williams & Wilkins, pp 1633-1648.
18. Shuman M. Hemorrhagic disorders: abnormalities of platelet and vascular function. In Goldman L, Ausiello D, editors: *Cecil textbook of medicine*, ed 22, Philadelphia, 2004, Saunders, pp 1060-1069.
19. Lebrin F, et al: Thalidomide stimulates vessel maturation and reduces epistaxis in individuals with hereditary hemorrhagic telangiectasia, *Nat Med* 16:420-428, 2010.
20. Nurden AT: Qualitative disorders of platelets and megakaryocytes, *J Thromb Haemost* 3:1773-1782, 2005.
21. Freson K, et al: What's new in using platelet research? To unravel thrombopathies and other human disorders, *Eur J Pediatr* 166:1203-1210, 2007.
22. Eckstein JD, Filip DJ, Watts JC: Hereditary thrombocytopenia, deafness, and renal disease, *Ann Intern Med* 82:639-645, 1975.
23. Greinacher A, Mueller-Eckhardt C: Hereditary types of thrombocytopenia with giant platelets and inclusion bodies in the leukocytes, *Blut* 60:53-60, 1990.
24. Doubek M, et al: [Hereditary thrombocytopenia. Differential diagnosis of a case.], *Cas Lek Cesk* 142:683-686, 2003.
25. Salles II, et al: Inherited traits affecting platelet function, *Blood Rev* 22:155-172, 2008.
26. Tefre KL, Ingerslev J, Sorensen B: Clinical benefit of recombinant factor VIIa in management of bleeds and surgery in two brothers suffering from the Bernard-Soulier syndrome, *Haemophilia* 15:281-284, 2009
27. Karimi M, et al: Spectrum of inherited bleeding disorders in southern Iran, before and after the establishment of comprehensive coagulation laboratory, *Blood Coagul Fibrinolysis* 20:642-645, 2009.
28. Noris P, et al: Platelet size distinguishes between inherited macrothrombocytopenias and immune thrombocytopenia, *J Thromb Haemost* 7:2131-2136, 2009.
29. Streif W, Knofler R, Eberl W: Inherited disorders of platelet function in pediatric clinical practice: a diagnostic challeng, *Klin Padiatr* 222:203-208, 2010.
30. Pham A, Wang J: Bernard-Soulier syndrome: an inherited platelet disorder, *Arch Pathol Lab Med* 131:1834-1836, 2007.
31. Mezzano D, Quiroga T, Pereira J: The level of laboratory testing required for diagnosis or exclusion of a platelet function disorder using platelet aggregation and secretion assays, *Semin Thromb Hemost* 35:242-254, 2009.
32. Bennett JS: Inherited and acquired disorders of platelet function. In Young NS, Gerson SL, High KA, editors: *Clinical hematology*, St. Louis, 2006, Mosby, pp 767-781.
33. Depner C, et al: Perioperative management of Glanzmann's syndrome: how we did it! *Blood Coagul Fibrinolysis* 21:283-284, 2010.
34. Di Minno G, et al: Glanzmann's thrombasthenia (defective platelet integrin alphaIIb-beta3): proposals for management between evidence and open issues, *Thromb Haemost* 102: 1157-1164, 2009.
35. Kannan M, Saxena R: Glanzmann's thrombasthenia: an overview, *Clin Appl Thromb Hemost* 15:152-165, 2009.
36. Sebastiano C, et al: Glanzmann's thrombasthenia: report of a case and review of the literature, *Int J Clin Exp Pathol* 3:443-447, 2010
37. Erduran E, Aksoy A, Zaman D: The use of recombinant FVIIa in a patient with Glanzmann thrombasthenia with uncontrolled bleeding after tonsillectomy, *Blood Coagul Fibrinolysis* 20(3):215-217, 2009.
38. Javed A, et al: Control of severe bleeding episode in case of Glanzmann's thrombasthenia refractory to platelet transfusion therapy by administering recombinant factor VIIa, *J Ayub Med Coll Abbottabad* 21:171-173, 2009.
39. Lozier JN, Kessler GM: Clinical aspects and therapy of hemophilia. In Hoffman R, et al, editors: *Hematology: basic principles and practice*, ed 4, Philadelphia, 2005, Churchill Livingstone, pp 2047-2071.
40. McVey JH: Coagulation factors. In Young NS, Gerson SL, High KA, editors: *Clinical hematology*, St. Louis, 2006, Mosby, pp 103-123.

41. Ragni MV: The hemophilias: factor VIII and factor IX deficiencies. In Young NS, Gerson SL, High KA, editors: *Clinical hematology*, St. Louis, 2006, Mosby, pp 814-830.
42. Rodgers GM, Greenberg CS: Inherited coagulation disorders. In Lee GR, et al, editors: *Wintrobe's clinical hematology*, ed 10, Philadelphia, 1999, Lippincott Williams & Wilkins, pp 1682-1733.
43. Feinstein DI: Inhibitors in hemophilia. In Hoffman R, et al, editors: *Hematology: basic principles and practice*, ed 4, Philadelphia, 2005, Churchill Livingstone, pp 2071-2081.
44. Shord SS, Lindley CM: Coagulation products and their uses, *Am J Health-Syst Pharm* 57:1403-1418, 2000.
45. Metjian A, Konkle BA: Inhibitors in hemophilia A and B. In Hoffman R, et al, editors: *Hematology: basic principles and practice*, ed 5, Philadelphia, 2009, Churchill Livingstone, pp 1931-1938.
46. Hedner U: History of rFVIIa therapy, *Thromb Res* 125(Suppl 1):S4-S6, 2010.
47. Hedner U, Lee CA: First 20 years with recombinant FVIIa (NovoSeven), *Haemophilia* 17:e172-e182, 2011.
48. Perez Bianco R, et al: Secondary prophylaxis with rFVIIa in hemophilia and inhibitors: recommendations from an experts committee from Argentina, *Medicina (B Aires)* 70:209-214, 2010.
49. Margaritis P, High KA: Gene therapy in haemophilia—going for cure? *Haemophilia* 16(Suppl 3):24-28, 2010.
50. Schwaab R, Oldenburg J: Gene therapy of hemophilia, *Semin Thromb Hemost* 27:417-424, 2001.
51. Scott DW: Gene therapy for immunological tolerance: using "transgenic" B cells to treat inhibitor formation, *Haemophilia* 16:89-94, 2010.
52. Kessler CM: Hemorrhagic disorders: coagulation factor deficiencies. In Goldman L, Ausiello D, editors: *Cecil textbook of medicine*, Philadelphia, 2004, Saunders, pp 1069-1078.
53. Roberts HR, Escobar MA: Other clotting factor deficiencies. In Hoffman R, et al, editors: *Hematology: basic principles and practice*, ed 4, Philadelphia, 2005, Churchill Livingstone, pp 2081-2097.
54. Handin RI: Bleeding and thrombosis. In Fauci AS, et al, editors: *Harrison's principles of internal medicine*, ed 14, New York, 1998, McGraw-Hill, pp 339-345.
55. Schafer AI: Thrombotic disorders: hypercoagulable states. In Goldman L, Ausiello D, editors: *Cecil medicine*, ed 23, Philadelphia, 2008, Saunders, pp 1318-1323.
56. Bauer KA: Hypercoagulable states. In Hoffman R, et al, editors: *Hematology: basic principles and practice*, ed 5, Philadelphia, 2009, Churchill Livingstone, pp 2021-2042.
57. Scully C, Cawson RA: *Medical problems in dentistry*, ed 5, Edinbugh, 2005, Elsevier.
58. Reding MT, Kay NS: Hematologic problems in the surgical patient: bleeding and thrombosis. In Hoffman R, et al, editors: *Hematology: basic principles and practice*, ed 5, Philadelphia, 2009, Churchill Livingstone, pp 2369-2385.
59. Lee APH, et al: Effectiveness in controlling haemorrhage after dental scaling in people with haemophilia by using tranexamic acid mouthwash, *Br Dent J* 198:33-38, 2005.
60. Federici AB, et al: Optimising local therapy during oral surgery in patients with von Willebrand disease: effective results from a retrospective analysis of 63 cases, *Haemophilia* 6:71-77, 2000.

CHAPTER

26

Cancer and Oral Care of the Cancer Patient

Collectively, all cancers combined account for about 23% of deaths in the United States, thereby placing cancer second only to heart disease as a leading cause of death.[1] Cancer is a major public health problem in the United States and other developed countries. Concordant with improvements in health and medical care resulting in increased longevity, the prevalence of cancer has increased over the past 50 years. Currently, one in four deaths in the United States is due to cancer. In 2006, the probability of developing cancer from birth to death in the United States in men was 46% and in women, 38%.[2,3]

A total of 1.5 million new cancer cases and over 600,000 deaths from cancer are expected in the United States in 2011 (Table 26-1). When deaths are aggregated by age, cancer has surpassed heart disease as the leading cause of death for those younger than age 85 since 1999.[1,2]

The death rate from all cancers combined has decreased slightly in the past 10 years.[1,2] The mortality rate has also continued to decrease for the three most common cancer sites in men (lung and bronchus, colon and rectum, and prostate) and for breast and colon and rectum cancers in women.[2] Lung cancer mortality among women continues to increase slightly. As with many diseases, ethnic disparities exist. In analyses by race and ethnicity, African American men and women have 40% and 18% higher death rates from all cancers combined than white men and women, respectively. Cancer incidence and death rates are lower in other racial and ethnic groups than in whites and African Americans for all sites combined and for the four major cancer sites. However, these groups generally have higher rates for stomach, liver, and cervical cancers than those reported for whites. Furthermore, minority populations are more likely than whites to be diagnosed with advanced-stage disease. Progress in reducing the burden of suffering and death from cancer can be accelerated by applying existing cancer control knowledge across all segments of the population.[2,3]

Because patients diagnosed with cancer are experiencing increased survival as a result of improved diagnostics and advances in antineoplastic therapy, an increased likelihood exists of dentists treating patients in various phases of cancer therapy. For optimum oral health, the dentist should be an integral part of the cancer patient's health care team. The characteristic clinical course, cancer progression status, treatment modalities, the location of cancer therapy (hospital or outpatient facility), and the likely outcome all will affect the dental treatment plan. Maintenance of proper oral hygiene is critical for limiting local and systemic complications associated with chemotherapy, radiation therapy, and marrow and stem cell transplantation. In addition, dentists have the unique opportunity to reduce the risk of cancer by providing advice regarding cancer screening, a healthy diet, counseling patients as appropriate regarding smoking cessation and risks associated with alcohol consumption, and performing cancer screening procedures.

This chapter focuses on common cancers that may affect patients who require dental care. No attempt is made here to include all cancers; instead, an overview of cancer is presented first, followed by a discussion of common cancers, along with relevant considerations regarding oral care of patients with cancer. A discussion of lymphoma and leukemia can be found in Chapter 23.

DEFINITION AND SCOPE OF THE PROBLEM

Cancer is characterized by uncontrolled growth of aberrant neoplastic cells.[4] Cancerous cells kill by destructive invasion of tissues—that is, direct extension and spread to distant sites by metastasis through blood, lymph, or serosal surfaces. Malignant cells arise from genetic and acquired mutations, chromosomal translocations, and over- or underexpression of factors (oncogenes, growth factor receptors, signal transducers, transcription factors) that cause cells to lose their ability to regulate deoxyribonucleic acid (DNA) synthesis and the cell cycle. Cellular abnormalities of malignancy result in three common features: uncontrolled proliferation, ability to recruit blood vessels (i.e., neovascularization), and ability to spread.[4]

TABLE 26-1 Estimated New Cancer Cases and Deaths by Sex, United States, 2010*

	Estimated New Cases			Estimated Deaths		
Primary Tumor Location	**Both Sexes**	**Male**	**Female**	**Both Sexes**	**Male**	**Female**
All sites	1,529,560	789,620	739,940	569,490	299,200	270,290
Oral cavity and pharynx	36,540	25,420	11,120	7880	5430	2450
Tongue	10,990	7690	3300	1990	1300	690
Mouth	10,840	6430	4410	1830	1140	690
Pharynx	12,660	9880	2780	2410	1730	680
Other oral cavity	2050	1420	630	1650	1260	390
Digestive system	274,330	148,540	125,790	139,580	79,010	60,570
Esophagus	16,640	13,130	3510	14,500	11,650	2850
Stomach	21,000	12,730	8270	10,570	6350	4220
Small intestine	6960	3680	3280	1100	610	490
Colon	102,900	49,470	53,430	51,370	26,580	24,790
Rectum	39,670	22,620	17,050	—	—	—
Anus, anal canal, anorectum	5260	2000	3260	720	280	440
Liver/intrahepatic bile duct	24,120	17,430	6690	18,910	12,720	6190
Gallbladder, other biliary cancers	9760	4450	5310	3320	1240	2080
Pancreas	43,140	21,370	21,770	36,800	18,770	18,030
Other digestive organs	4880	1660	3220	2290	810	1480
Respiratory system	240,610	130,600	110,010	161,670	89,550	72,120
Larynx	12,720	10,110	2610	3600	2870	730
Lung and bronchus	222,520	116,750	105,770	157,300	86,220	71,080
Other respiratory organs	5370	3740	1630	770	460	310
Bones and joints	2650	1530	1120	1460	830	630
Soft tissue (including heart)	10,520	5680	4840	3920	2020	1900
Skin (excluding basal and squamous)	74,010	42,610	31,400	11,790	7910	3880
Melanoma—skin	68,130	38,870	29,260	8700	5670	3030
Other nonepithelial skin cancers	5880	3740	2140	3090	2240	850
Breast	209,060	1970	207,090	40,230	390	39,840
Genital system	311,210	227,460	83,750	60,420	32,710	27,710
Uterine cervix	12,200	—	12,200	4210	—	4210
Uterine corpus	43,470	—	43,470	7950	—	7950
Ovary	21,880	—	21,880	13,850	—	13,850
Vulva	3900	—	3900	920	—	920
Vagina and other genital, female	2300	—	2300	780	—	780
Prostate	217,730	217,730	—	32,050	32,050	—
Testis	8480	8480	—	350	350	—
Penis and other genital, male	1250	1250	—	310	310	—
Urinary system	131,260	89,620	41,640	28,550	19,110	9440
Urinary bladder	70,530	52,760	17,770	14,680	10,410	4270
Kidney and renal pelvis	58,240	35,370	22,870	13,040	8210	4830
Ureter and other urinary organs	2490	1490	1000	830	490	340
Eye and orbit	2480	1240	1240	230	120	110
Brain and other nervous system	22,020	11,980	10,040	13,140	7420	5720
Endocrine system	46,930	11,890	35,040	2570	1140	1430
Thyroid	44,670	10,740	33,930	1690	730	960
Other endocrine structures	2260	1150	1110	880	410	470

TABLE 26-1 Estimated New Cancer Cases and Deaths by Sex, United States, 2010*—cont'd

	Estimated New Cases			Estimated Deaths		
Primary Tumor Location	Both Sexes	Male	Female	Both Sexes	Male	Female
Lymphoma	74,030	40,050	33,980	21,530	11,450	10,080
Hodgkin lymphoma	8490	4670	3820	1320	740	580
Non-Hodgkin lymphoma	65,540	35,380	30,160	20,210	10,710	9500
Myeloma	20,180	11,170	9010	10,650	5760	4890
Leukemia	43,050	24,690	18,360	21,840	12,660	9180
Acute lymphocytic leukemia	5330	3150	2180	1420	790	630
Chronic lymphocytic leukemia	14,990	8870	6120	4390	2650	1740
Acute myeloid leukemia	12,330	6590	5740	8950	5280	3670
Chronic myeloid leukemia	4870	2800	2070	440	190	250
Other leukemia	5530	3280	2250	6640	3750	2890
Other and unspecified primary sites	30,680	15,170	15,510	44,030	23,690	20,340

*Excludes basal and squamous cell skin cancers and in situ carcinoma except urinary bladder. Estimates are rounded to the nearest 10.
These data are for the most common cancers expected to occur in men and women in 2010. Among men, cancers of the prostate, lung and bronchus, and colon and rectum account for over 56% of all newly diagnosed cancer. Prostate cancer alone accounts for about 33% (218,000) of incident cases in men. Based on cases diagnosed between 1995 and 2001, an estimated 91% of these new cases of prostate cancer are expected to be diagnosed at local or regional stages, for which 5-year relative survival approaches 100%.
About 54,010 cases of female carcinoma in situ of the breast and 46,770 cases of melanoma in situ will be newly diagnosed in 2010.
Estimated deaths for colon and rectum cancers are combined.
More deaths than cases may reflect lack of specificity in recording underlying cause of death on death certificates or an undercount in the case estimate.
NOTE: Percentages may not total to 100% because of rounding. *(From Jamal A, et al: Cancer statistics, 2010,* CA Cancer J Clin *60;277-300, 2010. © 2010 American Cancer Society.)*

Epidemiology: Incidence and Prevalence

Figure 26-1 indicates the most common cancers expected to occur in men and women in 2010.[1,2] Among men, cancers of the prostate, lung and bronchus, and colon and rectum account for more than 56% of all newly diagnosed cancers. In women the most common cancers are breast, lung, colon, and uterine.[3]

Etiology and Prevention

Carcinogenesis is a complex multistep process that involves the accumulation of mutations and the loss of regulatory control over cell division, differentiation, apoptosis, and adhesion[4] (Figure 26-2). The process originates at the level of gene and cell cycle control, either by a hereditary mutation, acquired mutation or inappropriate expression of a transcription factor. Some syndromes which predispose individuals to cancer can be seen in Table 26-2.

The aggregation of cancer in a family can be due to genetic or nongenetic causes, the former through mendelian (single-gene mutation) or nonmendelian (polygenic or multifactorial) inheritance of genes that predispose to cancer and the latter related to common exposure to carcinogenic agents or lifestyle, or simple coincidence. The modern understanding of familial aggregation of cancer has required increasingly sophisticated epidemiologic and statistical methods in combination with genetic concepts and technologies.[4]

Although mendelian inheritance accounts for a small minority of all cancers, mutations that predispose to cancer have provided some of the most penetrating insights into the understanding of the genetic basis of normal as well as abnormal development; these mutations manifest the classical recessive or dominant modes of inheritance. Nonmendelian inheritance, which also plays a major role in the overall incidence of cancer, has been more difficult to characterize. In addition, the interaction of mutated genes with the environment adds another level of complexity in deciphering the role of genetics of cancer in individual patients as well as in families.[4] Some of the genetic associations with cancer are shown in Table 26-2.

At least three to six somatic mutations are needed to transform a normal cell into a malignant cell. Acquired mutations can arise from exposure to hazardous chemicals and pathogens that lead to activation of oncogenes, inactivation of tumor suppressor genes (*pRb* and *TP53*), and chromosomal abnormalities (translocations, deletions, insertions). The accumulation of these abnormalities leads to a cell that becomes functionally independent and aggressive. Natural killer cells provide surveillance for cancerous cells. Reduction in numbers or function of natural killer cells, which occurs during immunosuppression, increases the risk for cancer.[5]

National efforts currently focus on the reduction or elimination of factors known to be associated with cancer. Recommendations from the American Cancer Society (ACS) are to minimize exposure to tobacco

Cancer Statistics, 2010

Estimated New Cases*

Males			Females		
Prostate	217,730	28%	Breast	207,090	28%
Lung & bronchus	116,750	15%	Lung & bronchus	105,770	14%
Colon & rectum	72,090	9%	Colon & rectum	70,480	10%
Urinary bladder	52,760	7%	Uterine corpus	43,470	6%
Melanoma of the skin	38,870	5%	Thyroid	33,930	5%
Non-Hodgkin lymphoma	35,380	4%	Non-Hodgkin lymphoma	30,160	4%
Kidney & renal pelvis	35,370	4%	Melanoma of the skin	29,260	4%
Oral cavity & pharynx	25,420	3%	Kidney&renal pelvis	22,870	3%
Leukemia	24,690	3%	Ovary	21,880	3%
Pancreas	21,370	3%	Pancreas	21,770	3%
All sites	**789,620**	**100%**	**All sites**	**739,940**	**100%**

Estimated Deaths

Males			Females		
Lung & bronchus	86,220	29%	Lung & bronchus	71,080	26%
Prostate	32,050	11%	Breast	39,840	15%
Colon & rectum	26,580	9%	Colon & rectum	24,790	9%
Pancreas	18,770	6%	Pancreas	18,030	7%
Liver & intrahepatic bile duct	12,720	4%	Ovary	13,850	5%
Leukemia	12,660	4%	Non-Hodgkin lymphoma	9,500	4%
Esophagus	11,650	4%	Leukemia	9,180	3%
Non-Hodgkin lymphoma	10,710	4%	Uterine corpus	7,950	3%
Urinary bladder	10,410	3%	Multiple myeloma	6,190	2%
Kidney & renal pelvis	8,210	3%	Brain & other nervous system	5,720	2%
All sites	**299,200**	**100%**	**All sites**	**270,290**	**100%**

FIGURE 26-1 Ten leading cancer types in estimated new cancer cases and deaths, by gender, United States, 2006. Indicated are the most common cancers that were expected to occur in men and women in 2006. Among men, cancers of the prostate, lung and bronchus, and colon and rectum account for more than 56% of all newly diagnosed cancers. Prostate cancer alone accounts for about 33% (234,460) of incident cases in men. On the basis of cases diagnosed between 1995 and 2001, an estimated 91% of new cases of prostate cancer were expected to be diagnosed at local or regional stages, for which relative 5-year survival approaches 100%. (*From Jamal A, et al: Cancer statistics, 2010,* CA Cancer J Clin *60;277-300, 2010.* © 2010 American Cancer Society.)

smoke and to environmental and occupational carcinogens (e.g., asbestos fibers, arsenic compounds, chromium compounds, pesticides); decrease intake of fat and exposure to ultraviolet light; moderate the intake of alcohol; obtain an adequate intake of dietary fiber and antioxidants (vitamins C and E, selenium); and perform moderate levels of physical activity.[5]

Pathophysiology and Complications

The loss of regulatory control in a cell destined to become a cancer cell results in a series of pathologic changes that eventuate in hyperproliferative epithelium, dysplasia, and finally carcinoma. Dysplastic tissue is characterized by atypical cell proliferation, nuclear enlargement, failure of maturation, and differentiation short of malignancy (see Figure 26-2).

Cytogenetic studies of various leukemias established four cardinal attributes of genetic change in cancer: (1) Specific or nonrandom chromosomal changes may characterize individual cancer types; (2) tumor genomes are genetically unstable and subject to continuing change, a feature now recognized as genomic instability; (3) all cells in a given tumor trace back to a single progenitor cell and therefore are clonal; and (4) tumor progression often is associated with additional specific or nonrandom chromosomal changes, presumably "selected" from the genomic instability, in subpopulations of tumor cells that lead clonal diversity and evolution. Chromosomal changes are of many types, the most common being gain of an entire chromosome (aneuploidy) or a region of it (duplication), loss of an entire chromosome (monosomy) or a region of it (deletion), translocation or inversion (rearrangement), and amplification (Figure 26-3).

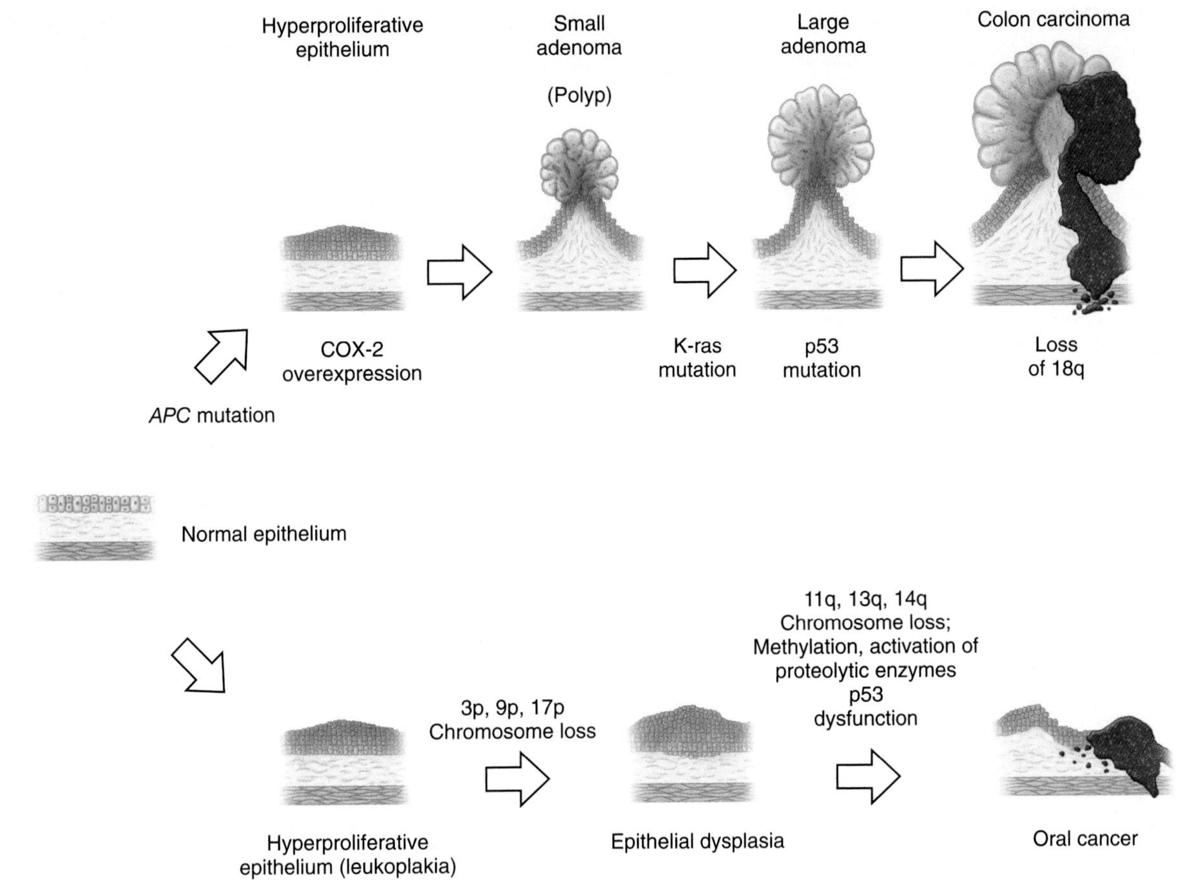

FIGURE 26-2 Carcinogenesis: pathologic sequence in gastrointestinal mucosa. Examples in colon and oral mucosa. *(Adapted from Jänne PA, Mayer RJ: Chemoprevention of colorectal cancer,* N Engl J Med *342:1960-1968, 2000.)*

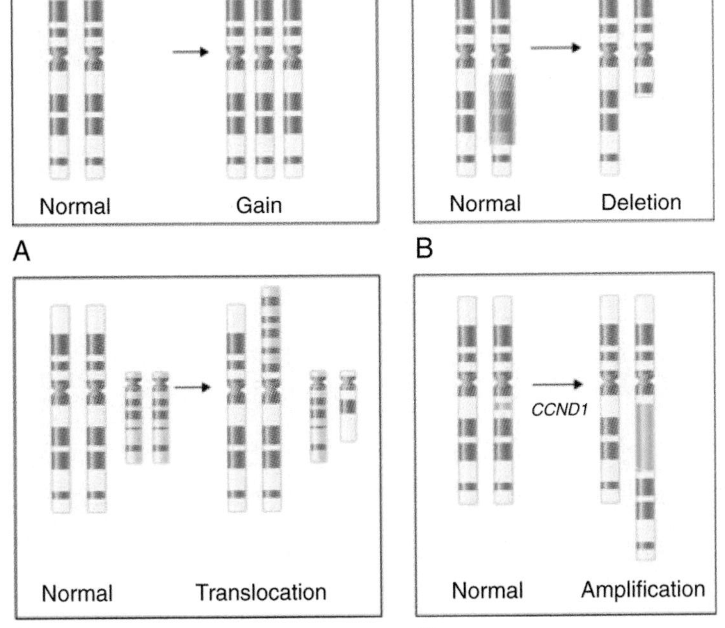

FIGURE 26-3 Common cytogenetic changes in cancer. The chromosome (at metaphase) is traditionally distinguished by its short and long arms separated by a centromere. Stylized bands (*dark and light stripes* along the length of the chromosome) produced by special treatments are also shown. The abnormality (*right*) and the corresponding normal image of the chromosome are illustrated in each panel. **A,** Gain of a chromosome leading to aneuploidy. **B,** Deletion of a chromosomal segment from one of the two homologues. **C,** Translocation showing exchange of segments between nonhomologous chromosomes. **D,** Amplification, with an increase in a region of a chromosome by replicating many times in place. *(From Goldman L, Ausiello D, editors:* Cecil textbook of medicine, *ed 23, Philadelphia, 2008, Saunders.)*

TABLE 26-2 Syndromes of Inherited Cancer Predisposition in Clinical Oncology Syndrome

Syndrome	Mode of Inheritance	Gene(s)
Hereditary Breast Cancer Syndromes		
Hereditary breast and ovarian cancer syndrome	Dominant	*BRCA1*
		BRCA2
Li-Fraumeni syndrome	Dominant	*TP53*
Cowden's syndrome	Dominant	*PTEN*
Bannayan-Riley-Ruvalcaba syndrome	Dominant	*PTEN*
Hereditary Gastrointestinal Malignancies		
Hereditary nonpolyposis colon cancer	Dominant	*MLH1*
		MLH2
		MSH6
Familial polyposis	Dominant	*APC*
Hereditary gastric cancer	Dominant	*CDH1*
Juvenile polyposis		*SMAD4/DPC4*
		BMPR1A
Peutz-Jeghers syndrome	Dominant	*STK11*
Hereditary melanoma–pancreatic cancer syndrome	Dominant	*CDKN2A*
Hereditary pancreatitis	Dominant	*PRSS1*
Turcot's syndrome	Dominant	*APC*
		MLH1
		PMS2
Familial gastrointestinal stromal tumor	Dominant	*KIT*
Genodermatoses With Cancer Predisposition		
Melanoma syndromes	Dominant	*CDKN2A*
		CDK4
		CMM
Basal cell cancer, Gorlin's syndrome	Dominant	*PTCH*
Cowden's syndrome	Dominant	*PTEN*
Neurofibromatosis 1	Dominant	*NF1*
Neurofibromatosis 2	Dominant	*NF2*
Tuberous sclerosis	Dominant	*TSC1*
		TSC2
Carney's complex	Dominant	*PRKAR1A*
Muir-Torre syndrome	Dominant	*MLH1*
		MSH2
Xeroderma pigmentosum	Recessive	*XPA,B,C,D,E,F,G*
		POLH
Rothmund-Thomson syndrome	Recessive	*RECOL4*
Leukemia/Lymphoma Predisposition Syndromes		
Bloom's syndrome	Recessive	*BLM*
Fanconi's anemia	Recessive	*FANCA,B,C*
		FANCA,D2
		FANCE,F,G
		FANCL
Ataxia-telangiectasia	Recessive	*ATM*
Shwachman-Diamond syndrome	Recessive	*SBDS*
Nijmegen breakage syndrome	Recessive	*NBS1*
Canale-Smith syndrome	Dominant	*FAS*
		FASL
Wiskott-Aldrich syndrome	X-linked recessive	*WAS*
Common variable immune deficiency	Recessive	
Severe combined immune deficiency	X-linked recessive	*IL2RG*
	Recessive	*ADA*
		JAK3
		RAG1
		RAG2
		IL7R
		CD45
		Artemis
X-linked lymphoproliferative syndrome	X-linked recessive	*SH2D1A*

TABLE 26-2 Syndromes of Inherited Cancer Predisposition in Clinical Oncology Syndrome—cont'd

Syndrome	Mode of Inheritance	Gene(s)
Genitourinary Cancer Predisposition Syndromes		
Hereditary prostate cancer	Dominant	*HPC1* *HPCX* *HPC2/ELAC2* *PCAP* *PCBC* *PRCA*
Simpson-Golabi-Behmel syndrome	X-linked recessive	*GPC3*
von Hippel–Lindau syndrome	Dominant	*VHL*
Beckwith-Wiedemann syndrome	Dominant	*CDKN1C* *NSD1*
Wilms' tumor syndrome	Dominant	*WT1*
Wilms' tumor, aniridia, genitourinary abnormalities, mental retardation (WAGR) syndrome	Dominant	*WT1*
Birt-Hogg-Dub? syndrome	Dominant	*FLCL*
Papillary renal cancer syndrome	Dominant	*MET,PRCC*
Constitutional t(3;8) translocation	Dominant	*TRCB*
Hereditary bladder cancer	Sporadic	
Hereditary testicular cancer	Possibly X-linked	
Rhabdoid predisposition syndrome	Dominant	*SNF5INI1*
Central Nervous System/Vascular Cancer Predisposition Syndromes		
Hereditary paraganglioma	Dominant	*SDHD* *SDHC* *SDHB*
Retinoblastoma	Dominant	*RB1*
Rhabdoid predisposition syndrome	Dominant	*SNF5/INI1*
Sarcoma/Bone Cancer Predisposition Syndromes		
Multiple exostoses	Dominant	*EXT1* *EXT2*
Leiomyoma/renal cancer syndrome	Dominant	*FH*
Carney's complex	Dominant	*PRKAR1A*
Werner's syndrome	Recessive	*WRN*
Endocrine Cancer Predisposition Syndromes		
Multiple endocrine neoplasia 1	Dominant	*MEN1*
Multiple endocrine neoplasia 2	Dominant	*RET*
Familial papillary thyroid cancer	Dominant	Multiple loci

Adapted from Garber JE, Offit K: Hereditary cancer predisposition syndromes, J Clin Oncol *23:276-292, 2005.*

Malignant cells exhibit antigenic, karyotypic, biochemical, and membrane changes that cause loss of contact inhibition, changes in chromosomal morphology, and increased permeability. Malignant tumors lack cell cycle control and replicate rapidly, becoming clinically detectable after about 30 cell doublings, when the mass contains about 10^9 cells (1 g). A three-log increase to 10^{12} cells produces a tumor that weighs 1 kg and often is lethal. After reaching clinically detectable size, tumors slow in growth as they reach anatomic boundaries and begin to outgrow their blood supply. Malignant tumors overcome the limitation of anatomic boundaries by losing cell adherence and by metastasizing. Metastasis is a distinct form of cancerous spread that occurs when malignant cells enter blood or lymphatic vessels and travel to distant sites. Metastasis is related to factors produced by tumors cells that allow individual cells to invade tissues and endothelium. It often results in end-organ failure and death.[5]

CLINICAL PRESENTATION

Screening

Each year the ACS publishes a summary of its recommendations for early cancer detection. Obviously, the earlier any form of cancer is diagnosed, the more expeditiously and effectively it can be treated in order to minimize adverse outcomes: morbidity and mortality.

TABLE 26-3 Screening Recommendations of the American Cancer Society

Cancer Site	Population	Test/Procedure	Frequency
Breast	Women aged ≥20 years	Self exam (is an option)	Every month
	aged 20-39 years	Clinical exam	Every 3 years
	aged ≥40 years	Clinical exam	Every year
	aged 40-49 years	Mammography	Every year
	aged ≥50 years	Mammography	Every year
Colon	Men and women, aged ≥50 years	Sigmoidoscopy	Every 3-5 years
		Fecal occult blood test	Every year
	Men and women, aged ≥40 years	Digital rectal exam	Every year
Cervix	Women aged ≥18 years	Pelvic exam Papanicolaou test	Every year*
Prostate	Men, aged ≥50 years (if average risk); aged ≥45 years (if high risk); aged ≥40 years (if very high risk)	Prostate examination Blood tests for prostate-specific antigen (PSA)	Every year
Health counseling and cancer checkups	Men and women, aged ≥20 years	To include examination cancers of the thyroid, testicles, ovaries, lymph nodes, oral cavity, and skin, as well as health counseling about tobacco, sun exposure, diet and nutrition, risk factors, sexual practices, and environmental and occupational exposures.	Every year

*With 3 or more consecutive satisfactory normal annual examinations, screening may be performed less frequently.
These recommendations often are applied 5 to 10 years earlier for specific cancers in persons with a family history of cancer and when specific racial (e.g., African American) populations are at increased risk.
Data from Smith RA, et al: Cancer screening in the United States, 2011: a review of current American Cancer Society guidelines and issues in cancer screening, CA Cancer J Clin *61:8-30, 2011.*

Table 26-3 outlines the most recent ACS recommendations for early cancer detection for several cancers. Further information can be found at http://cacancerjournal.org.

Signs and Symptoms

Cancers often manifest as a palpable mass that increase in size over time. Preceding the development of the tumor are subtle changes that are dependent on the anatomic site involved and the cell type of origin. Initial features can include a change in surface color, a lump, enlarged lymph node, or altered organ function. Symptoms include pain and paresthesia. Tumors permitted to increase in size often result in a reddened epithelial surface (due to increased blood vessels) that ulcerates.[6]

Staging

Most cancers are assigned a stage (I, II, III, or IV) by the medical team on the basis of the size of the tumor and how far it has spread (Box 26-1). Generically speaking, stage I disease is localized and confined to the organ of origin. Stage II disease is regional, affecting nearby structures. Regional head and neck lymph node anatomy can be seen in Figure 26-4. Stage III disease extends beyond the regional site, crossing several tissue planes, and stage IV disease is widely disseminated. This system often is supplemented by detailed and specific staging systems

BOX 26-1 International Tumor-Node-Metastasis (TNM) System of Classification and Staging of Oral Carcinomas

T: Tumor Size
- T_{IS}, carcinoma in situ
- T_1, tumor up to 2 cm in size
- T_2, tumor >2 cm up to 4 cm in size
- T_3, tumor >4 cm in size
- T_4, massive tumor with deep invasion into bone, muscle, skin

N: Regional Lymph Node Involvement
- N_0, no palpable nodes
- N_1, single, homolateral palpable node up to 3 cm in diameter
- N_2, single, homolateral palpable node, 3 to 6 cm *or* multiple, homolateral nodes, none >6 cm
- N_3, single or multiple, homolateral nodes, one >6 cm, *or* bilateral nodes (stage each side of neck), *or* contralateral nodes

M: Metastases
- M_0, no known distant metastasis
- M_1, distant metastasis—PUL (pulmonary), OSS (osseous), HEP (liver), BRA (brain)

Stage Classification

0 (carcinoma in situ)	T_{IS}, N_0, M_0
I	T_1, N_0, M_0
II	T_2, N_0, M_0
III	T_3, N_0, M_0 *or* T_1, T_2 *or* T_3, N_1, M_0
IVA	T_4, N_0, M_0 *or* T_4, N_1, M_0 *or* any T, N_2, M_0
IVB	Any T, N_3, M_0
IVC	Any T, any N, M_1

Adapted from Sobin L, Gospodarowicz M, Wittekind C, editors: UICC TNM classification of malignant tumours, *ed 7, Hoboken, NJ, 2010, Wiley-Blackwell.*

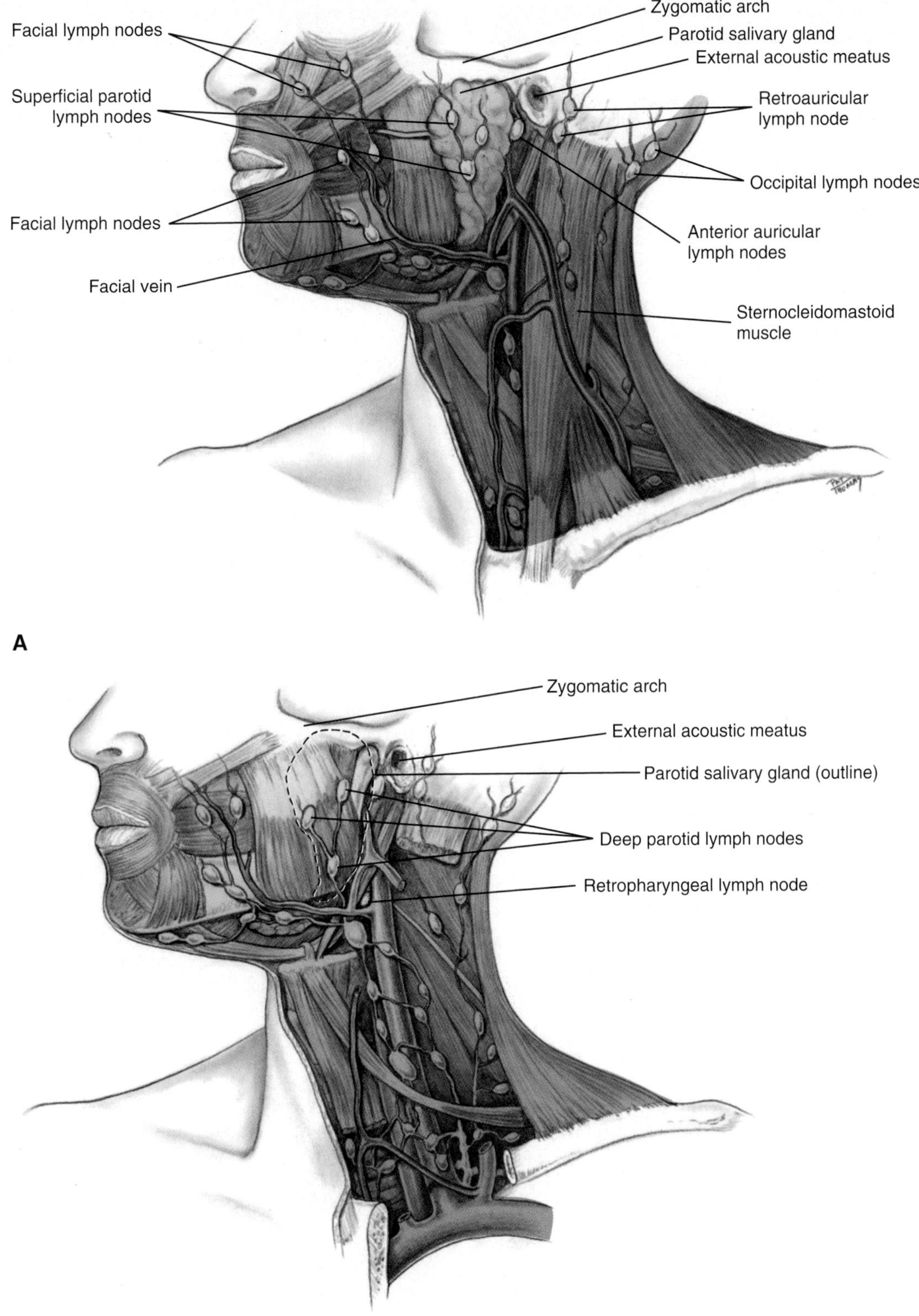

FIGURE 26-4 Regional lymph node anatomy. *(From Fehrenbach MJ, Herring SW:* Illustrated anatomy of the head and neck, *ed 4, St. Louis, 2012, Saunders.)*

BOX 26-2 Microscopic Criteria for Malignancy

Cytoplasm Scant cytoplasm, increased nucleus to cytoplasm ratio, tight molding of cytoplasmic membrane around nucleus

Nucleus Enlargement with variation in size, irregular membrane with sharp angles, hyperchromasia, irregular chromatin distribution with clumping, prominent nucleoli, abundant or abnormal mitotic figures

Relationships Variation in cell size and shape, abnormal stratification, decreased cohesiveness

developed for particular cancers and generally does not apply to leukemia (because leukemia is a disease of the blood cells that does not usually form a solid mass or tumor). The tumor-node-metastasis (TNM) system frequently is used for this purpose (see Box 26-1). The patient's prognosis depends in large part on the stage of disease at the time of diagnosis.[6]

Laboratory Findings

The diagnosis of cancer is dependent on microscopic examination of an adequate sample of tissue taken from the lesion (Box 26-2). Tissue can be obtained by cytologic smears, needle biopsy, or incisional or excisional biopsy. Cells also can be subjected to flow cytometry, chromosomal analyses, in situ hybridization, or other molecular procedures to identify specific cancer markers, ploidy, and DNA analysis. Serum tumor markers such as carcinoembryonic antigen (CEA) for colorectal carcinoma (CA 15-3 or CEA in breast cancer and CA 125 for ovarian cancer) have low sensitivity for the detection of early-stage cancers but are useful in monitoring disease progression and response to therapy.

MEDICAL MANAGEMENT

Treatment strategies for cancer are based on eliminating fast multiplying cancer cells without killing the host. Therapeutic modalities include surgery; irradiation (by external beam or implants); regimens based on cytotoxic, chemotherapeutic, and endocrine drugs; and possibly stem cell or bone marrow transplantation. Surgery often is used when anatomy permits to debulk a tumor or if the cancer is limited in size. Radiation therapy (often at doses greater than 50 grays [Gy][7]) kills cells by damaging cancer cell DNA and chromosomes needed for cell replication and is used when the tissue cannot be excised and when cells are most susceptible to this form of therapy. Chemotherapeutic agents are most effective against rapidly growing tumors by adversely affecting the DNA synthesis or protein synthesis of cancerous cells. A wide range of cancer chemotherapeutic compounds exist. They are divided into several categories: alkylating agents, antimetabolites, hormones, antibiotics, mitotic inhibitors, and miscellaneous drugs (Table 26-4). Tumoricidal efficacy is gained with use of these various agents in combination. High-dose multidrug protocols are employed in hospital settings to induce myelosuppression for patients with leukemia, lymphoma (see Chapter 23), and more recently, breast cancer who are scheduled to undergo bone marrow transplantation. Opportunistic infections are a major concern during the myelosuppressive period. Patients who receive outpatient chemotherapy are administered

TABLE 26-4 Chemotherapy Drugs of Choice for Common Cancers

Cancer	Drugs of Choice
Breast	*Risk reduction*: Tamoxifen *Adjuvant*: Doxorubicin + cyclophosphamide ± fluorouracil followed by paclitaxel; cyclophosphamide + methotrexate + fluorouracil; tamoxifen for receptor-positive and hormone-responsive tumors *Metastatic*: Doxorubicin + cyclophosphamide ± fluorouracil; cyclophosphamide + methotrexate + fluorouracil Tamoxifen or toremifene for receptor-positive and/or hormone-responsive tumors Paclitaxel + trastuzumab for tumors that overexpress HER2 protein
Cervix	*Locally advanced*: Cisplatin ± fluorouracil *Metastatic:* Cisplatin; ifosfamide with mesna; bleomycin + ifosfamide with mesna + cisplatin
Colorectal	*Adjuvant*: Fluorouracil + leucovorin *Metastatic*: Fluorouracil + leucovorin + irinotecan
Head and neck	Cisplatin + fluorouracil or paclitaxel
Kaposi sarcoma	Liposomal doxorubicin or daunorubicin; doxorubicin + bleomycin + vincristine
Leukemia and lymphoma	See Table 24-2
Liver	Hepatic intraarterial floxuridine, cisplatin, doxorubicin or mitomycin
Lung	
Non–small cell	Paclitaxel + cisplatin or carboplatin; cisplatin + vinorelbine; gemcitabine + cisplatin; cisplatin or carboplatin + etoposide (PE)
Small cell	
Melanoma	*Adjuvant*: Interferon alfa *Metastatic*: Dacarbazine
Multiple myeloma	Melphalan or cyclophosphamide + prednisone; vincristine + doxorubicin (Adriamycin) + dexamethasone (VAD)
Prostate	Gonadotropin-releasing hormone (GnRH) agonists (leuprolide or goserelin) ± antiandrogen (flutamide, bicalutamide, or nilutamide)
Renal	Interleukin-2

Adapted from Drugs for cancer, Med Lett Drugs Ther *42:83-92, 2000.*

a lower-dose regimen on a 3- to 4-week schedule and are at lower risk for opportunistic infections.[8]

Breast Cancer

Breast cancer is the most common type of cancer in the United States, with 98% of cases occurring in women. In 2010, approximately 207,000 cases of breast cancer were reported in the United States, with about 40,000 persons dying of the disease in that year.[2] The incidence increases with age. Risk factors include early menarche, late menopause, and nulliparity (women who do not bear children). All breast cancers are the result of somatic genetic abnormalities. The most important risk factor of breast cancer is family history of the disease with 5% to 10% of cases arising in high-risk families. The most common mutations identified in breast cancer cells are in the *BRCA1* and *BRCA2* genes. These mutations confer a 50% to 85% lifetime risk of breast cancer. Abnormalities also have been identified in genes (*bcl*-2, c-*myc,* c-*myb* and *TP53*) and gene products (Her2/neu and cyclin D1) that regulate the cell cycle and DNA replication. Gonadal steroid hormones, growth factors, and various chemokines (such as IL-6) influence the behavior and dissemination of the disease. Cancer in one breast increases the risk for cancer development in the other.[7,9,10]

Breast cancer often is detected as a lump in the breast with or without nipple discharge, breast skin changes and breast pain. Mammography detects the mass in only 75% to 85% of patients (Figure 26-5). Although mammography recently has been controversial, it is still a valuable screening technique as considered by the ACS.[11] In a small percentage of patients, the first sign is an axillary mass. Diagnosis is made from a tissue core biopsy of breast tissue. Most breast cancers are infiltrating ductal carcinomas, whereas a smaller percentage of tumors are infiltrating lobular carcinomas, medullary carcinomas, mucinous carcinoma, or tubular carcinoma. Metastasis occurs after the cancer becomes clinically detectable and is primarily to regional lymph nodes and within the chest wall, bone, lung, and liver.[12]

Treatment of breast cancer depends on the histologic type of cancer and stage. Cellular markers such as the Her2/*neu* molecule (target of drug herceptin) and the sodium-iodide symporter (NIS) aid in the diagnosis and treatment planning. Lumpectomy (when the tumor is less than 5 cm) or lumpectomy plus radiotherapy is preferred over radical mastectomy. Axillary node dissection is performed if the regional sentinel node is positive for malignancy. Hormone therapy (tamoxifen) and chemotherapy combined with local therapy is recommended when invasive carcinoma exceeding 1 cm in diameter or axillary lymph nodes are positive. The combination of fluorouracil, doxorubicin, and cyclophophamide usually is administered for 4 to 6 months, given at 3- to 4-week intervals. At present, metastatic breast cancer is incurable. Accordingly, the ACS recommends a mammogram and professional clinical examination every year for women 40 years of age and older (Box 26-3; see also Table 26-3). Women 20 to 39 years of age should have a professional breast examination at least every 3 years. Breast self-examination is an option for women starting in their 20s. The American Geriatrics Society recommends mammography every 2 or 3 years for healthy women between the ages of 65 and 85.[12]

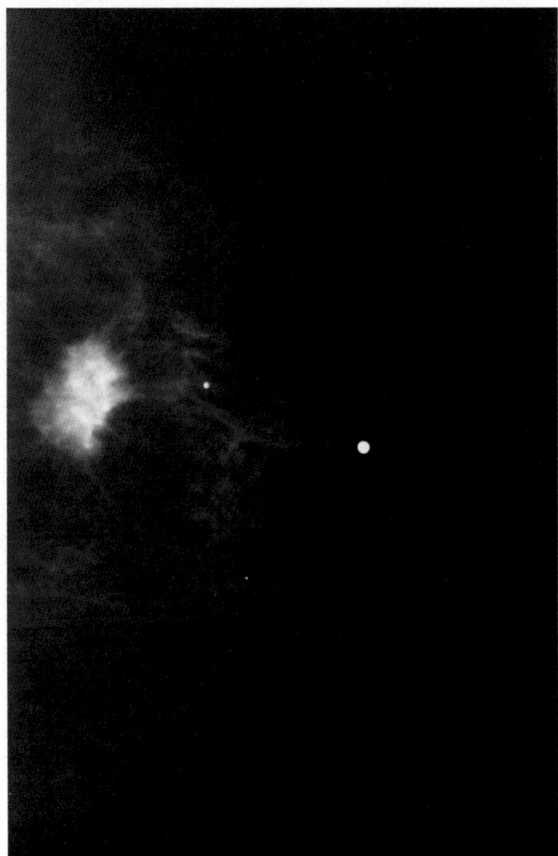

FIGURE 26-5 Mammogram showing a radiodense area in the breast suggestive of a malignancy that should be recommended for biopsy. *(Courtesy A.R. Moore, Lexington, Kentucky.)*

Cervical Cancer

Cancer of the uterine cervix occurred in nearly 12,000 women in the United States in 2010, and more than 4000 women died of the disease.[8] Cervical cancer is relatively uncommon in developed countries because of the intensive screening programs in place. Since the widespread use of screening Papanicolaou (Pap) smears, which detect asymptomatic cancerous precursor lesions at early stages, the incidence of cervical cancer has decreased dramatically, from 32 cases per 100,000 women in the 1940s to 8.3 cases per 100,000 women at present. However, approximately 30% of these patients die of the disease

BOX 26-3 American Cancer Society Recommendations for Early Breast Cancer Detection

- Women age 40 and older should have a mammogram every year and should continue to do so for as long as they are in good health.
- Women in their 20s and 30s should have a clinical breast exam (CBE) as part of a periodic (regular) health exam by a health professional preferably every 3 years. Starting at age 40, women should have a CBE by a health professional every year.
- Breast self-examination (BSE) is an option for women starting in their 20s. Women should be told about the benefits and limitations of BSE. Women should report any breast changes to their health professional right away.
- Women at high risk (greater than 20% lifetime risk) should get an MRI and a mammogram every year. Women at moderately increased risk (15% to 20% lifetime risk) should talk with their doctors about the benefits and limitations of adding MRI screening to their yearly mammogram. Yearly MRI screening is not recommended for women whose lifetime risk of breast cancer is less than 15%.

MRI, Magnetic resonance imaging.

From the American Cancer Society: Recommendations for early breast cancer detection in women without breast symptoms (Web site): http://www.cancer.org/Cancer/BreastCancer/MoreInformation/BreastCancerEarlyDetection/breast-cancer-early-detection-acs-recs. Accessed December 20, 2011.

within 5 years, and the death rate for African Americans is more than twice the national average.[13]

Human papillomaviruses (HPVs), which are epitheliotropic sexually transmitted DNA viruses, are the major etiologic agent of cervical carcinogenesis. These viruses dysregulate the cell cycle and tumor suppressor genes (*TP53* and *pRb*) through overexpression of viral early genes E6 and E7. Certain HPV strains (HPV serotypes 16, 18, 45, and 56) are classified as high-risk types, because they are associated with a majority of cases. HPV types 30, 31, 33, 35, 39, 51, 52, 58, and 66 are classified as intermediate oncogenic risk. In addition to viral infection, chronic cigarette smoking, multiple sexual partners, and immunosuppression increase the risk of cervical cancer[14,15] (see Figure 26-6).

Cervical cancer typically has a long asymptomatic period before the disease becomes clinically evident. The cancer classically manifests in women who are between 40 and 60 years of age. The earliest preinvasive changes are diagnosed by Pap smear. Further evaluation is made by colposcopy and colposcopy-directed biopsy. If neoplastic cells penetrate the underlying basement membrane of the uterine cervix, widespread dissemination can occur. Metastases often affect renal tissues, resulting in ureteral obstruction and azotemia. Treatment is based on the stage of the disease and involves hysterectomy in the early stages and radiation therapy for disease that extends to or invades local organs. The 5-year survival rate is relatively high (see Table 26-1) but drops below 50% when the cancer extends to and beyond the pelvic wall.[15]

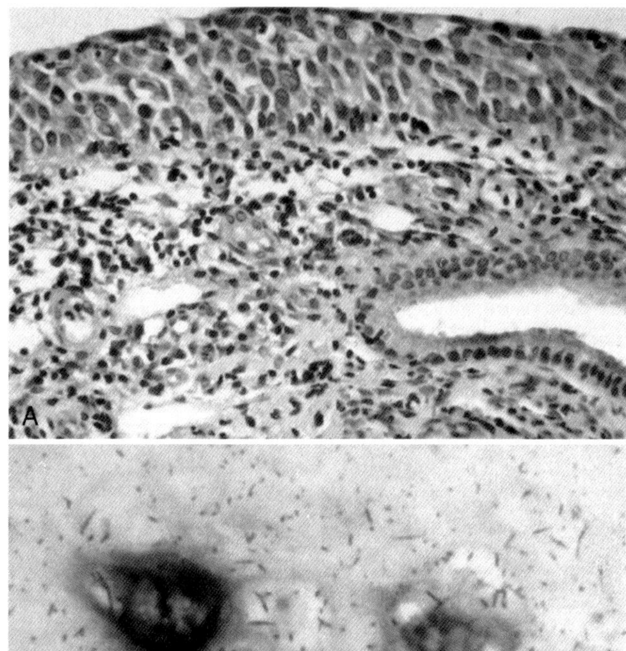

FIGURE 26-6 A, Biopsy specimen revealing cancerous epithelium of the uterine cervix (hematoxylin and eosin stain). **B,** Human papillomavirus DNA detected in cervical epithelium by in situ hybridization. *(Courtesy Dr. Michael Cibull, Lexington, Kentucky.)*

The ACS recommends that a Pap smear and professional pelvic examination be performed in women at the onset of sexually activity or at 18 years of age. Because cervical cancer is associated with immunosuppression, the Centers for Disease Control and Prevention (CDC) advises all women who are seropositive for human immunodeficiency virus (HIV) to receive semiannual screening beginning the first year after diagnosis. Health care providers may elect to screen less often when three annual examinations in a row are negative.[16]

Colorectal Cancer

Cancer of the large bowel (colon and rectum) is the most common malignancy of the gastrointestinal tract and overall the fourth most common cancer of persons living in the United States. This cancer was diagnosed in approximately 160,000 persons in the United States in 2010, and nearly 60,000 people died of the disease in that year.[8] Colorectal cancer accounts for about 10% of all cancers in the United States and carries a 5-year survival rate of 61%. Over the past 2 decades, mortality has decreased for white women and men but increased in African American men and women.[8,17]

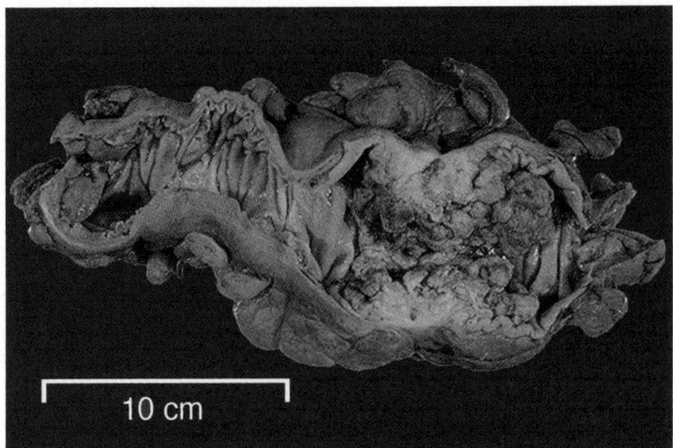

FIGURE 26-7 Destructive effects of colon cancer. *(From Klatt ED: Robbins and Cotran atlas of pathology, ed 2, Philadelphia, 2010, Saunders.)*

The vast majority of colorectal cancers are adenocarcinomas (Figure 26-7). Inherited predisposition and environmental factors contribute to their development. Genetic abnormalities in chromosome 5 (in familial adenomatous polyposis), chromosome 17 (*TP53* gene), and chromosome 18 (DCC gene) are contributory. An initiating and probably obligatory event is the oncogenic activation of the adhesion protein, beta-catenin, resulting from its overexpression, or loss of its negative regulator, the adenomatous polyposis cancer protein (APC). These abnormalities result in an upregulation in cell cycle signaling. Patients with chronic inflammation (ulcerative colitis) have approximately 10 to 20 times the risk of colorectal cancer as in the general population. The risk also increases with high-fat diet (40% of total calories), low dietary fiber intake, and smoking cigarettes for 20 years or more. By contrast, use of nonsteroidal antiinflammatory drugs (NSAIDs) and folate supplementation reduces the risk for colorectal cancer. Colonic adenomas (polyps) have malignant potential; however, less than 5% develop into carcinomas. The exception to this rule is in Gardner's syndrome, in which virtually all affected patients develop malignant polyposis by age 40 unless treated.[18-20]

Colorectal cancer often is not diagnosed until age 40 and increases in incidence after age 50. Risk rises sharply by age 60 and doubles every decade until it peaks at age 75 years. Spread is by direct extension through the bowel wall and invasion of adjacent organs by lymphatics and the portal vein to the liver. The major signs and symptoms of colorectal cancer are rectal bleeding, abdominal pain, and change in bowel habits (constipation). Presenting symptoms may include those referable to invasion of adjacent organs (kidney, liver, vagina).[18-20] Screening for colorectal cancer as recommended by the ACS is summarized in Box 26-4 and also Table 26-3.

Colonoscopy is the preferred approach for evaluating a patient for colorectal cancer. This approach permits tissue and brush biopsy to be performed. Staging of the patient is aided by endoscopic ultrasonography and computed tomography (CT) scanning. Surgical excision is the treatment of choice with lesions encroaching the distal 5 cm of the colon, resulting in colostomy. Radiation therapy is used for treatment of rectal and anal cancer. Chemotherapy (fluorouracil and leucovorin for up to 6 months or, more recently, topoisomerase I inhibitors [camptothecins] and oxaliplatin) are used when metastatic spread occurs. Liver metastases have been treated with hepatic arterial therapy using implantable pumps and injection ports to deliver chemotherapeutic agents.[18-20]

The poor prognosis with advanced colorectal cancer (stage III or IV) emphasizes the need for annual screening of at-risk adults. Digital rectal examination, fecal occult blood test, stool DNA testing, sigmoidoscopy, colonoscopy, and barium enema with air contrast are the screening procedures for colorectal cancer. The ACS recommends that screening start at age 50 for both men and women and even earlier if a family history exists, especially among first-degree relatives of colorectal cancer, preexisting inflammatory bowel disease, a personal history

BOX 26-4 American Cancer Society (ACS) Colorectal Cancer Screening Guidelines

Beginning at age 50, both men and women at average risk for developing colorectal cancer should use one of the screening tests below:

Tests that find polyps and cancer
- Flexible sigmoidoscopy every 5 years*
- Colonoscopy every 10 years
- Double-contrast barium enema every 5 years*
- CT colonography (virtual colonoscopy) every 5 years*

Tests that mainly find cancer
- Fecal occult blood test (FOBT) every year*,†
- Fecal immunochemical test (FIT) every year*,†
- Stool DNA test (sDNA), interval uncertain*

If you are at an increased or high risk of colorectal cancer, you should begin colorectal cancer screening before age 50 and/or be screened more often.

The following conditions make your risk higher than average:
- A personal history of colorectal cancer or adenomatous polyps
- A personal history of inflammatory bowel disease (ulcerative colitis or Crohn's disease)
- A strong family history of colorectal cancer or polyps (see "Risk factors for colorectal cancer")
- A known family history of a hereditary colorectal cancer syndrome such as familial adenomatous polyposis (FAP) or hereditary non-polyposis colon cancer (HNPCC)

*Colonoscopy should be done if test results are positive.

†For FOBT or FIT used as a screening test, the take-home multiple sample method should be used. An FOBT or FIT done during a digital rectal exam in the doctor's office is not adequate for screening.

From the American Cancer Society: Recommendations for colorectal cancer early detection (Web site): http://www.cancer.org/Cancer/ColonandRectumCancer/MoreInformation/ColonandRectumCancerEarlyDetection/colorectal-cancer-early-detection-acs-recommendations. Accessed December 20, 2011.

of colorectal cancer or adenomatous polyp, or a family history of hereditary colorectal cancer syndromes (e.g., familial adenomatous polyposis, Peutz-Jeghers syndrome, Gardner's syndrome). Digital rectal examination and a test for occult blood should be performed once a year. Sigmoidoscopy is recommended every 5 years and colonoscopy every 10 years. A barium enema can be performed in place of the sigmoidoscopy and colonoscopy.[21]

Lung Cancer

Lung cancer is the cause of 14% of cancer cases and is the leading cause of cancer deaths (almost 157,000 deaths annually) in the United States (see Table 26-1).[8] Although it maintains a similar incidence with breast and prostate cancer, the number of deaths caused by lung cancer exceeds the two combined. The number of new cases has been declining in men since 1984; by contrast, the incidence in women increased in the 1980s and 1990s and only recently declined. Lung cancer is more prevalent in industrialized countries, but increased incidence in nonindustrialized countries has resulted from the introduction of cigarettes into these regions. Overall, more than 85% of cases are related to smoking tobacco with a dose-dependent effect. In 60% of human lung cancers, the p53 tumor suppressor gene is mutated. Current evidence suggests that polycyclic aromatic hydrocarbons (e.g., benzopyrene metabolite) of tobacco smoke form adducts within the *TP53* gene that contribute to an abnormally functioning p53. Deletions in chromosomal 3p and 9p and overexpression of the *ras* and *myc* oncogenes and growth factor receptor c-erbB-2 appear to be important steps in malignant transformation. Risk of lung cancer increases in persons who are exposed to certain inorganic minerals (asbestos and crystalline silica), metals (arsenic, chromium, and nickel), and ionizing radiation (e.g., radon).[7]

Histologically, lung cancers are divided into two groups. About 80% are non–small cell lung cancers (large cell undifferentiated 10%; squamous cell carcinoma [SCC] 30%; and adenocarcinoma 40%) (Figure 26-8), and 20% are small cell lung cancers (i.e., oat cell carcinoma). Small cell cancers have a rapid growth rate and metastasize early.[22]

Lung cancer is a clinically silent disease until late in its course. Tumors that grow locally can produce a cough or change the nature of a chronic cough or manifest as dyspnea on exertion. Cancers that invade adjacent structures can produce chest pain and dyspnea, hemoptysis or produce syndromes (e.g., Horner's syndrome) from disruption of nerves in the chest and neck or endocrine, cutaneous, or neurologic manifestations. Metastases to the brain, bone, adrenal gland, and liver produce features associated with malfunction of these organs and lymphadenopathy. With advanced disease, patients present with anorexia, weight loss, weakness, and profound fatigue.[22]

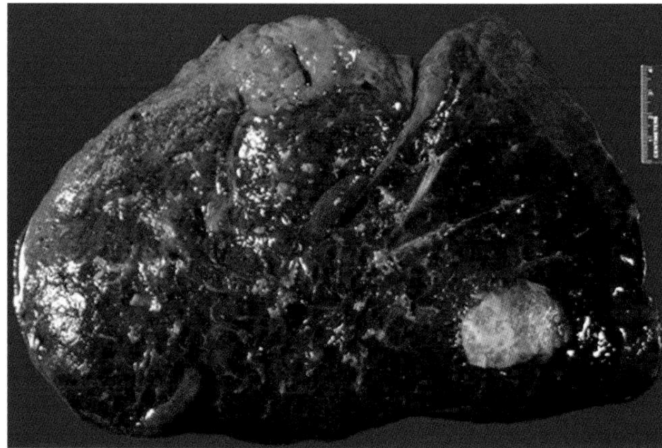

A

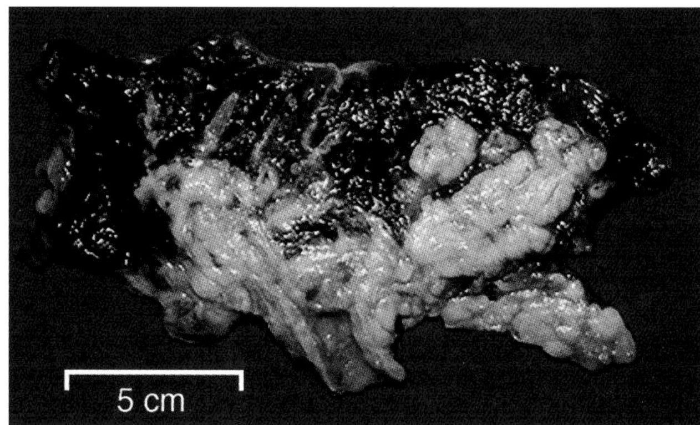

B

FIGURE 26-8 Large cell undifferentiated carcinoma infiltrating the entire lung shown in cross section. *(From Klatt ED:* Robbins and Cotran atlas of pathology, *ed 2, Philadelphia, 2010, Saunders.)*

Unfortunately, so far there is not any lung cancer screening test that has been shown to prevent people from dying of this disease. The use of chest x-ray imaging and sputum cytology (evaluating phlegm microscopically for abnormal cells) has been studied for several years. The recently updated studies have not yet yielded any value in screening programs for the early detection of lung cancer. Lung cancer screening is not recommended even for persons at high risk such as smokers.

The diagnosis of lung cancer is made by imaging studies, bronchoscopy, bronchial washings, brush and tissue biopsies, and histologic examination of the cells and tissue. Stage I and stage II non–small cell lung cancers are treated by surgical resection. Radiotherapy is used for more advanced non–small cell lung cancers and when patients with stage I or II disease refuse or are medically unfit for surgery. Chemotherapy using two or three agents (e.g., cisplatin, carboplatin, etoposide, vinblastine, vindesine) is employed in combination with radiotherapy for stage III and stage IV non–small cell lung cancers. Chemotherapy is the mainstay of treatment for small cell lung cancer. Adjuvant radiotherapy is used in patients with limited disease. Stage I lung cancer and stage II squamous cell lung cancers are associated with 5-year survival rates of more than 50%. The current 5-year survival rate for all stages of lung cancer is just 15.8%.[23] Despite the poor prognosis, national recommendations have not been made in the United States to deploy diagnostic image screening for the detection of lung cancer even in high-risk persons.[22]

Prostate Cancer

Prostate cancer is the second most common cancer (approximately 234,000 cases per year) and the most common cancer of men in the United States (see Table 26-1). It is the second leading cause of cancer deaths among men (nearly 28,000 per year).[8] Prostate cancer develops in approximately 9% of white men and in 11% of African American men. Family history and race (African American) are definitive risk factors for the development of this disease.[24]

At present, the etiologic factors for prostate cancer remain unknown. High dietary fat intake and mutations in chromosome 1 (1q24-25) and X (Xq27-28) appear to increase the risk for prostate cancer. Overexpression of the *c-myc* oncogene also is commonly detected in solid tumors such as prostate cancer.[24]

More than 90% of all prostate carcinomas are adenocarcinomas. They typically arise at multiple locations within the gland. Cancer of the prostate produces few signs and symptoms other than problems in urination (hesitancy, decreased force of urination) that, if present, occur late in the course of the disease. Thus screening procedures are paramount to the successful management of this disease. Methods used to screen for prostate cancer include the digital rectal examination (DRE) in combination with blood tests for prostate-specific antigen (PSA), and endorectal ultrasound imaging (Box 26-5; see also Table 26-3). The PSA velocity (change in the PSA level over time) aid in the diagnosis. The upper normal level for the PSA is 4 ng/mL. Transrectal ultrasound–guided needle biopsy is recommended for patients with the following findings[24]:

- PSA value greater than 10 ng/mL
- A positive DRE (palpable nodule or abnormality); even if the PSA value is less than 4 ng/mL, a positive DRE represents about 25% of all prostate cancer
- PSA value between 4 and 10 ng/mL, a negative DRE
- PSA value less than 4 ng/mL, a negative DRE, and a PSA value that has increased from 1 year to the next by 0.75 ng/mL (PSA velocity) or more

Radionuclide scanning or pelvic magnetic resonance imaging (MRI) is recommended for men diagnosed with prostate cancer with a PSA greater than 10 ng/mL to determine the extent of the disease. Metastasis occurs by lymphatic or hematogenous dissemination. Lymphatic spread is usually to thoracic and pelvic regions. Hematogenous spread is usually to bone. Bony metastasis is often identified in the pelvis, spine, and femur (Figure 26-9).

Treatment options include radical prostatectomy, external-beam radiation, interstitial seed radiation, and cryosurgery. Androgen deprivation therapy is offered in cases of more advanced disease. Prognosis correlates with the histologic grade and stage of the tumor, with persons who have limited disease (stage I) having the best prognosis.

BOX 26-5 American Cancer Society Recommendations for the Early Detection of Prostate Cancer

Tests to Detect Prostate Cancer

Prostate-specific antigen (PSA) blood test

Prostate-specific antigen (PSA) is a substance made by cells in prostate gland (it is made by both normal cells and cancer cells). Although PSA is mostly found in semen, a small amount is also found in the blood. Most healthy men have levels under 4 nanograms per milliliter (ng/mL) of blood. The chance of having prostate cancer goes up as the PSA level goes up.

When prostate cancer develops, the PSA level usually goes above 4. Still, a level below 4 does not mean that cancer isn't present – about 15% of men with a PSA below 4 will have prostate cancer on biopsy. Men with a PSA level in the borderline range between 4 and 10 have about a 1 in 4 chance of having prostate cancer. If the PSA is more than 10, the chance of having prostate cancer is over 50%.

Digital rectal exam (DRE)

For a digital rectal exam (DRE), the doctor inserts a gloved, lubricated finger into the rectum to feel for any bumps or hard areas on the prostate that might be cancer. The prostate gland is located just in front of the rectum, and most cancers begin in the back part of the gland that can be reached by a rectal exam. This exam is uncomfortable, but it's not painful and only takes a short time. It is more uncomfortable in men who have hemorrhoids.

Transrectal ultrasound (TRUS)

Transrectal ultrasound (TRUS) uses sound waves to make an image of the prostate on a video screen. For this test, a small probe that gives off sound waves is placed in the rectum. The sound waves enter the prostate and create echoes that are picked up by the probe. A computer turns the pattern of echoes into a black and white image of the prostate.

From the American Cancer Society: Recommendations for prostate cancer early detection and What tests can detect prostate cancer? (Web sites): http://www.cancer.org/Cancer/ProstateCancer/MoreInformation/ProstateCancerEarlyDetection/prostate-cancer-early-detection-acs-recommendations and http://www.cancer.org/Cancer/ProstateCancer/MoreInformation/ProstateCancerEarlyDetection/prostate-cancer-early-detection-tests. Accessed December 20, 2011.

Skin Cancer

Of the three primary types of skin cancer, basal cell carcinoma is the most common type, followed by SCC (discussed under "Oral Cancer") and melanoma. Basal

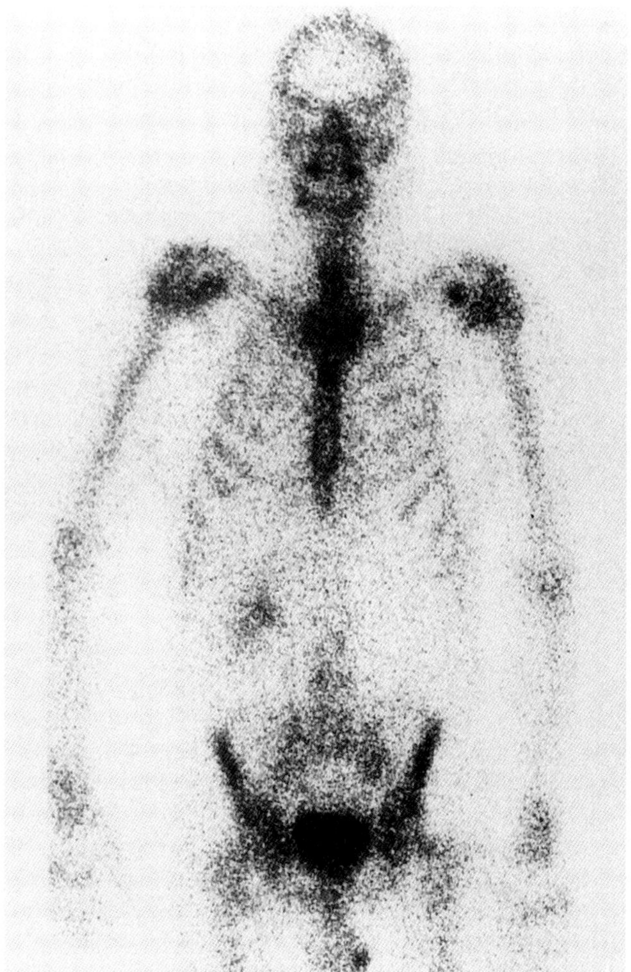

FIGURE 26-9 Radionuclide scan showing increased uptake of technetium at sites of bony metastasis from prostate cancer. *(Courtesy Dale A. Miles, DDS, Fountain Hills, Arizona.)*

cell carcinoma occurs in about 70,000 new persons annually in the United States. They are slow-growing, locally invasive tumors that arise in the basal layer of epithelium, generally as a result of chromosomal changes caused by chronic exposure to ultraviolet light (particularly UVB radiation). Evidence suggests that mutation plus inactivation of the human "patched" gene located in chromosome 9 (9q22.3) probably is a requirement for the development of basal cell carcinoma.

Basal cell carcinomas are more common in older persons with lighter skin and blond or red hair. However, diagnosis in the second and third decades of life is becoming more common. About 85% of these lesions appear on sun-exposed surfaces of the head and neck (including the lip). Four types of basal cell carcinomas are recognized: nodular, superficial, sclerosing (morpheiform), and pigmented. Each type manifests as a gradually evolving local growth. Classically, the nodular basal cell carcinoma is a pearly papule with telangiectasias, a rolled waxy border, and a central ulceration ("rodent ulcer") (Figure 26-10). A history of intermittent

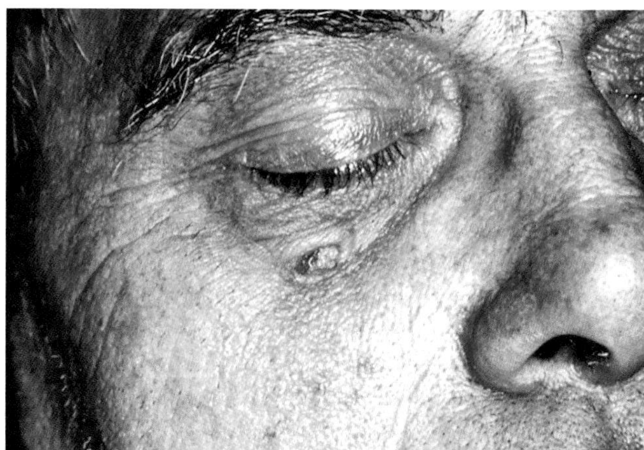

FIGURE 26-10 Basal cell carcinoma manifesting as a facial lesion in a dental patient.

encrustation and bleeding is common. The less common types appear reddish, pigmented, or scarlike. Basal cell carcinomas are readily removed with cryotherapy and surgical excision. Contemporary therapy results in greater than a 95% cure rate. Because basal cell carcinomas are locally invasive and destructive, preventive measures that include reduced sun exposure and frequent examination of sun-exposed skin by a health care provider is important in preventing recurrences. Inadequate treatment results in spread to deeper structures, but rarely do these tumors metastasize.[25]

Melanoma is a malignant neoplasm arising from melanocytes. This cancer occurs primarily in skin but can occur at any site where melanocytes are found, including the oral cavity. The incidence of melanoma is increasing faster than any other cancer, with approximately 70,000 new cases of melanoma reported in the United States annually.[8] Ultraviolet light sun exposure is the major etiologic factor. Because of increased time spent outdoors and thinning of the earth's atmosphere, the rate of melanoma has increased, from 1 in 1500 persons in 1935 to 1 in 75 persons in 2000. Increased risk also is associated with light skin color, history of severe sunburns in childhood, overall nevus count greater than 50, light and red hair color, extensive freckling, and regular use of tanning beds. Men are more commonly affected, as are persons over age 50. Cytogenetic studies have implicated chromosomal regions 1p and 9p as possible locations for genetic alterations associated with predisposition to melanoma.[26,27]

Approximately 30% of melanomas arise from previously existing pigmented lesions, particularly ones with a history of trauma. Clinical features of melanoma are characterized by the mnemonic ABCD—that is, **A**symmetry, irregular **B**order, **C**olor variegation, and **D**iameter greater than 6 mm. The color usually is deep and may be brown, gray, blue, or jet black (Figure 26-11). Multiple colors is a prominent sign. Bleeding, ulceration, firmness, and satellite lesions are characteristic of established

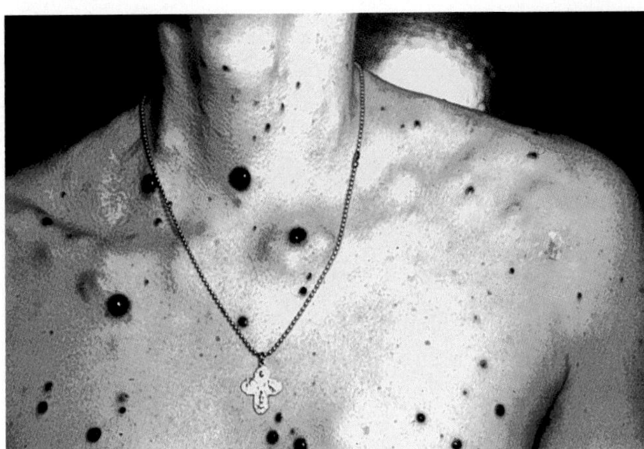

FIGURE 26-11 Malignant melanoma of the chest. The arms, face, and neck are readily visible surfaces that can be examined by the dentist.

lesions. Early diagnosis and complete resection are critical to long-term survival, because cure rates approach 100% for those persons with melanoma with a depth of 0.75 mm or less. By contrast, a depth of 1.6 mm or greater confers only a 20% to 30% 10-year survival. Vaccine therapies for melanoma are currently under clinical trial.[27]

Prevention of skin cancer is achieved from the use of sun protection measures (sunscreens and clothing) and periodic screening. The ACS recommends self-examination once a month using a full-length mirror and a hand mirror to view the back and other hard-to-see areas of the body. Professional examination of the skin should be done every 3 years from 20 to 40 years of age, and after 40 years of age it should be done every year.[27]

Oral Cancer

Oral cancer includes a variety of malignant neoplasms that occur within the mouth (Box 26-6). More than 90% of cases are attributed to SCC. About 9% are carcinomas that arise from salivary gland tissues and other tissue types such as sarcomas and lymphomas. The remaining 1% or so are metastatic from elsewhere in the body, most commonly from lung, breast, prostate, and kidney. In 2005, the ACS reported almost 31,000 cancers of the oral cavity and pharynx and 7500 deaths attributable to this disease in the United States.[28,29]

Oropharyngeal cancer represents about 3% of all cancers in the United States. The vast majority of oral cancers occur in patients older than 45 years of age, and the incidence increases with each decade beyond age 40 for men and women until age 65. Cancer incidence in African American men and women is increasing faster than in whites and other racial groups. Since 1985, little change has occurred in incidence and 5-year survival rates (see Table 26-1). The 5-year survival rates for all stages of oral cavity and pharyngeal cancer (53%) remain lower for African Americans (34%) than for whites (56%).[6,30]

The biochemical factors in the pathogenesis of oral SCC has not been fully elucidated. At least 80% of cases are associated with the multiple cellular abnormalities resulting from chronic and excessive exposure to carcinogens found in smoking tobacco, alcohol (including mouthwashes with high alcohol content), smokeless tobacco, and, in Southeast Asian cultures, paan, consisting of betel leaf plus areca nut. Ultraviolet light exposure and immunodeficiency (e.g., HIV infection, solid organ transplantation) are associated with approximately 10% of cases, particularly of the lip. HPV infection (with high-risk types) can be detected in about 30% of cases, particularly those involving the base of the tongue and tonsils. Plummer-Vinson syndrome and a vitamin A deficiency also increase the risk for cancers of the oral cavity and oropharynx. Other factors suggested to play a minor role in the cause of oral cancer include arsenic compounds used in the treatment of syphilis, nutritional deficiencies, heavy exposure to materials such as wood and metal dusts, and *Candida* infection.[6,30]

The cellular changes and contributory processes that result in SCC are shown in Figure 26-2. At the subcellular level, chronic exposure of mucosal cells to carcinogens results in activation of oncogenes and gene mutations and deletions. The most common deletion in smoking tobacco-related oral SCCs (66% of SCCs of the aerodigestive tract) occurs in chromosome 9 (9p21-22). The most frequently detected mutation occurs in p53.[6,30]

Overexpression of epidermal growth factor receptor (EGFR) and activation of the *ras* and c-*myc* oncogenes play contributory roles. HPV's involvement appears to be the result of its early gene (E6 and E7) products that increase the degradation of the p53 protein and protect

BOX 26-6 Features of Some Common Cancers of the Oral Cavity, Head, and Neck

Basal cell carcinoma Slightly raised lesion with rolled waxy border and central ulceration on sun-exposed surface

Squamous cell Nonhealing white, red-white carcinoma lesion; ulcer; or fungating mass of the lateral tongue, floor of the mouth, lip

Kaposi sarcoma Purple plaques or nodules of the palate, gingiva, or face

Melanoma Brown or black enlarging plaque on skin or palate (satellite lesions)

Mucoepidermoid Dome-shaped swelling with carcinoma central ulceration of palate, retromolar region, or lytic osseous lesion

Leukemia Gingival enlargement, and bleeding, skin pallor, small hemorrhages of the skin and mucous membranes and bruising

Lymphoma Enlarged, nonpainful lymph nodes, palatal or pharyngeal swellings, retromolar ulcerations

Advanced breast, prostate, and renal cancer Lytic osseous metastases in the mandible

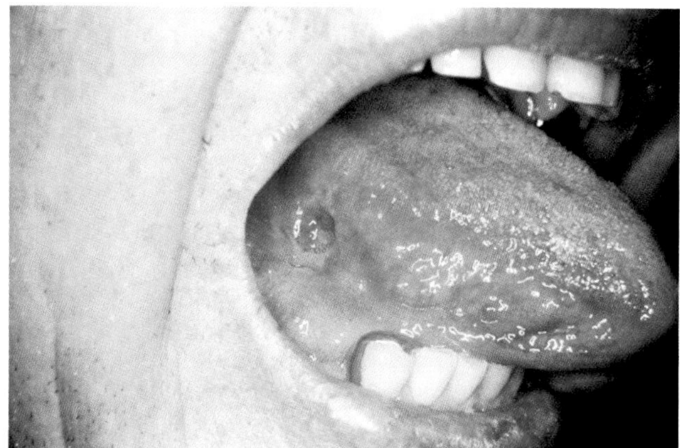

FIGURE 26-12 A clinical cause for this tongue lesion could not be identified, and its appearance was not highly suggestive of cancer. Nevertheless, it was diagnosed as early squamous cell carcinoma (SCC) by histopathologic analysis. In such cases, it would be appropriate for the dentist to request a biopsy of the lesion.

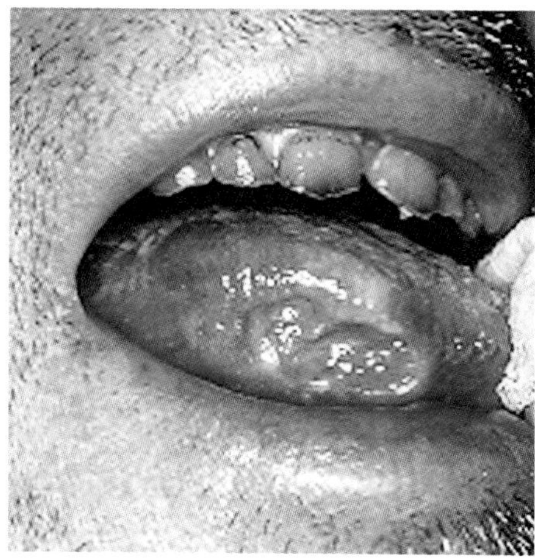

FIGURE 26-14 Tongue lesion with a high chance of being cancerous, as indicated by its clinical appearance (size, margins, induration). Direct referral of the patient to a cancer treatment center for diagnosis and therapy is indicated. This lesion was diagnosed as squamous cell carcinoma.

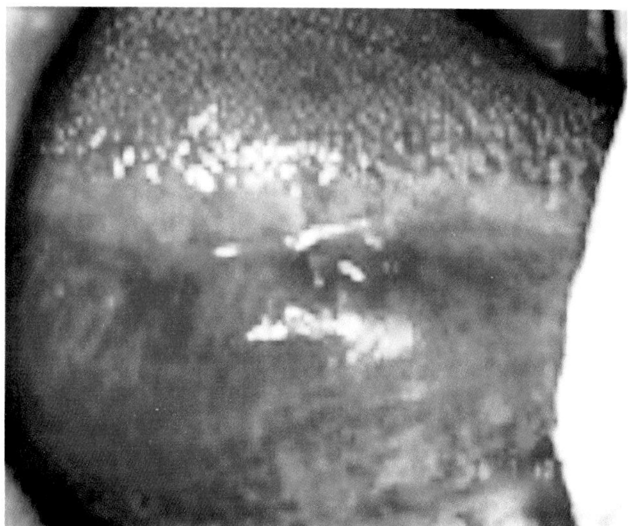

FIGURE 26-13 Squamous cell carcinoma appearing as erythroleukoplakia (a red patch in a diffuse white lesion).

TABLE 26-5 Color Characteristics of Oral Squamous Cell Carcinomas (SCCs)*

Color	% of Total SCCs
Only white lesions	24.8
White lesions with erythroplakia	60.0
Only erythroplakic (red) lesions	33.3
Other	1.9

*Data for 207 asymptomatic intraoral SCCs.
Adapted from Mashberg A, Samit A: Early diagnosis of asymptomatic oral and oropharyngeal squamous cancers, CA Cancer J Clin *45:328-345, 1995.*

cells from p53-induced apoptosis/tumor suppression. The result of these processes alters a normal cell into a dysplastic cell that eventually develops increased DNA content, functional independence, and loss of adherence. Eventually these cells also promote angiogenesis (i.e., a malignant cell).[6,30] Oral SCC is variable in appearance. It may be a white or red patch, an exophytic mass, an ulceration, or a granular raised lesion, or any combination of these (Figures 26-12 and 26-13). White lesions that cannot be scraped off and are clinically nonspecific, called *leukoplakia,* are potential precursor lesions. About 19% of leukoplakias are dysplastic, and about 4% are considered SCC at initial biopsy. Leukoplakias that are not cancerous when first biopsied have about a 6% chance of developing into cancer over time. Thus, the overall incidence of SCC in oral leukoplakia approximates 10% (Table 26-5). The malignant transformation rates for phenotypically heteromorphic leukoplakias are higher (as high as 17.5%).[28] Lesions with a histologic diagnosis of epithelial dysplasia have an even greater likelihood of becoming SCC (as high as 42% if dysplasia is severe).[6] Compared with homogeneous leukoplakias, leukoplakias with areas of erythema have a three- to five-fold greater chance of being cancerous at initial biopsy or developing into cancer. Nonspecific red lesions involving the oral mucosa (erythroplakia), although less common than white lesions (see Table 26-5), are malignant in more than 60% of cases at initial biopsy.[28-30]

A majority of early carcinomas are asymptomatic and have an erythroplastic component (see Table 26-5). Advanced lesions are more often ulcerated with raised margins and induration (Figure 26-14). Pain often is absent until late in the course of the disease. High-risk sites include the floor of the mouth; lateral (posterior) and ventral (anterior) surfaces of the tongue (Figure 26-15; see also Figure 26-14); soft palate; and surrounding tissues. These areas are less keratinized and more susceptible to carcinogens. The buccal mucosa and gingivae also are common sites, especially in regions where social oral habits result in carcinogens being placed in

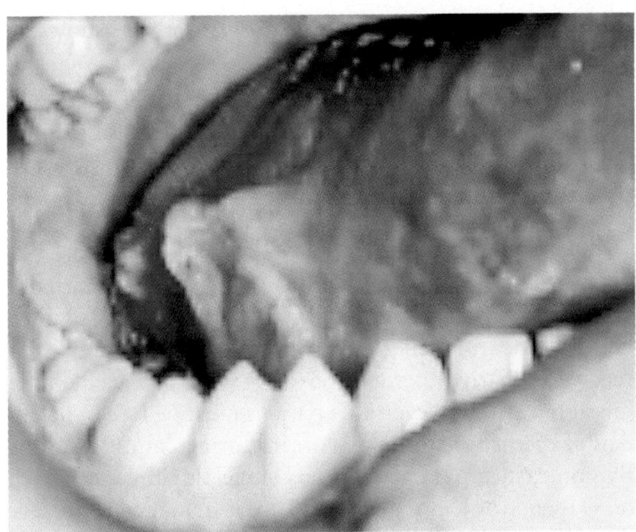

FIGURE 26-15 Squamous cell carcinoma appearing as an ulcerated lesion on the tongue with induration and raised margins.

close proximity to these tissues. Carcinoma of the upper lip and dorsum of the tongue (e.g., due to use of arsenic compounds) are rare.[6,30]

Oral SCC spreads by local infiltration into surrounding tissues or metastasis to regional lymph nodes through lymphatic channels. Spread to local structures results in induration, fixation, and lymphadenopathy. Routes of lymph node metastasis are through first-station drainage nodes (buccinator, jugulodigastric, submandibular, and submental) and then second-stage nodes (parotid, jugular, and the upper and lower posterior cervical nodes). Distant metastasis is rare but occurs more commonly to the lung, liver, and bone. Lesions of the floor of the mouth, tongue, and posterior sites tend to metastasize earlier than carcinomas located in anterior oral sites such as the lip. Moreover, about 40% of patients with SCC of the tongue and floor of the mouth lack evidence of metastases at the time of treatment but develop metastatic disease later. Lesions in the maxillary region have a greater tendency to metastasize than do those in the mandibular region. Oral cancer can lead to death by (1) local obstruction of the pathway for food and air; (2) infiltration into major vessels of the head and neck (resulting in significant blood loss); (3) secondary infections; (4) impaired function of other organs through distant metastases; (5) general wasting; or (6) complications of therapy.[6,30]

In advanced cases of oral carcinoma, the patient may complain of weight loss and difficulty in breathing or nerve involvement that may cause local musculature to become atrophic or result in unilateral paralysis (e.g., loss of the gag reflex when soft palate involved). Other symptoms include hoarseness, dysphagia, intractable ulcers, bleeding, numbness, loosening of teeth, difficulty opening, and a change in the fit of a denture. The diagnosis of oral cancer is made using microscopic examination of tissue or cells taken from the lesion. Vital staining with toluidine blue can aid in identifying the location from which to biopsy. The international tumor-node-metastasis (TNM) system of classification and staging is used to evaluate and classify a tumor's status (see Box 26-1).[6,30]

Most early oral SCCs are amenable to surgery, whereas stage III or IV cancers, (and those involving bone, vascular structures, and multiple lymph nodes) are usually treated with combination therapy (irradiation and surgery). Irradiation is by (1) interstitial, (2) implantation, or more commonly, (3) external beam methods, usually within 6 weeks of surgical resection. The tumoricidal dose of external beam radiation ranges from 5000 to 7000 centigrays (cGy), given in separate doses of 150 to 200 cGy over a 6- to 7-week period, with 4 or 5 treatment days followed by 2 or 3 nontreatment days. Hyperfractionation employs slightly lower daily doses and is delivered twice a day. "Prophylactic" neck dissection is performed to minimize the development of metastases after treatment of the primary tumor. Radiosensitizers, topical 5-fluorouracil, laser surgery photodynamic therapy (PDT) using a photosensitizing drug, Photofrin II, and 630-nm light from an argon dye laser also have been used as alternative treatment methods. A combination of radiotherapy and chemotherapy (cisplatin, 5-fluorouracil, or taxanes) is reserved for patients when the chance of cure is poor. Selective intraarterial infusion of a chemotherapeutic agent (cisplatin) also has been used successfully in a select group of patients.[31]

The overall 5-year survival rate (53%) for oral SCC has been virtually unchanged since 1980. Higher survival rates are associated with early diagnosis, younger age, early cancers (stages I and II), anterior sites, cancer depth of 5 mm or less, and carcinomas that do not infiltrate bone. Recurrences are frequent, especially if patients fail to stop using tobacco and alcohol products.[30]

DENTAL MANAGEMENT

Recognition of Cancer and Medical Considerations

The dentist has an important role in the management of the patient with cancer. A primary role is early recognition of the disease. Accordingly, dentists are advised to take a consistent approach for ascertaining pertinent medical, historical, and clinical information from the patient. The dentist should question the patient carefully for signs and symptoms of cancer, particularly those in the head and neck region. Matters involving cancer can be approached by asking the patient questions such as "Have you experienced any change in your health since your last visit?" or "Are you aware of a lump or bump developing under your arm or in your neck for no apparent reason, a lesion changing color, pain in any body region, or abnormal bleeding from any site, such as blood in the stool?" Such questions allow patients to recall events and situations pertinent to the pathogenesis of disease and may permit them to discuss the condition with the practitioner. Questions in the social history regarding overall health, exercise, diet, vitamin intake, tobacco and alcohol use, and cancer in family members also are important and permit a global assessment of the risk of cancer in the patient. The dentist also is in a prime position to discuss the benefits of cancer screening of organ systems (e.g., breast, colon, rectum, cervix, mouth, ovary, prostate, and skin) and its impact on survival (see Table 26-3). Certain medical centers and programs offer free cancer screening and patients should be encouraged to take advantage of these services.

After the interview, clinical examination is mandatory to reveal clues of underlying cancer. A head and neck and intraoral soft tissue examination should be performed on each person on entry into the patient roster. This examination, which can be life-saving in the patient with an early cancerous lesion, should be repeated on a regular basis as often as possible, but at least during dental recall visits. It is important to remember that the early stages of cancer are often subtle, and cancer is most amenable to treatment when the lesion is small or asymptomatic and has not spread. The dentist also should remember that the clinical features vary with the type of cancer and location. Lesions clinically suspicious for cancer and those that fail to heal within 14 days despite alleviating measures should be biopsied by a skilled clinician. In addition, patients with hard, fixed, and/or matted lymph nodes should be referred directly to a head and neck surgeon or a cancer treatment center. Each patient should be advised of the concern in a frank and open manner. Patients with other signs and symptoms suggestive of cancer should undergo workup with laboratory tests and imaging studies. Screening laboratory tests can be obtained by sending the patient to a hospital, a commercial clinical laboratory, or a physician. Blood tests should include a total red blood cell (RBC) and white blood cell (WBC) count; a differential white cell count; a smear for cell morphologic study; hemoglobin; hematocrit count; and a platelet count. If the screening tests are ordered by the dentist and one or more are abnormal, the patient should be referred for medical evaluation and treatment.

Treatment Planning Modifications

Dental treatment planning for the patient with cancer begins with the establishment of the diagnosis. Planning involves (1) pretreatment evaluation and preparation of the patient; (2) oral health care during cancer therapy, which includes hospital and outpatient care; and (3) post-treatment management of the patient, including long-term considerations. Cancers that are amenable to surgery and do not affect the oral cavity require few treatment plan modifications. However, certain cancers affect oral health either directly because of surgery or indirectly due to chemotherapy or immunosuppression. The focus of the remainder of this chapter is on those treatments and complications that can affect the oral cavity.

Pretreatment Evaluation and Considerations

The dentist should be aware of the type of treatment selected for the patient and whether the cancer stands a good chance of being controlled. A patient who is to receive palliative therapy may not want replacement of missing teeth; however, this patient must be free of active dental disease that could worsen during cancer therapy. By contrast, a patient who has stage I or II cancer with no evidence of regional spread can be managed for future dental care as a normal patient. In such cases, however, more frequent recall appointments to examine the patient for evidence of metastases, recurrence of the lesion, or presence of a new cancer may be advisable. Careful follow-up is particularly important in patients with oral cancer, who are at increased risk for a second primary cancer in the respiratory system, upper digestive tract, or oral cavity. The risk for a second oral cancer in smokers whose habits remained unchanged is about 30%, as compared with 13% for those who quit.[3,23]

A pretreatment oral evaluation is recommended for all cancer patients before the initiation of cancer therapy to (1) rule out oral disease that may exacerbate during cancer therapy, (2) provide a baseline for comparison and monitoring sequelae of radiation and chemotherapy damage, (3) detect metastatic lesions, and (4) minimize oral discomfort during cancer therapy. The evaluation should include a thorough clinical and radiographic examination and review of findings on blood laboratory studies. Edentulous regions should be surveyed to rule out impacted teeth, retained root tips, and latent osseous disease that could be exacerbated with immunosuppressive cancer therapy. A panoramic film is acceptable; however, supplemental bitewing and periapical films may be required for adequate visualization of dental and osseous structures.[3,23]

Pretreatment care should include oral hygiene instructions, the encouragement of a noncariogenic diet, calculus removal, prophylaxis and fluoride treatment, and elimination of all sources of irritation and infection. In children undergoing chemotherapy, mobile primary teeth and those expected to be lost during chemotherapy should be extracted, and gingival opercula should be evaluated for surgical removal to prevent entrapment of food debris. Box 26-7 presents some guidelines for extracting questionable teeth before radiation therapy. Orthodontic bands should be removed before initiation of chemotherapy.

If head and neck radiation therapy and immunosuppressive chemotherapy are scheduled, the following recommendations should be considered[3,23]:

BOX 26-7 Guidelines for Tooth Extraction in Patients Scheduled to Receive Head and Neck Irradiation (Including the Mouth) or Chemotherapy

Indicators of Extraction

- Pocket depths 6 mm or greater, excessive mobility, purulence on probing
- Presence of periapical inflammation
- Broken-down, nonrestorable, nonfunctional, or partially erupted tooth in a patient who is noncompliant with oral hygiene measures
- Patient lack of interest in saving tooth/teeth
- Inflammatory (e.g., pericoronitis), infectious, or malignant osseous disease associated with questionable tooth

Extraction Guidelines

- Extraction should be performed with minimal trauma, with timing as follows:
  - At least 2 weeks,* ideally 3 weeks, before initiation of radiation therapy
  - At least 5 days (in maxilla) before initiation of chemotherapy
  - At least 7 days (in mandible) before initiation of chemotherapy
- Trim bone at wound margins to eliminate sharp edges.
- Obtain primary closure.
- Avoid intraalveolar hemostatic packing agents, which can serve as a nidus for microbial growth.
- Transfuse if the platelet count is less than 50,000/mm^3.
- Delay extraction if the white blood count is less than 2000/μm or the absolute neutrophil count is less than 1000/μm or expected to be this level within 10 days; alternatively, prophylactic antibiotics (cephalosporin) can be used with extractions that are mandatory.

*In *select* circumstances in which healing will not be compromised, a minimum of 10 days is acceptable. Biologic modifiers that promote healing (e.g., vitamin C) may be useful in these circumstances. Alternatively, if these time recommendations cannot be met before initiation of chemotherapy, a root canal procedure can be performed to reduce the number of viable microbes; then the extraction can be performed after the white blood cell count returns to sufficient levels.

Data from Rankin KB, Jones DL, Redding SW, editors: Oral health care in cancer therapy: a guide for health care professionals, ed 3, Dallas, Baylor Oral Health Foundation/Cancer Prevention & Research Institute of Texas, *2008.*

- Reduce radiation exposure to noncancerous tissues (salivary glands) with lead-lined stents, beam-sparing procedures, or the management of salivary flow with the of anticholinergic (biperiden) or parasympatheticomimetic (pilocarpine HCl, Salagen) drugs during and after radiotherapy should be discussed with the radiation oncologist and the patient.
- Nonrestorable teeth with poor or hopeless prognosis, acute infection or severe periodontal disease that may predispose the patient to complications (e.g., sepsis, osteoradionecrosis) should be extracted; sharp, bony edges trimmed and smoothed; and primary closure obtained (Box 26-8). Chronic inflammatory lesions in the jaws and potential sources of infection should be examined and treated or eradicated before radiation or chemotherapy.

BOX 26-8 Complications of Head and Neck Radiotherapy and Myelosuppressive Chemotherapy

- Nausea and vomiting—acute onset
- Mucositis—starts about second week
- Ulceration (C)
- Taste alteration—starts about second week
- Xerostomia (R)—starts about second week
- Secondary infections: fungal, bacterial, viral
- Bleeding (C)
- Radiation caries (R)—delayed onset
- Hypersensitive teeth—acute and delayed onset
- Muscular dysfunction (R)—delayed onset
- Osteoradionecrosis (R)—delayed onset (more common in mandible, less common in maxilla)
- Pulpal pain and necrosis—delayed onset (R): (orthovoltage-related; not found with cobalt-60)

C, limited to or more prominent with chemotherapy; *R,* limited to or more prominent with radiotherapy.

From Rhodus NL: Pretreatment management of oral complications from chemotherapy and/or radiation therapy for head and neck cancer, News from SPOHNC, 18(4):1-3, November 2008.

- Adequate time for wound healing before the induction of radiation therapy or myelosuppressive chemotherapy should be provided for extractions and surgical procedures (see Box 26-8).
- Symptomatic nonvital teeth should be endodontically treated at least 1 week before initiation of head and neck radiation or chemotherapy. However, dental treatment of asymptomatic teeth even with periapical involvement can be delayed.
- Prioritize treatment of infections, extractions, periodontal care, and irritations before treatment of carious teeth, root canal therapy, and replacement of faulty restorations. Temporary restorations can be placed and certain treatment (cosmetic, prosthodontic, endodontic) can be delayed when time is limited.
- Tooth scaling and prophylaxis should be provided before initiation of cancer therapy to optimize oral health and reduce the risk of oral complications such as mucositis and infection. Removable prosthodontic appliances should be removed during therapy.
- Patients who will be retaining their teeth and undergoing head and neck radiation therapy must be informed concerning the problems associated with decreased salivary function, which includes xerostomia and increased risk of oral infections, including radiation caries, and osteoradionecrosis (Box 26-9).

Dental preparation in the cancer patient who is going to be treated by surgery is not as critical as in the patient undergoing head and neck irradiation and chemotherapy. However, active oral infection should be treated,

BOX 26-9 Radiation Effect on Normal Tissues in the Path of the External Beam

Tissue	Effect
Mucosa and lamina propria	Epithelial changes (atrophy), mucositis, vascular changes, intimal thickening, luminal stenosis, obliteration, decreased blood flow
Muscle	Fibrosis, vascular changes
Bone	Decreased number of osteocytes, decreased numbers of osteoblasts, decreased blood flow
Salivary glands	Atrophy of acini, vascular changes, fibrosis
Pulp	Necrosis (orthovoltage)

Data from Rhodus NL: Management of oral complications from radiation and chemotherapy, Northwest Dent *89:39-42, 2010.*

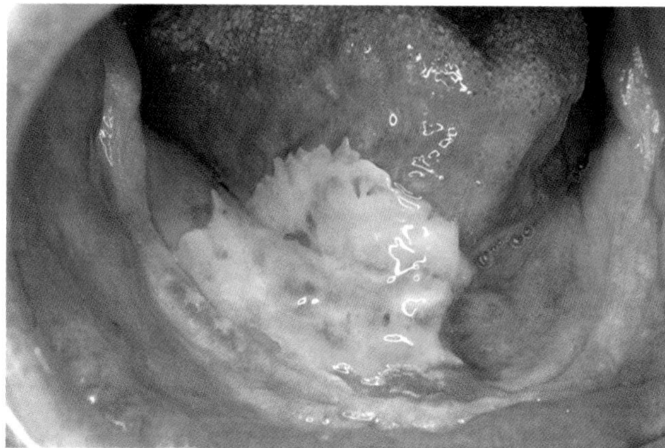

FIGURE 26-16 Extensive mucositis that developed from the effects of radiation on the oral mucosa. *(From Neville BW, et al:* Oral and maxillofacial pathology, *ed 3, St. Louis, 2009, Saunders.)*

teeth that are broken down should be removed, and teeth that may be needed for retention of a prosthetic appliance can be restored as required. The better the dental health of the patient, the lower will be the risk of dental infection complicating the healing process. For all patients with oral cancer, the dentist should consider consultation with the maxillofacial prosthodontist so that proper coordination of the patient's dental and tooth replacement needs can be accomplished during the presurgical and postsurgical phases.

Oral Care During Cancer Therapy. Maintenance of oral health during cancer therapy is very important to outcome, because oral complications develop in a significant proportion of patients who undergo cancer irradiation and chemotherapy. Patients whose treatment will include head and neck irradiation or inpatient chemotherapy should have oral infections and potential problems eliminated before initiation of cancer therapy, with routine dental care delayed until after cancer therapy is complete. Outpatient chemotherapy requires dental treatment to be provided at appropriate times between cycles. Discussed next are oral complications that occur during and after chemotherapy and irradiation of head and neck structures that may require modifications in oral health care management.[32]

Management of Complications of Radiation Therapy and Chemotherapy. General management considerations with radiation therapy and chemotherapy are presented in Box 26-10. Acute toxic reactions occur during and immediately after radiation therapy and chemotherapy. The severity of such toxicity is directly proportional to the amount of radiation or cytotoxic drug to which the tissues are exposed, and toxic effects are more evident in rapidly dividing cells. Delayed toxicity can occur several months to years after radiation therapy.[33]

Radiation therapy induces cell necrosis, microvascular damage, parenchymal and stromal damage. The production of oxygen free radicals from ionizing radiation is one of the leading causes of cell damage. Cells that undergo rapid turnover are more susceptible to such damage. For this reason, hypoxic cells and slowly replicative cells are more resistant to radiation than those that are well oxygenated and mitotically active. Box 26-9 lists the effects of radiotherapy on different oral tissues. Box 26-11 lists the recommendations for performing invasive dental treatment on these patients.

Most chemotherapeutic agents will cause alopecia, breakdown of the mucous membranes (mucositis), depression of the bone marrow (infection, bleeding, anemia), gastrointestinal changes (diarrhea, malabsorption), and altered nutritional status, and such agents also can induce cardiac and pulmonary dysfunctions. Bone marrow suppression and mucositis associated with chemotherapy are predictable, dose-dependent, and usually manageable. Patients receiving chemotherapy may manifest erythema and ulceration of the oral mucosa, infection of the surrounding tissues, excessive bleeding with minor trauma, xerostomia, anemia, and neurotoxicity.

Mucositis. Mucositis, inflammation of the oral mucosa, results from the direct cytotoxic effects of radiation or antineoplastic agents on rapidly dividing oral epithelium, and from the upregulation of proinflammatory cytokine expression (see Appendix C). Mucositis occurs in up to 40% of patients undergoing chemotherapy and often is a dose-limiting factor for chemotherapy and a cause of dose interruption of radiation therapy. It develops more often in nonkeratinized mucosa (buccal and labial mucosa, ventral tongue) and adjacent to metallic restorations by the end of the second week of radiation therapy (if the dose is 200 cGy per week). Mucositis develops most often between days 7 and 14 after chemotherapy (especially VP16, epotoside, methotrexate), when the effects of the drugs produce an extremely low WBC count (*nadir*). It generally subsides 1 to 2 weeks after the completion of treatment (see Figure 26-16). Young cancer patients with higher

BOX 26-10 Management of the Patient with Oral Complications of Radiotherapy and Chemotherapy

Complication	Recommended Management
Mucositis	Eliminate infection, irritations, establish good oral hygiene Mouth rinses (three choices of similar efficacy in controlling mucositis): 1. Salt plus sodium bicarbonate mouthwash (1 tsp. each in 1 pint of water) 2. Elixir of diphenhydramine (Benadryl) or viscous lidocaine 0.5% in Milk of Magnesia, Kaopectate, or sucralfate 3. Chlorhexidine 0.12% (can be formulated in water by pharmacist) Antiinflammatory: topical steroids, Kamillosan Liquidum Protectants: Orabase Avoid tobacco, alcohol, carbonated drinks Soft diet, maintain hydration Use humidifier, vaporizer Consider topical and systemic antimicrobials if severe Biologic response modifiers (under investigation)
Xerostomia	Sugarless lemon drops, sorbitol-based chewing gum, buffered solution of glycerine and water, salivary substitutes
Radiation caries	Educate patient concerning the risks and motivate to maintain optimum oral hygiene Custom trays for the daily application of fluoride constructed of soft flexible mouth guard material. Trays hold 5 to 10 drops of a 1% to 2% acidulated fluoride gel, applied 5 minutes each day. If the 1% to 2% acidulated gel is found to be irritating to the tissues; 0.5% neutral sodium fluoride gel can be substituted. Alternative: A single brush-on application of 5000 ppm fluoride (PrevDent) may be more effective for some patients. Frequent dental recall Patient compliance confirmed by monthly recall during first year. Restoration for early carious lesions
Secondary infection	Culture, cytologic study, antibiotics, antifungal agents, antiviral agents
Sensitivity of teeth	Topical fluorides
Loss of taste	Zinc supplementation
Osteoradionecrosis	Prevention, caution with surgery, hyperbaric oxygen therapy
Muscular dysfunction	Use of tongue blades to help retain maximum opening of jaws and access to oral cavity

Adapted from Rhodus NL: Pretreatment management of oral complications from chemotherapy and/or radiation therapy for head and neck cancer, News from SPOHNC, 18(4):1-3, November 2008.
See Appendix B for medications, dosage, and duration of use.

BOX 26-11 Recommendations for Invasive Oral Procedures in the Cancer Patient Undergoing Chemotherapy in an Outpatient Setting

Provide routine care when:
- The patient feels best—generally 17 to 20 days after chemotherapy session
- Granulocyte count* is greater than 2000 cells/μmPlatelet count*† is greater than 50,000 cells/μm

If indwelling catheter (or port) is present, administer antimicrobial prophylaxis:
- Amoxicillin 2 g 1 hour before procedure *or,* for patients allergic to penicillin:
- Clindamycin 600 mg 1 hour before procedure

*Consultation with physician is recommended when values are lower than those listed.
†Platelet values below 50,000/μm may be associated with significant bleeding.

cell division rates exhibit a greater prevalence of chemotherapy-induced mucositis than older cancer patients.[34]

Mucositis produces red, raw, and tender oral mucosa with epithelial sloughing similar to a severe oral burn. Oral ulcerations can result from breakdown of the epithelial barrier and infection by viral, bacterial, or fungal organisms. Patients typically complain of ulceration, pain, dysphagia, loss of taste, and difficulty in eating, and the risk for oral and systemic infection is increased. If the major salivary glands have been irradiated, xerostomia (Figure 26-17) comes after the initial onset of mucositis. The complications of mucositis and xerostomia make the patient extremely uncomfortable, increasing the difficulty of maintaining proper nutritional intake.[32,34]

During this acute phase, the goal is to maintain mucosal integrity and oral hygiene. Mucositis generally is well managed with use of the following: (1) a bland mouth rinse (salt and soda water) to keep ulcerated areas as clean as possible; (2) topical anesthetics (viscous lidocaine 0.5%) and/or an antihistamine solution (benzydamine HCl [Tantum rinse], diphenhydramine [Benadryl],

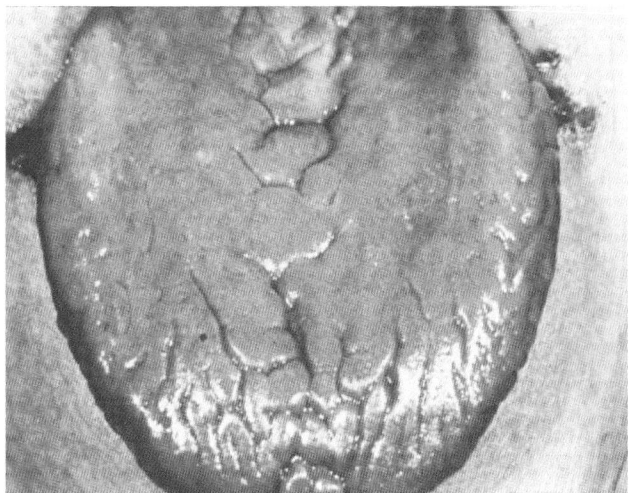

FIGURE 26-17 Severe xerostomia that developed from the effects of radiation on the oral mucosa. Note the angular cheilitis.

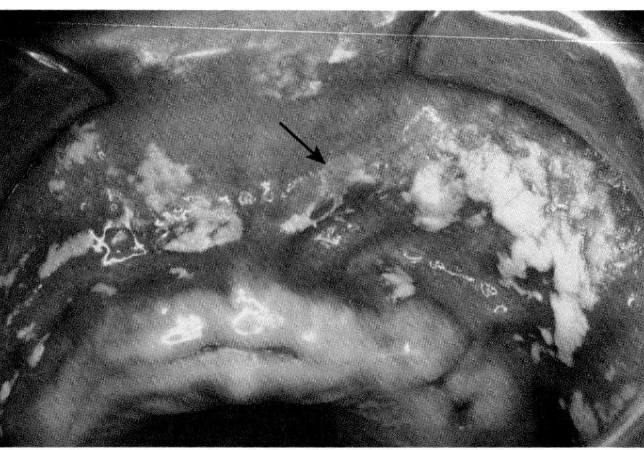

FIGURE 26-18 Oral candidiasis (pseudomembranous form) in a patient undergoing chemotherapy. *(From Allen CM, Blozis GG: Oral mucosal lesions. In Cummings CW, et al, editors:* Otolaryngology: head and neck surgery, *ed 3, St. Louis, 1998, Mosby.)*

promethazine [Phenergan]) to provide pain control or, when combined with milk of magnesia, Kaopectate, or sucralfate, to serve as a coating agent (for protection of the ulcerated areas); (3) antimicrobial rinses such as chlorhexidine; (4) antiinflammatory agents (e.g., Kamillosan Liquidum or topical steroids [dexamethasone]); (5) adequate hydration; (6) a diet consisting of soft foods, protein, and vitamin supplementation at therapeutic levels; (7) oral lubricants and lip balms with a water base, beeswax base, or vegetable oil base (e.g., Surgi-Lube); (8) humidified air (humidifiers or vaporizers); and (9) avoidance of alcohol, tobacco, and irritating foods (e.g., citrus fruits and juices and hot, spicy dishes)[33] (see Box 26-10 and Appendix C). Dentures should not be worn until the acute phase of mucositis resolves. Dentures should be cleaned and soaked in an antimicrobial solution daily to prevent infections.[35]

Secondary Infections. During radiation therapy and chemotherapy, patients are prone to secondary infections. Because of the quantitative decrease in actual salivary flow and compositional alterations in saliva, various microbial organisms (bacterial, fungal, and viral) can cause opportunistic infections of the oral cavity. Moreover, if the patient is immunosuppressed from chemotherapy, and the white blood count falls below 2000 cells/μm^3, the immune system is less able to manage such infections. Opportunistic infections also are common in patients who receive chemotherapy and broad-spectrum antibiotics.

The organism most frequently implicated in opportunistic infections of the oral cavity in patients undergoing cancer therapy (in whom hyposalivation and immunosuppression are common) is *Candida albicans*. Cytologic study, potassium hydroxide (KOH) staining, microscopic examination, and *Candida*-specific cultures are often performed to provide a definitive diagnosis. Candidal infections can produce pain, burning, taste alterations, and intolerance to certain foods, especially acidic citrus fruits or spicy foods. They manifest clinically in four different forms ranging from denuded epithelium to hyperplastic lesions. During cancer therapy, the most common type is *pseudomembranous* candidiasis, which produces white plaques that are easily scraped off, leaving behind tiny petechial hemorrhages (Figure 26-18). Slightly less prevalent is the *erythematous*, atrophic form, which manifests as a red patch accompanied by a burning sensation (see Appendix C). The other forms of candidiasis—*angular cheilosis* and the less common *hypertrophic* form, which manifests as a thick, white plaque that cannot be scraped off—are more commonly detected in patients with chronic hyposalivation.

Candidiasis is best managed with topical oral antifungal agents. These include nystatin (oral suspension 100,000 international units [IU]/mL 4 to 5 times daily), clotrimazole (Mycelex lozenges 10 mg 5 times day), and other preparations such as vaginal topical antifungal agents. Prophylactic use of antifungal agents may be required in patients undergoing chemotherapy who have frequent recurrent infections. Ketoconazole (Nizoral), fluconazole (Diflucan), or itraconazole (Sporanox) may be used if systemic therapy is warranted or if patients develop unusual oral fungal infections (torulopsis, aspergillosis, mucormycosis) or fungal septicemia (possibly from the oral cavity) (Box 26-12; see also Appendix C). Alternatively, the physician may prescribe granulocyte (monocyte) colony-stimulating factor (G[M]-CSF), which elevates the neutrophil count to normal levels and can contribute to resolution of the lesions.[35]

Bacteria and viruses may be the cause of other secondary infections. Oral bacterial infections may appear with typical signs of swelling, erythema, and fever. Alternatively, these features can be masked in patients with low WBC counts due to chemotherapy. In immunosuppressed

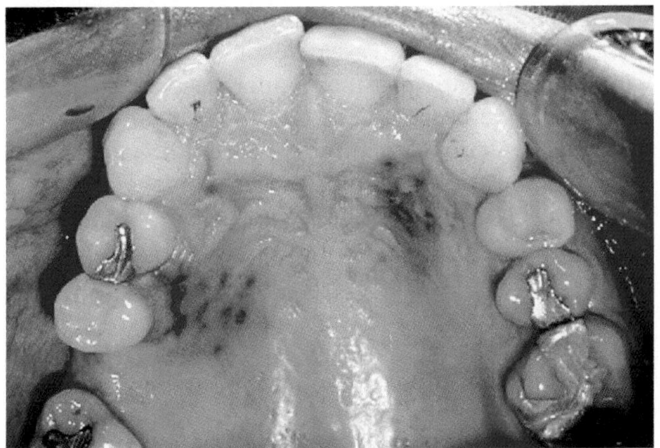

FIGURE 26-19 Recurrent herpes simplex virus infection manfesting as a large ulcer on the palate of a patient undergoing chemotherapy.

patients, a shift occurs in the oral flora to gram-negative organisms that normally inhabit the gastrointestinal or respiratory tract such as *Pseudomonas, Klebsiella, Proteus, Escherichia coli,* or *Enterobacter.* The most common presentation is an oral ulceration. Dentists should therefore culture all nonhealing oral ulcerations in such patients, and these specimens should be sent for diagnosis and antibiotic sensitivity testing. If a bacterial infection is suspected, appropriate antibacterial therapy should be initiated. Antimicrobial sensitivity data are important for the selection of an effective antibiotic when little or no clinical improvement occurs after several days.

Recurrent herpes simplex virus eruptions often develop during chemotherapy if antivirals are not prophylactically prescribed. They are infrequent during radiation therapy. HSV recurrences in patients with cancer undergoing chemotherapy tend to be larger and take longer to heal than herpetic lesions found in nonimmunocompromised patients (Figure 26-19). Antiviral agents (acyclovir, famciclovir, or valacyclovir) are recommended prophylactically for HSV antibody–seropositive patients who are undergoing chemotherapy to prevent recurrences. A daily dose of at least 1 g acyclovir equivalent is needed to suppress HSV recurrences. Because these ulcers can mimic the appearance of aphthous and can occur on nonkeratinized mucosa in immunocompromised cancer patients, obtaining a culture or use of an enzyme-linked immunoassay is important for accurate diagnosis. Laboratory tests also help distinguish the infection from other oral herpesvirus infections, such as varicella zoster and cytomegalovirus infections, that can occur in these patients. Antiviral sensitivity testing should be considered for patients with unresolving or extensive infections and those in poor general health.[36]

Bleeding. Cancer patients who undergo total body irradiation or high-dose chemotherapy or have bone marrow involvement due to disease also are susceptible

BOX 26-12 Management of Salivary Dysfunction*

1. Moisture–Lubrication

General

- Drink **or** sip water, liquids (that lack fermentable carbohydrate and carbonic acid).
- Avoid ethanol, tobacco, coffee, tea, hot spicy foods.
- Use sugarless candy/gum(Spry gum).

Products (Over-the-Counter [OTC] and Prescription)

Artificial salivas: Glandosane spray, Moi-Stir, Mouthkote, Optimoist, Roxane Saliva Substitute, Salivart spray, Salix lozenges or generic (sodium carboxymethylcellulose 0.5% aqueous solution)

OTC Oral Balance: apply ½ tsp. 5 to 6 times daily

Rx Pilocarpine HCl 2% (Salagen)† 5 mg, 3 or 4 times daily

Rx Anethole trithione (Sialor)† 25 mg 3 times a day

Rx Bethanechol chloride (Urecholine)† 25 mg 3 times a day

Rx Cevimeline (Evoxac)† 30 mg caps 3 times a day

2. Soft Tissue Lesions–Soreness

OTC

- Oral Balance
- Biotene

Rx "Magic Mouthwash": diphenhydramine (Benadryl) + Maalox + nystatin elixir‡ (± Sucralfate) (±0.5% viscous lidocaine) (± guafenesin)

Rx Dexamethasone (Decadron Elixir) 0.5 mg/5 mL§

Rx Triamcinolone 0.1% (in hydrocortisone acetate [Orabase] Orabase-HCA)

Rx Clotrimazole (Mycelex) 60-mg troches

Rx Nystatin plus triamcinolone ointment (Mycolog II, Tristatin II, Mytrex)

3. Prevention of Caries–Periodontal Disease

- Meticulous personal oral hygiene
- Avoidance of acidic drinks
- Fluoridated toothpaste (Biotene)
- Regular hygiene recalls and dental prophylaxis (at 3-month intervals)
- Mechanical brushes, Waterpik, $NaHCO_4$ rinses
- Fluoride varnishes

Rx Neutral sodium fluoride (NaF) 1.0%–trays (Prevident 5000)

Rx Chlorhexidine gluconate (Peridex, Periguard—alcohol-free)

*Salivary gland dysfunction, hyposalivation, or xerostomia should be managed by the diagnosis and according to the signs, symptoms, and severity of its manifestations in the oral cavity. Decreases in the quantity and alterations in the composition of beneficial constituents of saliva render the patient susceptible to many problems. The strategies for management will vary from patient to patient according to severity and are divided into three major areas, as listed.

†Caution is indicated with use in patients who have chronic obstructive pulmonary disease (COPD) and patients at risk for myocardial infarction (MI).

‡*Rx*: Benadryl 25 mg/10 mL, nystatin 100,000 IU/mL, Maalox 4 mL, to equal 15 mL.

§*Rx*: Decadron Elixir 0.5%/5 mL. *Disp*: 100 mL. *Sig*: 1 tsp. tid swish-swallow.

Adapted from Rhodus NL: Post treatment management of oral complications from chemotherapy and/or radiation therapy for head and neck cancer, News from SPOHNC, 18(4):1-3, December 2008.

to thrombocytopenia. Gingival bleeding and submucosal hemorrhage can occur as a result of minor trauma (e.g., tongue biting or toothbrushing) when the platelet count drops below 50,000 cells/mm^3. Palatal petechiae, purpura on the lateral margin of the tongue, and gingival bleeding or oozing are common features. Gingival hemorrhage is aggravated by poor oral hygiene. When gingival tissues bleed easily and the platelet count is severely reduced, the patient should avoid vigorous brushing of the teeth and begin using softer devices such as Toothettes or gauze wrapped around a finger and dampened in warm water or an antimicrobial solution (chlorhexidine in water, prepared by the pharmacist). During this stage, patients should be instructed not to use toothpicks, water-irrigating appliances, or dental floss. To control gingival bleeding, local measures, such as application of pressure with a gelatin sponge with thrombin or microfibrillar collagen placed over the area or use of an oral antifibrinolytic rinse (aminocaproic acid [Amicar] syrup 250 mg/mL) placed in a soft vinyl mouthguard can be used to control bleeding. If local measures fail, medical help should be obtained and platelet transfusion considered.

Neural and Chemosensory Changes. Many patients receiving radiation therapy experience diminished sense of taste, probably as a result of damage to the microvilli of the taste cells. Patients receiving chemotherapeutic agents typically complain of bitter taste in the mouth, unpleasant odors, and aversions to certain foods. To minimize sensory stimulation, the dentist should avoid use of scented body care products, including cologne, before contact with patients undergoing radiation therapy or chemotherapy.

In most patients, the ability to taste returns in 3 to 4 months after completion of radiotherapy. In cases of chronic loss of taste, zinc supplementation has been reported to improve taste perceptions. Silverman recommends 220 mg of zinc two times a day for patients with severe chronic loss of taste.[35] However, currently, no effective treatment is available for complete restoration of damaged taste.

Neurotoxicity is a side effect of chemotherapeutic agents, particularly vincristine and vinblastine. Although this complication more commonly arises in the peripheral nerves, patients treated with these agents can experience odontogenic pain that mimics irreversible pulpitis. The pain is more frequently described in the molar region and can be bilateral. Proper diagnosis requires the clinician to be familiar with the chemotherapy drug regimen and is aided by the absence of clinical or radiographic abnormalities.

Other Considerations in Dental Management

Many cancer patients have indwelling catheters (Hickman catheters or ports) that are susceptible to infection. The CDC does not recommend antibiotic prophyaxis for these patients before invasive dental procedures.[37] Likewise, patients with prosthetic implants (breast, penile, oral) that have been placed to restore esthetics or function after resection of cancerous tissue or cancer treatment are not considered to be at risk for bacterial seeding from oral invasive procedures and do not require antibiotic coverage.[39]

Patients who are neutropenic should not undergo invasive dental procedures without special preparation and precautions. The patient's physician may select to use recombinant human granulocyte-stimulating factor to promote growth and differentiation of neutrophils before surgical procedures. After necessary treatment is cleared with the patient's physician, the use of prophylactic antibiotics is dictated by WBC and neutrophil counts. Prophylactic antibiotics are often recommended if the WBC count is less than 2000, or the neutrophil count is less than 500 (or 1000 at some institutions). Antibiotic regimens are empiric. Penicillin VK 2 g given 1 hour before the procedure and 500 mg given 4 times daily for 1 week is a reasonable selection, when needed. There is no evidence that antibiotic prophylaxis is effective under these circumstances, but it is often recommended (see Chapter 23).

Whether a patient is receiving inpatient or outpatient chemotherapy, the dentist should be familiar with the patient's WBC count and platelet status before dental care. In general, routine dental procedures can be performed if the granulocyte count is greater than 2000/mm^3, the platelet count is greater than 50,000/µm, and the patient feels capable of withstanding dental care. For outpatient care, this is generally 17 days after chemotherapy or a few days before the next chemotherapy cycle (see Box 26-11). If urgent care is needed and the platelet count is below 50,000/mm^3, consultation with the patient's oncologist is required. Platelet replacement may be indicated if invasive or traumatic dental procedures are to be performed and topical therapy using pressure, thrombin, microfibrillar collagen, and splints may be required (see Chapter 23).[39]

If urgent dental care is needed and the granulocyte count is less than 2000 cells/mm^3, consultation with the physician is recommended and antibiotic prophylaxis may be provided (see Box 26-11). The dentist should recognize that use of prophylactic antibiotics for these patients is rational but without scientific evidence of effectiveness. The potential adverse effects of antibiotics should be kept in mind in making the decision to use them. No standard antibiotic regimen is recommended for prophylaxis. The drug(s), duration, and dosage to be used for prophylaxis should be established in consultation with the patient's oncologist. Penicillin V, 500 mg, every 6 hours starting at least 1 hour before any invasive procedure that involves bone, pulp, or periodontium and continuing for at least 3 days is a reasonable regimen. Periodontal infections and patients who are allergic to penicillin will require the selection of alternative antibiotics.[26-28]

Post–Cancer Treatment Management

After cancer therapy, consultation with the physician is recommended to determine whether the patient is cured or in remission or is completing palliative care. If cancer therapy is completed and remission or a cure is the outcome, the cancer patient should be placed on an oral recall program. Usually, the patient is seen once every 1 to 3 months during the first 2 years and at least every 3 to 6 months thereafter. After 5 years, the patient should be examined at least once per year. This recall program is important for the following reasons: (1) a patient with cancer tends to develop additional lesions; (2) latent metastases may develop; (3) the initial lesions may recur; and (4) complications related to therapy can be detected and managed. The usual long-term complications associated with the cancer and its therapy include chronic xerostomia, loss of taste, altered bone, and related problems. Recall appointments also are important, to ensure that the dentate patient continues to maintain good oral hygiene (including daily brushing, flossing, and fluoride gel applications), and to promote early detection of oral soft tissue and hard tissue disease, before inflammation and infection involves the underlying bone leading to necrosis. Patients who have completed palliative care should be afforded any preventive oral care and dental procedures they desire and can withstand.

Hyposalivation and Its Sequelae. Salivary gland tissue is moderately sensitive to radiation damage. Because of this, acinar tissue that is in the field of radiation can be permanently damaged during head and neck radiation therapy, resulting in hyposalivation. The degree of hyposalivation is directly related to the radiation field and dose (i.e., the dose delivered to the major salivary glands) and to baseline salivary function. Dosages in excess of 3000 cGy are the most damaging, especially if shielding or medication is not provided to the patient during delivery of radiation. Irradiated salivary glands become dysfunctional as a consequence of acinar atrophy, vascular alterations, chronic inflammation, and loss of salivary parenchymal tissue. Usually, a 50% to 60% reduction in salivary flow occurs in the first week after radiation therapy. As a sequela of radiotherapy, saliva is reduced in volume and altered in consistency, pH, and immunoglobulin concentration. The consistency is mucinous, thick, sticky, and ropy because the serous acini are more sensitive to radiation than mucous acini. Unfortunately, the pathologic changes often progress over several months after radiotherapy has ceased, and the radiation-induced salivary gland damage and dysfunction may be permanent. In most cases, no recovery of salivary gland function occurs.[32,33]

The direct effects of hyposalivation include extreme dryness of the oral mucosa (see Figure 26-17). Of major significance are the discomfort, inconvenience, and substantial diminution of quality of life that accompanies oral dryness. Clearly, saliva is an important host defense mechanism against oral disease, serving a variety of important functions in the oral cavity. In a healthy mouth, copious saliva containing essential electrolytes, glycoproteins, immunoglobulins, hydrolytic enzymes (amylase), antimicrobial enzymes, and a number of other important factors continually lubricates and protects the oral mucosa. Saliva in normal quantities and composition serves to cleanse the mouth, clear potentially toxic substances, regulate acidity, buffer decalcifying acids, neutralize bacterial toxins and enzymes, destroy microorganisms, and remineralize enamel with inorganic elements (e.g., calcium and phosphorus), thereby maintaining the integrity of the teeth and soft tissues.[32,33]

When the normal environment of the oral cavity is altered because of a decrease in or total absence of salivary flow or as a consequence of alterations in salivary composition, a healthy mouth becomes susceptible to painful deterioration and decay. Dry, atrophic, and fissured oral mucosa and soft tissues are the usual results of the hyposalivary condition, along with accompanying ulcers and desquamation, opportunistic bacterial and fungal infections, inflamed and edematous tongue, caries, and periodontal disease. Extreme difficulty in lubricating and masticating food (sticking to the tongue or hard palate) and difficulty swallowing food (dysphagia) are common and among the most devastating clinical consequences of hyposalivation, with the potential for profound systemic changes affecting the overall health of the patient. Additionally, lack of or altered taste perception (hypogeusia or dysgeusia) and tolerance for certain acidic foods (e.g., citrus fruits, acetic acid, vinegar) are substantially altered in the absence of adequate saliva. As a result, nutritional intake may be impaired.[3,40]

The manifestations of salivary hypofunction in patients having undergone radiation therapy for head and neck cancer include severe xerostomia (unstimulated salivary flow less than 0.2 mL/minute); mucositis; cheilitis; glossitis; fissured tongue; glossodynia; dysgeusia; dysphagia; and a severe form of caries called *radiation caries* (Figure 26-20). The incidence of such severe caries is estimated to be 100 times higher in patients who have received head and neck radiation than in normal, healthy persons. Radiation caries can progress within months, advancing toward pulpal tissues and resulting in periapical infection that extends to involve the surrounding irradiated bone; extensive infection and necrosis can result. A prescription for concentrated fluoride toothpaste (5000 ppm) should be provided to these patients for use in custom trays or brush-on application (see Box 26-12), and an assessment of salivary flow should be made.[33,40]

After a proper diagnostic assessment that determines the level of unstimulated and stimulated salivary flow, xerostomia is managed according to the three categories

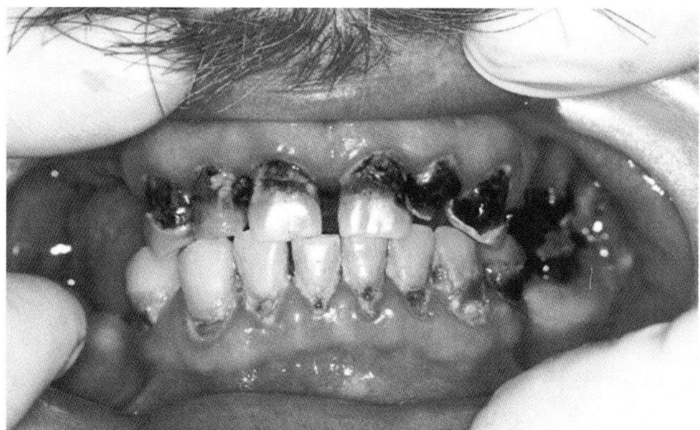

FIGURE 26-20 Note the extensive cervical caries in a patient who received radiotherapy. (*Courtesy R. Gorlin, Minneapolis, Minnesota.*)

delineated in Box 26-12. First is the provision of additional moisture and lubrication to the oral cavity and oropharynx. This may be accomplished by either simulation of oral fluids or stimulation of endogenous saliva. Several artificial salivas are available, some of which provide a modicum of symptomatic relief from oral dryness. However, synthetic saliva solutions alone do not appear to be satisfactory for relief of the complaints associated with chronic xerostomia. Generally, they are compounded from carboxymethylcellulose or hydroxymethylcellulose. Some contain fluoride and supersaturated calcium and phosphate ions. An artificial saliva that has been particularly effective but is available only in Europe is AS Saliva-Orthana (AS Pharma, Hampshire, United Kingdom), which contains some natural animal mucins. Mouthkote (Parnell Pharmaceuticals, San Rafael, California) contains a plant glycoprotein that reproduces the lubricating mucosal protection normally provided by saliva. Xero-Lube (Colgate-Palmolive, NY), Optimoist (Colgate-Palmolive), Glandosane (Fresenius Medical Care, St. Wendel, Germany), and Salivart (Gebauer Co., Cleveland, Ohio) are other examples of artificial salivas that are primarily compounds of carboxymethylcellulose and may be effective. A gel form of artificial saliva that provides long-lasting relief, especially at night, is Oral Balance (Laclede, Inc., Rancho Dominguez, California). This product contains two antimicrobial enzymes, lactoperoxidase and glucose oxidase, that normally are found in saliva.[33,40]

Patients should be encouraged to drink plenty of water and other fluids with the exception of diuretics such as coffee or tea. Ethanol and tobacco should be avoided or minimized, because these dry the oral mucosa. Also, patients who have undergone irradiation for cancer treatment may sip drinks constantly to keep the oral mucosa moist; suche drinks should not be products containing a fermentable carbohydrate or carbonic acid, which may cause exposed cementum and dentin to break down rapidly (in less than 6 months), resulting in radiation caries. Sucking on sugarless mints or hard candies and chewing gum are beneficial in producing some additional moisture.[41]

Considerable research has been performed with various sialagogue drugs such as pilocarpine HCl (Salagen), anethole trithione (Sialor), and recently, cevimeline (Evoxac). Pilocarpine is the prototype parasympathomimetic drug derived from the pilocarpus plant. It is an alkaloid, muscarinic-cholinergic agonist and is known to stimulate smooth muscle and exocrine secretions. Pilocarpine has been extensively tested in safety and efficacy trials, and it appears to be very promising as a sialagogue. These parasympathomimetic drugs appear to be effective for stimulating salivary flow in most patients who have some residual salivary acinar function. However, certain side effects occur, and patients have to be carefully screened (i.e., for cardiovascular disease, diabetes, and concomitant medications) before being placed on these drugs. Of particular note is that approximately half of the patients who used pilocarpine and experienced increased salivary flow noticed symptomatic improvement in their dry mouth. Therefore, although the drug increases salivary flow and provides endogenous beneficial constituents to the oral cavity, patients may still need adjunctive artificial salivas in order to feel more comfortable.[42]

Fungal Infection. Opportunistic infection with *Candida albicans* is very prevalent among patients who have undergone radiation therapy, with more than 80% of such patients exhibiting infection with the fungus if proper diagnostic testing is used (see earlier under "Secondary Infections").

Tooth Sensitivity. During and after radiotherapy, the teeth may become hypersensitive, which could be related to the decreased secretion of saliva and the lowered pH of secreted saliva. The topical application of a fluoride gel, dentinal tubule–blocking agents including fluoride solution, oxalate-containing resin and resin-based desensitizers, and yttrium-aluminum-garnet (YAG) laser treatment may be of benefit in reducing these symptoms.[43]

Muscle Trismus. Radiation therapy of the head and neck can cause damage to the vasculature of muscles (obliterative endoarteritis) and consequent trismus of the masticatory muscles and joint capsule. To minimize the effects of radiation on the muscles around the face and the muscles of mastication, a mouth block should be placed when the patient is receiving external beam irradiation. The patient also should perform daily stretching exercises to relieve trismus and apply local warm moist heat. One exercise is for the patient to place a given number of tongue blades in the mouth at least three times a day for 10-minute intervals. By slowly increasing the number of tongue blades, muscle stretching will occur, and more normal function will ensue.

Prosthodontics. Patients should avoid wearing their dentures during the first 6 months after completion of the radiotherapy, because even mild trauma to the altered mucosa can result in ulcerations and possible necrosis of underlying bone (see "Osteoradionecrosis," next). Once patients start to wear their dentures, they must be instructed to return to the dentist if any sore spots develop, so that the dentures can be adjusted. Ill-fitting dentures should be replaced by new ones. In severe cases of chronic xerostomia, a small amount of petrolatum can be applied to the mucosal surface of the denture to help with adhesion. Implants can be placed 12 to 18 months after radiation therapy, but the procedure will require knowledge of tissue irradiation fields, degree of healing and vascularity of the region. For example, implants placed in the maxilla and the anterior mandible are associated with less of a risk for osteoradionecrosis than those placed in the posterior mandible.

Osteoradionecrosis. Osteoradionecrosis is a condition characterized by exposed bone that fails to heal (present for 6 months) after high-dose radiation to the jaws (Figure 26-21). Osteoradionecrosis results from radiation-induced changes (hypocellularity, hypovascularity, and ischemia) in the jaws. Most cases result from damage to tissues overlying the bone as opposed to direct damage to the bone. Accordingly, soft tissue necrosis usually precedes involvement of bone and is variably present at the time of diagnosis. Risk for development of this complication is greatest in posterior mandibular sites and in patients who have received radiation doses in excess of 6500 cGy to the jaw, those who continue to smoke, and those who have undergone a traumatic (e.g., extraction) procedure. Risk is greater for dentate patients than for edentulous patients and for those with periodontal disease. Nonsurgical procedures associated with tissue trauma (e.g., curettage) or with reduction in blood supply to the region (e.g., use of vasoconstrictors) can result in osteoradionecrosis. Spontaneous osteoradionecrosis also occurs. The risk remains throughout the patient's lifetime.[44,45]

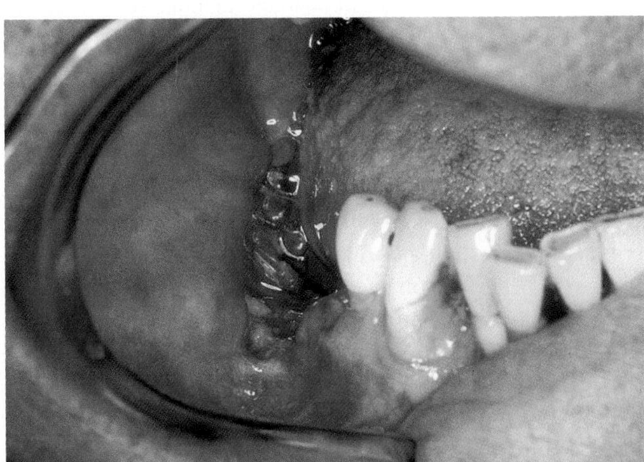

FIGURE 26-21 Osteoradionecrosis. Exposed necrotic bone is evident in the posterior mandible edentulous ridge of a patient who previously received radiation therapy to the head and neck region.

If the dentist is unsure of the amount of radiation received and invasive procedures are planned, the radiation oncologist should be contacted to determine the total dose to the head and neck region before dental care is initiated (Box 26-13). Clinicians should be aware that risk of osteoradionecrosis increases with increasing dose to the jaws (e.g., 7500 cGy is associated with greater risk than 6500 cGy). Patients determined to be at risk should be provided with the appropriate preventive measures. Protocols to reduce the risk of osteoradionecrosis include selection of endodontic therapy over extraction, use of non-lidocaine local anesthetics that contain no or a very

BOX 26-13 Recommendations to Prevent Osteoradionecrosis in the Patient Undergong Irradiation of the Head and Neck

1. Extract teeth with questionable and hopeless prognosis at least 2 weeks before radiotherapy.
2. Avoid extractions during radiotherapy.
   - Mandible is at greater risk than maxilla.
   - Posterior sites are at greater risk than anterior sites.
3. Minimize infection:
   - Prophylactic antibiotic use: Give 2 g penicillin VK orally 1 hour before surgical procedure.
   - After surgery: continue with penicillin VK 500 mg four times a day for 1 week.
4. Minimize hypovascularity after radiotherapy:
   - Use non-lidocaine local anesthetic (e.g., prilocaine plain or forte) for dental procedures.
   - Minimize or avoid use of vasoconstrictor; if necessary, consider low-concentration epinephrine (1:200,000 or less).
   - Consider hyperbaric oxygen therapy.*
5. Minimize trauma:
   - Endodontic therapy is preferred over extraction (if the tooth is at all restorable).
   - Atraumatic surgical technique is essential.
   - Avoid periosteal elevations.
   - Limit extractions to two teeth per quadrant per appointment.
   - Irrigate with saline, obtain primary closure, eliminate bony edges or spicules.
6. Maintain good oral hygiene:
   - Use oral irrigators.
   - Use antimicrobial rinses (chlorhexidine).
   - Use daily fluoride gels.
   - Eliminate smoking.
   - Schedule frequent postoperative recall appointments.

*Alternatives include referral of patient in need of extractions to an oral-maxillofacial surgeon who has experience with such cases and use of hyperbaric oxygen (HBO) therapy after consultation with a medical specialist. HBO treatments often consist of 20 preextraction dives and 10 postsurgical dives.

low concentration of epinephrine; atraumatic surgical technique (if surgery is necessary); prophylactic antibiotics plus antibiotics during the week of healing (penicillin VK for 7 days); and hyperbaric oxygen therapy before invasive procedures (see Box 26-13). Hyperbaric oxygen therapy involves sequential daily "dives" under 2 atmospheres of oxygen pressure in a chamber.[45]

The use of prophylactic antibiotics to prevent infection after surgical procedures in postradiation patients minimizes bacterial invasion of the surgical site.[38] The effectiveness of such coverage, however, can be greatly reduced because of altered blood flow to the affected bone. The dentist should be aware that reduction in blood flow after radiotherapy is much greater in the mandible than in the maxilla because of the limited source and lack of collateral circulation, which accounts for the greater frequency and severity of osteoradionecrosis in the mandible. The use of hyperbaric oxygen treatment at the time of extraction is gaining more support but is costly and cannot be repeated later with the same effect.[45]

Once necrosis occurs, conservative management usually is indicated. The exposed bone (see Figure 26-21) should be irrigated with a saline or antibiotic solution, and the patient should be directed to use oral irrigating devices to clean the involved area. However, extreme pressures should be avoided when use of these devices is prescribed. Bony sequestrum should be removed to allow for epithelialization. If swelling and suppuration are present, broad-spectrum antibiotics are indicated. Severe cases benefit from hyperbaric oxygen treatment (60- to 90-minute dives, 5 days per week, for a total of 20 to 30 dives). Cases that do not respond to conservative measures may require surgical resection of involved bone.[45]

Bisphosphonate-Associated Osteonecrosis. In the past decade, a potentially serious oral complication of cancer treatment was identified: bisphosphonate-associated osteonecrosis (BON) (Figure 26-22). Bisphosphonates are synthetic analogues of inorganic pyrophosphate that have a high affinity for calcium. Bisphophonates also are potent inhibitors of osteoclastic activity. All bisphosphonate compounds accumulate over extended periods of time in mineralized bone matrix. Depending on the duration of the treatment and the specific bisphosphonate prescribed, the drug may remain in the body for years.[46-49]

Bisphosphonates are used to treat osteoporosis, Paget's disease of bone, multiple myeloma (which is discussed in Chapter 23), and hypercalcemia of malignancy. In patients with osteoporosis, it is expected that bisphosphonates will arrest bone loss and increase bone density, decreasing the risk of pathologic fracture resulting from progressive bone loss. Bisphosphonates are given to patients with cancer to help control bone loss resulting from metastatic skeletal lesions. Use of these agents has been shown to reduce skeletal-related events associated with multiple myeloma (such as fractures) and metastatic solid tumors, (such as breast, lung, and prostate cancers) in the bones. The physician's decision regarding which type of bisphosphonate to use depends on the type of medical condition being treated and the potency of the drug required. For example, orally administered bisphosphonates often are used in patients with osteoporosis, while the injectable bisphosphonates are used in patients with cancer who develop primary lesions of bone or skeletal metastasis.[47] BON can occur with the oral administration of bisphosphonates but is rare. In

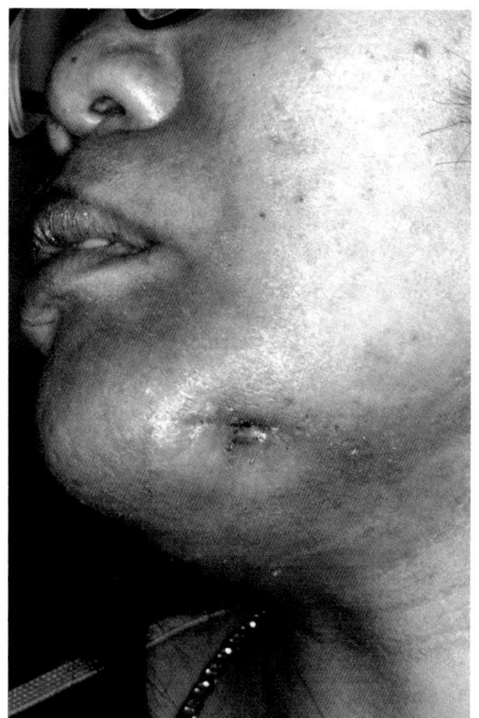

A

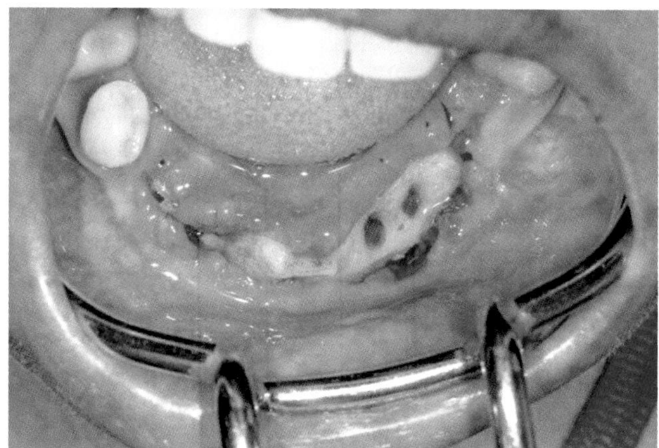

B

FIGURE 26-22 Extraoral (**A**) and intraoral (**B**) views of bisphosphonate-associated osteonecrosis of the mandible in a patient with metastatic breast cancer. (*Courtesy Dr. Denis Lynch, Milwaukee, Wisconsin.*)

contrast BON is a much more common complication of injected bisphosphonates.[49] The exact mechanism that leads to the induction of BON is unknown. However, risk factors have been recognized and may be classified as systemic and local. These include previous use of intravenous bisphosphonates (i.e., etidronate [Didronel], pamidronate [Aredia], zoledronic acid [Zometa]), diabetes mellitus, overall cancer stage and tumor burden, overall systemic and immue health, immunosuppressive drug use, any periodontal or other oral infection, and history of radiation to the jaws. Also, posterior sites are at higher risk than anterior sites, and the mandible is more often affected than the maxilla.[40-43]

Bone remodeling is a physiologic function that occurs in normal bone. During bone remodeling, the drug is taken up by osteoclasts and internalized in the cell cytoplasm, where it inhibits osteoclastic function and induces apoptotic cell death. It also inhibits osteoblast-mediated osteoclastic resorption and has antiangiogenic properties. As a result, bone turnover becomes profoundly suppressed, and over time, the bone shows little physiologic remodeling. The bone becomes brittle and unable to repair physiologic microfractures that occur in the human skeleton with daily activity (e.g., common masticatory forces). In the oral cavity, the maxilla and mandible are subjected to constant stress from masticatory forces.[46,47]

Physiologic microdamage and mircofractures occur daily in the oral cavity. Although the exact cause of BON is not known, it is theorized that in a patient taking a bisphosphonate, the resulting microdamage is not repaired, setting the stage for oral osteonecrosis to occur. Therefore, BON results from a complex interplay of bone metabolism, local trauma, increased demand for bone repair, infection, and hypovascularity.[47]

In the early stages of oral BON, no radiographic manifestations can be seen. Patients usually are asymptomatic but may develop severe pain because of the necrotic bone becoming infected secondarily after it is exposed to the oral environment. The osteonecrosis often is progressive, potentially leading to extensive areas of bony exposure and dehiscence. When tissues are acutely infected, patients may complain of severe pain or lack of sensory sensation (paresthesia). Either symptom may be an indication of peripheral nerve compression (see Figure 26-22).[47,48]

In patients in whom BON develops spontaneously, the most common initial complaint is the sudden presence of intraoral discomfort and the presence of roughness that may progress to traumatize the oral soft tissues surrounding the area of necrotic bone. Therefore, the diagnosis of BON is based on the medical and dental history or each patient, as well as the observation of clinical signs and symptoms of this pathologic process.[48,49]

According to the most recent recommendations from the American Association of Oral and Maxillofacial Surgeons (AAOMS),[49] the working definition of BON (or BRONJ [bisphosphonate-related osteonecrosis of the jaw]) is based on the following criteria:

1. Current or previous treatment with a bisphosphonate
2. Exposed bone in the maxillofacial region that has persisted for more than 8 weeks
3. No history of radiation therapy to the jaws

The AAOMS staging (four stages) for BON (BRONJ), is summarized in Box 26-14.

In the early stage (stage 0) of BON, no clinical or radiographic manifestations are evident. Patients usually are asymptomatic but may complain of nonspecific pain. Exposed bone becomes apparent in stage 1, during which the patient is asymptomatic but may develop severe pain secondary to development of infection of the necrotic bone after exposure to the oral environment. In stage 2, the osteonecrosis often progresses, as evidenced by pain and erythema. Stage 3 is characterized by extension of exposed and necrotic bone beyond the region of alveolar bone, resulting in pathologic fracture, extraoral fistula formation, and establishment of oral antral–oral nasal communication. Patients with stage 2 or 3 BON may complain of severe pain and lack of sensory sensation (paresthesia). As noted previously, such changes may be an indication of peripheral nerve compression (see Figure 26-14).[47,48]

Treatment Strategies. Effective treatment strategies would be those that would yield consistent resolution and healing of BON. However, to date those have been elusive.[49] In fact, many cases had poor outcomes in spite of therapy, progressing to extensive dehiscence and exposure of bone. Treatment strategies included local surgical débridement, bone curettage, local irrigation with antibiotics, and hyperbaric oxygen therapy. However, none of these therapeutic modalities has proved successful. Therefore, the inability to manage lesions of BON compromises the oncologic, nutritional, and oral management of affected patients. Prevention of this condition is of paramount importance for these patients so that they can receive the anticancer therapies required for the best possible outcome of their neoplastic disease.[47] The most current recommendations for the dental management of patients with BON (BRONJ) are summarized in Box 26-15.[49]

Accordingly, the dental management program for patients taking oral bisphosphonates should include the following elements:

1. Medical consultation to determine the medical diagnoses and type of drugs taken and ideally performance of all necessary dental treatments performed before administration of the drug(s) (similar to the approach indicated for patients undergoing head and neck radiation therapy).

BOX 26-14 AAOMS Staging for BON (BRONJ)

Stage 0: No clinical evidence of necrotic bone in patients who nevertheless present with nonspecific symptoms or clinical and radiographic findings, including:

Symptoms
- Odontalgia not explained by an odontogenic cause
- Dull, aching bone pain in the body of the mandible that may radiate to the temporomandibular joint region
- Sinus pain, which could be associated with inflammation and thickening of the maxillary sinus wall
- Altered neurosensory function

Clinical findings
- Loosening of teeth not explained by chronic periodontal disease
- Periapical/periodontal fistula that is not associated with pulpal necrosis due to caries

Radiographic findings
- Alveolar bone loss or resorption not attributable to chronic periodontal disease changes to trabecular pattern—dense woven bone and persistence of unremodeled bone in extraction sockets
- Thickening or obscuring of periodontal ligament (thickening of the lamina dura and decreased size of the periodontal ligament space)
- Inferior alveolar canal narrowing

These nonspecific findings, which characterize stage 0, also may be seen in patients with a history of stage 1, 2, or 3 disease whose lesions have healed and who have no clinical evidence of exposed bone.

Stage 1: Exposed and necrotic bone in patients who are asymptomatic and have no evidence of infection

Stage 2: Exposed and necrotic bone in patients with pain and clinical evidence of infection

Stage 3: Exposed and necrotic bone in patients with pain, infection, and one or more of the following:
- Exposed necrotic bone extending beyond the region of alveolar bone (i.e., inferior border and ramus in the mandible, maxillary sinus, and zygoma in the maxilla)

Pathologic fracture
- Extraoral fistula
- Oral antral–oral nasal communication
- Osteolysis extending to the inferior border of the mandible or sinus floor

AAOMS, American Association of Oral and Maxillofacial Surgeons; *BON,* Bisphosphonate-associated osteonecrosis; *BRONJ,* Bisphosphonate-related osteonecrosis of the jaw.

From Ruggiero SL, et al: American Association of Oral and Maxillofacial Surgeons position paper on bisphosphonate-related osteonecrosis of the jaw—2009 update, Aust Endod J *35:119-130, 2009.*

BOX 26-15 Treatment Strategies for BON (BRONJ)

At risk: Patients who are at risk for the development of BRONJ subsequent to exposure to a bisphosphonate do not require any immediate treatment. However, these patients should be informed of the associated risk, as well as the signs and symptoms of this disease process.

Stage 0: Provide symptomatic treatment, with conservative management for other local factors, such as caries and periodontal disease. Systemic management can include the use of medication for chronic pain and the control of infection with antibiotics, when indicated.

Stage 1: These patients benefit from the use of oral antimicrobial rinses, such as chlorhexidine 0.12%. No surgical treatment is indicated.

Stage 2: These patients benefit from the use of oral antimicrobial rinses combined with antibiotic therapy. It has been hypothesized that the pathogenesis of BRONJ might be related to factors adversely influencing bone remodeling. Additionally, the etiology of BRONJ does not include a primary infectious process. Most of the isolated microbes have been sensitive to the penicillin group of antibiotics. Quinolones, metronidazole, clindamycin, doxycycline, and erythromycin have been used with success in those patients allergic to penicillin. Microbial cultures also should be analyzed for the presence of *Actinomyces* bacteria. If this microbe is isolated, the antibiotic regimen should be adjusted accordingly. In some refractory cases, patients may require combination antibiotic therapy, long-term antibiotic maintenance, or a course of intravenous antibiotic therapy.

Stage 3: These patients benefit from débridement, including resection, combined with antibiotic therapy, which may offer long-term palliation, with resolution of acute infection and pain.

Regardless of disease stage, mobile segments of bony sequestrum should be removed without exposing uninvolved bone. The extraction of symptomatic teeth within exposed, necrotic bone also should be considered, because it is unlikely that the extraction will exacerbate the established necrotic process.

BON, Bisphosphonate-associated osteonecrosis; *BRONJ,* Bisphosphonate-related osteonecrosis of the jaw.

From Ruggiero SL, et al: American Association of Oral and Maxillofacial Surgeons position paper on bisphosphonate-related osteonecrosis of the jaw—2009 update, Aust Endod J *35:119-130, 2009.*

2. Protocol for prevention of complications from cancer chemo- or radiation therapy:
   a. Comprehensive examination
   b. Establishment of excellent periodontal health (through eradication of any infection or inflammation)
   c. Immediate extraction of all nonrestorable or questionable teeth
   d. Elimination of dental caries
   e. Maintenance of excellent oral hygiene and oral health
3. Routine dental care can and should be provided, using routine local anesthetics.
4. All procedures should be performed as atraumatically as possible with little tissue trauma, bleeding and risk for postoperative infection.
5. Specific precautions may be necessary for special types of procedures (i.e., orthodontic, endodontic, prosthodontic, others). Of course, oral surgery or periodontal procedures involving the manipulation of bone will present the greatest risk.[50]

6. Should BON occur, no definitive treatment is available at this time; however, some recommendations are as follows:
   a. Antimicrobial rinses (e.g., chlorhexidine 0.12%)
   b. Surgical treatment should be conservative or delayed and be limited to (1) removal of sharp bony edges to prevent trauma to adjacent soft tissues; (2) removal of loose segments of bony sequestra without exposing uninvolved bone; and (3) segmental jaw resection for symptomatic patients with large segments of necrotic bone or pathologic fracture.
   c. There is no empirical evidence to inform the decision of whether to cease bisphosphonate therapy in the event of development of BON. The AAOMS guidelines recommend that the indication for bisphosphonate therapy be considered and bisphosphonate therapy stopped only if the systemic condition permits. Hence, management is interdisciplinary and involves ongoing close monitoring. Recommencement of bisphosphonate therapy should with either oral non-NBPs or a reduced frequency of intravenous NBPs, clinical condition permitting.[50]
7. In the instance of any infection, aggressive use of systemic antibiotics is indicated.[50]

As noted, prevention of this condition is of paramount importance for optimal outcomes for these patients.[47,48]

See also Chapter 23.

Carotid Atheroma. Patients who have received neck irradiation (at a total dose of 45 Gy or more) are more likely to develop carotid artery atheromas (calcified atherosclerotic plaques) after treatment than are risk-matched control patients who have not undergone irradiation. These lesions can be detected by panoramic radiography and constitute a risk factor for stroke that warrants referral of the patient to the physician for evaluation.[51]

REFERENCES

1. Thun M: Epidemiology of cancer. In Goldman L, Ausiello D, editors: *Cecil textbook of medicine*, ed 23, Philadelphia, 2007, Saunders.
2. Jemal A, et al: Cancer statistics 2010, *CA Cancer J Clin* 60:277-300, 2010.
3. Jemal AL, et al: Cancer statistics, 2006, *CA Cancer J Clin* 56:100-130, 2006.
4. Chaganti R: Genetics of cancer. In Goldman L, Ausiello D, editors: *Cecil textbook of medicine*, ed 23, Philadelphia, 2007, Saunders.
5. Simone SL: Oncology. In Goldman L, Bennett JC, editors: *Cecil textbook of medicine*, ed 21, Philadelphia, 2000, WB Saunders, p 1498.
6. Rhodus NL, Vibeto BM, Hamamoto DT: Glycemic control in patients with diabetes mellitus upon admission to a dental clinic: considerations for dental management, *Quintessence Int* 36:474-482, 2005.
7. Hortobagyi GN: Treatment of breast cancer, *N Engl J Med* 339:974-984, 1998.
8. Fox RI: Clinical features, pathogenesis, and treatment of Sjögren's syndrome, *Curr Opin Rheum* 8:438-445, 1996.
9. McKenzie K, Sukumar S: Molecular genetics of human breast cancer, *Prog Clin Biol Res* 394:183-194, 1997.
10. Chu KC, et al: Recent trends in U.S. breast cancer incidence, survival, and mortality rates, *J Natl Cancer Inst* 88:1571-1579, 1996.
11. *ACS responds to study saying mammography benefit limited* (article online), 2010, American Cancer Society; http://pressroom.cancer.org/index.php?item=234&s=43; accessed on August 10, 2011.
12. D'Angelo PC, Galliano DE, Rosemurgy AS: Stereotactic excisional breast biopsies utilizing the advanced breast biopsy instrumentation system, *Am J Surg* 174:297-302, 1997.
13. Canavan TP, Doshi NR: Cervical cancer, *Am Family Phys* 61:1369-1376, 2000.
14. Southern SA, Herrington CS: Differential cell cycle regulation by low- and high-risk human papillomaviruses in low-grade squamous intraepithelial lesions of the cervix, *Cancer Res* 58:2941-2945, 1998.
15. Hausen Z: Papillomaviruses in human cancers, *Proc Assoc Am Physicians* 111:581-587, 1999.
16. Guidelines for treatment of sexually transmitted diseases. Centers for Disease Control and Prevention, *MMWR Morb Mortal Wkly Rep* 47:101-111, 1998.
17. *Statistics on colorectal cancer*, SEER (web site), 2010; http://seer.cancer.gov/statfacts/html/colorect.html; accessed on March 23, 2010.
18. Hill MJ: Molecular and clinical risk markers in colon cancer trials, *Eur J Cancer* 36:1288-1291, 2000.
19. Fuchs CS, et al: Dietary fiber and the risk of colorectal cancer and adenoma in women, *N Engl J Med* 340:169-176, 1999.
20. Chao A, et al: Cigarette smoking and colorectal cancer mortality in the cancer prevention study II, *J Natl Cancer Inst* 92:1888-1896, 2000.
21. Ahlquist DA, et al: Colorectal cancer screening by detection of altered human DNA in stool: feasibility of a multitarget assay panel, *Gastroenterology* 119:1219-1227, 2000.
22. Hoffman PC, Mauer AM, Vokes EE: Lung cancer, *Lancet* 355:479-485, 2000.
23. *Statistics on lung cancer*, SEER (web site), 2010; http://seer.cancer.gov/statfacts/html/lungb.html; accessed on March 23, 2010.
24. Ozen M, Pathak S: Genetic alterations in human prostate cancer: a review of current literature, *Anticancer Res* 20:1905-1912, 2000.
25. Green A, et al: Sun exposure, skin cancers and related skin conditions, *J Epidemiol* 9(S7):7-13, 1999.
26. Rigel DS, Friedman RJ, Kopf AW: The incidence of malignant melanoma in the United States: issues as we approach the 21st century, *J Am Acad Dermatol* 34:839-847, 1996.
27. Parker F: Skin diseases of general importance. In Goldman L, Bennett JC, editors: *Cecil textbook of medicine*, ed 21, Philadelphia, 2000, WB Saunders.
28. Rhodus NL: Oral cancer: leukoplakia and squamous cell carcinoma, *Dent Clin North Am* 49:143-165, ix, 2005.
29. Rhodus NL: Oral cancer and precancer: improving outcomes, *Compend Contin Educ Dent* 30:486-488, 490-494, 496-498, 2009.
30. Brennan JA, et al: Association between cigarette smoking and mutation of the p53 gene in squamous cell carcinoma of the head and neck, *N Engl J Med* 332:712-717, 1999.
31. Suntharalingam M: Principles and complications of radiation therapy. In Ord RA, Blanchaert R Jr, editors: *Oral cancer: the dentist's role in diagnosis, management, rehabilitation, and prevention*, Chicago, 2000, Quintessence.

32. Eisbruch A, et al: The prevention and treatment of radiotherapy-induced xerostomia, *Semin Radiat Oncol* 13:302-308, 2003.
33. Rhodus NL: Management of oral complications from radiation and chemotherapy, *Northwest Dent* 89:39-42, 2010.
34. Dodd MJ, et al: Randomized clinical trial of the effectiveness of 3 commonly used mouthwashes to treat chemotherapy-induced mucositis, *Oral Surg Oral Med Oral Pathol Oral Radiol Endod* 90:39-47, 2000.
35. Silverman S Jr: *Oral cancer*, ed 4, Hamilton, Ontario, Canada, 1998, BC Decker.
36. Miller CS, Redding SW: Diagnosis and management of orofacial herpes simplex virus infections, *Dent Clin North Am* 36:879-895, 1992.
37. O'Grady NP, et al: Guidelines for prevention of intravascular catheter-related infections, *MMWR Morb Mortal Wkly Rep* 51(RR-10):1-29, 2002.
38. Baddour LM, et al: Nonvalvular cardiovascular device-related infections, *Circulation* 108:2015-2031, 2003.
39. Robbins MR: Oral care of the patient receiving chemotherapy. In Ord RA, Blanchaert R Jr, editors: *Oral cancer: the dentist's role in diagnosis, management, rehabilitation, and prevention*, Chicago, 2000, Quintessence.
40. Rhodus NL, et al: Dysphagia in patients with three different etiologies of salivary gland dysfunction, *Ear Nose Throat J* 74:39-42, 45-48, 1995.
41. Rhodus NL: Dysphagia in post-irradiation therapy head and neck cancer patients, *J Cancer Res Ther Control* 4:49-54, 1994.
42. LeVeque FG, et al: A multicenter, randomized, double-blind, placebo-controlled, dose-titration study of oral pilocarpine for treatment of radiation-induced xerostomia in head and neck cancer patients, *J Clin Oncol* 114:1141-1149, 1995.
43. Proceedings of the International Conference on Novel Anti-caries and Remineralizing Agents. Vina del Mar, Chile, January 10-12, 2008, *Adv Dent Res* 21:3-89, 2009.
44. McKenzie MR, et al: Hyperbaric oxygen and postradiation osteonecrosis of the mandible, *Eur J Cancer B Oral Oncol* 29B:201-207, 1993.
45. Epstein J, et al: Postradiation osteonecrosis of the mandible: a long-term follow-up study, *Oral Surg Oral Med Oral Pathol Oral Radiol Endod* 83:657-662, 1997.
46. Melo MD, Obeid G: Osteonecrosis of the jaws in patients with a history of receiving bisphosphonate therapy, *J Am Dent Assoc* 136:1675-1681, 2005.
47. Migliorati CA, et al: Managing the care of patients with bisphosphonate-associated osteonecrosis: an American Academy of Oral Medicine position paper, *J Am Dent Assoc* 136:1658-1668, 2005.
48. Markiewicz MR, et al: Bisphosphonate-associated osteonecrosis (BON) of the jaws: a review, *J Am Dent Assoc* 136:1669-1676, 2005.
49. Ruggiero SL, et al: American Association of Oral and Maxillofacial Surgeons position paper on bisphosphonate-related osteonecrosis of the jaw—2009 update, *Aust Endod J* 35:119-130, 2009.
50. Borromeo GL, et al: A review of the clinical implications of bisphosphonates in dentistry, *Aust Dent J* 56:2-9, 2011.
51. Freymiller EG, Sung EC, Friedlander AH: Detection of radiation-induced cervical atheromas by panoramic radiography, *Oral Oncol* 36:175-180, 2000.

PART IX

Neurologic, Behavioral, and Psychiatric Disorders

CHAPTER

27

Neurologic Disorders

Neurologic diseases are common in the general population and therefore are commonly encountered in dental patients. Several diseases affecting the nervous system are of clinical significance in dental practice. Such diseases may vary in severity and consequences. The focus of this chapter is on five of the more important neurologic diseases—epilepsy, stroke, Parkinson's disease, Alzheimer's disease, and multiple sclerosis (MS). Also discussed are cerebrospinal fluid shunts, because of the assumed risk of bacterial seeding after an invasive dental procedure in patients with such shunts.

EPILEPSY

DEFINITION

The term *epilepsy* includes disorders or syndromes with widely variable pathophysiologic findings, clinical manifestations, treatments, and outcomes.[1] *Epilepsy* is not a specific diagnosis but rather a term that refers to a group of disorders characterized by chronic and recurrent, paroxysmal changes in neurologic function (seizures), altered consciousness, or involuntary movements caused by abnormal and spontaneous electrical activity in the brain. Seizures may be convulsive (i.e., accompanied by motor manifestations) or may occur with other changes in neurologic function (i.e., sensory, cognitive, and emotional).[2]

Seizures are characterized by discrete episodes, which tend to be recurrent and often are unprovoked, in which movement, sensation, behavior, perception, and consciousness are disturbed. Symptoms are produced by excessive temporary neuronal discharging, which may result from intracranial or extracranial causes.[3]

Although seizures are required for the diagnosis of epilepsy, not all seizures imply presence of epilepsy. Seizures may occur during many medical or neurologic illnesses, including stress, sleep deprivation, fever, alcohol or drug withdrawal, and syncope.[3] A list of epilepsy syndromes and the currently accepted classification of seizure types are presented in Box 27-1. This seizure classification, based on clinical behaviors and electroencephalographic changes, consists of two major groups: partial and generalized. *Partial* seizures are limited in scope (to a part of the cerebral hemisphere) and clinical manifestations and involve motor, sensory, autonomic, or psychic abnormalities.[3] Partial seizures are subdivided into *simple,* in which consciousness is preserved, and *complex,* in which consciousness is impaired. *Generalized* seizures are more global in scope and manifestations. They begin diffusely, involve both cerebral hemispheres, are associated with alteration in consciousness, and frequently produce abnormal motor activity.[3] Discussion in this section is limited to generalized tonic-clonic seizures (idiopathic grand mal), because these represent the most severe expression of epilepsy that the dentist is likely to encounter.

EPIDEMIOLOGY

Epilepsy, which is the most common chronic neurologic condition, affects people of all ages, with a peak incidence in childhood and old age. In the United States, the incidence of all types of epilepsy is 35 to 52 cases per 100,000 population, varying by age: 60 to 70 per 100,000 per year in young children (younger than 5 years of age), 45 per 100,000 in adolescents, as low as 30 per 100,000 in the early adult years, but rising through the sixth and seventh decades back to 60 to 70 per 100,000 and reaching as high as 150 to 200 per 100,000 in persons older than 75 years. The incidence in males is higher at every age. Estimates of the prevalence of epilepsy range from 4.7 to 6.9 per 1000, but its prevalence is much higher in less developed countries for all age groups.[3]

Approximately 10% of the population will have at least one epileptic seizure in a lifetime, and 2% to 4% will experience recurrent seizures at some point.[2,3] The overall incidence of seizures is 0.5%.[2,3] Seizures are most common during childhood, with as many as 4% of children experiencing at least one seizure during the first 15 years of life. Most children outgrow the disorder. About 4 in 1000 children do not outgrow the disorder and will require medical care. Seizures also are common in old age, with an estimated annual incidence of 134 per 100,000. In a typical dental practice of 2000 patients, 3 or 4 can be expected to have a seizure disorder. Cerebrovascular disease is the most common factor underlying seizures occurring in elderly persons.[2,3]

BOX 27-1 Classification of Epileptic Syndromes and Seizure Types*

Epileptic Syndromes

Primary/Idiopathic

Localization-Related

Benign epilepsy with centrotemporal spikes
Autosomal dominant nocturnal frontal lobe epilepsy

Generalized

Juvenile myoclonic epilepsy
Juvenile absence epilepsy
Severe myoclonic epilepsy of infancy
Progressive myoclonic epilepsies
Generalized epilepsy with febrile seizures

Secondary/Symptomatic

Localization-Related

Mesial temporal lobe epilepsy
Neoplasm (primary, metastatic)
Infection (abscess, encephalitis, meningitis, syphilis, cysticercosis, Lyme disease, tuberculosis, fungal disease, herpes)
Vascular (stroke, transient ischemic attack, migraine, hemorrhage)
Developmental (migrational)
Perinatal
Traumatic
Degenerative (e.g., Alzheimer's disease)
Immunologic (e.g., multiple sclerosis)

Generalized

West's syndrome
Lennox-Gastaut syndrome
Tuberous sclerosis
Sturge-Weber syndrome

Seizure Types*

I. Partial (Focal, Local)

- Simple partial seizures
- Complex partial seizures
- Partial seizures evolving to secondarily generalized seizures

II. Generalized (Convulsive or Nonconvulsive)

- Absence seizures (petit mal)
- Myoclonic seizures
- Tonic-clonic seizures (grand mal)
- Tonic seizures
- Atonic seizures

III. Unclassified Epileptic Seizures

*International classification of epileptic syndromes (condensed).
Data from Commission on Classification and Terminology of the International League Against Epilepsy. Proposal for revised clinical and electroencephalographic classification of epileptic seizures, Epilepsia *22:489-501, 1981.*

Etiology

Epileptic seizures are idiopathic in more than half of all affected patients.[2,3] Vascular (cerebrovascular disease) and developmental abnormalities (cavernous malformation), intracranial neoplasms (gliomas), and head trauma are causative in about 35% of adult cases. Other common causes include hypoglycemia, drug withdrawal, infection, and febrile illness (e.g., meningitis, encephalitis). Seizures occur with genetic conditions such as Down syndrome, tuberous sclerosis, and neurofibromatosis and are associated with several genetic abnormalities that result in neuronal channel dysfunction.[2,3]

Seizures sometimes can be evoked by specific stimuli. Approximately 1 of 15 patients reports that seizures occurred after exposure to flickering lights, monotonous sounds, music, or a loud noise.[2,4] Syncope and diminished oxygen supply to the brain also are known to trigger seizures. It is valuable for the dentist to know what factors have the potential to exacerbate a seizure in a particular patient, so that certain stimuli can be avoided.[2]

Pathophysiology and Complications

The basic event underlying an epileptic seizure is an excessive focal neuronal discharge that spreads to thalamic and brain stem nuclei. The cause of this abnormal electrical activity is not precisely known, although a number of theories have been put forth.[2,3] These include altered sodium channel function, altered neuronal membrane potentials, altered synaptic transmission, diminution of inhibitory neurons, increased neuronal excitability, and decreased electrical threshold for epileptic activity. During the seizure, blood becomes hypoxic, with consequent development of lactic acidosis.[2,3]

Approximately 60% to 80% of patients with epilepsy achieve complete control over their seizures within 5 years; the remainder achieve only partial or poor control.[2,3,5] A significant problem in the medical management of epileptic patients is one of compliance (i.e., adherence to prescribed treatment regimens including medication). This problem is common to many chronic disorders, such as hypertension, because patients may have to take medication for the rest of their lives, even though they remain asymptomatic. Evidence suggests that patients who have epilepsy from an early age have a higher incidence of future complications and die at an earlier age. Noncompliance may be a clinically important consideration in dental patients because it is associated with a higher risk of later complications that may lead to death.[4] Complications of seizures include trauma (as a result of falls) to the head, neck, and mouth and aspiration pneumonia. Also, frequent and severe seizures are associated with altered mental function, dullness, confusion, argumentativeness, and increased risk of sudden death (about 1 in 75 persons in this group die annually).[2,3]

Status Epilepticus. A serious acute complication of epilepsy (especially the tonic-clonic type) is the occurrence of repeated seizures over a short time without a recovery period, called *status epilepticus.* This condition most frequently is caused by abrupt withdrawal of anticonvulsant medication or an abused substance but may be triggered by infection, neoplasm, or trauma. Status epilepticus constitutes a medical emergency.[2,3] Patients may become seriously hypoxic and acidotic during this event and suffer permanent brain damage or death. Patients with epilepsy also are at increased risk for sudden death and death due to accident.[2,3]

CLINICAL PRESENTATION

Signs and Symptoms

The clinical manifestations of generalized tonic-clonic convulsions (grand mal seizures) are classic. An aura (a momentary sensory alteration that produces an unusual smell or visual disturbance) precedes the convulsion in one third of patients. Irritability is another premonitory signal. After the aura warning, the patient emits a sudden "epileptic cry" (caused by spasm of the diaphragmatic muscles) and immediately loses consciousness. The tonic phase consists of generalized muscle rigidity, pupil dilation, rolling of the eyes upward or to the side, and loss of consciousness. Breathing may stop because of spasm of respiratory muscles.[2,3] This phase is followed by clonic activity consisting of uncoordinated beating movements of the limbs and head, forcible jaw closing, and up and down head rocking.[2,3] Urinary incontinence is common, but fecal incontinence is rare. The seizure (ictus) usually does not last longer than 90 seconds; thereafter, movement ceases and muscles relax, with a gradual return to consciousness, accompanied by stupor, headache, confusion, and mental dulling. Several hours of rest or sleep may be needed for the patient to regain full cognitive and physical abilities.[2,3]

Laboratory Findings

The diagnosis of epilepsy generally is based on the history of seizures and presence of abnormalities on the electroencephalogram (EEG).[2,3] Seizures produce characteristic spike and sharp wave patterns on the EEG tracing. Serial recordings during sleep deprivation, which can induce seizures, may help to establish the diagnosis. Other diagnostic procedures that are useful for ruling out other causes of seizures include computed tomography (CT), magnetic resonance imaging (MRI), single-photon emission computed tomography (SPECT), lumbar puncture, serum chemistry profiles, and toxicology screening.[2,3]

Medical Management

The medical management of epilepsy usually is based on long-term drug therapy. Phenytoin (Dilantin), carbamazepine (Tegretol), and valproic acid are considered first-line agents for treatment of this disease. Several other drugs are available for control of generalized tonic-clonic seizures[5,6] (Table 27-1). These drugs reduce the frequency of seizures by elevating the seizure threshold of motor cortex neurons, depressing abnormal cerebral electrical discharge, and limiting the spread of excitation from abnormal foci. Phenytoin and carbamazepine are efficient at blocking sodium or calcium channels of motor neurons.[5-7] Many of the other antiepileptic drugs augment γ-aminobutyric acid (GABA), which inhibits glutamate activity—the major determinant of brain excitability. Adverse effects of phenytoin include anemia, ataxia, gingival overgrowth, cosmetic changes (coarsening of facial features, hirsutism, facial acne), lethargy, skin rash, and gastrointestinal disturbances. Phenobarbital, which is considered a second-line drug, can induce hepatic microsomal enzymes that promote the metabolism of concurrently used drugs.[8] Several antiseizure medications (see Table 27-1) may cause drowsiness, sedation, ataxia, weight gain, cognitive impairment, and hypersensitivity reactions.[5-7] Adverse effects are more common at the start of therapy, when drugs are administered rapidly or at high dose. For these reasons, and to facilitate compliance, single-drug therapy and a slow increase in dose are recommended. Unfortunately, the use of combination therapy frequently is necessary for seizure control.[5-7] Drug therapy usually is continued in children until a 1- to 2-year seizure-free period is attained, or until around age 16 years. Attempts to taper the antiepileptic drug regimen are made thereafter.

Vagus nerve stimulation (VNS) is reserved for patients who have been unable to achieve satisfactory seizure control with several medications, and it is an option for some before brain surgery. The mechanism of VNS is similar to that of an implantable cardiac pacemaker, in which a subcutaneous pulse generator is implanted in the left chest wall and delivers electrical signals to the left vagus nerve through a bipolar lead. The stimulated vagus nerve provides direct projection to regions in the brain potentially responsible for the seizure. The VNS device generally is used in combination with antiepileptic medications.[5-7]

DENTAL MANAGEMENT

Medical Considerations

The first step in the management of an epileptic dental patient is identification of the patient as having the disorder (Box 27-2). This is best accomplished by the medical history and by discussion with the patient or family members. Once a patient with epilepsy has been identified, the dental practitioner must learn as much as possible about the seizure history, including the type of seizures, age at onset, cause (if known), current and regular use of medications, frequency of physician visits, quality of seizure control, frequency of seizures, date of last seizure, and any known precipitating factors. In addition, a history of previous injuries associated with seizures and their treatment may be helpful.

TABLE 27-1 Anticonvulsants Used in the Management of Generalized Tonic-Clonic (Grand Mal) Seizures

Drug	Trade Name(s)	Mechanism of Action	Dental Treatment Considerations
Drugs of Choice			
Phenytoin*	Dilantin	Blocks sodium channels	Gingival hyperplasia, increased incidence of microbial infection, delayed healing, gingival bleeding (leukopenia), osteoporosis, Stevens-Johnson syndrome
Carbamazepine*	Tegretol	Blocks sodium channels	Xerostomia, microbial infection, delayed healing, gingival bleeding (leukopenia and thrombocytopenia), ataxia, osteoporosis, Stevens-Johnson syndrome *Drug interactions*: propoxyphene, erythromycin
Valproic acid*	Depakene, Depakote	GABA augmentation and *N*-methyl-D-aspartate (NMDA) receptor	Excessive bleeding and petechiae, decreased platelet aggregation, increased incidence of microbial infection, delayed healing, drowsiness, gingival bleeding (leukopenia and thrombocytopenia), hepatotoxicity *Drug interactions*: aspirin and other NSAIDs
Lamotrigine*	Lamictal	Blocks sodium and calcium channels, reduces glutamate	Ataxia; may require help getting into and out of the dental chair; risk for development of Stevens-Johnson syndrome
Alternatives			
Clonazepam*	Klonopin	Augments inhibitory GABAergic system	*Drug interactions*: CNS depressants
Ethosuximide	Zarontin	Blocks sodium and calcium channels	Risk for development of Stevens-Johnson syndrome, blood dyscrasias
Felbamate	Felbatol	Blocks sodium channels, reduces glutamate	Risk for development of aplastic anemia, Stevens-Johnson syndrome
Gabapentin	Neurontin	Modulates calcium channel; augments GABAergic system	Dizziness
Oxcarbazepine	Trileptal	Blocks sodium channels	Liver enzyme induction but less than with carbamazepine
Phenobarbital*	Luminal	Blocks calcium channel; augments inhibitory GABAergic system	Sedation, liver enzyme induction *Drug interactions*: CNS depressants
Primidone*	Mysoline	Blocks calcium channel; augments inhibitory GABAergic system	Ataxia, vertigo—increased risk of falls
Topiramate	Topemax	Blocks sodium channels; augments inhibitory GABAergic system	Impaired cognition
Vigabatrin	Sabril	Augments inhibitory GABAergic system	*Drug interactions*: CNS depressants

*Preexisting liver disease can exacerbate adverse effects associated with antiepileptics. Drugs of choice for absence (petit mal) seizures: ethosuximide (Zarontin), valproate, lamotrigine, clonazepam. Drugs of choice for status epilepticus: lorazepam 4 to 8 mg, diazepam 10 mg, intravenously.
CNS, Central nervous sytem; *GABA*, γ-aminobutyric acid; *NSAIDs*, Nonsteroidal antiinflammatory drugs.

Fortunately, most epileptic patients are able to attain good control of their seizures with anticonvulsant drugs and are therefore able to receive normal routine dental care. In some instances, however, the history may reveal a degree of seizure activity that suggests noncompliance or a severe seizure disorder that does not respond to anticonvulsants. For these patients, a consultation with the physician is advised before dental treatment is rendered. A patient with poorly controlled disease may require additional anticonvulsant or sedative medication, as directed by the physician.

Patients who take anticonvulsants may suffer from the toxic effects of these drugs, and the dentist should be aware of these manifestations. In addition to the more common adverse effects (see Table 27-1), allergy may be seen occasionally as a rash, erythema multiforme, or worse (e.g., Stevens-Johnson syndrome). Phenytoin, carbamazepine, and valproic acid can cause bone marrow suppression, leukopenia, and thrombocytopenia, resulting in an increased incidence of microbial infection, delayed healing, and gingival and postoperative bleeding. Valproic acid can decrease platelet aggregation, leading to spontaneous hemorrhage and petechiae.[8]

Propoxyphene and erythromycin should not be administered to patients who are taking carbamazepine because of interference with metabolism of carbamazepine, which could lead to toxic levels of the anticonvulsant drug.[5-7] Aspirin and other nonsteroidal

BOX 27-2 Dental Management
Considerations in Patients with Seizure Disorders

P

Patient Evaluation/Risk Assessment (see Box 1-1)

- Evaluate to determine the nature, severity, control, and stability of disease.

Potential Issues/Factors of Concern

- Well-controlled seizure disorders pose no specific management problems.

	A
Analgesics	Clinicians should provide good pain control to avoid stress, which may precipitate a seizure.
Antibiotics	There is no need for antibiotic prophylaxis.
Anesthesia	It is very important to obtain adequate anesthesia to reduce stress as possible precipitant for a seizure. Epinephrine (1:100,000 and no more than two carpules) in local anesthetics generally is well tolerated.
Anxiety	Paatients with untreated or poorly controlled seizure-associated disorders may appear very anxious and stressed, increasing the risk for a seizure. Use of special anxiety and stress reduction techniques may be indicated.
Allergy	Allergic skin changes (rash, erythema multiforme) may signify a reaction to antiepileptic medications.

	B
Bleeding	The possibility of a bleeding tendency has been noted in patients taking valproic acid (Depakene) or carbamazepine (Tegretol) as the result of platelet interference.
Blood pressure	Monitor blood pressure, because it may significantly increase or decrease with onset of a seizure.

	C
Chair position	This usually is not a problem if the patient is under good medical management; with symptoms of impending syncope associated with cardiac stress or pulmonary congestion, however, a supine position may not be tolerated. In patients at risk for seizure, the chair back should be in supported supine position.
Consultation	Once the patient is under good medical management, the dental treatment plan is unaffected. However, consultation with the patient's physician to establish the level of control is recommended as part of the management program.

	D
Devices	No issues.
Drugs	These patients typically are on anticonvulsant drugs, which may have adverse effects including drowsiness, slow mentation, dizziness, others.

	E
Equipment	No issues.
Emergencies	Be prepared for occurrence of a grand mal seizure: • Placement of a ligated mouth prop at the beginning of the procedure may be considered. • The dental chair should be in supported supine position. *During a seizure:* • Clear the area. • Turn the patient to the side (to avoid aspiration). • Do not attempt to use a padded tongue blade. • Passively restrain. *After a seizure:* • Examine for traumatic injuries. • Discontinue treatment; arrange for patient transport. Most commonly seizures are self-limited, but rarely a seizure may progress to cardiac arrest, necessitating emergency medical treatment; call 911. A patient who is ambulatory and stable should seek urgent medical care. Ongoing vital signs must be monitored and cardiopulmonary resuscitation initiated if necessary; transport patient to emergency medical facilities.

	F
Follow-up	Follow-up with the patient (and physician) is indicated. after any seizure event in the dental office. In patients who have undergone surgery, a follow-up phone call within the next day or two is advised.

antiinflammatory drugs (NSAIDs) (see Table 27-1) should not be administered to patients who are taking valproic acid, because these agents can further decrease platelet aggregation, leading to hemorrhagic episodes. No contraindication has been identified to the use of local anesthetics in proper amounts in these patients. Patients who have a VNS device implanted in the chest do not need antibiotic prophylaxis before undergoing invasive dental procedures.[5-7]

Seizure Management. Despite consistent use of appropriate preventive measures by both dentist and patient, the possibility always exists that an epileptic patient may experience a generalized tonic-clonic convulsion in the dental office. The dentist and office staff members should anticipate and be prepared for such events. Preventive measures include knowing the patient's history, scheduling the patient at a time within a few hours of taking the anticonvulsant medication, using a mouth prop, removing dentures, and discussing with the patient the urgency of mentioning an aura as soon as it is sensed. The clinician also should be aware that irritability often is a symptom of impending seizure. With a premonitory stage of sufficient duration, 0.5 to 2 mg of lorazepam can be given sublingually, or diazepam 2 to 10 mg can be given intravenously.[9]

If the patient has a seizure while in the dental chair, the primary task of management is to protect the patient and try to prevent injury. No attempt should be made to move the patient to the floor. Instead, the instruments and instrument tray should be cleared from the area, and the chair should be placed in a supported supine position (Figure 27-1). The patient's airway should be maintained patent. No attempt should be made to restrain or hold the patient down. Passive restraint should be used only to prevent injury that may result when the patient hits nearby objects or falls out of the chair.[10,11]

If a mouth prop (e.g., a padded tongue blade between the teeth to prevent tongue biting) is used, it should be inserted at the beginning of the dental procedure (see Box 27-2). Trying to insert a mouth prop is not advised during the seizure, because doing so may damage the patient's teeth or oral soft tissue and may be nearly impossible. An exception is the case in which the patient senses an impending seizure and can cooperate.[10,11]

A grand mal seizure generally does not last longer than a few minutes. Afterward, the patient may fall into a deep sleep from which he or she cannot be aroused. Oxygen (100%), maintenance of a patent airway, and mouth suction should be provided during this phase. Alternatively, the patient can be turned to the side to control the airway and to minimize aspiration of secretions. Within a few minutes, the patient gradually regains consciousness but may be confused, disoriented, and embarrassed. Headache is a prominent feature during this period. If the patient does not respond within a few minutes, the seizure may be associated with low serum glucose, and delivery of glucose may be needed.[10,11]

No further dental treatment should be attempted after a generalized tonic-clonic seizure, although examination for sustained injuries (e.g., lacerations, fractures) should be performed. In the event of avulsed or fractured teeth (Figure 27-2) or a fractured appliance, an attempt should be made to locate the tooth or fragments to rule out aspiration. A chest radiograph may be required to locate a missing fragment or tooth.[10,11]

In the event that a seizure becomes prolonged (status epilepticus) or is repeated, intravenous lorazepam (0.05 to 0.1 mg/kg) 4 to 8 mg, or 10 mg diazepam, generally is effective in controlling it. Lorazepam is preferred by many experts because it is more efficacious and lasts longer than diazepam.[2,3] Oxygen and respiratory support should be provided, because respiratory function may become depressed. If the seizure lasts longer than 15 minutes, the following protocol should be implemented: secure intravenous access, repeat lorazepam dosing, administer fosphenytoin, and activate the emergency medical services (EMS) system.[10,11]

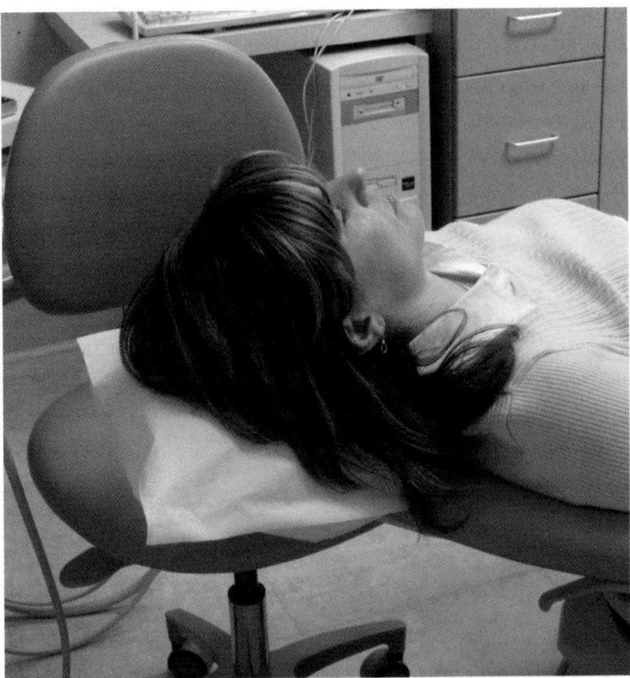

FIGURE 27-1 Dental chair in the supine position with the back supported by the operator's or assistant's stool.

Treatment Planning Considerations

Because gingival overgrowth is associated with phenytoin administration, every effort should be made to maintain a patient at an optimal level of oral hygiene. This

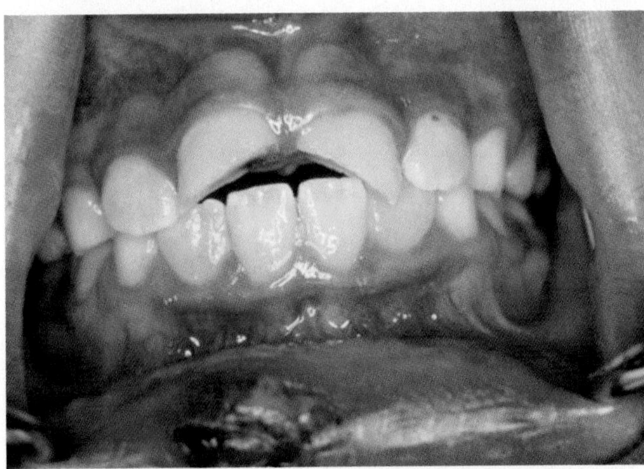

FIGURE 27-2 Fracture of teeth and laceration of lower lip sustained during a grand mal seizure. *(Courtesy Gerald A. Ferretti, DDS, Lexington, Kentucky.)*

may require frequent visits for monitoring of progress. If gingival overgrowth is significant, surgical reduction will be necessary. This correction must be accompanied by an increased awareness of oral hygiene needs and a positive commitment by the patient to maintain oral cleanliness.

A missing tooth or teeth should be replaced if possible to prevent the tongue from being caught in the edentulous space during a seizure (as commonly happens). Generally, a fixed prosthesis or implant is preferable to a removable one. (The removable prosthesis becomes dislodged more easily.) For fixed prostheses, all-metal units should be considered when possible, to minimize the chance of fracture. When placing anterior castings, the dentist may wish to consider using three-quarter crowns or retentive nonporcelain facings.

Removable prostheses are, nevertheless sometimes constructed for epileptic patients. Metallic palates and bases are preferable to all-acrylic ones. If acrylic is used, it should be reinforced with wire mesh.

Oral Complications and Manifestations

The most significant oral complication seen in epileptic patients is gingival overgrowth, which is associated with phenytoin (Figure 27-3) and rarely with valproic acid and vigabatrin.[7,10] The incidence of phenytoin-induced gingival overgrowth in epileptic patients ranges from 0% to 100%, with an average rate of approximately 42%. A greater tendency to develop gingival overgrowth occurs in youngsters than in adults. The anterior labial surfaces of the maxillary and mandibular gingivae are most commonly and severely affected.[7,10]

Meticulous oral hygiene is important for preventing overgrowth and significantly decreasing its severity. Good home care must always be combined with the removal of irritants, such as overhanging restorations and calculus. Frequently, enlarged tissues interfere with function or appearance, and surgical reduction may become necessary.

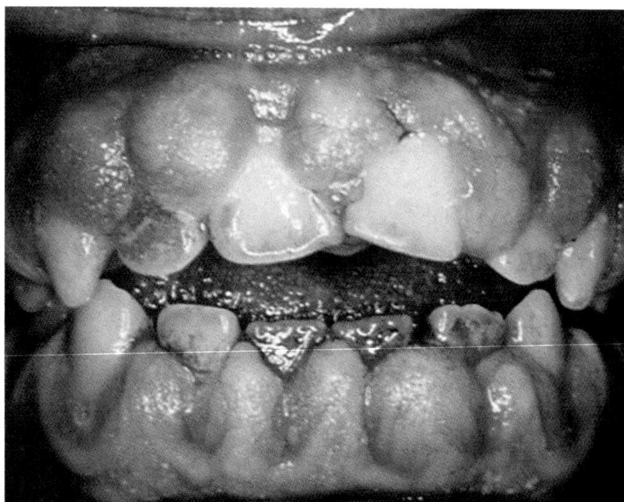

FIGURE 27-3 Phenytoin-induced gingival overgrowth. *(Courtesy H. Abrams, Lexington, Kentucky.)*

Traumatic injuries such as broken teeth, tongue lacerations, and lip scars also are common in patients who experience generalized tonic-clonic seizures. Stomatitis, erythema multiforme, and Stevens-Johnson syndrome are rare adverse effects associated with the use of phenytoin, valproic acid, lamotrigine, phenobarbital, and carbamazepine. These complications are more common during the first 8 weeks of treatment.[7,10]

STROKE (CEREBROVASCULAR ACCIDENT)

DEFINITION

Stroke is a generic term that is used to refer to a cerebrovascular accident (CVA)—a serious and often fatal neurologic event caused by sudden interruption of oxygenated blood to the brain. The associated ischemic injury results in focal necrosis of brain tissue, which may be fatal if the damage is catastrophic. Even if a stroke is not fatal, the survivor often is to some degree debilitated in motor function, speech, or cognition. The scope and gravity of stroke are reflected in the fact that stroke is the leading cause of serious, long-term disability in the United States; 5% of the population older than 65 years of age has had one stroke.[2,3]

EPIDEMIOLOGY

Incidence and Prevalence

Stroke is one of the most significant health problems in the United States. Stroke is the third leading cause of death (behind heart disease and cancer) in the United States, with 275,000 Americans dying of stroke annually.[12] Each year in the United States, about 700,000 people experience new or recurrent stroke. This figure translates to the occurrence of one stroke about every minute, and 75% of persons survive their stroke.[12,13]

Hypertension is the most important risk factor for ischemic and hemorrhagic stroke.[12,13] The incidence of stroke increases directly in relation to the degree of elevation of systolic and diastolic arterial blood pressure above threshold values. More important, conclusive evidence accrued since 1980 indicates that control of hypertension prevents strokes. Metaanalyses of randomized controlled trials confirm an approximate 30% to 40% reduction in stroke risk with lowering of blood pressure.[12,13]

Approximately 7% to 10% of men and 5% to 7% of women older than 65 years have asymptomatic carotid stenosis of greater than 50%. Epidemiologic studies suggest that the rate of unheralded stroke evolving ipsilateral to a stenosis is about 1% to 2% annually.[12,13]

Nonvalvar atrial fibrillation carries a 3% to 5% annual risk for stroke, with the risk becoming even higher in the presence of advanced age, previous transient ischemic attack (TIA) or stroke, hypertension, impaired left ventricular function, and diabetes mellitus.[12,13]

In epidemiologic studies, the risk for stroke in smokers is almost double that in nonsmokers, but the risk becomes essentially identical to that in nonsmokers by 2 to 5 years after quitting. The relative risk for stroke is two to six times greater for patients with insulin-dependent (type 1) diabetes.[12,13] An association with race has been recognized: Compared with whites, African Americans are at 38% greater risk for a first stroke. Also, 40,000 more women than men have a stroke each year. Risk of stroke increases with age; however, on average, 28% of people who have a stroke are younger than 65 years.[12-14] A total of 4.7 million stroke survivors live in the United States, and an average dental practice of 2000 adult patients will include about 31 patients who have had or will experience a stroke.

Etiology

Stroke is caused by the interruption of blood supply and oxygen to the brain as a result of ischemia or hemorrhage. The most common type is ischemic stroke induced by thrombosis (in 60% to 80% of cases) of a cerebral vessel. Ischemic stroke also can result from occlusion of a cerebral blood vessel by distant emboli. Hemorrhage causes about 15% of all strokes and carries a 1-year mortality rate greater than 60%.[12,13]

Cerebrovascular disease is the primary factor associated with stroke. Atherosclerosis and cardiac pathosis (myocardial infarction, atrial fibrillation) increase the risk of thrombolic and embolic strokes, whereas hypertension is the most important risk factor for intracerebral hemorrhagic stroke.[12,13] Approximately 10% of persons who have had a myocardial infarction will have a stroke within 6 years.[12,13] Additional factors that increase the risk for stroke include the occurrence of transient ischemic attacks, a previous stroke, high dietary fat, obesity and elevated blood lipid levels, physical inactivity, uncontrolled hypertension, cardiac abnormalities, diabetes mellitus, elevated homocysteine levels, elevated hematocrit, elevated antiphospholipid antibodies, heavy tobacco smoking, increasing age (risk doubles each decade after the age of 65 years), and periodontal disease.[12,13] Increased risk for hemorrhagic stroke also occurs with use of phenylpropanolamine, an α-adrenergic agonist.[12,13]

Pathophysiology and Complications

Pathologic changes associated with stroke result from infarction, intracerebral hemorrhage, or subarachnoid hemorrhage. Cerebral infarctions most commonly are caused by atherosclerotic thrombi or emboli of cardiac origin. The extent of an infarction is determined by a number of factors, including site of the occlusion, size of the occluded vessel, duration of the occlusion, and collateral circulation. The production and circulation of proinflammatory cytokines, the occurrence of clotting factors, and arterial inflammation contribute to platelet aggregation. Neurologic abnormalities result from excitotoxicity, free radical accumulation, inflammation, mitochondrial and DNA damage, and apoptosis of the region supplied by the damaged artery.[12,13]

The most common cause of intracerebral hemorrhage is hypertensive atherosclerosis, which results in microaneurysms of the arterioles (Figure 27-4). Vessels within the circle of Willis often are affected (Figure 27-5).

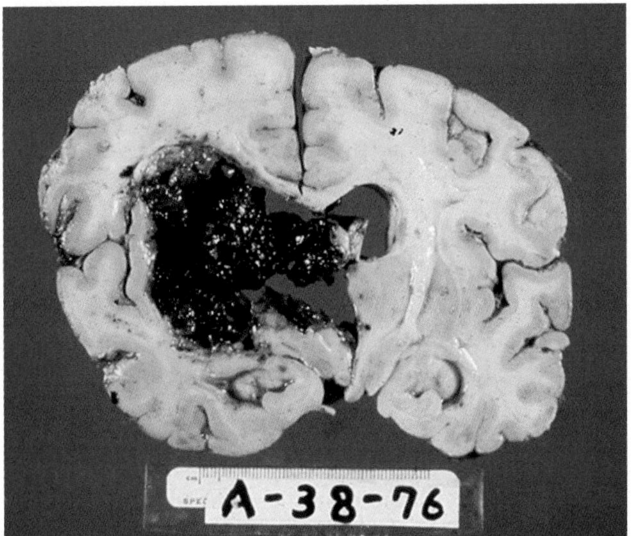

FIGURE 27-4 Cerebral infarction in a patient who had chronic hypertension.

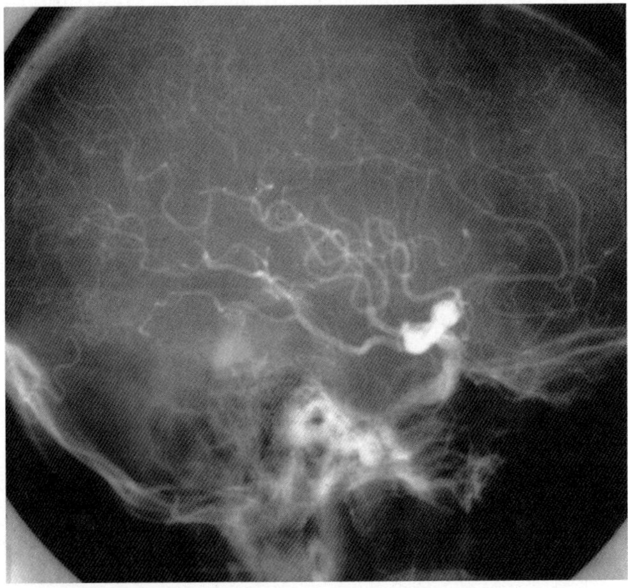

FIGURE 27-5 Aneurysm of the middle cerebral artery.

Rupture of these microaneurysms within brain tissue leads to extravasation of blood, which displaces brain tissue, causing increase in intracranial volume until resultant tissue compression halts bleeding. Hemorrhagic strokes also may be caused by subarachnoid hemorrhage. The most common cause of subarachnoid hemorrhage is rupture of a saccular aneurysm at the bifurcation of a major cerebral artery.[15,16]

The most serious outcome of stroke is death, which occurs in 8% of those who experience ischemic strokes and 38% to 47% of those with hemorrhagic strokes within a month of the event. Overall, about 23% of patients die within 1 year.[15-17] Mortality rates are directly related to type of stroke, with 80% of patients dying after an intracerebral hemorrhage, 50% after a subarachnoid hemorrhage, and 30% after occlusion of a major vessel by a thrombus. Death from stroke may not be immediate (sudden death) but rather may occur hours, days, or even weeks after the initial stroke episode.[15-17]

If the victim survives, it is highly likely that a neurologic deficit or disability of varying degree and duration will remain. Of those who survive the stroke, 10% recover with no impairment, 50% have a mild residual disability, 15% to 30% are disabled and require special services, and 10% to 20% require institutionalization. Approximately 50% of those who survive the acute period (the first 6 months) are alive 7 years later.[15-17]

The type of residual deficit that results from a stroke is directly dependent on the size and location of the infarct or hemorrhage. Deficits include unilateral paralysis, numbness, sensory impairment, dysphasia, blindness, diplopia, dizziness, and dysarthria. Return of function is unpredictable and usually takes place slowly, over several months. Even with improvement, patients frequently are left with some permanent residual problem, such as difficulty in walking, using the hands, performing skilled acts, or speaking. Dementia also may be an outcome of stroke.[15-19]

CLINICAL PRESENTATION

Signs and Symptoms

Familiarity with the warning signs and symptoms and the phases of stroke can lead to appropriate action that may be lifesaving. Four events associated with stroke are (1) the transient ischemic attack (TIA), (2) reversible ischemic neurologic deficit (RIND), (3) stroke-in-evolution, and (4) the completed stroke. These events are defined principally by their duration.[12,13]

A TIA is a "mini" stroke that is caused by a temporary disturbance in blood supply to a localized area of the brain. A TIA often is associated with numbness of the face, arm, or leg on one side of the body (hemiplegia); weakness, tingling, numbness, or speech disturbances that usually last less than 10 minutes. Most commonly, a major stroke is preceded by one or two TIAs within several days of the first attack.[15-17]

A RIND is a neurologic deficit that is similar to a TIA but does not clear within 24 hours. Eventual recovery is the rule, however.[15-17]

Stroke-in-evolution is a neurologic condition that is caused by occlusion or hemorrhage of a cerebral artery in which the deficit has been present for several hours and continues to worsen during a period of observation. Signs of stroke include hemiplegia, temporary loss of speech or trouble in speaking or understanding speech, temporary dimness or loss of vision, particularly in one eye (may be confused with migraine), unexplained dizziness, unsteadiness, or a sudden fall.[15-17]

Clinical manifestations that remain after a stroke vary in accordance with the site and size of residual brain deficits; these include language disorders, hemiplegia, and paresis, a form of paralysis that is associated with loss of sensory function and memory and weakened motor power. Box 27-3 presents the different behavioral manifestations of right-sided brain damage versus left-sided brain damage. Of note, in most patients with stroke, the intellect remains intact; however, massive left-sided stroke has been associated with cognitive decline.[15-18,20]

Laboratory Findings

Patients suspected of having had a stroke usually undergo a variety of laboratory tests and diagnostic imaging procedures to rule out conditions that can produce neurologic alterations, such as diabetes mellitus, uremia, abscess, tumor, acute alcoholism, drug poisoning, and extradural hemorrhage.[12,13] Such investigations often include urinalysis, blood sugar level, complete blood count, erythrocyte sedimentation rate, serologic tests for syphilis, blood cholesterol and lipid levels, chest radiographs, and electrocardiogram (ECG). Various abnormalities may be disclosed by the test results, depending

BOX 27-3 Manifestations of Right-Sided Versus Left-Sided Brain Damage

Right-Sided Brain Damage
- Paralyzed left side
- Spatial-perceptual deficits
- Impaired thought process
- Quick, impulsive behavior
- Inability to use mirror
- Difficulty performing tasks (toothbrushing)
- Memory deficits—for events or people, generalized
- Neglect of left side

Left-Sided Brain Damage
- Paralyzed right side
- Language and speech problems
- Decreased auditory memory (inability to remember long instructions)
- Slow, cautious, disorganized behavior
- Memory deficits—language-based
- Anxiety

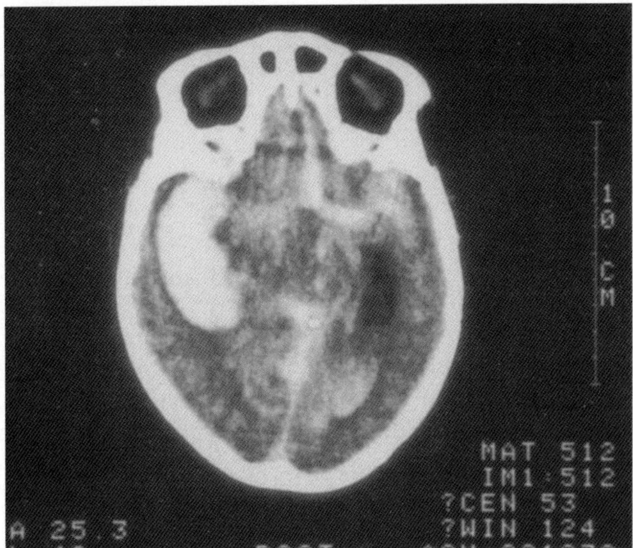

FIGURE 27-6 Computed tomography (CT) scan of the brain demonstrating a cerebrovascular accident (stroke) lesion that extended from the midbrain to the temporal lobe.

on the type and severity of stroke and its causative factors. A lumbar puncture also may be ordered by the physician to check for blood or protein in the cerebrospinal fluid (CSF) and for altered CSF pressure, which would be suggestive of subarachnoid hemorrhage.[12,13] Doppler blood flow studies, EEG, cerebral angiography, CT (Figure 27-6), and MRI, including diffusion and perfusion studies of the brain, are important for determining the extent and location of arterial injury.[12-14,21]

MEDICAL MANAGEMENT

Prevention

The first aspect of stroke management is prevention. This is accomplished by identifying specific risk factors (e.g., hypertension, diabetes, atherosclerosis, cigarette smoking) and attempting to reduce or eliminate as many of these as possible. Blood pressure lowering (see Chapter 3), antiplatelet therapy (see Chapter 24), and statin therapy are primary stroke prevention methods. Carotid endarterectomy is a secondary stroke prevention method.[12,13]

The benefit of lowering blood pressure is evident in the fact that a reduction of systolic blood pressure by 10 mm Hg is associated with a one-third reduction in risk for stroke.[12,13] Regimens of aspirin, ticlopidine, or extended-release dipyridamole are accepted preventive therapies for ischemic stroke in patients who have experienced TIAs, or who have had a stroke. Aspirin dosed at 81 to 325 mg daily redo, surgical intervention through endarterectomy reduces the risk by about 1% per year, such that one stroke is prevented for every 20 patients who undergo surgery over a 5-year period.[16-19]

Stroke Treatment

Treatment for stroke generally has three components. The immediate task is to sustain life during the period immediately after the stroke. This is done by means of life support measures and transport to a hospital. The second task involves emergency efforts to prevent further thrombosis or hemorrhage, and to attempt to lyse the clot in cases of thrombosis or embolism. Thrombolysis and improved neurologic outcomes have been achieved with intravenous recombinant tissue-type plasminogen activator (rt-PA) and intraarterial prourokinase.[22-24] Of the two, intravenous administration of rt-PA within 3 hours of ischemic stroke onset is the only approved therapy in the United States.[22-25]

After the initial period, efforts to stabilize the patient continue with anticoagulant medications such as heparin, coumarin, aspirin, and dipyridamole combined with aspirin (Aggrenox) in cases of thrombosis or embolism. Heparin is administered intravenously during acute episodes, whereas coumarin, dipyridamole, aspirin, subcutaneous low-molecular-weight heparin, or platelet receptor antagonists (clopidogrel, abciximab, ticlopidine) are employed for prolonged periods to reduce risk of thrombosis (e.g., deep vein thrombosis). Corticosteroids may be used acutely after a stroke to lessen the cerebral edema that accompanies cerebral infarction. Such therapy can markedly reduce the likelihood of complications. Surgical intervention may be indicated for removal of a superficial hematoma or management of a vascular obstruction. The latter usually is accomplished by thromboendarterectomy or by use of bypass grafts in the neck or thorax. Diazepam, phenytoin, and other anticonvulsants are prescribed in the management of seizures that may accompany the postoperative course of stroke.[22-24]

If the patient survives, the third and final task consists of institution of preventive therapy, administration of medications that reduce the risk of another stroke (statins and antihypertensive drugs), and initiation of rehabilitation. Rehabilitation generally is accomplished by intense physical, occupational, and speech therapy (if indicated). Although marked improvement is common, many patients are left with some degree of permanent deficit.[16-19]

Emerging and Experimental Therapies

Numerous strategies are being evaluated for treating acute ischemic stroke (AIS). These include intraarterial thrombolysis (IAT); augmentation of rt-PA with other medications, thereby enlarging the therapeutic window (i.e., lengthening the period of efficacy); and neuroprotection.[26] IAT may be a treatment option for selected patients. Possible selection criteria include presentation between 3 and 6 hours from symptom onset, major cerebral artery occlusion, severe neurologic deficits, and high risk of systemic hemorrhage with intravenous rt-PA (e.g., recent surgery). In most circumstances, the availability of IAT should not preclude the use of intravenous rt-PA in patients meeting appropriate criteria. IAT requires access to emergent cerebral angiography, experienced stroke physicians, and neurointerventionalists; it should be performed only at a clinical center with considerable expertise in this technique.[26]

The MERCI (Mechanical Embolus Removal in Cerebral Ischemia) retrieval system (Concentric Medical, Inc., Mountain View, California) has been FDA-approved for recanalizing acutely occluded cerebral arteries. In the Multi-MERCI study, patients who did not improve immediately after intravenous rt-PA underwent mechanical embolectomy within 8 hours of symptom onset. Partial or complete recanalization occurred in 74% of patients, with a symptomatic intracerebral hemorrhage (sICH) rate of 6.7%.[25]

Another, newer FDA-approved device for AIS is the Penumbra stroke system (Penumbra, Inc., Alameda, California).[26] This device combines two methods of clot extraction, aspiration and mechanical extraction. First the clot is aspirated; then a thrombus removal ring can be used if necessary to remove remaining clot.[26]

DENTAL MANAGEMENT

Medical Considerations

Important public health roles of the dentist are that of educator in stroke prevention and as an identification of the stroke-prone patient. Patients with a history or clinical evidence of hypertension, congestive heart failure, diabetes mellitus, previous stroke or TIA, and advancing age are predisposed to stroke, as well as to myocardial infarction. As these factors increase in frequency, so does the level of risk[12,13] (Box 27-4). The dentist should assess patient risk, encourage persons with risk factors to seek medical care, and eliminate or control all possible risk factors[27] (see Box 27-4).

Assessment of risk aids in the decision-making process regarding the timing and type of dental care to be provided. For example, the risk of stroke is greater in a patient who has had a previous stroke or TIA than in a person who has not had either.[20,27] In fact, up to one third of strokes recur within 1 month of the initial event, and risk remains elevated for at least 6 months.[27] A degree of caution is therefore indicated in the approach to dental treatment of persons with a history of stroke or TIA, and deferral of treatment is advised for 6 months. Although risk decreases after 6 months, it continues to be present; 14% of those who survive a stroke or TIA have a recurrence within 1 year.[20,27] In addition, patients who have recently experienced a TIA or RIND are clinically unstable and should not undergo elective dental care. Medical consultation and referral to a physician are mandatory[20,27] (Box 27-5).

A patient who takes coumarin or antiplatelet drugs is at risk for abnormal bleeding (see Box 27-4). The status of coumarin anticoagulation is monitored by assessment of the international normalized ratio (INR). An INR level of 3.5 or less is acceptable for performance of most invasive and noninvasive dental procedures. If the INR is greater than 3.5 and oral surgery is planned, significant bleeding may occur, and the physician should be consulted regarding a decrease in dosage of the anticoagulant. In such cases, a reduction in dose of the anticoagulant is recommended over interruption of anticoagulation therapy, because the risk for significant adverse outcomes is minimized by this approach (see Chapter 24).[20,27]

Recent data indicate that post-CVA patients in whom the usual anticoagulant regimen is altered before undergoing dental treatment are at risk for adverse events.[27,28] Therefore, it is advisable to not adjust the anticoagulant regimen unless close consultation with the physician occurs.[27] Also, metronidazole and tetracycline may increase the INR by inhibiting the metabolism of warfarin (Coumadin); therefore, concurrent use of these drugs probably should be avoided.[20,27] Postoperative pain should be managed with acetaminophen-containing products and not any aspirin[21] (see Box 27-5).

Patients whom have recently undergone a stroke may be safely and effectively managed in the dental clinic without complications as long as the patient is carefully monitored.[21] Management of stroke-prone patients or patients with a history of stroke includes the use of short, midmorning appointments that are as stress-free as possible. Assisted transfer to the dental chair may be needed. It is important not to overestimate the patient's abilities, especially because good verbalization skills may mask a surprising lack of self-awareness regarding the extent of paresis that is present, reflecting a "neglect" syndrome. Dental care providers should move slowly around the patient and should speak clearly, with the mask off, while facing the patient. Effective communication techniques are listed in Box 27-6.[21]

Blood pressure should be monitored to ensure good control. Pain control is important. Nitrous oxide–oxygen may be given if good oxygenation is maintained

BOX 27-4 Risk Factors for Stroke

- Hypertension*
- Congestive heart failure*
- Diabetes mellitus*
- History of TIAs or previous CVA*
- Age >75 years*
- Hypercholesterolemia
- Coronary atherosclerosis
- Smoking tobacco

*NOTE: The risk of stroke increases by a factor of 1.5 for each of these conditions. With the combination of several factors, the risk obviously becomes much greater.

CVA, Cerebrovascular accident [stroke]; *TIA*, Transient ischemic attack.

BOX 27-5 Dental Management
Consideraations in the Patient with History of a Stroke

P

Patient Evaluation/Risk Assessment (see Box 1-1)
- Evaluate to determine the nature, severity, control, and stability of disease.

Potential Issues/Factors of Concern

A	
Antibiotics	Avoid use of metronidazole and tetracyclines in patients taking warfarin (Coumadin) because of its decreased metabolism.
Anesthetics	Good pain control should be achieved during the procedure, but dose of epinephrine should be limited to two carpules; no epinephrine- containing retraction cord should be used.
Analgesics	Use of acetaminophen as pain reliever is recommended; avoid the use of ASA and other NSAIDs (including for postoperative pain) due to increased bleeding
B	
Bleeding	Patients taking an anticoagulant or on antiplatelet therapy are at increased risk for bleeding: • Aspirin ± dipyridamole (Aggrenox), clopidogrel (Plavix), abciximab (ReoPro), or ticlopidine (Ticlid) • Coumarin—pretreatment INR ≤3.5. Higher levels require consultation with physician to reduce dose. • Heparin, intravenous—use palliative emergency dental care only, or 6-12 hours before surgery, discontinue heparin and start another anticoagulant (e.g., warfarin [Coumadin]) with physician's approval. Then restart heparin after clot forms (6 hours later). Heparin, subcutaneous (low-molecular-weight)—generally, no changes required. Use measures that minimize hemorrhage (atraumatic surgery, pressure, Gelfoam, suturing), as needed. Have available nonadrenergic hemostatic agents and devices (stents, electrocautery unit). Additional steps should be taken to achieve hemostasis in patients on an anticoagulant or antiplatelet therapy.
Blood pressure	Monitor blood pressure and oxygen saturation.
C	
Cardiac	Blood pressure should be monitored throughout appointment during dental procedures
Chair position	Deficits from a previous stroke may warrant assistance for patient transfer to the chair, effective oral evacuation and airway management, and rigorous oral hygiene measures delivered by a health care provider.
D	
Drugs	Use minimum amount of anesthetic containing a vasoconstrictor. Avoid use of epinephrine-impregnated retraction cord. Also avoid the use of metronidazole and tetracyclines in patients taking warfarin (Coumadin), because these agents cause decreased warfarin metabolism.
E	
Emergencies	Only emergency treatment procedures should be done within 6 months of TIA, RIND, or stroke. Appointments should be short and stress-free, with good anesthesia achieved using nitrous oxide–oxygen. Monitoring of blood pressure and oxygen saturation is indicated throughout the procedure. Recognize signs and symptoms of a stroke, provide emergency care, and activate EMS system as needed.
Equipment	No issues.

EMS, Emergency medical services; *INR,* International normalized ratio; *IV,* Intravenous; *RIND,* Reversible ischemic neurologic deficit; *TIA,* Transient ischemic attack.

at all times. Pulse oximeter monitoring is indicated to ensure that oxygenation is adequate. A local anesthetic with 1:100,000 or 1:200,000 epinephrine may be used in judicious amounts (4 mL or less). Gingival retraction cord impregnated with epinephrine should not be used.[20,21,27]

A patient who develops signs or symptoms of a stroke in the dental office should receive oxygen, and the EMS system should be activated. Transport to a medical facility should not be delayed (minutes count in the treatment of patients with acute stroke). For ischemic stroke, thrombolytic agents should be administered within 3 hours if they are to be maximally effective in reestablishing arterial flow; the earlier subjects receive these agents, the better the outcome.[29] The phrase "time is brain" emphasizes the urgency of the situation. Finally, the dental staff should recognize that patients who have had a stroke typically experience feelings of grief, loss, and depression and should be treated with compassion.

Treatment Planning Modifications

Technical modifications may be required for patients with residual physical deficits who have difficulty in practicing adequate oral hygiene. For these patients, extensive bridgework is not a good choice. However, fixed prostheses may be more desirable than removable ones because of difficulties associated with daily placement and removal. Individualized treatment plans are important. All restorations should be placed with ease

BOX 27-6 Effective Communication Techniques for the Patient Who Has Suffered a Stroke

- Face the patient.
- Use a slower, more deliberate, less complex pattern of speech.
- Communicate at eye level.
- Be positive.
- Ask "yes-or-no" questions—be simple and brief.
- Give frequent, accurate, and immediate feedback.
- Use simple drawings to explain procedures.
- Do not underestimate or overestimate abilities.
- Do not raise voice or use baby talk.
- Do not wear a mask when talking to the patient.
- Communicate also with significant other or personal care provider.

Data from Henry R, personal communication, 1995; and Ostuni E: Stroke and the dental patient, J Am Dent Assoc *125:721-727, 1994.*

of cleansability in mind. Hygiene often is facilitated by an electric toothbrush, a large-handled toothbrush, or a water irrigation device. Flossing aids should be prescribed, and family members and personal care providers should be instructed on how and when these services should be provided. Frequent professional prophylaxis and the provision of topical fluoride and chlorhexidine are advisable.[20,27]

Oral Complications and Manifestations

A stroke-in-evolution may become apparent as slurred speech, weak muscles, or difficulty swallowing. After a stroke, complete loss of or difficulty in speech, unilateral paralysis of the orofacial musculature, and loss of sensory stimuli of oral tissues may occur. The tongue may be flaccid, with multiple folds, and may deviate on extrusion. Dysphagia is common, along with difficulty in managing liquids and solids. Patients with right-sided brain damage may neglect the left side. Thus, food and debris may accumulate around teeth, beneath the tongue, or in alveolar folds. Patients may need to learn to clean teeth or dentures with only one hand, or they may require assistance to maintain oral hygiene; otherwise, caries, periodontal disease, and halitosis occur commonly.

Calcified atherosclerotic plaques have been demonstrated in the carotid arteries of elderly and diabetic patients on panoramic films[30-34] (Figure 27-7). This radiographic feature indicates a risk for stroke and warrants referral to the patient's physician for evaluation. Also of note, severe periodontal bone loss is associated with carotid artery plaques and increased risk for stroke. However, the exact causative relationship between periodontal disease and stroke remains to be defined. Although periodontal treatment can reduce serum inflammatory markers potentially involved in stroke, evidence that periodontal therapy reduces the risk for stroke is lacking.[20-27]

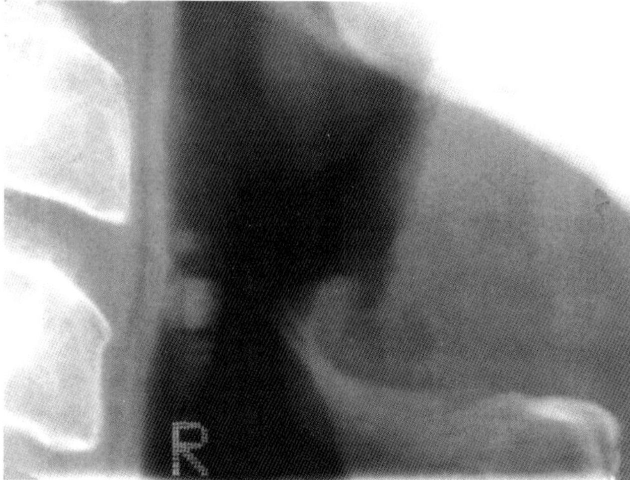

FIGURE 27-7 Carotid atheroma in an elderly patient at risk for stroke. The calcification usually is located near cervical vertebrae 3 and 4, generally at a 45-degree angle from the angle of the mandible.

PARKINSON'S DISEASE

DEFINITION

Parkinson's disease is a progressive neurodegenerative disorder of neurons that produce dopamine. Loss of these neurons results in characteristic motor disturbances—resting tremor, muscular rigidity, bradykinesia, and postural instability.[35-37] Dopaminergic neurons are found in the nigrostriatal pathway of the brain. Approximately 80% of the dopamine in these neurons must be depleted before symptoms of the disease emerge. This disease is chronic and progressive.[35-37]

EPIDEMIOLOGY

Incidence and Prevalence

Parkinson's disease, which is the second most common neurodegenerative disorder after Alzheimer's disease, occurs in approximately 1 in 1000 people in the general population and in 1% of persons older than 65 years. Each year, this disease is diagnosed in 50,000 persons. Men are affected slightly more often than women.[35-37] In keeping with the aging phenomenon in the United States, a three- to four-fold increase in Parkinson's disease frequency is predicted over the next 50 years. Parkinson's disease has a peak age at onset between 55 and 66 years, but a particular form of the disease can strike teenagers. An average dental practice of 2000 adult patients is predicted to include about 4 patients who have Parkinson's disease.[35-37]

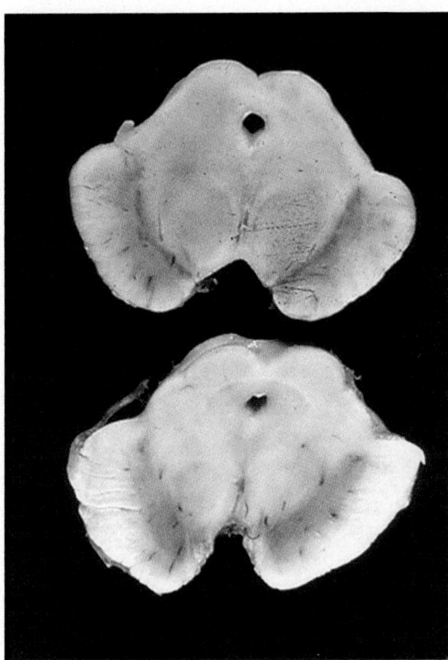

FIGURE 27-8 **Parkinson's Disease.** Normal pigmentation of dopaminergic neurons in the substantia nigrans of a healthy patient (*top*), in contrast with depleted and depigmented dopaminergic neurons of the substantia nigrans in a patient who has Parkinson's disease (*bottom*).

Etiology

Parkinson's disease is caused by death and depletion of dopaminergic neurons, which are manufactured in the substantia nigra (Figure 27-8) and released in the caudate nucleus and putamen (the nigrostriatal pathway).[35-37]

The etiology of Parkinson's disease is believed to be a variable combination of poorly understood genetic and environmental factors. Both autosomal dominant and recessive genes can cause classic Parkinson's disease. The protein α-synuclein, which is the chief constituent of the hallmark cytoplasmic inclusion, the Lewy body, is critical in the pathogenesis of Parkinson's disease. Abnormal aggregation of the protein, either from mutations in the α-synuclein gene or occurring as a result of excessive production of the normal protein due to gene duplications or triplications, is associated with various disease phenotypes. Other defined genetic abnormalities may be associated with classic later-onset Parkinson's disease, including *LRRK2,* which is currently the most common cause of autosomal dominantly inherited Parkinson's disease, or with early-onset parkinsonism, typically found in the autosomal recessive forms associated with *parkin,* DJ-1, and *PINK1.* Other genes in which mutations may increase the risk for development of Parkinson's disease include the glucocerebrosidase gene (*GBA*) in Ashkenazi Jews.[35]

More recent studies also have implicated oxidative stress in the pathogenesis of Parkinson's disease. Other proposed pathogenetic factors include excitotoxicity and inflammation.[35]

Other causes include stroke, brain tumor, and head injury (e.g., boxing) that damage cells in the nigrostriatal pathway.[35] Exposure to manganese (in miners and welders), mercury, carbon disulfide, certain agricultural herbicides (rotenone), and street heroin contaminated with a meperidine analogue (1-methyl-4-phenyl-1,2,3,6-tetrahydropyridine) can be neurotoxic, giving rise to Parkinson's disease symptoms. Also, neuroleptic drugs (phenothiazines, butyrophenones) may cause parkinsonian symptoms and rigidity.[35]

Pathophysiology and Complications

Parkinson's disease is thought to be caused by environmental and genetic factors that trigger failure in proteasome-mediated protein turnover in susceptible neurons, resulting in accumulation of toxic proteins.[35] This toxicity leads to degeneration and loss of pigmented neurons, primarily those of the substantia nigra, and destructive lesions in the circuitry to the limbic system, motor system, and centers that regulate autonomic functions. Damaged neurons display neuronal cytoskeleton changes including eosinophilic intraneuronal inclusion bodies (called Lewy bodies) and Lewy neurites in their neuronal processes.[38,39] Inclusion bodies contain compacted aggregates of presynaptic protein α-synuclein.[38,39] The course of the disease is complicated by degeneration of other regions in the brain such as the cholinergic nucleus basalis, which can result in depression.[40,41]

CLINICAL PRESENTATION

Signs and Symptoms

A major manifestation of Parkinson's disease is resting tremor (that is attenuated during activity), muscle rigidity, slow movement (bradykinesia, shuffling gait), and facial impassiveness (mask of Parkinson's disease)[42] (Figure 27-9). The tremor, which is rhythmic and fine and is best seen in the extremity at rest, produces a "pill-rolling rest tremor" and handwriting changes. Cogwheel-type rigidity (decreased arm swing with walking and foot dragging), stooped posture, unsteadiness, imbalance (gait instability), and falls also are common features. In addition, pain, (musculoskeletal, sensory [burning, numbness, tingling][42] or akathisia—subjective feeling of restlessness—restless leg syndrome), orthostatic hypotension, and bowel and bladder dysfunction occur in approximately 50% of patients.[36] Cognitive impairment of memory and concentration occurs to a variable degree, depending on the extent of destruction of the cortical–basal ganglia–thalamic neural loops. Mood disturbances (depression, dysthymia, apathy, anxiety), insomnia, and fatigue occur in approximately 40% of patients; dementia occurs in approximately 25%. Psychosis, related to dopaminergic medications, occurs in approximately 20% of patients.[36,38,41,43,44]

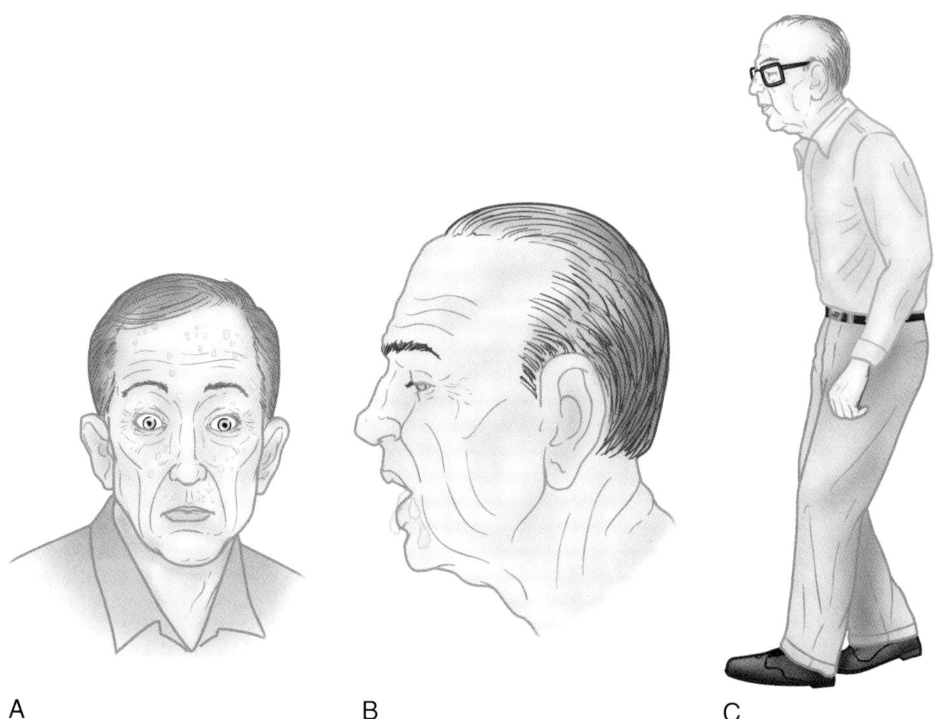

FIGURE 27-9 Characteristic features of Parkinson's disease. **A,** Masklike appearance, stare, and excessive sweating. **B,** Drooling with excessive saliva. **C,** Parkinsonian gait with rapid, short, shuffling steps and reduced arm swinging. *(From Seidel HM, et al: Mosby's guide to physical examination, ed 7, St. Louis, 2011, Mosby.)*

Laboratory Findings

Because no diagnostic test is available to detect Parkinson's disease, the diagnosis requires a thorough history, clinical examination, and specific tests and imaging procedures to rule out diseases that can produce similar clinical manifestations, such as Wilson's disease, arteriosclerotic pseudoparkinsonism, multiple stem atrophy, and progressive supranuclear palsy.[42]

MEDICAL MANAGEMENT

Therapy is begun with the goal of increasing dopamine levels in the brain. Because no optimal drug treatment is available for Parkinson's disease, each person is treated on an individual basis with a variety of drugs. The six classes of drugs used to manage the symptoms of Parkinson's disease are shown in Table 27-2.[35] Drug therapy generally is not initiated until lifestyle impairment such as slowness or imbalance occurs. Drug selection is based on anticipated adverse effects and complications, and therapy is initiated at the lowest effective dose.

The mainstay of treatment for advanced Parkinson's disease is carbidopa-levodopa (Sinemet), an immediate precursor of the neurotransmitter dopamine. Use of this agent generally is reserved for later in the course of the disease, because its activity wanes after about 5 to 10 years, and when given over the long term, it produces complicating adverse effects (dyskinesia—involuntary rapid, flowing movements of limbs, trunk, or head). Management of progressive disease requires a careful balance between the beneficial effects of Sinemet or controlled-release levodopa (Sinemet CR) and the use of adjunctive medications such as (1) dopamine agonists and (2) catechol-O-methyltransferase (COMT) inhibitors (entacapone) used to diminish motor fluctuations, as well as (3) serotonin reuptake inhibitors used to manage depression and (4) acetylcholinesterase inhibitors given for dementia.[35] Dosage adjustments are required when dyskinesias, immobility, psychosis, or other adverse effects occur. Physical therapy is important for providing patients with safe methods for rising from a chair, walking around a room, navigating stairs, and combating immobility and contractures.[35]

If symptoms progress despite drug therapy, surgery involving replacement of dopamine neurons by grafting of fetal nerve tissue appears to be an encouraging alternative for patients with advanced Parkinson's disease.[45] Newer modalities are focusing on halting neuronal loss with the use of antioxidants, or introducing (injecting) trophic factors through lentiviral delivery of a gene that encodes glial cell line–derived neurotrophic factor. Deep

TABLE 27-2 Drugs Used in the Management of Parkinson's Disease

Drug/Class	Reason Used	Adverse Effects	Dental Treatment Considerations
Anticholinergic	Blocks the effect of another brain neurotransmitter (acetylcholine) to rebalance its levels with dopamine		
Trihexyphenidyl HCl (Artane)		Sedation, urinary retention, constipation	Dry mouth
Benztropine mesylate (Cogentin)			
Dopamine Precursor	Provides a drug that is metabolized into dopamine (dopamine replacement)		
Levodopa			
Carbidopa-levodopa (Sinemet CR, Madopar CR)		Dyskinesia, fatigue, headache, anxiety, confusion, insomnia, orthostatic hypotension	If choreiform movements, dyskinesias, or tremors are present, sedation techniques may be required to perform dentistry; caution on getting up from the dental chair
Dopamine Agonist	Mimics the action of dopamine		
Bromocriptine mesylate (Parlodel)*		Dopaminergic effects: psychosis (hallucinations, delusions), orthostatic hypotension, dyskinesia, nausea	Caution on getting up from the dental chair
Pramipexole (Mirapex)			Mirapex adversely interacts with erythromycin.
Ropinirole HCl (Requip)			
Catechol-*O*-Methyltransferase (COMT) Inhibitor†	Used along with levodopa. This medication blocks the enzyme COMT, to prevent levodopa breakdown in the intestine, thus allowing more of levodopa to reach the brain		
Tolcapone (Tasmar)*† Entacapone (Comtan)		Potentiate levodopa effects: dyskinesia, psychosis, or orthostatic hypotension; nausea and diarrhea, abnormal taste	Caution with use of vasoconstrictors Monitor vital signs during and after administration of first capsule; limit dose to two capsules containing 1:100,000 epinephrine (36 μg) or less, depending on vital signs and patient response; aspirate to avoid intravascular injection.
Monoamine Oxidase B Inhibitor†	Prevents metabolism of dopamine within the brain		
Selegiline†		Dizziness, orthostatic hypotension, nausea	Select adrenergic agents (i.e., amphetamine, pseudoephedrine, tyramine) may cause increased pressor response. However, this does not appear to occur with epinephrine or levonordefrin.
Neurotransmitter Inhibitor	Has anticholinergic properties that enhance dopamine transmission		
Amantadine		Sedation, urinary retention, peripheral edema, nausea, constipation, confusion	

*May cause significant hepatic toxicity.
†Also has adverse vasoconstrictive properties.

brain stimulation of subthalamic nuclei, thalamotomy, or pallidotomy is reserved for patients with advanced disease and severe disabling or intractable tremor.[36,46]

DENTAL MANAGEMENT

Medical Considerations

The dentist who treats adult patients can play an important role in recognizing the features of Parkinson's disease and making a referral to a physician for thorough evaluation of persons who exhibit features of the disease. Once the diagnosis has been made, concerns in dental management are two-fold: (1) minimizing the adverse outcomes of muscle rigidity and tremor and (2) avoiding drug interactions (Box 27-7).

Because the muscular defect and tremor can contribute to poor oral hygiene, the dentist should assess the patient's ability to cleanse their dentition by demonstration. For patients unable to provide adequate home care, alternative solutions should be provided, such as the introduction of the Collis curve toothbrush, mechanical toothbrushes, assisted brushing, or chlorhexidine rinses.

Drug interactions of concern in dentistry are outlined in Table 27-2.[36] Although no adverse interactions have been reported between COMT inhibitors (tolcapone [Tasmar], entacapone [Comtan]) and epinephrine at dosages typically used in dentistry, they can potentially interact, and it is advisable to limit the dose of epinephrine to two carpules containing 1:100,000 epinephrine (36 μg) in patients who take COMT inhibitors. Erythromycin should not be given to patients who take the

BOX 27-7 Dental Management
Considerations in the Patient with Parkinson's Disease

P
Patient Evaluation/Risk Assessment (see Box 1-1)
- Evaluate to determine the nature, severity, control, and stability of disease.

Potential Issues/Factors of Concern
- Well-controlled Parkinson's disease poses no specific management problems.

A	
Analgesics	Clinicians should provide good pain control.
Antibiotics	There is no need for antibiotic prophylaxis.
Anesthesia	It is very important to obtain adequate anesthesia to reduce stress, which may worsen the movement disturbance. Epinephrine (1:100,000) in local anesthetics generally is well tolerated.
Anxiety	Patients with untreated or poorly controlled disease may experience exaggerated trembling and involuntary shaking movements and appear very anxious and stressed. Use of special anxiety and stress reduction techniques may be indicated.
Allergy	No issues.
B	
Bleeding	Generally, no bleeding problems are expected.
Blood pressure	Monitor blood pressure, because dopamine may cause hypotension.
C	
Chair position	This usually is not a problem if the patient is under good medical management; with symptoms of impending syncope, however, a supine position may not be tolerated. The patient taking dopamine may experience hypotension, warranting precautions with getting seated or on arising. The chair may need adjustment for adequate support to help reduce unnecessary movement or to stabilize the patient in a comfortable position.
Consultation	Once the patient is under good medical management, the dental treatment plan is unaffected. However, consultation with the patient's physician to establish the level of control is recommended as part of the management program.
D	
Devices	No issues.
Drugs	These patients typically are on anticholinergic and dopamine agonist drugs, which may have adverse effects including sedation, drowsiness, slow mentation, fatigue, confusion, and dizziness (see Table 27-2).
E	
Emergencies	Tremors most commonly are self-limited, but rarely the movement disturbance may be severe enough to interrupt dental treatment or to necessitate cessation of treatment.
Equipment	No issues.
F	
Follow-up	Routine follow-up is recommended.

dopamine agonist pramipexole (Mirapex). The clinician should be aware that antiparkinsonian drugs can be CNS depressants, and a dentally prescribed sedative may have an additive effect to those of such agents.[36]

Orthostatic hypotension and rigidity are common in patients who have Parkinson's disease. Orthostatic hypotension is an adverse effect associated with COMT inhibitors. To reduce the likelihood of a fall from the dental chair, the patient should be assisted to and from the chair. At the end of the appointment, the chair should be inclined slowly to allow for reequilibration.[36]

Treatment Planning Modifications

The treatment plan for the patient with Parkinson's disease may require modification based on the patient's ability to cleanse the oral cavity. When communicating the treatment plan and other advice, the dentist should directly face the patient. This provides effective communication with a person who has the potential for cognitive impairment.

Patients should receive dental care during the time of day at which their medication has maximum effect (generally, 2 to 3 hours after taking it). The presence of tremors or choreiform movements may warrant use of soft arm restraints or sedation procedures.

Oral Complications and Manifestations

Parkinson's disease is associated with staring, excess salivation and drooling, and decreased frequency of blinking and swallowing.[35] Muscle rigidity makes repetitive muscle movement and maintenance of good oral hygiene difficult. By contrast, the drugs used to manage the disease (anticholinergics, dopaminergics, amantadine, and L-dopa) often result in xerostomia, nausea, and tardive dyskinesia.[35] Dental recall visits should be more frequent for this population, and specific measures (specialized toothbrushes—e.g., Collis curve toothbrush, mechanical brushes) should be devised to maintain adequate oral hygiene. If the patient is experiencing xerostomia, dysphagia and poor denture retention are likely to result. Salivary substitutes are beneficial in alleviating symptoms. Topical fluoride should be considered for use in dentate patients with xerostomia, to prevent root caries. Personal care providers should be educated about their role in assisting and maintaining the oral hygiene of these patients.

DEMENTIA AND ALZHEIMER'S DISEASE

DEFINITION

Dementia is a disorder of cognition that consequently interferes with daily functions and results in a loss of independence.[42] Dementia consists of a slow, progressive, chronic decline in intellectual abilities that includes impairment in memory, abstract thinking, and judgment. It is primarily a disease of aging; 1% of cases appear by age 60, and more than 40% of cases occur by age 85. Overall, the course of dementia is chronic in 65% of cases, partially treatable in 25% of cases, and reversible in only 10% of cases.[42] The most common causes of dementia are Alzheimer's disease, vascular dementia, and dementia caused by Parkinson's disease. Other causes include hepatic encephalopathy, acid-base and electrolyte disturbances, hypoglycemia, head trauma, thyroid disease (involving either low or high levels of hormone), uremia, primary or metastatic brain lesions, acquired immunodeficiency syndrome (AIDS), trauma, syphilis, MS, stroke, and drugs. A small subset of dementias, such as Creutzfeldt-Jakob disease, may have a very rapid onset with a clinical course of less than a year.[42]

Because of its relatively high prevalence, Alzheimer's disease serves as the prototype for discussion of dementia in this chapter. This disease, which was first described by Alois Alzheimer in 1907, predominantly affects elderly persons. However, the process may occur in younger adults as well.[42]

EPIDEMIOLOGY

Incidence and Prevalence

The prevalence of dementia increases with age. Among persons older than 65 years of age, the prevalence is about 7%. From age 70 years on, the prevalence doubles every 5 years. By age 85, more than 40% of persons will have developed Alzheimer's disease. With the aging of the population in the United States, the prevalence of this disease is predicted to double by 2020.[42] Approximately 6 to 8 million people in the United States experience dementia, and more than half of these cases are of the Alzheimer's type. Women are at greater risk for developing the disease, primarily because women live longer than men. An average dental practice of 2000 adult patients is predicted to include about 20 patients who experience Alzheimer's disease.[42]

Etiology

The cause of Alzheimer's disease is unknown but appears to involve the loss of cholinergic neurons. Unidentified factors trigger the deposition of beta-amyloid plaques that initiate an inflammatory response, oxidative damage, progressive neuritic injury, and loss of cortical neurons. As a result, levels of neurotransmitters important for learning and memory decrease. Genetic predisposition contributes to less than 20% of all cases. In these cases, the disease appears to be inherited by way of the apolipoprotein E4 (ApoE4) allele located on chromosome 19. Three other chromosomes have been implicated to a lesser degree in the transmission of Alzheimer's disease—an amyloid precursor gene on chromosome 21, a presenilin-1 gene on chromosome 14, and a presenilin-2 gene on chromosome 1.[42] Inasmuch as chromosome 21 contains a gene that expresses a cleavage product of the amyloid precursor protein, it is not surprising that adults with trisomy 21 (Down syndrome) consistently develop neuropathologic hallmarks of Alzheimer's disease if they survive beyond the age of 40 years. Risk factors for Alzheimer's disease comprise age, family history of dementia, and the presence of both ApoE4 alleles.[42,47-49]

Pathophysiology and Complications

Alzheimer's disease is characterized by beta-amyloid plaques and neuroinflammation that results in neurofibrillary tangles and loss of cortical neurons.[42] The process begins in the hippocampus and the entorhinal cortex. Over time, it spreads to specific regions of the brain (temporal, parietal, and frontal lobes) that are important for learning and memory. Affected neurons make up part of the cholinergic system and use acetylcholine and glutamate as their primary neurotransmitters. These neurotransmitters are intimately involved in cognition. Progressive destruction of the neurons leads to atrophy of the cerebral cortex and enlargement of the ventricles. Motor, visual, and somatosensory portions of the cerebral cortex typically are spared. Resultant cognitive defects and associated memory loss cause significant impairment in social and occupational functioning.[42]

CLINICAL PRESENTATION

Signs and Symptoms

The onset of Alzheimer's disease occurs subtly and insidiously; the first sign is loss of recent memory, orientation, or language, or a change in personality (apathy) or behavior. Slowly, cognitive problems at the early stage begin to interfere with daily activities such as keeping track of finances, following instructions on the job, driving, shopping, and housekeeping.[42] Some patients remain unaware of these developing problems; others are aware of them and become frustrated and anxious. At the middle stage of the disease, the patient is unable to work, is easily lost and confused, and requires daily supervision. Patients may become lost while taking walks or driving. Social graces, routine conversation, and superficial conversation may be maintained for variable periods. Language may be impaired, especially comprehension and naming of objects. Motor skills such as eating, dressing, or solving simple puzzles are eventually lost. Patients are unable to do simple calculations or to tell time. Loss of inhibitions and belligerence may occur, and nighttime wandering may become a problem with some patients. Anxiety and depression become more of a problem as the disease progresses.[50] At the advanced stage of Alzheimer's disease, patients may become rigid, mute, incontinent, and bedridden, often requiring a nursing facility. Generalized seizures may occur. Death usually results from malnutrition, secondary infection, or heart disease. The typical duration of Alzheimer's disease is 5 to 15 years. However, the course of the illness can range from 1 to 20 years. Some patients exhibit a steady downhill course; others may have prolonged plateaus without major deterioration.[42]

Laboratory Findings

Although the definitive diagnosis of Alzheimer's can be made only by brain biopsy or at autopsy, the clinical diagnosis of Alzheimer's disease can be made on the basis of patient history and clinical findings.[42] Criteria for making this diagnosis include (1) progressive functional decline and dementia established by clinical examination and mental status testing, (2) the presence of at least two cognitive deficits, (3) normal level of consciousness at presentation, (4) onset between the ages of 40 and 90 years, and (5) absence of any other condition that could account for the deficits. The battery of tests useful in ruling out other correctable causes of dementia include a complete blood count, electrolyte panel, screening metabolic panel, thyroid function tests, determination of vitamin B_{12} and folate levels, tests for syphilis and human immunodeficiency virus (HIV) antibodies, urinalysis, ECG, chest radiograph, and noncontrast CT scan or MRI of the brain.[42]

At autopsy, characteristic macroscopic changes include cerebral cortical atrophy and ventricular enlargement. Microscopic features include neurofibrillary tangles, neuritic plaques that contain beta-amyloid, and accumulation of beta-amyloid in the walls of cerebral vessels (amyloid angiopathy). On a biochemical level, a deficiency of acetylcholine and its associated enzymes has been confirmed.[42,47-49]

The Alzheimer's Association and the National Institutes of Health/National Institute on Aging have developed new criteria for categories of Alzheimer's. These criteria divide the disease into three stages: preclinical Alzheimer's, marked by no outward symptoms and only measurable changes in biomarkers such as spinal fluid chemistry; mild cognitive impairment, in which changes in memory and thinking appear but do not yet compromise everyday activities and functioning; and dementia, the defining trait of late-stage disease. The previous criteria offer no way to diagnose Alzheimer's in a preclinical state, because appropriate biomarkers are still being investigated and standardized, which means that "preclinical Alzheimer's" remains mainly for future studies to define.

However, the publication of these new criteria makes it official that the middle stage, measurable mild cognitive impairment, can be considered part of the disease spectrum for Alzheimer's. In other words, Alzheimer's can now be defined by subtle brain changes, rather than exclusively by dementia.[88]

MEDICAL MANAGEMENT

The management of Alzheimer's disease remains difficult. Standard medications used in the treatment of mild to moderate disease have been the cholinesterase inhibitors. These drugs—donepezil (Aricept), rivastigmine (Exelon), galantamine (Reminyl), and tacrine (Cognex)—increase acetylcholine levels in the brain by inhibiting hydrolysis of cholinesterase (Table 27-3).[42] Clinical trials indicate that these agents perform better than placebo but have limited effectiveness in preventing disease progression and in reversing memory deficits. Less than 50% of patients appear to benefit from these medications.[42] Common adverse effects of the cholinesterase inhibitors include gastrointestinal disturbance and headache. Tacrine, the first of the cholinesterase inhibitors to be marketed, is infrequently prescribed today because it requires frequent dosing and can be hepatotoxic.[46,57]

To slow the progression of disease, the American Academy of Neurology recommends that vitamin E be considered as an additional medication.[42] Studies have shown that vitamin E and selegiline (two antioxidants) each can delay the development of dementia in patients with Alzheimer's disease.[42]

For the management of moderate to severe Alzheimer's disease, memantine (Axura), an *N*-methyl-D-aspartate (NMDA) receptor antagonist—has been approved by the U.S. Food and Drug Administration (FDA).[51,52] This drug works by selectively blocking the excitotoxic effects of abnormal glutamate transmission. Initial studies suggest that it may preserve or improve memory and learning and, when given with the cholinesterase inhibitors, appears to produce additive beneficial effects. Memantine-related adverse effects are mild and include headache and confusion.[51,52]

Noncognitive symptoms of Alzheimer's disease are manageable. Although efforts are made to use nonpharmacologic approaches to manage symptoms such as anxiety, depression, irritability, and sleep disturbances, medications inevitably are generally required. Antidepressants, sedative-hypnotics, and antipsychiatric agents all are used, with varying degrees of success. A small percentage of patients experience seizures, which are treated with standard anticonvulsant agents. Nursing home care often is provided during the latter stages of the disease.[51,52]

DENTAL MANAGEMENT

Medical Considerations

Dental management requires knowledge of the stage of disease, medications taken, and the cognitive abilities of the patient (Box 27-8). Patients with mild to moderate disease generally maintain normal systemic organ function and can receive routine dental treatment. As the disease progresses, antipsychotics, antidepressants, and anxiolytics frequently are used to manage behavioral disturbances. These medications, however, contribute to xerostomia with increased risk for dental caries.[53]

There is no cure for Alzheimer's disease. However, several prescription drugs are currently approved by the FDA (see Table 27-3) for use in people diagnosed with this condition. Treating the symptoms of Alzheimer's disease can maximize the comfort, dignity, and independence of these patients for a longer period of time, thereby providing support and assistance for their caregivers as well.[42] It is important to recognize that none of these medications stops the disease itself.

Several cholinesterase inhibitors are prescribed for mild to moderate Alzheimer's disease. These drugs may help delay or prevent symptoms from becoming worse for a limited time and may help control some behavioral symptoms. The medications include galantamine (Razadyne), rivastigmine (Exelon), and donepezil (Aricept). Another drug, tacrine (Cognex), was the first approved cholinesterase inhibitor but is rarely prescribed today owing to safety concerns.[42] No one fully understands how cholinesterase inhibitors work to treat Alzheimer's disease, but research indicates that these agents prevent the breakdown of acetylcholine, believed to be important for memory and thinking. As Alzheimer's progresses, the brain produces less and less acetylcholine; therefore, cholinesterase inhibitors may eventually lose their effect.[42]

Another medication, memantine (Namenda®), an *N*-methyl-D-aspartate (NMDA) antagonist, is prescribed to treat moderate to severe Alzheimer's disease (see Table 27-3). This drug's main effect is to delay progression of some of the symptoms of moderate to severe disease. It may allow patients to maintain certain daily functions a little longer than they would without the medication. For example, memantine may help a patient in the later stages of the disease maintain the ability to use the bathroom independently for several more months, a benefit for both patients and caregivers.[42]

Memantine is believed to work by regulating glutamate, an important brain chemical. When produced in excessive amounts, glutamate may lead to brain cell death. Because NMDA antagonists work very differently from cholinesterase inhibitors, the two types of drugs can be prescribed in combination.[42]

TABLE 27-3 Drugs Used in the Management of Alzheimer's Disease

Drug	Drug Type and Use	How It Works
Memantine (Namenda)	*N*-methyl-D-aspartate (NMDA) antagonist prescribed to treat symptoms of moderate to severe Alzheimer's	Blocks the toxic effects associated with excess glutamate and regulates glutamate activation
Galantamine (Razadyne)	Cholinesterase inhibitor prescribed to treat symptoms of mild to moderate Alzheimer's	Prevents the breakdown of acetylcholine and stimulates nicotinic receptors to release more acetylcholine in the brain
Rivastigmine (Exelon)	Cholinesterase inhibitor prescribed to treat symptoms of mild to moderate Alzheimer's	Prevents the breakdown of acetylcholine and butyrylcholine (a brain chemical similar to acetylcholine) in the brain
Donepezil (Aricept)	Cholinesterase inhibitor prescribed to treat symptoms of mild to moderate, and moderate to severe Alzheimer's	Prevents the breakdown of acetylcholine in the brain

*Available as a generic drug.

From the Alzheimer's Disease Education and Referral (ADEAR) Center, a Service of the National Institute on Aging: Alzheimer's disease medications fact sheet, *NIH Publication No. 08-3431, (updated December 2010), Bethesda, Maryland, National Institutes of Health, U.S. Department of Health and Human Services, 2008.*

The FDA also has approved donepezil for the treatment of moderate to severe Alzheimer's disease.[42]

Dosage and Side Effects

Patients usually are started at low drug doses, with gradual increases in dosage based on how well the drug is tolerated. Some evidence suggests that certain patients may benefit from higher doses of the cholinesterase inhibitors. However, the higher the dose, the more likely are side effects.[42]

The recommended effective dosages of drugs prescribed to treat the symptoms of Alzheimer's disease, along with possible side effects, are summarized in Table 27-3.

Patients should be monitored when a drug is started. Any unusual symptoms should be reported right away to the prescribing doctor. It is important to follow the physician's instructions for taking any medication, including vitamins and herbal supplements. Also, any additions to or changes in medications should be cleared beforehand with the patient's physician.[42]

Testing New Alzheimer's Drugs

Clinical trials are the best way to find out if promising new treatments are safe and effective in humans. Volunteer participants are needed for many Alzheimer's trials conducted around the United States. To learn more, patients can be advised to talk with their doctor or to visit the Alzheimer's Disease Education and Referral (ADEAR) Center's listing of clinical trials on the National Institute on Aging Web site (www.nia.nih.gov/Alzheimers/ResearchInformation/ClinicalTrials).

Treatment Planning Considerations

Patients with Alzheimer's are best managed with use of an understanding and empathetic approach. The dental team should communicate a positive, hopeful attitude regarding maintenance of the patient's oral health to both the patient and family members (see Box 27-8). The dental team should determine whether the patient is legally able to make rational decisions. This issue should be discussed with the patient and family. Treatment

Common Side Effects	Manufacturer's Recommended Dosage	For More Information
Dizziness, headache, constipation, confusion	*Tablet*: Initial dose of 5 mg once a day May increase dose to 10 mg/day (5 mg twice a day), 15 mg/day (5 mg and 10 mg as separate doses), and 20 mg/day (10 mg twice a day) at minimum 1-week intervals if well tolerated *Oral solution*: same dosage as above *Extended-release tablet*: Initial dose of 7 mg once a day; may increase dose to 14 mg/day, 21 mg/day, and 28 mg/day at minimum 1-week intervals if well tolerated.	For current information about this drug's safety and use, visit www.namenda.com. Click on "Prescribing Information" to see the drug label.
Nausea, vomiting, diarrhea, weight loss, loss of appetite	*Tablet**: initial dose of 8 mg/day (4 mg twice a day) May increase dose to 16 mg/day (8 mg twice a day) and 24 mg/day (12 mg twice a day) at minimum 4-week intervals if well tolerated *Oral solution**: same dosage as above *Extended-release capsule**: same dosage as above but taken once a day	For current information about this drug's safety and use, visit www.razadyneer.com. Click on "Important Safety Information" to see links to prescribing information.
Nausea, vomiting, diarrhea, weight loss, loss of appetite, muscle weakness	*Capsule**: initial dose of 3 mg/day (1.5 mg twice a day) May increase dose to 6 mg/day (3 mg twice a day), 9 mg (4.5 mg twice a day), and 12 mg/day (6 mg twice a day) at minimum 2-week intervals if well tolerated *Patch*: Initial dose of 4.6 mg once a day; may increase to 9.5 mg once a day after minimum of 4 weeks if well tolerated *Oral solution*: same dosage as for capsule	For current information about this drug's safety and use, visit www.fda.gov/cder. Click on "Drugs@FDA," search for Exelon, and click on drug name links to see "Label Information."
Nausea, vomiting, diarrhea	*Tablet**: Initial dose of 5 mg once a day May increase dose to 10 mg/day after 4-6 weeks if well tolerated, then to 23 mg/day after at least 3 months *Orally disintegrating tablet**: same dosage as for regular tablet 23-mg dose available as brand-name tablet only	For current information about this drug's safety and use, visit www.fda.gov/cder. Click on "Drugs@FDA," search for Aricept, and click on drug name links to see "Label Information."

planning often involves input and permission from a family member so that appropriate decisions can be made. Before initiation of any procedure, the patient's attention should be engaged and the dentist should explain what is going to happen.[50] The dentist should communicate using short words and sentences and should repeat instructions and explanations. Nonverbal communication can be very helpful. Facial motion and body posture of the dentist should show support—cues that the patient is understood and that the dentist is attentive to the patient's well-being. Positive nonverbal communication includes direct eye contact, smiling, touching the patient on the arm, and so forth. Patients with Alzheimer's disease should be placed on an aggressive preventive dentistry program, including 3-month recall, oral examination, prophylaxis, fluoride gel application, oral hygiene education, and adjustment of prostheses.[50,54,55]

In a patient with mild dementia, good oral health should be quickly restored because of the progressive nature of the disease. Subsequent care should concentrate on preventing dental disease as dementia progresses. A patient with moderate dementia may not be as amenable to dental treatment as in earlier stages of the disease. In such cases, treatment consists of maintaining dental status and minimizing deterioration. Complex dental procedures should be performed, if at all, before the disease has reached the moderate to advanced stage.[50,54,55]

Patients with advanced dementia often are anxious, hostile, and uncooperative in the dental office and very difficult to treat. These patients are best served with short appointments and noncomplex procedures; use of sedation may be required for more complex and tedious procedures. Sedative medication should be selected in consultation with the patient's physician. Chloral hydrate and benzodiazepines can be used to provide the level of sedation required for performance of routine dental procedures.[50,54,55]

In advanced cases, removable prosthetic devices may have to be taken from the patient because of the danger of self-injury. All treatment should be provided with the knowledge that these patients have memory loss, lack of drive, and slowed thinking. Thus, their ability to

BOX 27-8 Dental Management
Considerations in Patients with Alzheimer's Disease or Other Dementias

P

Patient Evaluation/Risk Assessment (see Box 1-1)

- Evaluate to determine the nature, severity, control, and stability of disease.

Potential Issues/Factors of Concern

- Well-controlled Alzheimer's disease/dementia poses no specific management problems.

A

Analgesics	Clinicians should provide good pain control.
Antibiotics	There is no need for antibiotic prophylaxis.
Anesthesia	Local anesthesia obtained with epinephrine (1:100,000) in local anesthetics generally is not associated with any problems.
Anxiety	Patints with untreated or poorly controlled disease may experience difficulty in understanding commands or instructions and appear very anxious or stressed. Use of special anxiety or stress reduction techniques may be indicated.
Allergy	No issues.

B

Bleeding	Generally, no bleeding problems are expected.
Blood pressure	Monitor blood pressure, because some medications may cause hypotension.

C

Chair position	This usually is not a problem if the patient is under good medical management: with symptoms of impending syncope, however, a supine position may not be tolerated. The chair may need adjustment to address patients' concerns or fears.
Consultation	Once the patient is under good medical management, the dental treatment plan is unaffected. However, consultation with the patient's physician to establish the level of control is recommended as part of the management program.

D

Devices	No issues.
Drugs	These patients typically are on anticholinergic drugs, which may have adverse effects including sedation, drowsiness, slow mentation, fatigue, confusion, and dizziness (see Table 27-3).

E

Emergencies	Most commonly, cognitive problems are self-limited, but rarely the patient's condition may progress acutely to warrant interruption of dental treatment or to necessitate cessation of treatment.
Equipment	No issues.

F

Follow-up	In patients who have undergone surgery or other complex dental procedures, a follow-up call within the next day or two is advisable to check on clinical status.

maintain proper daily oral hygiene can become severely compromised.

Oral Complications and Manifestations

Patients with moderate to severe Alzheimer's disease may not have an interest in caring for themselves, and they may lack the ability to do so. Hence, oral hygiene is poor, and dental problems are increased. Most of the medications used to treat psychiatric disorders contribute to increased dental problems in such patients because xerostomia is one of their primary adverse effects. Patients with Alzheimer's disease have a greater incidence of dry mouth, mucosal lesions, candidiasis, plaque and calculus buildup, periodontal disease, and smooth surface (root) and coronal caries, along with an increased risk for aspiration pneumonia.[50,54,55]

These patients often sustain oral injuries from falls and ulcerations of the tongue, cheeks, and alveolar mucosa as the result of accidents with forks or spoons or with mastication, attrition and abrasion of teeth, missing teeth, and migration of teeth. Edentulous patients with dementia may misplace or lose their dentures and at times may even attempt to wear the upper denture on the lower arch and vice versa.[50,54,55]

Antipsychotic drugs sometimes taken by these patients can cause agranulocytosis, leukopenia, or thrombocytopenia. Additional adverse effects of antipsychotic agents include muscular problems such as dystonia, dyskinesia, and tardive dyskinesia in the oral and facial regions.[51,52]

MULTIPLE SCLEROSIS

DEFINITION

Multiple sclerosis (MS) is the most common autoimmune disease of the nervous system. MS is characterized by chronic and continuous demyelination of the corticospinal tract neurons in two or more regions of the brain and spinal cord. MS typically manifests in young adults with episodic neurologic dysfunction, and 85% of patients present with relapsing and remitting symptoms.[56] Demyelinated regions are limited to the white

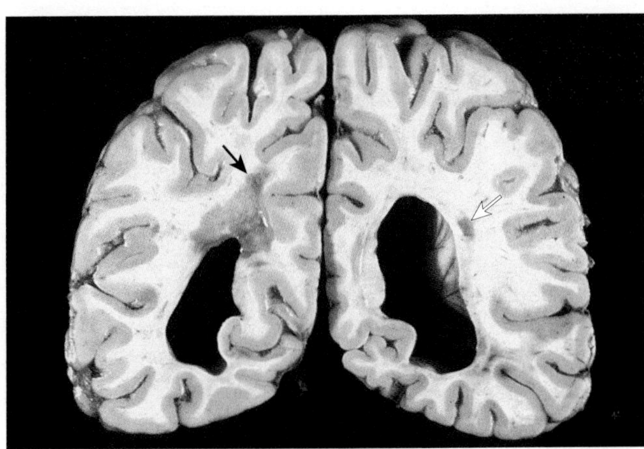

FIGURE 27-10 Multiple Sclerosis. Large periventricular "demyelinated plaque" (*dark region* above left ventricle, *black arrow*) and smaller "demyelinated plaque" (*white arrow*) lateral to right ventricle, shown in a coronal section of the brain of a patient who had multiple sclerosis. (*Courtesy Daron G. Davis, MD, Lexington, Kentucky.*)

matter of the CNS and are randomly located and multiple (Figure 27-10). The peripheral nervous system is not affected.[56]

EPIDEMIOLOGY

Incidence and Prevalence

MS is second only to head trauma as the leading cause of neurologic disability in young adults. Approximately 400,000 people in the United States and more than 1 million worldwide have the disease, for a prevalence rate of about 1 case per 850 persons.[56] The incidence of MS has been increasing beginning in the past century. The disease typically manifests between the ages of 15 to 50 years and affects women twice as often as men. Its prevalence is highest in the temperate regions of the world (i.e., Northern and Southern latitudes), and it is infrequently seen along the Equator.[56] Dentists who manage 2000 adult patients can expect to have about 3 patients in their practice in whom this condition has been diagnosed.

Etiology

MS involves autoimmune-mediated inflammation that leads to demyelination and axonal injury. The cause of MS remains unknown; however, it is widely held that the disease is triggered by an infectious agent. Initial support for this association arises from cluster studies of MS outbreaks in small geographic regions. Over the past century, several microbes (e.g., rabies virus, measles virus, herpesviruses, *Chlamydia pneumoniae*) have been purported to be associated with MS. In recent years, human herpesvirus type 6 has been identified in active demyelinated regions of the CNS in patients who have MS.[57,58] It is hypothesized that this neurotropic virus, in combination with host genetic factors, mediates processes that cause immune-mediated attacks on myelin. However, not all persons who are infected with human herpesvirus type 6 develop MS, suggesting that genetic factors and other environmental factors also are important.[57] Consistent with the role of genetic factor involvement, the concordance rate among monozygotic twins is 30%. Risk is increased when human leukocyte antigen DR2 is carried by a person of Northern European ancestry.[51,52]

Pathophysiology and Complications

Demyelination of MS occurs in scattered white matter regions in the brain. Areas of myelin loss range in size from 1 mm to several centimeters in diameter.[56,59,60] Affected regions show inflammatory demyelination and axonal damage with accumulation of macrophages, B and T lymphocytes, and plasma cells. Specifically, myelin-reactive type 1 helper T cells (T_H1) that produce lymphotoxin and interferon-γ, but little interleukin-4 (IL-4), appear to be central to the pathogenesis of this disease.[56,59,60] The acute MS lesion is accompanied by generation of inflammatory cytokines and antimyelin immunoglobulins that influence macrophages to attack myelin, resulting in tissue destruction, swelling, and breakdown of the blood-brain barrier. Demyelinated disease areas or "plaques" show impairment in axonal conduction; such changes constitute the basic pathophysiologic defect. The most commonly affected regions are the optic nerve, periventricular cerebral white matter, and cervical spinal cord.[56,59,60]

A significant complication of the axonal damage associated with MS is that 50% of patients need help to walk within 15 years of onset of the disease. Continued muscle atrophy can lead to restriction to a wheelchair or a bed, thus increasing the chances for development of pneumonia. The life expectancy for patients with MS is calculated to be 82.5% of normal (approximately 58 years).[56,59,60]

CLINICAL PRESENTATION

Signs and Symptoms

The first clinical signs of MS often appear in young adulthood. Clinical manifestations vary according to which region of the CNS is involved (motor or sensory region) and what degree of disruption occurs in the myelin sheath. Disturbances in visual function (sometimes resulting in blindness) and abnormal eye movements (nystagmus and double vision) are the most common presenting manifestations. Motor disturbances that affect walking and use of the hands (incoordination, spasticity, difficulty in walking, loss of balance and vertigo, coordination or weakness, tremor or paralysis of a limb) and that cause bowel and bladder incontinence, spastic paresis of skeletal muscles (imprecise speech or tremor), and sensory disturbances, including loss of touch, pain, temperature, and proprioception (numbness, pins and needles sensations), are common.[56,59,60] Fatigue is a major symptom (occurring in up to 90%), and worsening fatigue occurs in the afternoon. Symptoms are exacerbated by heat (hot baths, sun exposure) and dehydration and generally emerge over a few days before stabilizing and subsiding a few weeks later. Problems with concentration also occur.[56,59,60]

A typical presentation consists of attacks and relapses that recur for several years. The course is unpredictable and depends on the frequency of attacks and the extent of recovery. Four categories have been used to describe the course of the disease: relapsing-remitting (occurs in 85% of patients), primary progressive, secondary progressive, and progressive-relapsing. Recovery in most cases is temporary, because remyelination is only transient. Repeated attacks can cause permanent physical damage; however, intellectual function remains intact. Depression and emotional instability are features that commonly accompany this disease.[56,59,60]

Laboratory Findings

The diagnosis of MS usually is made on the basis of information derived from the history, clinical examination, CSF analysis, sensory evoked potential studies, and magnetic resonance imaging (MRI) performed over time.[57,61,62] The relapsing-remitting variant is diagnosed when two or more clinical attacks occur in a patient who has two or more affected CNS locations, or when a new MRI lesion appears after a second clinical attack.[56,59,60] The disease also is diagnosed after one clinical attack when a new MRI lesion appears. MRI scans typically reveal multiple hypodense demyelinated regions (plaques) in white matter, usually near the ventricles (see Figure 27-10), brain stem cerebellum, and optic nerves.[56,59,60] The CSF shows signs of low-grade inflammation, and protein and immunoglobulin levels are increased in 80% to 90% of patients. Antibodies to myelin basic protein also can be detected in the CSF. Myelin destruction causes slowing of conduction velocity. The conduction response to visual stimuli (visual evoked potential) or to somatosensory evoked stimuli usually is delayed and altered in amplitude.[56,59,60]

MEDICAL MANAGEMENT

Patients with relapsing forms of MS are given antiinflammatory medications in the form of intravenous corticosteroids (methylprednisolone) for acute attacks or interferon beta-1a (Avonex) or interferon beta-1b (Betaseron) injections.[63,64] The interferons reduce antigen presentation, proliferation of T cells, and production of tumor necrosis factor and have been shown to slow the progression of disease[63,64] (Table 27-4). Corticosteroids have many antiinflammatory functions, including the ability to block eicosanoid and cytokine release and endothelial cell expression of intracellular and extracellular adhesion molecules (ICAMs and ELAMs, respectively), which attract neutrophils. Interferons and glatiramer acetate (Copaxone), a myelin-like polypeptide that suppresses T cell attacks on the myelin sheath, are used during periods of remission to reduce the rate of clinical relapse.[63-65] Use of mitoxantrone, an antineoplastic medication that arrests cell cycle and reduces T_H1 cytokines, is reserved for patients who have aggressive disease and whose symptoms are worsening despite therapy. This agent is used on a short-term basis with glatiramer. However, mitoxantrone use is associated with cardiac complications and risk for leukemia.[66,67]

Some of the newer biologic agents, such as natalizumab, ustekinumab, and rituximab, have shown promise in treating MS.[63-66,68,69] Additionally, clinical trials with cladribine have shown promise, particularly in cases of relapsing MS.[70] Other more recent studies indicate that treatment with vitamin D and the hydroxymethylglutaryl–coenzyme A (HMG-CoA) reductase inhibitors (statins) may be effective for management of MS.[59,71-73]

TABLE 27-4 Drugs Used in the Management of Multiple Sclerosis

Drug	Dental Management Considerations	Local Anesthetic/ Vasoconstrictor
Primary Drugs		
Interferon beta-1a (Avonex, Rebif) injection	Transient flulike symptoms, anemia uncommon; may increase anticoagulant effects of warfarin	No information to suggest that any special precautions are required
Interferon beta-1b (Betaseron) injection	Transient flulike symptoms, anemia uncommon	No information to suggest that any special precautions are required
Natalizumab, ustekinumab, rituximab	Transient flulike symptoms, anemia uncommon, lymphoma	
Alternatives		
Glatiramer acetate (Copaxone) injection	Ulcerative stomatitis, lymphadenopathy, and salivary gland enlargement	No information to suggest that any special precautions are required
Mitoxantrone (Vovantrone) infusion	Leukopenia, risk for cardiac complications and leukemia, mucositis, and stomatitis	No information to suggest that any special precautions are required

Many complications of MS require management with several drugs. Spasticity is managed with antispastic drugs such as baclofen (a GABA agonist), benzodiazepines (GABA receptor activators), dantrolene (modifier of calcium release in muscle fibers), and tizanidine (Zanaflex) (an α_2-adrenergic agonist). An implantable pump for intrathecal administration of baclofen sometimes is used. Poor bladder control is managed with anticholinergics such as oxybutynin (Ditropan) or tolterodine tartrate (Detrol). Fatigue is managed with afternoon naps, exercise, and amantadine (Symmetrel) or modafinil. Paroxysmal events respond to carbamazepine, phenytoin, gabapentin, and pergolide. Serotonin reuptake inhibitors (e.g., fluoxetine [Prozac]) and tricyclic antidepressants are used to manage the depression that accompanies MS in about half the patients. Associated conditions (e.g., trigeminal neuralgia, headache, optic neuritis) often are managed by experts in chronic pain clinics.[57,67,74-76]

DENTAL MANAGEMENT

Medical Considerations

The dentist can play an important role in directing the patient with clinical findings suggestive of MS to the appropriate health care provider for definitive diagnosis. Reports of abnormal facial pain (mimicking trigeminal neuralgia), numbness of an extremity, visual disturbance, or muscle weakness require the dentist to perform a neuromuscular examination to rule out MS. The disease should be suspected if onset is progressive over several days, the patient is between 20 and 35 years of age, and afternoon fatigue is a feature. Referral to a neurologist is the next step in confirming the diagnosis.[56,60]

Patients experiencng a relapse are unfit to receive routine dental care. Emergency dental care can be provided but is affected by the medications these patients take. In particular, corticosteroids are immunosuppressive, and during stressful surgical procedures, an increase in dose may be required (see Chapter 15). The physician should be consulted before emergency dental care is provided to these patients.

The optimal time for treating patients with MS is during periods of remission. The dental care plan should take into consideration the potential effects on oral health of the medications used in management of MS. In particular, the anticholinergics (oxybutynin, tolterodine tartrate) and tricyclic antidepressants can cause a dry or burning mouth, which may require the use of salivary substitutes for relief.[77,78] If additional relief is needed, the use of pilocarpine (see Appendix C) should be discussed with the physician. Several of the medications used in the treatment of MS are immunosuppressants, thus placing patients at risk for opportunistic and community-acquired infections and for the development of cancers.[79]

Treatment Planning Modifications

Treatment planning changes are dictated by levels of motor impairment and fatigue. Patients with stable disease and little motor spasticity or weakness can receive routine dental care. Patients with more advanced disease may require help in transferring to and from the dental chair, may have difficulty maintaining oral hygiene, and may be poor candidates for reconstructive and prosthetic procedures. Because fatigue is often worse in the afternoon, short morning appointments are advised.

Oral Complications and Manifestations

Oral manifestations of MS are reported to occur in 2% to 3% of affected persons.[60,75,80] These features may serve as the presenting symptoms of MS. The most common features include dysarthria, paresthesia, numbness of the orofacial structures, and trigeminal neuralgia. Dysarthria produces slow, irregular speech with unusual separation of syllables of words, referred to as *scanning speech*. During an attack, the patient may experience facial paresthesia, and muscles of facial expression (especially the periorbital) can undulate in a wavelike motion. The term *myokymia* is used to describe these unusual muscle movements, which have been said to feel like a "bag of worms" on palpation. Referral to a physician is advised if the condition has not been diagnosed.[60,75,80]

Trigeminal neuralgia is 400 times more likely among persons with MS than among the general population. Relief of trigeminal neuralgia pain can be obtained with the use of carbamazepine, clonazepam, or amitriptyline or surgery.[60,75,76,80]

CEREBROSPINAL FLUID SHUNTS

Within the spectrum of neurologic disorders is the condition known as *hydrocephalus,* characterized by an increasing accumulation of CSF within the cerebral ventricles. Management of this condition often requires placement of a shunt within cerebral ventricles and peripheral cavities to reduce increased CSF pressure. Several types of shunts are used to reduce fluid pressure; ventriculoperitoneal, ventriculoatrial, and lumboperitoneal are the most common types.[81-84] In the United States, around 75,000 CSF shunts are placed each year.[81-84]

With respect to dentistry, the most significant concern is the risk of CSF shunt infection. Overall, shunt infection rates range from about 5% to 15%, with most infections resulting from wound contamination. Almost 70% of infections are caused by skin flora staphylococcal organisms.[1,83-86] CSF shunt infections usually occur within 2 months after implantation. The infection rate is higher for ventriculoperitoneal shunts than for ventriculoatrial shunts. However, other types of complications include thromboemboli, severe complications of infection, and shunt malfunctions.[1,83-86]

CSF shunts do not appear to increase the risk for infection produced by hematogenous seeding of bacteria after dental procedures. Thus, the American Heart Association has issued a statement indicating that antibiotic prophylaxis is not recommended for patients with CSF shunts who are undergoing dental procedures.[87]

REFERENCES

1. Drucker MH, et al: Thromboembolic implications of cerebrovascular shunts, *Surg Neurol* 22:444-448, 1984.
2. Lowenstein DH: Seizures and epilepsy. In Fauci AS, et al, editors: *Harrison's principles of internal medicine*, ed 17, New York, 2008, McGraw-Hill.
3. Spencer S: Seizures and epilepsy. In Goldman L, Ausiello D, editors: *Cecil textbook of medicine*, ed 23, Philadelphia, 2007, Saunders.
4. Sillanpaa M, Shinnar S: Long-term mortality in childhood-onset epilepsy, *N Engl J Med* 363:2522-2227, 2010.
5. Sperling MR, et al: Seizure control and mortality in epilepsy, *Ann Neurol* 46:45-50, 1999.
6. Dichter M, Brodie MJ: New antiepileptic drugs, *N Engl J Med* 334:1583-1589, 1996.
7. Greenwood RS: Adverse effects of antiepileptic drugs, *Epilepsia* 41(Suppl 2):S42-S52 , 2000.
8. Camfield C, Camfield P: Management guidelines for children with idiopathic generalized epilepsy, *Epilepsia* 46(Suppl 9): 112-116, 2005.
9. Ford PJ, Amazaki K, Seymour GJ: Cardiovascular and oral disease interactions: what is the evidence? *Prim Dent Care* 14:59-66, 2007.
10. Guerrini R: Epilepsy in children, *Lancet* 367:499-506, 2006.
11. Lewandowski L, Osmola K, Grodzki J: [Dyskinesias of the tongue and other face structures.] *Ann Acad Med Stetin* 52(Suppl 3):61-63, 2006.
12. Zivin J: Hemorrhagic cerebrovascular disease. In Goldman L, Ausiello D, editors: *Cecil textbook of medicine*, ed 23, Philadelphia, 2007, Elsevier.
13. Zivin J: Ischemic cerebrovascular disease. In Goldman L, Ausiello D, editors: *Cecil textbook of medicine*, ed 23, Philadelphia, 2007, Elsevier.
14. Feigin VL, et al: A review of population-based studies of incidince, prevalence, and case-fatality in the late 20th century, *Lancet Neurol* 2:43-53, 2003.
15. Caplan L: Cerebrovascular disease, *Med Clin North Am* 93:353-369, 2009.
16. Smith WS, Easton JD: Cerebrovascular diseases. In Fauci AS, et al, editors: *Harrison's principles of internal medicine*, ed 17, New York, 2008, McGraw-Hill.
17. American Heart Association: *Heart disease and stroke statistics, 2007 update* (website), http://www.americanheart.org/presenter.jhtml?identifier=2007; accessed on March 5, 2010.
18. Tonarelli SB, Hart RG: What's new in stroke? *J Am Geriatr Soc* 54:674-671, 2006.
19. Konecny P, Elfmark M, Urbanek K: Facial paresis after stroke and its impact on patients' facial movement and mental status, *J Rehabil Med* 43:73-75, 2011.
20. Fatahzadeh M, Glick M: Stroke: epidemiology, classification, risk factors, complications, diagnosis, prevention, and medical and dental management, *Oral Surg Oral Med Oral Pathol Oral Radiol Endod* 102:180-191, 2006.
21. Elad S, et al: A new management approach for dental treatment after a cerebrovascular event: a comparative retrospective study, *Oral Surg Oral Med Oral Pathol Oral Radiol Endod* 110:145-150, 2010.
22. Tissue plasminogen activator for acute ischemic stroke. The National Institute of Neurological Disorders and Stroke rt-PA Stroke Study Group, *N Engl J Med* 333:1581-1587, 1995.
23. Furlan A, et al: Intra-arterial prourokinase for acute ischemic stroke, *JAMA* 282:2003-2011, 1999.
24. Caplan L: Tissue plasminogen activator for acute ischemic stroke, *N Engl J Med* 341:1240-1241, 1999.
25. Albers GW, et al: Intravenous tissue-type plasminogen activator for treatment of acute stroke, *JAMA* 283:1145-1150, 2000.
26. Khaja A: Acute ischemic stroke management, *Neurol Clin North Am* 26:224-232, 2008.
27. Minassian C, et al: Invasive dental treatment and risk for vascular events: a self-controlled case series, *Ann Intern Med* 153:499-506, 2010.
28. Shobha N, Bhatia R, Barber PA: Dental procedures and stroke: a case of vertebral artery dissection, *J Can Dent Assoc* 76: a82, 2010.
29. Hacke W, et al: Association of outcome with early stroke treatment, *Lancet* 363:768-773, 2005.
30. Kumagai M, et al: Carotid artery calcification seen on panoramic dental radiographs in the Asian population in Japan, *Dentomaxillofac Radiol* 36:92-96, 2007.
31. Mupparapu M, Kim IH: Calcified carotid artery atheroma and stroke: a systematic review, *J Am Dent Assoc* 138:483-492, 2007.
32. Ramesh A, Pabla T: Panoramic radiographs: a screening tool for calcified carotid atheromatous plaque, *J Mass Dent Soc* 56:20-21, 2007.
33. Friedlander AH: Calcified carotid artery atheromas, *J Am Dent Assoc* 138:1191-1192, 2007.
34. Masood F, et al: Presence of carotid artery calcification on panoramic radiographs of patients with chronic diseases, *Gen Dent* 57:39-44, 2009.
35. Lang A: Parkinson's disease. In Goldman L, Ausiello D, editors: *Cecil textbook of medicine*, ed 23, Philadelphia, 2007, Elsevier.
36. Friedlander AH, et al: Parkinson disease: systemic and orofacial manifestations, medical and dental management, *J Am Dent Assoc* 140:658-669, 2009.
37. Hawkes CH, Del Tredici K, Braak H: A timeline for Parkinson's disease, *Parkinsonism Relat Disord* 16: 79-84, 2010.
38. Ravina B, et al: Diagnostic criteria for psychosis in Parkinson's disease: report of an NINDS, NIMH work group, *Mov Disord* 22:1061-1068, 2007.
39. Yokota O, et al: Lewy body variant of Alzheimer's disease or cerebral type Lewy body disease? Two autopsy cases of presenile onset with minimal involvement of the brainstem, *Neuropathology* 27:21-35, 2007.
40. Ravina B, et al: A longitudinal program for biomarker development in Parkinson's disease: a feasibility study, *Mov Disord* 24:2081-2090, 2009.
41. Ravina B, et al: The course of depressive symptoms in early Parkinson's disease, *Mov Disord* 24:1306-1311, 2009.
42. Knopman DS: Alzheimer's disease and other dementias. In Goldman L, Ausiello D, editors: *Cecil textbook of medicine*, ed 23, Philadelphia, 2007, Elsevier.
43. Katsoulis J, Huber S, Mericske-Stern R: [Gerodontology consultation in geriatric facilities: general health status (I).], *Schweiz Monatsschr Zahnmed* 119:12-18, 2009.
44. Ravina B, et al: The impact of depressive symptoms in early Parkinson disease, *Neurology* 69:342-347, 2007.
45. Hallet M, Litvan I: Evaluation of surgery for Parkinson's disease, *Neurol Res* 53:1910-1921, 1999.
46. Kordower JH, et al: Neurogeneration prevented by lentiviral vector, *Science* 290:767-772, 2000.

47. Yoshida H, et al: An autopsy case of Creutzfeldt-Jakob disease with a V180I mutation of the PrP gene and Alzheimer-type pathology, *Neuropathology* 30:159-164, 2010.
48. Hu Z, et al: Inflammation: a bridge between postoperative cognitive dysfunction and Alzheimer's disease, *Med Hypotheses* 74:722-724, 2010.
49. Levin EC, et al: Neuronal expression of vimentin in the Alzheimer's disease brain may be part of a generalized dendritic damage-response mechanism, *Brain Res* 1298:194-207, 2009.
50. Henry RG, Smith BJ: Managing older patients who have neurologic disease: Alzheimer disease and cerebrovascular accident, *Dent Clin North Am* 53:269-294, ix, 2009.
51. Wilkinson DG, et al: Cholinesterase inhibitors used in the treatment of Alzheimer's disease: the relationship between pharmacological effects and clinical efficacy, *Drugs Aging* 21:453-459, 2004.
52. Doody RS, et al: Practice parameter: management of dementia (an evidence-based review). Report of the Quality Standards Subcommittee of the American Academy of Neurology, *Neurology* 56:1154-1166, 2001.
53. Kamer AR, et al: Alzheimer's disease and peripheral infections: the possible contribution from periodontal infections, model and hypothesis, *J Alzheimers Dis* 13:437-449, 2008.
54. Sacco D, Frost DE: Dental management of patients with stroke or Alzheimer's disease, *Dent Clin North Am* 50:625-633, viii, 2006.
55. Rejnefelt I, Andersson P, Renvert S: Oral health status in individuals with dementia living in special facilities, *Int J Dent Hyg* 4:67-71, 2006.
56. Calabresi P: Multiple sclerosis and demyelinating conditions of the CNS. In Goldman L, Ausiello D, editors: *Cecil textbook of medicine*, ed 23,Philadelphia, 2007, Elsevier.
57. Bermel RA, Cohen JA: Multiple sclerosis: advances in understanding pathogenesis and emergence of oral treatment options, *Lancet Neurol* 10:4-5, 2011.
58. Sloka S, et al: A quantitative analysis of suspected environmental causes of MS, *Can J Neurol Sci* 38:98-105, 2011.
59. Prat A: Special issue on molecular basis of multiple sclerosis, *Biochim Biophys Acta* 1812:131, 2011.
60. Bähr M: Special issue on multiple sclerosis, *Exp Neurol* 225:1, 2010.
61. Sormani M, et al: Magnetic resonance imaging as surrogate for clinical endpoints in multiple sclerosis: data on novel oral drugs, *Mult Scler* 17:630-633, 2011.
62. Sastre-Garriga J, et al: A functional magnetic resonance proof of concept pilot trial of cognitive rehabilitation in multiple sclerosis, *Mult Scler* 17:457-467, 2011.
63. Popova NF, et al: [Omaron in the complex treatment of patients with multiple sclerosis.] *Zh Nevrol Psikhiatr Im S S Korsakova* 110:17-20, 2010.
64. Oliver BJ, Kohli E, Kasper LH: Interferon therapy in relapsing-remitting multiple sclerosis: a systematic review and meta-analysis of the comparative trials, *J Neurol Sci* 302:96-105, 2011.
65. Oliver B, et al: Kinetics and incidence of anti-natalizumab antibodies in multiple sclerosis patients on treatment for 18 months, *Mult Scler* 17:368-371, 2011.
66. Yeh EA, Weinstock-Guttman B: Natalizumab in pediatric multiple sclerosis patients, *Ther Adv Neurol Disord* 3:293-299, 2010.
67. Kieseier BC, Jeffery DR: Chemotherapeutics in the treatment of multiple sclerosis, *Ther Adv Neurol Disord* 3:277-291, 2010.
68. Scherl EJ, Kumar S, Warren RU: Review of the safety and efficacy of ustekinumab, *Therap Adv Gastroenterol* 3: 321-328, 2010.
69. Taupin P: Antibodies against CD20 (rituximab) for treating multiple sclerosis: US20100233121, *Expert Opin Ther Pat* 21:111-114, 2011.
70. Giovanni G, et al: A placebo-controlled clinical trial of cladribine for relapsing multiple sclerosis, *N Engl J Med* 362: 416-422, 2010.
71. Wang J, et al: Statins for multiple sclerosis, *Cochrane Database Syst Rev* 12:CD008386, 2010.
72. Neau JP, et al: [Vitamin D and multiple sclerosis. A prospective survey of patients of Poitou-Charentes area.] *Rev Neurol (Paris)* 167:317-323, 2011.
73. Smolders J: Vitamin D and multiple sclerosis: correlation, causality, and controversy, *Autoimmune Dis* 2011:629538, 2010.
74. Haacke EM: Chronic cerebral spinal venous insufficiency in multiple sclerosis, *Expert Rev Neurother* 11:5-9, 2011.
75. Mollaoğlu M, Fertelli TK, Tuncay FÖ: Disability in elderly patients with chronic neurological illness: stroke, multiple sclerosis and epilepsy, *Arch Gerontol Geriatr* 53:e227-e231, 2011.
76. Grau-López L, et al: [Analysis of the pain in multiple sclerosis patients.] *Neurologia* 26:208-213, 2011.
77. Danhauer SC, et al: Impact of criteria-based diagnosis of burning mouth syndrome on treatment outcome, *J Orofac Pain* 16:305-311, 2002.
78. Rhodus NL, Carlson CR, Miller CS: Burning mouth (syndrome) disorder, *Quintessence Int* 34:587-593, 2003.
79. Berger JR, Houff S: Drugs for the treatment of multiple sclerosis, *Ann Neurol* 64:367-377, 2009.
80. Marchiondo K: Multiple sclerosis, *Medsurg Nurs* 19:303-304, 2010.
81. Walker ML: Shunt survival, *J Neurosurg Pediatr* 6:526, 2010.
82. Paulsen AH, Lundar T, Lindegaard KF: Twenty-year outcome in young adults with childhood hydrocephalus: assessment of surgical outcome, work participation, and health-related quality of life, *J Neurosurg Pediatr* 6:527-535, 2010.
83. Lundkvist B, et al: Cerebrospinal fluid dynamics and long-term survival of the Strata((R)) valve in idiopathic normal pressure hydrocephalus, *Acta Neurol Scand* 124:115-121, 2011.
84. Chern JJ, et al: Effectiveness of a clinical pathway for patients with cerebrospinal fluid shunt malfunction, *J Neurosurg Pediatr* 6:318-324, 2010.
85. Aoki N: Lumboperitoneal shunt: clinical implications, complications, and comparison with ventriculoperitoneal shunt, *Neurosurgery* 26:998-1003, 1990.
86. Gardner P, Leipzig TJ, Sadigh M: Infections of cerebrovascular shunts, *Curr Clin Top Infect Dis* 9:185-189, 1989.
87. Baddour LM, et al: Nonvalvular cardiovascular device related infections, *Circulation* 108:2015-2023, 2003.
88. Albert MS, et al: The diagnosis of mild cognitive impairment due to Alzheimer's disease: recommendations from the National Institute on Aging and Alzheimer's Association workgroups on diagnostic guidelines for Alzheimer's disease, *Alzheimers Dement* 7:270-279, 2011.

CHAPTER

28

Anxiety, Eating Disorders, and Behavioral Reactions to Illness

Problems may be encountered in the dental practice that stem from a patient's behavioral patterns, rather than from physical conditions. A good dentist-patient relationship can reduce the number of behavioral problems encountered in practice and can modify the intensity of emotional reactions. A positive dentist-patient relationship is based on mutual respect, trust, understanding, cooperation, and empathy. Role conflicts between the dentist and the patient should be avoided or should be identified and dealt with effectively. The anxious patient should be offered support that minimizes the damaging effects of anxiety, and the angry or uncooperative patient should be accepted and encouraged to share reasons for feelings and behavior, allowing emergence of a more peaceful and cooperative state of mind. Patients with emotional factors that contribute to oral or systemic diseases or symptoms and patients with more serious mental disorders can be managed in an understanding, safe, and empathetic manner.

The dentist may treat patients with a variety of behavioral and mental disorders. The fourth edition of *Diagnostic and Statistical Manual of Mental Disorders*, text revision (DSM-IV-TR),[1] presents a classification system with which the dentist should be familiar to be better able to understand psychiatric diagnoses and associated symptoms. This system consists of five axes (axis I through axis V), or categories, used to describe mental disorders. Table 28-1 lists the five specific areas used to evaluate the psychosocial health of the patient. Box 28-1 lists the clinical conditions encountered in an axis I disorder.[1]

The American Psychiatric Association plans to publish the new edition of the *Diagnostic and Statistical Manual of Mental Disorders* (i.e., DSM-5) in 2013.[2] Thirteen work groups began meeting in late 2007. The progress of these efforts can be followed at the Web site http://www.dsm5.org/ProgressReports/pages/default.aspx.

This chapter discusses anxiety disorders (panic, phobias, posttraumatic stress disorder, and generalized anxiety disorder), eating disorders, and behavioral reactions to illness (Box 28-2). Adverse reactions and drug interactions associated with drugs used to treat anxiety states are covered, with an emphasis on the dental implications of these reactions. The dental management of the patient with anxiety and eating disorders is covered in detail. Chapter 29 is devoted to mood disorders (depression and bipolar disorders), somatoform disorders (conversion, hypochondriasis, pain, somatization), and schizophrenia. Dementia is discussed in Chapter 27 and substance abuse in Chapter 30. A dental practice of 2000 adults can be expected to include more than 200 patients with a behavioral or psychiatric disorder.

ANXIETY DISORDERS

DEFINITION

Anxiety is a natural response and a necessary warning adapatation in humans. Anxiety becomes a pathologic disorder when it is excessive and uncontrollable, requires no specific external stimulus, and results in physical and affective symptoms and changes in behavior and cognition.[3] Anxiety disorders occur in two patterns: (1) chronic, generalized anxiety and (2) episodic, panic-like anxiety.[4] Several related psychiatric disorders often coexist with anxiety disorders, including posttraumatic stress disorder, substance abuse, and depression.[4]

Anxiety is a sense of psychological distress that may not have a focus. It is a state of apprehension that may involve an internal psychological conflict, an environmental stress, a physical disease state, or a medicine or drug effect, or combinations of these. Anxiety can be a purely psychological experience, with few somatic manifestations. Alternatively, it can be experienced as a purely physical phenomenon encompassing tachycardia, palpitations, chest pain, indigestion, headaches, and so forth, with no psychological distress other than concern about the physical symptoms. The reason for the variability in physical responses is not clear.[3-6]

An understanding of anxiety requires definitions of some related entities, phobia and panic attack. A *phobia* is defined as an irrational fear that interferes with normal behavior. Phobias are fears of specific objects, situations,

TABLE 28-1 System for Classification of Psychosocial Health

Type	Description
Axis I	Clinical disorders Other conditions that may be the focus of clinical attention
Axis II	Personality disorders Mental retardation
Axis III	General medical conditions
Axis IV	Psychosocial and environmental problems
Axis V	Global assessment of functioning

From American Psychiatric Association: Diagnostic and statistical manual of mental disorders, *fourth ed, text rev, Washington, DC, American Psychiatric Association, 2000.*

BOX 28-1 Axis I: Clinical Disorders and Other Conditions That May Be a Focus of Clinical Attention

- Disorders usually first diagnosed in infancy, childhood, or adolescence (excluding Mental Retardation, which is diagnosed on Axis II)
- Delirium, dementia, and amnestic and other cognitive disorders
- Mental disorders due to a general medical condition
- Substance-related disorders
- Schizophrenia and other psychotic disorders
- Mood disorders
- Anxiety disorders
- Somatoform disorders
- Factitious disorders
- Dissociative disorders
- Sexual and gender identity disorders
- Eating disorders
- Sleep disorders
- Impulse control disorders not elsewhere classified
- Adjustment disorders
- Other conditions that may be a focus of clinical attention

From American Psychiatric Association: *Diagnostic and statistical manual of mental disorders,* fourth ed, text rev, Washington, DC, American Psychiatric Association, 2000.

or experiences. The feared object, situation, or experience has taken on a symbolic meaning for the patient. Unconscious wishes and fears have been displaced from an original goal onto an external object.[7]

A *panic attack* consists of a sudden, unexpected, overwhelming feeling of terror with symptoms of dyspnea, palpitations, dizziness, faintness, trembling, sweating, choking, flushes or chills, numbness or tingling sensations, and chest pains. The panic attack peaks in about 10 minutes and usually lasts for about 20 to 30 minutes.[7] A person who has repeated panic attacks is described as having a panic disorder.

Epidemiology: Incidence and Prevalence

Anxiety disorders constitute the most frequently found psychiatric problem in the general population. Simple phobia is the most common of the anxiety disorders (up to 25% of the population will experience a phobia); however, panic disorder is the most common anxiety disorder in people who seek medical treatment (lifetime prevalence of 3.5%).[3] Generalized anxiety disorder has a lifetime prevalence of 5% to 6%.[6] Posttraumatic stress disorder (PTSD) has a lifetime prevalence of 5% to 10%, with a point prevalence of 3% to 4%.[8,9] Panic disorder, phobic disorders, and obsessive-compulsive disorders occur more frequently among first-degree relatives of people with these disorders than in the general population.[3,4]

Etiology

Anxiety represents a threatened emergence into consciousness of painful, unacceptable thoughts, impulses, or desires (anxiety may result from psychological conflicts of the past and present). These psychological conflicts or feelings stimulate physiologic changes that lead to clinical manifestations of anxiety.[5,7] Anxiety disorders may occur in persons who are under emotional stress, in those with certain systemic illnesses, or as a component of various psychiatric disorders. Panic disorders tend to occur in families: First-degree relatives of a person with a panic disorder have about an 18% increased risk for development of a similar disorder.[5,7]

The cause of panic disorder is unknown but appears to involve a genetic predisposition, altered autonomic responsivity, and social learning. Panic disorder shows a familial aggregation; the disorder is concordant in 30% to 45% of monozygotic twins, and genome-wide screens have identified suggestive risk loci on 1q, 7p15, 10q, 11p, and 13q. Acute panic attacks appear to be associated with increased noradrenergic discharges in the locus coeruleus.[9]

No single theory fully explains all anxiety disorders. No single biologic or psychological cause of anxiety has been identified. Psychosocial and biologic processes together may best explain anxiety. The locus coeruleus, a brain stem structure that contains most of the noradrenergic neurons in the central nervous system (CNS), appears to be involved in panic attacks and anxiety. Panic and anxiety may be correlated with dysregulated firing of the locus coeruleus caused by input from multiple sources, including peripheral autonomic afferents, medullary afferents, and serotonergic fibers.[4-6]

Anxiety states also may be associated with organic diseases, other psychiatric disorders, use of certain drugs, hyperthyroidism, and mitral valve prolapse. Anxiety also is associated with mood disorders, schizophrenia, or personality disorders.[3,4,6]

BOX 28-2 Classification of Behavioral and Psychiatric Disorders

Anxiety Disorders
Specifics
- Panic disorders
- Agoraphobia
- Phobias
- Obsessive-compulsive disorder*
- Posttraumatic stress disorder
- Acute stress disorder
- Generalized anxiety disorder
- Anxiety disorder due to a general medical condition*
- Substance-induced anxiety disorder*

Mood Disorders
Specifics
- Depressive disorders
- Major depression
- Dysthymic disorder
- Depression not otherwise specified
- Bipolar disorders
- Bipolar I—manic, mixed, depressed
- Bipolar II—hypomanic, depressed
- Cyclothymic disorder
- Bipolar not otherwise specified

Somatoform Disorders
Specifics
- Body dysmorphic disorder*
- Conversion disorder
- Hypochondriasis
- Somatization disorder
- Pain disorder

Factitious Disorders
Specifics
- Predominantly psychological signs and symptoms
- Predominantly physical signs and symptoms
- Combined psychological and physical signs and symptoms

Psychological Factors That Affect Medical Conditions*
Specifics
- Mental disorder affecting medical condition*
- Stress-related physiologic response affecting medical condition*

Substance Abuse Disorders*
Specifics
- Alcohol and other sedatives (barbiturates, benzodiazepines, others)*
- Opiates*
- Stimulants (amphetamine, cocaine)*
- Cannabis*
- Hallucinogens (lysergic acid diethylamide [LSD], phencyclidine [PCP])*
- Nicotine*
- Others (steroids; inhalants such as paint, glue, and gasoline)*

Cognitive Disorders*
Specifics
- Delirium*
- Dementia*
  - Primary (Alzheimer's type)*
  - Vascular*
  - Human immunodeficiency virus (HIV) infection–related (AIDS dementia)*
- Parkinson's disease*
- Amnestic disorder*

Schizophrenia
Specifics
- Catatonic type
- Disorganized type
- Paranoid type
- Undifferentiated type

Delusional (Paranoid) Disorder*
- Erotomania, grandiosity, jealousy, persecution complex, somatic delusions*

*Conditions not covered in this chapter or in Chapter 29.
Data from American Psychiatric Association: Diagnostic and statistical manual of mental disorders, *fourth ed, text rev, Washington, DC, American Psychiatric Association, 2000.*

CLINICAL PRESENTATION AND MEDICAL MANAGEMENT

From a psychological perspective, *anxiety* can be defined as emotional pain or a feeling that all is not well—a feeling of impending disaster. The source of the problem usually is not apparent to persons with anxiety. The feeling is the same in anxious patients as that in patients with fear, but the latter are aware of what the problem is and why they are "fearful."[10]

Physiologic reactions to anxiety and to fear are the same and are mediated through the autonomic nervous system. Sympathetic and parasympathetic components may be involved. Signs and symptoms of anxiety caused by overactivation of the *sympathetic* nervous system include increased heart rate, sweating, dilated pupils, and muscle tension. Signs and symptoms of anxiety resulting from stimulation of the *parasympathetic* system include urinary frequency and episodic diarrhea.[3,4,6]

Most people periodically experience some degree of anxiety in one or more aspects of their lives. Anxiety can be a strong motivator; low levels of anxiety can increase attention and improve performance. Anxiety leads to dysfunction when it is constant, or it may result in episodes of extreme vigilance, excessive motor tension, autonomic hyperactivity, and impaired concentration. Anxiety is part of the clinical picture in many patients with psychiatric disorders. Patients with mood disorders, dementia, psychosis, panic disorder, adjustment disorders, and toxic and withdrawal states often report feelings of anxiety.[3,4,6,11,12]

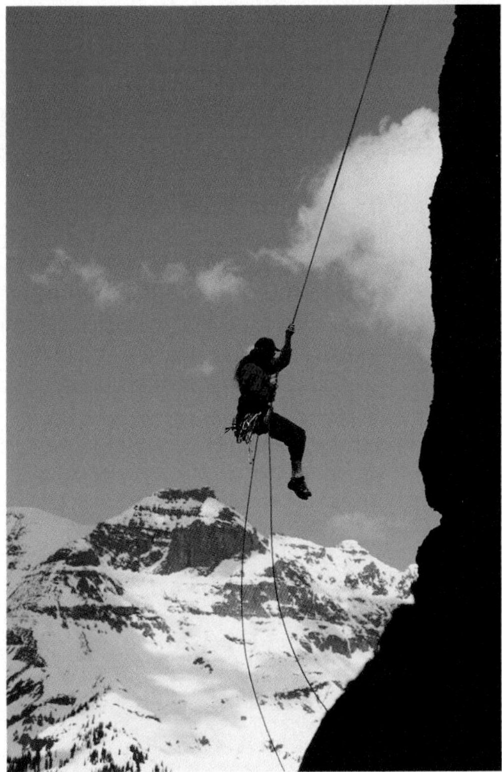

FIGURE 28-1 A specific phobia is acrophobia, the fear of heights.

Phobias

Phobias consist of three major groups: agoraphobia, social, and simple. Agoraphobia is a fear of having distressful or embarrassing symptoms on leaving home. It often accompanies panic disorder. Social phobias may be specific, such as fear of public speaking, or general, such as fear of being embarrassed when with people. Simple phobias include fear of snakes, heights (Figure 28-1), flying, darkness, and needles. The two phobias that may affect medical or dental care are needle phobia and claustrophobia, the latter during magnetic resonance imaging (MRI) or radiation therapy.[5] Dental "phobia" is associated with more extreme anxiety than the "usual" level attending a visit to the dentist.[13] Previous frightening dental experiences are cited as the major cause. Patients may specifically fear the noise and vibration of the drill, the sight of the injection needle, and the act of sitting in the dental chair, and they may experience muscle tension, fast heart rate, accelerated breathing, sweating, and/or stomach cramps. True phobic neurosis about dental treatment is rare.[13]

Panic Attack

About 15% of patients who are seen by cardiologists come to the doctor because of symptoms associated with a panic attack. Onset usually is between late adolescence and the mid-30s, but it may occur at any age. A key feature of panic is the adrenergic surge, which results in the fight-or-flight response. This response is an exaggerated sympathetic response (Table 28-2). Panic attacks may be cued or uncued. An example of a cued attack is that occurring in a person who is fearful of flying. Many patients report that they are unaware of any life stressors preceding the onset of panic disorder; such attacks are classified as uncued. The major complication of repeated panic attacks is a restricted lifestyle adopted to avoid situations that might trigger an attack. Some patients develop agoraphobia, an irrational fear of being alone in public places, which can cause them to be housebound for years. Sudden loss of social supports or disruption of important interpersonal relationships appears to predispose the affected person to development of panic disorder.[4,7,9]

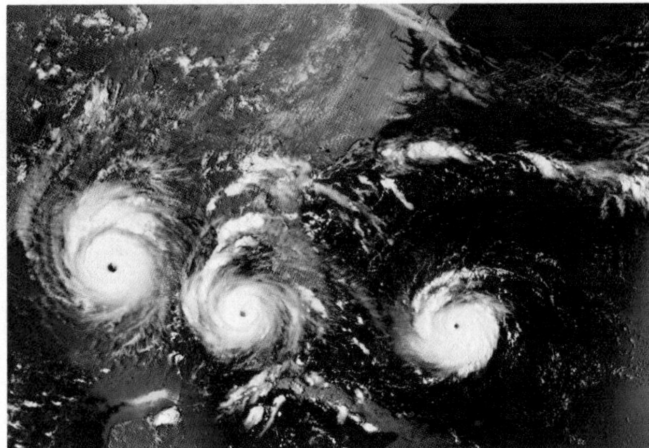

FIGURE 28-2 Time lapse photo of Hurricane Andrew, which hit southern Florida in August 1992. During past years, a number of major hurricanes hit the United States. Hurricane Katrina, which hit the Gulf Coast states in August 2005, was the most destructive in recent history in terms of number of deaths and extent of property damage.

Generalized Anxiety Disorder

Some patients present with a persistent, diffuse form of anxiety characterized by signs and symptoms of motor tension, autonomic hyperactivity, and apprehension (see Table 28-2). No familial or genetic basis for this *generalized anxiety disorder* has been found. Outcomes typically are better than those with panic disorder; however, the persistent anxiety may lead to depression and substance abuse.[4,6,7,9]

Posttraumatic Stress Disorder

Posttraumatic stress disorder (PTSD) is a syndrome of psychophysiologic signs and symptoms that develop after exposure to a traumatic event outside the usual range of human experience, such as combat exposure, a holocaust experience, rape, or a civilian disaster such as a hurricane (Figure 28-2) or eruption of a volcano

TABLE 28-2 Anxiety, Panic Attack, Generalized Anxiety Disorder, and Posttraumatic Stress Disorder

Anxiety Disorder	Signs/Symptoms	Major Diagnostic Criteria
Anxiety	Motor tension • Trembling, twitching, or feeling shaky • Muscle tension, aches, or soreness • Restlessness • Easy fatigability Autonomic hyperactivity • Shortness of breath or smothering sensations • Palpitations or accelerated heart rate (tachycardia) • Sweating or cold, sweaty hands • Dry mouth • Dizziness or lightheadedness • Nausea, diarrhea, or other manifestation of abdominal distress • Flashes (hot flashes) or chills • Frequent urination • Trouble swallowing or "lump in throat" Vigilance and scanning • Feeling "keyed up" or on edge • Exaggerated startle response • Difficulty concentrating, or episodes in which the patient's "mind goes blank" • Trouble falling or staying asleep • Irritability	Some of the signs and symptoms of anxiety may be noted in persons who are under the daily stresses of life. This form of anxiety can be helpful in the sense of focusing necessary attention on a specific task, such as a school examination, driver's test, or athletic event. Anxiety becomes a negative factor when signs and symptoms are present for longer periods and start having an effect on the person's emotional and physical well-being.
Panic disorder	Sudden onset of intense fear, arousal, and cardiac and/or respiratory symptoms without provocation (panic attack); often confused with systemic medical illness such as angina pectoris or epilepsy Symptoms of anxiety listed above Fear of dying Fear of "going crazy" or doing something uncontrolled	One or more panic attacks have occurred that were unexpected and were not triggered by situations in which the person was the focus of another's attention. Either four attacks have occurred within a 4-week period, or one or more attacks have been followed by a period of at least 1 month of persistent fear of having another attack.
Generalized anxiety disorder	At least six of the symptoms of anxiety listed above must be present over a period of 6 months or longer.	Presence of unrealistic or excessive worry and apprehension about two or more life circumstances, for a period of 6 months or longer, during which the person has been bothered more days than not by these concerns
Posttraumatic stress disorder (PTSD)	Symptoms of PTSD arise only after an exceptionally threatening event that is outside the normal range of experience (e.g., combat, rape, attempted murder or torture, acts of terrorism, natural disasters): • Marked irritability • Hyperarousal • Hypervigilance • Insomnia • Secondary drug and alcohol abuse is common.	Repeated reliving of trauma as daydreams, intrusive memories, flashbacks, or nightmares Persistent psychic numbness or "emotional bloating" Avoidance of thoughts about or reminders of the trauma, which may lead to marked detachment from personal involvement or relationships Symbols, anniversaries, or similar events often prompt exacerbation of symptoms.

Data from Schiffer RB: Psychiatric disorders in medical practice. In Goldman L, Ausiello D, editors: *Cecil textbook of medicine,* ed 23, Philadelphia, Saunders, 2008; and Lucey JV, Corvin A: Anxiety disorders. In Wright P, Stern J, Phelan M, editors: *Core psychiatry,* ed 2, Edinburgh, Elsevier, 2005.

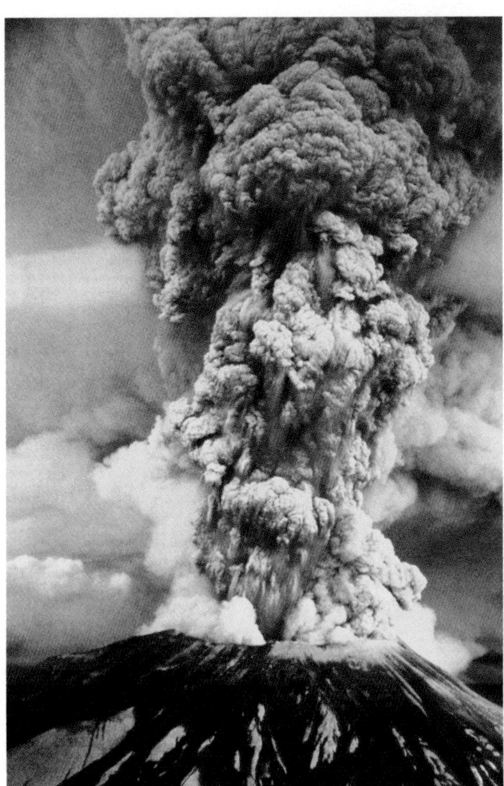

FIGURE 28-3 The 1980 eruption of Mount St. Helens resulted in an increased incidence of posttraumatic stress disorder among residents of the Pacific Northwest.

(Figure 28-3). The traumatic event may represent a serious threat to the person's life or physical integrity; a serious threat to children, spouse, or other loved ones; or sudden destruction of home or community; alternatively, it may result when the person views an accident or an act of physical violence that seriously injures or kills another person(s).[3,4,6,7,9] Other experiences that have resulted in PTSD or are associated with increased risk for the disorder include child abuse,[14] weaning from mechanical ventilation,[15] traumatic experience of myocardial infarction,[16] and loss of a close relative or loved one to cancer.[17]

Most men with PTSD have been in combat (Figure 28-4), and most women give a history of sexual or physical abuse. The three cardinal features of PTSD are hyperarousal; intrusive symptoms, or flashbacks to the initial trauma; and psychic numbing.[3,4,6,7,9] PTSD may follow traumatic or violent events that are anticipated or not anticipated, constant or repetitive, natural or malevolent. For this reason, terrorist attacks often lead to PTSD[18-24] (Figures 28-5 and 28-6). PTSD is further defined by onset of symptoms at least 6 months after the trauma, or duration of more than 3 months (see Table 28-2).

Diagnostic criteria for PTSD consist of a history of a traumatic experience and reexperiencing of the event through intrusive memories, disturbing dreams, "flashbacks," and psychological or physical distress in response to reminders of the event; another criterion is avoidance of things associated with the trauma (see Table 28-2). Signs and symptoms include sleep problems, irritability, trouble concentrating, hypervigilance, startle

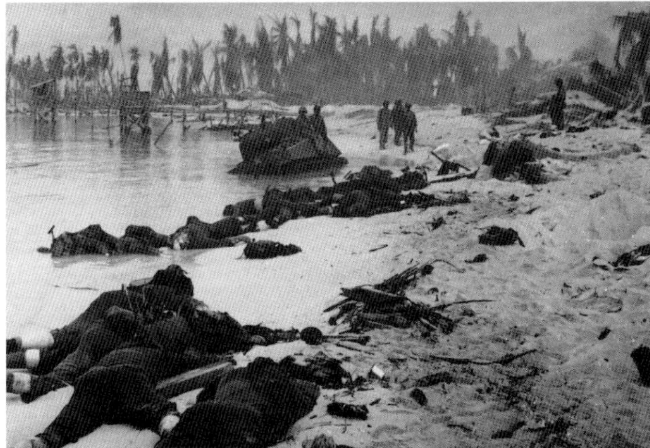

FIGURE 28-4 Combat during World War II on the island of Tarawa.

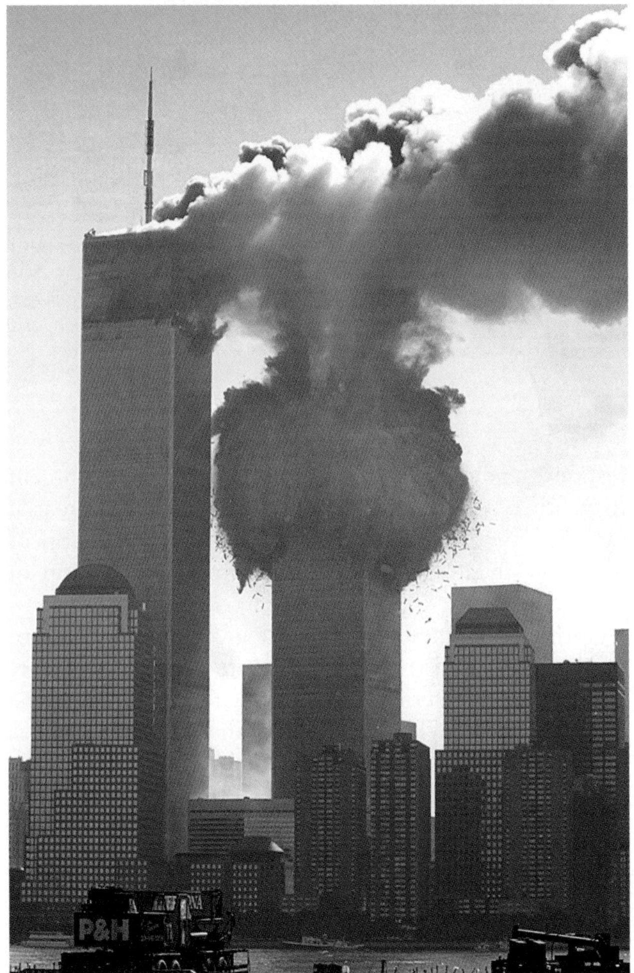

FIGURE 28-5 Attack on the Twin Towers of the World Trade Center in New York City on September 11, 2001. *(Courtesy Getty Images.)*

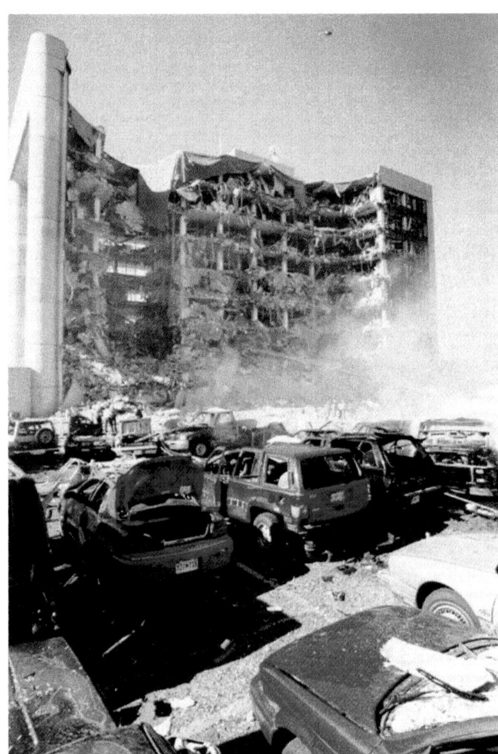

FIGURE 28-6 The 1995 bombing of the Alfred P. Murrah Federal Building in Oklahoma City, Oklahoma, resulted in a greater than 33% incidence of posttraumatic stress disorder among survivors. *(Courtesy NASA Ames Research Center, Disaster Assistance and Rescue Team, Mountain View, California.)*

responses, and psychic numbing, seen as detachment from others, reduced capacity for intimacy, and decreased interest in sex.[3-6,7,9] Avoidance and numbing appear to be the most specific symptoms for identification of PTSD.[25]

Although women generally are given the diagnosis of PTSD more often than men, the rate of PTSD is higher among male veterans than among female veterans; however, some evidence suggests that the condition is underdiagnosed in female veterans.[21] Pereira[21] found that (1) men experienced higher levels of combat stress, (2) greater exposure to stress was associated with increased symptoms of PTSD, (3) men and women exposed to similar levels of stress were equally likely to experience PTSD symptoms, and (4) men were more likely to be given the diagnosis of PTSD. Unit cohesion may protect from PTSD regardless of the level of stress exposure.[24] Drug treatment of men and persons with combat trauma–induced PTSD (men and women) is less effective than that provided to other veteran women or women with civilian trauma–induced PTSD.[20]

Acute Stress Disorder

Acute stress disorder is a more recent addition to the DSM-IV category of anxiety disorder. This disorder also develops after exposure of the patient to a traumatic event, and specific signs and symptoms resemble those of PTSD. In acute stress disorder, however, symptoms are of shorter duration and emerge more rapidly after the trauma. The symptomatic reaction is limited to the period during which the stressful event is occurring and its immediate aftermath.[6,7]

Treatment of Anxiety Disorders

Psychological, behavioral, and drug modalities are used to treat anxiety disorders. Psychological treatment involves psychotherapy, which, in general, is used in more severe cases. Behavioral treatment includes cognitive approaches (anxiety management, relaxation, and cognitive restructuring), biofeedback, hypnosis, relaxation imaging, desensitization, and flooding. Drug treatment includes the use of tricyclic antidepressants, selective serotonin reuptake inhibitors (SSRIs), monoamine oxidase inhibitors (MAOIs), benzodiazepines, antihistamines, β-adrenergic receptor antagonists, and sedative-hypnotics.[23] The most commonly used drugs are the benzodiazepines and the SSRI buspirone, or a combination of medications (Table 28-3). Most patients benefit maximally from a combination of therapies such as cognitive therapy plus medication.[3,4,6,7]

Systemic desensitization (whereby the patient is gradually exposed to the feared situation) and flooding (by which the patient is exposed directly to the anxiety-provoking stimulus) are techniques used in the treatment of phobias. Claustrophobia associated with MRI can be managed with a low dose of benzodiazepines and behavioral therapy.[5,18,19]

First-line treatment for PTSD consists of psychotherapy (exposure therapy, group therapy, patient and family education), cognitive-behavioral therapy, and eye movement desensitization and reprocessing (EMDR).[22] EMDR is a newer, relatively novel treatment in which the patient focuses on movements of the clinician's finger while maintaining a mental image of the traumatic experience.[22]

Second-line treatment consists of a combination of psychotherapy and pharmacologic therapy.[22] In cases with comorbid psychiatric disorders or with especially severe symptoms of PTSD, a combination of psychotherapy and pharmacologic treatment is recommended as the first line of treatment. The U.S. Food and Drug Administration (FDA) has approved the SSRIs paroxetine and sertraline for the treatment of PTSD. Bupropion or other antidepressants are used when depression is a component of the clinical picture.

Benzodiazepines are used when anxiety is part of the symptom complex. Early intervention in patients with PTSD can shorten the duration and severity of anxiety.[22] In some complex and treatment-resistant cases, mood stabilizers such as valproate or carbamazepine are indicated.[22]

TABLE 28-3 Drugs Used to Treat Patients with Anxiety and Panic Attacks

Drug Class	Drug	Trade Name	Comments
Sedative-hypnotics	Chloral hydrate	Noctel	Seldom appropriate
	Meprobamate	Miltown	Seldom appropriate
Antihistamines	Hydroxyzine	Atarax	Most useful at bedtime for associated sleep
	Diphenhydramine	Benadryl	Most useful at bedtime for associated sleep
Benzodiazepines	Lorazepam	Ativan	Also effective for generalized anxiety
	Diazepam	Valium	
	Triazolam	Halcion	Abuse potential with many of the benzodiazepines!
	Chlordiazepoxide	Librium	
	Temazepam	Restoril	
	Alprazolam	Xanax	
	Clorazepate	Tranxene	
	Flurazepam	Dalmane	Higher risk of abuse potential with flurazepam
	Oxazepam	Serax	
	Clonazepam	Klonopin	Long duration of action permits once-daily dosing
	Buspirone	Buspar	No dependence with prolonged use
	Zolpidem	Ambien	Most useful on an as-needed basis
Beta blockers	Propranolol	Inderal	Does not block the fear component of anxiety or panic

Data from Schiffer RB: Psychiatric disorders in medical practice. In Goldman L, Ausiello D, editors: Cecil textbook of medicine, *ed 23, Philadelphia, Saunders, 2008, p 2633.*

EATING DISORDERS

DEFINITION

The two major eating disorders are anorexia nervosa and bulimia nervosa (Table 28-4). *Anorexia nervosa* is characterized by severe restriction of food intake, leading to weight loss and the medical sequelae of starvation (Figure 28-7). *Bulimia nervosa* is characterized by attempts to restrict food intake, but in a different form from that seen in anorexia nervosa. In bulimia, attempts at restriction are interspersed with binge eating followed by various methods of trying to rid the body of food. These include induced vomiting (often by means of a finger in the throat or with syrup of ipecac), laxatives, and diuretics.[26-28]

Binge eating disorder (BED) is a more recently described syndrome characterized by repeated episodes of binge eating, similar to those of bulimia nervosa, in the absence of inappropriate compensatory behavior. Patients with BED typically are middle-aged men or women with significant obesity.[29]

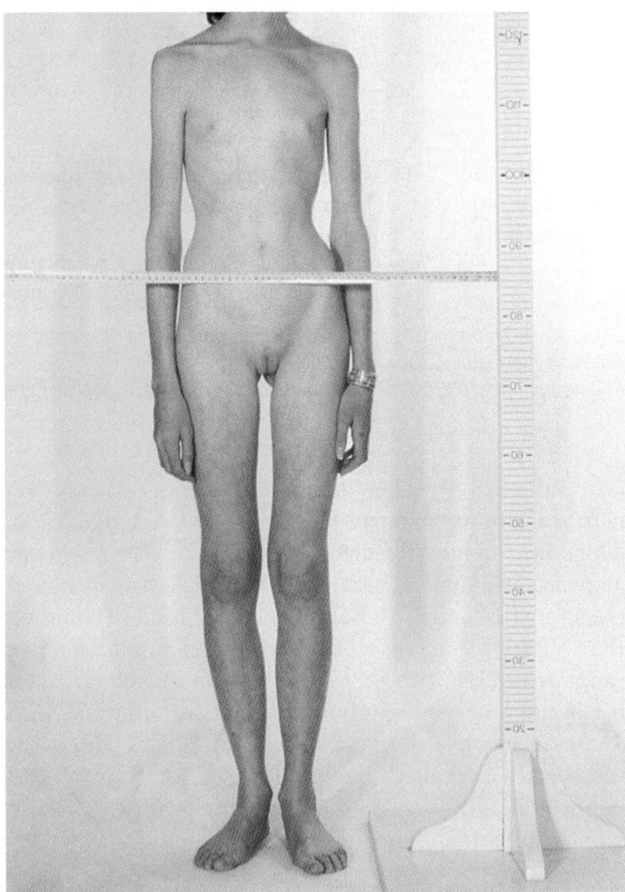

FIGURE 28-7 Anorexia nervosa in a young woman. Note the low body weight and the preservation of breast tissue. (*From Moshang T: Pediatric endocrinology: the requisites in pediatrics, St. Louis, 2005, Mosby.*)

Epidemiology: Incidence and Prevalence

These disorders cause psychological and physical morbidity in women (90% to 95% of cases) and, to a much lesser extent, in men (5% to 10% of cases).[30,31] Anorexia nervosa affects an estimated 1% of women between 12 and 25 years of age.[30,31] It is more common in white women and women from higher socioeconomic groups

TABLE 28-4 Clinical Findings and Epidemiology of Eating Disorders

Condition	Clinical Findings*	Epidemiology**
Anorexia nervosa	Individual refuses to maintain a minimally normal body weight (the individual weigh less than 85% of that weight that is considered normal for the person's age and height) • Intense fear of gaining weight or becoming fat • Significant disturbance in the perception of the shape or size of his or her body Postmenarcheal females with this disorder are amenorrheic The most obvious findings on physical examination is emaciation. There may also be hypotension, hypothermia, and dryness of skin. Most individuals with Anorexia Nervosa exhibit bradycardia.	Prevalence: 0.5-3.7% Mean age at onset: bimodal, with peaks at 14 and 18 years Rare after 40 years of age Females, 90-95% of cases More common in women in higher socioeconomic groups and among white women Mortality: 5-20% • Starvation • Suicide • Electrolyte imbalance
Bulimia nervosa	Recurrent episodes of binge eating characterized by both of the following: (1) eating, in a discrete period of time (e.g., within any 2-hour period), an amount of food that is definitely larger than most people would eat during a similar period of time and under similar circumstances (2) a sense of lack of control over eating during the episode (e.g., a feeling that one cannot stop eating or control what or how much one is eating) The binge eating and inappropriate compensatory behaviors both occur, on average, at least twice a week for 3 months. Recurrent inappropriate compensatory behavior in order to prevent weight gain, such a self-induced vomiting; misuse of laxatives, diuretics, enemas, or medications; fasting; or excessive weight gain. Self-evaluation is unduly influenced by body shape and weight.	Prevalence: 1.1-4.2% of women and 0.1% of men develop the condition during their lifetime. Average age at onset: ~ 20 years Females, 90-95% of cases More than 30% abuse alcohol and stimulants. Half have personality disorders. Rates are similar in high- and lower-income groups, but treatment is sought more often by women in higher-income groups. Higher rate in white women, but more cases are beginning to appear in ethnic minority groups. Long-term outcome not known but appears to have a more optimistic prognosis than for anorexia nervosa; the death rate from anorexia nervosa due to cardiac arrest and suicide is much higher than the death rate for bulima.
Eating disorders not otherwise specified	The eating disorder not otherwise specified category is for disorders of eating that do not meet the criteria for any specific eating disorder For example, for females, all the criteria for Anorexia Nervosa are met except that, the individual has regular menses.	Difficult to establish the prevalence of this more newly recognized group of eating disorders

*From American Psychiatric Association: Eating disorders. In Diagnostic and statistical manual of mental disorders, fourth edition, text rev, Washington, DC, American Psychiatric Association, 2000.
**Data from Franco KN: Eating disorders. In Carey WD, et al, editors: Current clinical medicine 2009—Cleveland Clinic, Philadelphia, Saunders, 2009.

(see Table 28-4). The lifetime prevalence of anorexia nervosa among women ranges from 0.5% to 3.7%, depending on how the disease is defined.[28] The mean age at onset of anorexia nervosa is bimodal, with peaks at the ages of 14 and 18.[30] Bulimia nervosa is more common than anorexia nervosa. Its prevalence among women range from 1.1% to 4.2%.[28] The average age at onset for bulimia nervosa is about 20 years. In contrast with anorexia nervosa, bulimia nervosa occurs at about the same rate in higher- and in lower-income groups of women. It is more common in white women than in women of ethnic minority groups.[30]

Etiology

The cause of eating disorders is unknown. Genetic, cultural, and psychiatric factors appear to play a role in the origin of these disorders.[28,29] In addition, primary dysfunction of the hypothalamus has been suggested to play a causative role in eating disorders. However, recognized hypothalamic abnormalities revert to normal with weight gain and thus appear to be secondary in nature.[29] Some evidence indicates that dysfunction in serotonin-mediated neurotransmission may contribute to the development of eating disorders.[31] Elevated homocysteine levels have been reported in patients with eating disorders and may be involved in the pathophysiology of these conditions.[32] Lack of self-esteem appears to play an important role in eating disorders.[33] Genetic factors are recognized to contribute to the risk of development of anorexia nervosa: Its incidence is greater in families with one affected member, and the concordance in monozygotic twins is greater than in dizygotic twins. Specific genes, however, have not been identified.[29] Linkage studies have found an association of anorexia nervosa with chromosome 1 and an association of bulimia nervosa with chromosome 10.[31]

Cultural issues are important in the origin of eating disorders. The quest for health and slimness is a powerful force in modern society and may reinforce the fear of fatness in patients with an eating disorder or may tip the borderline case into overt disease. Certain hobbies and occupations (e.g., modeling, skating, gymnastics, wrestling, track, ballet dancing) that emphasize body shape, weight, and appearance also may play a role in eating disorders.[26-29]

CLINICAL PRESENTATION AND MEDICAL MANAGEMENT

The diagnosis of an eating disorder is made on clinical grounds, as set forth in Box 28-3. The weight criterion for diagnosis of anorexia is 85% or less of expected ideal weight. An expressed intense fear of gaining weight or becoming fat, even when underweight, and a disturbance in body image complete the diagnostic triad.[26-29] The diagnosis of bulimia is made with a history of binge eating without major weight gain, evidence of purging (induced vomiting or regular use of laxatives or diuretics), obsessive-compulsive behavior, and antisocial activity or self-mutilation.[26-29]

Anorexia nervosa usually begins around puberty but may appear later, usually by the mid-20s. Despite severe weight loss, patients deny hunger, thinness, or fatigue. They often are physically active and participate in ritualized exercise. Constipation and cold intolerance are common. Amenorrhea usually accompanies or comes after weight loss. In advanced cases, bradycardia, hypothermia, and hypotension occur. Little or no body fat is evident, and bony protrusions (e.g., at the hips or shoulder blades) are pronounced. Parotid glands may become enlarged. The skin may be dry and scaly and often is yellow because of carotenemia. Patients with eating disorders may show other dermatologic abnormalities; alopecia, xerosis, hypertrichosis, and nail fragility may be clinical manifestations of starvation.[26-29] Peripheral edema may occur in up to 20% of adolescent patients with anorexia nervosa and can be misinterpreted as weight gain by the patient, making acceptance of treatment difficult.[34]

Patients with bulimia ("ox-hunger") nervosa engage in episodic, compulsive ingestion of large amounts of food (see Box 28-3). They are aware that this eating is abnormal; they have a fear that they cannot stop eating and have feelings of depression at the completion of eating. Bulimic patients also have a morbid fear of becoming fat. Secrecy about the eating-vomiting sequence is common. Episodes of binge eating are followed by

BOX 28-3 DSM-IV Diagnostic Criteria for Anorexia Nervosa and Bulimia Nervosa

Anorexia Nervosa

A. Refusal to maintain body weight at or above minimally normal weight for age and height (e.g., weight loss leading to maintenance of body weight less than 85% of that expected; or failure to make expected weight gain during period of growth, leading to body weight less than 85% of that expected)
B. Intense fear of gaining weight or becoming fat, even though underweight
C. Disturbance in the way in which one's body weight or shape is experienced, undue influence of body shape on self-evaluation, or denial of the seriousness of the current low body weight
D. In postmenarcheal females, amenorrhea, i.e., the absence of at least three consecutive menstrual cycles. (A woman is considered to have amenorrhea if her periods occur only following hormone, e.g., estrogen, administration).

Specify Type

- *Restricting type:* During the current episode of anorexia nervosa, the person has not regularly engaged in binge eating or purging behavior (i.e., self-induced vomiting or misuse of laxatives, diuretics, or enemas).
- *Binge eating/purging type:* During the current episode of anorexia nervosa, the person has regularly engaged in binge eating or purging behavior (i.e., self-induced vomiting or misuse of laxatives, diuretics, or enemas).

Bulimia Nervosa

A. Recurrent episodes of binge eating; an episode of binge eating is characterized by both of the following:
   (1) Eating, in a discrete period of time (e.g., within any 2-hour period), an amount of food that is definitely larger than most people would eat during a similar period of time and under similar circumstances
   (2) A sense of lack of control over eating during the episode (e.g., a feeling that one cannot stop eating or control what or how much one is eating)
B. Recurrent inappropriate compensatory behavior in order to prevent weight gain, such as self-induced vomiting; misuse of laxatives, diuretics, enemas, or other medication; fasting; or excessive exercise
C. Binge eating and inappropriate compensatory behaviors both occur, on average, at least twice a week for 3 months.
D. Self-evaluation is unduly influenced by body shape and weight.
E. The disturbance does not occur exclusively during episodes of anorexia nervosa.

Specify Type

- *Purging type:* During the current episode of bulimia nervosa, the person has regularly engaged in self-induced vomiting or the misuse of laxatives, diuretics, or enemas.
- *Nonpurging type:* During the current episode of bulimia nervosa, the person has used other inappropriate compensatory behaviors, such as fasting or excessive exercise, but has not regularly engaged in self-induced vomiting or the misuse of laxatives, diuretics, or enemas.

From American Psychiatric Association: Diagnostic and statistical manual of mental disorders, *fourth ed, text rev, Washington, DC, American Psychiatric Association, 2000.*

vomiting induced by means of a finger or another object, or with a drug such as ipecac, with or without subsequent ingestion of laxatives or diuretics. Bloating, constipation, esophagitis, abdominal pain, and nausea are common. Binge eating generally occurs daily; large amounts of food, usually high-carbohydrate foods such as ice cream, bread, candy, and doughnuts, are consumed at each episode. Dental caries becomes a problem because of the high carbohydrate content of the diet.[26-29]

Serum amylase has been reported to be elevated in 45% of bulimic patients.[35] In the same study, serum amylase was found to be elevated in pregnant women with hyperemesis but not in nonvomiting pregnant women. The authors of the study[35] concluded that vomiting, rather than binge eating, increases serum amylase in bulimic patients. They speculated that increased amylase came from the salivary gland. Another study[36] found that parotid gland size was enlarged in 36% of bulimic patients and was correlated with frequency of bulimic symptoms and with serum amylase concentrations.

Patients with anorexia nervosa are vulnerable to sudden death from ventricular tachyarrhythmias. The risk of death becomes greater when weight declines to below 35% of ideal weight. Complications of bulimia include aspiration of vomitus, esophageal or gastric rupture, hypokalemia with cardiac arrhythmias, pancreatitis, and ipecac-induced myopathy and cardiomyopathy.[26-29]

Long-term follow-up evaluation of patients with anorexia nervosa shows recovery rates of 44% to 76%, with a recovery time of 57 to 59 months. Mortality rates of up to 20% have been reported, with cardiac arrest and suicide the primary causes of death.[28] The long-term mortality associated with anorexia nervosa is among the highest for any psychiatric disorder. Approximately 5% of patients die per decade of follow-up, primarily from the physical effects of chronic starvation or by suicide.[29] Long-term follow-up data for bulimia nervosa are less comprehensive. Short-term success rates range from 50% to 70%, with relapse rates between 30% and 50% after 6 months. Patients with bulimia nervosa have an overall better prognosis than those with anorexia nervosa.[28]

The treatment of anorexia nervosa cannot proceed in a meaningful way in the absence of weight gain. The patient's nutritional status and medical stability are first evaluated. Patients with electrolyte disturbances or with abnormalities on electrocardiogram (ECG) may require hospitalization. Once the patient is medically stable, psychiatric treatment can begin. Behavior modification techniques are used to assist the patient in weight gain. The efficacy of psychotherapy has not been established. A recent report showed that yoga may be an effective adjunctive treatment for eating disorders.[37] Drug therapy (antipsychotics, cyproheptadine, antidepressants) has not significantly improved the outcomes for patients with anorexia nervosa. The antidepressant fluoxetine has been shown to be useful in preventing relapse in patients who have gained back their weight.[27-29]

Antidepressant medication, cognitive-behavioral therapy, and interpersonal therapy all are effective in bulimia nervosa. Most patients are treated on an outpatient basis. Those patients with medical complications such as extreme electrolyte imbalance or severe bulimic symptoms may require hospitalization.[27-29] The supportive care of a knowledgeable but sympathetic physician also may be helpful for the bulimic patient. Attempts should be made to stop the gorging-regurgitation cycle, or at least to limit the load of food ingested, to minimize the chance of aspiration or gastric rupture. Potassium supplementation may be needed in patients who vomit and in those who use laxatives.[27-29]

DRUGS USED TO TREAT ANXIETY DISORDERS

Benzodiazepines are used to treat various anxiety states (see Table 28-3). These drugs selectively but indirectly enhance γ-aminobutyric acid neurotransmission. The mechanism for this effect may involve an increase in neuronal receptor sensitivity to γ-aminobutyric acid. The benzodiazepines are very effective for short-lived reactive states of tension and anxiety and are the drugs of choice for generalized anxiety disorder. Tricyclic antidepressants and MAOIs are the drugs of choice for the management of panic disorders. Benzodiazepines are used for the treatment of anticipatory anxiety associated with panic disorder. They also are used in the treatment of other forms of anxiety associated with panic disorder and for anxiety symptoms in patients with phobic disorder.[3,4,6]

Diazepam is the standard agent for antianxiety therapy. No other anxiolytic drug has shown better antianxiety efficacy. Treatment with anxiolytic drugs should continue for a period of only 4 weeks or less. To avoid the development of drug tolerance, these agents often are given for 7 to 10 days; a 2- to 3-day period without the drug follows. An early sign of drug tolerance is the requirement for increased dosage to obtain the same effects. Signs and symptoms of drug withdrawal include muscle aches, agitation, restlessness, insomnia, confusion, delirium, and, on rare occasion, grand mal seizures. Some patients may experience rebound anxiety after the drug has been stopped.[9,22,38,39]

Adverse effects of the benzodiazepines include daytime sedation, mild cognitive impairment, and aggressive and impulsive behavioral responses. Use of any of this group of agents, which can potentiate the CNS effects of opioids, barbiturates, and alcohol, is hazardous or is contraindicated in the following groups of patients: those who drive or operate machinery, patients with depressive mood disorders or psychosis, and moderate to heavy drinkers, pregnant women, and elderly persons. Tolerance and habitual and physical dependence may occur with therapeutic doses. Actions of the benzodiazepines are additive and usually are synergistic with psychotropic agents. Drug interactions have been reported with cimetidine and erythromycin.[9,22,38,39]

Buspirone has mixed agonist-antagonist actions at serotonergic receptors that are thought to be involved in anxiety. It appears to have anxiolytic effects that are comparable with those of benzodiazepines, without sedative, anticonvulsant, or muscle relaxant effects. These anxiolytic effects are delayed in onset, taking up to 3 weeks before becoming clinical obvious. The drug is recommended for short-term use only. At this time, buspirone is not a first-line drug for the treatment of anxiety.[9,22,38,40]

Several tricyclics and other antidepressants have additional sedative or anxiolytic effects. They appear to be as effective as benzodiazepines for generalized anxiety and superior for panic disorder and agoraphobia. SSRIs and MAOIs also are effective in phobic states and panic disorders.[23] Disadvantages of these drugs include slow rate of onset of effect, potential for initial exacerbation of anxiety symptoms, toxicity in overdose, and numerous adverse effects.[9,22,38]

DENTAL MANAGEMENT

Patients' Attitudes Toward Dentists

Childhood experiences and learned social roles of the patient are important factors in the development of feelings and attitudes toward dentists. Children learn role expectations through the teachings of physicians, dentists, parents, and peers. The patient may come to believe that the physician and the dentist are powerful and dangerous, eliciting feelings of awe and envy. Other emotions, attitudes, and behaviors associated with the patient's relationships with one or both parents also may be transferred to the dentist. Those of respect and politeness can be helpful. By contrast, those associated with a need for unending love, a demand for unceasing attention, and feelings of resentment and hate can be destructive. The dentist can take steps to help deflect such unrealistic expectations and inappropriate behaviors. From the initial patient encounter, maintaining a respectful, genuine, and open demeanor is less likely to encourage misplaced attitudes and feelings. In addition, these and related issues should be open for discussion between the dentist and the patient, to clarify any impediments to development of a solid relationship.

Behavioral Reactions to Illness

The DSM-IV calls attention to the interplay of psychological and behavioral factors with medical illness under the diagnostic category of psychological factors that affect medical conditions. All patients with medical illness experience psychological reactions to being ill. Specific reactions may vary according to the nature of the illness and the nature of the affected person. Significant aspects of the illness include severity, chronicity, and the site and nature of symptoms. Relevant patient characteristics include age, level of maturity, personality style, previous experience with illness, and social supports.[1,41]

Regression, denial, anxiety, depression, and anger are general responses to illness that are common to all human beings. These responses originate in the various meanings that people attribute to physical illness, the fears that typically are raised by being ill, and the means used to cope with illness.[1,41]

Depressive thoughts and feelings are common psychological reactions to medical illness. Being ill usually is perceived as a loss, which may be experienced as impairment of physical abilities and compromise of bodily integrity through the loss of organs or limbs. Feelings of loss of control are very common among hospitalized patients. Patients may feel that they cannot do some of the things they have always done that are an important part of the pre-illness identity. Such activities typically include being unable to fulfill family roles, taking care of professional responsibilities, and participating in recreational and social events. Many medical patients experience loss of a sense of well-being. Transient depressed thoughts and feelings are common in medically ill patients. Major depression in medically ill patients is not normal, however, and must be aggressively identified and treated.[1,41]

Patients commonly experience anger about being ill. In occasional cases, as part of an effort to feel less helpless, guilty, or afraid, the patient may lash out at others, becoming hostile, suspicious, and accusatory toward family members and health care providers alike. The most common causes of anger, irritability, and suspiciousness in medically ill patients are medications and substances of abuse. Patient groups at high risk for paranoid reactions include elderly persons, people with depression or cognitive impairment, and patients with a previous history of psychotic illness.[1,41]

Severe and chronic illnesses foster a type of dependency of the patient on others. Severely disabled patients have a greater need to rely on others. Some people cannot accept this dependency and become anxious and try to deny the need for help. Feelings of resentment, anger, and hostility may develop toward persons in contact with such a patient. Once again, an understanding of this process will allow those who care for such a patient to be empathetic and supportive.[1,41]

Sick people tend to view the world around them as very limited in scope, and they develop a preoccupation with their sickness, needs, and fears. They may retreat to a highly personal interpretation of their illness, or to magical notions about its cause. For example, patients with cancer may believe that the illness is a punishment for previous "unacceptable" behaviors or thoughts.[1,41]

Patient Management

Anxiety. Anxiety related to dental treatment is fairly common. Severe dental fear or anxiety, however, is far less common. The origin of this anxiety may lie in negative personal dental experiences, or in cognitive perceptions of what it may be like to go to the dentist. Armfield, in a study of Australian adult dental patients, found that the patients' perceptions were stronger predictors of dental fear than negative dental experiences.[42] In another study, Fuentes and associates concluded that dental anxiety is specific, with its own features and is not necessarily associated with so-called trait anxiety.[43] Van Wijk and Hoogstraten reported that pain felt during dental injections is dependent on dental anxiety, fear of dental pain, fear of the injection, and the amount of injection fluid.[44] Binkley and colleagues reported that dental care–related anxiety, fear of dental pain, and avoidance of dental care may be influenced by genetic variations such as red hair color (caused by variants of the melanocortin-1 receptor gene).[45] By taking a comprehensive dental history (including negative dental experiences and the patient's perception of dental treatment) and observing the patient for signs of anxiety, the dentist can identify the patient who may need additional supportive care during dental treatment.

The dentist may detect anxiety in persons by observing their physical appearance, speech, and dress and checking for the presence of certain signs and symptoms. The anxious person looks overly alert and exhibits various restless-appearing postures and behaviors such as sitting forward in a chair; moving fingers, arms, or legs; getting up and moving; pacing around the room; checking certain portions of clothing; straightening ties or scarves; and so forth. Conversely, sloppy dress habits and other signs that convey just the opposite of a concern with perfection may be seen instead. Anxious persons may appear especially watchful of possessions, always trying to keep them in sight.[10]

The anxious person may speak mechanically and rapidly and at times may seem to block out or not connect thoughts. The anxious person may respond quickly, often not allowing the dentist to finish a question.[10]

Sweating, tension in the muscles, increased breathing, and rapid heart rate are other frequent manifestations of anxiety. The patient may report an inability to sleep or may awaken at an early hour and not be able to go back to sleep. Attacks of diarrhea and increased frequency of urination are not uncommon. In general, anxious persons are overly alert and tense, feel apprehensive, and have a sense of impending disaster that has no apparent cause. Insomnia, tension, and apprehension lead to fatigue, which may further impair efforts to deal with anxiety or its causes.[10]

In interactions with the patient, the dentist should convey an appropriate level of personal interest. Verbal and nonverbal components of communication must be consistent (Box 28-4). An often helpful approach is to begin by mentioning that the patient appears anxious and then to invite the patient to talk about relevant feelings, which may include attitudes toward the dentist. During these discussions, tension-free pauses between expressions of ideas should be permitted, allowing a temporary state of regression to occur that will help the patient to restore a more anxiety-free state. Some patients may respond well to this approach without ever indicating why they were anxious.[10]

If the patient remains anxious, the dentist may elect to use hypnosis, oral or parenteral sedation agents, or nitrous oxide plus oxygen to better manage the dental treatment (see Box 28-4). A recent study demonstrated a beneficial effect of acupuncture on the level of anxiety in patients with dental anxiety.[46]

Anxiety or a history of panic attacks also may be associated with mitral valve prolapse.[5,7,47] In the past, patients with mitral valve prolapse and valvular regurgitation were given antibiotic prophylaxis for invasive dental procedures. In accordance with the 2007 AHA guidelines, these patients no longer require prophylaxis (see Chapter 2).

Patients with uncontrolled hyperthyroidism also may experience increased levels of anxiety; in such patients, therefore, it is important to avoid the use of epinephrine, including even the small amounts present in local anesthetics (see Chapter 16). Patients who display signs and symptoms of hyperthyroidism should be referred for medical evaluation and treatment.[48]

Posttraumatic Stress Disorder. Veterans with PTSD may view the dentist as a representative authority figure who misled them and sent them to war.[10] They may associate dental treatment with loss of control; hence, the dentist must attempt to establish communication and trust with these patients. Patients with intravenous drug habits may be carriers of the hepatitis B virus (hepatitis B surface antigen [HBsAg]-positive) and of human immunodeficiency virus (HIV). Those who are heavy drinkers may have liver and bone marrow involvement and may be at increased risk for infection, excessive bleeding, delayed healing, and altered drug metabolism. During the depressive stage of PTSD, patients often show a total disregard for oral hygiene procedures and are at increased risk for development of dental caries, periodontal disease, and pericoronitis. They may report atypical facial pain, glossodynia, temporomandibular joint (TMJ) disorder, and bruxism.[10]

Stress-Related Disorders. Oral diseases that are thought to have a psychological component in their clinical presentation (the older term was *psychophysiologic disorders*) include aphthous ulcers, lichen planus, TMJ dysfunction, myofascial pain, and geographic tongue. Examples of some of these lesions are shown in Figures 28-8 to 28-10.

In these disorders, an identifiable lesion with an emotional component is part of the clinical presentation. The

BOX 28-4 Dental Management
Considerations in the Anxious Patient

P

Patient Evaluation/Risk Assessment (see Box 1-1)

- Evaluate to determine whether anxiety is present.
- Obtain medical consultation if clinical signs and symptoms point to an undiagnosed problem, or if diagnosis is uncertain.

Potential Issues? Factors of Concern

A	
Analgesics	The control of postoperative pain is extremely important in the anxious patient. In accordance with the procedure performed, the dentist should select the most appropriate drug for pain control (nonsteroidal antiinflammatory drugs, salicylates, acetaminophen, codeine, oxycodone, fentanyl, morphine, and others). Also, adjunctive medications such as antidepressants, muscle relaxants, steroids, and antibiotics may be indicated.
Antibiotics	Not indicated unless acute infection is present.
Anesthesia	Effective local anesthesia is essential, and oral sedation provided on the night before and just before the dental appointment with a fast-acting benzodiazepine (alprazolam, 0.5 mg tab; diazepam, 2, 5, or 10 mg tab; or triazolam, 0.125 or 0.25 mg tab) will aid in the management of anxiety in a majority of cases. For the more anxious patient, inhalation sedation with nitrous oxide, intramuscular sedation (midazolam, promethazine, or meperidine), or intravenous sedation (diazepam, midazolam, or fentanyl) can be used.
Anxiety	Establish effective communication, maintain an open and honest demeanor with appropriate level of genuine personal revelation, be consistent in verbal and nonverbal components of communication, provide explanations of procedures with short "question-and-answer" breaks to address the patient's concerns, and finally, if discomfort is anticipated, reassure the patient that all possible measures for a "pain-free" procedure will be used. If the patient appears overly anxious, confirmation of/attentiveness to this distress may be helpful (e.g., "You seem tense today—would you like to talk about it?"). During the procedure, it is important to signal the patient when any discomfort may be expected, and also to let the patient know that things are going well. Advise the patient beforehand of what usually occurs after the procedure, what drugs and measures will be prescribed to minimize any discomfort, and any activities or medications to be avoided. Describe any complications that could occur, such as pain, bleeding, infection, or allergic reactions to any medications that may have been prescribed. Instruct the patient to contact the dental office if any complication occurs or, in the event of severe bleeding or allergic reaction, to go to the nearest hospital emergency department.
Allergy	No issues.
B	
Bleeding	No issues.
Breathing	No issues.
Blood pressure	No issues.
C	
Chair position	No issues.
Cardiovascular	Many patients experiencing a panic attack think that they are having a heart attack.
Consultation	With severe anxiety associated with any of the anxiety states such as PTSD or panic disorder, the patient's physician should be consulted regarding any special management considerations.
D	
Devices	No issues.
Drugs	No issues.
E	
Equipment	No issues.
Emergencies	Patients with PTSD who make comments about suicidal thoughts should be referred for psychiatric care.
F	
Follow-up	Routine follow-up evaluation is recommended.

pathologic process is potentially dangerous to the patient. The disorder does not reduce the level of anxiety or depression but rather increases it, and increased anxiety or depression can aggravate the condition. These disorders can be treated through the regimen provided in Appendix C. The anxious patient can be sedated with the use of one of the agents shown in Box 28-4. Patients with atypical facial pain, TMJ dysfunction, or myofascial pain often are treated with an antidepressant medication.

Eating Disorders. The main task of the dentist in the management of patients with bulimia nervosa is to deal with the results of improper diet (dental caries) and the effects of chronic vomiting on the teeth (erosion).[49] One

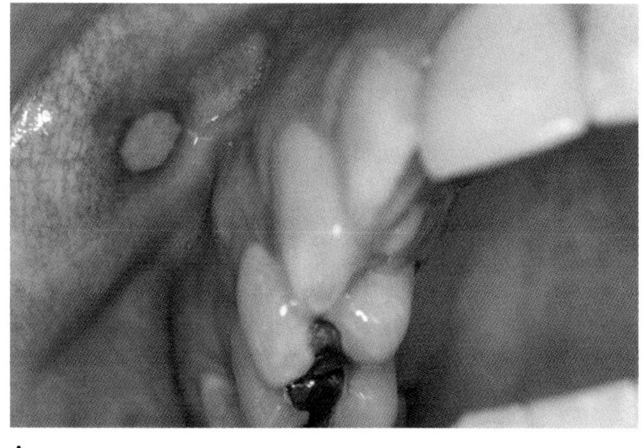

A

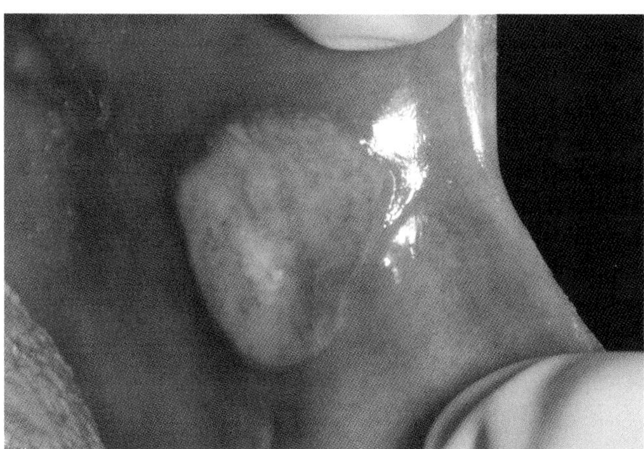

B

FIGURE 28-8 A, A single minor aphthous ulceration of the anterior buccal mucosa. **B,** A large major aphthous ulceration of the left anterior buccal mucosa. (*From Neville BW, et al:* Oral and maxillofacial pathology, *ed 3, Philadelphia, 2009, Saunders.*)

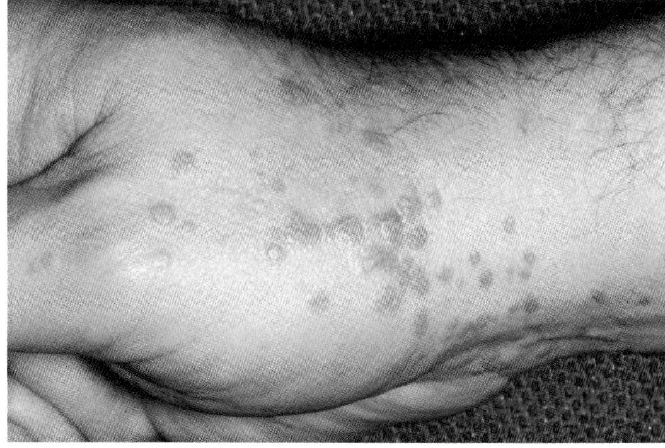

A

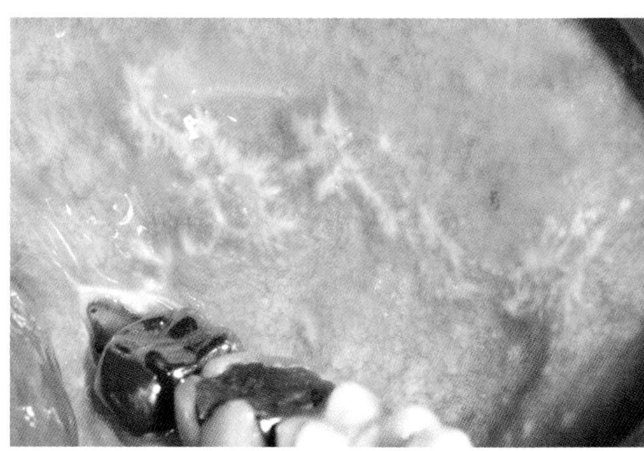

B

FIGURE 28-9 A, Lichen planus on the skin of the wrist. **B,** Lichen planus on the buccal mucosa. (*From Neville BW, et al:* Oral and maxillofacial pathology, *ed 3, Philadelphia, 2009, Saunders.*)

study[50] found that the average pH of vomitus was 3.8; chronic exposure can therefore lead to severe erosion of teeth. The dentist has an important public health role as a case finder. On the dental examination, the finding of a pattern of tooth erosion that is consistent with habitual regurgitation of stomach contents may be the first indication of the presence of an eating disorder (Figure 28-11). Subsequent referral can lead to medical diagnosis and appropriate treatment; however, patients often deny the pathologic behaviors. The erosive pattern involves the lingual surfaces of the teeth, primarily the maxillary teeth because the tongue protects the mandibular teeth. This particular type of erosion is known as *perimylolysis*. In some cases, erosion also can affect the occlusal surfaces of molar and premolar teeth, where the process can be accelerated by attrition.[50-52] The potential for serious medical complications of bulimia nervosa (gastric rupture, esophageal tears, cardiac arrhythmia, and death) must be pointed out to the patient, along with the fact that these can be avoided with proper medical and psychological therapy.[31,53,54]

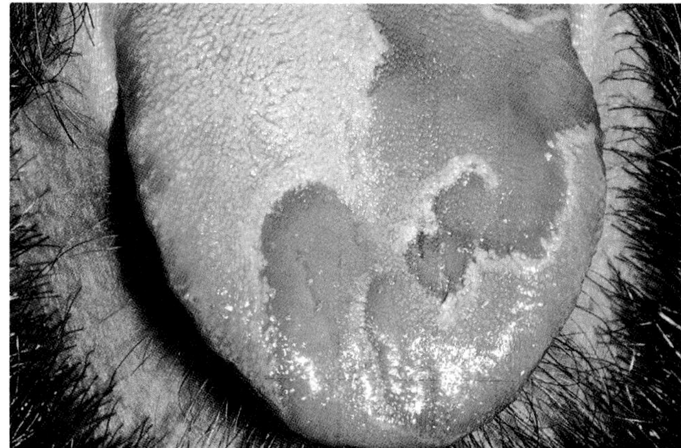

FIGURE 28-10 Geographic tongue (benign migratory glossitis, erythremia migrans) consists of erythematous, well-demarcated areas of papillary atrophy, with a tendency to involve the lateral aspects of the tongue. (*From Neville BW, et al:* Oral and maxillofacial pathology, *ed 3, Philadelphia, 2009, Saunders.*)

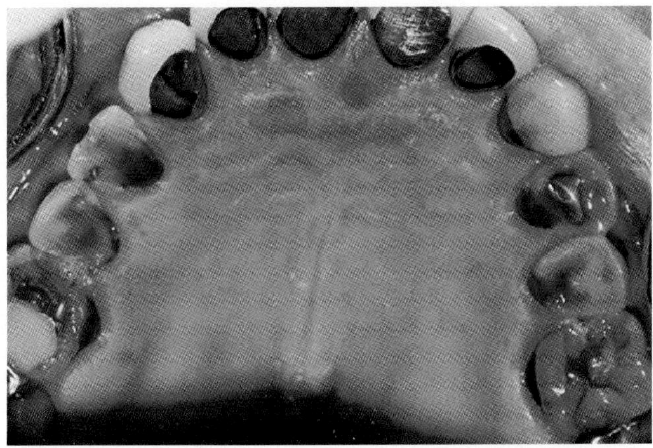

A

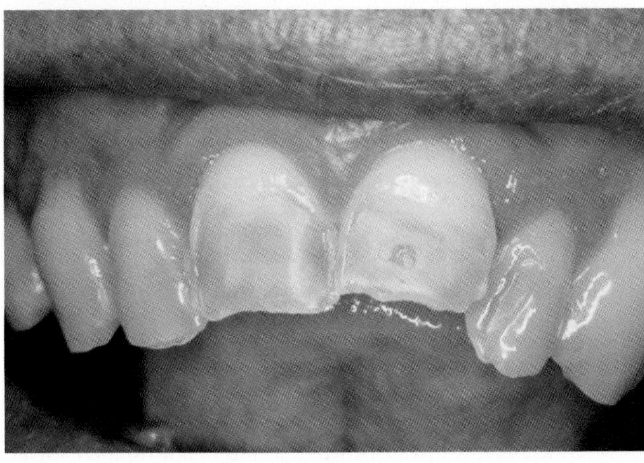

B

FIGURE 28-11 **A,** Lingual erosion of enamel in a patient with bulimia, due to regurgitation of stomach contents. **B,** Labial erosion of enamel in a patient who habitually sucked on citrus products.

The diet of some bulimic patients is rich in carbohydrates and carbonated liquids, which can lead to extensive dental caries and additional erosion of the teeth. An increase in dental caries most often is seen in patients with poor oral hygiene. Accordingly, an important goal of dental care is to improve oral hygiene practices.[49] To this end, the dentist should provide instruction on toothbrushing, use of dental floss, and application of topical fluoride. The patient is instructed to use a baking soda mouth rinse and to brush the teeth after induced vomiting.[49] Tooth sensitivity can be managed with the use of desensitizing toothpastes, fluoride applications, and other means.[49]

Patients with anorexia nervosa may be difficult to identify and deal with in a dental practice. About 40% to 50% of patients with anorexia nervosa also are bulimic and may show dental signs of bulimia.[31,54] Young patients who appear to be anorexic should be confronted about the weight loss. If the initial exam and history reveal no evidence of serious medical disease such as cancer or diabetes mellitus, the possibility of self-starvation should be discussed with the patient. Serious medical complications of anorexia nervosa, including death (reported mortality rates are as high as 15% to 20%), must be discussed in a straightforward manner. Again, when young patients are involved, parents must be informed. Every attempt should be made to refer patients to a physician for evaluation and treatment.

Drug Interactions and Adverse Effects

The potential for clinically significant drug interactions between benzodiazepines—the mainstay of treatment for anxiety—and barbiturates, opioids, psychotropic agents, cimetidine, and erythromycin is well recognized. In general, these agents potentiate the CNS depressant effects of benzodiazepines. Regarding the concomitant use of these agents and benzodiazepines, two situations are of clinical concern in dental treatment:

- Barbiturates (not used often now in dentistry) and opioids used for dental sedation or pain control must be administered with caution and in decreased dosages in patients who are taking a benzodiazepine for an anxiety disorder.
- The dentist may prescribe a benzodiazepine for sedation to control dental treatment–related anxiety, but care must be taken with use of these drugs in patients receiving psychotropic agents for a psychiatric disorder.

Usually, the dosage of the medication can be reduced to avoid overdepression of the CNS. The dentist should consult with the patient's physician before using these drug combinations. During treatment, the patient can be monitored with the use of a pulse oximeter.[8-10,55]

Treatment Planning Considerations

Goals of treatment planning for patients with psychiatric disorders are to maintain oral health, comfort, and function and to prevent and control oral disease. Without an aggressive approach to prevention, the incidence of dental caries and periodontal disease can be expected to increase. Susceptibility to these problems stems from the adverse effects of xerostomia associated with most of the medications used in treatment, coupled with the characteristically reduced interest in or impaired ability to perform oral hygiene procedures seen in many of these psychiatric disorders. In addition, the diet of persons with such disorders often contains significant amounts of foods or drinks associated with increased risk for dental disease.[10,56]

The dental treatment plan should contain the following elements: (1) Daily oral hygiene procedures must be identified; (2) the treatment plan must be realistic in terms of the patient's psychiatric disorder and physical status; and (3) the plan must be dynamic to take into account changes in the acuity or severity of the psychiatric disorder and in the patient's physical status.[57]

The dental team should communicate to the patient and family members a positive, hopeful attitude toward maintenance of the patient's oral health. The dental team should determine whether the patient is legally able to make rational decisions. This should be discussed with the patient and a loved one. Treatment planning often involves input and permission from a loved one so that decisions can be made.[57]

The last aspect of the treatment plan deals with the selection of medications to be used in providing dental treatment to the patient. Some agents may have to be avoided; others may require a reduction in the usual dosage. Medical consultation is suggested to establish the patient's current status, ascertain the medications the patient is taking, identify complications that may be present, and confirm dental medications and doses that will minimize possible drug interactions.[57]

In bulimic patients, complex restorative procedures should not be planned until the gorging and vomiting cycle has been broken. In a few cases, crowns may be required in an attempt to save teeth. Once the patient's overall health status is stable, restoration of teeth with severe erosion can begin. The dentist and the patient must be aware, however, that relapse is common and that complex restorations may fail with recurrence of chronic vomiting.[49] Fortunately, with the development of resin composite and adhesive systems, it is now possible to reconstruct damaged teeth with minimal dental preparation and with less expense. Thus, it has become more practical to restore teeth even when the pathologic vomiting has not yet been curtailed.[58]

Oral Complications and Manifestations

Patients with bulimia may present with severe erosion of the lingual and occlusal surfaces of the teeth (see Figure 28-11). Severe erosion can be associated with increased tooth sensitivity to touch and to cold temperature. Dental caries may be more prevalent among these patients. The amount of saliva produced may be decreased. Patients often report dry mouth. Those with poor oral hygiene exhibit increased periodontal disease. The parotid gland may become enlarged. Patients with anorexia nervosa also may demonstrate decreased salivary flow, dry mouth, atrophic mucosa, and an enlarged parotid gland.[49]

REFERENCES

1. American Psychiatric Association: *Diagnostic and statistical manual of mental disorders*, fourth ed, text rev, Washington, DC, 2000, American Psychiatric Association.
2. American Psychiatric Association: *Publication date for the diagnostic and statistical manual of mental disorders V*, Washington, DC, 2010, American Psychiatric Association.
3. Rowney J: Anxiety disorders. In Carey WD, et al, editors: *Current clinical medicine 2009—Cleveland Clinic*, Philadelphia, 2009, Saunders, pp 983-988.
4. Schiffer RB: Psychiatric disorders in medical practice. In Goldman L, Ausiello D, editors: *Cecil medicine*, ed 23, Philadelphia, 2008, Saunders, pp 2628-2638.
5. Vogel LR, Muskin PR: Anxiety disorders. In Cutler JL, Marcus ER, editors: *Saunders text and review series: psychiatry*, Philadelphia, 1999, WB Saunders, pp 105-127.
6. Reus VI: Mental disorders. In Fauci AS, et al, editors: *Harrison's principles of internal medicine*, ed 17, New York, 2008, McGraw-Hill, pp 2710-2723.
7. American Psychiatric Association: Anxiety disorders. In *Diagnostic and statistical manual of mental disorders*, fourth ed, text rev, Washington, DC, 2000, American Psychiatric Association, pp 429-485.
8. Reus VI: Mental disorders. In Kasper DL, et al, editors: *Harrison's online principles of medicine*, ed 16, New York, 2005, McGraw-Hill, pp 2547-2562.
9. Saver DF, et al: *Anxiety*, 2006, Elsevier.
10. Little JW: Anxiety disorders: dental implications, *J Gen Dent* 51:562-570, 2003.
11. Pollack EF, et al: *Schizophrenia*, Elsevier, available at http://www.firstconsult.com/schizophrenia, accessed March, 2006.
12. Scherger J, Sudak D, Alici-Evciment Y: *Depression, Elsevier*, available at http://www.firstconsult.com/schizophrenia, accessed March, 2006.
13. Scully C, Cawson RA: *Medical problems in dentistry*, ed 5, Edinburgh, 2005, Churchill Livingstone.
14. Cantón-Cortés D, Cantón J: Coping with child sexual abuse among college students and post-traumatic stress disorder: the role of continuity of abuse and relationship with the perpetrator, *Child Abuse Negl* Jun 1, 2010. [Epub ahead of print.]
15. Jubran A, et al: Post-traumatic stress disorder after weaning from prolonged mechanical ventilation, *Intensive Care Med* 36:2030-2037, 2010.
16. Hari R, Begre S, et al: Change over time in posttraumatic stress caused by myocardial infarction and predicting variables, *J Psychosom Res* 69:143-150, 2010.
17. Elklit A, et al: Posttraumatic stress disorder among bereaved relatives of cancer patients, *J Psychosoc Oncol* 28:399-412, 2010.
18. Judd LL, Britton KT, Braff DL: Mental disorders. In Isselbacher KJ, et al, editors: *Harrison's principles of internal medicine*, ed 13, New York, 1994, McGraw-Hill, pp 2400-2420.
19. Goldberg RJ: *Practical guide to the care of the psychiatric patient*, St Louis, 1995, Mosby.
20. Davis LL, et al: Pharmacotherapy for post-traumatic stress disorder: a comprehensive review, *Expert Opin Pharmacother* 2:1583-1595, 2001.
21. Pereira A: Combat trauma and the diagnosis of post-traumatic stress disorder in female and male veterans, *Mil Med* 167:23-27, 2002.
22. Kabongo ML, et al: *Posttraumatic stress disorder*, 2006, Elsevier.
23. Healy D: *Psychiatric drugs explained*, ed 5, St. Louis, 2009, Churchill Livingstone.
24. Dickstein BD, et al: Unit cohesion and PTSD symptom severity in Air Force medical personnel, *Mil Med* 175:482-486, 2010.
25. North CS, et al: Toward validation of the diagnosis of posttraumatic stress disorder, *Am J Psychiatry* 166:34-41, 2009.
26. American Psychiatric Association: Eating disorders. In *Diagnostic and statistical manual of mental disorders*, fourth ed, text rev, Washington, DC, 2000, American Psychiatric Association, pp 583-597.
27. Marcus DM: Eating disorders. In Goldman L, Ausiello D, editors: *Cecil medicine*, ed 23, Philadelphia, Saunders, 2008, pp 1640-1642.

28. Franco KN: Eating disorders. In Carey WD, et al, editors: *Current clinical medicine 2009—Cleveland Clinic*, Philadelphia, 2009, Saunders, pp 1013-1018.
29. Walsh BT: Eating disorders. In Fauci AS, et al, editors: *Harrison's principles of internal medicine*. ed 17, New York, 2008, McGraw-Hill, pp 473-478.
30. West DS: The eating disorders. In Goldman L, Ausiello D, editors: *Cecil textbook of medicine*, ed 22, Philadelphia, 2004, Saunders, pp 1336-1338.
31. Majid SH, Treasure JL: Eating disorders. In Wright P, Stern J, Phelan M, editors: *Core psychiatry*, ed 2, Edinburgh, 2005, Elsevier, pp 217-241.
32. Wilhelm J, et al: Elevation of homocysteine levels is only partially reversed after therapy in females with eating disorders, *J Neural Transm* 117:521-527, 2010.
33. Vanderlinden J, et al: Be kind to your eating disorder patients: the impact of positive and negative feedback on the explicit and implicit self-esteem of female patients with eating disorders, *Eat Weight Disord* 14:e237-e242, 2009.
34. Derman O, Kilic EZ: Edema can be a handicap in treatment of anorexia nervosa, *Turk J Pediatr* 51:593-597, 2009.
35. Robertson C, Millar H: Hyperamylasemia in bulimia nervosa and hyperemesis gravidarum, *Int J Eat Disord* 26:223-227, 1999.
36. Metzger ED, et al: Salivary gland enlargement and elevated serum amylase in bulemia nervosa, *Biol Psychiatry* 45:1520-1522, 1995.
37. Carei TR, et al: Randomized controlled clinical trial of yoga in the treatment of eating disorders, *J Adolesc Health* 46:346-351, 2010.
38. Ashton CH: Insomnia and anxiety. In Walker R, Edwards C, editors: *Clinical pharmacy and therapeutics*, ed 2, Edinburgh, 1999, Churchill Livingstone, pp 393-408.
39. Pratt JP: Affective disorders. In Walker R, Edwards C, editors: *Clinical pharmacy and therapeutics*, ed 2, Edinburgh, 1999, Churchill Livingstone, pp 409-425.
40. Horwath E, Courinos F: Schizophrenia and other psychotic disorders. In Cutler JL, Marcus ER, editors: *Saunders text and review series: psychiatry*, Philadelphia, 1999, WB Saunders, pp 64-80.
41. Caligor E: Psychological factors affecting medical conditions. In Cutler JL, Marcus ER, editors: *Saunders text and review series: psychiatry*, Philadelphia, 1999, WB Saunders, pp 221-246.
42. Armfield JM: Towards a better understanding of dental anxiety and fear: cognitions vs. experiences, *Eur J Oral Sci* 118:259-264, 2010.
43. Fuentes D, Gorenstein C, Hu LW: Dental anxiety and trait anxiety: an investigation of their relationship, *Br Dent J* 206:E17, 2009.
44. van Wijk AJ, Hoogstraten J: Anxiety and pain during dental injections, *J Dent* 37:700-704, 2009.
45. Binkley CJ, et al: Genetic variations associated with red hair color and fear of dental pain, anxiety regarding dental care and avoidance of dental care, *J Am Dent Assoc* 140:896-905, 2009.
46. Rosted P, et al: Acupuncture in the management of anxiety related to dental treatment: a case series, *Acupunct Med* 28:3-5, 2010.
47. Friedlander AH, Gorelick DA: Panic disorder: its association with mitral valve prolapse and appropriate dental management, *Oral Surg Oral Med Oral Pathol* 63:309-312, 1987.
48. Little JW: Thyroid disorders: part I, hyperthyroidism, *Oral Surg Oral Med Oral Path Oral Radiol Endod* 101:276-284, 2006.
49. Little JW: Eating disorders, *Oral Surg Oral Med Oral Path Oral Radiol Endod* 93:138-144, 2002.
50. Milosevic A, Brodie DA, Slade PD: Dental erosion, oral hygiene, and nutrition in eating disorders, *Int J Eat Disord* 21:195-199, 1997.
51. Scheutzel P: Etiology of dental erosion—intrinsic factors, *Eur J Oral Sci* 104:178-190, 1996.
52. Milosevic A: Eating disorders and the dentist, *Br Dent J* 186:109-113, 1999.
53. Foster DW: Anorexia nervosa and bulimia nervosa. In Fauci AS, et al, editors: *Harrison's principles of internal medicine*, ed 14, New York, 1998, McGraw-Hill, pp 462-472.
54. Devlin MJ: Eating disorders. In Cutler JL, Marcus ER, editors: *Saunders text and review series: psychiatry*, Philadelphia, 1999, WB Saunders, pp 170-185.
55. Feinstein RE: Cognitive and mental disorders due to general medical conditions. In Cutler JL, Marcus ER, editors: *Saunders text and review series: psychiatry*, Philadelphia, 1999, WB Saunders, pp 81-104.
56. Little JW: Dental implications of mood disorders, *J Gen Dent* 52:442-450, 2004.
57. Little JW: Alzheimer's disease, *J Gen Dent* 53:289-298, 2005.
58. Spreafico RC: Composite resin rehabilitation of eroded dentition in a bulimic patient: a case report, *Eur J Esthet Dent* 5:28-48, 2010.

CHAPTER

29

Psychiatric Disorders

Mental disorders are common in today's society. Approximately one third of the population in the United States will have at least one psychiatric disorder during their lifetime, and 20% to 30% of adults in the United States will experience one or more psychiatric disorders during a 1-year period. About 5% of the population suffers from serious affective or mood disorders. Schizophrenic disorders are reported in 1.1%.[1-4]

Psychiatric problems, which can affect the clinical course in various medical illnesses, increase required duration of treatment, decrease the patient's functional level, and have a negative impact on overall prognosis and outcome. Disorders related to drug and alcohol use account for a significant proportion of the treatment-related psychiatric issues. In the elderly population, a high prevalence of psychiatric complications is associated with medical illness. About 11% to 15% of these patients experience depressive symptoms, and between 10% and 20% have anxiety disorders, including phobias. Phobia is the most common psychiatric disorder in women older than 65 years of age. Approximately 20% of elderly persons have a substance abuse disorder.[5] The prevalence of psychiatric disorders among adult dental patients seeking treatment at the Virginia Commonwealth University School of Dentistry was found to be 28% of a randomly selected patient group of 442.[6] The most common disorder reported was depression.[6]

This chapter provides an overview of mood disorders, somatoform disorders, and schizophrenia, with an emphasis on drugs used to treat these conditions and their significant adverse reactions and interactions with drugs used in dentistry. Also discussed are specific considerations in the dental management of patients with these disorders.

MOOD DISORDERS

DEFINITION

Mood disorders represent a heterogeneous group of mental disorders that are characterized by extreme exaggeration and disturbance of mood and affect. These disorders are associated with physiologic, cognitive, and psychomotor dysfunction. Mood disorders, which tend to be cyclic, include depression and bipolar disorder.[3,4,7,8]

EPIDEMIOLOGY

Incidence and Prevalence

About 5% of the adults in the United States have a significant mood disorder. Mood disorders are more common among women (Table 29-1). Major depression may begin at any age, but the prevalence is highest among elderly persons, followed by those 30 to 40 years of age and, in recent years, an increased number of 15- to 19-year-olds.[9] Lifetime prevalence rates for major depressive disorders are 15% to 20%.[4] Point prevalence rates for major depression in urban U.S populations are 2% to 4% for men and 4% to 6% for women.[4] After the age of 55 years, depression starts to occur more commonly in men.[9] About one third of depressed persons require hospitalization; 30% follow a chronic course with residual symptoms and social impairment.[3,4,9,10]

The prevalence of major depression is fairly consistent across races and cultures. However, this disorder occurs with greater frequency among recent immigrants and the displaced.[9] No evidence suggests significant geographic variability, except in seasonal affective disorder, which is due to limited exposure to the sun during the winter in the northern states. No clear association with social class has been found, but major depression is associated with poverty and unemployment as significant stressors.[9] Risk factors include current stress burden; history of early trauma, neglect, abuse, or deprivation; personal and family history of mood and anxiety disorders; medical and psychiatric disorders; and personality disorder.[10]

The lifetime prevalence of dysthymia, a chronic, milder form of depression, is 2.2% in women and 4.1% in men.[2] Approximately 0.4% to 1.6% of adults in the United States have bipolar disorder.[2] In contrast with major depression, which is more than twice as common in women as in men, bipolar disorder occurs almost with equal frequency in both sexes. Bipolar disorders are much less common than major depression (see Table 29-1).[4,8,10]

TABLE 29-1 Epidemiology of Mood Disorders

Variable	Depressive Disorders	Bipolar Disorders
Prevalence	Major depression • Point prevalence: Men: 2.0-4.0% Women: 4.0-6.0% Older adults: 11-15% • Lifetime prevalence: Overall rate: 15-20% • More common in divorced or separated persons Dysthymia • Point prevalence: Men: 5.0% Women: 8.0%	Bipolar illness • Lifetime prevalence: 0.6-0.9% • May be as high as 1-10% if all subtypes are included • Annual incidence: Men: 9-15 cases per 100,000 Women: 7.4-32 cases per 100,000 • More common in upper socioeconomic groups • Equal among races • High rates of divorce Cyclothymia • Lifetime prevalence: 0.4-3.5%
Age at onset	Late 20s or 30s Childhood possible May have much later onset Higher rate and earlier onset for persons born after 1940 than for those born before	Late teens or early 20s Childhood possible Cyclothymia may precede late onset of overt mania or depression
Family and genetic studies	Unipolar patients tend to have relatives with major depression and dysthymic disorder and fewer with bipolar disorder. Early onset, recurrent course, and psychotic depression appear to be heritable.	Bipolar patients have many relatives with bipolar disorder, cyclothymia, unipolar depression, and schizoaffective disorder
Twin studies	Concordance in monozygotic twins: • Recurrent depression: 59% • Single episode only: 33% Concordance rate for identical (monozygotic) twins is 4 times greater than for fraternal (dizygotic) twins	72% concordance in monozygotic twins, 19% in same sex dizygotic twins

Data from Schiffer RB: Psychiatric disorders in medical practice. In Goldman L, Ausiello D, editors: Cecil textbook of medicine, *ed 23, Philadelphia, Saunders, 2008; and Kahn DA: Mood disorders. In Cutler JL, Marcus ER:* Saunders text and review: psychiatry, *Philadelphia, Saunders, 1999.*

Etiology

Several theories have been presented to explain the origin of mood disorders. Reduced brain concentrations of norepinephrine and serotonin (neurotransmitters) for some time have been believed to cause depression. Increased levels of these neurotransmitters have contributed to the onset of mania. The causes of depression and mania now appear to be complex.[4,8,10] Current research focuses on the interactions of norepinephrine and serotonin with a variety of other brain systems and on abnormalities in the function or quantity of receptors for these transmitters. Thyrotropin release of thyroid-stimulating hormone and cortisol release by corticotropin-releasing factor and adrenocorticotropin over a long period may be associated with the development of depression. This model suggests that depression is the result of a stress reaction that has gone on too long.[3,4,9,10]

Evidence for a genetic predisposition to bipolar disorder is significant. The concordance rate for monozygotic twin pairs approaches 80%, and segregation analyses are consistent with autosomal dominant transmission. Multiple genes are likely to be involved, with strongest evidence for loci on chromosomal arms 18p, 18q, 4p, 4q, 5q, 8p, and 21q.[3]

Positron emission tomography (PET) studies show decreased metabolic activity in the caudate nuclei and frontal lobes in depressed patients that returns to normal with recovery. Single-photon emission computed tomography (SPECT) studies show comparable changes in blood flow.[3]

Psychosocial theory focuses on loss as the cause of depression in vulnerable persons. Mania receives much less attention because it is thought to be more of a biologically caused disorder.[3,4,8,10]

CLINICAL PRESENTATION AND MEDICAL MANAGEMENT

Depressive Disorders

The *Diagnostic and Statistical Manual of Mental Disorders*, fourth edition, text revision (DSM-IV-TR), lists three types of depressive disorders: *major depression*, *dysthymic disorder*, and *depression not otherwise specified* (NOS).[11] Major depression (unipolar) is one of the primary mood disorders. Patients with major depression are depressed most of the day, show a marked decrease in interest or pleasure in most activities, exhibit a marked

BOX 29-1 Diagnostic Criteria for Depressive Disorders

Major Depressive Episode

- At least five of the following symptoms have been present during the same 2-week period (one of the symptoms must be depressed mood or loss of interest or pleasure):
  - Depressed mood most of the day
  - Marked loss of interest or pleasure in most or all activities most of the day
  - Significant weight gain or loss when not dieting, or change in appetite
  - Insomnia or hypersomnia nearly every day
  - Psychomotor agitation or retardation nearly every day that is observable by others
  - Fatigue or loss of energy nearly every day
  - Feelings of worthlessness or excessive guilt feelings
  - Inability to think or concentrate, or indecisiveness
  - Recurrent thoughts of death, or suicidal ideation without a specific plan, or with a plan, or attempted
- An organic factor did not initiate or maintain the disturbance.
- The disturbance is not a normal reaction to the death of a loved one.
- At no time during the disturbance have there been delusions or hallucinations for as long as 2 weeks in the absence of prominent mood symptoms (i.e., before the mood symptoms developed or after they have remitted.)
- Not superimposed on schizophrenia, schizophreniform disorder, delusional disorder, or psychotic disorder; no other specific diagnosis

Dysthymia

- Depressed mood for most of the day for at least 2 years
- Presence, while depressed, of two or more of the following:
  - Poor appetite
  - Insomnia or hypersomnia
  - Low energy or fatigue
  - Low self-esteem
  - Poor concentration or difficulty making decisions
  - Feelings of hopelessness
- During the 2-year period, the person has never been without the symptoms for more than 2 months at a time.
- No major depressive episode has been present during the first 2 years of the disturbance.
- There has not been an intermixed manic episode.
- The disturbance does not occur during the course of a psychotic disorder.
- The symptoms are not caused by the physiologic effects of a substance.
- The symptoms cause significant distress or functional impairment.

From Schiffer RB: Psychiatric disorders in medical practice. In Goldman L, Ausiello D, editors: Cecil textbook of medicine, *ed 23, Philadelphia, 2008, Saunders.*

gain or loss in weight, and suffer from insomnia or hypersomnia (Box 29-1). These symptoms must be present for at least 2 weeks before a diagnosis of major depression can be made. About 50% to 80% of persons who have had a major depressive episode will have at least one more depressive episode; 20% of these people will have a subsequent manic episode and should be reclassified as bipolar. A major depression usually will last about 8 to 9 months if the patient is not treated. Dysthymia represents a chronic, milder form of depression with symptoms that last at least 2 years (see Box 29-1). Depression NOS is a form of depression that falls short of the diagnostic criteria for major depression and has been too brief for dysthymic disorder.[9,12] A form of depression called *seasonal affective disorder* may occur in areas of the country that have limited amounts of sunlight during the winter.[9]

Bipolar Disorder

The DSM-IV lists four types of bipolar disorder: bipolar I, bipolar II, cyclothymic, and bipolar disorder NOS (Figure 29-1).[11] Figure 29-2, *A* shows the normal variation in moods. Bipolar I disorder consists of recurrences of mania and major depression or mixed states that occur at different times in the patient, or a mixture of symptoms that occur at the same time (see Figure 29-2, *B*). The essential feature of a manic episode is a distinct period during which the affected person's mood is elevated and expansive or irritable (Table 29-2). Associated symptoms of the manic syndrome include inflated self-esteem, grandiosity, a decreased need for sleep, excessive speech, flight of ideas, distractibility, psychomotor agitation, and excessive involvement in pleasurable activities. During a manic episode, the mood often is described as euphoric, cheerful, or "high." The expansive quality of the mood is characterized by unceasing and unselective enthusiasm for interacting with people. However, the predominant mood disturbance may be irritability and anger. Speech often is loud, rapid, and difficult to interpret, and behavior may be intrusive and demanding. Style of dress often is colorful and strange, and long periods without sleep are common. Poor judgment may lead to financial and legal problems. Drug and alcohol abuse also are commmon in this patient population.[3,4,11,13]

Bipolar II disorder (see Figure 29-2, *C*) consists of recurrences of major depression and hypomania (mild

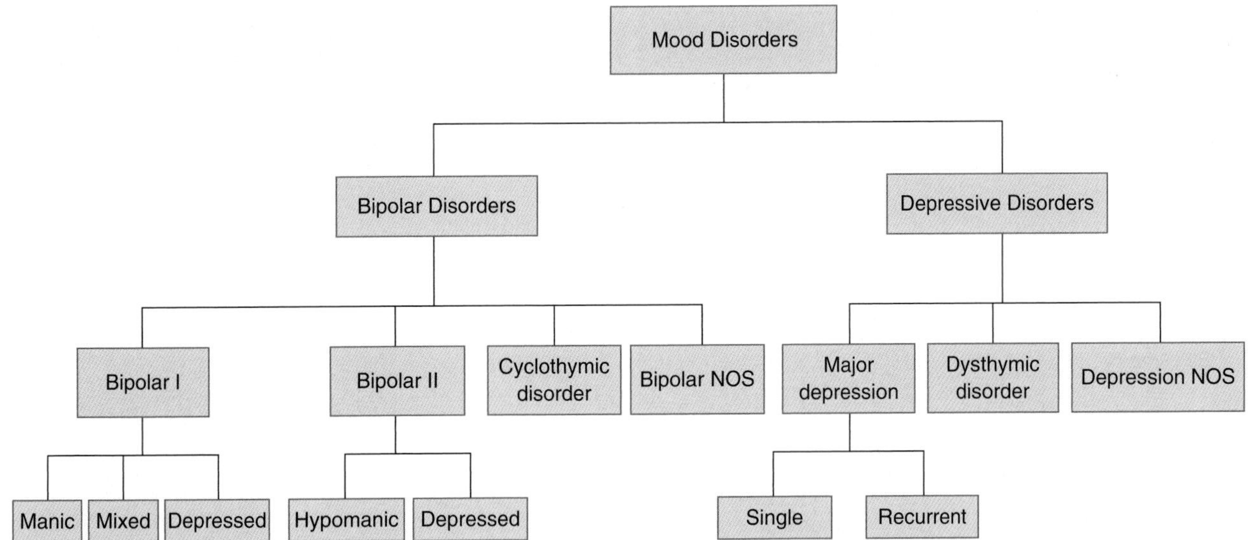

FIGURE 29-1 Mood disorders listed in the *Diagnostic and Statistical Manual of Mental Disorders,* fourth edition (DSM-IV-TR). Patients with bipolar disorder have had at least one episode of mania or hypomania. Cyclothymic disorder consists of recurrent brief episodes of hypomania and mild depression. Major depression usually is recurrent but sometimes happens as a single lifetime episode. Dysthymic disorder is mild depression that lasts at least 2 years.

TABLE 29-2 Clinical Features of Hypomania and Mania

Feature	Hypomania	Mania
Appearance	May be unremarkable Demeanor may be cheerful	Often striking Clothes may reflect mood state Demeanor may be cheerful Disordered and fatigued in severe states
Behavior	Increased sociability and loss of inhibition	Overactivity and excitement Social loss of inhibition
Speech	May be talkative Mild elation or irritability	Often pressured, with flight of ideas Elated or irritable Boundless optimism Typically, no diurnal pattern May be labile
Vegetative signs	Increased appetite Reduced need for sleep Increased libido	Increased appetite Reduced need for sleep Increased libido
Psychotic symptoms	Not present Thoughts may have an expansive quality	Thoughts may have an expansive quality Delusions and second-person auditory hallucinations may be present, often grandiose in nature Schneiderian First Rank (symptoms associated with schizophrenia) symptoms found in 10-20%
Cognition	Mild distractibility	Marked distractibility More marked disturbances in severe states
Insight	Usually preserved	Insight often lost, especially in severe states

From Mackin P, Young A; Bipolar disorders. In Wright P, Stern J, Phelan M, editors: Core psychiatry, *ed 2, Edinburgh, 2005, Elsevier.*

mania). Cyclothymic disorder manifests as recurrent brief episodes of hypomania (see Table 29-2) and mild depression. Bipolar disorder NOS refers to partial syndromes, such as recurrent hypomania without depression. Patients with bipolar disorder have at least one episode of mania or hypomania.[3,8,11,13]

The diagnosis of bipolar disorder is made as soon as the patient has one manic episode, even if that person has never had a depressive episode. Most patients who become manic will eventually experience depression. However, about 10% of patients in whom bipolar disorder is diagnosed appear to have only manic episodes.[14]

Men tend to have a greater number of manic episodes and women, more numerous depressive episodes. Untreated patients with bipolar disorder will experience a mean of nine affective episodes during their lifetime.

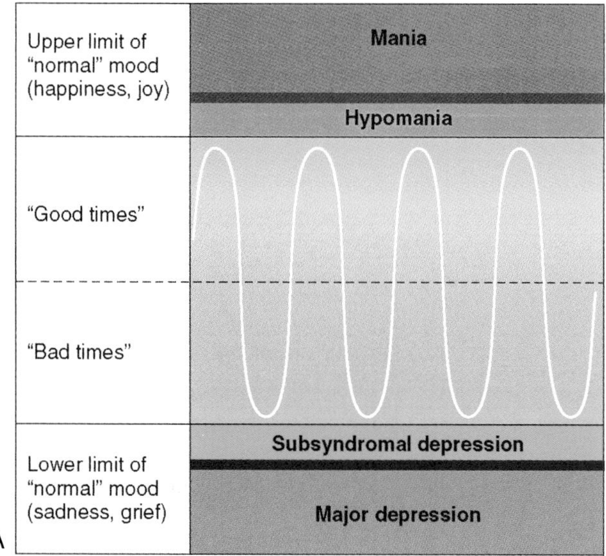

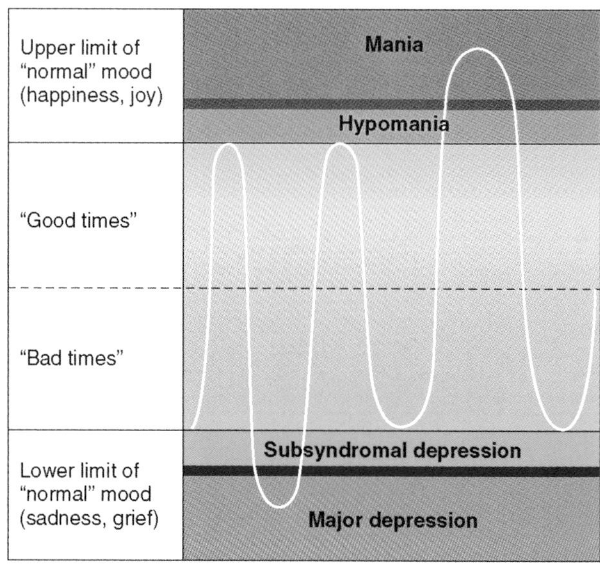

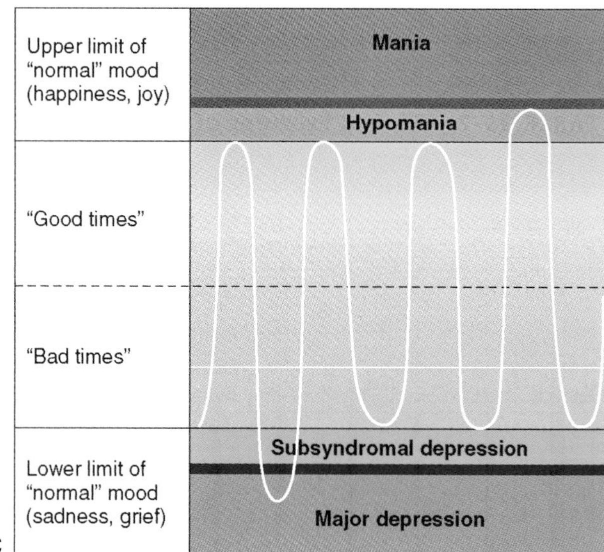

FIGURE 29-2 A, Normal mood cycles. **B,** Bipolar type I disorder. **C,** Bipolar type II disorder. *(From Khalife S: Bipolar disorder. In Carey WD, et al, editors:* Current clinical medicine 2009—Cleveland Clinic, *ed 2, Philadelphia, 2010, Saunders.)*

The length of each cycle tends to decrease, although the number of cycles increases with age (Figure 29-3). Each affective episode lasts about 8 to 9 months. Bipolar patients have a greater number of episodes, hospitalizations, divorces, and suicides compared with unipolar patients.[15]

Treatment of Mood Disorders

Table 29-3 shows commonly used antidepressants. The first-line medication for major depression is a selective serotonin reuptake inhibitor (SSRI) such as citalopram. Sertraline, venlafaxine, and bupropion are second-line drugs that may be used in patients who fail to achieve remission with citalopram.[3,4,9-11] These agents are used primarily to treat major depression, dysthymic disorder, and depression NOS and have a limited role in depression associated with bipolar disorder that responds to an antipsychotic medication and the standard antidepressant medication fluoxetine. Drug therapy is essential in bipolar disorder for achieving two goals: (1) rapid control of symptoms in acute episodes of mania and depression and (2) prevention of future episodes or reduction in their severity and frequency. Mood disorders have a tendency to recur. Affective episodes may occur spontaneously or may be triggered by adverse events. Persons with mood disorders and their families must become aware of the early signs and symptoms of affective episodes, so that treatment can be initiated. These patients also must be made aware of the need for medication compliance and of the medication's adverse effects and possible complications.[3,4,8,10]

The mainstays of drug therapy for bipolar disorders are the mood-stabilizing drugs, which generally act on

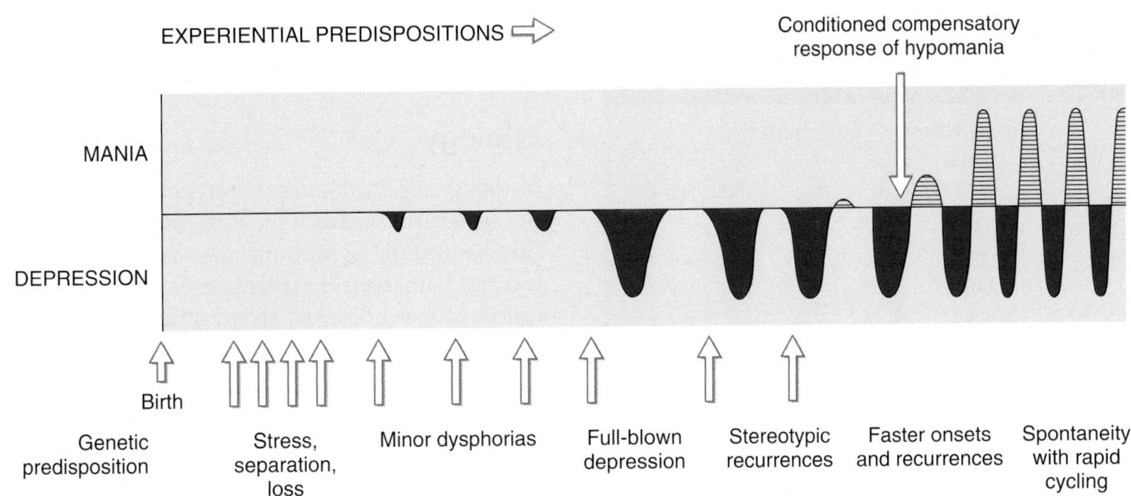

FIGURE 29-3 Natural history of recurrent mood disorders: an integrated model. Genetic factors and early environmental stress may predispose to development of a mood disorder. Early episodes are likely to be precipitated by environmental stress; later episodes are more likely to occur closer together and spontaneously, without precipitants.

both mania and depression (Table 29-4). Drugs used are lithium, valproic acid or divalproex (valproate semisodium), lamotrigine, and carbamazepine.[16] The most widely used mood stabilizer is lithium carbonate. Lithium is most helpful in patients with euphoric mania. When lithium is ineffective, or when medical problems prevent its use, one of the anticonvulsants (valproic acid or divalproex, lamotrigine, or carbamazepine), with mood stabilizing effects, can be used.[8]

Mixed depressive and manic episodes are difficult to manage. First the manic behavior needs to be stabilized, and then the depression is addressed. An atypical antipsychotic (olanzapine) or a mood stabilizer is administered to stabilize the manic behavior, and depression is addressed with a standard antidepressant drug (fluoxetine). Another approach is to use a mood stabilizer and a combination agent consisting of an antidepressant plus an atypical antipsychotic—the olanzapine-fluoxetine combination (OFC) drug available as Symbyax.[8]

Electroconvulsive therapy is an effective antimanic treatment.[17] It may be used in cases of manic violence, delirium, or exhaustion. It also is appropriate for use with patients who do not respond to medication taken for many weeks. When antidepressant drugs are given for bipolar depression, they may cause a switch to mania or a mixed state, or they may induce rapid cycling. The most common treatment for bipolar depression is an antidepressant combined with a mood stabilizer to prevent a manic switch or rapid cycling.[3,4,8]

It takes about 7 to 10 days for lithium to reach full therapeutic effectiveness. With most antidepressant drugs, a delay (10 to 21 days) is noted before full therapeutic benefits are achieved.[3,4]

Patients who have had two or three episodes of bipolar disorder, including depressive episodes, usually are treated indefinitely because of the near certainty of relapse. Lithium is the treatment of choice. About one third of patients will not experience additional episodes and are considered cured; a third of those who take lithium will experience less frequent or less severe episodes and will function well; and the remaining third of patients will continue to have frequent and severe episodes with ongoing disability.[3,4,8]

An estimated 30,000 suicides occur each year in the United States. About 70% of these involve persons with major depression. The physician must consider suicidal lethality in the management of patients with depression. In general, the risk for suicide is increased in association with the following factors: alcoholism, drug abuse, social isolation, elderly male status, terminal illness, and undiagnosed or untreated mental disorders. Patients at greatest risk are those with a history of previous suicide attempts, drug or alcohol abuse, recent diagnosis of a serious condition, loss of a loved one, or recent retirement, and those who live alone or lack adequate social support. Persons with a suicide plan and the means to carry out that plan are at greatest risk for suicide. Once medical control is attained in the patient with a mood disorder, insight-oriented psychotherapy often is initiated as an adjunct for management of the patient's condition.[4,11,17,18]

SOMATOFORM DISORDERS

DEFINITION

Persons with somatoform disorders have physical complaints for which no general medical cause is present. Associated unconscious psychological factors contribute to the onset, exacerbation, or maintenance of physical symptoms. The following conditions are regarded as somatoform disorders: somatization, conversion disorder, pain disorder, and hypochondriasis (Table 29-5).

TABLE 29-3 Commonly Used Antidepressants (by Structural Group)

Drug	Trade Name	Comments
Tricyclic		
Amitriptyline	Elavil	
Trimipramine	Surmontil	
Desipramine	Norpramin	
Doxepin	Sinequan	
Imipramine	Tofranil	
Nortriptyline	Pamelor	
Protriptyline	Vivactil	
Tetracyclic		
Maprotiline	Ludiomil	
Selective Serotonin Re-uptake Inhibitors		
Escitalopram	Lexapro	
Fluoxetine	Prozac	
Fluvoxamine	Luvox	
Paroxetine	Paxil	
Sertraline	Zoloft	
MAOIs		Patients taking these drugs must be on a tyramine-free diet.
Phenelzine	Nardil	
Tranylcypromine	Parnate	
Atypical or Nontricyclic		
Nefazodone	Serzone	As effective as imipramine
Venlafaxine	Effexor	SNRI; may be effective in treatment of resistant depression
Amoxapine	Asendin	
Bupropion	Wellbutrin	May be especially helpful for atypical depression
Mirtazapine	Remeron	Increase at 1- to 2-week intervals.
Trazodone	Desyrel	Helpful as a second drug for sleep disturbance
Duloxetine	Cymbalta	Additionally useful in pain syndromes

MAOIs, Monoamine oxidase inhibitors; *SNRI,* Serotonin-norepinephrine reuptake inhibitor.
Data from Schiffer RB: Psychiatric disorders in medical practice. In Goldman L, Ausiello D, editors: Cecil textbook of medicine, *ed 23, Philadelphia, 2008, Saunders.*

Patients with a somatization disorder experience multiple, unexplained somatic symptoms that may last for years.[3,4,19]

EPIDEMIOLOGY

Incidence and Prevalence

The prevalence of somatoform disorders is 5%.[3] Most of these occur in women. Patients with symptoms that do not meet the full criteria for somatization disorder are much more common. Conversion disorder, pain disorder, and hypochondriasis appear to be more common than somatization disorder.[3]

Etiology

In this group of disorders, physical symptoms suggest a physical disorder for which no underlying physical basis can be found. Symptoms are linked to psychological factors. Somatization therefore is defined as the manifestation of psychological stress in somatic symptoms.

A conversion reaction results when a psychological conflict or need is expressed as an alteration or loss of physical function, suggesting a physical disorder. A person who views a traumatic event, for example, but has a conflict about acknowledging that event may develop a conversion disorder of blindness. In this instance, the symptom of blindness has symbolic value and is a representation of and a partial solution to the underlying psychological conflict. By contrast, patients with hypochondriasis or a factitious (self-inflicted) disorder are aware of the nature of their problem but may be unable to control it. Many patients with pain disorder describe a history of a physical injury that precedes later onset of pain. The onset of pain is accompanied by environmental stress or emotional conflict.[3,4,19]

CLINICAL PRESENTATION AND MEDICAL MANAGEMENT

Somatization Disorder

Somatization consists of multiple signs and symptoms and usually begins before the age of 30 years. Patients experience multiple, unexplained physical manifestations of illness or disease, which may include pain, diarrhea, bloating, vomiting, sexual dysfunction, blindness, deafness, weakness, paralysis, or coordination problems. Somatization disorder is a serious psychiatric illness. Many patients have concurrent anxiety, depression, or personality disorder.[3,4,19]

Conversion Disorder

Conversion disorder is a monosymptomatic somatoform disorder that affects the voluntary motor system or sensory functions. The patient may experience blindness, deafness, paralysis, or an inability to speak or to walk. Symptoms suggest a physical condition, but the cause is psychological. The somatic manifestation, which is not intentionally produced, typically is a symbolic representation that relieves an underlying emotional conflict.[3,4,19]

Pain Disorder

Pain disorder causes the patient significant distress in important areas of functioning such as social and

TABLE 29-4 Initial Treatment Guidelines for Bipolar Disorder

Drug/Indication Category	Step 1		Step 2		Step 3
	Starting Dose	Target	Drug	Starting Dose	Additional Options
Depression					
Lithium	300-450 mg twice daily	Serum level >0.8 mEq/L	OFC*	6 mg/25 mg at bedtime	Combinations of lithium, OFC, quetiapine
Lamotrigine	25 mg once a day Initial and target doses may be affected by concomitant medications	Dose 50-200 mg/day	Quetiapine (pending FDA approval for bipolar disorder type 1 and type 2 depression)	100 mg at bedtime; increase to 300 mg at bedtime by day 3	Add traditional antidepressant† to one or more of these (Step 1 or Step 2) ECT
Mania					
Lithium	300-450 mg three times a day	Serum level generally 1.0-1.5 mEq/L	Choose two of the following in combination: Lithium VPA or divalproex AAP (excluding olanzapine and clozapine)		Other two-drug combinations (choose from lithium, VPA, AAPs, carbamazepine, oxcarbamazepine, topiramate)
VPA	500 mg three times a day				
Divalproex	750 mg at bedtime				
AAP (excluding clozapine and aripiprazole)	Initial dosing varies				ECT Clozapine Triple-drug therapy

*FDA-approved for bipolar disorder type 1 depression.
†Traditional antidepressants include selective serotonin reuptake inhibitors, serotonin-norepinephrine uptake inhibitors, bupropion, venlafacine, and mirtazapine.
AAP, Atypical antipsychotic [agent]; *ECT,* Electroconvulsive therapy; *FDA,* U.S. Food and Drug Administration; *OFC,* Olanzapine-fluoxetine combination; *VPA,* Valproic acid.
From Khalife S, Singh V, Muzina DJ: Bipolar disorder. In Carey WD, et al, editors: *Current clinical medicine 2009—Cleveland Clinic,* Philadelphia, 2009, Saunders.

occupational activities. In patients with pain disorder, no organic disease can be identified. Often, a stressful event precedes the onset of pain. Pain often results in secondary gain in the form of increased attention and sympathy from others.[3,4,19]

Hypochondriasis

Patients with hypochondriasis are preoccupied with the fear or belief that they have a serious disease. Their misinterpretations of normal bodily functions generally are to blame.[3,4,19]

Factitious Disorder

Factitious disorder consists of intentional self-harm that is produced by infliction of physical, chemical, or thermal injury. It involves the voluntary production of signs and symptoms (physical injury or psychological symptoms) without external incentives such as avoidance of responsibility or financial gain. Factitious disorder is more common among men and occurs more often in health care workers. The skin is the most common site for injury.

Treatment

Treatment of patients with somatoform disorders often requires multiple therapeutic modalities, including psychotherapy for their interpersonal and psychological problems. Medication for the treatment of underlying depressive disorder also may be needed. Group therapy is beneficial in some cases. Unneeded medical or surgical treatment must not be rendered and will not correct the problem. Such treatment is costly and may lead to significant associated complications.[3,4,19]

SCHIZOPHRENIA

DEFINITION

Disordered thinking, inappropriate emotional responses, hallucinations, delusions, and bizarre behavior characterize schizophrenia. The lifetime prevalence rate for schizophrenic disorders is about 1% to 1.5% (across all cultures and both genders). Worldwide, the prevalence is 0.85%.[3] Onset usually is during adolescence or early adulthood. Studies have suggested an earlier onset in men than in women.[3]

TABLE 29-5 Somatoform Disorders

Somatoform Disorder	Features
Somatization disorder	Chronic multisystem disorder characterized by complaints of pain, and gastrointestinal and sexual dysfunction. Onset usually is early in life, and psychosocial and vocational achievements are limited. Rarely affects men. Diagnostic criteria include four pain symptoms plus two gastrointestinal symptoms, plus one sexual-reproductive symptom, plus one pseudoneurologic symptom.
Conversion disorder	Syndrome of symptoms or deficits mimicking neurologic or medical illness in which psychological factors are judged to be of etiologic importance. Patients report isolated symptoms that have no physical cause (blindness, deafness, stocking anesthesia) and that do not conform to known anatomic pathways or physiologic mechanisms. In a group of such patients followed over time, a physical disease process will become apparent in 10% to 50%.
Pain disorder	Clinical syndrome characterized predominantly by pain in which psychological factors are judged to be of etiologic importance
Hypochondriasis	Chronic preoccupation with the idea of having serious disease. This preoccupation usually is poorly amenable to reassurance. May consist of a morbid preoccupation with physical symptoms or bodily functions. Can be described as "illness is a way of life."
Body dysmorphic disorder	Preoccupation with an imagined or exaggerated defect in physical appearance
Other somatoform-like disorders	
Factitious disorder	Intentional production or feigning of physical or psychological signs when external reinforcers (e.g., avoidance of responsibility, financial gain) are not clearly present Voluntary production of symptoms without external incentive More common in men and seen in health care workers more often Skin lesions more common than oral (oral lesions cannot be seen) Oral lesions include those associated with self-extraction of teeth, picking at the gingiva with fingernails, nail file gingival injury, and application of caustic substances to the lips.
Malingering	Intentional production or feigning of physical or psychological signs when external reinforcers (e.g., avoidance of responsibility, financial gain) are present
Dissociative disorders	Disruptions of consciousness, memory, identity, or perception judged to be due to psychological factors

From Schiffer RB: Psychiatric disorders in medical practice. In Goldman L, Ausiello D, editors: Cecil textbook of medicine, *ed 23, Philadelphia, 2008, Saunders, and Scully C, Cawson RA:* Medical problems in dentistry, *ed 5, Edinburgh, 2005, Churchill Livingstone.*

EPIDEMIOLOGY

Etiology

The cause of schizophrenia is not known, but it appears to involve the interaction of genetic and environmental factors. Evidence for a genetic relationship has come from family, twin, and adoption studies. Family studies have shown a 13% risk for schizophrenia in children with one parent with schizophrenia. If both parents are schizophrenic, the risk increases to 46%.[20] The risk of developing schizophrenia for first-degree relatives is 5% to 10%, and for second-degree relatives, it is 2% to 4%. Concordance in twins for schizophrenia is 46% for identical twins and 14% for nonidentical twins. However, 89% of persons with schizophrenia do not have a parent with the disease, and 81% do not have a parent or a sibling with the disease.[3,4,21] Despite evidence for a genetic causation, the results of molecular genetic linkage studies in schizophrenia are inconclusive. Major gene effects appear to be unlikely.[3]

The predominant biologic hypothesis for a neurophysiologic defect in schizophrenia is the dopamine hypothesis, which states that symptoms of schizophrenia are caused in part by a disturbance in dopamine-mediated neuronal pathways in the brain. This theory is supported by the blocking effect that most antipsychotic drugs have on postsynaptic dopamine receptors. The disease is more common among persons of lower socioeconomic status. A separate risk factor is the chronic stress of poverty, which may have an adverse effect on the outcomes of the illness.[20]

Schizophrenia appears to be triggered by certain environmental events in a genetically predisposed person. Drugs, medical illness, stressful psychosocial events, viral infection, and family situations characterized by conflicting and self-contradictory forms of communication have been reported to precipitate schizophrenia in susceptible people.[20] A hypothesis that has gained support relates to the cytokine activity associated with inflammatory immune processes, the cytokine hypothesis.[22]

CLINICAL PRESENTATION AND MEDICAL MANAGEMENT

According to the DSM-IV definition, schizophrenia can be diagnosed in patients who have two or more of the following symptoms for at least 1 month: hallucinations,

TABLE 29-6 Schizophrenia and Other Psychotic Disorders

Diagnostic Features of Schizophrenia			Schizoaffective and Mood Disorder Exclusion	Substance/General Medical Condition Exclusion
Characteristic Symptoms	**Social/Occupational Dysfunction**	**Duration**		
At least two of the following, each present for a major portion of the time during a 1-month period (or less if successfully treated):* Delusions Hallucinations Disorganized speech (e.g., frequent derailment, "jumping from one topic to another," or incoherence) Grossly disorganized or catatonic behavior Negative symptoms (i.e., affective flattening, alogia, or avolition)	For a significant portion of the time since the onset of the disturbance, one or more major areas of functioning (e.g., work, interpersonal relationships, self-care) are markedly below the level achieved before onset (or, when onset is in childhood or adolescence, failure to realize the expected level of interpersonal, academic, or occupational achievement).	Continuous signs of the disturbance persist for at least 6 months. This 6-month period must include at least 1 month of characteristic symptoms as described above (i.e., active-phase symptoms) and may include periods of prodromal or residual symptoms. During these prodromal or residual periods, signs of the disturbance may be manifested by only negative symptoms or two or more of the characteristic symptoms present in an attenuated form (e.g., odd beliefs, unusual perceptual experiences).	Schizoaffective disorder and mood disorder with psychotic features have been ruled out because (1) no major depressive or manic episodes have occurred concurrently with the active-phase symptoms or (2) if mood episodes have occurred during active-phase symptoms, their total duration has been brief in relation to the duration of the active and residual periods.	The disturbance is not due to the direct effects of a substance (e.g., drugs of abuse, medication) or a general medical condition.

*NOTE: Only one characteristic symptom is required if delusions are bizarre or hallucinations consist of a voice keeping a running commentary on the person's behavior or thoughts or involve two or more voices conversing with each other.
From Schiffer RB: Psychiatric disorders in medical practice. In Goldman L, Ausiello D, editors: Cecil textbook of medicine, *ed 23, Philadelphia, 2008, Saunders.*

delusions, disorganized speech, grossly disorganized or catatonic behavior, or negative symptoms such as affective flattening, alogia (poverty of speech, lack of additional unprompted content), or avolition (lack of desire, drive, or motivation). In addition, the patient's social or occupational functioning must have deteriorated.[21]

Patients with schizophrenia show psychotic symptoms consisting of delusions, hallucinations, incoherence, catatonic behavior, or flat or grossly inappropriate affect. Delusions and hallucinations are referred to as "positive" symptoms, and withdrawal and reduction of affective expression as "negative" symptoms. Delusions, such as thought broadcasting or being controlled by a deceased person, usually are bizarre. Hallucinations are prominent and occur throughout the day for several days or several times a week for several weeks (Table 29-6). The four types of schizophrenic disorders are *catatonic, disorganized, paranoid,* and *undifferentiated.* Patients with schizophrenic disorders show deterioration in their level of functioning at work and in social relations and self-care. They often are confused, depressed, withdrawn, anxious, and without emotion. Physically, they may grimace and pace about, or they may be rigid and catatonic. Vulnerability to a schizophrenic disorder is inherited, and life stresses appear to trigger the disorder.[20,21]

In schizophrenia, two types of thought disturbances are seen: formal thought disorder and disorder of thought content. *Formal thought disorders* affect relationships and associations among the words used to express thought. Thoughts may be strung together by incidental associations, or they may be completely unrelated. Thought blocking is common with psychotic patients. *Disorders of thought content* involve the development of delusions, which are fixed ideas that are based on incorrect perceptions of reality. Delusions, which commonly are paranoid or persecutory, also may be bizarre, somatic, grandiose, or referential (as to events that the patient believes have special significance). Perceptual disturbances in schizophrenic patients include auditory, visual, tactile, olfactory, and gustatory hallucinations. Auditory hallucinations consist of sounds heard by the patient in the absence of any real auditory stimulus. Patients may hear sounds of bells, whistles, whispers, rustlings, and other noises. The most commonly heard sound is that of voices talking. Often, visual, tactile, or olfactory hallucinations occur.[20,21]

The most common emotional change in schizophrenia is a general "blunting" or "flattening" of affect. The patient seems to be emotionally detached or distant, may appear wooden and robot-like, and may lack warmth or spontaneity. Paranoid patients may feel frightened or enraged in response to a perceived threat or a delusion of persecution. They can be very hostile and guarded to any perceived slight.[20,21]

The long-term course of illness is variable. About 25% of patients experience full remission of symptoms. Another 25% have mild residual symptoms. The remaining 50% continue to have moderate to severe symptoms.[23]

DRUGS USED TO TREAT PSYCHIATRIC DISORDERS

Drug treatment has had the most dramatic impact on control of symptoms and improvement in quality of life of patients with schizophrenia. Psychotherapy and other psychosocial treatments also are important because they provide patients with the human connection that helps them develop social skills, educates them about their illness and what to expect, and offers support throughout a long, difficult course of illness. Drug treatment of schizophrenic disorders consists of antipsychotic medications that act selectively against specific target symptoms. These drugs are effective for "positive" symptoms such as hallucinations and psychotic agitation but are noneffective for "negative" symptoms such as social withdrawal or anhedonia (inability to get pleasure from or find interest in activities). The newer atypical antipsychotic medications (clozapine, olanzapine, risperidone, and quetiapine) are quite effective for control of both "positive" and "negative" symptoms of schizophrenia and are associated with minimal movement adverse effects. Antipsychotic drugs are described later in this chapter.[20,21]

Antidepressant Medications (Excluding Those for Bipolar Depression)

Tricyclic Antidepressants. The group of drugs that are used primarily to treat depression are the tricyclic antidepressants (see Table 29-3). The first tricyclic used to treat depression was imipramine. Tricyclics inhibit neural reuptake of norepinephrine and 5-hydroxytryptamine (5-HT), resulting in downregulation of their respective receptors. All tricyclics are equally effective in the management of depression, but these agents differ in their associated adverse effects.[16] Amitriptyline and doxepin are the most sedating, and this adverse effect is put to advantage by patients who take these drugs just before bedtime. Two combinations of drugs are available for treating depression and other psychotic symptoms. Triavil (amitriptyline plus perphenazine) is used to treat patients with depression and agitation or psychotic behavior. Limbitrol (amitriptyline plus chlordiazepoxide) is used to treat patients with depression and anxiety.[2-4] Table 29-3 summarizes the drugs used to treat depression.

Adverse effects associated with tricyclics include dry mouth, constipation, blurred vision, cardiac dysrhythmias such as tachycardia, hypotension, blurred vision, allergic reactions, and important drug interactions (Table 29-7). Tricyclic drugs should be used with caution in patients with cardiac conditions because of the associated risk for atrial fibrillation, atrial ventricular block, or ventricular tachycardia. Tricyclics can lower the seizure threshold and must be used with care in patients with a history of seizures. They can increase intraocular pressure in patients with glaucoma. Urinary retention may be increased in patients with prostate hypertrophy. Erectile or ejaculatory disturbances occur in up to 30% to 40% of patients. If used in some patients with bipolar disorder, tricyclics can reduce the time between episodes, induce manic episodes, and cause rapid cycling of the clinical course of the disorder.[2-4]

Drug interactions reported with the use of tricyclic antidepressants include the following: (1) Tricyclics may potentiate the effects of other central nervous system (CNS) depressants such as ethanol and benzodiazepines; (2) they may potentiate the actions of anticholinergic drugs such as antihistamines; (3) their levels are reduced with use of oral contraceptives, alcohol, barbiturates, and phenytoin sodium (Dilantin); and (4) they may cause other drug interactions, including potentiation of the pressor effects of sympathomimetic agents such as epinephrine and levonordefrin, blockade of the antihypertensive effects of guanethidine, and induction of a hypertensive crisis if taken with or soon after an MAO inhibitor (see Table 29-7). Overdosage with a tricyclic antidepressant can cause death from cardiac arrhythmia or respiratory failure.[2-4]

Monoamine Oxidase Inhibitors. Traditional monoamine oxidase (MAO) inhibitors, which are both nonselective and irreversible, were the first effective drugs used for the treatment of depression. Only two drugs now on the market are included in the group of MAO inhibitors: phenelzine (Nardil) and tranylcypromine (Parnate). These drugs act by inhibiting the two forms of MAO—type A and type B. Inhibition of type A MAO results in the antidepressant effects seen with MAO inhibitors. More than 80% of type A MAO must be bound to serum proteins before adverse effects can be seen clinically. Resynthesis of new enzymes takes 10 to 14 days. If a patient is changing from an MAO inhibitor drug to a tricyclic drug, 2 weeks or more must elapse after the MAO inhibitor is stopped and the tricyclic agent is begun. Significant drug interactions may occur between MAO inhibitors and opioids and sympathomimetic amines. MAO inhibitors potentiate the depressant activity of opioids. They can produce a hypertensive crisis if combined with specific sympathomimetic amines (see Table 29-7).[4,10,24]

Phenylethylamine and phenylephrine must not be given to patients who are taking MAO inhibitors. MAO metabolizes these agents, and their use with an MAO inhibitor could lead to significant potentiation of their pressor effects (see Chapter 4). These adverse effects are not seen with epinephrine and levonordefrin. Many OTC cold remedies contain phenylephrine and should

TABLE 29-7 Adverse Effects and Drug Interactions of Antidepressant Drugs

Category of Complications	Tetracyclics	MAO Inhibitors	SSRIs	SNRIs
Adverse effects	Dry mouth Nausea and vomiting Constipation Urinary retention Postural hypotension Nervousness Insomnia Drowsiness Sleepiness Reflux Anorgasmia (women) Erectile problems (men) Loss of libido Gynecomastia (men)	Dry mouth Nausea and vomiting Constipation Urinary retention Drowsiness Confusion Anorexia Weight gain Tremor Fatigue Insomnia Anorgasmia (women) Erectile problems (men)	Dry mouth Nausea and vomiting Diarrhea Anorexia Weight loss Blurred vision Insomnia Nervousness Sexual dysfunction Sweating Sedation (paroxetine) Akathisia	Dry mouth Nausea and vomiting Constipation Somnolence Weight loss/ gain Blurred vision Dizziness Anorexia Impotence Loss of libido
Serious adverse effects	Mania Seizures Obstructive jaundice Leukopenia Tachycardia Arrhythmias Myocardial infarction Stroke	Mania Hypertensive crisis Orthostatic hypotension Peripheral edema Anemia Leukopenia Thrombocytopenia Agranulocytosis	Mania Seizures Orthostatic hypotension Anemia Bleeding (platelet effect) Hypothyroidism	Mania Hypertension (venlafaxine)
Drug interactions				
Barbiturates	CNS depression	CNS depression		
Benzodiazepines	CNS depression	CNS depression	CNS depression	
SSRIs	Dangerous—do not use	Dangerous—do not use		Serotonin syndrome Seizures
SNRIs	Dangerous—do not use	Dangerous—do not use	Dangerous—do not use	
MAO inhibitors	Anticholinergic toxicity	Do not use two or more agents		Dangerous—do not use
Heterocyclics	Dangerous—do not use	Dangerous—do not use		Dangerous—do not use
Anticonvulsants	Interferes with action of anticonvulsants	Interferes with action of anticonvulsants		
Antihistamines	CNS depression	CNS depression		
Beta blockers	Anticholinergic toxicity	Sinus bradycardia	Bradycardia	
Warfarin	Warfarin metabolism inhibited—can lead to increased INR values		Warfarin metabolism inhibited—can lead to increase in INR values	
Cimetidine	Inhibits clearance—can lead to toxicity		Inhibits clearance—can lead to overdosage	
Erythromycin	Interferes with action of the antibiotic			
Opioid analgesics	Increase sedative effect			
Vasoconstrictors	Actions are enhanced	Actions are enhanced		
• Epinephrine	Use with caution	Use with caution		
• Levonordefrin		Best to avoid		
• Phenylephrine		Avoid		
Interactions involving foods and beverages				
Tyramine	Avoid	Hypertension/arrhythmias; must avoid these agents		
Caffeine	Avoid			
Ethanol	CNS depression	CNS depression		

CNS, Central nervous system; *INR,* International normalized ratio; *MAO,* Monoamine oxidase; *SNRIs,* Serotonin-norepinephrine reuptake inhibitors; *SSRIs,* Selective serotonin reuptake inhibitors.

not be prescribed for patients who are taking MAO inhibitors (see Table 29-7).

Tyramine is a naturally occurring amine that releases norepinephrine from sympathetic nerve endings. Dietary tyramine is deaminated by gastrointestinal MAO-A. In the presence of MAO inhibitors, dietary tyramine is rapidly absorbed into the circulation, and a hypertensive crisis may result. Patients taking these agents must therefore avoid foods that contain high concentrations of tyramine. Such foods include aged foods such as cheeses, red wines, and pickled fish, as well as bananas and chocolate.[4,10,24]

Second-Generation Antidepressant Drugs.

Selective Serotonin Reuptake Inhibitors. The group of drugs known as selective serotonin reuptake inhibitors (SSRIs) includes fluoxetine (Prozac), sertraline (Zoloft), paroxetine (Paxil), escitalopram (Lexapro), and fluvoxamine (Luvox); these agents now are considered first-line drugs for the treatment of depression. As a group, these drugs are just as effective as the tricyclics, but they are not more effective. These drugs typically are better tolerated than the tricyclics. The tricyclics generally are more lethal in overdose than the newer antidepressants. The SSRIs are considerably more expensive than the traditional tricyclic agents. Nausea, which occurs in up to 25% of patients who use these drugs, is the most frequent problem associated with their use. Higher doses of the SSRIs more often are associated with nervousness and insomnia (see Table 29-7). Many physicians consider SSRIs to be first-line drugs for the treatment of depression.[2-4,10]

Atypical or Nontricyclic Antidepressant Agents. Amoxapine (Asendin), bupropion (Wellbutrin), trazodone (Desyrel), maprotiline (Ludiomil), nefazodone (Serzone), mirtazapine (Remeron), venlafaxine (Effexor), and duloxetine (Cymbalta) are other nontricyclics that are used as antidepressants.[16] Bupropion has a greater tendency to produce seizures than the other antidepressants. Nefazodone does not cause sexual adverse effects. Mirtazapine was one of the first antidepressants to demonstrate a significantly improved toxicity profile after overdose. However, blood dyscrasias have been reported with its use. Venlafaxine and duloxetine are drugs that belong to a newer class of antidepressants—the serotonin-norepinephrine reuptake inhibitors (see Tables 29-3 and 29-7). Venlafaxine has an adverse effect profile similar to that for the SSRIs. It also has been reported to increase blood pressure at higher doses. Duloxetine and SSRIs have been shown to cause sexual side effects in some patients, both male and female. Although usually reversible, these sexual side effects can sometimes last for months, or years, even after the drug has been completely withdrawn. This disorder is known as post-SSRI sexual dysfunction.[2-4,10] Table 29-3 shows some of the second-generation antidepressant drugs.

Bipolar Depression Drugs. There are many more FDA-approved options for the treatment of mania than for treatment of bipolar depression.[8] The combination agent OFC (i.e., the atypical antipsychotic olanzapine plus the antidepressant fluoxetine) is the only FDA-approved drug for treatment of acute bipolar depression.[8] Antidepressants, when prescribed alone, are not effective in bipolar depression. Olanzapine has been associated with weight gain and hyperglycemia. Dosing of OFC as Symbyax starts with the 6/25 formulation (olanzapine 6 mg and fluoxetine 25 mg) daily and is adjusted as needed to the 12/50 formulation (see Table 29-4).[8] Other atypical antipsychotics may serve as potential antidepressant agents for management of bipolar depression.[8]

Mood-Stabilizing Drugs

Lithium. Lithium has some antidepressant effects, but it is primarily used for the treatment of patients with bipolar disorder. Its mode of action is unclear. Lithium is used to treat acute manic episodes and to prevent manic episodes in patients with bipolar disorder. It is effective when used alone in 60% to 80% of patients with classic bipolar disorder (see Table 29-4). Lithium should not be used if renal disease is present. Lower doses must be used in older patients. The dose ranges from 600 to 3000 mg/day, and full therapeutic effect is attained in 7 to 10 days. The patient who is on maintenance therapy should be evaluated every 3 to 6 months for serum levels of lithium, sodium, potassium, creatinine, thyroxine (T_4), thyroid-stimulating hormone, and free T_4 index. Medical complications associated with long-term lithium use include nontoxic goiter and hypothyroidism, arrhythmia, T wave depression, and vasopressin-resistant nephrogenic diabetes insipidus. All of these complications are related to the effects of lithium on adenylate cyclase activity. Drugs that interact with lithium include erythromycin and nonsteroidal anti-inflammatory drugs (NSAIDs), which increase serum lithium levels, possibly leading to toxicity.[3,4,8,13]

Carbamazepine. Carbamazepine, an anticonvulsant drug, has been successfully used in the treatment of manic episodes in bipolar patients who do not respond to lithium or who cannot take lithium because of associated complications. The dose is 600 to 1600 mg/day. Adverse effects include nausea, blurred vision, ataxia, leukopenia, and aplastic anemia.[3,4,8,13]

Valproic Acid and Divalproex. Valproic acid is used as an anticonvulsant and mood-stabilizing drug, primarily in the treatment of epilepsy and bipolar disorder. It is marketed under the brand names Depakote, Depakote ER, Depakene, Depacon, Depakine, and Stavzor. It is used when lithium cannot be tolerated by the patient. Starting dosage for valproic acid is 500 mg three times a day.[8] Common side effects are dyspepsia and weight gain. Less common are fatigue, peripheral edema, acne, dizziness, drowsiness, hair loss, headaches, nausea, sedation, and tremors. Rarely, valproic acid can cause blood dyscrasias, impaired liver function, jaundice, and thrombocytopenia. Valproic acid should not be used with the benzodiazepine clonazepam and aspirin, to avoid adverse effects.[8] Divalproex sodium consists of valproate semisodium, a compound of sodium valproate, and valproic acid in a 1:1 molar relationship in an enteric-coated tablet form.

Lamotrigine. Lamotrigine is a anticonvulsant drug used to treat epilepsy and bipolar disorder. It is marketed as Lamictal. It is an effective mood stabilizer and is the only drug approved for this purpose since the FDA approved lithium about 30 years ago.[8] Lamotrigine is approved by the FDA for the maintance treatment of bipolar disorder type 1. The starting dosage of lamotrigine ranges from 25 mg to 300 mg daily.[8] Common side effects include headaches, body aches and cramps, hysteria, muscle aches, abdominal pain, back pain; dizziness and lack of coordination; acne, rash and skin irritation; sleepiness, insomnia, vivid dreams or nightmares, night sweats; dry mouth, mouth ulcers, damage to tooth enamel; fatigue, memory and cognitive problems; blurred or double vision; irritability, weight changes, hair loss, changes in libido, frequent urination, nausea, fever, tremor, appetite changes, and other side effects. In rare cases, lamotrigine has been known to cause the dangerous drug eruptions, Stevens-Johnson syndrome and toxic epidermal necrolysis. Drug interactions include those with hormonal forms of birth control, carbamazepine, divalproex, oxcarbazepine, phenobarbital, phenytoin, rifampin, and valproic acid.

Antipsychotic (Neuroleptic) Drugs. The introduction of chlorpromazine in the 1950s revolutionized the practice of psychiatry. Other agents have been introduced since chlorpromazine, but none represents any real improvement beyond this prototypical agent.[16] The popularity of these drugs is highlighted by the fact that two thirds of all prescriptions for antidepressant and antipsychotic (neuroleptic) drugs are written by physicians other than psychiatrists. Antipsychotic drugs appear to work by antagonizing the effects of dopamine in the basal ganglia and limbic portions of the forebrain. Because of significant adverse reactions associated with their use, these agents should be used only when they are clearly the drugs of choice[4,24,25]

The antipsychotic drugs are categorized as first-generation (typical) or second-generation (atypical). The following are examples of typical antipsychotic drugs: chlorpromazine (Thorazine), thioridazine (Mellaril), fluphenazine (Prolixin), and haloperidol (Haldol). Clozapine (Clozaril), risperidone (Risperdal), olanzapine (Zyprexa) and quetiapine (Seroquel) are examples of atypical antipsychotic drugs.[16] In general, the typical antipsychotic drugs are more likely to cause extrapyramidal symptoms of all types. Although the atypical drugs are much less likely to cause such symptoms, their use is not without risk for these and other adverse effects.[26]

Antipsychotic drugs sedate, tranquilize, blunt emotional expression, attenuate aggressive and impulsive behavior, and cause disinterest in the environment. They leave higher intellectual functions intact but ameliorate the bizarre behavior and thinking of psychotic patients. All of these drugs have significant anticholinergic adverse effects and produce dystonias and extrapyramidal symptoms. Commonly used antipsychotic drugs are shown in Table 29-8.[4,24,25]

Adverse effects of the antipsychotic drugs are numerous and often significant (Table 29-9). Patients become sedated, lethargic, and drowsy when first placed on these drugs; however, after several days, tolerance to these effects emerges. The anticholinergic actions produced by these drugs include dry mouth, postural hypotension, constipation, and urinary retention. Other adverse effects observed are obstructive jaundice, retinal pigmentation, lenticular opacity, skin pigmentation, and male impotence.[3,4,13]

The extrapyramidal adverse effects (motor or movement disorders) include acute and chronic conditions. During the first 5 days of treatment with an antipsychotic agent, acute muscular dystonic reactions or a Parkinson-like syndrome may occur. Akathisia, or extreme motor restlessness, also may develop early in treatment. Clinical manifestations consist of involuntary repetitive movements of the lips (lip smacking), the tongue (tongue thrusting), the extremities, and the trunk. This risk increases for patients older than 60 years of age and for those with preexisting CNS disease (70% risk). Many of the acute extrapyramidal adverse effects are reversible if the drug is stopped, or if anticholinergic agents are given.[3,4,26]

Tardive dyskinesia is the most common late extrapyramidal adverse effect associated with the use of antipsychotic drugs.[3,4,26] It usually occurs after antipsychotic medication has been used for several years. The chief sign is involuntary movements of the lips, tongue, mouth, jaw, upper and lower extremities, or trunk. Classic tardive dyskinesia affects the buccal, lingual, and masticatory muscles, leading to "flycatcher's tongue," "bon-bon sign," grimaces, or chewing movements. Flycatcher's tongue refers to darting of the tongue into and out of the mouth. The bon-bon sign is the pushing of the tongue against the cheek wall, so that it looks as though a piece of candy is pressed against the cheek. An early sign of tardive dyskinesia is wormlike movement of the tongue within the mouth. Tardive dyskinesia develops in about 20% of schizophrenic patients who receive antipsychotics over a period of years. Patients treated with such agents will develop tardive dyskinesia at the rate of about 4% per year. Elderly patients appear to be at much higher risk for the development of tardive dyskinesia early in their treatment.[23,27,28]

Additional adverse effects of the anticholinergic antipsychotic drugs include hormone-related changes, postural hypotension, and photosensitivity (see Table 29-9). These hormonal changes are primarily the result of the effect of these drugs on prolactin and may include

TABLE 29-8 Commonly Used Antipsychotic Medications

Class	Drug	Trade Name	Side Effect(s)
Phenothiazine/aliphatic	Chlorpromazine	Thorazine	EPMD
Phenothiazine/piperazine	Perphenazine	Trilafon	EPMD
	Fluphenazine	Prolixin	EPMD
	Trifluoperazine	Stelazine	EPMD
Phenothiazine/piperidine	Thioridazine	Mellaril	EPMD, risk for retinal degeneration
	Mesoridazine	Serentil	EPMD, risk for retinal degeneration
Butyrophenone	Haloperidol	Haldol	EPMD, dysphoria
			EPMD, dysphoria
Thioxanthene	Chlorprothixene	Taractan	
	Thiothixene	Navane	
Dibenzoxazepine	Loxapine	Loxitane	
Dihydroindole	Molindone	Moban	Less likely to reduce seizure threshold
Benzisoxazole	Risperidone	Risperdal	Low incidence of EPMD effects
Dibenzodiazepine	Olanzapine	Zyprexa	Fewer EPMD effects, agranulocytosis
	Clozapine	Clozaril	Fewer EPMD effects, agranulocytosis
Diphenylbutylpiperidine	Pimozide	Orap	
Phenylindole	Quetiapine	Seroquel	Low incidence of EPMD effects
	Ziprasidone	Geodon	Low incidence of EPMD effects
Piperazinil/dihydrocarbostyril	Aripirazole	Abilify	Hyperglycemia

EPMD, Extrapyramidal movement disorder.
Data from Schiffer RB: Psychiatric disorders in medical practice. In Goldman L, Ausiello D, editors: Cecil textbook of medicine, *ed 23, Philadelphia, 2008, Saunders.*

TABLE 29-9 Adverse Reactions of Antipsychotic Drugs Based on Type of Neuroreceptor Affected

Neuroreceptor	Adverse Effects
Anticholinergic	Dry mouth Urinary hesitancy Constipation Urinary retention Dry eyes Sexual dysfunction Blurred vision Mild tachycardia Closed angle glaucoma Impaired memory and confusion
Antiserotonergic	Weight gain (antihistaminergic mechanisms also proposed)
Antiadrenergic	Dizziness Postural hypotension (may lead to falls and hip fractures in older patients) Sexual dysfunction
Antidopaminergic	Hyperprolactinemia (causes hypoestrogenemia) • *In men:* gynecomastia, impotence, loss of libido, impaired spermatogenesis • *In women:* amenorrhea, altered ovarian function, loss of libido, risk for osteoporosis Extrapyramidal syndromes (least frequent with atypical drugs—olanzapine, quetiapine, risperidone, and ziprasidone) Acute dystonia: • Parkinsonism • Akathisia • Tardive dyskinesia
Combination of receptors	Neuroleptic malignant syndrome—rigidity, fluctuating consciousness (delirium, stupor), and autonomic lability (hyperthermia, tachycardia, hypotension or hypertension, sweating, pallor, salivation, and urinary incontinence)
Other adverse effects	Agranulocytosis Cholestatic jaundice Seizures With some agents, increased risk of suicide/suicidal behavior (during induction of drug)

From Wright P, Perahia D: Psychopharmacology. In Wright P, Stern J, Phelan M, editors: Core psychiatry, *ed 2, Edinburgh, 2005, Elsevier.*

galactorrhea, missed menstrual periods, and loss of libido. Orthostatic hypotension is a potentially serious adverse effect that is most common with low-potency agents. Dehydrated patients are at greatest risk for this complication.[3,4,27]

Several atypical antipsychotic drugs, including clozapine (Clozaril), risperidone (Risperdal), olanzapine (Zyprexa), and quetiapine (Seroquel), are available for the treatment of schizophrenia. Clozapine does not cause extrapyramidal adverse effects or carry a risk for tardive dyskinesia. It also can be effective for decreasing the negative symptoms of schizophrenia. Unfortunately, use of clozapine is associated with a 1% to 2% incidence of agranulocytosis. Patients treated with clozapine must be monitored weekly with complete blood cell counts. Clozapine is effective in some schizophrenic patients who do not respond to standard antipsychotic drugs. Risperidone is a combined serotonin-dopamine antagonist. In contrast with the standard neuroleptics, which have little or no effect on the "negative" symptoms, risperidone is effective for both "negative" and "positive" symptoms of schizophrenia. All of the atypical antipsychotics have a lower affinity for binding to D_2 dopamine receptors and a lower risk for extrapyramidal adverse effects.[20,26,27]

Important drug interactions may occur in patients who are being treated with antipsychotic drugs (Table 29-10). Antacids can diminish the absorption of neuroleptic drugs from the gut. Neuroleptic drugs can decrease blood levels of warfarin sodium. Neuroleptics and tricyclic antidepressants reduce the metabolism of each other, allowing for increased plasma concentrations of both drugs. Thioridazine can prevent the metabolism of phenytoin, allowing buildup of toxic blood levels. Smoking can decrease the blood levels of antipsychotic agents. When neuroleptic drugs are used with tricyclic antidepressants or antiparkinsonian drugs, a powerful anticholinergic effect may result. Sympathomimetics such as epinephrine can result in hpotension when given to patients taking antipsychotic drugs.[3,20,21,27]

Malignant neuroleptic syndrome represents a rare but very serious adverse effect of antipsychotic drugs. This syndrome combines autonomic dysfunction, extrapyramidal dysfunction, and hyperthermia. The patient develops tachycardia, labile blood pressure, dyspnea, masked facies, tremors, muscle rigidity, catatonic behavior, dystonia, and marked elevation in temperature (up to 106° F). The syndrome was first reported in 1960; since that time, more than 200 cases have been described. It occurs after neuroleptic drugs are given in therapeutic doses. Malignant neuroleptic syndrome is most common in young male adults with mood disorders. Symptoms continue 5 to 10 days after the drug has been stopped. Reported mortality rates range from 10% to 20%. Treatment consists of stopping all neuroleptic medication, body cooling, rehydration, and treatment with bromocriptine (a dopamine agonist).[3,20,21,27]

TABLE 29-10 Significant Drug Interactions with Antipsychotic (AP) Agents

Interacting Drug/ Drug Class	Complication
Alcohol	Increases risk of hypotension and respiratory depression
Anesthetics	Increase risk of hypotension
Antiarrhythmics	Increase risk of arrhythmias
Anticonvulsants	Reduce effects of AP drug
Tricyclic antidepressants	The AP drug will increase the serum level of the tricyclic agent
Antihypertensives	Increase risk of hypotension
Anxiolytics	Increase risk of sedation Increase risk of respiratory depression
Cimetidine	Increases the antipsychotic effects of the AP drug
Opioids	Increase the sedative effects of the opioids Increase risk of respiratory depression
Erythromycin	Increases the serum level of the AP drug, risk of convulsions
Sympathomimetics (epinephrine)	Increase risk of hypotension

DENTAL MANAGEMENT

Medical Considerations

Depression. During a deep depressive episode, significant impairment of all personal hygiene, including a total lack of oral hygiene, is likely. Salivary flow may be reduced, and patients may report dry mouth, with an increased rate of dental caries and periodontal disease. In addition, complaints of glossodynia and various facial pain syndromes are common.[29]

Signs of low-grade chronic depression include tiredness even after getting enough sleep; difficulty getting up in the morning; restlessness; loss of interest in family, work, and sex; inability to make decisions; anger and resentment; chronic complaining; self-criticism; feelings of inferiority; and excessive daydreaming. Signs of more severe depression include excessive crying, change in sleeping habits, a sense of nausea precipitated by thoughts of food, weight loss without dieting, strong feelings of guilt, nightmares, thoughts about suicide, feeling unreal or in a "fog," and an inability to concentrate.[29]

Depressed patients often have poor oral hygiene because they lack interest in caring for themselves. The effects of poor oral hygiene may be compounded by xerostomia, which is an adverse effect of medications that the patient may be taking. Only small amounts of epinephrine should be used in local anesthesia, because more concentrated forms of epinephrine can cause severe hypertension when given to patients on antidepressive drugs. Sedative medication may have to be given in reduced dosages to avoid overdepression of the CNS. No medical contraindication to dental treatment during a depressive episode has been recognized. Most depressed patients, however, may be best served by addressing only their immediate dental needs during the depressive episode. Once the patient has responded to medical treatment, more complex dental procedures can be performed[29] (Box 29-2).

Patients with severe depression must be referred for medical evaluation and treatment. If the patient is not responsive to this recommendation, the problem should be shared with a family member and every attempt made to get the affected person in for medical attention. During severe depression, suicide is an ever-possible outcome; however, medical treatment can reduce this possibility.[29]

Bipolar Disorder. From a dental standpoint, lithium, which is used to manage bipolar disorders, can cause xerostomia and stomatitis. However, no adverse drug interactions occur between lithium and other agents used in dentistry other than NSAIDs and erythromycin, which can cause lithium toxicity.[24]

Patients who do not respond to lithium and those who can no longer take lithium usually are treated with a phenothiazine type of drug. Phenothiazines can cause

BOX 29-2 Dental Management

Considerations in Patients with Depression, Bipolar Disorder, and Schizophrenia

P

Patient Evaluation/Risk Assessment (see Box 1-1)

- Evaluate and determine whether psychiatric disorder exists.
- Obtain medical consultation if patient's condition is poorly controlled, if signs and symptoms point to undiagnosed condition, or if diagnosis is uncertain.

Potential Issues/Factors of Concern

A	
Allergy	No issues.
Analgesics	Avoid sedative agents or use in reduced dosage (see drugs) in patients taking antidepressant and/or antipsychotic drugs.
Anesthesia	The use of epinephrine should be limited in patients taking antidepressants or antipsychotic drugs, because hypertensive reaction (with antidepressants) or hypotensive reaction (with antipsycotics) can occur. Limit to two cartridges of 1:100,000 epinephrine (also avoid more concentrated forms of epinephrine in retraction cord or used to control bleeding).
Antibiotics	Not indicated unless acute infection is present.
Anxiety	No issues.
B	
Bleeding	Thrombocytopenia and leukopenia may occur as side effects of medications used to treat these patients. Examine for signs of these conditions.
Breathing	No issues.
Blood pressure	Check blood pressure, because hypotension may occur as result of some medications (antidepressant and antipsychotic drugs).
C	
Cardiovascular	No issues.
Chair position	Patients taking tricyclic antidepressants or MAOIs may be prone to postural hypotension with sudden changes in chair position. Support patient getting out of the dental chair.
Consultation	Patient's physician should be consulted to confirm medications and the status of control of the illness. Elective dental treatment may have to be deferred for patients with severe symptoms of mania, depression, or schizophrenia until the condition is better controlled. Confirm the need to reduce the dosage of drugs required in management of the patient's dental problems. If severe xerostomia is found, request the physician to change medication if possible. Refer patients found to be developing chronic extramedullary movement complications related to antipsychotic medications.
D	
Devices	No issues.
Drugs	Avoid or, use in reduced dosage, sedatives, hypnotics, and narcotic agents in patients taking antidepressants or antipsychotic drugs. Avoid NSAIDs, tetracycline, and metronidazole in patients taking lithium, because lithium toxicity may occur. Also, diazepam should be avoided, because hypothermia may occur. Some psychiatric drugs may cause xerostomia.
E	
Emergencies	With patients who are depressed and have shared thoughts of suicide, a relative and the patient's physician should be contacted immediately.
Equipment	No issues.
F	
Follow-up	Ensure that patient is seeking routine follow-up for the condition.

bone marrow suppression and fluctuations in blood pressure. The dentist must be aware of these adverse effects and should examine the patient for signs of thrombocytopenia and leukopenia (see Chapters 23 and 24), which can lead to serious problems with infection and/or excessive bleeding. Phenothiazine drugs potentiate the sedative action of sedative medications, and serious respiratory depression may result with use of these agents at normal dosage. Therefore, if these agents must be used, the dosage must be reduced. The dentist should consult with the patient's physician regarding this point. Epinephrine used in normal amounts in local anesthetic solutions (1:100,000) usually will not produce adverse effects in patients who are taking phenothiazine-type drugs (see Box 29-2). The primary effect of epinephrine-phenothiazine interaction—hypotension—should be a consideration in management; monitoring of blood pressure is therefore indicated.[24,30]

Somatoform Disorder. The characteristics of a somatoform disorder include the following:

- No identifiable lesion or pathologic condition can be found.
- The disorder or reaction has an emotional cause.
- The disorder is not dangerous to the patient.
- The disorder is a defense for the patient in terms of reducing the level of anxiety.

Reducing anxiety by converting it into a symptom is called *primary gain*. Patients also may have *secondary gains* as a result of their condition—for example, because of their symptoms, they may not be able to work, or they may receive increased attention from their family.

Examples of oral symptoms that can be produced by somatoform disorders are burning tongue, painful tongue, numbness of soft tissue, tingling sensations of oral tissues, and pain in the facial region. The diagnosis of a somatoform disorder should be made only after the following criteria have been met: (1) A thorough search from a clinical standpoint has failed to provide any evidence of a disease process that could explain the symptoms; (2) the symptoms have been present long enough that if they were related to a disease process, a lesion would have developed; (3) symptom localization does not reflect known anatomic distribution of nerves; and (4) underlying systemic conditions that could produce the symptoms have been ruled out by laboratory tests or by referral to a physician. Systemic conditions that must be ruled out are anemia, diabetes, cancer, and a nutritional deficiency (vitamin B complex).[19,30]

The process of establishing the diagnosis of somatoform disorders is slow and time-consuming. Dental treatment should not be provided on the basis of a patient's symptoms unless a dental cause can be found. Many patients have undergone needless extractions, root canal treatments, and other procedures in an attempt to address somatoform symptoms. Complex dental care should not be attempted until the somatoform problem has been appropriately managed. The diagnosis of a somatoform disorder should not be reached until a thorough search has been made over time that fails to uncover pathologic findings that could explain the symptoms.

After the diagnosis of an oral somatoform disorder has been established, the following management approach is recommended: First, the findings should be discussed with the patient in the presence of a close relative or spouse. During this discussion, the dentist should point out that no organic source for the patient's problem could be found, that the patient does not have oral cancer, and that the pain or symptom is real to the patient. Next, the possibility that feelings of unhappiness or other distress are the source of the symptoms should be pointed out; this correlation often will be difficult for the patient to understand and accept, but it is important to establish this "groundwork." Complex or unnecessary dental procedures should not be performed, even if the patient demands them in the belief that this will cause the symptoms to disappear.

Dentists should pay close attention to their feelings toward the patient. Symptoms may be viewed only as a device to gain attention and sympathy, and this may cause feelings of hostility and anger on the part of the dentist, which will not enhance proper management of the patient. The dentist should try to feel empathy toward the patient and to understand the cause of the problem and then should react in a positive manner.

An attempt should be made by the dentist to provide effective management for the patient with a mild somatoform disorder (mild in the sense that the patient remains able to function at a reasonable level, the patient's psychoaffective status appears to be stable, and the patient has shown or expressed no suicidal tendencies). Such patients should be assured that they do not have a life-threatening disease such as cancer. A series of regular short appointments should be scheduled to reexamine the patient for possible signs of disease, to discuss symptoms, and to provide reassurance that tissue changes are not clinically evident.

Patients with a severe somatoform disorder should be referred to a psychiatrist; however, once a patient has been referred, the dentist should be willing to remain involved. The patient may need to be reexamined and the psychiatrist consulted regarding the findings. If patients feel that the dentist only wants to "get rid of them," the suggestion of referral will not be helpful or effective.

Schizophrenia. Consultation with the patient's physician is recommended before dental treatment is started, to establish the patient's current status, medications the patient is taking, and the ability of the patient to give a valid consent for treatment.[31] It is suggested that the dentist ask the psychiatrist's opinion regarding the patient's medicolegal competence to sign a consent form.[31] Also, the dentist should inquire about the ability of the patient to perform preventive hygiene procedures.[31]

Routine dental treatment of the schizophrenic patient should not be attempted unless the patient is under medical management. Even then, these patients may be difficult to manage. An attendant or family member should accompany the patient to maximize comfort and familiarity. Patients should be scheduled for morning appointments. Preventive dental education is important, although the importance of good oral hygiene and appropriate technique is more difficult to convey to this group of patients. Oral instructions, modeled demonstrations (hygienist brushes and flosses his or her own teeth), and descriptive posters showing proper toothbrushing and flossing techniques can be used to communicate to the patient what needs to be done and how.[31] For patients who are not able to perform oral hygiene procedures, or who lack the motivation, a family member or attendant should be instructed on the procedures. The dentist may use artificial saliva products, antimicrobial agents (chlorhexidine gluconate), and fluoride mouth products to promote good oral hygiene.[31] Patients should be recalled at 3-month intervals for examination, oral prophylaxis, and application of a fluoride gel or varnish.[31]

Confrontation and an authoritative attitude on the part of the dentist should be avoided. If the standard approach does not allow for proper dental management, the dentist should consider sedation or tranquilization, which should be provided in consultation with the patient's physician. Chlorpromazine (Thorazine), chloral hydrate, diazepam (Valium), or oxazepam may be considered.[32,33] Antipsychotic medications may add to or potentiate the actions of other CNS depressants such as narcotic analgesics and barbiturates. When these agents are used, caution must be exercised to avoid excessive CNS depression, hypotension, orthostatic hypotension, and respiratory depression. Epinephrine must be used with caution in patients taking antipsychotic drugs as severe hypotension may result. The small amount of epinephrine used in local anesthetics is safe, however more concentrated forms of the drug should not be used. Patients who are treated with clozapine can develop bone marrow suppression; the most recent white blood cell count should be reviewed before dental treatment is started.[31]

Suicidal Patient. Suicide is one of the leading causes of death among persons younger than 45 years of age. It also is far too common in the elderly population. Since 1980, a dramatic increase has occurred in the rate of suicide in persons 5 to 19 years of age and in persons 65 years or older. In fact, in some countries, the suicide rate has increased by 60% during the past 45 years.[18] Men are three times more successful in their suicide attempts than women. However, women are 10 times more likely to attempt suicide. The most common methods of suicide include hanging, overdose of medication or poison, carbon monoxide poisoning through car exhaust systems, jumping from a height (building, cliff), jumping in front of a moving vehicle, and the use of firearms[18] (Figure 29-4).

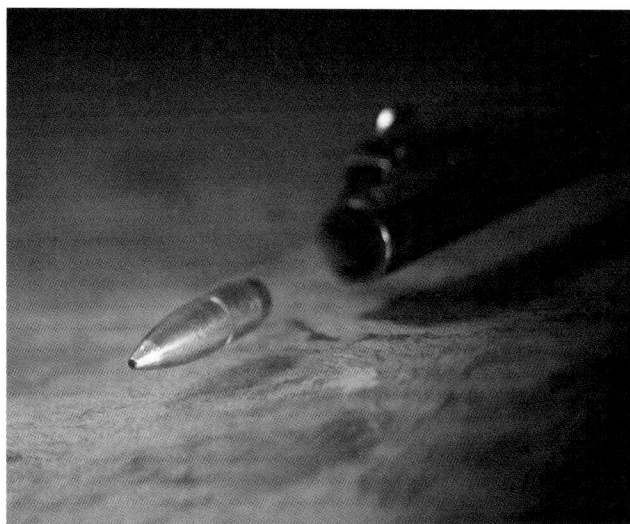

FIGURE 29-4 In the United States during 2001, about 55% of all suicides were committed with the use of firearms.

Physician-assisted suicide occurs when a physician administers an agent that will end the patient's life. The patient has given previous consent for the procedure and usually has a terminal condition such as advanced cancer that is not responding to treatment. Only a very few countries in the world (Belgium, Luxembourg, Netherlands, and Switzerland) and three states (Oregon, Washington, and Montana) in the United States have endorsed this practice.[18,34,35]

Patients with suicidal symptoms often say that they feel frustrated, helpless, or hopeless. They frequently are angry, self-punishing, and harshly self-critical. The potential for suicide is high among persons who suffer from any of the following conditions: chronic physical illness, alcoholism, drug abuse, and depression. Suicide statistics show that men, adolescents, and elderly persons are at greatest risk. A history of a previous suicide attempt greatly increases the risk, as does a history of recent psychiatric hospitalization. Recent diagnosis of a serious condition such as cancer or AIDS also may increase the risk of suicide. The recent loss of a loved one or recent retirement may increase this risk as well. Occurrence of any of these events is associated with increased risk for suicide in people who live alone or have little or no social support. Patients most likely to attempt or complete suicide are those who are perturbed, who state a plan for suicide, and who have the means to carry it out.[18,36]

The dentist should ask whether the very depressed patient has had any thoughts about suicide. Studies have shown that questions about suicide do not prompt the act in these patients. Patients who state they have had these thoughts must be referred for immediate medical care. If possible, members of the family should get involved.[18,29]

Drug Interactions and Adverse Effects

Tricyclic Antidepressants. Many of the heterocyclic antidepressants can cause hypotension, orthostatic hypotension, tachycardia, and cardiac arrhythmia. When sedatives, hypnotics, barbiturates, and narcotics are used together with the heterocyclic antidepressants, severe respiratory depression may result. If these agents must be used, the dosage should be reduced. Atropine should be used with care in these patients because it may increase intraocular pressure. Small amounts of epinephrine (1:100,000) can be used in patients who are taking heterocyclic antidepressants if the dentist aspirates before injecting and injects the anesthetic slowly. No more than two cartridges should be injected at any appointment (see Box 29-2). Other, more concentrated forms of epinephrine must be avoided.[9,28,37]

Monoamine Oxidase Inhibitors. Patients who are taking MAO inhibitors can receive small amounts of epinephrine in local anesthetics, as described previously. Other forms of epinephrine (retraction cord, topical for control of bleeding) are best avoided. Phenylephrine must not be used in patients who are taking MAO inhibitors. MAO inhibitors may interact with sedatives, narcotics, nonnarcotic analgesics, antihistamines, and atropine to prolong and intensify their effects on the CNS (see Table 29-7).[9,28,37]

Antipsychotic Drugs. Several important drug interactions may occur in patients who are taking neuroleptic drugs. Extreme care is indicated with use of sedatives, hypnotics, antihistamines, and opioids in patients who are taking neuroleptic agents, which will increase the respiratory depressant effects of these drugs. This potentiation can be dangerous, particularly in patients with compromised respiratory function. If these types of drugs must be used, the dosage must be reduced. The dentist should always consult with the patient's physician before using these agents.[25,28,37]

Epinephrine must be used with great care in patients who are receiving a neuroleptic drug because a severe hypotensive episode may result. Small amounts of epinephrine (1:100,000) can be used in patients who are taking neuroleptic drugs if the dentist aspirates before injecting, injects the anesthetic solution slowly, and, in general, uses no more than two cartridges. Use of epinephrine-impregnated retraction cord or as a topically applied agent for control of bleeding is contraindicated (see Box 29-2).

With older patients who are taking antipsychotic drugs, several important problems arise in terms of drug usage. These patients usually have decreased levels of serum albumin; hence, many of them have a higher percentage of the drug in an unbound state. This free drug increases the risk for toxic reactions. In addition, many of these patients have marginal liver function; hence, drugs metabolized by the liver may remain in the circulation for longer periods and in increased concentrations.

Treatment Planning Considerations

The goals of treatment planning for patients with psychiatric disorders are to maintain oral health, comfort, and function, and to prevent and control oral disease. Without an aggressive approach to prevention, many of these patients will be susceptible to dental caries and periodontal disease. Susceptibility to such diseases increases because of the adverse effect of xerostomia, which is associated with most of these medications, and the fact that some of the psychiatric conditions for which these patients are being treated are associated with reduced interest in performing or impaired ability to perform oral hygiene procedures. Also, many of these patients, consume an improper diet containing foods or drinks that increase the risk for dental disease.[29]

The dental treatment plan should contain the following elements. Daily oral hygiene procedures must be identified. The treatment plan must be realistic for the patient's psychiatric disorder and physical status. The plan must be both flexible and dynamic, to take into account variability in energy level and other uncertainties associated with major depression or bipolar disorder. During affective episodes, emphasis should be placed on maintenance and prevention. Complex dental procedures should be performed only when the patient is in a stable condition in terms of the mood disorder. The treatment plan should minimize any stress associated with the dental visit. This can best be accomplished through effective patient management efforts and the use of nonverbal communication.

The dental team should communicate to the patient and family members a positive, hopeful attitude toward maintenance of the patient's oral health. The dental team should determine whether the patient is legally able to make rational decisions. This issue should be discussed with the patient and a close relative or spouse. Treatment planning often involves input and permission from a significant other so that decisions can be made.

The last aspect of the treatment plan deals with selection of medications to be used in dental treatment. Certain agents may have to be avoided, and others may require a reduction in their usual dosage. Medical consultation is suggested to establish the patient's current status, confirm medications the patient is taking, identify possible complications, and confirm dental medications and doses that will minimize the chance or severity of drug interactions.

Oral Complications and Manifestations

Antipsychotic drugs may cause agranulocytosis, leukopenia, or thrombocytopenia. Oral lesions associated with these reactions may occur. If the dentist notes oral lesions, fever, or sore throat in a patient who is taking antipsychotic drugs, the patient must be evaluated for possible agranulocytosis. The mood-stabilizing

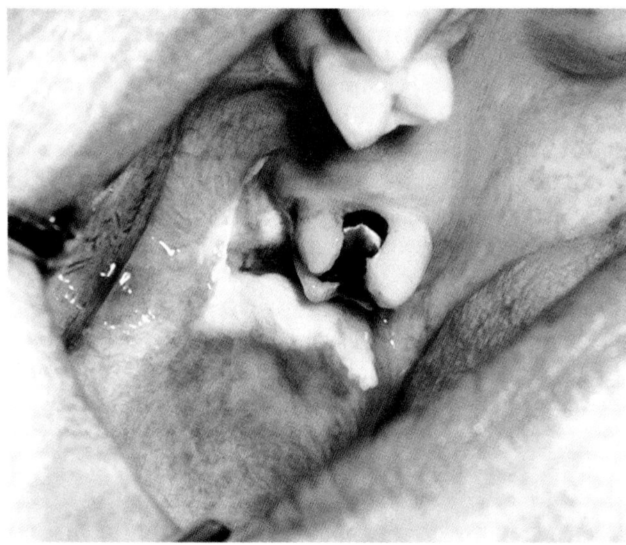

FIGURE 29-5 Agranulocytosis. The dentist should be aware that agranulocytosis may be associated with the drugs used to treat psychoses. *(From Sapp JP, Eversole LR, Wysocki GP:* Contemporary oral and maxillofacial pathology, *ed 2, St. Louis, 2004, Mosby.)*

drugs—carbamazepine and valproate—also may cause agranulocytosis, leukopenia, or thrombocytopenia (Figure 29-5).

Patients who are taking antipsychotic agents may develop muscular problems (dystonia, dyskinesia, or tardive dyskinesia) in the oral and facial regions. If the dentist observes such initial symptoms of dysfunction, the patient should be referred to the primary care physician or psychiatrist for evaluation and appropriate management.[25]

Patients with psychiatric disorders may engage in painful self-destructive acts. Acts of orofacial mutilation such as eye gouging, pushing sharp objects into the ear canal, lip biting, cheek biting, tongue biting, burning of oral tissues with the tip of a cigarette, and mucosal injury with a sharp or blunt object have been reported.

Patients with severe psychiatric disorders may not have an interest in caring for themselves or the ability to do so. Hence, oral hygiene is poor, and increased dental problems develop. Most of the medications used to treat psychiatric disorders contribute to increased dental problems in such patients because xerostomia is one of their primary adverse effects. This unfavorable oral environment may create conditions leading to an increased incidence of smooth-surface caries and candidiasis. Stiefel and colleagues[38] reported on the oral health of persons with and without chronic mental illness in community settings. Patients with chronic mental illness were found to have a significantly greater incidence of dry mouth, mucosal lesions, and coronal smooth-surface caries, as well as increased severity of plaque and calculus buildup.

REFERENCES

1. Schiffer RB: Psychiatric disorders in medical practice. In Goldman L, Ausiello D, editors: *Cecil textbook of medicine*, ed 22, Philadelphia, 2004, Saunders, pp 2212-2122.
2. Cleare A: Unipolar depression. In Wright P, Stern J, Phelan M, editors: *Core psychiatry*, ed 2, Edinburgh, 2005, Elsevier, pp 271-295.
3. Reus VI: Mental disorders. In Fauci AS, et al, editors: *Harrison's principles of internal medicine*, ed 17, New York, 2008, McGraw-Hill, pp 2710-2723.
4. Schiffer RB: Psychiatric disorders in medical practice. In Goldman L, Ausiello D, editors: *Cecil textbook of medicine*, ed 23, Philadelphia, 2008, Saunders, pp 2628-2638.
5. Shah A, Tovey E: Psychiatry of old age. In Wright P, Stern J, Phelan M, editors: *Core psychiatry*, ed 2, Edinburgh, 2005, Elsevier, pp 481-493.
6. Giglio JA, Laskin DM: Prevalence of psychiatric disorders in a group of adult patients seeking general dental care, *Quintessence Int* 41:433-437, 2010.
7. American Psychiatric Association: DSM-IV classification. In *Diagnostic and statistical manual of mental disorders*, fourth ed, text rev, Washington, DC, 2000, American Psychiatric Association, pp 13-24.
8. Khalife S: Bipolar disorder. In Carey WD, et al, editors: *Current clinical medicine 2009—Cleveland Clinic*, Philadelphia, 2009, Saunders, pp 1007-1012.
9. Scherger J, Sudak D, Alici-Evciment Y: *Depression*, 2006, Elsevier.
10. Tesar GE: Recognition and treatment of depression. In Carey WD, et al, editors: *Current clinical medicine 2009—Cleveland Clinic*, Philadelphia, 2009, Saunders, pp 997-1006.
11. American Psychiatric Association: Schizophrenia and other psychotic disorders. In *Diagnostic and statistical manual of mental disorders*, fourth ed, text rev, Washington, DC, 2000, American Psychiatric Association, pp 345-428.
12. American Psychiatric Association: *Diagnostic and Statistical Manual of Mental Disorders*, fourth ed, text rev, Washington, DC, 2000, American Psychiatric Association.
13. Scherger JE, et al: *Bipolar disorders*, Elsevier, available at http://firstconsult.com/depression, accessed March, 2006.
14. Kahn DA: Mood disorders. In Cutler JL, Marcus ER, editors: *Saunders text and review series: psychiatry*, Philadelphia, 1999, WB Saunders, pp 34-63.
15. Rush AJ, et al: Bupropion-SR, sertraline, or venlafaxine-XR after failure of SSRIs for depression, *N Engl J Med* 354:1231-1142, 2006.
16. Healy D: *Psychiatric drugs explained*, ed 5, St. Louis, Churchill Livingstone, 2009.
17. Trevino K, McClintock SM, Husain MM: A review of continuation electroconvulsive therapy: application, safety, and efficacy, *J ECT* 26:186-195, 2010.
18. Srinath S: Suicide and deliberate self-harm. In Wright P, Stern J, Phelan M, editors: *Core psychiatry*, ed 2, Edinburgh, 2005, Elsevier, pp 319-335.
19. American Psychiatric Association: Schizophrenia and other psychotic disorders. In *Diagnostic and statistical manual of mental disorders*, fourth ed, text rev, Washington, DC, 2000, American Psychiatric Association, pp 485-513.
20. Wright P: Schizophrenia and related disorders. In Wright P, Stern J, Phelan M, editors: *Core psychiatry*, ed 2, Edinburgh, 2005, Elsevier, pp 241-267.
21. American Psychiatric Association: Schizophrenia and other psychotic disorders. In *Diagnostic and statistical manual of mental disorders*, fourth ed, text rev, Washington, DC, 2000, American Psychiatric Association, pp 297-345.
22. Watanabe Y, Someya T, Nawa H: Cytokine hypothesis of schizophrenia pathogenesis: evidence from human studies

and animal models, *Psychiatry Clin Neurosci* 64:217-230, 2010.
23. Horwath E, Courinos F: Schizophrenia and other psychotic disorders. In Cutler JL, Marcus ER, editors: *Saunders text and review series: psychiatry*, Philadelphia, 1999, WB Saunders, pp 64-80.
24. Wright P, Perahia D: Psychopharmacology. In Wright P, Stern J, Phelan M, editors: *Core psychiatry*, ed 2, Edinburgh, 2005, Elsevier, pp 579-611.
25. Pollack EF, et al: *Schizophrenia*, Elsevier, available at http://firstconsult.com/schizophrenia, accessed March 2006.
26. Mathews M, et al: Schizophrenia and acute psychosis. In Carey WD, et al, editors: *Current clinical medicine 2009—Cleveland Clinic*, Philadelphia, 2009, Saunders, pp 1027-1036.
27. Branford D: Schizophrenia. In Walker R, Edwards C, editors: *Clinical pharmacy and therapeutics*, ed 2, London, 1999, Churchill Livingstone, pp 425-435.
28. Russakoff LM: Psychopharmacology. In Cutler JL, Marcus ER, editors: *Saunders text and review series: psychiatry*, Philadelphia, 1999, WB Saunders, pp 308-331.
29. Little JW: Dental implications of mood disorders, *J Gen Dent* 52:442-450, 2004.
30. Goldberg RJ: *Practical guide to the care of the psychiatric patient*, St. Louis, 1995, Mosby.
31. Friedlander AH, Marder SR: The psychopathology, medical management and dental implications of schizophrenia, *J Am Dent Assoc* 133:603-610, 2002.
32. Friedlander AH, Brill NQ: Dental management of patients with schizophrenia, *Spec Care Dent* 6:217-219, 1986.
33. Scully C, Cawson RA: *Medical problems in dentistry*, ed 5, Edinburgh, 2005, Churchill Livingstone.
34. Dyer C: Washington follows Oregon to legalise physician assisted suicide, *BMJ* 337:A2480, 2008.
35. Gouras M: Montana lawmakers punt on physician-assisted suicide, *National on Sunday*, Associated Press, 2011.
36. Feinstein RE: Suicide and violence. In Cutler JL, Marcus ER, editors: *Saunders text and review series: psychiatry*, Philadelphia, 1999, WB Saunders, pp 201-221.
37. Felpel LP: Psychopharmacology: antipsychotics and antidepressants. In Yagiela JA, Neidle EA, Dowd FJ, editors: *Pharmacology and therapeutics for dentistry*, ed 4, St. Louis, 1998, Mosby, pp 151-168.
38. Stiefel DJ, et al: A comparison of oral health of persons with and without chronic mental illness in community settings, *Spec Care Dent* 10:6-12, 1990.

CHAPTER

30

Drug and Alcohol Abuse

The abusive use of drugs and alcohol is a huge and growing public health problem in the United States, as well as in many other countries worldwide. Drug and alcohol abuse has far-reaching effects on persons engaging in such activity, as well as their families and communities, with a consequent heavy impact on law enforcement, the judicial system, politics, and health care. It is inevitable that dental practitioners will encounter abusers of drugs and/or alcohol among their patients, and unfortunately, some practitioners will themselves turn to such abuse. This chapter discusses the effects of drug and alcohol abuse as they pertain to dental management. Another legal drug of abuse, nicotine, is discussed in Chapter 8.

DEFINITIONS

According to the *Diagnostic and Statistical Manual of Mental Disorders,* fourth edition (DSM-IV), of the American Psychiatric Association,[1,2] a diagnosis of *substance abuse* requires the recurrent use of a substance over the past 12 months with subsequent adverse consequences (e.g., failure to fulfill a major role at work, school, or home; legal problems; persistent interpersonal problems) or placement of the affected person in high-risk physically hazardous situations. *Dependence* involves tolerance and withdrawal in addition to certain patterns of drug use, the effect on life activities, and the uncontrollable need for use of the substance in spite of adverse consequences. *Tolerance* is defined as either a need for increased amounts of a substance to achieve the desired effect or a diminished effect with continued use of the same amount of the substance. *Withdrawal* is manifested by a characteristic syndrome emerging upon abstinence from a habitually used substance. There is confusion over the use of the term addiction. *Addiction* is equated with *dependence* in the DSM-IV. Some authors, however, advocate separating the terms dependence and addiction, with addiction being a distinct disease characterized by compulsive substance use despite serious negative consequences.[3] Tolerance, dependence, and withdrawal all *may* occur with addiction but are not necessary for the diagnosis. In addition, addicted persons remain at high risk for relapse long after detoxification and the cessation of withdrawal symptoms.

Alcoholism is a term commonly used to describe a condition of substance abuse focused on consumption of alcohol. A more precise definition, however, has been proposed by O'Conner: "a primary chronic disease with genetic, psychosocial, and environmental factors ... often progressive and fatal ... characterized by impaired control over drinking, preoccupation with the drug alcohol, use of alcohol despite future consequences, and distortions of thinking, most notably denial."[4]

EPIDEMIOLOGY

Incidence and Prevalence

Illicit drugs of abuse include marijuana and hashish, heroin, cocaine (including crack), methamphetamine and its analogues, so-called club drugs, hallucinogens, and dissociative drugs (Table 30-1). Legally prescribed opioids and sedative/hypnotics are abused when used nonmedically. Alcohol is legal but is abused when consumed inappropriately or in excessive amounts. According to the 2009 National Survey on Drug Use and Health (NSDUH),[5] an estimated 21.8 million Americans 12 years of age and older were current illicit drug users, which is higher than in 2008. This number represents approximately 8.7% of the population. Illicit drug use is highest among young persons 18 to 25 years of age. In a dental practice of 2000 patients, it can be expected that approximately 175 of them abuse at least one type of drug or other substance.

Marijuana is the most commonly used illicit drug. In 2009, there were 16.7 million past-month users. Among persons aged 12 or older, the rate of past-month marijuana use and the number of users in 2009 (6.6%, or 16.7 million) were higher than in 2008 (6.1%, or 15.2 million) and in 2007 (5.8%, or 14.4 million). In 2009, there were 1.6 million current cocaine users aged 12 or older, comprising 0.7% of the population. These estimates were similar to the number and rate in 2008

TABLE 30-1 Most Common Illicit Drugs of Abuse

Substance of Abuse	Street Names	How Administered	Acute Effects
Cannabinoids			
Marijuana	Blunt, dope, ganja, grass, herb, joint, bud, Mary Jane, pot, reefer, green, trees, smoke, sinsemilla, skunk, weed	Smoked, swallowed	Euphoria; relaxation; slowed reaction time; distorted sensory perception; impaired balance and coordination; increased heart rate and appetite; impaired learning, memory; anxiety; panic attacks; psychosis/cough, frequent respiratory infections; possible mental health decline; addiction
Opioids			
Heroin	Smack, horse, brown sugar, dope, H, junk, skag, skunk, white horse, China white; cheese (with OTC cold medicine and antihistamine)	Injected, smoked, snorted	Euphoria; drowsiness; impaired coordination; dizziness; confusion; nausea; sedation; feeling of heaviness in the body; slowed or arrested breathing/constipation; endocarditis; hepatitis; HIV; addiction; fatal overdose
Stimulants			
Cocaine	Blow, bump, C, candy, Charlie, coke, crack, flake, rock, snow, toot	Snorted, smoked, injected	Increased heart rate, blood pressure, body temperature, metabolism; feelings of exhilaration; increased energy, mental alertness; tremors;
Amphetamine	Bennies, black beauties, crosses, hearts, LA turnaround, speed, truck drivers, uppers	Swallowed, snorted, smoked, injected	reduced appetite; irritability; anxiety; panic; paranoia; violent behavior; psychosis/weight loss, insomnia; cardiac or cardiovascular complications; stroke; seizures; addiction
Methamphetamine	Meth, ice, crank, chalk, crystal, fire, glass, go fast, speed	Swallowed, snorted, smoked, injected	*Cocaine*—also nasal damage from snorting *Methamphetamine*—also severe dental problems
Club Drugs			
MDMA	Ecstasy, Adam, clarity, Eve, lover's speed, peace, uppers	Swallowed, snorted, injected	*MDMA*—mild hallucinogenic effects; increased tactile sensitivity; empathic feelings; lowered inhibition; anxiety; chills; sweating; teeth clenching; muscle
Flunitrazepam	Forget-me pill, Mexican Valium, R2, roach, Roche, roofies, roofinol, rope, rophies	Swallowed, snorted	cramping/sleep disturbances; depression; impaired memory; hyperthermia; addiction *Flunitrazepam*—sedation; muscle relaxation;
GHB	G, Georgia home boy, grievous bodily harm, liquid ecstasy, soap, scoop, goop, liquid X	Swallowed	confusion; memory loss; dizziness; impaired coordination/addiction *GHB*—drowsiness; nausea; headache; disorientation; loss of coordination; memory loss/unconsciousness; seizures; coma
Dissociative Drugs			
Ketamine	Cat, Valium, K, Special K, vitamin K	Injected, snorted, smoked	Feelings of being separate from one's body and environment; impaired motor function/anxiety; tremors; numbness; memory loss; nausea
PCP and analogues	Angel dust, boat, hog, love boat, peace pill	Swallowed, smoked, injected	*Ketamine*—also analgesia; impaired memory; delirium; respiratory depression and arrest; death *PCP and analogues*—also analgesia; psychosis; aggression; violence; slurred speech; loss of coordination; hallucinations
Hallucinogens			
LSD	Acid, blotter, cubes, microdot yellow sunshine, blue heaven	Swallowed, absorbed through oral mucosa	Altered states of perception and feeling; hallucinations; nausea *LSD and mescaline*—also increased body temperature, heart rate, blood pressure; loss of
Mescaline	Buttons, cactus, mesc, peyote	Swallowed, smoked	appetite; sweating; sleeplessness; numbness, dizziness, weakness, tremors; impulsive behavior; rapid shifts in emotion *LSD*—also flashbacks, hallucinogen, persisting perception disorder

Adapted from the National Institutes of Health, National Institute on Drug Abuse (Web site), http://www.drugabuse.gov/DrugPages/DrugsofAbuse.html; accessed on March 3, 2011.

(1.9 million, or 0.7%) but were lower than the estimates in 2006 (2.4 million, or 1.0%). An estimated 3.7 million people have reported previous use of heroin, with an estimated 150,000 persons becoming new users every year.[2] The level of heroin use is relatively stable, with an approximate 1.5% annual increase. Methamphetamine is a synthetic drug that is easily manufactured, and its use is spreading across the United States at alarming rates. The number of past-month methamphetamine users decreased between 2006 and 2008 but then increased in 2009. The reported figures were 731,000 (0.3%) in 2006, 529,000 (0.2%) in 2007, 314,000 (0.1%) in 2008, and 502,000 (0.2%) in 2009.

The use of prescription opioids (e.g., OxyContin) for nonmedical reasons is currently one of the fastest-growing dimensions of drug abuse in the United States, with a 225% increase from 1992 to 2000.[2] The lifetime nonmedical use of OxyContin increased from 1.9 million to 3.1 million in the 2-year period from 2002 to 2004.[6] From 2002 to 2009, there was an increase among young adults 18 to 25 years of age in the rate of current nonmedical use of prescription-type drugs (from 5.5% to 6.3%), driven primarily by an increase in pain reliever misuse (from 4.1% to 4.8%). The nonmedical use of opioids has become epidemic in certain parts of the nation, especially in regions on the east coast.

According to the 2009 NSDUH,[5] slightly more than half (51.9%) of Americans aged 12 or older reported being current drinkers of alcohol. This translates to an estimated 130.6 million people, which is similar to the 2008 estimate of 129.0 million people (51.6%). In 2009, nearly one quarter (23.7%) of persons aged 12 or older participated in binge drinking. This translates to about 59.6 million people. The rate in 2009 is similar to the estimate in 2008. *Binge drinking* is defined as consumption of five or more drinks on the same occasion on at least 1 day in the 30 days prior to the survey. In 2009, heavy drinking was reported by 6.8 percent of the population aged 12 or older, or 17.1 million people. This rate was similar to the rate of heavy drinking in 2008. *Heavy drinking* is defined as binge drinking on at least 5 days in the past 30 days. The highest rates of alcohol use, heavy or binge use, and alcohol use disorders occur between the ages of 18 and 29 years.[5]

The prevalence of problem drinking in general outpatient and inpatient medical settings has been estimated to be between 15% and 40%.[4] The lifetime prevalence of an alcohol use disorder in the United States is about 18.6% (13.2% for abuse and 5.4% for dependence).[7] Surveys assessing past-year prevalence of these disorders indicate that nearly 8.5% (18 million) of American adults meet standard diagnostic criteria for one of the DSM-IV alcohol use disorders. Of these, 4.7% (10 million) meet criteria for alcohol abuse, and 3.8% (8 million), for dependence. Gender-specific rates of abuse and dependence differ within the general population, with men exhibiting higher rates of both abuse and dependence (8.5%) than those reported for women (4%).[8] Although problem drinking is seen primarily in adults, the prevalence among teenagers is alarmingly high. Alcoholism among elderly persons also is a significant problem. A dental practice comprising 2000 adult patients could include as many as 170 patients who have a problem with alcohol.

Etiology

The neurobiology of addiction and dependence is complex and involves a unique set of variables. Disruption of the endogenous reward systems in the brain is a common feature of all of the major drugs of abuse; most of these drugs act by disrupting dopamine circuits in the brain.[6] Acute changes increase synaptic dopamine and disrupt circuits that mediate motivation and drive, conditioned learning, and inhibitory controls. This enhancement of synaptic dopamine is particularly rewarding for persons with abnormally low density of the D_2 dopamine receptor (D_2DR).[6] A complex neural circuitry underlies the valuation and pursuit of rewards[3] (Figure 30-1). Although dopamine is the primary neurotransmitter involved in drug abuse and addiction, many other neurotransmitters are involved, depending on the drug of abuse (Figure 30-2). Evidence suggests that inherited genetic factors are involved in alcoholism. Psychological factors such as depression, self-medication (to relieve psychic distress), personality disorder, and poor coping skills appear to be involved in addictive behavior. Social factors that may be involved include interpersonal, cultural, and societal influences.[1]

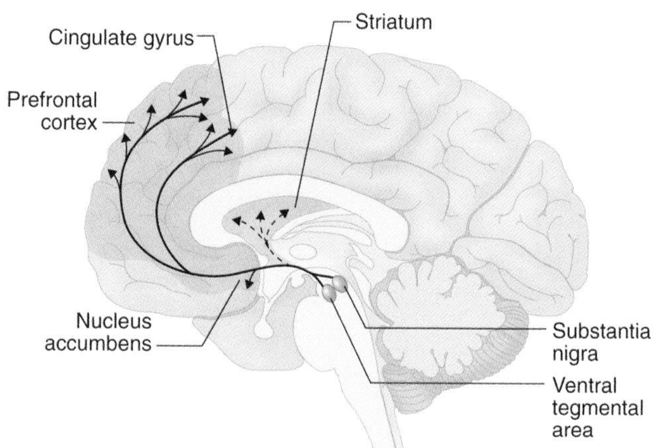

FIGURE 30-1 Brain reward circuits. The major dopaminergic projections to the forebrain that underlie brain reward are shown superimposed on a diagram of the human brain: projection from the ventral tegmental area to the nucleus accumbens, and prefrontal cerebral cortex. Also shown are projections from the substantia nigra to the dorsal striatum, which play a role in habit formation and in well-rehearsed motor behavior, such as drug seeking and drug administration. *(From Hyman SE: Biology of addiction. In Goldman L, Ausiello D, editors:* Cecil medicine, *ed 23, Philadelphia, 2008, Saunders.)*

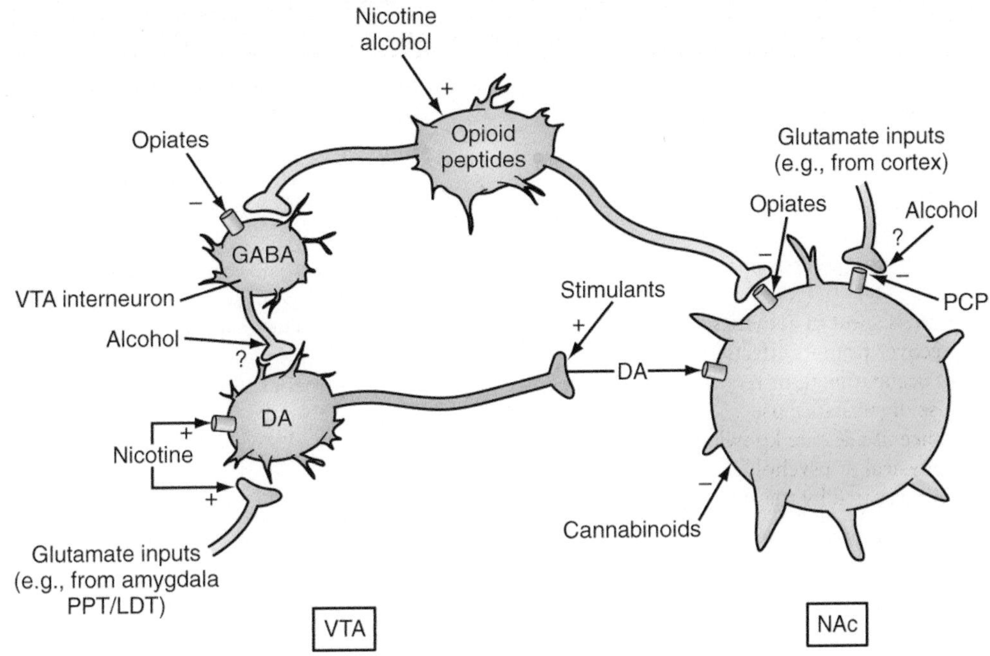

FIGURE 30-2 Converging acute actions of drugs of abuse on the ventral tegmental area and nucleus accumbens. *DA,* Dopamine; *GABA,* γ-aminobutyric acid; *LDT,* Laterodorsal tegmentum; *NAc,* Nucleus accumbens; *PCP,* Phencyclidine; *PPT,* Pedunculopontine tegmentum; *VTA,* Ventral tegmental area. *(From Renner JA, Ward EN: Drug addiction. In Stern TA, et al, editors:* Massachusetts General Hospital comprehensive clinical psychiatry, *Philadelphia, 2008, Mosby.)*

CLINICAL PRESENTATION AND MEDICAL MANAGEMENT

Substance *dependence* occurs when the person using the substance takes it in larger amounts or over a longer period than was originally intended. A great deal of time may be spent in activities needed to procure the substance, take it, or recover from its effects. The person gives up important social, occupational, and recreational activities because of substance use. Marked tolerance to the substance may develop; therefore, progressively larger amounts are needed to achieve intoxication or to produce the desired effect. The person with the disorder continues to take the substance, despite persistent or recurrent social, psychological, and physical problems that result from its use.[1,2]

Substance *abuse* denotes substance use that does not meet the criteria for dependence (Table 30-2). This diagnosis is most likely to be applicable to persons who have just started to take psychoactive substances. Examples of substance abuse are that of a middle-aged man who repeatedly drives his car while intoxicated (the man has no other symptoms) and that of a woman who keeps drinking even though her physician has warned her that alcohol is responsible for exacerbating the symptoms of a duodenal ulcer (she has no other symptoms).[1]

Withdrawal occurs when the person with substance dependence stops or reduces intake of the substance. Withdrawal symptoms vary in accordance with the substance involved. Physiologic signs of withdrawal are common after prolonged use of alcohol, opioids, sedatives, hypnotics, and anxiolytics. Such signs are less obvious in withdrawal from cocaine, nicotine, amphetamines, and cannabis.[1,2]

Marijuana

Marijuana is the common name for cannabis, which is the most commonly used illicit drug in the world.[2] Delta-9-tetrahydrocannabinol (THC) is the major psychoactive ingredient in substances that causes cannabis dependence. Several different preparations of marijuana are available. These preparations—bhang, charas, ganja, and hashish—are known to vary in potency and quality. They usually are smoked but can be taken orally and are sometimes mixed with food. With inhalation, peak effects occur within 20 to 30 minutes; with oral ingestion, peak effects occur within 2 to 3 hours.[2] Currently available marijuana supplies are much more potent than those that were available in the 1960s. Most users describe an altered sense of time and distance perception. Acute intoxication may result in anxiety and paranoid ideation or frank delusions. Tolerance and physical dependence can occur, but clinical presentation of these symptoms is not common.[2] Marijuana use can destabilize patients whose schizophrenia is in remission. Social and occupational impairment occurs but is less severe than that seen with alcohol and cocaine use.[1] Marijuana use rarely requires medical treatment. Anxiety reactions may require treatment with benzodiazepines. Of note, some states allow the use of marijuana for medicinal purposes.

TABLE 30-2 Diagnostic Criteria for Dependence and Drug Abuse

Dependence (3 or more needed for diagnosis)	Abuse (1 or more for 12 months needed for diagnosis)
• Tolerance • Withdrawal • The substance is often taken in larger amounts over a longer period than intended • Any unsuccessful effort or a persistent desire to cut down or control substance use • A great deal of time is spent in activities necessary to obtain the substance or to recover from its effects • Important social, occupational, or recreational activities given up or reduced because of substance use • Continued substance use despite knowledge of having had persistent or recurrent physical or psychological problems that are likely to be caused or exacerbated by the substance	• Recurrent substance use resulting in failure to fulfill major role obligations at work, school, and home • Recurrent substance use in situations in which it is physically hazardous • Recurrent substance-related legal problems • Continued substance use despite having persistent or recurrent social or interpersonal problems caused or exacerbated by the effects of the substance • Never met criteria for dependence

From Samet JH: Drug abuse and dependence. In Goldman L, Ausiello D, editors: Cecil textbook of medicine, *ed 23, Philadelphia, 2008, Saunders.*

Opioids

The primary effects of the opioids (opiate-like drugs) are to decrease pain perception, cause modest levels of sedation, and produce euphoria. Drugs in this category include those derived from naturally occurring alkaloids morphine and codeine. Semisynthetic drugs produced from morphine or thebaine molecules include hydrocodone, hydromorphone, heroin, and oxycodone. Synthetic opioids include meperidine, propoxyphene, diphenoxylate, fentanyl, buprenorphine, methadone, and pentazocine. Tolerance to any single opioid is likely to generalize to other drugs in the group.

Through direct effects on the central nervous system (CNS), opiates may produce nausea and vomiting, decreased pain perception, euphoria, and sedation. Additives in street drugs can cause permanent damage to the nervous system, including peripheral neuropathy and CNS dysfunction. Users of such drugs may experience constipation and anorexia. Respiratory depression occurs as the result of a decreased response of the brain stem to carbon dioxide tension. This effect is part of the toxic reaction to opiates,as described later on, but it also can be significant in patients with compromised lung function.

Complications are common among abusers of narcotics, especially when administered intravenously. Cardiovascular effects of the opiates are mild, and no direct effect on heart rhythm or myocardial contractility has been noted with their use. Orthostatic hypotension, probably caused by dilation of peripheral vessels, may occur. The major complication with intravenous use of these drugs involves the use of contaminated or shared needles; pathogens introduced in this manner can cause hepatitis B and C and bacterial endocarditis, and an association with increased risk for infection with human immunodeficiency virus (HIV) also has been noted.[2,6] The bacterial endocarditis is unusual in that it predominantly affects the right side of the heart (the location of the tricuspid valve), with *Staphlococcus aureus* being the most common causative organism.

Dependence on opiates can be seen in at least three groups of patients. The first group is the minority of patients with chronic pain syndromes who misuse their prescribed drugs. The second group at high risk consists of physicians, dentists, nurses, and pharmacists. These persons have easy access to drugs with abuse potential.[9] Members of the third and largest group buy their drugs on the street to get high. Once persistent opiate use has been established, the outcome is often very serious. According to statistics from the Centers for Disease Control and Prevention (CDC), in 2007 pain killers killed twice as many people as cocaine and five times as many as heroin.[10] From 1999 to 2007, the number of U.S. poisoning deaths involving any opioid analgesic (e.g., oxycodone, methadone, hydrocodone) more than tripled, from 4041 to 14,459.

Toxic reactions (overdose) are seen with all opiates. These reactions are more frequent and dangerous with more potent drugs such as fentanyl, which is 80 to 100 times more powerful than morphine. Intravenous overdose can lead immediately to slow, shallow respirations, bradycardia, a drop in body temperature, and lack of responsiveness to external stimulation. Emergency treatment includes support of vital signs with the use of a respirator and administration of a reversal agent such as naloxone by intramuscular or intravenous injection.[2]

In contrast with sedative withdrawal, withdrawal from opiates is an unpleasant but not life-threatening experience. Gastrointestinal upset, muscle cramps, rhinorrhea, and irritability are the prominent signs and symptoms. Opiate users with memory impairment or cognitive dysfunction should be assessed for HIV infection by evaluation of risk factors and blood screening of the patient after appropriate counseling has been provided.[6]

Cocaine

Cocaine is a stimulant and a local anesthetic with potent vasoconstrictor properties. After alcohol, it is the leading drug of abuse in terms of frequency of emergency department (ED) visits, general hospital admissions, family violence, and other social problems.[11] Cocaine is used medically in otolaryngologic procedures as a potent topical anesthetic and is used to treat some patients with attention deficit–hyperactivity disorders.[2] The drug produces physiologic and behavioral effects when administered orally, intranasally (snorting), topically on mucous membranes, intravenously, or by smoking. "Crack" cocaine, which is inhaled by "freebasing" or smoking, results in much higher blood levels of cocaine than those achievable with "snorting" and is particularly addictive. Cocaine has potent pharmacologic effects on dopamine, norepinephrine, and serotonin neurons in the CNS. Cocaine has an elimination half-life of 30 minutes to 1 hour.[2]

Cocaine intoxication produces a sense of well-being, a heightened awareness of sensory input, anorexia, a decreased desire to sleep, restlessness, elation, grandiosity, agitation, and psychotic states (panic attack, paranoid ideation, delusions, and auditory and visual hallucinations). Acute users (people who aren't major addicts but have just recently taken the drug) experience intense euphoria often associated with increased sexual desire along with improved sexual function. These rewards often are followed by a moderate to severe post–cocaine use depression that provides a strong compulsion for further cocaine use.[6] Physical findings in cocaine intoxication consist of tachycardia, cardiac arrhythmias, papillary dilation, and elevated blood pressure. Affected persons may experience headache, as well as chills, nausea, and vomiting. Needle tracks (from "skin popping") may be found on the arms of intravenous users of cocaine and heroin. Frequent, chronic, or high-dose use of cocaine can produce psychiatric states similar to acute schizophrenic episodes. Pregnant women who are chronic users of cocaine or heroin may give birth to infants who are "addicted."

Cocaine overdose can be life-threatening. Myocardial infarction, arrhythmia, stroke, respiratory arrest, and symptoms consistent with neuroleptic malignant syndrome have been associated with cocaine use. Depression is common in cocaine addicts, particularly during periods of withdrawal, and under these conditions, the drug may be taken in an attempt to commit suicide.

Cocaine abuse is treated using psychotherapy, behavioral therapy, and 12-step programs.[2] Acupuncture may be used for detoxification and prevention of relapse. Cocaine overdose constitutes a medical emergency requiring resuscitation in an intensive care unit. Intravenous diazepam has been shown to be effective for control of seizures. Ventricular arrhythmias can be managed with intravenous propranolol. Medication is not available that is both safe and effective for cocaine detoxification or for maintenance of abstinence.[6] Intravenous cocaine abusers are at increased risk for acquiring hepatitis B and hepatitis C and for exposure to HIV. Some intravenous cocaine abusers develop a pruritic rash on the chest (as an allergic reaction to a benzoic acid ester), and ester-type local anesthetics must be avoided in these patients.

Amphetamines

Amphetamine, methamphetamine, and related drugs are CNS stimulants. The primary action of these drugs is to increase synaptic dopamine by causing the release of dopamine stores into the synapse, which produces a dopamine "high" that is both more intense and longer-lasting than that afforded by cocaine, lasting anywhere from 8 to 24 hours.[6] Amphetamines are used clinically for weight loss and for treatment of attention deficit disorder, narcolepsy, and treatment-resistant depression. Many people develop dependence when they first use amphetamines for their appetite suppressant effects in an attempt at weight control. Intravenous administration of amphetamine can lead to rapid development of dependence. Progressive tolerance is common in amphetamine dependence. Amphetamine use may result in the same symptoms and complications that are seen with cocaine abuse.[2]

Methamphetamine ("meth") is a potent synthetic psychostimulant form of amphetamine. It is highly addictive, and chronic use has been associated with violent behavior. On the street, methamphetamine is referred to as "speed," "crank," "go," and "zip." The smokable form is called "ice" or "crystal." The biologic half-life of methamphetamine is much longer than that of cocaine. Symptoms of withdrawal from methamphetamine may be more intense than those associated with cocaine. Cessation after daily use may result in severe depression with suicidal or homicidal ideation, hypersomnia, or sleeping difficulty.[2,6]

Amphetamine analogues produce very similar signs and symptoms. Those associated with normal dosage include hyperalertness, euphoria, hyperactivity, and increased physical endurance. Higher doses of these drugs may be associated with dysphonia, headache, tachycardia, and confusion. When methamphetamine is introduced intravenously or by inhalation, a rapid, prolonged rush may result. When abused, methamphetamine can induce psychotic symptoms very similar to those of acute schizophrenia.

Amphetamines were widely abused during the 1960s by persons in the so-called counterculture movement.

Amphetamine sulfate was known on the street as "speed," "whiz," "blues," "bennies," "pep pills," "uppers," or "splash." It was inhaled, snorted, smoked, taken orally, or injected intravenously. In the 1980s and 1990s, cocaine became the drug of choice and methamphetamine abuse declined. However, use of methamphetamine ("meth") and MDMA ("ecstasy") has undergone a major resurgence among adolescents and people in their early 20s. Stimulants (including amphetamine and methamphetamine) were involved in 10% of all illicit drug–related ED visits in 2004.[5] Methamphetamine was made illegal in 1971, and ecstasy in 1985.[12] Methamphetamine is widely used in California and in some Midwestern states, where it is synthesized in "home laboratories," putting the building's occupants at risk for inhaling toxic fumes and combustible fires. Methamphetamine is the most widely illegally manufactured, distributed, and abused type of amphetamine.[6]

Medications that contain pseudoephedrine (over-the-counter [OTC] decongestants, such as Sudafed) are used by illegal home laboratory operators to produce methamphetamine. As a result, many states passed laws to make it more difficult to purchase OTC medicines that contain pseudoephedrine. In 2006, President Bush signed into law a bill that imposed strict standards on products made with pseudoephedrine and required that products be placed behind the counter; it also required that customers show identification and sign a log book, and set limitations on how much of the medicine can be sold at one time.

Sedative-Hypnotics

The primary psychoactive substances used as sedatives and hypnotics are benzodiazepines (diazepam, lorazepam, temazepam) and, less commonly, barbiturates (phenobarbital, secobarbital, mephobarbital). Sedatives, hypnotics, and anxiolytic drugs are frequently abused and are estimated to account for 35% of ED visits due to the nonmedical use or misuse of pharmaceuticals.[13] The benzodiazepines are now the most frequently abused of the sedative and hypnotic drugs, replacing the barbiturates, which are no longer extensively used in the clinical setting.

The proportion of users of benzodiazepines who become dependent is a function of dose, type, and duration of use. Longer use or higher dosage is more likely to lead to dependence; however, dependence also can occur when the drug is used in low doses for prolonged periods of time, as may be seen in clinical practice.[2] Usage that lasts between 3 and 12 months leads to dependence in 10% to 20% of users. The rate of dependency increases to 20% to 45% when benzodiazepines are used for periods longer than a year.[14] Benzodiazepines should be prescribed cautiously for dependence-prone persons with other risk factors for drug abuse, in whom the use of these agents should be limited to no longer than 2 weeks when possible.[14] Patients who are dependent on benzodiazepines are managed with gradual reduction in dose of the abused drug, or by substitution of another long-acting sedative-hypnotic with gradual reduction in dosage.[6]

Withdrawal symptoms produced by benzodiazepines are similar to those caused by withdrawal from alcohol. They can occur after several weeks or longer of moderate use of the drug. Signs and symptoms of withdrawal from benzodiazepines include nausea and vomiting, weakness, autonomic hyperactivity (tachycardia and sweating), anxiety, orthostatic hypotension, tremor, loss of appetite and weight loss, tinnitus, delirium with delusions, and hallucinations.[6]

Alcohol

The behavioral and physiologic effects of alcohol depend on the amount of intake, its rate of increase in plasma, the presence of other drugs or medical problems, and the past experience with alcohol. Chronic use of heavy alcohol intake can result in clinically significant cognitive impairment (even when the person is sober) or distress. The pattern displayed usually is one of intermittent relapse and remission. If the disease is allowed to progress untreated, many affected persons develop other psychiatric problems (anxiety, antisocial behavior, and affective disorders), whereas some develop alcohol amnestic disorder and are unable to learn new material or to recall known material. Alcoholic blackouts may occur. In some patients, alcohol-induced dementia and severe personality changes develop.

The DSM-IV[1] defines *alcohol dependence* as repeated alcohol-related difficulties in at least three of seven areas of functioning. These include any combination of tolerance, withdrawal, increased intake of alcohol in greater amounts and over longer periods than intended, an inability to control use, giving up important activities to drink, spending a great deal of time pursuing alcohol use, and continued use of alcohol despite physical or psychological consequences. Thus, a clinical diagnosis of alcohol dependence rests on the documentation of a pattern of difficulties associated with alcohol use and is not based on the quantity and frequency of alcohol consumption.

Treatment for alcohol dependence consists of three basic steps. The first is identification and intervention. A thorough physical examination is performed to evaluate organ systems that could be impaired. This includes a search for evidence of liver failure, gastrointestinal bleeding, cardiac arrhythmia, and glucose or electrolyte imbalance. Hemorrhage from esophageal varices and hepatic encephalopathy require immediate treatment. Ascites mandates measures to control fluids and electrolytes; alcoholic hepatitis often is treated with glucocorticoids; and infection or sepsis is managed with antimicrobial agents. During this phase, the patient may refuse to accept the diagnosis and deny that a problem exists.[4]

The second step is withdrawal from alcohol, or in cases of severe dependence, reduction of alcohol consumption. Abrupt alcohol withdrawal results in loss of appetite, tachycardia, anxiety, insomnia, and delirium tremens ("DTs")—characterized by shaking tremors, hallucinations, disorientation, impaired attention and memory, and extreme agitation. Physical findings include severe sweating, elevated blood pressure, and tachycardia. Management goals are to minimize the severity of withdrawal symptoms. Strict dietary modifications are required, including a high-protein, high-calorie, low-sodium diet and possibly fluid restriction. Patients should receive adequate nutrition and rest, oral multiple B vitamins, including 50 to 100 mg of thiamine daily for at least 1 to 2 weeks, and iron replacement and folic acid supplementation as needed to correct any anemia present.[4]

The third step is to manage the CNS depression resulting from rapid removal of the ethanol. Administration of a benzodiazepine, such as diazepam or chlordiazepoxide, in gradually decreasing doses to achieve downward titration of the serum drug levels over a 3- to 5-day period, alleviates alcohol withdrawal symptoms. The beta blockers clonidine and carbamazepine are more recent additions to the pharmacotherapeutic management of withdrawal.[4]

Once treatment of withdrawal has been completed, the patient is educated about alcoholism. This aspect of management includes teaching the family and friends to stop protecting the patient from the problems caused by alcohol. Attempts are made to help the patient with alcoholism achieve and maintain a high level of motivation toward abstinence. Steps also are taken to help the patient with alcoholism readjust to life without alcohol and to reestablish a functional lifestyle. The drug disulfiram has been used for some patients during alcohol rehabilitation. Disulfiram inhibits aldehyde dehydrogenase causing accumulation of acetaldehyde blood levels and thus sweating, nausea, vomiting, and diarrhea when taken with ethanol. Naltrexone (an opioid antagonist) and acamprosate (an inhibitor of the γ-aminobutyric acid [GABA] system) may be used to decrease the amount of alcohol consumed or to shorten the period during which alcohol is used in cases of relapse.[4]

DENTAL MANAGEMENT

Medical Considerations (Box 30-1)

The dentist should be on the alert for signs and symptoms that may indicate substance abuse (see Table 30-2). Telltale cutaneous lesions often indicate parenteral abuse of

BOX 30-1 Dental Management

Considerations in Patients with Drug/Alcohol Abuse or Dependence

P

Patient Evaluation/Risk Assessment (see Box 1-1)

- Evaluate to determine whether drug/alcohol abuse or dependence is present.
- Obtain medical consultation if clinical signs and symptoms point to an undiagnosed problem, or if the diagnosis is uncertain.

Potential Issues/Factors of Concern

A	
Antibiotics	No issues.
Analgesics	Avoid prescribing narcotic analgesics, if possible. However, if needed, consult with patient's primary care physician who is managing the substance abuse program. Prescribe an adequate-strength medication and only a limited number of doses with specific instructions, with no refills. It may be appropriate to have a third party (such as a "12-step program" sponsor) monitor and dispense the medication.
Anesthesia	For cocaine and methamphetamine abusers, avoid the use of epinephrine for 24 hours after the last dose of drug.
Allergies	No issues.
Anxiety	If the patient requires an anxiolytic for treatment, contact the patient's physician to discuss options. Consider using a short-acting benzodiazepine, and prescribe only enough for one appointment. Also, consider intraoperative use of nitrous oxide–oxygen.
B	
Bleeding	For patients with alcohol abuse, excessive bleeding secondary to liver disease is possible. Lab tests may be needed for confirmation.
Breathing	No issues.
Blood pressure	For cocaine and methamphetamine abusers, monitor blood pressure and pulse during appointment.
C	
Chair position	No issues.
Cardiovascular	Cocaine and methamphetamine abusers are at increased risk for cardiac arrhythmias, myocardial infarction, and stroke.
D	
Drugs	Epinephrine can potentiate the adverse cardiovascular effects of cocaine and amphetamines.
Devices	No issues.
E	
Equipment	No issues.
Emergencies	For cocaine and methamphetamine abusers, cardiovascular emergencies are possible, especially with the use of epinephrine within 24 hours of last drug use.
F	
Follow-up	If narcotic analgesics are prescribed, the patient should be monitored to ensure proper drug use.

drugs. Findings may include subcutaneous abscesses, cellulitis, thrombophlebitis, skin "tracks" (chronic inflammation from multiple injections), and infected lesions. Skin tracks usually appear as linear or bifurcated erythematous lesions, which become indurated and hyperpigmented. An ill-defined febrile illness also may indicate a possible problem with parenteral drug abuse.[2,15]

Drug abusers may try to obtain drugs from dentists by demanding pain medication for a dental problem (e.g., toothache) instead of problem-specific treatment. Likewise, pain medication may be requested (or demanded) after minor, nonsurgical procedures that typically would not be a cause of significant postoperative pain (e.g., small restoration). The opioid abuser also may claim to be allergic to codeine or intolerant to nonsteroidal anti-inflammatory drugs, in an attempt to obtain a stronger drug such as hydrocodone or oxycodone. Prescription pads should not be left out in clear view, nor should they be kept where patients can easily find and take them. The practitioner also should avoid the use of prewritten or presigned prescription forms for controlled drugs.

Drug abuse is found more often in dentists and other dental office personnel than in the general population because of the ready access to opioid analgesics and sedative-hypnotic drugs. Abusive use of nitrous oxide inhalation is another form of drug abuse that is found among dentists.

Marijuana. Chronic use of marijuana can lead to chronic bronchitis, airway obstruction, poor oral health due to neglect and xerostomia, and squamous metaplasia. The autonomic effects of marijuana include tachycardia, reduced peripheral resistance, and, with large doses, orthostatic hypotension.[15] Thus, marijuana use may be harmful to persons with ischemic heart disease or cardiac failure. Care should be taken in providing dental treatment to such patients, and if such an association is identified, dental treatment should be postponed until the patient is stable.

Cocaine. Patients who are "high" on cocaine should not receive any local anesthetic containing epinephrine for at least 6 hours after the last administration of cocaine, because cocaine potentiates the response of sympathomimetic amines.[16] Use of epinephrine-impregnated retraction cord should be avoided. The danger of significant myocardial ischemia and cardiac arrhythmia is the primary concern in patients with cocaine intoxication. Peak blood levels of cocaine occur within 30 minutes, and effects usually dissipate within 2 hours.

Before treating a patient who is participating in a cocaine treatment program, the dentist should consult the patient's physician regarding medications that the patient may be taking and how best to manage procedure-related pain. Patients with substance abuse should rarely be prescribed addictive substances, and then only with great caution.[2]

Methamphetamine. Patients who are "high" on methamphetamine should not receive dental treatment for at least 8 hours after the last administration of the drug, and for maximum safety, dental treatment probably should not occur until at least 24 hours after the last administration. Peak blood levels occur within 30 to 60 minutes, and effects usually dissipate within 8 hours; however, depending on the compound, the serum half-life of the various amphetamines can last between 7 and 34 hours.[2,17] Significant myocardial ischemia and cardiac arrhythmia are the primary concerns in patients with methamphetamine intoxication. Local anesthetics with epinephrine or levonordefrin must not be used during the 8-hour waiting period after methamphetamine administration, because methamphetamine potentiates the response of sympathomimetic amines, which could result in a hypertensive crisis, stroke, or myocardial infarction.[18]

Alcohol. The dentist has an opportunity to assist patients who have, or may have, alcohol-abuse problems. It has been shown that even brief advice or discussions in a clinical setting by a health care provider can have positive effects. Research indicates that brief interventions for alcohol problems are more effective than no intervention and, in some cases, can be as effective as more extensive intervention.[19,20] On the basis of these findings, the Center for Substance Abuse Treatment (CSAT) has devised a new initiative known as Screening, Brief Intervention, Referral, and Treatment (SBIRT), summarized next.

Screening. The patient with alcohol-related problems often can be recognized from examination of health problems and behaviors, such as medical signs and symptoms, noncompliance, exacerbated anxieties and fears, failure to fulfill obligations, and emotional fluctuations. Features suggestive of alcohol abuse include missed appointment, enlargement of the parotid glands (Figure 30-3), and spider angiomas (Figure 30-4). A common

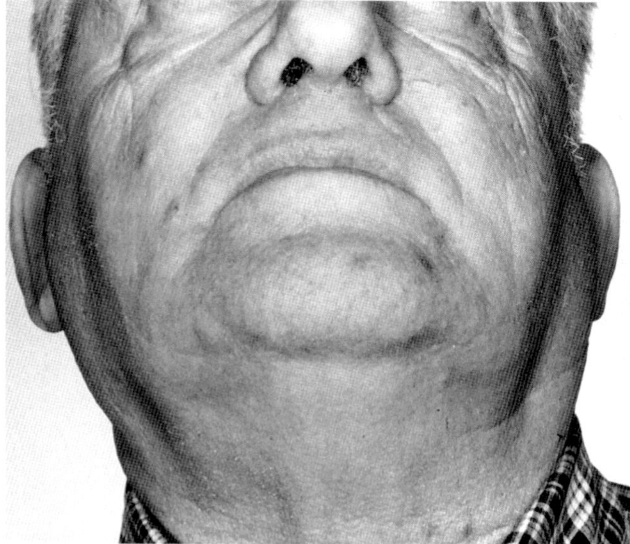

FIGURE 30-3 Painless enlargement of the parotid glands associated with alcoholism. *(Courtesy Valerie Murrah, Chapel Hill, North Carolina.)*

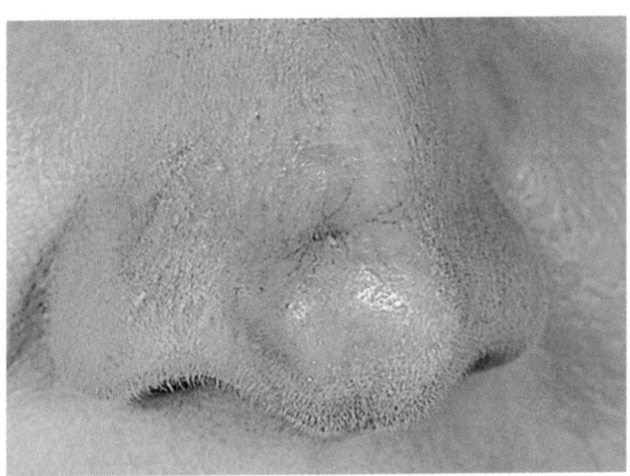

FIGURE 30-4 Spider angiomas, which may be a sign of alcoholism. *(From Seidel HM, et al:* Mosby's guide to physical examination, *ed 6, St. Louis, 2006, Mosby.)*

scenario that should raise a red flag is that in which the patient presents for treatment with alcohol on the breath. Of note, problems with alcohol transcend age, gender, and socioeconomic spectrum, and many patients are skilled at masquerading their dependence.

During the medical history, the dentist should obtain information from all adolescent and adult patients about the type, quantity, frequency, pattern of alcohol use, as well as consequences of its use, and family history of alcoholism. The National Institute on Alcohol Abuse and Alcoholism (NIAAA) has recommended either the use of a single alcohol screening question (SASQ) or administration of the Alcohol Use Disorders Identification Test (AUDIT) self-report questionnaire (Table 30-3) as the standard screening approach to detection of alcohol-related problems. An alternative screening approach is the use of the CAGE questionnaire, which only asks four questions that are designed to identify problem drinkers. The use of either the AUDIT or CAGE questionnaire is ideal but in most dental practices would be too time-consuming and probably impractical, so the SASQ approach is a recommended alternative. When using the SASQ, clinicians are advised to ask if the patient has consumed five or more standard drinks (for a man) on one occasion during the last year (four drinks for women). The questioning should be done in an objective, nonjudgmental manner. A positive response may indicate an alcohol-related problem and requires more detailed assessment.[8]

Brief Intervention. It is important that the patient understand the adverse consequences of alcohol abuse in all aspects of the problem—medical, dental, psychological, and social. The dentist can point out destructive patterns of alcohol use and identify future health issues and other difficulties expected if alcohol abuse continues. Also important to review with the patient are the possibilities and successes of treatment. After a review of key ingredients in several brief intervention protocols, Miller and Sanchez[21] proposed six critical elements that they summarized with the acronym FRAMES: Feedback, Responsibility, Advice, Menu, Empathy, and Self-efficacy. The clinician completes some assessment and provides *feedback* on the patient's alcohol-related problems, stresses the patient's *responsibility* to address the problem, gives clear *advice* to change drinking behavior, provides a *menu* of treatment options, expresses *empathy* for the patient's problem, and stresses *self-efficacy*—the expectation that the patient has the skills and information needed to successfully resolve the drinking problems. Additional components of goal setting, follow-up, and timing also have been identified as important to the effectiveness of brief interventions.

Referral. Assisting a patient into a treatment program requires that the dentist share concerns obtained from the medical assessment. Accordingly, the dentist will need to be familiar with treatment options within the local community such as detoxification, inpatient programs, outpatient programs, halfway houses, and continuing care. Consultation with or referral to the patient's primary care provider (if the person has one) is advised.

Treatment. Treatment of nondependent but at-risk problem drinkers may be accomplished by counseling, motivational techniques, and setting drinking limits below at-risk limits (e.g., less than one drink per day for women and two drinks per day for men).[4] Treatment of alcohol dependence can occur informally without professional assistance; however, chances of a successful outcome are greater with an organized program based on professional help. The first step is complete withdrawal and abstinence from alcohol. Most often, this step can be accomplished on an outpatient basis, although for more severe dependence, inpatient treatment may be necessary. The major goals of medical management of alcohol withdrawal are to minimize the severity of withdrawal-related symptoms, to prevent specific withdrawal-related complications such as seizures and delirium tremens, and to provide referral to relapse prevention treatment.[4] Relapse prevention is accomplished using psychotherapeutic techniques (motivational enhancement techniques, "12-step program" facilitation, cognitive-behavioral coping skills), self-help groups (e.g., Alcoholics Anonymous [AA]), and pharmacotherapy. Three drugs are currently approved for the treatment of alcohol dependence: disulfiram, naltrexone, and acamprosate.[4]

To minimize risk for relapse, the dentist should avoid the use of psychoactive drugs, narcotics, sedatives, and alcohol-containing medications in patients who are recovering from alcoholism. If a potentially mood-altering drug is required, the patient's primary care physician (or substance abuse advisor) should be consulted about its use. If approved for use, the drug should be prescribed only in the amount needed without refills. Designating a family member

TABLE 30-3 Alcohol Use Disorders Identification Test (AUDIT) Self-Report Questionnaire

PATIENT: Because alcohol use can affect your health and can interfere with certain medications and treatments, it is important that we ask some questions about your use of alcohol. Your answers will remain confidential so please be honest. Place an X in one box that best describes your answer to each question.

Questions	0	1	2	3	4	Score
1. How often do you have a drink containing alcohol?	Never	Monthly or less	2 to 4 times a month	2 to 3 times a week	4 or more times a week	
2. How many drinks containing alcohol do you have on a typical day when you are drinking?	1 or 2	3 or 4	5 or 6	7 to 9	10 or more	
3. How often do you have five or more drinks on one occasion?	Never	Less than monthly	Monthly	Weekly	Daily or almost daily	
4. How often during the last year have you found that you were not able to stop drinking once you had started?	Never	Less than monthly	Monthly	Weekly	Daily or almost daily	
5. How often during the last year have you failed to do what was normally expected of you because of drinking?	Never	Less than monthly	Monthly	Weekly	Daily or almost daily	
6. How often during the last year have you needed a first drink in the morning to get yourself going after a heavy drinking session?	Never	Less than monthly	Monthly	Weekly	Daily or almost daily	
7. How often during the last year have you had a feeling of guilt or remorse after drinking?	Never	Less than monthly	Monthly	Weekly	Daily or almost daily	
8. How often during the last year have you been unable to remember what happened the night before because of your drinking?	Never	Less than monthly	Monthly	Weekly	Daily or almost daily	
9. Have you or has someone else been injured because of your drinking?	No		Yes, but not in the last year		Yes, during the last year	
10. Has a relative, friend, doctor, or other health care worker been concerned about your drinking or suggested you cut down?	No		Yes, but not in the last year		Yes, during the last year	
					Total:	

NOTE: This self-report questionnaire (the Alcohol Use Disorders Identification Test [AUDIT]) is from the World Health Organization. To reflect standard drink sizes in the United States, the number of drinks in question 3 was changed from 6 to 5. A free AUDIT manual with guidelines for use in primary care is available online at http://www.who.org.

From Babor TF, et al: AUDIT: the alcohol use disorders identification test: guidelines for use in primary health care. Geneva: World Health Organization, *2001, WHO/MSD/MSB/01.6a.*

to fill and dispense the drug can minimize the risk of abuse.

Treatment Planning Considerations

(see Box 30-1)

The goals of dental treatment for patients with substance and alcohol abuse disorders are to maintain oral health, comfort, and function and to prevent and control oral disease. Without an aggressive approach to prevention, dental caries and periodontal disease will occur with increased frequency. Susceptibility to these problems stems from a reduced interest in performing or the inability to perform oral hygiene procedures. Also, in many of these patients, the diet typically relies heavily on foods and drinks that increase the risk for dental disease.[22]

The dental treatment plan should contain the following elements (see Box 30-1). Daily oral hygiene procedures must be identified. Complex dental procedures should be performed only when the patient is in a stable condition in the context of the substance abuse disorder. The dental team should communicate to the patient a positive, hopeful attitude toward maintenance of the patient's oral health. The last aspect of the treatment plan deals with selection of pain or anxiolytic medications to be used in dental treatment procedures. It is critical that appropriate pain and anxiolytic medication be provided to the patient; however, certain agents may have to be avoided, and others may require a reduction in their usual dosage. Consultation with the physician who is overseeing the management of the substance or alcohol abuse problem is advisable, to discuss drug selection and administration. It also may be necessary to involve a third party, such as a "12-step program" sponsor, to monitor the taking of medication.[23]

In addition to the above considerations, three specific problems of major clinical importance in patients with alcoholic liver disease are recognized: (1) bleeding tendencies, (2) unpredictable metabolism of certain drugs, and (3) risk for spread of infection. These conditions may require the dentist to change usual drug dosages. Chapter 10 presents specific management recommendations for these problems.

Oral Complications and Manifestations

Patients with drug and alcohol abuse disorders tend to have more plaque, calculus, caries, and gingival inflammation than is typical for patients without such disorders. These problems are related primarily to oral neglect, rather than to any inherent property of the abused substance. Depending on the degree of neglect, caries, and periodontal disease, the dentist should not provide extensive care until the patient demonstrates an interest in and ability to care for the dentition. With intraoral use of cocaine, gingival recession and erosion of the facial aspects of the maxillary teeth may result from persistent rubbing of the powder over these surfaces. Chronic methamphetamine use causes xerostomia and rampant caries with subjective reports of a bad taste in the mouth, bruxism (grinding of the teeth), and muscle trismus (jaw clenching).[18] Xerostomia significantly increases the risks for dental caries, enamel erosion, and periodontal disease. Neglect of personal oral hygiene, high intake of refined carbohydrates and sucrose, and increased acidity from gastrointestinal regurgitation, bulimia, or vomiting also contribute to exaggerated caries and erosion problems in meth abusers. The combination of these effects is referred to as "meth mouth" (Figure 30-5). Meth users are "wired" and exhibit extremely high levels of energy and neuromuscular activity, often leading to parafunctional jaw activity and bruxism. Bruxism and muscle trismus can compound the effects of periodontal disease. Patients who use ecstasy demonstrate "bruxing" activity during use of the drug. To combat the tooth clenching, pacifiers have been used.

A variety of oral abnormalities may be found in patients with alcohol abuse. Patients with cirrhosis have been reported to have impaired gustatory function and are malnourished. Nutritional deficiencies can result in glossitis and loss of tongue papillae along with angular

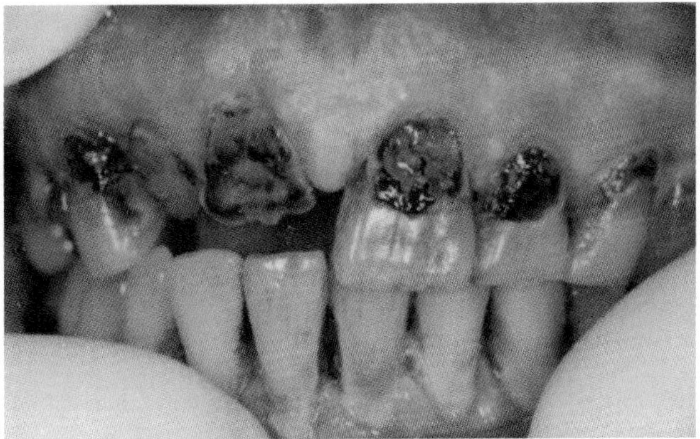

FIGURE 30-5 "Meth mouth."

or labial cheilitis, which is complicated by concomitant candidal infection. Vitamin K deficiency, disordered hemostasis, portal hypertension, and splenomegaly (causing thrombocytopenia) can result in spontaneous gingival bleeding, mucosal ecchymoses, and petechiae. In some instances unexplained gingival bleeding has been the initial complaint of alcoholic patients. Also, a sweet, musty odor to the breath is associated with liver failure, as is jaundiced mucosal tissue. A bilateral, painless enlargement of the parotid glands (sialadenosis) is a frequent finding in patients with cirrhosis.[24-27]

Alcohol abuse and tobacco use are strong risk factors for the development of oral squamous cell carcinoma, and the dentist must be aggressive (as with all patients) in the detection of unexplained or suspicious soft tissue lesions (especially leukoplakia, erythroplakia, or ulceration) in chronic alcoholics. High-risk sites for development of oral squamous cell carcinoma include the lateral border of the tongue and the floor of the mouth (see Chapter 26).

REFERENCES

1. American Psychiatric Association: *Diagnostic and statistical manual of mental disorders*, ed 4, text rev, Washington, DC, 2000, American Psychiatric Association.
2. Samet JH: Drug use and dependence. In Goldman L, Ausiello D, editors: *Cecil medicine*, ed 23, Philadelphia, 2008, Saunders, pp 174-182.
3. Hyman SE: Biology of addiction. In Goldman L, Ausiello D, editors: *Cecil medicine*, ed 23, Philadelphia, 2008, Saunders, pp 159-161.
4. O'Conner PG: Alcohol abuse and dependence. In Goldman L, Ausiello D, editors: *Cecil medicine*, ed 23, Philadelphia, 2008, Saunders, pp 167-174.
5. Substance Abuse and Mental Health Services Administration, Office of Applied Studies: *The NSDUH report*, Rockville, Md, 2009, U.S. Department of Health and Human Services.
6. Renner JA, Ward N: Drug addiction. In Stern TA, et al, editors: *Massachusetts General Hospital comprehensive clinical psychiatry*, Philadelphia, 2008, Mosby.
7. Grant BF, et al: Prevalence and co-occurrence of substance use disorders and independent mood and anxiety disorders: results from the National Epidemiologic Survey on Alcohol and Related Conditions, *Arch Gen Psychiatry* 6:807-816, 2004.

8. National Institute on Alcohol Abuse and Alcoholism: *Helping patients who drink too much: a clinician's guide and related professional support resources*, Rockville, Md, 2005, U.S. Department of Health and Human Services.
9. Kenna GA, Lewis DC: Risk factors for alcohol and other drug use by healthcare professionals, *Subst Abuse Treat Prev Policy* 3:3, 2008.
10. Painkillers fuel growth in drug addiction. Opioid overdoses now kill more people than cocaine or heroin, *Harv Ment Health Lett.* 27:4-5, 2011.
11. Volkow ND, Fowler JS, Wang GJ: The addicted human brain: insights from imaging studies, *J Clin Invest* 111:1444-1451, 2003.
12. Cho AK, Melega WP: Patterns of methamphetamine abuse and their consequences, *J Addict Dis* 21:21-34, 2002.
13. Substance Abuse and Mental Health Services Administration, Office of Applied Studies: *Drug abuse warning network, 2004: national estimates of drug-related emergency department visits*, Rockville, Md, 2004, U.S. Department of Health and Human Services.
14. Winstock A: Psychoactive drug misuse. In Wright P, Stern J, Phelan M, editors: *Core psychiatry*, Edinburgh, 2005, Elsevier, pp 431-455.
15. Bockman CS, Abel PW: Drugs of abuse. In Yagiella JA, et al, editors: *Pharmacology and therapeutics for dentistry*, St. Louis, 2011, Mosby, pp 799-813.
16. Blanksma CJ, Brand HS: Cocaine abuse: orofacial manifestations and implications for dental treatment, *Int Dent J* 55: 365-369, 2005.
17. Albertson TE, Kenyon NJ, Morrissey B: Amphetamines and derivatives. In Shannon MW, Borron SW, Burns MJ, editors: *Haddad and Winchester's clinical management of poisoning and drug overdose*, Philadelphia, 2007, Saunders.
18. Hamamoto DT, Rhodus NL: Methamphetamine abuse and dentistry, *Oral Dis* 15:27-37, 2009.
19. Fleming MF: Brief interventions and the treatment of alcohol use disorders: current evidence, *Recent Dev Alcohol* 16: 375-390, 2003.
20. Bien T, Miller WR, Tonigen JS: Brief interventions for alcohol problems: a review, *Addiction* 88:315-336, 1993.
21. Miller WR, Sanchez V: Motivating young adults for treatment and lifestyle change. In Howard G, Nathan P, editors: *Alcohol use and misuse by young adults*, 1994, University of Notre Dame Press: Notre Dame, Ind.
22. Little JW: Dental implications of mood disorders, *Gen Dent* 52:442-450, 2004.
23. Lindroth JE, Herren MC, Falace DA: The management of acute dental pain in the recovering alcoholic, *Oral Surg Oral Med Oral Pathol Oral Radiol Endod* 95:432-436, 2003.
24. McCullough AJ, O'Shea RS, Dasarathy S: Diagnosis and management of alcoholic liver disease, *J Dig Dis* 12:257-262, 2011.
25. Bergasa NV: Approach to the patient with liver disease. In Goldman L, Ausiello D, editors: *Cecil medicine*, ed 23, Philadelphia, 2008, Saunders, pp 1087-1090.
26. Friedman LS: Surgery in the patient with liver disease, *Trans Am Clin Climatol Assoc* 121:192-204, 2010.
27. Brennan MT, et al: Utility of an international normalized ratio testing device in a hospital-based dental practice, *J Am Dent Assoc* 139:697-703, 2008.

APPENDICES

APPENDIX A

Guide to Management of Common Medical Emergencies in the Dental Office*

GENERAL CONSIDERATIONS

The best management of a dental office medical emergency is prevention. Dental practitioners must be prepared to treat the seemingly well but chronically ill patient whose condition is managed by a variety of drugs. Prevention begins with the dental professional's awareness of the patient's medical condition at the outset of the dental visit. Knowledge of the type of condition, its severity, and level of control provides a strong indicator of the patient's risk for experiencing a medical emergency. Proper assessment that includes review of the medical history, physical evaluation, and medical consultation gives the practitioner the opportunity to take measures that could prevent such emergencies. If an emergency does occur, an informed dentist will have a better idea of the type of medical problem the patient is experiencing. The dentist must also understand the pathophysiologic factors regulating disease processes and the pharmacodynamics of drug action and interaction.

Patients frequently experience physical reactions during treatment. Accordingly, considerable responsibility rests on the dentist first to recognize the signs and symptoms of the problem and then to respond to any emergency quickly, efficiently, and competently with adequate resuscitative procedures. Obviously, important precepts of good medical emergency management include (1) being well prepared, (2) having confidence in selected interventions, and (3) remaining calm in difficult circumstances. The health professional is responsible for knowing and using techniques that are recognized to be up to date, safe, and efficient. An unfamiliar or unreliable maneuver should never be attempted. The dentist must be trained in providing basic cardiac life support (BCLS) and in managing emergencies in the dental office. Advanced cardiac life support (ACLS) training to include intravenous (IV) drug administration may be useful in dental practices that more often encounter medically complex cases. The dental practitioner also should be aware of the changes in basic cardiopulmonary resuscitation (CPR) guidelines introduced in 2010.

Although dentists should be prepared to provide resuscitation procedures in the dental setting, even more consideration should be directed at preventing such situations. Prevention begins with obtaining an adequate medical history of the patient, making an appropriate physical evaluation, and ensuring that both patient and environment are properly prepared before treatment begins. Sometimes a potentially catastrophic event may be prevented through recognition of physical conditions or limitations before treatment begins.

Management of emergencies must begin long before the point of occurrence. Preparation should include a designated plan of action and an adequate armamentarium to meet emergencies. To minimize largely unhelpful emotional responses, the actions of the dental team must be based on a thorough background in relevant subject matter, continued study, and carefully prepared and rehearsed emergency procedures in which each person has specific duties and responsibilities. This approach will require the availability of appropriate resuscitative equipment and drugs to permit the team to work together calmly and precisely. This teamwork must be based on knowledge, practice, sound judgment, and confidence. To this end, all members of the dental office (dentist, hygienist, assistant, receptionist) should be

*Much of the material contained herein is modified from Malamed SF: *Medical emergencies in the dental office*, ed 6, St Louis, 2007, Mosby; Malamed SF: *Emergency medicine in the dental office* (DVD), Edmonds, WA, HealthFirst Corporation, 2008, Joseph Massad Productions; 2005 American Heart Association guidelines for cardiopulmonary resuscitation and emergency cardiovascular care, *Circulation* 112(Suppl 24):IV1-203, 2005; and Part 1: executive summary: 2010 American Heart Association guidelines for cardiopulmonary resuscitation and emergency cardiovascular care, *Circulation* 122(Suppl 3):S640-S656, 2010.

trained in and be able to perform BCLS procedures properly when needed. Also, every dental office should have a written plan that spells out specific duties for each member of the office staff, covering areas such as who will activate the emergency medical services (EMS) system (i.e., call 911), start CPR, place an intravenous line, and administer drugs. A staff member should be designated to assist in necessary tasks during the emergency situation, such as getting and preparing drugs and recording every event and the time of each action.

Dental offices should have up-to-date emergency drugs, oxygen, a pulse oximeter, and an automated external defibrillator (AED). Electrocardiography is an additional important adjunct modality for monitoring the patient's vital signs.

GENERAL PRINCIPLES OF EMERGENCY CARE

Most life-threatening office emergencies are caused by the patient's inability to withstand physical or emotional stress or the patient's reaction to drugs. Emergencies also can originate with a complication of a preexisting systemic disease. Cardiopulmonary systems can be involved, thereby necessitating some emergency supportive therapy.

Algorithms (i.e., standardized step-by-step procedures) are recommended to be performed during emergencies after the signs and symptoms of the condition are recognized. Most often, the algorithm for medical emergencies follows the sequence P-A-B-C-D, where P is for *positioning,* A is for *airway,* B is for *breathing,* C is for *circulation,* and D is for *definitive care* (e.g., diagnosis, drugs and defibrillator and other equipment). Of note, however, in 2010, the American Heart Association recommended use of a slightly different algorithm for cardiac arrest, that is, P-C-A-B-D. Our own contribution has been to add an E, for *ensure proper patient response,* and an F, for *facilitate next steps in medical/dental care,* for a more specific approach to this aspect of dental management.

This appendix presents recommended management protocols, following the algorithms just described, for various medical emergencies likely to be encountered in the dental office.

Key Points

The following elements are essential to the successful treatment of medical emergencies:

1. Quick recognition of signs and symptoms and early diagnosis of the underlying problem
2. Fast response time (4 to 6 minutes without oxygen leads to irreversible brain damage)
3. Systematic monitoring of the patient's well-being using an algorithm such as P-A-B-C-D-E-F or, for cardiac arrest, P-C-A-B-D-E-F

TYPES OF EMERGENCIES AND THEIR TREATMENT

Unconsciousness

Syncope and Psychogenic Shock

Signs and Symptoms. Pallor, sweating, nausea, anxiety, pupillary dilation, yawning, decreased blood pressure, bradycardia (slow pulse), convulsive movements, unconsciousness.

Cause. Cerebral hypoxia (reduced blood flow to brain), sitting or standing stiff, anxiety.

Treatment

P: Positioning: Place patient in supine position; lower head slightly and elevate legs (for pregnant women, roll on left side)—assess consciousness.
A: Airway: Ensure open airway.
B: Breathing: Check breathing—should be adequate.
C: Circulation: Check carotid pulse—should be adequate.
D: Dispense/administer:
- Oxygen at flow rate of 5-6 L/minute
- Aromatic ammonia (e.g., Vaporole)—"smelling salts" (optional)
- Cold compresses applied to forehead

E: Ensure that vital signs, drug administration, and patient responses are properly monitored and recorded.
F: Facilitate next steps in medical/dental care and reassure patient.

Low Blood Pressure/Slow Pulse

For low blood pressure or pulse (systolic is less than previous diastolic), the following protocol is indicated:

Treatment: Low Blood Pressure

P: Positioning: Place patient in supine position; lower head and raise legs.
A: Airway: Ensure open airway.
B: Breathing: Check breathing—should be adequate.
C: Circulation: Check pulse and ensure adequate circulation, which may be weak.
D: Dispense/administer:
- Intravenous drip of 5% dextrose in lactated Ringer's solution
- In *unresponsive patient*: a vasopressor drug such as phenylephrine 10 mg/mL (1 ampule), or epinephrine 0.3-0.5 mg given subcutaneously (SC) or intramuscularly (IM), or intravenously (IV) with ACLS training

E: Ensure that vital signs, drug administration, and patient responses are properly monitored and recorded.

F: Facilitate next steps in medical/dental care; reassure patient.

Treatment: Slow Pulse. (Less than 60 beats/minute)

P: Positioning: Place patient in supine position; lower head and raise arms and legs.

A: Airway: Ensure and maintain patent airway.

B: Breathing: Check breathing—should be adequate.

C: Circulation: Check—should be adequate in this situation.

D: Dispense/administer:

- Oxygen at flow rate of 5-6 L/minute (if patient is hypoxemic)
- Atropine 0.5 mg IV (to increase heart rate). Repeat dose up to 3 mg; then consider use of additional vasopressors (dopamine or epinephrine).

E: Ensure that vital signs, drug administration, and patient responses are properly monitored and recorded.

F: Facilitate next steps in medical/dental care; reassure patient.

Cardiac Arrest

Signs and Symptoms. No pulse or blood pressure, sudden cessation of respiration (apnea), cyanosis, dilated pupils.

Cause. Abrupt interruption of blood supply and oxygen to the coronary arteries and heart muscle due to ischemia (clot).

Treatment

For *unresponsive cardiac arrest victim* (adult):

P: Positioning: Place patient in supine position and establish unresponsiveness (tap and shout). Call for help, activate EMS (call 911), and get defibrillator.

C: Circulation and compressions: Health care provider should assess pulse (carotid) for no more than 10 seconds. If no pulse is detected, and victim is not breathing and is unresponsive, promptly initiate chest compressions.

One operator: 30 compressions per every 2 ventilations for a rate of 100 compressions/minute (depth of 2 inches), until advanced airway is placed

A: Airway: Establish airway by head tilt–chin lift, or by jaw thrust if neck injury is suspected. *Suction mouth/pharynx if vomitus is blocking the airway.*

B: Breathing: Ventilate lungs with mask Ambubag–delivered positive-pressure oxygen (or mouth-to-mask resuscitation); breathe every 6 to 8 seconds (8 to 10 breaths/minute).

If rescuer is ACLS-trained, perform endotracheal intubation and provide positive-pressure oxygen.

NOTE: As of 2010: Ventilation technique uses slower breaths with inspiration time of 1.5 to 2 seconds.

Two operators: 15 compressions per every 2 ventilations (without pause for compressions), for a rate of 100 compressions/minute. Continue resuscitation until spontaneous pulse returns.

NOTE: The importance of technique for chest compressions cannot be overemphasized; they must be hard, fast, and maximally effective, with minimal interruptions.

D: Defibrillator: Attach and use automated external defibrillator (AED) as soon as available (ideally within 3 to 5 minutes of collapse).

- Check rhythm and shock if indicated (repeated every 2 minutes).
- Resume CPR beginning with compressions immediately after each shock.

NOTE: With intravenous drugs: Start normal saline solution (with ACLS-trained rescuer).

- Epinephrine 1.0 mg 1:1000; repeat every 3 to 5 minutes as needed.
- Vasopressin 40 units can replace first or second dose of epinephrine.
- Amiodarone—*first dose*: 300 mg bolus; *second dose*: 150 mg

Other drugs used for treatment of cardiac arrest (with ACLS-trained rescuer)

- Lidocaine (antiarrhythmic agent)
- Calcium chloride (increases myocardial contractility)
- Morphine sulfate (for pain relief)
- Thrombolytic agents

E: Ensure that vital signs, drug administration, and patient responses are properly monitored and recorded.

F: Facilitate/ensure next steps in medical care (transport to hospital); reassure patient.

Hypoglycemia (Insulin Shock)

Signs and Symptoms. Hunger, weakness, trembling, tachycardia, pallor, sweating, paresthesias, uncooperative, mental confusion (headache), incoherent, uncooperative, belligerent, unconscious, tonic-clonic movements, hypotension, hypothermia, rapid thready pulse, coma.

Cause. Lack of blood glucose to the brain; taking insulin and not eating.

Treatment

P: Position:

In *conscious patient*: place in upright sitting position.

In *unconscious patient*: place in supine position.

A: Airway: Ensure open airway.

B: Breathing: Ensure that patient is breathing.

C: Circulation: Check pulse and confirm adequate circulation; pulse could be weak.

D: Dispense:
In *conscious patient*: Give a drink with high sugar content such as orange juice, or a glucose paste (cake icing) applied to the buccal mucosa.
In *unconscious patient*: Activate EMS by calling 911; then administer:
- Oxygen at flow rate of 5-6 L/minute
- 5% dextrose in Ringer's lactate (D5LR) IV: Run the intravenous drip as fast as possible.
- Alternatively, give glucagon 1 mg SC or IM (or IV), or epinephrine (for transient relief).

E: Ensure that vital signs, drug administration, and patient responses are properly monitored and recorded.
F: Facilitate/ensure next steps in medical care (transport to hospital, if some improvement is not fairly rapid). When patient regains consciousness, provide reassurance and information about what happened, because person is likely to have little memory of the incident.

Acute Adrenal Insufficiency

Signs and Symptoms. Altered consciousness, wet, clammy, confusion, weakness, fatigue, headache, pain in abdomen or legs, nausea and vomiting, hypotension and syncope, coma.
Cause. Adrenal suppression (low adrenocorticotropic hormone) by exogenous steroids. The patient may be medicated with steroids for many medical problems, or the cause may be primary or secondary malfunction of the adrenal cortex.

Treatment

P: Positioning: Place patient in semireclined position, and raise feet slightly; call for help.
A: Airway: Ensure open airway.
B: Breathing: Should be adequate (i.e., predicted to be adequate in this situation).
C: Circulation: Check pulse and confirm adequate circulation.
D: Dispense:
In *conscious patient*:
- Provide oxygen at flow rate of 5-6 L/minute.
- Give hydrocortisone 100 mg, or dexamethasone 4 mg (IV).

In *unconscious patient*:
- Place in supine position.
- Activate EMS by calling 911.
- Administer oxygen at flow rate of 5-6 L/minute.
- Confirm diagnosis from review of medical history, signs, and symptoms.
- Then start intravenous administration of 5% dextrose in Ringer's lactate (D5LR) and run the intravenous drip as fast as possible.
- Also provide hydrocortisone 100 mg, or dexamethasone 4 mg (IV).
- Give a vasopressor drug (e.g., epinephrine 1:1000, 0.5 mL).

E: Ensure that vital signs, drug administration, and patient responses are properly monitored and recorded.
F: Facilitate/ensure next steps in medical care (transport to hospital); reassure patient.

Cerebrovascular Accident (Stroke)

Signs and Symptoms. Dizziness (patient may fall), vertigo and vision changes, nausea and vomiting, transient paresthesia, unilateral weakness or paralysis, headache, nausea, vomiting, convulsions, coma.

NOTE: Blood pressure and pulse generally are normal. Raised blood pressure and body temperature and lowered pulse and respiration indicate increased intracranial pressure.
Cause. Interruption of blood supply and oxygen to the brain occurring as a result of ischemia or hemorrhage.

Treatment

P: Positioning: Place patient in reclined, semisitting position with the head elevated. Call for help and activate EMS (call 911).
A: Airway: Ensure that airway is open and maintained open.
B: Breathing: Ensure that breathing is adequate.
C: Circulation: Check pulse and confirm adequate circulation.
D: Dispense/administer:
- Use pulse oximeter to determine oxygenation.
- Administer oxygen at flow rate of 5-6 L/minute if needed.

E: Ensure that vital signs, drug administration, and patient responses are properly monitored and recorded.
- Keep patient quiet and still.

F: Facilitate/ensure next steps in medical care (transport to hospital); reassure patients. (Seizure)

Convulsions (Seizure)

Signs and Symptoms. Aura (flash of light or sound, a unusual smell), mental confusion, excessive salivation, rolling back of eyes, loss of consciousness, tonic phase (contractions—clenching of teeth) followed by clonic phase (tremors, convulsive movements of extremities).
Causes. There are several potential causes of convulsions and seizures including syncope, drug reactions (local anesthetic overdose), hypoglycemia, hyperventilation, cerebrovascular accident, and convulsive seizure disorder.

Treatment

P: Positioning: Place patient in supine position; clear instruments and protect patient from injury (i.e., lightly restrain arms and legs from gross movements). Call for help.

After convulsion ceases:

A: Airway: Ensure that airway is open. Suction mouth along buccal surfaces of teeth if excessive secretions are making breathing difficult.

B: Breathing: Ensure that breathing is adequate.

C: Circulation: Check pulse and confirm adequate circulation.

D: Dispense/administer:

- Oxygen at flow of 5-6 L/minute

For status epilepticus (a seizure lasting more than 5 minutes):

- Activate EMS (call 911).
- For adult, give diazepam (Valium) 5-20 mg IV *or* intranasal lorazepam 2-4 mg *or* intranasal midazolam 5 mg, one-half volume per nostril (may not be readily available—ask pharmacist)

If convulsions persist for 5 minutes after treating, repeat with one-half dose.

E: Ensure that vital signs, drug administration, and patient responses are properly monitored and recorded.

- Support respiration (seizure may precipitate respiratory arrest).

F: Facilitate/ensure next steps in medical care (transport to hospital, if needed), and reassure patient.

Local Anesthesia Drug Toxicity

Signs and Symptoms. Confusion, talkative, restless, apprehensive state, excited manner, headache, lightheadness, convulsions, increase in blood pressure and pulse rate. NOTE: Stimulation is followed by depression of the central nervous system.

Late features can include drowsiness, disorientation, convulsions followed by depression, drop in blood pressure, weak or rapid pulse or bradycardia, apnea, unconsciousness, death. NOTE: Lidocaine toxicity is documented to occasionally exhibit depression only, without the usual prodromal of the excitatory phase.

Causes. Too-large a dose of local anesthetic per body weight, rapid absorption of drug or inadvertent intravenous injection, slow detoxification or elimination of drug

Treatment

P: Positioning: Place patient in comfortable position; convulsing or unconscious patient should be in supine position.

If patient is convulsing:

- Clear instruments and protect patient from injury.
- Call for help.

After convulsion ceases:

A: Airway: ensure airway is open.

B: Breathing: Ensure that breathing is adequate.

C: Circulation: Check pulse and confirm adequate circulation.

D: Dispense/administer:

- Oxygen at flow rate of 5-6 L/minute
- If local anesthesia overdose results in seizure, a benzodiazepine (diazepam, lorazepam, or midazolam) as described in the seizure algorithm may be administered.

E: Ensure vital signs, drug administration are properly monitored and recorded; maintain blood pressure

F: Facilitate/ensure next steps in medical care (provide supportive therapy):

- Treat bradycardia (0.4 mg atropine IV, with ACLS-trained rescuer).
- Transport to hospital.
- Reassure patient.

NOTE: If patient becomes unconscious, maintain airway, administer CPR, and activate EMS (call 911).

Respiratory Difficulty

Hyperventilation

Signs and Symptoms. Rapid and shallow breathing, confusion, dizziness, paresthesias, cold hands, carpal-pedal spasms; can progress to seizure.

Cause. Anxiety-induced excessive loss of CO_2 from deep and rapid breathing; also respiratory alkalosis.

Treatment

P: Positioning: Place patient in an upright position. Explain the problem and reassure the patient.

A: Airway: Maintain open airway by talking with patient.

B: Breathing: Instruct the patient to be calm and breathe slowly into a paper bag or into the cupped hands over the nose and mouth (i.e., rebreathe carbon dioxide).

C: Circulation: No treatment required.

D: Dispense (i.e., provide) reassurance.

E: Ensure that vital signs, drug administration, and patient responses are properly monitored and recorded.

F: Facilitate/ensure next steps in medical/dental care: Consider rescheduling appointment with antianxiety measures/presedation.

Aspiration or Swallowing a Foreign Object

Signs and Symptoms. Coughing or gagging associated with a foreign object; inability to speak; possible cyanosis from airway obstruction; violent respiratory effort; suprasternal retraction; rapid pulse.

Cause. Foreign body in larynx or pharynx.

Treatment. *With conscious victim*:

P: Positioning: Keep the patient standing, or sitting leaning forward. Ask: "Can you speak?" or "Are you choking?" Patient may indicate need for help by demonstrating the "universal choking sign"—clutching hands wrapping around the neck or nodding.

A: Airway: Open airway by placing arms around patient and applying Heimlich maneuver.

B: Breathing: Repeat maneuver until object is cleared and breathing is reestablished, or until patient becomes unconscious.

With unconscious or unresponsive victim:

P: Positioning: Place victim in supine position. Activate EMS (call 911); then initiate CPR in C-A-B sequence.

C: Circulation: Check pulse; begin CPR if no pulse is felt. Provide chest compressions in ratio of 30 per 2 ventilations. (NOTE: Chest compressions provide pressure to dislodge foreign object.)

A: Airway: Open airway by administering quick upward abdomen thrusts (up to 5).

B: Breathing: Check airway for breathing and attempt to ventilate. Each time the airway is opened, the rescuer should look for an object in the victim's mouth and remove it if found.

- Do not delay the 30 chest compressions for longer than 10 sec while looking for object.
- Continue chest compressions and ventilation attempts until EMS unit arrives.

NOTE: If cricothyrotomy is necessary (i.e., rescuer is unable to ventilate for 4 to 5 minutes), refer to "Cricothyroid Membrane Puncture" procedure that follows.

Once breathing has been reestablished:

D: Dispense/administer:

- Oxygen at flow rate of 5-6 L/minute

E: Ensure that vital signs, drug administration, and patient responses are properly monitored and recorded.

F: Facilitate/ensure next steps in medical care (maintain supine position and transport to hospital); reassure patient.

- Inform patient and request radiographs to locate foreign object or trauma to chest cavity is suspected, if needed (posterior-anterior chest view, lateral chest view, flat plane abdominal).

NOTE: If foreign object is in gastrointestinal tract, track with x-ray examination. Foreign object in trachea or lung requires removal using bronchoscopy or thoracotomy. If foreign object has occluded the airway, the Heimlich maneuver may be of benefit before initiation of a cricothyrotomy.

Cricothyroid Membrane Puncture

The approach to a patient with acute airway obstruction should consist of the following steps:

- Recognition of obstruction
- Use of nonsurgical maneuvers to relieve obstruction (i.e., back blows, Heimlich maneuver).
- Administration of mouth-to-mouth breathing to bypass obstruction or to diagnose obstruction
- Activation of EMS with 911 call
- Establishment of an emergency surgical airway (cricothyrotomy) if Heimlich maneuver is unsuccessful

Cricothyrotomy

1. Place patient in head-down position with neck hyperextended.
2. Ensure that chin and sternal notch are held in median plane.
3. Cut skin or puncture with very-large-bore needle over cricothyroid cartilage.
4. Insert cricothyrotomy canula (Portex Mini-Trach II) or very-large-bore needle through skin over cricothyroid cartilage. Insert pointed end caudally to avoid damage to the vocal cords.
   If cannula is not available:
   a. Insert small scissors or hemostats through cricothyroid membrane and into the tracheal space, or use large (8-gauge) needle.
   b. Expand instrument and dilate transversely.
   c. Insert tube into trachea between beaks of dilating instrument.
   d. Remove scissors or hemostats.
   e. Tape tube into place.
5. Use positive pressure or enriched oxygen flow if patient is breathing independently.
6. Arrange for rapid transfer of patient to the hospital.

Bronchial Asthma

Signs and Symptoms. Sense of suffocation, pressure in chest, nonproductive cough, expiratory wheezes, prolonged expiratory phase, increased respiratory effort, chest distension, thick, stringy mucous sputum, cyanosis (in severe cases).

Causes. Can be induced by allergy, infection, exercise, anxiety leading to bronchial inflammation, bronchoconstriction, vascular permeability, occlusion of bronchioles by thick mucous plugs, and bronchospasm.

Treatment

P: Positioning: Place patient in an upright comfortable position.

A: Airway: Ensure that airway is open by removing dental materials and listening to breath sounds.

B: Breathing: Encourage relaxed slow breathing.

C: Circulation and communication: generally circulation is adequate if patient is conscious. Communicate with patient and/or staff to get a rapid bronchodilator for use. Calm the patient and the staff.

D: Dispense/administer:
- Two deep inhalations of fast-acting, β_2-agonist bronchodilator (e.g., albuterol, Isuprel mistometer)
- Repeat with two additional deep inhalations of bronchodilator if attack persists 5 minutes.
- Oxygen at flow rate of 5-6 L/minute, if needed

E: Ensure that vital signs are properly monitored and recorded.
- If attack persists, activate EMS (call 911).

F: Facilitate next steps in medical care (transport to hospital); reassure patient.
- Maintain oxygen at flow rate of 5-6 L/minute.
- With *unresponsive Patient*: administer epinephrine 1:1000 (0.3-0.5 mL SC); repeat every 20 minutes as needed.

If transport to hospital is pending:
- Give theophylline ethylenediamine (aminophylline) 250-500 mg IV slowly over a 10-minute period.
- Administer hydrocortisone sodium succinate (Solu-Cortef), 100 mg IV.

NOTE: Because aminophylline may cause hypotension, it should be given with extreme caution to patients with asthma who are hypotensive.

Mild (Delayed Onset) Allergic Reaction

Signs and Symptoms. Mild pruritus (itching)—slow appearance; and mild urticaria (rash)—slow appearance.
Cause. Overreaction to allergens such as drugs, pollens, or food in which mast cells degranulate and release histamine, often in skin or mucosa.

Treatment

P: Positioning: Place patient in comfortable position (upright).

A: Airway: Ensure that airway is open by talking with patient.

B: Breathing: Ensure that breathing is adequate.

C: Circulation and communication: Should be adequate in this situation. Request blood pressure cuff. There should be no tachycardia, hypotension, dizziness, dyspnea, or wheezing. Inform the patient that an antihistamine drug will be administered.

D: Dispense/administer:
- Diphenhydramine (Benadryl) 25-50 mg PO, or IM (or IV if dentist has ACLS or advanced training).
- Repeat dose up to 50 mg every 6 hours orally for 2 days, if needed.

E: Ensure that vital signs, drug administration, and patient responses are properly monitored and recorded.

F: Facilitate/ensure next steps in medical care.
- In this case, allergy testing should be considered, and dentist should initiate discussion with physician to withdraw offending drug.

Severe (Immediate Onset) Allergic Reaction

Signs and Symptoms. Skin reactions—rapid appearance such as severe pruritus (itching of skin, throat, palate); severe urticaria (rash); swelling of lips, eyelids, cheeks, pharynx, and larynx (angioneurotic edema); and anaphylactic shock (cardiovascular—fall in blood pressure), (respiratory—wheezing, choking, cyanosis, hoarseness), (central nervous system—loss of consciousness, dilation of pupils).
Cause. Overreaction to allergens such as drugs, pollens, food where mast cells degranulate and release histamine in cardiopulmonary system.

Treatment

P: Positioning

With *conscious patient*: place in upright (most comfortable) position.

With *unconscious patient*: place in supine position and activate EMS (call 911).

A: Airway: Assess to ensure that airway is open.

B: Breathing: Ensure breathing is adequate by talking to and reassuring patient.

C: Circulation: No immediate requirement. Apply blood pressure cuff (pulse oximeter) to assess circulation within 5 minutes.

D: Dispense/administer:
- Epinephrine 0.3-0.5 mg 1:1000 SC or IM, or IV if dentist has ACLS training
- Oxygen maintained at flow rate of 5-6 L/minute
- Repeat epinephrine 0.3-0.5 mg 1:000 SC or IM, every 5-10 minutes as needed.

E: Ensure that vital signs, drug administration, and patient responses are properly monitored and recorded. NOTE: *Monitor blood pressure to ensure hypertension is not occurring.*

F: Facilitate/ensure next steps in medical care (transport to hospital); reassure patient.

If transport to hospital is pending:
- Give repeat doses of epinephrine 0.3-0.5 mg 1:1000 SC or IM, every 5-10 minutes as needed.
- Also administer 25 to 50 mg diphenhydramine (Benadryl), once patient's life is no longer in danger.

If dentist has ACLS training and laryngeal edema is involved:

- Provide steroids—hydrocortisone sodium succinate (Solu-Cortef), 100 mg SC or IM or IV
- Perform CPR if patient stops breathing and has no pulse, including use of automated external defibrillator (AED).
- Use cricothyrotomy if needed.

NOTE: Aminophylline may cause hypotension and should be used with extreme caution in patients with asthma who also are hypotensive.

Respiratory Arrest

Signs and Symptoms. Cessation of breathing, cyanosis.
Cause. Physical obstruction of airway (tongue or foreign object), drug-induced apnea.

Treatment

P: Positioning: Place patient in supine position, and activate EMS (call 911).
A: Airway: Maintain open airway, tilting the patient's head back as indicated.
B: Breathing: Respirations will be absent.
- Open mouth to see if foreign object is readily accessible; remove object if visible (in adult).
- If foreign object cannot be removed, perform *Heimlich maneuver* (abdominal thrusts) until object is removed or no pulse is detected. If no pulse is felt, initiate CPR (using the C-A-B sequence) and chest compressions in a ratio of 30 per 2 ventilations.
- Once airway is open, ventilate patient 12 to 15 times per minute.

C: Circulation: Support blood pressure through position of patient, parenteral fluids, and vasopressors.
D: Dispense/administer appropriate drug:
- Give oxygen or artificial respiration.

If apnea is secondary to sedative/benzodiazepine (e.g., diazepam) overdose: administer reversal agent:
- Flumazenil (0.2 mg IV over 15 sec) if diazepam was used to sedate (with ACLS-trained rescuer); repeat 0.2 mg every minute up to 1 mg.

If apnea is secondary to narcotic/opioid overdose: administer reversal agent:
- 0.4 mg naloxone hydrochloride (Narcan) IV, IM, or SC plus oxygen
- Keep patient awake.

E: Ensure that vital signs, drug administration, and patient responses are properly monitored and recorded.
F: Facilitate/ensure next steps in medical/dental care (transport to hospital, if necessary); reassure patient.

NOTE: Monitor patient carefully for the duration of action of reversal agent (e.g., naloxone), which may be less than that of the narcotic. No reversal agent exists for barbiturate overdose.

Chest Pain

Angina Pectoris

Signs and Symptoms. Substernal myocardial pain that can radiate to arms, neck, jaw, or abdomen; myocardial pain lasting less than 15 minutes and possibly radiating to the left shoulder; pain relieved by nitroglycerin; patient usually has a history of the condition.

NOTE: Vital signs are normal; no hypotension, sweating, or nausea occurs.
Cause. Blood supply to the cardiac muscle is insufficient for oxygen demand (atherosclerosis or coronary artery spasm). Angina episode may be precipitated by stress, anxiety, or physical activity.

Treatment

P: Positioning: Place patient in sitting-up or semi-sitting-up (comfortable) position with head elevated.
A: Airway: Ensure open airway.
B: Breathing: Ensure that breathing is adequate.
C: Circulation and communication: Check pulse and communicate with patient and staff to get the nitroglycerin.
D: Dispense/administer:
- Nitroglycerin 0.4-mg tablet sublingually or one or two metered spray doses (0.3-0.6 mg) of nitroglycerin sublingually
- Repeat 1 nitroglycerin tablet every 5 minutes up to a total of 3 tablets or 3 sprays in 15-minute period.
- Oxygen at flow rate of 5-6 L/minute
- If pain is not relieved with 3 doses of nitroglycerin, give one aspirin 325 mg, and call 911.

E: Ensure that vital signs, drug administration, and patient responses are properly monitored and recorded.
F: Facilitate next steps in medical care (transport to hospital if needed); reassure patient.

NOTE: If any doubt exists about whether angina or myocardial infarction exists (i.e., pain continues, worsens or subsides but then returns), activate EMS (call 911) or transport patient to hospital. Once the nitroglycerin tablet container has been opened, the remaining tablets have a poor shelf life (30 days); a new supply should be stocked.

Myocardial Infarction

Signs and Symptoms. Development of chest pain, sometimes manifested as a crushing, squeezing, or heavy feeling, that is more severe than with angina, possibly radiating to the neck, shoulder, or jaw; lasting longer than 15 minutes; and not relieved by nitroglycerin tablets, in a conscious patient. Cyanotic, pale, or ashen appearance; weakness, cold sweat, nausea, vomiting, air hunger and sense of impending death; increased, irregular pulse beat of poor quality with palpitations, feeling of impending doom.

Cause. Interruption of blood supply to the heart, most commonly due to occlusion of coronary vessels. Anoxia, ischemia, and infarct are present.

Treatment. (For adult victim who is conscious and responsive)

P: Positioning: Place patient in a comfortable position. Call for help and activate EMS (call 911).
A: Airway: Ensure open airway.
B: Breathing: Ensure that breathing is adequate by communicating with and reassuring patient.
C: Circulation: Request equipment to check pulse and blood pressure.
D: Dispense/administer:
- Aspirin 325-mg tablet in conscious patient
- Oxygen at flow rate of 5-6 L/minute

E: Ensure that vital signs, drug administration, and patient responses are properly monitored and recorded.
F: Facilitate/ensure next steps in medical/dental care (transport to hospital); reassure patient.

NOTE: Maintain patient in most comfortable position; this may not be the supine position, because the air hunger may be associated with orthopnea.

- Administer nitrous oxide–oxygen (N_2O 30%, O_2 70%), if available.
- Alternatively, demerol (50 mg IV) or morphine (10 mg IV) may be administered if the dentist has ACLS training.

The condition may progress to cardiac arrest.

With *unresponsive patient*: Initiate CPR, including use of automated external defibrillator (AED).

Other Reactions

Intraarterial Injection of Drug into the Arm

Signs and Symptoms. Pain and burning sensation distal to the injection site; cold and blanching skin on hand or fingers distal to the injection site.

Cause. Intraarterial injection of drug into the arm.

Treatment

P: Positioning: Place patient in supine position.
A: Airway: Administer oxygen at flow rate of 5-6 L/minute.
B: Breathing: Ask patient to breathe slowly.
C: Circulation and communication: Leave needle in place and communicate next steps to patient.
D: Dispense:
- 40-60 mg 2% lidocaine (2-3 mL)
- 100 mg hydrocortisone sodium succinate (Solu-Cortef) IM

E: Ensure that vital signs (obtained on other arm), drug administration, and patient responses are properly monitored and recorded.
F: Facilitate/ensure next steps in medical care (transport to hospital), which may include heparinization and brachial plexus block.

Extrapyramidal Reactions

Antipsychotic Drugs Producing Side Reactions. Phenothiazines (Compazine, Thorazine, Phenergan, Sparine, Stelazine, Trilafon, Mellaril); butyrophenones (Haldol, Innovar [general anesthetic]); thioxanthenes (Navane, Taractan).

Signs and Symptoms. Acute dystonic reaction (more frequent in young people, women): rapid onset, involuntary movement of tongue, muscles of mastication, and muscles of facial expression; neck muscles affected frequently (torticollis), arms and legs less frequently; akathisia (constant motion); parkinsonism, tardive dyskinesia (involving buccolinguomasticatory triad—sucking, smacking, chewing, fly-catching movements of tongue).

Cause. Adverse effects of drug.

Treatment

P: Positioning: Place patient in semiupright position.
A: Airway: Ensure open airway.
B: Breathing: Ensure that breathing is adequate by talking with and reassuring patient.
C: Circulation: Request blood pressure equipment or pulse oximeter to check circulation.
D: Dispense/administer:
- Diphenhydramine HCl (Benadryl) 25-50 mg orally, or IV if dentist has ACLS training
- Oxygen at flow rate of 5-6 L/minute

E: Ensure that vital signs, drug administration, and patient responses are properly monitored and recorded.
F: Facilitate/ensure next steps in medical care (transport to hospital); reassure patient.

Response to Unknown Cause

When a likely cause for the patient's response cannot be identified, a period of observation is justified.

P: Positioning: Place patient in supine position and activate EMS (call 911).
A: Airway: Ensure open airway, support respiration, and administer oxygen.
B: Breathing: Ensure that breathing is adequate.

C: Circulation: Request blood pressure equipment or pulse oximeter to check blood pressure and circulation.
D: Dispense/administer intravenous 5% dextrose with lactated Ringer's solution.
E: Ensure that vital signs, drug administration, and patient responses are properly monitored and recorded.
F: Facilitate/ensure next steps in medical/dental care:
- Keep patient off all medication.
- Reassure patient.
- Transfer to hospital if patient's condition is serious.
- Be prepared to do CPR and use the AED, if needed.

Emergency Kit

Review contents, expiration date, and appearance of all drugs periodically (at least monthly). Ensure that kit contains the following:

1. Oxygen tank and setup
2. Blood pressure cuff
3. Stethoscope
4. Syringes (1, 5, 10, and 20 mL)
5. Lacrimal pocket mask
6. Disposable airway, No. 2, 3, and 4
7. Butterfly needles, No. 3, 21 gauge
8. 22-gauge needles
9. Intravenous tubing set, long No. 880-35
10. 250 mL dextrose, lactated Ringer's solution
11. Paper tape roll
12. Alcohol sponges
13. Drugs
    a. Atropine: 0.5 mg/1-mL ampule
    b. Aspirin: 325-mg tablets
    c. Benadryl (diphenhydramine): 50-mg tablets or 50 mg/1 mL syringe/22 gauge, 1-inch needle
    d. Aminophylline (theophylline ethylenediamine): 250 mg/1 mL syringe/22 gauge, 1-inch needle
    e. Hydrocortisone sodium succinate (Solu-Cortef): 100 mg/2 mL syringe/22 gauge, 1-inch needle
    f. Epinephrine 1:1000
        i. Twinject: two doses of 0.3 mg
        ii. EpiPen: auto-injector 0.3 mg
        iii. 1.0-mL ampules
    g. Glucagon: 1 mg/mL ampule
    h. Naloxone hydrochloride (Narcan): 0.4 mg/1-mL ampule/tuberculin syringe
    i. Nitroglycerin: 0.4-mg tabs (packed as 30/bottle), or nitroglycerin pump spray (400 μg/spray)
    j. Phenylephrine: 10 mg/mL (two or three 1-mL ampules)
    k. Two ammonia inhalant buds (Vaporole)
    l. Orange juice, glucose paste, or dextrose 50%: 100 mL
    m. Diazepam (Valium): 5 mg/mL (Alternatively, stock lorazepem 2 mg/mL or midazolam 1 mg/mL)
    n. Lidocaine 2%, 2-mL ampules
14. Curved cricothyrotomy cannula
15. Padded tongue blade
16. Pulse oximeter/ECG unit (medical resources)
17. Automated external defibrillator (AED) (e.g., Heartstream FR-2, Medtronic Physio-control, Survivalink)

NOTE: Commercial medical emergency kits for dentistry are available from companies such as Banyan International (Abilene, Texas), Dixie Medical Inc. (Franklin, Tennessee), and HealthFirst (Mountlake Terrace, Washington).

Pediatric Drug Doses

Pediatric doses are presented on a weight basis, which can be simply multiplied based on the patients weight. Although nomograms using weight, surface area, and other factors may be more accurate, use of the following method is suggested in an emergency situation.

1. Diphenhydramine HCl (Benadryl): 1-1.25 mg/kg, up to 50 mg maximum, IV; then 1-1.25 mg/kg q6h orally or parenterally
2. Atropine sulfate: 0.01 mg/kg, up to 0.4 mg maximum, IV or SC
3. Theophylline ethylenediamine (aminophylline): 3-5 mg/kg IV slowly—20 mg/minute maximum
4. Epinephrine (adrenaline) 1:1000
    a. 0.05 mg-0.3 mg maximum SC or IM (diluted to 1:10,000 for intravenous administration)
    b. EpiPen Junior—autoinjector 0.15 mg
5. Ammonia inhalants (e.g., Vaporole): Same as for adults
6. Hydrocortisone sodium succinate:: Adult dose IV—50 mg, 100 mg, and above
7. Naloxone HCl (Narcan): No pediatric doses clearly established; 0.01 mg/kg IV (preferably) every 2-3 minutes for 2-3 doses maximum
8. 50% dextrose injection: 0.5 mg/kg or 1 mL/kg
9. Diazepam (Valium): Dose not clearly established in patients younger than 12 years of age but in the range of 0.1-0.5 mg/kg for intractable seizures

Record of Emergency Treatment Patient Name ____________ Chart #				
Time	BP	Pulse	Drug(s) delivered, amount, concentration	Patient Response (comments)

APPENDIX B

Guidelines for Infection Control in Dental Health Care Settings

Presented in this appendix are the most recent (2011) recommendations from the Centers for Disease Control and Prevention (CDC) for infection control in dental health care settings. Most of these recommendations are essentially the same as in the 2003 guidelines, with some updates in the prevention of H1N1 influenza transmission in dental health care settings, which were updated in 2009. Also included are a few summary statements (and tables) regarding recommendations for tuberculosis (TB) infection control (2009).

The CDC believes that dental offices that follow these new recommendations will strengthen an already admirable record of safe dental practice. Patients and providers alike can be assured that oral health care can be delivered and received in a safe manner.

OVERVIEW[1]

Although the principles of infection control remain unchanged, new technologies, materials, equipment, and data require continuous evaluation of current infection control practices. The unique nature of many dental procedures, instrumentation, and patient care settings also may require use of specific strategies directed at preventing the transmission of pathogens among dental health care workers and their patients. Recommended infection control practices are applicable to all settings in which dental treatment is provided.

Prevention of 2009 H1N1 Influenza Transmission in Dental Health Care Settings (Updated on November 23, 2009)[1]

CDC provides updated guidance on preventing 2009 H1N1 influenza transmission in dental health care settings. Guidance includes new recommendations on using airborne infection isolation rooms, N95 respirators (i.e., those that filter at least 95% of airborne particles), and infection control measures for personnel with influenza-like illness.

Tuberculosis Infection Control Recommendations[1]

The changing epidemiology of TB and discovery of new diagnostic methods prompted a revision of CDC's *Guidelines to Prevent TB Transmission in Healthcare Settings.* The revised CDC's TB infection control recommendations for dental settings, as well as information on how they should be incorporated into an infection control program, are available online (see "Additional Resources" later on).

Educational Materials[1]

Slide Presentation for Infection Control Guidelines. A slide set and accompanying speaker notes that provide an overview of many of the basic principles of infection control in the CDC's *Guidelines for Infection Control in Dental Health-Care Settings* can be downloaded as a PowerPoint presentation or viewed on the CDC Web site.

If Saliva Were Red: A Visual Lesson on Infection Control.* The video training system *If Saliva Were Red* features an 8-minute video (VHS, CD-ROM) that shows dental professionals at work to highlight common infection control and safety flaws; the cross-contamination in everyday clinical practice that would be evident if saliva were red; and how controlling contamination by using personal barrier protection, safe work practices, and effective infection control products reduces the risk of exposure.

From Policy to Practice: OSAP's Guide to the Guidelines*. The Organization for Safety & Asepsis Procedures (OSAP) has produced a 170-page workbook that contains practical information to help health care professionals put the infection control recommendations into practice. These resources were produced by OSAP through a CDC cooperative agreement.

Related Organizations

- American Dental Association Infection Control Resources*
- National Institute for Occupational Safety and Health
- Organization for Safety and Asepsis Procedures*
- Safety and Health Topics for Dentistry from the Occupational Safety and Health Administration (OSHA)
- U.S. Air Force (USAF) Dental Evaluation and Consultation Service

PREVENTION OF H1N1 INFLUENZA TRANSMISSION IN DENTAL HEALTH CARE SETTINGS[2]

Exposures to 2009 H1N1 influenza virus occurs in household, community, and occupational settings, and transmission is thought to occur through droplet exposure of mucosal surfaces; through indirect contact, usually via the hands, with respiratory secretions from an infectious patient or contaminated surface; and through inhalation of small particle aerosols in the vicinity of the infectious individual.

Symptoms of Influenza

Persons with influenza, including 2009 H1N1 influenza, may have some or all of these symptoms*:

- Fever
  Note: not everyone with a influenza will have a fever.
- Cough
- Sore throat
- Runny or stuffy nose
- Body aches
- Headache
- Chills
- Fatigue
- Sometimes diarrhea and vomiting

Control of 2009 H1N1 Influenza

A hierarchy of control measures should be applied to prevent transmission of 2009 H1N1 influenza in all health care settings. To apply the hierarchy of control measures, facilities should take the following steps, ranked according to their likely effectiveness:

1. Elimination of potential exposures (e.g., deferral of treatment for ill patients and source control by masking persons who are coughing)
2. Engineering controls that reduce or eliminate exposure at the source without placing primary responsibility of implementation on individual employees
3. Administrative controls including sick leave policies and vaccination that depend on consistent implementation by management and employees
4. Personal protective equipment (PPE) for exposures that cannot otherwise be eliminated or controlled

(PPE includes gloves, surgical face masks, respirators, protective eyewear, and protective clothing such as gowns.)

Vaccination. Vaccination, an administrative control, is one of the most important interventions for preventing transmission of influenza to health care personnel. More information on this hierarchy of controls is available in the CDC's *Interim Guidance on Infection Control Measures for 2009 H1N1 Influenza in Healthcare Settings, Including Protection of Healthcare Personnel* (see CDC: H1N1 Flue Clinical and Public Health Guidance, http://www.cdc.gov/h1n1flu/guidance/).

Specific Recommendations for Dental Health Care

- Encourage all dental health care personnel to receive seasonal influenza and 2009 H1N1 influenza vaccinations.
- Use patient reminder calls to identify patients reporting influenza-like illness, and reschedule nonurgent visits until 24 hours after the patient is free of fever without the use of fever-reducing medicine.
- Identify patients with influenza-like illness at check-in; offer a face mask or tissues to symptomatic patients; follow *respiratory hygiene/cough etiquette*[3] and reschedule nonurgent care. Separate ill patients from others whenever possible if evaluating for urgent care.
- Urgent dental treatment can be performed without the use of an airborne infection isolation (AII) room, because transmission of 2009 H1N1 influenza is thought not to occur over longer distances through the air, such as from one patient room to another.
- Use a treatment room with a closed door, if available. If not, use one that is farthest from other patients and personnel.
- Wear recommended PPE before entering the treatment room.
- Dental health care personnel should wear a NIOSH fit-tested, disposable N95 respirator when entering the patient room and when performing dental procedures on patients with suspected or confirmed 2009 H1N1 influenza.

*Links to nonfederal organizations do not constitute an endorsement of any organization by CDC or the federal government, and none should be inferred. The CDC is not responsible for the content of the individual organization Web pages found at such links.

- If N95 respirators and/or fit-testing is not available despite reasonable attempts to obtain, the dental office should switch over to a prioritized use mode (i.e., non–fit-tested disposable N95 respirators or surgical face masks can be considered as a lower level of protection for personnel at lower risk of exposure or lower risk of complication from influenza until fit-tested N95 respirators are available). Detailed information can be found in the CDC's *Interim Guidance on Infection Control Measures for H1N1 Influenza in Healthcare Settings, Including Protection of Healthcare Personnel* (see later under "Additional Resources"). Additional guidance, including recommendations regarding fit-testing issues, can be found in the related question and answer document regarding respiratory protection (see under "Additional Resources").
- As customary, minimize spray and spatter (e.g., use a dental dam and high-volume evacuator).

Dental Health Care Personnel

- Dental health care personnel should self-assess daily for symptoms of febrile respiratory illness (fever plus one or more of the following: nasal congestion or runny nose, sore throat, or cough).
- Personnel who develop fever and respiratory symptoms should promptly notify their supervisor and should not report to work.
- Personnel should remain at home until at least 24 hours after they are free of fever (100° F/37.8° C), or signs of a fever, without the use of fever-reducing medications.
- Personnel with a family member who is diagnosed with 2009 H1N1 influenza can still go to work but should self-monitor for symptoms so that any illness is recognized promptly.

Additional Resources

For comprehensive information on CDC 2009 H1N1 influenza infection control guidelines, visit Infection Control and Clinician Guidance at http://www.cdc.gov/h1n1flu/guidance/, for access to the following:

- *Interim Guidance on Infection Control Measures for 2009 H1N1 Influenza in Healthcare Settings, Including Protection of Healthcare Personnel*
- *Questions and Answers about CDC's Interim Guidance on Infection Control Measures for 2009 H1N1 Influenza in Healthcare Settings, Including Protection of Healthcare Personnel*
- *Questions and Answers Regarding Respiratory Protection for Infection Control Measures for 2009 H1N1 Influenza Among Healthcare Personnel*
- *10 Steps You Can Take: Actions for Novel H1N1 Influenza Planning and Response for Medical Offices and Outpatient Facilities*

Information on swine flu also is available at this Web site:

- *2009 H1N1 Flu (Swine Flu) (http://www.cdc.gov/h1n1flu)*

COMPARISON OF SELECTED CHANGES BETWEEN 1994 AND 2005 EDITIONS OF CDC GUIDELINES FOR PREVENTING TUBERCULOSIS IN DENTAL HEALTH CARE SETTINGS[4]

Although rates of tuberculosis (TB) in the United States have decreased in recent years, disparities in TB incidence still exist between U.S.-born and foreign-born people (people living in the United States but born outside it) and between white people and nonwhite people. In addition, the number of TB outbreaks among health care personnel and patients has decreased since the implementation of the 1994 CDC guidelines to prevent transmission of *Mycobacterium tuberculosis.* Therefore, there are a few updates on the epidemiology of TB, advances in TB diagnostic methods and TB infection control guidelines for dental settings.

Clinical Implications

Although the principles of TB infection control have remained the same, the changing epidemiology of TB and the advent of new diagnostic methods for TB led to the development of the 2005 update to the 1994 guidelines. Dental health care personnel should be aware of the modifications that are pertinent to dental settings and incorporate them into their overall infection control programs.

Tuberculosis Risk Categories and Recommended Testing Frequency[5]

Low—fewer than three patients with unrecognized TB treated in past year: Baseline screening at hiring; further testing not needed unless exposure occurs

Medium—three or more patients with unrecognized TB treated in past year: Baseline screening, then annual testing

Potential of ongoing transmission—evidence of ongoing person-to-person transmission: Baseline screening, then testing every 8 to 10 weeks until evidence of transmission has ceased

Baseline screening should be conducted by a qualified health care professional using a two-step tuberculin skin test or a single blood assay for interferon gamma release

Tuberculosis Precautions for Outpatient Dental Settings[5]

Administrative Controls

- Assign responsibility for managing TB infection control program.
- Conduct annual risk assessment.
- Develop written TB infection control policies for promptly identifying and isolating patients with suspected or confirmed TB disease for medical evaluation or urgent dental treatment.
- Instruct patients to cover mouth when coughing and/or wear a surgical mask.
- Ensure that dental health care personnel (DHCP) are educated regarding signs and symptoms of TB.
- When hiring DHCP, ensure that they are screened for latent TB infection and TB disease.
- Postpone urgent dental treatment.

Environmental Controls

- Use airborne infection isolation room to provide urgent dental treatment to patients with suspected or confirmed infectious TB.
- In settings with high volume of patients with suspected or confirmed TB, use high-efficiency particulate air filters or ultraviolet germicidal irradiation.

Respiratory Protection Controls

- Use respiratory protection—at least an N95 filtering face piece (disposable)—for DHCP when they are providing urgent dental treatment to patients with suspected or confirmed TB.
- Instruct patients with TB to cover the mouth when coughing and to wear a surgical mask.
- Respiratory hygiene and cough etiquette measures[3]:
  - Use tissues to cover the nose and mouth and to contain respiratory secretions when coughing or sneezing.
  - Dispose of tissues in no-touch receptacles (such as those with foot pedal–operated lids or an open, plastic-lined wastebasket).
  - When coughing or sneezing, if tissues are not available, cover the mouth and nose with the inner surface of the arm and forearm, to keep pathogenic organisms away from the hands; although *Mycobacterium tuberculosis* cannot be spread by the hands, other respiratory pathogens such as rhinoviruses can be spread in this manner.
  - Practice hand hygiene (such as hand washing with nonantimicrobial soap and water, alcohol-based hand rub or antiseptic hand wash) after contact with respiratory secretions or contaminated objects and materials; hand hygiene is recommended to prevent transmission of all respiratory illnesses in general but will not affect TB transmission.

CLINICAL IMPLICATIONS

The CDC *Guidelines for Infection Control in Dental Health Care Settings—2003*[6] is a major update and revision of the CDC's *Recommended Infection Control Practices for Dentistry—1993*.[7] As of 2011, these guidelines still apply (along with the previous updates on H1N1 and TB). As the nation's disease prevention agency, the CDC develops a broad range of guidelines intended to improve the effect and effectiveness of public health interventions and to inform key audiences, most often clinicians, public health practitioners, and the public, about applicable findings.

Why are guidelines needed that are specific for dentistry? More than a half-million dental health care personnel (DHCP) work in the United States—approximately 168,000 dentists, 112,000 registered dental hygienists, 218,000 dental assistants,[8] and 53,000 dental laboratory technicians.[4] Most dentists are solo practitioners who work in outpatient, ambulatory care facilities. In these settings, no epidemiologists or other hospital infection control experts track possible health care–associated (i.e., nosocomial) infections or monitor and recommend safe practices. Instruments frequently used in dental practice generate spatter, mists, aerosols, or particulate matter. Unless precautions are taken, the possibility is great that patients and DHCP will be exposed to blood and other potentially pathogenic infectious material. Fortunately, by understanding certain principles of disease transmission and using infection control practices based on those principles, dental personnel can prevent disease transmission.

The CDC's first set of infection control recommendations for dentistry was published as an article in the *Morbidity and Mortality Weekly Report* in 1986.[10] At that time, a position paper from the American Association of Public Health Dentistry commented on the state of dental infection control, noting: "Dental practitioners are virtually the only health care providers who routinely place an ungloved hand into a body cavity."[11] Reports published from 1970 through 1987 described nine clusters of patients who were believed to be infected with hepatitis B virus (HBV) through treatment by an infected DHCP.[1] However, since 1987, no transmission of HBV from dentist to patient has been reported. This good statistic possibly is the result of widespread acceptance of the hepatitis B vaccine and the adoption of standard (formerly universal) precautions, including routine glove use. HBV seroprevalence among dentists has fallen from about 14% in 1983 to about 9% today—a proportion that is expected to decline to below that for the general population as older dentists retire (because older dentists are more likely than young dentists to be infected) (personal communication, C. Siew, PhD, American Dental Association, 2003).

In early 1988, a published report described a dentist who was seropositive for human immunodeficiency virus

(HIV) but had no admitted risk factors for HIV infection, which suggests the possibility of occupational transmission.[7,9] In addition, during the early 1990s, the health care community was shaken when six cases of transmission from an HIV-infected dentist to his patients were reported.[12,13,14] No additional reports have described HIV transmission from HIV-infected DHCP to patients, and since the CDC began surveillance for occupationally acquired HIV, no cases of occupationally acquired HIV have been documented among DHCP.[9,12]

In 1991, OSHA released the bloodborne pathogen standard that mandated certain practices for all dental offices.[15] For example, employers must provide hepatitis B vaccine for their employees, and all employees must use appropriate personal protective equipment (e.g., gloves, protective eyewear, gowns). After OSHA published its standards, the CDC published Recommended Infection Control Practices for Dentistry in 1993.[7] Those recommendations, which focused on preventing transmission of disease due to bloodborne pathogens, were based primarily on health care precedent, theoretical rationale, and expert opinion. In contrast with OSHA (which is a regulatory agency), the CDC cannot mandate certain practices; it can only recommend. Nevertheless, many dental licensing boards have adopted the CDC's recommendations, or variations of them, as the infection control standard for dental practice in their states.

The following introductory commentary has been adapted from Kohn WG, et al: Guidelines for infection control in dental health care settings—2003, J Am Dent Assoc *135:33-47, 2004. American Dental Association.*

Ten years after the 1993 recommendations, new technologies and issues have emerged; the CDC has answered thousands of questions from concerned dental providers and patients about appropriate infection control practices in dental offices. In addition, the CDC has updated or created major guidelines on specific topics such as hand hygiene, environmental infection control, *Mycobacterium tuberculosis,* disinfection and sterilization, prophylaxis after exposure to bloodborne pathogens, prevention of surgical site infection, immunization for health care workers, and infection control for health care personnel. Regulatory directives from OSHA, the U.S. Food and Drug Administration (FDA), and the U.S. Environmental Protection Agency (EPA) also affect dental practice.

This new set of CDC recommendations discusses portions of the numerous federal guidelines and regulatory mandates that are relevant to dentistry. It also consolidates previous recommendations and adds new ones specific to infection control in dental health care settings. The new dental guidelines are longer than the 1993 version, principally because they provide more background information and the scientific rationale for the recommendations.

The recommendations cover a broad range of topics and include a number of major updates and additions. Most recommendations are familiar to DHCPs and already are practiced routinely. They are designed to prevent or reduce the potential for disease transmission from patient to DHCP, from DHCP to patient, and from patient to patient. The document emphasizes the use of "standard precautions" (which replaces the term "universal precautions") for the prevention of exposure to and transmission not only of bloodborne pathogens but also of other pathogens encountered in oral health care settings. Although the guidelines focus mainly on practices in outpatient, ambulatory dental health care settings, the recommended infection control practices are applicable to all settings in which dental treatment is provided.

In the recommendations, the term *DHCP* refers to all paid and unpaid personnel in dental health care who could experience occupational exposure to infectious materials, including body substances and contaminated supplies, equipment, environmental surfaces, water, or air. DHCP include dentists, dental hygienists, dental assistants, dental laboratory technicians (in-office and commercial), students and trainees, contract personnel, and other persons who are not directly involved in patient care but who could be exposed to infectious agents (such as administrative, clerical, housekeeping, maintenance, or volunteer personnel).

The guidelines have two parts. The first part provides the background and scientific evidence on which recommendations are based. More than 450 articles are referenced. From the CDC online version (www.cdc.gov/oralhealth/infectioncontrol), readers who want more information on particular topics can link to key reference documents such as the OSHA Bloodborne Pathogen Standard and other CDC infection control guidelines. The second part lists the recommendations and explains the ranking system for the level of scientific evidence for each recommendation.

Varying levels of scientific evidence support infection control practices in health care settings—and in dental settings specifically. Whenever possible, recommendations in the guidelines are based on data from well-designed scientific studies. However, only a limited number of studies have characterized the risk factors for contracting an infection in a dental office and the effectiveness of measures to prevent infection. Certain infection control practices routinely used by health care practitioners cannot be examined rigorously for ethical or logistical reasons. Because there are no scientific studies to support certain recommended practices, they are based instead on strong theoretical rationale, suggestive evidence, or the opinions of respected authorities. Those authorities base their opinions on clinical experience, descriptive studies, or committee reports. Some recommendations are derived from federal regulations. No recommendations are offered for practices for which insufficient scientific evidence exists or for which there is a lack of consensus to support their effectiveness in dental settings.

The full recommendations and ranking system follow. Reference numbers that appear in parentheses in the Recommendations section of this [Appendix] relate to the first part of the full set of guidelines. Although the reference list is omitted from this [Appendix] in the interest of [saving] space, reference numbers were left in the text to allow readers who copy this [Appendix] to match it later with the full document.

The CDC's new guidelines for infection control in dental health care settings should provide dental practitioners with the information needed to make informed and intelligent choices when they select infection control processes, methods, and products. Although most dental practices will find that they already are carrying out most of the recommendations in the guidelines, they now will have the scientific rationale that underlies these recommendations. The practice of infection control in dentistry has made remarkable progress since the 1980s, and the CDC believes that dental offices that follow these new recommendations will strengthen an already admirable record of safe dental practice. Patients and providers alike can be assured that oral health care can be delivered and received in a safe manner.

The CDC plans to distribute these guidelines broadly to the dental community through organizational mailing lists. In addition, the guidelines will be accessible at www.cdc.gov/oralhealth. Soon, the CDC oral health website also will include a PowerPoint slide series that can be downloaded for the purpose of staff education.

The following recommendations are from the Centers for Disease Control and Prevention. Guidelines for Infection Control in Dental Health-Care Settings—2003. MMWR 52(No. RR-17): 39-48, 2003. See also http://www.cdc.gov/mmwr/pdf/rr/rr5217.pdf

Each recommendation is categorized on the basis of existing scientific data, theoretical rationale, and applicability. Rankings are based on the system used by the CDC and the Healthcare Infection Control Practices Advisory Committee (HICPAC) to categorize recommendations:

- *Category IA*—strongly recommended for implementation and strongly supported by well-designed experimental, clinical, or epidemiologic studies
- *Category IB*—strongly recommended for implementation and supported by experimental, clinical, or epidemiologic studies and a strong theoretical rationale
- *Category IC*—required for implementation as mandated by federal or state regulations or standards. When IC is used, a second rating can be included to provide the basis of existing scientific data, theoretical rationale, and applicability. Because of state differences, readers should not assume that the absence of a IC recommendation implies the absence of any state regulations.
- *Category II*—suggested for implementation and supported by suggestive clinical or epidemiologic studies or a theoretical rationale
- *Unresolved issue*—no recommendation. Insufficient evidence or no consensus regarding efficacy exists.

I. PERSONNEL HEALTH ELEMENTS OF AN INFECTION CONTROL PROGRAM
   A. General Recommendations
      1. Develop a written health program for DHCP that includes policies, procedures, and guidelines for education and training; immunizations; exposure prevention and postexposure management; medical conditions, work-related illness, and associated work restrictions; contact dermatitis and latex hypersensitivity; and maintenance of records, data management, and confidentiality (IB) (5,16-18,22).
      2. Establish referral arrangements with qualified health care professionals to ensure prompt and appropriate provision of preventive services, occupationally related medical services, and postexposure management with medical follow-up (IB, IC) (5,13,19,22).
   B. Education and Training
      1. Provide DHCP (1) on initial employment, (2) when new tasks or procedures affect the employee's occupational exposure, and (3) at a minimum, annually, education and training regarding occupational exposure to potentially infectious agents and infection control procedures/protocols appropriate for and specific to assigned duties (IB, IC) (5,11,13,14,16,19,22).
      2. Provide educational information appropriate in content and vocabulary to the educational level, literacy, and language of DHCP (IB, IC) (5,13).
   C. Immunization Programs
      1. Develop a written comprehensive policy on immunizing DHCP, including a list of all required and recommended immunizations (IB) (5,17,18).
      2. Refer DHCP to a prearranged qualified health care professional or to their own health care professional to receive all appropriate immunizations based on the latest recommendations, as well as their medical history and risk for occupational exposure (IB) (5,17).
   D. Exposure Prevention and Postexposure Management
      1. Develop a comprehensive postexposure management and medical follow-up program (IB, IC) (5,13,14,19).
         a. Include policies and procedures for prompt reporting, evaluation, counseling, treatment, and medical follow-up of occupational exposures.
         b. Establish mechanisms for referral to a qualified health care professional for medical evaluation and follow-up.
         c. Conduct a baseline tuberculin skin test (TST), preferably through a 2-step test, for all DHCP who might have contact with persons with suspected or confirmed infectious TB, regardless of the risk classification of the setting (IB) (20).
   E. Medical Conditions, Work-Related Illness, and Work Restrictions
      1. Develop and have readily available to all DHCP comprehensive written policies on work restriction and exclusion that include a statement of authority defining who can implement such policies (IB) (5,22).
      2. Develop policies for work restriction and exclusion that encourage DHCP to seek appropriate preventive and curative care and report their illnesses, medical conditions, or treatments that can render them more susceptible to opportunistic infection or exposure; do not penalize DHCP with loss of wages, benefits, or job status (IB) (5,22).

3. Develop policies and procedures for evaluation, diagnosis, and management of DHCP with suspected or known occupational contact dermatitis (IB) (32).
4. Seek definitive diagnosis by a qualified health care professional for any DHCP with suspected latex allergy to carefully determine its specific etiology and appropriate treatment, as well as work restrictions and accommodations (IB) (32).

F. Maintenance of Records, Data Management, and Confidentiality

1. Establish and maintain confidential medical records (e.g., immunization records, documentation of tests received as a result of occupational exposure) for all DHCP (IB, IC) (5,13).
2. Ensure that the practice complies with all applicable federal, state, and local laws regarding medical record keeping and confidentiality (IC) (13,34).

II. PREVENTING TRANSMISSION OF BLOODBORNE PATHOGENS

A. HBV Vaccination

1. Offer the HBV vaccination series to all DHCP with potential occupational exposure to blood or other potentially infectious material (IA, IC) (2,13,14,19).
2. Always follow U.S. Public Health Service/CDC recommendations for hepatitis B vaccination, serologic testing, follow-up, and booster dosing (IA, IC) (13,14,19).
3. Test DHCP for anti-HBs 1 to 2 months after completion of the three-dose vaccination series (IA, IC) (14,19).
4. DHCP should complete a second three-dose vaccine series or be evaluated to determine if HBsAg-positive if no antibody response occurs to the primary vaccine series (IA, IC) (14,19).
5. Retest for anti-HBs at completion of the second vaccine series. If no response to the second three-dose series, nonresponders should be tested for HBsAg (IC) (14,19).
6. Counsel nonresponders to vaccination who are HBsAg negative regarding their susceptibility to HBV infection and precautions to take (IA, IC) (14,19).
7. Provide employees appropriate education regarding the risks of HBV transmission and availability of the vaccine. Employees who decline the vaccination should sign a declination form to be kept on file with the employer (IC) (13).

B. Preventing Exposures to Blood and Other Potentially Infectious Material (OPIM)

1. General recommendations
   a. Use standard precautions (OSHA's bloodborne pathogen standard retains the term *universal precautions*) for all patient encounters (IA,IC) (11,13,19,53).
   b. Consider sharp items (e.g., needles, scalers, burs, laboratory knives, and wires) that are contaminated with patient blood and saliva as potentially infective, and establish engineering controls and work practices to prevent injuries (IB, IC) (6,13,113).
   c. Implement a written, comprehensive program designed to minimize and manage DHCP exposures to blood and body fluids (IB, IC) (13,14,19,97).
2. Engineering and work practice controls
   a. Identify, evaluate, and consider devices with engineered safety features at least annually and as they become available on the market (e.g., safer anesthetic syringes, blunt suture needle, retractable scalpel, or needleless IV systems) (IC) (13,97,110-112).
   b. Place used disposable syringes and needles, scalpel blades, and other sharp items in appropriate puncture-resistant containers located as close as feasible to the area in which the items are used (IA, IC) (2,7,13,19,113,115).
   c. Do not recap used needles by using both hands or any other technique that involves directing the point of a needle toward any part of the body. Do not bend, break, or remove needles before disposal (IA, IC) (2,7,8,13,97,113).
   d. Use a one-handed scoop technique or a mechanical device designed for holding the needle cap when recapping needles (e.g., between multiple injections, before removing from a nondisposable aspirating syringe) (IA, IC) (2,7,8,13,14,113).
3. Postexposure management and prophylaxis
   a. Follow current CDC recommendations after percutaneous, mucous membrane, or nonintact skin exposure to blood or other potentially infectious material (IA, IC) (13,14,19).

III. HAND HYGIENE

A. General Considerations

1. Perform hand hygiene with a nonantimicrobial or antimicrobial soap and water when hands are visibly dirty or are contaminated with blood or other potentially infectious material. If hands are not visibly soiled, an alcohol-based handrub can also be used. Follow the manufacturer's instructions (IA) (123).
2. Indications for hand hygiene include the following:
   a. When hands are visibly soiled (IA, IC)

b. After barehanded touching of inanimate objects likely to be contaminated by blood, saliva, or respiratory secretions (IA, IC)
c. Before and after treating each patient (IB)
d. Before donning gloves (IB)
e. Immediately after removing gloves (IB, IC) (7-9,11,13,113,120-123,125,126, 138).

3. For oral surgical procedures, perform surgical hand antisepsis before donning sterile surgeon's gloves. Follow the manufacturer's instructions by using an antimicrobial soap and water, or soap and water followed by drying of hands and application of an alcohol-based surgical hand scrub product with persistent activity (IB) (121-123,127-133,137, 144,145).
4. Store liquid hand care products in disposable closed containers or closed containers that can be washed and dried before refilling. Do not add soap or lotion (i.e., top off) to a partially empty dispenser (IA) (9,120,122,149, 150).

B. Special Considerations for Hand Hygiene and Glove Usage
1. Use hand lotions to prevent skin dryness associated with handwashing (IA) (153,154).
2. Consider the compatibility of lotion and antiseptic products and the effects of petroleum or other oil emollients on the integrity of gloves during product selection and glove usage (IB) (2,14,122,155).
3. Keep fingernails short with smooth, filed edges to allow thorough cleaning and to prevent glove tears (II) (122,123,156).
4. Do not wear artificial fingernails or extenders when having direct contact with patients at high risk (e.g., those in intensive care units or operating rooms) (IA) (123,157-160).
5. Use of artificial fingernails usually is not recommended (II) (157-160).
6. Do not wear hand or nail jewelry if it makes donning gloves more difficult or compromises the fit and integrity of the glove (II) (123,142,143).

IV. PERSONAL PROTECTIVE EQUIPMENT (PPE)

A. Masks, Protective Eyewear, Face Shields
1. Wear a surgical mask and eye protection with solid side shields or a face shield to protect mucous membranes of the eyes, nose, and mouth during procedures likely to generate splashing or spattering of blood or other body fluids (IB, IC) (1,2,7,8,11,13,137).
2. Change masks between patients or during patient treatment if the mask becomes wet (IB) (2).
3. Clean with soap and water or, if visibly soiled, clean and disinfect reusable facial protective equipment (e.g., clinician and patient protective eyewear or face shields) between patients (II) (2).

B. Protective Clothing
1. Wear protective clothing such as a reusable or disposable gown, laboratory coat, or uniform that covers personal clothing and skin (e.g., forearms) likely to be soiled with blood, saliva, or OPIM (IB, IC) (7,8,11,13,137).
2. Change protective clothing if visibly soiled (134); change immediately or as soon as feasible if penetrated by blood or other potentially infectious fluids (IB, IC) (13).
3. Remove barrier protection, including gloves, mask, eyewear, and gown, before departing work area (e.g., dental patient care, instrument processing, laboratory areas) (IC) (13).

C. Gloves
1. Wear medical gloves when the potential exists for contacting blood, saliva, OPIM, or mucous membranes (IB, IC) (1,2,7,8,13).
2. Wear a new pair of medical gloves for each patient, remove them promptly after use, and wash hands immediately to avoid transfer of microorganisms to other patients or environments (IB) (1,7,8,123).
3. Remove gloves that are torn, cut, or punctured as soon as feasible, and wash hands before regloving (IB, IC) (13,210,211).
4. Do not wash surgeon's or patient examination gloves before use or wash, disinfect, or sterilize gloves for reuse (IB, IC) (13,138,177, 212,213).
5. Ensure that appropriate gloves in the correct size are readily accessible (IC) (13).
6. Use appropriate gloves (e.g., puncture- and chemical-resistant utility gloves) when cleaning instruments and performing housekeeping tasks involving contact with blood or OPIM (IB, IC) (7,13,15).
7. Consult with glove manufacturers regarding the chemical compatibility of glove material and dental materials used (II).

D. Sterile Surgeon's Gloves and Double Gloving During Oral Surgical Procedures
1. Wear sterile surgeon's gloves when performing oral surgical procedures (IB) (2,8,137).
2. No recommendation is offered regarding the effectiveness of wearing two pairs of gloves to prevent disease transmission during oral surgical procedures. The majority of studies among HCP and DHCP have demonstrated a lower frequency of inner glove perforation and visible blood on the surgeon's hands when double gloves are worn; however, the

effectiveness of wearing two pair of gloves in preventing disease transmission has not been demonstrated (Unresolved issue).

V. CONTACT DERMATITIS AND LATEX HYPERSENSITIVITY

A. General Recommendations

1. Educate DHCP regarding the signs, symptoms, and diagnoses of skin reactions associated with frequent hand hygiene and glove use (IB) (5,31,32).
2. Screen all patients for latex allergy (e.g., take health history) and refer for medical consultation when latex allergy is suspected (IB) (32).
3. Ensure a latex-safe environment for patients and DHCP with latex allergy (IB) (32).
4. Have emergency treatment kits with latex-free products available at all times (II) (32).

VI. STERILIZATION AND DISINFECTION OF PATIENT CARE ITEMS

A. General Recommendations

1. Use only FDA-cleared medical devices for sterilization, and follow the manufacturer's instructions for correct use (IB) (248).
2. Clean and heat sterilize critical dental instruments before each use (IA) (2,243,244,246, 249,407).
3. Clean and heat sterilize semicritical items before each use (IB) (2,249,260,407).
4. Allow packages to dry in the sterilizer before they are handled, to avoid contamination (IB) (247).
5. Use of heat-stable semicritical alternatives is encouraged (IB) (2).
6. Reprocess heat-sensitive critical and semicritical instruments by using FDA-cleared sterilant/high-level disinfectants or an FDA-cleared low-temperature sterilization method (e.g., ethylene oxide). Follow manufacturer's instructions for use of chemical sterilants/ high-level disinfectants (IB) (243).
7. Single-use disposable instruments are acceptable alternatives, provided they are used only once and disposed of correctly (IB, IC) (243,383).
8. Do not use liquid chemical sterilants/high-level disinfectants for environmental surface disinfection or as holding solutions (IB, IC) (243,245).
9. Ensure that noncritical patient care items are barrier protected or cleaned, or, if visibly soiled, cleaned and disinfected after each use with an EPA-registered hospital disinfectant with an HIV/HBV effectiveness claim (low-level disinfectant) or a tuberculocidal claim (intermediate-level disinfectant) (i.e., intermediate level if visibly contaminated with blood or OPIM) (IB) (2,243,244).
10. Inform DHCP of all OSHA guidelines for exposure to chemical agents used for disinfection and sterilization. Using this report, identify areas and tasks that have potential for exposure (IC) (15).

B. Instrument Processing Area

1. Designate a central processing area. Divide the instrument processing area, physically or, at a minimum, spatially, into distinct areas for (1) receiving, cleaning, and decontamination; (2) preparation and packaging; (3) sterilization; and (4) storage. Do not store instruments in an area where contaminated instruments are held or cleaned (II) (174,247,248).
2. Train DHCP to employ work practices that prevent contamination of clean areas (II).

C. Receiving, Cleaning, and Decontaminating Work Area

1. Minimize handling of loose contaminated instruments during transport to the instrument processing area. Use work practice controls (e.g., carry instruments in a covered container) to minimize exposure potential (II). Clean all visible blood and other contamination from dental instruments and devices before sterilization or disinfection procedures (IA) (249-252).
2. Use automated cleaning equipment (e.g., ultrasonic cleaner or washer/disinfector) to remove debris to improve cleaning effectiveness and decrease worker exposure to blood (IB) (2,253).
3. Use work practice controls that minimize contact with sharp instruments, if manual cleaning is necessary (e.g., long-handled brush) (IC) (14).
4. Wear puncture- and chemical-resistant/heavy duty utility gloves for instrument cleaning and decontamination procedures (IB) (7).
5. Wear appropriate PPE (e.g., mask, protective eyewear and gown) when splashing or spraying is anticipated during cleaning (IC) (13).

D. Preparation and Packaging

1. Use an internal chemical indicator in each package. If the internal indicator cannot be seen from outside the package, also use an external indicator (II) (243,254,257).
2. Use a container system or wrapping compatible with the type of sterilization process used and that has received FDA clearance (IB) (243,247,256).
3. Before sterilization of critical and semicritical instruments, inspect instruments for cleanliness, then wrap or place them in containers

designed to maintain sterility during storage (e.g., cassettes, organizing trays) (IA) (2,247,255,256).

E. Sterilization of Unwrapped Instruments
   1. Clean and dry instruments prior to the unwrapped sterilization cycle (IB) (248).
   2. Use mechanical and chemical (place an internal chemical indicator among the instruments or items to be sterilized) indicators for each unwrapped sterilization cycle (IB) (258).
   3. Allow unwrapped instruments to dry and cool in the sterilizer before they are handled, to avoid contamination and thermal injury (II) (260).
   4. Semicritical instruments that will be used immediately or within a short time frame can be sterilized unwrapped on a tray or in a container system, provided that the instruments are handled aseptically during removal from the sterilizer and transport to the point of use (II).
   5. Critical instruments intended for immediate reuse can be sterilized unwrapped, provided that the instruments are maintained sterile during removal from the sterilizer and transport to the point of use (e.g., transported in a sterile, covered container) (IB) (258).
   6. Do not sterilize implantable devices unwrapped (IB) (243,247).
   7. Do not store critical instruments unwrapped (IB) (248).

F. Sterilization Monitoring
   1. Use mechanical, chemical, and biologic monitors according to the manufacturer's instructions to ensure the effectiveness of the sterilization process (IB) (248,278,279).
   2. Monitor each load with mechanical (e.g., time, temperature, pressure) and chemical indicators (II) (243,248).
   3. Place a chemical indicator on the inside of each package. If the internal indicator is not visible from the outside, also place an exterior chemical indicator on the package (II) (243,254,257).
   4. Place items/packages correctly and loosely into the sterilizer, so as not to impede penetration of the sterilant (IB) (243).
   5. Do not use instrument packs if mechanical or chemical indicators indicate inadequate processing (IB) (243,247,248).
   6. Monitor sterilizers at least weekly by using a biologic indicator with a matching control (i.e., biologic indicator and control from the same lot number) (IB) (2,9,243, 247,278,279).
   7. Use a biologic indicator for every sterilizer load that contains an implantable device. Verify results before using the implantable device, whenever possible (IB) (243,248).
   8. The following are recommended in the case of a positive spore test:
      a. Remove the sterilizer from service, and review sterilization procedures (e.g., work practices, use of mechanical and chemical indicators) to determine whether operator error could be responsible (II) (8)
      b. Retest the sterilizer by using biologic, mechanical, and chemical indicators after correcting any identified procedural problems (II)
      c. If the repeat spore test is negative, and mechanical and chemical indicators are within normal limits, put the sterilizer back in service (II) (9,243).
   9. The following are recommended if the repeat spore test is positive:
      a. Do not use the sterilizer until it has been inspected or repaired, or the exact reason for the positive test has been determined (II) (9,243)
      b. Recall, to the extent possible, and reprocess all items processed since the last negative spore test (IB) (9,283)
      c. Before placing the sterilizer back in service, rechallenge the sterilizer with biologic indicator tests in three consecutive empty chamber sterilization cycles after the cause of sterilizer failure has been determined and corrected (II) (9,283).
   10. Maintain sterilization records (i.e., mechanical, chemical, and biological) in compliance with state and local regulations (IB) (243).

G. Storage Area for Sterilized Items and Clean Dental Supplies
   1. Implement practices based on date- or event-related shelf-life for the storage of wrapped, sterilized instruments and devices (IB) (243,284).
   2. Even for event-related packaging, at a minimum, place the date of sterilization and, if multiple sterilizers are used in the facility, the sterilizer used on the outside of the packaging material to facilitate the retrieval of processed items in the event of a sterilization failure (IB) (243,247).
   3. Examine wrapped packages of sterilized instruments before opening them, to ensure the barrier wrap has not been compromised during storage (II) (243,284).
   4. Reclean, repack, and resterilize any instrument package that has been compromised (II).

5. Store sterile items and dental supplies in covered or closed cabinets, if possible (II) (285).

VII. ENVIRONMENTAL INFECTION CONTROL

A. General Recommendations

1. Follow the manufacturers' instructions for correct use of cleaning and EPA-registered hospital disinfecting products (IB, IC) (243-245).
2. Do not use liquid chemical sterilants/high-level disinfectants for disinfection of environmental (clinical contact or housekeeping) surfaces (IB, IC) (243-245).
3. Use PPE, as appropriate, when cleaning and disinfecting environmental surfaces. Such equipment might include gloves (e.g., puncture- and chemical-resistant utility), protective clothing (e.g., gown, jacket, lab coat), and protective eyewear/face shield and mask (IC) (13,15).

B. Clinical Contact Surfaces

1. Use surface barriers to protect clinical contact surfaces, particularly those that are difficult to clean (e.g., switches on dental chairs), and change surface barriers between patients (II) (1,2,260,288).
2. Clean and disinfect clinical contact surfaces that are not barrier protected, by using an EPA-registered hospital low- (i.e., HIV and HBV label claims) to intermediate-level disinfectant (i.e., tuberculocidal claim). Use an intermediate-level disinfectant if visibly contaminated with blood (IB) (2,243,244).

C. Housekeeping Surfaces

1. Clean housekeeping surfaces (e.g., floors, walls, sinks) with a detergent and water or an EPA-registered hospital disinfectant/detergent on a routine basis, depending on the nature of the surface and type and degree of contamination and, as appropriate, location in the facility, and when visibly soiled (IB) (243,244).
2. Clean mops and cloths after use and allow to dry before reuse, or use single-use, disposable mopheads or cloths (II) (244).
3. Prepare fresh cleaning or EPA-registered disinfecting solutions daily and as instructed by the manufacturer (II) (243,244).
4. Clean walls, blinds, and window curtains in patient care areas when they are visibly dusty or soiled (II) (9,244).

D. Spills of Blood and Body Substances

1. Clean spills of blood or OPIM, and decontaminate surface with an EPA-registered hospital disinfectant of low (i.e., HBV and HIV label claims) to intermediate level (i.e., tuberculocidal claim), depending on the size of the spill and surface porosity (IB, IC) (13,113).

E. Carpet and Cloth Furnishings

1. Avoid using carpeting and cloth-upholstered furnishings in dental operatories, laboratories, and instrument processing areas (II) (9,293-295).

F. Regulated Medical Waste

1. General recommendations
   a. Develop a medical waste management program. Disposal of regulated medical waste must follow federal, state, and local regulations (IC) (13,301).
   b. Ensure that DHCP who handle and dispose of potentially infective wastes are trained in appropriate handling and disposal methods and informed of possible health and safety hazards (IC) (13).
2. Management of regulated medical waste in dental health care facilities
   a. Use a color-coded or labeled container that prevents leakage (e.g., biohazard bag) to contain nonsharp, regulated medical waste (IC) (13).
   b. Place sharp items (e.g., needles, scalpel blades, orthodontic bands, broken metal instruments, burs) in an appropriate sharps container (i.e., puncture resistant, color coded, and leakproof). Close container immediately before removal or replacement to prevent spillage or protrusion of contents during handling, storage, transport, or shipping (IC) (2,8,13,113,115).
   c. Pour blood, suctioned fluids, or other liquid waste into a drain connected to a sanitary sewer system, if local sewage discharge requirements are met and the state has declared this an acceptable method of disposal. Wear appropriate PPE while performing this task (IC) (7,9,13).

VIII. DENTAL UNIT WATER LINES, BIOFILM, AND WATER QUALITY

A. General Recommendations

1. Use water that meets EPA regulatory standards for drinking water (i.e., 500 CFU]/mL of heterotropic water bacteria) for routine dental treatment output water (IB, IC) (341,342).
2. Consult with the dental unit manufacturer for appropriate methods and equipment to maintain the recommended quality of dental water (II) (339).
3. Follow recommendations for monitoring water quality provided by the manufacturer

of the unit or water line treatment product (II).

4. Discharge water and air for a minimum of 20-30 seconds after each patient, from any device connected to the dental water system that enters the patient's mouth (e.g., handpieces, ultrasonic scalers, air/water syringes) (II) (2,311,344).
5. Consult with the dental unit manufacturer the need for periodic maintenance of antiretraction mechanisms (IB) (2,311).

B. Boil-Water Advisories
1. The following apply while a boil-water advisory is in effect:
    a. Do not deliver water from the public water system to the patient through the dental operative unit, ultrasonic scaler, or other dental equipment that uses the public water system (IB, IC) (341,342,346, 349,350).
    b. Do not use water from the public water system for dental treatment, patient rinsing, or handwashing (IC) (341,342, 346,349,350).
    c. For handwashing, use antimicrobial-containing products that do not require water for use (e.g., alcohol-based hand-rubs). If hands are visibly contaminated, use bottled water, if available, and soap or an antiseptic towelette (IB, IC) (13,122).
2. The following apply when a boil-water advisory is canceled:
    a. Follow guidance given by the local water utility on adequate flushing of water lines. If no guidance is provided, flush dental water lines and faucets for 1 to 5 minutes before using for patient care (IC) (244,346,351,352).
    b. Disinfect dental water lines as recommended by the dental unit manufacturer (II).

IX. SPECIAL CONSIDERATIONS

A. Dental Handpieces and Other Devices Attached to Air and Water Lines
1. Clean and heat sterilize handpieces and other intraoral instruments that can be removed from the air and water lines of dental units between patients (IB, IC) (2,246,275,356,357,360,407).
2. Follow the manufacturer's instructions for cleaning, lubrication, and sterilization of handpieces and other intraoral instruments that can be removed from the air and water lines of dental units (IB) (361-363).
3. Do not surface-disinfect or use liquid chemical sterilants or ethylene oxide on handpieces and other intraoral instruments that can be removed from the air and water lines of dental units (IC) (2,246,250,275).
4. Do not advise patients to close their lips tightly around the tip of the saliva ejector to evacuate oral fluids (II) (364-366).

B. Dental Radiology
1. Wear gloves when exposing radiographs and handling contaminated film packets. Use other PPE (e.g., protective eyewear, mask and gown) as appropriate if spattering of blood or other body fluids is likely (IA, IC) (11,13).
2. Use heat-tolerant or disposable intraoral devices whenever possible (e.g., film-holding and positioning devices). Clean and heat sterilize heat-tolerant devices between patients. At a minimum, use high-level disinfectant on semicritical heat-sensitive devices, according to manufacturer's instructions (IB) (243).
3. Transport and handle exposed radiographs in an aseptic manner to prevent contamination of developing equipment (II).
4. The following apply for digital radiography sensors:
    a. Use FDA-cleared barriers (IB) (243).
    b. Clean and heat-sterilize, or high-level disinfect, barrier-protected semicritical items. If the item cannot tolerate these procedures, then, at a minimum, protect with an FDA-cleared barrier, and clean and disinfect with an EPA-registered hospital disinfectant product with intermediate-level (i.e., tuberculocidal claim) activity, between patients. Consult with the manufacturer for methods of disinfection and sterilization of digital radiology sensors and for protection of associated computer hardware (IB) (243).

C. Aseptic Technique for Parenteral Medications
1. Do not administer medication from a syringe to multiple patients even if the needle on the syringe is changed (IA) (378).
2. Use single-dose vials for parenteral medications when possible (II) (376,377).
3. Do not combine the leftover contents of single-use vials for later use (IA) (376,377).
4. The following apply if multiple-dose vials are used:
    a. Clean the access diaphragm with 70% alcohol before inserting a device into the vial (IA) (380,381).
    b. Use a sterile device to access a multiple-dose vial, and avoid touching the access diaphragm. Both the needle and syringe

used to access the multiple-dose vial must be sterile. Do not reuse a syringe even if the needle is changed (IA) (380,381).

c. Keep multiple-dose vials away from the immediate patient treatment area to prevent inadvertent contamination by spray or spatter (II).

d. Discard the multiple-dose vial if sterility is compromised (IA) (380,381).

5. Use fluid infusion and administration sets (i.e., IV bags, tubings, connections) for one patient only, and dispose of appropriately (IB) (378).

D. Single-Use (Disposable) Devices

1. Use single-use devices for one patient only, and dispose of them appropriately (IC) (383).

E. Preprocedural Mouthrinses

1. No recommendation is offered on using preprocedural antimicrobial mouth rinses to prevent clinical infection among DHCP or patients. Although studies have demonstrated that a preprocedural antimicrobial rinse (e.g., chlorhexidine gluconate, essential oils, povidone-iodine) can reduce the level of oral microorganisms in aerosols and spatter generated during routine dental procedures, and can decrease the number of microorganisms introduced into the patient's bloodstream during invasive dental procedures (391-399), scientific evidence is inconclusive that the use of these rinses prevents clinical infection among DHCP or patients (see discussion Special Considerations: Preprocedural Mouth Rinses) (Unresolved issue).

F. Oral Surgical Procedures

1. The following apply when performing oral surgical procedures:

a. Perform surgical hand antisepsis by using an antimicrobial product (e.g., antimicrobial soap and water, soap and water followed by alcohol-based hand scrub with persistent activity) (IB) (127-132,137).

b. Use sterile surgeon's gloves (IB) (2,7,121,123,137).

c. Use sterile saline or sterile water as a coolant/irrigator when performing oral surgical procedures. Use devices specifically designed for the delivery of sterile irrigating fluids (e.g., bulb syringe, single-use disposable products, sterilizable tubing) (IB) (2,121).

G. Handling of Biopsy Specimens

1. During transport, place biopsy specimens in a sturdy, leakproof container labeled with the biohazard symbol (IC) (2,13,14).

2. If a biopsy specimen container is visibly contaminated, clean and disinfect the outside of a container, or place it in an impervious bag labeled with the biohazard symbol (IC) (2,13).

H. Handling of Extracted Teeth

1. Dispose of extracted teeth as regulated medical waste unless returned to the patient (IC) (13,14).

2. Do not dispose of extracted teeth containing amalgam in regulated medical waste intended for incineration (II).

3. Clean and place extracted teeth in a leakproof container, labeled with a biohazard symbol, and maintain hydration, for transport to educational institutions or a dental laboratory (IB, IC) (13,14).

4. Heat-sterilize teeth that do not contain amalgam, before they are used for educational purposes (IB) (403,405,406).

I. Dental Laboratory

1. Use PPE when handling items received in the laboratory, until they have been decontaminated (IA, IC) (2,7,11,13,113).

2. Before they are handled in the laboratory, clean, disinfect and rinse all dental prostheses and prosthodontic materials (e.g., impressions, bite registrations, occlusal rims and extracted teeth) by using an EPA-registered hospital disinfectant having at least an intermediate level of activity (i.e., tuberculocidal claim) (IB) (2,249,252,407).

3. Consult with manufacturers regarding the stability of specific materials (e.g., impression materials) relative to disinfection procedures (II).

4. Include specific information regarding disinfection techniques used (e.g., solution used and duration) when laboratory cases are sent off-site and on their return (II) (2,407,409).

5. Clean and heat sterilize heat-tolerant items used in the mouth (e.g., metal impression trays and face-bow forks) (IB) (2,407).

6. Follow manufacturers' instructions for cleaning and sterilizing or disinfecting items that become contaminated but do not normally contact the patient (e.g., burs, polishing points, rag wheels, articulators, case pans, lathes). If manufacturer instructions are not available, clean and heat sterilize heat-tolerant items, or clean and disinfect with an EPA-registered hospital disinfectant with low- (HIV/HBV effectiveness claim) to intermediate-level (i.e., tuberculocidal claim) activity, depending on the degree of contamination (II).

J. Laser/Electrosurgery Plumes/Surgical Smoke
  1. No recommendation is offered on practices to reduce DHCP exposure to laser plumes/surgical smoke when using lasers in dental practice. Practices to reduce HCP exposure to laser plumes/surgical smoke have been suggested, including use of (a) standard precautions (e.g., high-filtration surgical masks, possibly full face shields) (437), (b) central room suction units with in-line filters to collect particulate matter from minimal plumes, and (c) dedicated mechanical smoke exhaust systems with a high-efficiency filter to remove substantial amounts of laser plume particles. The effect of exposure (e.g., disease transmission, adverse respiratory effects) to DHCP from dental applications of lasers has not been adequately evaluated (see previous discussion, Special Considerations: Laser/Electrosurgery Plumes or Surgical Smoke) (Unresolved issue).

K. *Mycobacterium tuberculosis*
  1. General recommendations
    a. Educate all DHCP regarding the recognition of signs, symptoms, and transmission of TB (IB) (20,21).
    b. Conduct a baseline tuberculin skin test (TST), preferably by using a two-step test, for all DHCP who might have contact with persons with suspected or confirmed active TB, regardless of the risk classification of the setting (IB) (20).
    c. Assess each patient for a history of TB as well as symptoms suggestive of TB, and document on the medical history form (IB) (20,21).
    d. Follow CDC recommendations for (1) developing, maintaining, and implementing a written TB infection control plan, (2) managing a patient with suspected or active TB, (3) completing a community risk assessment to guide employee TSTs and follow-up, and (4) managing DHCP with TB disease (IB) (2,21).
  2. The following apply for patients known or suspected to have active TB:
    a. Evaluate the patient away from other patients and DHCP. When not being evaluated, the patient should wear a surgical mask or be instructed to cover the mouth and nose when coughing or sneezing (IB) (20,21).
    b. Defer elective dental treatment until the patient is noninfectious (IB) (20,21).
    c. Refer patients requiring urgent dental treatment to a previously identified facility with TB engineering controls and a respiratory protection program (IB) (20,21).

L. Creutzfeldt-Jakob Disease and Other Prion Diseases
  1. No recommendation is offered regarding use of special precautions, in addition to standard precautions, when treating known CJD or vCJD patients. Potential infectivity of oral tissues in CJD or vCJD patients is an unresolved issue. Scientific data indicate the risk, if any, of sporadic CJD transmission during dental and oral surgical procedures is low to nil. Until additional information exists regarding the transmissibility of CJD or vCJD during dental procedures, special precautions in addition to standard precautions might be indicated when treating known CJD or vCJD patients; a list of such precautions is provided for consideration without recommendation (see Special Considerations: Creutzfeldt-Jakob Disease and Other Prion Diseases) (Unresolved issue).

M. Program Evaluation
  1. Establish routine evaluation of the infection control program, including evaluation of performance indicators, at an established frequency (II) (470-471).

HOW TO LEARN MORE

The American Dental Association (ADA) has posted on its Web site a "roadmap" to help the dental health professional navigate through the CDC guidelines and put the recommendations into practice. This roadmap (available at www.ada.org/prof/resources/topics/cdc/index.asp) provides a general overview of the guidelines and the major subjects covered and offers links to existing information about them.

This is an evolving document. Regular additions and updates will provide the information needed to understand and implement the new guidelines. Questions should be directed to the ADA Division of Science at 1-800-621-8099, extension 2878, or at science@ada.org.

Additional information on products and services for dental unit waterline cleaning and monitoring is available at www.ada.org, or from the ADA Division of Science, telephone: 1-800-621-8099, extension 2878, or e-mail: science@ada.org.

REFERENCES

1. Centers for Disease Control and Prevention, Division of Oral Health, Infection Control in Dental Settings (website), accessed on November 16, 2011.
2. Centers for Disease Control and Prevention, Division of Oral Health, Infection Control in Dental Settings: *Prevention of*

2009 H1N1 influenza transmission in dental health care settings (article online), http://www.cdc.gov/OralHealth/infectioncontrol/factsheets/2009_h1n1.htm; accessed on November 16, 2011.
3. Centers for Disease Control and Prevention: *Seasonal flu: respiratory hygiene/cough etiquette in healthcare settings* (article online), www.cdc.gov/flu/professionals/infectioncontrol/resphygiene.htm; accessed on November 16, 2011.
4. Cleveland JL, Robison VA, Panlilio AL: Tuberculosis epidemiology, diagnosis and infection control recommendations for dental settings: an update on the Centers for Disease Control and Prevention guidelines, *J Am Dent Assoc* 140:1092-1099, 2009.
5. Jensen PA, et al: Guidelines for preventing the transmission of *Mycobacterium tuberculosis* in health-care settings, 2005, *MMWR Recomm Rep* 54(RR-17):1-142, 2005.
6. Centers for Disease Control and Prevention: Guidelines for infection control in dental health-care settings—2003, *MMWR Morb Mortal Wkly Rep* 52(No. RR-17):1-66, 2003. [Medline].
7. Centers for Disease Control and Prevention: Recommended infection control practices for dentistry, 1993, *MMWR Morb Mortal Wkly Rep* 41(No. RR-8):1-12, 1993.
8. U.S. Census Bureau: *2001 statistical abstract of the United States: section 12—labor force, employment, and earnings* (article online), www.census.gov/prod/2002pubs/01statab/labor.pdf; accessed on December 2, 2003.
9. Health Resources and Services Administration: *U.S. health workforce personnel factbook*, Rockville, Md, 2000, Health Resources and Services Administration.
10. Centers for Disease Control and Prevention: Recommended infection control practices for dentistry, *MMWR Morb Mortal Wkly Rep* 35:237-242, 1986.
11. The control of transmissible disease in dental practice: a position paper of the American Association of Public Health Dentistry, *J Public Health Dent* 46:13-22, 1986.
12. Klein RS, et al: Low occupational risk of human immunodeficiency virus infection among dental professionals, *N Engl J Med* 318:86-90, 1988.
13. Ciesielski C, et al: Transmission of human immunodeficiency virus in a dental practice, *Ann Intern Med* 116:798-805, 1992.
14. Centers for Disease Control and Prevention: Epidemiologic notes and reports update: transmission of HIV infection during invasive dental procedures—Florida, *MMWR Morb Mortal Wkly Rep* 40:377-381, 1991.
15. U.S. Department of Labor, Occupational Safety and Health Administration: 29 CFR Part 1910: occupational exposure to blood-borne pathogens; needlestick and other sharps injuries; final rule, *Fed Reg* 66:5317-5325, 2001; available at www.osha.gov/FedReg_osha_pdf/FED20010118A.pdf; accessed on December 2, 2003.

APPENDIX C

Therapeutic Management of Common Oral Lesions

This Appendix is provided to the clinician as a guide to the management of oral lesions that may be commonly encountered in the dental practice. It is intended only as a reference and is based on correct diagnosis of the condition and background knowledge of how the recommended therapies can be properly used. This information also is provided as a courtesy of the American Academy of Oral Medicine (AAOM), which publishes a guide for clinicians (Siegel M, Silverman S, Sollecito T: *Clinician's guide: treatment of common oral lesions,* Hamilton, Ontario, Canada, BC Decker, 2006) that contains much of this same information. We (all members of the AAOM) acknowledge our deep appreciation for the authorization to publish this Appendix.

This Appendix is intended as a quick reference to the causative factors, clinical description, currently accepted therapeutic management, and patient education regarding the more common oral conditions. Some of the recommended treatments have been more thoroughly investigated than others, but all have been reported to be of clinical value.

No cure has been found for many of the oral conditions described here, but treatment modalities are available that can relieve discomfort, shorten clinical duration and frequency, and minimize recurrences.

Clinicians are reminded that an accurate diagnosis is imperative for clinical success. Every effort should be made to determine the diagnosis before treatment is initiated. Infection and malignancy must be ruled out. When signs and symptoms and microscopic and other laboratory evidence do not support a definitive diagnosis, empirical treatment may be initiated and evaluated on a therapeutic trial basis.

Patient management should be governed by the natural history of the oral condition and whether a palliative, supportive, or curative treatment exists. Appropriate referral is indicated when the clinical problem is beyond the scope of the clinician's practice. Further treatment can be determined by the patient's response. However, when healing of a lesion or an expected response to treatment is not attained within an expected length of time, biopsy is recommended.

Unless otherwise specified as over-the-counter (OTC) drugs, all therapeutic agents recommended for treatment of specific lesions and conditions are prescription drugs; particulars of the prescription (Rx) are given for each such agent. Of note, the U.S. Food and Drug Administration (FDA) has been active in recent years in allowing OTC status for drugs formerly available by prescription only. It is important to check the dosages of newly released OTC drugs, because they usually differ in strength from agents available by prescription.

SUPPORTIVE CARE

Management of oral mucosal conditions may require topical and systemic interventions. Therapy should address patient nutrition and hydration, oral discomfort, oral hygiene, management of secondary infection, and local control of the disease process. Depending on the extent, severity, and location of oral lesions, consideration should be given to obtaining a consultation from a dentist who specializes in oral medicine, oral pathology, or oral surgery. When a question arises involving a medical condition, a physician should be consulted.

Symptomatic relief of painful conditions can be provided with topical preparations such as 2% viscous lidocaine hydrochloride or 0.5% dyclonine hydrochloride. Topical anesthetic may be used as a rinse in adults but should be applied with a cotton swab in children so that they do not swallow the medication. Swallowing these anesthetics is contraindicated, in part because they may interfere with the patient's gag reflex. Symptomatic relief also can be attained by mixing equal parts of diphenhydramine hydrochloride elixir and magnesium hydroxid or aluminum hydroxide. Children's formula diphenhydramine hydrochloride elixir does not contain alcohol. Sucralfate suspension also may be used before meals. The diphenhydramine mixture and the sucralfate coat the ulcerated lesions, allowing the patient to eat more comfortably.

Meticulous oral hygiene is absolutely mandatory for these patients. Mucosal lesions that contact bacterial plaque present on the dentition are more likely to become secondarily infected. Patients should be seen by the dentist or the hygienist for scaling and root planing, with use of local anesthesia when necessary, in all cases in which oral hygiene is suboptimal. Patients must be encouraged to brush and floss their teeth after meals in a gentle yet efficient manner. This practice may be enhanced by use of a soft toothbrush that has been soaked briefly in hot water to further soften the bristles. Tartar control toothpastes that contain calcium pyrophosphate should be avoided because of their caustic nature and reported association with circumoral dermatitis.

HERPES SIMPLEX

Infection with the herpes simplex virus produces a disease that has a primary, or acute, phase and a secondary, or recurrent, phase.

PRIMARY HERPETIC GINGIVOSTOMATITIS

Etiology

A transmissible infection with herpes simplex virus, usually type I, less commonly type II.

Clinical Description

Clear, then yellowish vesicles develop intraorally and extraorally. These rupture within hours to form shallow, painful ulcers. Gingivae often are red, enlarged, and painful. The patient may have systemic signs and symptoms, including regional lymphadenitis, fever, and malaise. Usually, the eruption is self-limiting and heals in 7 to 10 days.

Rationale for Treatment

Relieve symptoms, prevent secondary infection, and support general health. Supportive therapy includes forced fluids, protein, vitamin and mineral food supplements, and rest. Systemic acyclovir is effective in treating herpes in immunocompromised patients. Topical steroids should be avoided because they tend to permit spread of the viral infection on mucous membranes, particularly ocular membranes. Patients should be cautioned to avoid touching the herpetic lesions and then touching the eyes, genitals, or other body areas, because of the possibility of self-inoculation.

Topical Anesthetics and Coating Agents

Rx:
Diphenhydramine (Benadryl) elixir 12.5 mg/5 mL (NOTE: elixir is Rx, and syrup [Benylin] is OTC) 4 oz, mixed with Kaopectate (OTC) 4 oz, to make a 50% mixture by volume
Disp: 8 oz
Sig: Rinse with 1 teaspoonful every 2 hours, and spit out.

Maalox OTC can be used in place of Kaopectate. Dyclonine (Dyclone) HCl 0.5%, 1 oz, may be added for greater anesthetic efficacy.

Rx:
Diphenhydramine (Benadryl) elixir 12.5 mg/5 mL (NOTE: elixir is Rx, and syrup [Benylin] is OTC)
Disp: 4-oz bottle
Sig: Rinse with 1 teaspoonful for 2 minutes, every 2 hours and before each meal, and spit out.

NOTE: This preparation can be mixed with 2% viscous lidocaine or dyclonine 0.5% for additional relief.

Rx:
Lidocaine (viscous) 2.0% or 1%
Disp: 1-oz bottle
Sig: Rinse with 1 teaspoonful for 2 minutes before each meal, and spit out.

Rx:
Dyclonine HCl (Dyclone) 0.5% or 1%
Disp: 1-oz bottle
Sig: Rinse with 1 teaspoonful for 2 minutes before each meal, and spit out.

Systemic Antiviral Therapy. Antiviral agent oral capsules may relieve and decrease the duration of symptoms.

Rx:
Acyclovir (Zovirax) capsules 200 mg
Disp: 50 (or 60) capsules
Sig: Take 1 capsule 5 times a day for 10 days (or 2 capsules 3 times a day for 10 days).

(Current FDA recommendation is that systemic acyclovir should be used to treat oral herpes only in immunocompromised patients.)

Rx:
Valacyclovir (Valtrex) caplets 500 mg
Disp: 20 caplets
Sig: Take 2 caplets twice a day for 5 days.

(This regimen is that currently recommended by the Centers for Disease Control and Prevention [CDC] for management of genital herpes.)

Systemic Antibiotics. (For secondary bacterial infection in susceptible patients—not for routine use.)

Rx:
Penicillin V tablets 500 mg
Disp: 40 tablets
Sig: Take 1 tablet 4 times a day.
For patients allergic to penicillin:

Rx:
Erythromycin tablets 250 mg
Disp: 40 tablets
Sig: Take 1 tablet 4 times a day.

If nausea or stomach cramps occur, prescribe enteric-coated preparations (E-Mycin, ERYC, PCE, etc.) or a second-generation erythromycin (e.g., clarithromycin [Biaxin]).

Nutritional Supplements

Rx:
Meritene—protein/vitamin/mineral food supplement (OTC)
Disp: 1-lb can (plain vanilla, chocolate, and eggnog flavors)
Sig: Take 3 servings daily. Prepare as indicated on the label. Serve cold.

Rx:
Ensure Plus—protein/vitamin/mineral food supplement (OTC)
Disp: 20 cans
Sig: Drink 3 to 5 cans in divided doses throughout the day as tolerated. Serve cold.

Analgesic

Rx:
Acetaminophen tablets 325 mg (OTC)
Sig: Take 2 tablets every 4 hours as needed for pain and fever. Limit 4 g per 24 hours.
For moderate to severe pain:
Acetaminophen 300 mg with codeine 30 mg (Tylenol #3)
Sig: Take 1 or 2 tablets every 4 hours for pain (requires Drug Enforcement Agency [DEA] number).

RECURRENT (OROFACIAL) HERPES SIMPLEX

Etiology

Reactivation of the latent virus that resides in the sensory ganglion of the trigeminal nerve. Precipitating factors include fever, stress, exposure to sunlight, trauma, and hormonal alterations.

Clinical Description

Intraoral—single or small clusters of vesicles that quickly rupture, forming painful ulcers. Lesions usually occur on the keratinized tissue of the hard palate and gingiva.
Labialis—clusters of vesicles on the lips that rupture within hours and then crust.

Rationale for Treatment

Treatment should be initiated as early as possible during the prodromal stage, with the objective of reducing duration and symptoms of the lesion. Oral acyclovir, given prophylactically and therapeutically, may be considered when frequent recurrent herpetic episodes interfere with daily function and nutrition.

(Current FDA recommendation is that systemic acyclovir should be used to treat oral herpes only in immunocompromised patients.)

Prevention

Rx:
PreSun 15 sunscreen lotion (OTC)
Disp: 4 fl oz
Sig: Apply to susceptible area 1 hour before sun exposure and every hour thereafter.

Rx:
PreSun 15 lip gel (OTC)
Disp: 15 oz
Sig: Apply to lips 1 hour before sun exposure and every hour thereafter.

If recurrence on the lips usually is precipitated by exposure to sunlight, the lesion may be prevented by the application to the area of a sunscreen with a high sunburn protection factor (SPF 15 or higher).

Topical Antiviral Agents. Antiviral creams and ointments are of minimal efficacy for recurrent herpes simplex. Their value may be attributable to coating of the lesion by the petrolatum vehicle, which reduces the possibility of self-inoculation. Constant or intermittent application of ice to the area for 90 minutes during the prodromal phase may result in abortion of the lesion. Cocoa butter ointment, lanolin-based lip preparations, or petrolatum (Vaseline) as an emollient may be palliative.

Rx:
Penciclovir (Denavir) topical ointment 5%
Disp: 15-g tube
Sig: Apply to the area every 2 hours during waking hours, beginning when symptoms first occur.

Rx:
Docosanol (Abreva) cream (OTC)
Disp: 2-g tube
Sig: Dab on lesion 5 times per day during waking hours for 4 days, beginning when symptoms first occur.

Systemic Antiviral Therapy. This is best implemented at the very onset of prodromal symptoms.

Rx:
Valacyclovir (Valtrex) caplets 500 mg
Disp: 8 caplets
Sig: Take 4 caplets at the very beginning of prodromal symptoms and 4 caplets 12 hours later.

VARICELLA ZOSTER (SHINGLES)

Etiology

Reactivation of latent herpesvirus–varicella virus present since an original varicella virus infection, typically chickenpox. Precipitating factors include thermal, inflammatory, radiologic, and mechanical trauma.

Clinical Description

Usually painful, segmental eruption of small vesicles that later rupture to form punctate or confluent ulcers. Acute zoster follows a portion of the trigeminal nerve distribution in approximately 20% of cases. It is rare in the young and more common in the elderly.

Rationale for Treatment

Promptly initiate antiviral therapy to reduce the duration and symptoms of lesions. Patients older than 60 years of age are particularly prone to postherpetic neuralgia. In the absence of specific contraindications, consideration should be given to prescribing short-term, high-dose corticosteroid prophylaxis for postherpetic neuralgia, in conjunction with oral acyclovir.

Rx:
Acyclovir (Zovirax) capsules 200 mg
Disp: 200 capsules
Sig: Take 4 capsules 5 times daily for 10 days.

Rx:
Valacyclovir (Valtrex) HCl caplets 500 mg
Disp: 42 capsules
Sig: Take 2 capsules 3 times daily for 7 days.
Use with caution in immunocompromised patients.

Rx:
Prednisone tablets 10 mg
Disp: 50 tablets
Sig: Take 6 tablets in the morning; then reduce the number by 1 on each successive day.

RECURRENT APHTHOUS STOMATITIS

Etiology

An altered local immune response is the predisposing factor. Patients with frequent recurrences should be screened for disease such as anemia, diabetes mellitus, vitamin deficiency, inflammatory bowel disease, and immunosuppression.

Precipitating factors include stress, trauma, allergies, endocrine alterations, and dietary components such as acidic foods and juices, and foods that contain gluten. Inspect the oral cavity closely for sources of trauma.

Clinical Description

Minor aphthae (canker sore), smaller than 0.6 cm—small, shallow, painful ulcerations covered by a gray membrane and surrounded by a narrow erythematous halo. They usually occur on nonkeratinized (movable) oral mucosa.

Major aphthae, greater than 0.6 cm—large, painful ulcers. A more severe form of aphthae that may last weeks or months. They may mimic other diseases such as granulomatous or malignant lesions.

Herpetiform ulcers—crops of small, shallow, painful ulcers. They may occur anywhere on nonkeratinized oral mucosa and resemble those of recurrent intraoral herpes simplex clinically but are of unknown origin.

Rationale for Treatment

Effective treatment involves barriers, amlexanox, topical or systemic corticosteroids, and immunosuppressants or combination therapy, when indicated. Treatment should be initiated as early in the course of the lesions as possible. Identification and elimination of precipitating factors may serve to minimize recurrent episodes. Medications such as mycophenolate mofetil, pentoxifylline, and thalidomide are useful for treating patients with severe, persistent recurrent aphthous ulcers but should not be routinely used.

Nonsteroidal Agents

Rx:
Amlexanox oral paste 5%
Disp: 5-g tube
Sig: Dab on affected area 4 times a day until healed.

Rx:
Orabase Soothe-N-Seal Protective Barrier (OTC)
Disp: 1 package
Sig: Apply according to the package directions every 6 hours, when necessary.

For mild to moderate relief:

"Special Mouthwash."* There is no "universal formula" for this preparation. Any of several variations can be concocted, depending on the diagnosis and the patient's symptoms. The Special Mouthwash must be made up for each individual patient.

Basic (OTC):

Benadryl	+	Carafate	+	Maalox elixir
160 mL		40 mL		40 mL

Optional:
± Kaopectate (OTC)
± nystatin
± anesthetic (dyclone, lidocaine)
± antibiotic (tetracycline, penicillin)

For example, for *glossitis, aphthous, mild lichen planus*:

*The Special Mouthwash is being considered for patent by the University of Minnesota under the name Rhodus Magical Mouthwash.

Special Mouthwash Rx:

Guafenesin	80 mL
Diphenhydramine (12.5/5 cc)	200 mL
Nystatin (100,000 IU/5 cc)	30 mL
Sucralfate	100 mL
Maalox	50 mL
2% viscous lidocaine	20 mL

Disp: 480 mL
Sig: Take 3 tsp (15 mL), swish for 3 minutes, gargle, and expectorate, t.i.d. for 2 weeks; then use daily prn for maintenance.

Topical Steroids. Therapies with steroids and immunomodulating drugs are presented to inform the clinician that such modalities are available. Because of the potential for adverse effects, close collaboration with the patient's physician is recommended if these medications are prescribed. These modalities may be beyond the scope of clinical experience of general dentists, and referral to a specialist in oral medicine or to an appropriate physician may be necessary.

Prolonged use of topical steroids (longer than 2 weeks of continuous use) may result in mucosal atrophy or secondary candidiasis and may increase the potential for systemic absorption. It may be necessary to prescribe antifungal therapy concomitantly with steroids.

Rx:
Triamcinolone acetonide (Kenalog) in Orabase 0.1%
Disp: 5-g tube
Sig: Coat the lesion with a thin film after each meal and at bedtime.

Other topical steroid preparations (cream, gel rinse, ointment) include the following:

Ultrapotent
- Clobetasol propionate (Temovate) 0.05%
- Halobetasol propionate (Ultravate) 0.05%

Potent
- Dexamethasone (Decadron) 0.5 mg/5 mL

Intermediate
- Betamethasone valerate (Valisone) 0.1%
- Triamcinolone acetonide (Kenalog) 0.1%

Low
- Hydrocortisone 1%

Note: Mixing ointments with equal parts of Orabase B paste promotes adhesion. Also, mixing with 2% lidocaine gel will help palliate symptoms.

Rx:
Dexamethasone (Decadron) elixir 0.5 mg/5 mL
Disp: 100 mL
Sig: Rinse with 1 teaspoon for 2 minutes 4 times a day, and expectorate. Discontinue when lesions become asymptomatic.

Some clinicians have had increased success by combining both topical rinses (dexamethasone) and ointments (triamcinolone) using them concomitantly for more severe cases.

Oral candidiasis may result from topical steroid therapy. The oral cavity should be monitored for emergence of fungal infection in patients who are placed on therapy. Prophylactic antifungal therapy should be initiated in patients with a history of fungal infection with previous steroid administration (see "Candidiasis").

System Steroids and Immunosuppressants

For severe cases:

Rx:
Dexamethasone (Decadron) elixir 0.5 mg/5 mL
Disp: 320 mL
Sig:
1. For 3 days, rinse with 1 tablespoon (15 mL) 4 times a day, and swallow. Then,
2. For 3 days, rinse with 1 teaspoonful (5 mL) 4 times a day, and swallow. Then,
3. For 3 days, rinse with 1 teaspoonful (5 mL) 4 times a day, and swallow every other time. Then,
4. Rinse with 1 teaspoonful (5 mL) 4 times a day, and spit out. Discontinue medication when mouth becomes comfortable.

If mouth discomfort recurs, restart treatment at Step 3. Rinsing should be done after meals and at bedtime. Refill one time.

Rx:
Prednisone tablets 5 mg
Disp: 40 tablets
Sig: Take 5 tablets in the morning for 5 days, then 5 tablets in the morning every other day until gone.

For very severe cases:

Rx:
Prednisone tablets 10 mg
Disp: 26 tablets
Sig: Take 4 tablets in the morning for 5 days: then decrease by 1 tablet on each successive day.

Therapy with medications such as systemic steroids, immunosuppressants, and immunomodulators is presented to inform the clinician that such modalities have been reported to be effective for patients with severe, persistent, recurrent aphthous stomatitis. Medications such as azathioprine, pentoxifylline, levamisole, colchicine, dapsone, and thalidomide are used to treat patients with severe, persistent, recurrent aphthous stomatitis but should not be routinely used because of the potential for adverse effects. Close collaboration with the patient's physician is recommended when these medications are prescribed.

CHEMICAL CAUTERY

In some instances, instant cautery of the ulcer, although it is temporarily painful, diminishes overall symptoms and eliminates the ulcer. The procedure involves professional application of an appropriate agent.

Rx:
Debacterol: One clinical application directly to the ulcer for 15 seconds; then rinse thoroughly.

Phased Therapy. In many cases of these oral erosive-ulcerative conditions (e.g., recurrent aphthous stomatitis, oral lichen planus), the therapy will only temporarily ameliorate the condition. Since the condition will remain (although less acute) or return over time, the clinician may choose to place the patient on a maintenance or less potent treatment during the remission (or less acute phase), thereby reducing the frequency and severity of flares.

CANDIDIASIS

Etiology

Candida albicans, a yeastlike fungus, is the infecting pathogen. *Candida* is an opportunistic organism that tends to proliferate with the use of broad-spectrum antibiotics, corticosteroids, medicines that reduce salivary output, and cytotoxic agents. Conditions that contribute to candidiasis include xerostomia, diabetes mellitus, poor oral hygiene, prosthetic appliances, and suppression of the immune system (e.g., acquired immunodeficiency syndrome [AIDS] or the adverse effects of some medications). It is important to ascertain the predisposing factors.

Clinical Description

The disease is characterized by soft, white, slightly elevated plaques that usually can be wiped away, leaving an erythematous area (pseudomembranous type). Candidiasis also may appear as generalized erythematous, sensitive areas (atrophic or erythematous type) or as confluent white areas (hypertrophic form). When the clinical diagnosis is questionable, it is advisable to culture for *C albicans* concurrent with the start of medication.

Rationale for Treatment

To reestablish a normal balance of oral flora and to improve oral hygiene. Medication should be continued for 48 hours after clinical signs have disappeared, to prevent immediate recurrence.

Topical Antifungal Agents

Rx:
Nystatin (Mycostatin, Nilstat) oral suspension 100,000 units/mL
Disp: 60 mL
Sig: Take 2 to 5 mL 4 times a day. Rinse for 2 minutes, and swallow. Nystatin suspension has a high sugar content; therefore, good oral hygiene should be reinforced. A few drops of nystatin oral suspension can be added to the water used for soaking acrylic prostheses.

Rx:
Nystatin ointment
Disp: 15-g tube
Sig: Apply a thin coat to the inner surface of the denture and to the affected area after each meal.

Rx:
Nystatin topical powder
Disp: 15 g
Sig: Apply a thin layer under the prosthesis after each meal.

Rx:
Nystatin pastilles (Mycostatin) 200,000 U
Disp: 50 pastilles
Sig: Let 1 pastille dissolve in the mouth 5 times a day.

Rx:
Nystatin vaginal suppositories 100,000 U
Disp: 40 suppositories
Sig: Let 1 suppository dissolve in the mouth 4 times a day. Do not rinse for 30 minutes.

Rx:
Clotrimazole (Mycelex) troches 10 mg
Disp: 70 troches
Sig: Let 1 troche dissolve in the mouth 5 times a day. If concern is expressed about the sugar content of nystatin and clotrimazole troches, vaginal tablets may be substituted.

Rx:
Ketoconazole (Nizoral) cream 2%
Disp: 15-g tube
Sig: Apply thin coat to inner surface of denture and affected areas after each meal.

Rx:
Clotrimazole (Gyne-Lotrimin, Mycelex-G) vaginal cream 1% (OTC)
Disp: 1 tube
Sig: Apply small dab to tissue side of denture or to infected oral mucosa 4 times a day.

Rx:
Miconazole (Monistat 7) vaginal cream 2% (OTC)
Disp: 1 tube
Sig: Apply small dab to tissue side of denture or to infected oral mucosa 4 times a day.

NOTE: In many cases, combinations of these antifungal preparations (liquids, troches, and ointments) may be used, depending on clinical considerations and response to therapy. Because patients presenting with candidiasis often have an underlying condition predisposing them to the disease (e.g., immunosuppression, xerostomia), it is important to keep in mind that as long as the predisposing condition is present, the candidiasis will persist or recur despite periodic treatment with these agents. Therefore, the clinican must consider removal of the etiologic factors or place the patient on maintenance therapy for recurrent candidiasis, or both.

Systemic Antifungal Agents. When topical therapy is not practical or is ineffective, ketoconazole (Nizoral) and fluconazole (Diflucan) are effective, well-tolerated, systemic drugs for mucocutaneous candidiasis. They should be used with caution in patients with impaired liver function (i.e., with a history of alcoholism or hepatitis). Liver function tests should be performed initially and then monthly when ketoconazole is prescribed for an extended period. Several drug interactions have been reported with ketoconazole.

Rx:
Ketoconazole (Nizoral) tablets 200 mg
Disp: 20 tablets
Sig: Take 1 tablet daily with a meal or with orange juice.

Rx:
Fluconazole (Diflucan) tablets 100 mg
Disp: 20 tablets
Sig: Take 2 tablets stat, then 1 tablet daily.

NOTE: Because patients often are susceptible to recurring *Candida* infection, some "burst" therapy with systemic and/or topical antifungals may be necessary, as well as ongoing maintenance therapy.

CHEILITIS AND CHEILOSIS

ANGULAR CHEILITIS AND CHEILOSIS

Etiology

Fissured lesions in the corners of the mouth are caused by a mixed infection of the microorganisms *C. albicans*, staphylococci, and streptococci. Predisposing factors include local habits, drooling, a decrease in intermaxillary space, anemia, immunosuppression, and extension of oral infection.

Clinical Description

Commissures may appear wrinkled, red, fissured, cracked, or crusted.

Rationale for Treatment

Identification and correction of predisposing factors and elimination of secondary infection and inflammation

Rx:
Nystatin plus triamcinolone acetonide (Mycolog II) ointment
Disp: 15-g tube
Sig: Apply to affected area after each meal and at bedtime. Concomitant intraoral antifungal treatment may be indicated.

Rx:
Ketoconazole (Nizoral) cream 2%
Disp: 15-g tube
Sig: Apply a small dab to corners of mouth daily at bedtime.

Rx:
Clotrimazole (Gyne-Lotrimin, Mycelex-G) vaginal cream 1% (OTC)
Disp: 1 tube
Sig: Apply small dab to corner of mouth 4 times a day.

Rx:
Miconazole (Monistat 7) nitrate vaginal cream 2% (OTC)
Disp: 1 tube
Sig: Apply a small dab to corner of mouth 4 times a day.

ACTINIC CHEILITIS AND SOLAR CHEILOSIS

Etiology

Prolonged exposure to sunlight results in irreversible degenerative changes in the vermilion of the lips, especially the everted lower lip.

Clinical Description

Normal red translucent vermilion with regular vertical fissuring of a smooth surface is replaced by a white flat surface that may exhibit periodic ulceration.

Rationale for Treatment

If exposure to ultraviolet light in the sun's rays is allowed to continue, degenerative changes may progress to malignancy. Sunscreens with a high SPF (greater than 15) should be used constantly.

Rx:
Several OTC sunscreen preparations are available (e.g., PreSun 15 lotion and lip gel). For those patients who are allergic to para-aminobenzoic acid, non–para-aminobenzoic acid sunscreens should be prescribed.

GEOGRAPHIC TONGUE (BENIGN MIGRATORY GLOSSITIS; ERYTHEMA MIGRANS)

Etiology

The cause of geographic tongue is unknown. Because the histologic appearance is similar to that of psoriasis, some investigators have associated it with psoriasis. This association may be purely coincidental. Oral lesions should not be attributed to psoriasis if no cutaneous signs of this disorder are evident. It also has been associated with Reiter's syndrome and atopy.

Clinical Description

Benign inflammatory condition caused by desquamation of superficial keratin and filiform papillae. It is characterized by red, denuded, irregularly shaped patches of the tongue dorsum and lateral borders surrounded by a raised white-yellow border.

Rationale for Treatment

Generally, no treatment is necessary because most patients are asymptomatic. When symptoms are present, they may be associated with secondary infection with *C. albicans* (see earlier under "Supportive Care"). Use of topical steroids, especially in combination with topical antifungal agents, is the treatment modality of choice. Patients must be educated regarding this condition and reassured that it does not indicate a more serious disease and that it is not contagious. In most cases, biopsy is not indicated, because of the pathognomonic clinical appearance.

Rx:
Nystatin-triamcinolone acetonide (Mycolog II, Mytrex) ointment
Disp: 15-g tube
Sig: Apply to affected areas after meals and at bedtime.

Rx:
Clotrimazole-betamethasone dipropionate (Lotrisone) cream
Disp: 15-g tube
Sig: Apply to affected area after each meal and at bedtime.

Rx:
Betamethasone valerate ointment 0.1%
Disp: 15-g tube
Sig: Apply to affected areas after meals and at bedtime.

Rx:
Nystatin ointment
Disp: 15-g tube
Sig: Apply to affected areas after meals and at bedtime.

For mild to moderate relief:
"Special Mouthwash"
Rx:
Refer to earlier section, "Recurrent Aphthous Stomatitis," for formulation.

XEROSTOMIA

Etiology

Acute or chronic reduced salivary flow may result from drug therapy, mechanical blockage, dehydration, emotional stress, infection of the salivary glands, local surgery, avitaminosis, diabetes, anemia, connective tissue disease, Sjögren syndrome, radiation therapy, and congenital factors (e.g., ectodermal dysplasia) (see Chapter 25).

Clinical Description

Tissues may be dry, pale, or red and atrophic. The tongue may be devoid of papillae and may be atrophic, fissured, and inflamed. Multiple carious lesions may be present, especially at the gingival margin and on exposed root surfaces.

Rationale for Treatment

Salivary stimulation or replacement therapy to keep the mouth moist, prevent caries and candidal infection, and provide palliative relief

Saliva Substitutes

Rx:
Sodium carboxymethyl cellulose 0.5% aqueous solution (OTC)
Disp: 8 fl oz
Sig: Use as a rinse as frequently as needed.

Saliva substitutes (OTC): Oasis, MouthKote, Sage Moist Plus, Xero-Lube, MedOral, Salivart, Moi-Stir, Orex
Commercial oral moisturizing gels (OTC): Sage Mouth Moisturizer, Oral Balance

Relief from oral dryness and accompanying discomfort may be attained conservatively by sipping water frequently all day long, letting ice melt in the mouth, restricting caffeine intake, not using mouth rinses that contain alcohol, humidifying the sleeping area, and coating lips with Blistex or Vaseline.

Saliva Stimulants. Chewing sugarless gum and sucking sugarless mints are conservative ways to temporarily stimulate salivary flow in patients with medication xerostomia or with salivary gland dysfunction. Patients should be cautioned against using products that contain sugar.

Rx:
Pilocarpine HCl solution 1 mg/mL
Disp: 100 mL

Sig: Take 1 teaspoonful 4 times a day. (Dosage should be adjusted to increase saliva while minimizing adverse effects [sweating, stomach upset].)

Rx:
Pilocarpine HCl 5-mg tablets (Salagen)
Disp: 100 tablets
Sig: Take 1 tablet 3 times a day. An extra tablet (10 mg) may be taken at bedtime.

Rx:
Cevimeline HCl (Evoxac) 30-mg tablets
Disp: 100 tablets
Sig: Take 1 tablet by mouth 3 or 4 times a day.

Rx:
Bethanechol (Urecholine) 25 mg
Disp: 21 tablets
Sig: Take 1 tablet 3 times a day.

Caries Prevention. Patients with hyposalivation are at significantly increased risk for development of caries, so an aggressive plan for prevention must be instituted as soon as possible. Frequent profession visits and prophylaxis are important, as is the application of fluoride varnishes.

Rx:
Stannous fluoride gel 0.4%
Disp: 4.3 oz
Sig: Apply to the teeth daily for 5 minutes; 5 to 10 drops in a custom tray. Do not swallow the gel.

Available stannous fluoride gels include IDP Gel-Oh, Stan-Gard, Perfect Choice, Flo Gel, True Gel, Nova Gel, Omni-Gel, Control, Gel-Pro, Perfect Choice, Basic Gel, Gel-Tin, IDP Gel-Oh, Gel-Kam, Stan-Gard, Easy-Gel, and Thera-Flur.

When the taste of acidulated stannous fluoride gels is poorly tolerated, or when etching of ceramic restorations occurs, neutral pH sodium fluoride gel 1% (Thera-Flur-N) should be considered.

Rx:
Neutral NaF gel (Thera-Flur-N) 1.0% or PreviDent (Colgate) 1.1% neutral NaF
Disp: 24 mL
Sig: Place 1 drop per tooth in custom tray; apply for 5 minutes daily. Avoid rinsing or eating for 30 minutes after treatment.

FDA regulations have limited the size of bottles of fluoride because of toxicity if ingested by infants. Because most preparations do not come in childproof bottles, the sizes of topical fluoride preparations vary; 24 mL is approximately a 2-week supply for application to full dentition in custom carriers. Xerostomia provides an excellent environment for overgrowth of *C. albicans*. The patient is likely to require treatment for candidiasis, along with treatment for dry mouth. In a dry oral environment, plaque control becomes more difficult. Scrupulous oral hygiene is essential.

ORAL LICHEN PLANUS

Etiology

Postulated to be a chronic mucocutaneous autoimmune disorder with a genetic predisposition that is initiated by a variety of factors, including emotional stress, hypersensitivity to drugs, dental products, or foods.

Clinical Description

Oral lichen planus varies in clinical appearance. Oral forms of this disorder include lacy white lines that represent Wickham's striae (reticular), an erythematous form (atrophic), and an ulcerating form that often is accompanied by striae peripheral to the ulceration (ulcerative).

Lesions are commonly found on the buccal mucosa, gingiva, and tongue but may be found on the lips and palate. Lichen planus lesions are chronic and also may affect the skin.

Any refractory lesion should be considered for a biopsy, to establish a diagnosis and to rule out a malignancy.

Rationale for Treatment

To provide oral comfort if lesions are symptomatic. No known cure exists. Systemic and local relief with antiinflammatory and immunosuppressant agents is indicated. Identification of any precipitating dietary component, dental product, or medication (lichenoid drug reaction) should be undertaken to ensure against a hypersensitivity reaction. Treatment or prevention of secondary fungal infection with a systemic antifungal agent also should be considered.

Therapies with steroids and immunomodulating drugs are presented to inform the clinician that such modalities are available. Because of the potential for adverse effects, close collaboration with the patient's physician is recommended when these medications are prescribed. These modalities may be beyond the scope of clinical experience of general dentists, and referral to a specialist in oral medicine or to an appropriate physician may be necessary.

Topical Steroids. Prolonged use of topical steroids (for a period of longer than 2 weeks of continuous use) may result in mucosal atrophy and secondary candidiasis and may increase the potential for systemic absorption. The prescribing of antifungal therapy with steroids may be necessary. Therapy with topical steroids, once the lichen planus is under control, should be tapered to alternate-day therapy, or treatment given less often, depending on level of control of the disease and its tendency to recur.

Rx:
Fluocinonide (Lidex) gel 0.05%
Disp: 30-g tube
Sig: Coat the lesion with a thin film after each meal and at bedtime.

Rx:
Dexamethasone (Decadron) elixir 0.5 mg/5 mL
Disp: 100 mL
Sig: Rinse with 1 teaspoonful for 2 minutes 4 times a day, and spit out. Discontinue when lesions become asymptomatic.

Other topical steroid preparations (cream, gel, ointment) include the following:

Ultrapotent
- Clobetasol propionate (Temovate) 0.05%
- Halobetasol propionate (Ultravate) 0.05%

Potent
- Dexamethasone (Decadron) 0.5 mg/5 mL
- Fluocinonide (Lidex) 0.05%
- Fluticasone propionate (Cutivate) 0.05%

Intermediate
- Betamethasone valerate (Valisone) 0.1%
- Alclometasone dipropionate (Aclovate) 0.05%
- Triamcinolone acetonide (Kenalog) 0.1%

Low
- Hydrocortisone 1%

Oral candidiasis may result from topical steroid therapy. The oral cavity should be monitored for emergence of fungal infection in patients who are placed on therapy. Prophylactic antifungal therapy should be initiated in patients with a history of fungal infection with prior steroid administration (see "Candidiasis").

Systemic Steroids and Immunosuppressants

For severe cases:

Rx:
Medrol Dose Pak
Disp: 1 dose pack
Sig: Follow directions on dose pack for number of tablets to take each day.

Rx:
Dexamethasone (Decadron) elixir 0.5 mg/5 mL
Disp: 320 mL
Sig:
1. For 3 days, rinse with 1 tablespoonful (15 mL) 4 times a day, and swallow. Then,
2. For 3 days, rinse with 1 teaspoonful (5 mL) 4 times a day, and swallow. Then,
3. For 3 days, rinse with 1 teaspoonful (5 mL) 4 times a day, and swallow every other time. Then,
4. Rinse with 1 teaspoonful (5 mL) 4 times a day, and expectorate.

Rx:
Prednisone tablets 10 mg
Disp: 26 tablets
Sig: Take 4 tablets in the morning for 5 days, then decrease by 1 tablet on each successive day.

Rx:
Prednisone tablets 5 mg
Disp: 40 tablets
Sig: Take 5 tablets in the morning for 5 days, then 5 tablets in the morning every other day until gone.

Rx:
Tacrolimus 0.03% ointment
Disp: 30-g tube
Sig: Apply to affected areas twice daily as directed.

Some clinicians have had increased success by combining both topical rinses (dexamethasone) and ointments (triamcinolone) using them concomitantly for more severe cases.

If oral discomfort recurs, the patient should return to the clinician for reevaluation.

Many studies suggest that oral lichen planus has an intrinsic property that predisposes to malignant transformation. However, the origin is complex, and interaction among genetic factors, infectious agents, and environmental and lifestyle factors is involved in its development. Prospective studies have shown that patients with lichen planus have a slightly increased risk for development of oral squamous cell carcinoma. All patients who exhibit intraoral lichen planus, particularly those who have had the ulcerative form, should undergo periodic follow-up evaluation.

Therapy with medications such as systemic steroids, immunosuppressants, and immunomodulators is presented to inform the clinician that such modalities have been reported to be effective for patients with ulcerative lichen planus. Medications such as azathioprine, mycophenolate mofetil, tacrolimus, hydroxychloroquine sulfate, acitretin, and cyclosporine are useful for treating patients with severe, persistent, ulcerative lichen planus but should not be routinely used because of the potential for adverse effects. Close collaboration with the patient's physician is recommended when these medications are prescribed.

Phased Therapy. In many cases of these oral erosive-ulcerative conditions (e.g., recurrent aphthous stomatitis, oral lichen planus), the therapy will only temporarily ameliorate the condition. Since the condition will remain (although less acute) or return over time, the clinician may choose to place the patient on a maintenance or less potent treatment during the remission (or less acute phase), thereby reducing the frequency and severity of flares.

For mild to moderate relief:
"Special Mouthwash"

Rx:

Refer to earlier section, "Recurrent Aphthous Stomatitis," for formulation.

PEMPHIGUS AND MUCOUS MEMBRANE PEMPHIGOID

Pemphigus and mucous membrane pemphigoid are relatively uncommon lesions. These should be suspected when chronic, multiple oral ulcerations and a history of oral and skin blisters are present. Often, they occur only in the mouth. Diagnosis is based on patient history and on the histologic and immunofluorescent characteristics of a biopsy specimen of the primary lesion.

Etiology

Both are autoimmune diseases with autoantibodies against antigens that appear in different portions of the epithelium (mucosa). In pemphigus, the antigens are found within the epithelium (desmosomes), and in pemphigoid, the antigens are located at the base of the epithelium within the hemidesmosomes.

Clinical Characteristics

In pemphigus, the lesion may stay in a single location for a long time, and small, placid bullae may develop. The bullae may rupture, leaving an ulcer. Approximately 80% to 90% of patients have oral lesions. In approximately two thirds of patients, oral manifestations are the first sign of disease. All parts of the mouth may become involved. The bullae rupture almost immediately in the mouth but may stay intact for some time on the skin. One of the classic signs, Nikolsky's sign (blister formation induced by gentle rubbing of an affected mucosal site), is present in pemphigus but is not pathognomic, because it also has been found to be present in other disorders. Because the vesicles or bullae are intraepithelial, they often are filled with clear fluid. On histologic examination, a cleavage (e.g., Tzanck cells, acantholytic cells) within the spinous layer of the epithelium is seen.

In pemphigoid, the cleavage or split is beneath the epithelium, resulting in formation of bullae that usually are blood-filled. Mucous membrane pemphigoid often is limited to the oral cavity, but some patients have ocular lesions (e.g., symblepharon, ankyloblepharon) that must be evaluated by an ophthalmologist. Gingiva is the oral site that is most commonly involved. Pemphigoid may appear clinically as a red, nonulcerated gingival lesion.

Rationale for Treatment

Because both pemphigus and pemphigoid are autoimmune disorders, the primary treatment consists of topical or systemic steroids or other immunomodulating drugs. Custom trays may be used to localize topical steroid medications on the gingival tissues (occlusive therapy). Because they may resemble other ulcerative bullous diseases, biopsy is necessary for a definitive diagnosis. Specimens should be submitted for light microscopic, immunofluorescent, and immunologic testing. Because of the potentially serious nature of the disorder, referral to a specialist in oral medicine, dermatology, and ophthalmology must be considered. When eye lesions are present, an ophthalmologist must be consulted immediately, in an effort to prevent blindness.

Therapy with medications such as systemic steroids, immunosuppressants, and immunomodulators is presented to inform the clinician that such modalities have been reported to be effective for patients with vesiculobullous disorders such as pemphigus vulgaris and mucous membrane pemphigoid. Therapies such as regimens based on dapsone, methotrexate, mycophenolate mofetil, cyclosporine, and niacinamide with tetracycline, as well as plasmapheresis, are useful for treating patients with vesiculobullous disorders such as pemphigus vulgaris and mucous membrane pemphigoid but should not be routinely used because of the potential for adverse effects. Close collaboration with the patient's physician is recommended when these medications are prescribed.

Injectable Steroids. Dexamethasone phosphate injectable, 1 ampule (4 mg/mL), may be used in the following manner. After the area is injected with lidocaine, 0.5 to 1 mL should be injected around the margins of the ulcer with a 25-gauge needle, twice a week until the ulcer heals. Therapy with systemic or injectable steroids should be coordinated with the patient's physician because of adverse effects and potential systemic complications.

ORAL ERYTHEMA MULTIFORME

Etiology

Oral erythema multiforme is believed to be an autoimmune condition that may occur at any age. Drug reactions to medications such as penicillin and sulfonamides may play a role in some cases. In a few patients who developed oral erythema multiforme, a herpetic infection immediately preceded the onset of clinical signs.

Clinical Description

Signs of oral erythema multiforme include "blood-crusted" lips, "targetoid" or "bull's-eye" skin lesions, and a nonspecific mucosal slough. The designation *multiforme* signifies that its appearance may take multiple forms.

A severe form of erythema multiforme is called *Stevens-Johnson syndrome,* or *erythema multiforme major.* Erythema multiforme, as a skin disease, occurs most often as the result of an allergic reaction.

Rationale for Treatment

Treatment is primarily antiinflammatory in nature. Steroids are initiated and then tapered. Because of the possible relationship of oral erythema multiforme with herpes simplex virus, suppressive antiviral therapy may be necessary before steroid therapy is initiated. Patients should be questioned carefully about a previous history of recurrent herpetic infection and prodromal symptoms that may have preceded the onset of erythema multiforme.

Dosing must be titrated to specific situations.

Steroid Therapy

Rx:
Prednisone tablets 10 mg
Disp: 100 tablets
Sig: Take 6 tablets in the morning until lesions recede; then decrease by 1 tablet on each successive day.

Suppressive Antiviral Therapy. Renew, as needed, the following:

Rx:
Acyclovir (Zovirax) 400-mg capsules
Disp: 90 capsules
Sig: Take 1 tablet 3 times a day.

Rx:
Valacyclovir (Valtrex) 500-mg capsules
Disp: 30 capsules
Sig: Take 1 tablet daily.

DENTURE SORE MOUTH

Etiology

Discomfort under oral prosthetic appliances may result from combinations of candidal infection, poor denture hygiene, an occlusive syndrome, overextension, and excessive movement of the appliance. This condition may be erroneously attributed to an allergy to denture material, which is a rare occurrence. Retention and fit of the denture should be idealized, and mechanical irritation should be ruled out.

Clinical Description

The tissue covered by the appliance, especially one made of acrylic, is erythematous and smooth or granular, and the condition may be asymptomatic or associated with burning.

Rationale for Treatment

Therapy is directed toward controlling all possible origins and improving oral comfort. If therapy is ineffective, underlying systemic conditions such as diabetes mellitus and poor nutrition should be considered.

The following protocol is recommended:

1. Institute appropriate antifungal medication (see "Candidiasis/Candidosis").
2. Improve oral and appliance hygiene. The patient may have to leave the appliance out for extended periods and should be instructed to leave out the denture overnight. The appliance should be placed in a commercially available denture cleanser, or it can be soaked in a 1% sodium hypochlorite solution (1 teaspoon of sodium hypochlorite in a denture cup of water) for 15 minutes and thoroughly rinsed for at least 2 minutes under running water.
3. Reline, rebase, or construct a new appliance.
4. Apply an artificial saliva or oral lubricant gel, such as Laclede Oral Balance or Sage Gel, to the tissue contact surface of the denture, to reduce frictional trauma.

If all of the foregoing measures fail to control symptoms, biopsy or a short trial of topical steroid therapy may be used to rule out contact mucositis (an allergic reaction to denture materials). If a therapeutic trial fails to resolve the condition, a biopsy should be performed to establish the diagnosis.

For mild to moderate relief:

"Special Mouthwash"

Rx:
Refer to earlier section, "Recurrent Aphthous Stomatitis," for formulation.

BURNING MOUTH SYNDROME

Etiology

Multiple conditions have been implicated in the causation of burning mouth syndrome. Current literature favors neurogenic, vascular, and psychogenic causes. However, other conditions such as xerostomia, candidiasis, referred pain from the tongue musculature, chronic infection, reflux of gastric acid, use of medications, blood dyscrasias, nutritional deficiency, hormonal imbalance, and allergic and inflammatory disorders must be considered.

Clinical Description

Burning mouth syndrome is characterized by the presence of oral burning symptoms and the absence of clinical signs.

Rationale for Treatment

To reduce discomfort by addressing possible causative factors.

Treatment begins with ruling out all possible organic causes on the basis of history, physical evaluation, and specific laboratory studies. Minimal blood studies should include complete blood count (CBC) and differential fasting, glucose, iron, ferritin, folic acid, B_{12}, and a thyroid profile (thyroid-stimulating hormone [TSH], triiodothyronine [T_3], and thyroxine [T_4]).

Rx:
Diphenhydramine (Children's Benadryl) elixir 12.5 mg/5 mL (OTC)
Disp: 1 bottle
Sig: Rinse with 1 teaspoon for 2 minutes before each meal, and swallow.
Children's Benadryl is alcohol-free.

For mild to moderate relief:

"Special Mouthwash"
Rx:
Refer to earlier section, "Recurrent Aphthous Stomatitis," for formulation.

When burning mouth is considered psychogenic or idiopathic, use of a tricyclic antidepressant or a benzodiazepine in low doses has been associated with properties of analgesia and sedation and frequently is successful in reducing or eliminating symptoms after several weeks or months. Dosage is adjusted according to patient reaction and clinical symptoms.

Rx:
Clonazepam (Klonopin) tablets 0.5 mg
Disp: 100 tablets
Sig: Take 1 tablet 3 times a day: then adjust dose after 3-day intervals.

This therapy probably is best managed by an appropriate specialist or by the patient's physician.

Rx:
Amitriptyline (Elavil) tablets 25 mg
Disp: 50 tablets
Sig: Take 1 tablet at bedtime for 1 week, then 2 tablets at bedtime. Increase to 3 tablets at bedtime after 2 weeks, and maintain at that dosage or titrate as appropriate.

Rx:
Chlordiazepoxide (Librium) tablets 5 mg
Disp: 50 tablets
Sig: Take 1 or 2 tablets 3 times a day.

Rx:
Alprazolam (Xanax) tablets 0.25 mg
Disp: 50 tablets
Sig: Take 1 tablet 3 times a day.

Rx:
Diazepam (Valium) tablets 2 mg
Disp: 50 tablets
Sig: Take 1 or 2 tablets.

Obviously, these are psychological therapies, so the clinician may prefer to make an appropriate referral, or to coordinate care with a behaviorial therapist professional. If the clinician elects to treat with these agents, the dosage should be adjusted according to the patient's response. Anticipated adverse effects are dry mouth and morning drowsiness. The rationale for the use of tricyclic antidepressant medications and other psychotropic drugs should be thoroughly explained to the patient, and the patient's physician should be made aware of the treatment. These medications have a potential for addiction and dependence.

Other agents that may provide relief:

Rx:
Tabasco sauce (Capsaicin) (OTC)
Disp: 1 bottle
Sig: Place 1 part Tabasco sauce in 2 to 4 parts water. Rinse for 1 minute 4 times a day, and expectorate.

Rx:
Capsaicin (Zostrix) cream 0.025% (OTC)
Disp: 1 tube
Sig: Apply sparingly to affected site(s) 4 times a day.
Wash hands after each application, and do not use near the eyes.

Topical capsaicin may serve to relieve the burning sensation in some patients. An increase in discomfort for a 2- to 3-week period should be anticipated.

CHAPPED OR CRACKED LIPS

Etiology

Alternate wetting and drying, resulting in inflammation and possible secondary infection.

Clinical Description

The surface of the vermilion is rough and peeling and may be ulcerated with crusting. Normal vertical fissuring may be lost.

Rationale for Treatment

A cracked or abraded and chronically inflamed surface invites secondary infection. Use of an antiinflammatory agent in a petrolatum or adhesive base will interrupt the cycle of surface irritation and damage, allowing healing.

Rx:

Betamethasone valerate (Valisone) ointment 0.1%
Disp: 15-g tube
Sig: Apply to the lips after each meal and at bedtime.

Prolonged use of corticosteroids can result in thinning of the tissue. Their use should be closely monitored.

For maintenance, frequent application of lip care products (e.g., Blistex, Chapstick, Vaseline, cocoa butter) should be suggested.

If lesions do not resolve with treatment, consider biopsy to rule out dysplasia or malignancy.

GINGIVAL ENLARGEMENT

Etiology

Phenytoin sodium (Dilantin), calcium channel blocking agents (nifedipine and others), and cyclosporine are drugs that are known to predispose some patients to gingival enlargement. Blood dyscrasias and hereditary fibromatosis should be ruled out by history and indicated laboratory tests.

Clinical Description

Gingival tissues, especially in the anterior region, are dense, resilient, insensitive, and enlarged but essentially of normal color.

Rationale for Treatment

Local factors, such as plaque and calculus accumulation, contribute to secondary inflammation and the hyperplastic process. This further interferes with plaque control. Specific drugs tend to deplete serum folic acid levels; this results in compromised tissue integrity. Folic acid and drug serum levels should be determined every 6 months. This assessment should be coordinated with the patient's physician.

Treatment consists of (1) meticulous plaque control, (2) gingivoplasty when indicated, and (3) folic acid oral rinse.

Rx:

Folic acid oral rinse 1 mg/mL
Disp: 16 oz
Sig: Rinse with 1 teaspoonful for 2 minutes 2 times a day, and spit out.

Rx:

Chlorhexidine gluconate (Peridex) 0.12%
Disp: 16 oz
Sig: Rinse with ½ oz 2 times a day for 30 seconds, and spit out.

TASTE DISORDERS

Etiology

Taste acuity may be affected by neurologic and physiologic changes and drugs. Diagnostic procedures should first rule out a neurologic deficiency, an olfactory deficit, and systemic influences such as malnutrition, metabolic disturbances, drugs, chemical and physical trauma, and radiation sequelae. Blood tests for trace elements should be conducted to identify any deficiencies.

Rationale for Treatment

A reduction in salivary flow may concentrate electrolytes in the saliva, resulting in a salty or metallic taste. (See treatment discussion under "Xerostomia.") A deficiency of zinc has been associated with a loss of taste (and smell) sensation.

For zinc replacement (in patients with proven zinc deficiency):

Rx:

Orazinc capsules 220 mg (OTC)
Disp: 100 capsules
Sig: Take 1 capsule with milk 3 times a day for at least 1 month.

Rx:

Z-Bec tablets (OTC)
Disp: 60 tablets
Sig: Take 1 tablet daily with food or after meals.

MANAGEMENT OF PATIENTS RECEIVING ANTINEOPLASTIC AGENTS AND RADIATION THERAPY

Etiology

Cancer chemotherapy and radiation to the head and neck tend to reduce the volume and alter the character of the saliva. The balance of the oral flora is disrupted, allowing overgrowth of opportunistic organisms (e.g., *C. albicans*). Also, anticancer therapy damages fast-growing tissues, especially in the oral mucosa.

Clinical Description

The oral mucosa becomes red and inflamed. The saliva is viscous or absent.

Rationale for Treatment

Treatment of these patients is symptomatic and supportive. Patient education, frequent monitoring, and close cooperation with the patient's physician are important.

Oral discomfort may be relieved by topical anesthetics such as diphenhydramine elixir (Benadryl) and dyclonine (Dyclone). Artificial salivas (e.g., Sage Moist Plus, Moi-Stir, Salivart, Xero-Lube) reduce oral dryness. Mouth moisturizing gels (e.g., Sage Mouth Moisturizer, Oralbalance Gel) also may be helpful. Nystatin and clotrimazole preparations control fungal overgrowth. Chlorhexidine rinses help control plaque and candidiasis. Fluorides are applied for caries control. A patient information sheet on this topic is presented in Box C-1, which can be reproduced as a patient handout.

Mouth Rinses

Rx:

Alkaline saline (salt/bicarbonate) mouth rinse—mix ½ teaspoonful each of salt and baking soda in a glass of water.

Sig: Rinse with copious amounts 4 times a day.

Commercially available as Sage Salt and Soda Rinse.

Gingivitis Control

Rx:

Chlorhexidine gluconate mouthwash (Peridex) 0.12%

Disp: 32 oz

Sig: Rinse with ½ oz 2 times a day for 30 seconds, and spit out. Avoid rinsing or eating for 30 minutes after treatment. (Rinse after breakfast and at bedtime.)

In xerostomic patients, chlorhexidine (Peridex) should be used concurrently with an artificial saliva to provide the needed protein binding agent for efficacy and substantivity.

Caries Control. (See "Xerostomia.")

Rx:

Neutral NaF gel (Thera-Flur-N) 1.0%

Disp: 24 mL

Sig: Place 1 drop per tooth in the custom tray; apply for 5 minutes daily. Avoid rinsing or eating for 30 minutes after treatment.

BOX C-1 Oral Care Patient Information Sheet

Listed here are general guidelines for oral care, to be individualized by your doctor. Follow your doctor's advice, or discuss any questions with your doctor if these guidelines differ from what you've been told or have heard.

A. Rinses

1. Rinse with warm, dilute solution of sodium bicarbonate (baking soda) or salt and bicarbonate every 2 hours to bathe the tissues and control oral acidity. Take 2 teaspoonfuls of bicarbonate (or 1 teaspoonful of table salt plus 1 teaspoonful of bicarbonate) per quart of water.
2. If you are experiencing pain, rinse with 1 teaspoonful of elixir of Benadryl before each meal. Be careful when eating while your mouth is numb, to avoid choking.
3. If your mouth is dry, sip cool water frequently (every 10 minutes) all day long. Allowing ice chips to melt in the mouth is comforting. Artificial salivas (e.g., Moi-Stir, Salivart, Xero-Lube, Orex) can be used as frequently as needed to make the mouth moist and "slick." Keep the lips lubricated with petrolatum or a lanolin-containing lip preparation. Commercial mouth rinses with alcohol and coffee, tea, and colas should be avoided as they tend to dry the mouth.
4. If an oral yeast infection develops, antifungal medications can be prescribed.
   a. Nystatin pastille,* let 1 dissolve in the mouth 5 times a day, or
   b. Let a 10-mg clotrimazole (Mycelex)* troche dissolve in the mouth 5 times a day.

B. Care of Teeth and Gums

1. Floss your teeth after each meal. Be careful not to cut the gums.
2. Brush your teeth after each meal. Use a soft, even-bristle brush and a bland toothpaste containing fluoride (e.g., Aim, Crest, Colgate). Brushing with a sodium bicarbonate–water paste also is helpful. Arm & Hammer Dental Care toothpaste and tooth powder are bicarbonate-based. If a toothbrush is too irritating, cotton-tipped swabs (Q-Tips) or foam sticks (Toothettes) can provide some mechanical cleaning.
3. A pulsating water device (e.g., Waterpik) will remove loose debris. Use warm water with a half-teaspoonful of salt and baking soda and low pressure to prevent damage to tissue.
4. Have custom, flexible vinyl trays made by your dentist for use in self-applying fluoride gel to the teeth for 5 minutes once a day after brushing.
5. Rinse with an antiplaque solution (Peridex) (if prescribed by your dentist) 2 or 3 times a day when you cannot follow other oral hygiene procedures.
6. Follow any alternative oral hygiene instructions prescribed by your dentist.

C. Nutrition

Adequate intake of nutrition and fluid is very important for oral and general health. Use diet supplements (e.g., Carnation Instant Breakfast, Meritene, Ensure). If your mouth is sore, a blender may be used to soften food.

D. Maintenance

Have your oral health status evaluated at regularly scheduled intervals by your dentist.

E. Supportive

A humidifier in the sleeping area will alleviate or reduce nighttime oral dryness.

*Drugs that must be prescribed by your dentist or physician.

NOTE: The oral regimen for patients receiving chemotherapy and radiotherapy is outlined in Chapter 26 of this textbook. This regimen also is applicable to patients with acquired immunodeficiency syndrome (AIDS).

Topical Anesthetics

Rx:

Diphenhydramine (Benadryl) elixir 12.5 mg/5 mL (NOTE: elixir is Rx, and syrup [Benylin] is OTC) 4 oz, mixed with Kaopectate (OTC) 4 oz, to make a 50% mixture by volume

Disp: 8 oz

Sig: Rinse with 1 teaspoonful every 2 hours, and spit out.

Maalox (OTC) can be used in place of Kaopectate. Dyclonine (Dyclone) HCl 0.5% 1 oz may be added to this preparation for greater anesthetic efficacy.

Rx:

Diphenhydramine (Benadryl) elixir 12.5 mg/5 mL (NOTE: elixir is Rx, and syrup [Benylin] is OTC)

Disp: 4-oz bottle

Sig: Rinse with 1 teaspoonful for 2 minutes before each meal, and spit out.

Rx:

Dyclonine HCl (Dyclone) 0.5% or 1%

Disp: 1-oz bottle

Sig: Rinse with 1 teaspoonful for 2 minutes before each meal, and spit out.

For mild to moderate relief:

"Special Mouthwash"

Rx:

Refer to earlier section, "Recurrent Aphthous Stomatitis," for formulation.

Antifungals.

(See "Candidiasis.")

Rx:

Clotrimazole (Mycelex) troches 10 mg

Disp: 70 troches

Sig: Let 1 troche dissolve in the mouth 5 times a day.

Rx:

Nystatin pastilles 200,000 U

Disp: 50 pastilles

Sig: Let 1 pastille dissolve in the mouth 5 times a day.

(See under "Candidiasis" for additional antifungal therapy.)

KEY POINTS TO REMEMBER

- When topical anesthetics are used, patients should be warned about a reduced gag reflex and the need for caution while eating and drinking to avoid possible airway compromise. Allergies are rare but may occur.
- In immunocompromised patients, herpes simplex virus lesions can occur on any mucosal surface and may have an atypical appearance. They may resemble major aphthae and allergic responses.
- Mixing ointments with equal parts of Orabase promotes adhesion.
- Therapy with systemic steroids and immunosuppressants is presented to inform the clinician that such modalities are available. Because of the potential for adverse effects, close collaboration with the patient's physician is recommended when these medications are prescribed.
- Although some consultants disagree with the intraoral use of vaginal creams, the clinical efficacy of these creams has been observed in selected cases in which other topical antifungal agents have failed.
- Generic carboxymethyl cellulose solutions may be prepared by a pharmacist. These cholinergics should be prescribed in consultation with a physician because of the potential for significant adverse effects.
- The rationale for use of tricyclic antidepressant medications and other psychotropic drugs should be thoroughly explained to patients, and the primary care physician also should be made aware of the treatment. These medications have a potential for addiction and dependency.
- When testing for serum folate level, it is judicious also to check the vitamin B_{12} level, because a B_{12} deficiency can be masked by the patient's use of a folic acid supplement. The phenytoin level also should be assessed for future reference.

SUGGESTED READING

Boger J, Araujo O, Flowers F: Sunscreens: efficacy, use and misuse, *South Med J* 77:1421-1427, 1984.

Brooke RI, Sapp JP: Herpetiform ulceration, *Oral Surg Oral Med Oral Pathol* 42:182-188, 1976.

Brown RS, Bottomley WK: Combination immunosuppressant and topical steroid therapy for treatment of recurrent major aphthae, *Oral Surg Oral Med Oral Pathol* 69:42-44, 1990.

Browning S, et al: The association between burning mouth syndrome and psychosocial disorders, *Oral Surg Oral Med Oral Pathol* 64:171-174, 1987.

Burns RA, Davis WJ: Recurrent aphthous stomatitis, *Am Fam Physician* 32:99-104, 1988.

Bystryn JC: Adjuvant therapy of pemphigus, *Arch Dermatol* 120:941-951, 1984.

Dilley D, Blozis G: Common oral lesions and oral manifestations of systemic illnesses and therapies, *Pediatr Clin North Am* 29:585-611, 1982.

Drew HJ, et al: Effect of folate on phenytoin hyperplasia, *J Clin Periodontol* 14:350-356, 1987.

Duxbury AJ, Hayes NF, Thakkar NS: Clinical trial of a mucin-containing artificial saliva, *IRCS Med Sci* 13:1197-1198, 1985.

Fardal O, Turnbull RS: A review of the literature on use of chlorhexidine in dentistry, *J Am Dent Assoc* 112:863-869, 1986.

Feinmann C: Pain relief by antidepressants: possible modes of action, *Pain* 23:1-8, 1985.

Fenske NA, Greenberg SS: Solar-induced skin changes, *Am Fam Physician* 25:109-117, 1982.
Fox PC: Systemic therapy of salivary gland hypofunction, *J Dent Res* 66:689-692, 1987 (special issue).
Gabriel SA, et al: Lichen planus: possible mechanisms of pathogenesis, *J Oral Med* 40:56-59, 1985.
Gorsku M, Silverman S, Chinn H: Clinical characteristics and management outcome in the burning mouth syndrome, *Oral Surg Oral Med Oral Pathol* 72:192-195, 1991.
Gorsline J, Bradlow HL, Sherman MR: Triamcinolone acetonide 21-oic acid methyl ester: a potent local anti-inflammatory steroid without detectable systemic effects, *Endocrinology* 116:263-273, 1985.
Greenberg MS: Oral herpes simplex infections in immunosuppressed patients, *Compendium* 9(suppl):289-291, 1988.
Grushka M: Clinical features of burning mouth syndrome, *Oral Surg Oral Med Oral Pathol* 63:30-36, 1987.
Hay KD, Reade PC: The use of an elimination diet in the treatment of recurrent aphthous ulceration of the oral cavity, *Oral Surg Oral Med Oral Pathol* 57:504-507, 1984.
Holst E: Natamycin and nystatin for treatment of oral candidiasis during and after radiotherapy, *J Prosthet Dent* 51:226-231, 1984.
Huff JC, et al: Therapy of herpes zoster with oral acyclovir, *Am J Med* 85:85-89, 1988.
Hughes WT, et al: Ketoconazole and candidiasis: a controlled study, *J Infect Dis* 147:1060-1063, 1983.
Katz S: The use of fluoride and chlorhexidine for the prevention of radiation caries, *J Am Dent Assoc* 104:164-169, 1982.
Lamey PJ, et al: Vitamin status of patients with burning mouth syndrome and the response to replacement therapy, *Br Dent J* 160:81-84, 1986.
Lang NP, Brecx MC: Chlorhexidine digluconate—an agent for chemical plaque control and prevention of gingival inflammation, *J Periodont Res* 43(suppl):74-89, 1986.
Lever WF, Schaumburg-Lever G: Treatment of pemphigus vulgaris: results obtained in 84 patients between 1961 and 1982, *Arch Dermatol* 120:44-47, 1984.
Lozada F, Silverman S Jr, Migliorati C: Adverse side effects associated with prednisone in the treatment of patients with oral inflammatory ulcerative diseases, *J Am Dent Assoc* 109:269-270, 1984.
Lucatorto FM, et al: Treatment of refractory oral candidiasis with fluconazole: a case report, *Oral Surg Oral Med Oral Pathol* 71:42-44, 1991.
Lundeen RC, Langlais RP, Terezhalmy GT: Sunscreen protection for lip mucosa: a review and update, *J Am Dent Assoc* 111:617-621, 1985.
O'Neil T, Figures K: The effects of chlorhexidine and mechanical methods of plaque control on the recurrence of gingival hyperplasia in young patients taking phenytoin, *Br Dent J* 152:130-133, 1982.
Owens NJ, et al: Prophylaxis of oral candidiasis with clotrimazole troches, *Arch Intern Med* 144:290-293, 1984.
Poland JM: The spectrum of HSV-1 infections in nonimmunosuppressed patients, *Compendium* 9(suppl):310-312, 1988.
Porter SR, Sculy C, Flint S: Hematologic status in recurrent aphthous stomatitis compared with other oral disease, *Oral Surg Oral Med Oral Pathol* 66:41-44, 1988.
Raborn GW, et al: Oral acyclovir and herpes labialis: a randomized, double-blind, placebo-controlled study, *J Am Dent Assoc* 11:38-42, 1987.
Rhodus NL, et al: *Candia albicans* levels in patients with Sjögren's syndrome before and after long-term use of pilocarpine hydrochloride, *Quintessence Int* 29:705-710, 1998.
Rhodus NL, Schuh MJ: The effects of pilocarpine on salivary flow in patients with Sjögren's syndrome, *Oral Surg Oral Med Oral Pathol* 72:545-549, 1991.
Rowe NJ: Diagnosis and treatment of herpes simplex virus disease. *Compendium* 9(suppl):292-295, 1988.
Schiffman SS: Taste and smell in disease (parts a and b), *N Engl J Med* 308:1275-1279, 1983.
Scully C, Mason DK: Therapeutic measures in oral medicine. In Jones JH, Mason DK, editors: *Oral manifestations of systemic disease*, London, 1980, Saunders.
Sharav Y, et al: The analgesic effect of amitriptyline on chronic facial pain, *Pain* 31:199-207, 1987.
Silverman S Jr, et al: A prospective study of findings and management in 214 patients with oral lichen planus, *Oral Surg Oral Med Oral Pathol* 72:665-670 1991.
Silverman S Jr, et al: Oral mucous membrane pemphigoid: a study of sixty-five patients, *Oral Surg Oral Med Oral Pathol* 61:233-237, 1986.
Sonis ST, Sonis AL, Lieberman A: Oral complications in patients receiving treatment for malignancies other than of the head and neck, *JAMA* 97:468-471, 1978.
Straus SE: Herpes simplex virus infection: biology, treatment, and prevention, *Ann Intern Med* 103:404-419, 1985.
Thompson PJ, et al: Assessment of oral candidiasis in patients with respiratory disease and efficacy of a new nystatin formulation, *BMJ* 292:699-700, 1986.
Vincent SD, et al: Oral lichen planus: the clinical, historical and therapeutic features of 100 cases, *Oral Surg Oral Med Oral Pathol* 70:165-171, 1990.
Wood MJ, et al: Efficacy of oral acyclovir treatment of acute herpes zoster, *Am J Med* 85:79-83, 1988.
Wright WE, et al: An oral disease prevention program for patients receiving radiation and chemotherapy, *J Am Dent Assoc* 110:43-47, 1985.

NOTE: The treatment protocols included herein were adapted with permission from Siegel MA, Silverman S, Sollecito TP, editors: *Clinician's Guide to Treatment of Common Oral Conditions*, ed 5, Baltimore, American Academy of Oral Medicine, 2001, and were provided as a courtesy of the American Academy of Oral Medicine (AAOM), which publishes a guide for clinicians: Siegel M, Silverman S, Sollecito T: *Clinician's Guide: Treatment of Common Oral Lesions*, Hamilton, Ontario, Canada, BC Decker, 2006. This guide contains much of this same information.

We (all members of the AAOM) acknowledge our deep appreciation for the authorization to publish this Appendix. Some portions of that text are reprinted here with permission of the AAOM. For further information, or to purchase a copy of the *Clinician's Guide to Treatment of Common Oral Conditions*, contact:

Jane Kantor, CMP
American Academy of Oral Medicine
P.O. Box 2016
Edmonds, WA 98020
Phone: 425 778-6162
Fax: 425 771-9588
www.aaom.com
www.jkantor@aaom.com

APPENDIX D

Drug Interactions of Significance in Dentistry

Dental Drug	Interacting Drug	Medical Condition/ Situation	Effect
Antibiotics			
Antibiotics	Oral contraceptives (birth control pills [BCPs])	Contraception	Decreased effectiveness of oral contraceptives has been suggested for several antibiotic classes because of the potential for lowering plasma levels of the contraceptive drug. However, most well-designed studies do not show any reduction in estrogen serum levels in patients taking antibiotics (except rifampin). **RECOMMENDATION: Okay to use dental antibiotics.** Provide advice to patient about potential risk and for consideration of additional contraceptive measures.
Beta-lactams (penicillins, cephalosporins)	Allopurinol (Lopurin, Zyloprim)	Gout	Incidence of minor allergic reactions to ampicillin is increased. Other penicillins have not been implicated. **RECOMMENDATION: Avoid ampicillin.**
	Beta blockers (e.g., Tenormin, Lopressor, Inderal, Corgard)	Hypertension	Serum levels of atenolol are reduced after prolonged use of ampicillin. Anaphylactic reactions to penicillins or other drugs may be more severe in patients taking beta blockers because of increased mediator release from mast cells. **RECOMMENDATION: Use ampicillin cautiously, advise patient of potential reaction.**
	Tetracyclines and other bacteriostatic antibiotics	Infection, acne, or periodontal disease	Effectiveness of penicillins and cephalosporins may be reduced by bacteriostatic agents. **RECOMMENDATION: Avoid interaction.**
Tetracyclines Fluoroquinolones	Antacids	Dyspepsia, gastroesophageal reflux, peptic ulcer	Antacids, dairy products, and other agents containing divalent (calcium, iron) and trivalent cations will chelate these antibiotics and limit their absorption. Doxycycline is least influenced by this interaction. **RECOMMENDATION: Avoid interaction.**
	Insulin	Diabetes mellitus	Doxycycline and oxytetracycline have been documented as enhancing the hypoglycemic effects of exogenously administered insulin. **RECOMMENDATION: Select a different antibiotic, or increase carbohydrate intake.**
Doxycycline	Methotrexate	Immunosuppression	In patients taking high-dose methotrexate, interaction can lead to increased methotrexate concentrations, making toxicity likely. **RECOMMENDATION: Select different antibiotic.**
Metronidazole	Ethanol	Alcohol use or abuse	Severe disulfiram-like reactions are well documented. **RECOMMENDATION: Avoid interaction.**
	Lithium	Manic depression	Inhibits renal excretion of lithium, leading to elevated/toxic levels of lithium. Lithium toxicity produces confusion, ataxia, and kidney damage. **RECOMMENDATION: Avoid interaction.**

Continued

Dental Drug	Interacting Drug	Medical Condition/ Situation	Effect
Antibiotics/ antifungals metabolized by CYP3A4 and CYP1A2 (e.g., macrolide antibiotics [erythromycin, clarithromycin], antifungals [ketoconazole, fluconazole, itraconazole])	Benzodiazepines	Anxiety	Delayed metabolism of benzodiazepine, increasing the pharmacologic effects, can result in excessive sedation and irrational behavior. **RECOMMENDATION: Reduce dose of benzodiazepine or avoid interaction.**
	Buspirone	Depression	Delayed metabolism of buspirone, increasing pharmacologic effect. **RECOMMENDATION: Avoid interaction.**
	Carbamazepine (Tegretol)	Seizure disorder	Increased blood levels of carbamazepine, leading to toxicity; symptoms include drowsiness, dizziness, nausea, headache, and blurred vision. Hospitalization has been required. **RECOMMENDATION: Avoid interaction.**
	Cisapride	Gastroesophageal reflux	Delayed metabolism of cisapride, increasing the pharmacologic effects and risk for cardiac arrhythmia and sudden death. **RECOMMENDATION: Avoid interaction.**
	Cyclosporine	Organ transplantation	Enhanced immunosuppression and nephrotoxicity. **RECOMMENDATION: Avoid interaction.**
	Disopyramide, Quinidine	Cardiac arrhythmias	Inhibits CYP3A4 metabolism, resulting in large increases in antiarrhythmia drug that can lead to arrhythmias. **RECOMMENDATION: Avoid interaction.**
	Lovastatin, pravastatin, simastatin, and other statins	Hyperlipidemia	Increases plasma concentration of statin drugs—may result in muscle (eosinophilia) myalgia and rhabdomyolysis (muscle breakdown and pain) and acute renal failure. **RECOMMENDATION: Avoid interaction.**
	Pimozide	Antipsychotic, used to control motor tics	May result in increased concentrations of pimozide and possibly prolongation of the QT interval. **RECOMMENDATION: Avoid interaction.**
	Prednisone, methylprednisolone	Autoimmune disorders, organ transplantation	Increased risk of Cushing's syndrome and immunosuppression **RECOMMENDATION: Monitor patient, and shorten duration of antibiotic administration if possible.**
	Theophylline (Theodur)	Asthma	Erythromycins inhibit the metabolism of theophylline, leading to toxic serum levels (symptoms of toxicity: headache, nausea, vomiting, confusion, thirst, cardiac arrhythmias, and convulsions). Conversely, theophylline reduces serum levels of erythromycin. **RECOMMENDATION: Avoid prescribing erythromycin.**
Antibiotics (especially erythromycin, clarithromycin, and tetracycline)	Digoxin (Lanoxin)	Congestive heart failure	Alters gastrointestinal flora and retards metabolism of digoxin in roughly 10% of patients, resulting in dangerously high digoxin serum levels that may persist for several weeks after discontinuation of antibiotic. Strongest documentation has been acquired for macrolide antibiotics and tetracycline. Patients should be cautioned to report any signs of digitalis toxicity (salivation, visual disturbances, and arrhythmias) during antibiotic therapy. **RECOMMENDATION: Safe in 90%, should have digoxin levels monitored during antimicrobial therapy.**
Antibiotics, cephalosporins, erythromycin, clarithromycin, metronidazole	Warfarin (Coumadin)	Atrial fibrillation, myocardial infarction, recent (postoperative) major surgery, stroke prevention	Anticoagulant effect of warfarin may be increased by several antibiotic classes. Reduced synthesis of vitamin K by gut flora is a putative mechanism, but several antibiotics have antiplatelet and anticoagulant activity. Cephalosporins, macrolide antibiotics, and metronidazole have the most convincing documentation, monitor INR. **RECOMMENDATION: Penicillins, tetracyclines, and clindamycin would be preferred choices but must be used cautiously.**
Analgesics			
Acetaminophen	Alcohol	Alcohol use and abuse	Increased risk of liver toxicity, especially during fasting state or ≥4 g of acetaminophen per day. **RECOMMENDATION: Use lower dose of acetaminophen and encourage discontinuation of alcohol use.**

Dental Drug	Interacting Drug	Medical Condition/ Situation	Effect
Acetaminophen	Warfarin (Coumadin)	Atrial fibrillation, thrombosis	*Data are somewhat conflicting:* Increased risk of bleeding if acetaminophen is given at a dose of >2 g/day for greater than 1 week. **RECOMMENDATION: Limit acetaminophen dosing and duration—monitor INR.**
Aspirin	Oral hypoglycemic (e.g., sulfonylureas: Glyburide, chlorpropamide, acetohexamide)	Diabetes type 2	Increased hypoglycemic effects. **RECOMMENDATION: Avoid interaction.**
Aspirin, other NSAIDs	Anticoagulants (Coumarin)	Atrial fibrillation, myocardial infarction, recent (postoperative) surgery, clot prevention	Increased risk of bleeding (GI, oral). **RECOMMENDATION: Avoid interaction.**
Aspirin, other NSAIDs	Alcohol	Alcohol use and abuse	Increases risk of gastrointestinal bleeding. **RECOMMENDATION: Lower dose; encourage discontinuation of alcohol use.**
Aspirin	Diltiazem	Hypertension, angina	Enhanced antiplatelet activity of aspirin. **RECOMMENDATION: Monitor for risk of prolonged bleeding. Advise patient to notify physician/dentist if they experience unusual bleeding or bruising.**
NSAIDs	Beta blockers, ACE inhibitors	Hypertension, recent myocardial infarction	Decreased antihypertensive effect. **RECOMMENDATION: Limit duration of NSAID dosage to about 4 days.**
NSAIDs	Lithium	Manic depression	Produces symptoms of lithium toxicity, including nausea, vomiting, slurred speech, and mental confusion. **RECOMMENDATION: NSAIDs should not be prescribed to patients who take lithium. It can result in toxic levels of lithium, or consult with physician to reduce lithium dose.**
NSAIDs (Naproxen)	Alendronate	Osteoporosis, multiple myeloma	Increased risk for gastric ulcers. **RECOMMENDATION: Use acetaminophen products.**
NSAIDs	SSRIs (Citalopram, Fluoxetine, Paroxetine, Sertraline)	Depression	Increased risk for peptic ulcers. **RECOMMENDATION: Avoid long-term use of NSAIDs; use acetaminophen products instead.**
NSAIDs	Methotrexate (MTX)	Connective tissue disease, cancer therapy	Toxic level of methotrexate may accumulate. **RECOMMENDATION: Avoid interaction if on high-dose MTX for cancer therapy.** **Low-dose MTX for arthritis is not a concern.**
Meperidine	MAO inhibitors (e.g., isocarboxazid, phenelzine)	Depressants (Note: MAO inhibitors often are last line of therapy)	May produce severe and potentially fatal adverse excitatory or depressive reactions **RECOMMENDATION: Avoid interaction.**
Propoxyphene	Carbamazepine	Seizure, trigeminal neuralgia	Can significantly increase the plasma concentrations of carbamazepine. **RECOMMENDATION: Avoid interaction.**
Anesthetics			
Lidocaine	Bupivacaine		Additive effect of these two local anesthetics increases the risk of central nervous system toxicity. **RECOMMENDATION: Limit dose of each.**
Mepivacaine	Meperidine (Demerol)		Sedation with opioids may increase risk of local anesthetic toxicity; especially in children. **RECOMMENDATION: Reduce anesthetic dose.**

Continued

Dental Drug	Interacting Drug	Medical Condition/ Situation	Effect
Sedatives			
Barbiturates	Digoxin, theophylline, corticosteroids, oral anticoagulants (coumarin)	Congestive heart failure, asthma, autoimmune disease, atrial fibrillation	Barbiturates bind P-450 cytochrome system in liver and enhance the metabolism of many drug, thus reducing effect of anticoagulant **RECOMMENDATION: Generally avoid. If necessary, limit dose, and observe for adverse effects.**
	Benzodiazepines, alcohol, antihistamines	Anxiety, alcohol use and abuse, seasonal allergies	Additive effects for sedation and respiratory depression **RECOMMENDATION: Reduce dose, and administer combination of sedatives with extreme caution.**
Benzodiazepines (BZDPs) (e.g., alprazolam, chlordiazepoxide, diazepam, triazolam)	Cimetidine, oral contraceptives, fluoxetine, isoniazid (INH), alcohol, azole antifungals (fluconazole, itraconazole, ketoconazole)	Peptic ulcer disease, depression, tuberculosis, alcohol use and abuse	Delayed metabolism of BZDP, increasing the systemic exposure and pharmacologic effects, can result in excessive sedation and adverse psychomotor effects. **RECOMMENDATION: Reduce dose of benzodiazepine or avoid interaction.**
	Digoxin (Lanoxin), phenytoin, theophylline (Theodur)	Congestive heart failure, epilepsy, asthma	Serum concentrations of digoxin and phenytoin may be increased, resulting in toxicity. Antagonize sedative effects of benzodiazepine **RECOMMENDATION: Avoid interaction.**
	Protease inhibitors (Indinavir, Nelfinavir)	HIV infection and AIDS	Increased bioavailability and effects of benzodiazepines, especially triazolam and oral midazolam **RECOMMENDATION: Avoid interaction.**
Vasoconstrictors			
Epinephrine and levonordephrine (Neocobefrin)	Nonselective beta blockers: Propranolol (Inderal), nadolol (Corgard), penbutolol (Levatol), pindolol (Visken), sotalol (Betapace), timolol (Blocadren)	Angina pectoris, hypertension, glaucoma, migraine, headache, hyperthyroidism, panic syndromes	Unopposed effects—Increased blood pressure with secondary bradycardia **RECOMMENDATION: Initial dose is one-half cartridge containing 1:100,000 epinephrine; aspirate to avoid intravascular injection, and inject slowly. Monitor vital signs, if no adverse cardiovascular changes occur, up to two cartridges containing a vasoconstrictor can be administered. Provide a 5-minute interval between the first and second cartridges, with continual monitoring. Avoid epinephrine-containing retraction cord and higher concentrations of epinephrine in the dental anesthetic.**
	Cocaine	Illicit use, topical anesthetic for mucous membrane procedures	Blocks reuptake of norepinephrine and intensifies postsynaptic response to epinephrine-like drugs. This potentiates the adrenergic effects on the heart, with the potential for a heart attack. **RECOMMENDATION: Recognize signs and symptoms of cocaine abuse; avoid use of vasoconstrictors in these patients until cocaine has been withheld for at least 24 hours.**
	Halothane	General anesthetic for surgical procedures	Stimulation of alpha and beta receptors, resulting in arrhythmia at doses that exceed 2 μg/kg. **RECOMMENDATION: Limit dose to remain below 2 μg/kg threshold; aspirate to avoid intravascular injection. Monitor vital signs. Avoid epinephrine-containing retraction cord and concentrations of epinephrine higher than 1:100,000.**

Dental Drug	Interacting Drug	Medical Condition/ Situation	Effect
	Tricyclic antidepressants* (amitriptyline [Elavil], amoxapine, clomipramine [Anafranil], desipramine [Norpramin], doxepin [Sinequan], imipramine [Tofranil], nortriptyline [Pamelor], protriptyline [Vivactil], trimipramine [Surmontil])	Depression, severe anxiety, neuropathic pain, attention deficit disorder	Blocks reuptake of norepinephrine, resulting in unopposed effects—increased pressor response (increased blood pressure, increased heart rate)—and potential cardiac arrhythmias; effect is greater with levonordefrin. **RECOMMENDATION: Avoid levonordefrin; limit dose to two cartridges containing 1:100,000 epinephrine (36 μg), aspirate to avoid intravascular injection. Monitor vital signs. Avoid epinephrine-containing retraction cord and higher concentrations of epinephrine in the dental anesthetic.**
	Monoamine oxidase (MAO) inhibitors (isocarboxazid [Marplan], phenelzine [Nardil], tranylcypromine [Parnate])	Depression	Although no reports have documented the effects on blood pressure or heart rate after dental procedures, the potential for increased pressor response is present. **RECOMMENDATION: Avoid levonordefrin; limit dose to two cartridges containing 1:100,000 epinephrine (36 μg), and aspirate to avoid intravascular injection. Monitor vital signs. Avoid epinephrine-containing retraction cord and higher concentrations of epinephrine in the dental anesthetic.**
	Antipsychotics Some examples: chlorpromazine (Thorazine), trifluoperazine (Stelazine), clozapine (Clozaril), olanzapine (Zyprexa)	Schizophrenia	Decrease blood pressure (hypotension) **RECOMMENDATION: Use only small amounts of epinephrine; limit dose to two cartridges containing 1:100,000 epinephrine (36 μg), and aspirate to avoid intravascular injection. Monitor vital signs.**
	Peripheral adrenergic antagonists (reserpine [Serpasil], guanethidine [Ismelin], guanadrel [Hylorel])	Hypertension	Potential for increased sensitivity of adrenergic receptors to epinephrine and levonordefrin. **RECOMMENDATION: Administer cautiously. Monitor vital signs during and after administration of first cartridge. Limit dose to two cartridges containing 1:100,000 epinephrine (36 μg) or less, depending on vital signs and patient response. Aspirate to avoid intravascular injection. Avoid epinephrine-containing retraction cord and higher concentrations of epinephrine in the dental anesthetic.**
	Catechol-*O*-methyltransferase inhibitors (tolcapone [Tasmar], entacapone [Comtan])	Parkinson's disease	Potential for increased sensitivity of adrenergic receptors to epinephrine and levonordefrin, resulting in increased heart rate, blood pressure, and arrhythmias **RECOMMENDATION: Administer cautiously. Monitor vital signs during and after administration of first cartridge. Limit dose to two cartridges containing 1:100,000 epinephrine (36 μg) or less, depending on vital signs and patient response. Aspirate to avoid intravascular injection. Avoid epinephrine-containing retraction cord and higher concentrations of epinephrine in the dental anesthetic.**

ACE, Angiotensin-converting enzyme; *AIDS,* Acquired immunodeficiency syndrome; *HIV,* Human immunodeficiency virus; *INR,* International normalized ratio; *NSAIDs,* Nonsteroidal antiinflammatory drugs; *SSRIs,* Selective serotonin reuptake inhibitors.

*Antidepressants, such as the SSRIs, do not interact with vasoconstrictors. However, antidepressants that block norepinephrine uptake (Venlafaxine [Effexor], Bupropion [Wellbutrin]) have the potential to interact with vasoconstrictors, resulting in pressor responses.

APPENDIX E

Drugs Used in Complementary and Alternative Medicine of Potential Importance in Dentistry

The term *alternative medicine* describes practices that are used instead of mainstream medical practice.[1,2] *Complementary medicine* refers to practices that are used as adjuncts to conventional medicine.[2] The combination of these practices has been referred to as *complementary and alternative medicine* (CAM) and, more recently, as *complementary and integrative medicine* (CIM).[3] These two systems are divided into five major categories[1,2]:

- Alternative medical systems (traditional Chinese medicine,[4] Ayurveda medicine of India,[5,6] and Native American healing approaches[7])
- Biologically based therapies (natural products)[8]
- Manipulative and body-based methods (chiropractic and osteopathic manipulation)[9]
- Mind–body interventions (hypnosis, cognitive therapies, and biofeedback), and
- Energy therapies (use of magnets and acupuncture[10])

Both alternative medicine and complementary medicine use treatments that often have no established efficacy. It is estimated that about 42% of Americans use alternative and complementary medicine therapies, which are supported by an estimated $30 billion industry.[2,11-14]

Complementary medicines are defined as herbal medicines, homoeopathic remedies, and essential oils.[15-19] The basic principle of homeopathy consists of selection of a remedy that, if given to a healthy person, will produce a range of symptoms similar to those observed in the ill patient ("like cures like").[16,20-22] Only minute amounts are given, to avoid toxicity. Only one remedy is used at any one time.[16,21] Dilute tinctures are used rather than concentrated ones. In homeopathic practice, it also is common to use medication in tablet form.[21]

Standard tinctures used in Western traditional herbal medicine are very different from those used in homeopathy.[16,18,23] Alcohol is used to dissolve the plant, and the final product is not diluted. Thus, these remedies are concentrated, highly potent preparations, and they usually are taken as the unmodified liquid tincture. Other preparations used in herbal remedies include lotions and creams for topical application. The tablet form of medication is not used very often (less than 5%).[21]

According to Eisenberg,[24] herbal remedies most commonly are used to treat patients with allergies, insomnia, lung problems, and digestive problems. These preparations also are used for the treatment of asthma, cancer, depression, dementia, schizophrenia, bipolar disorders, heart failure, rheumatologic conditions, and others.[24-36] A recent United States survey reported by Ernst found that 90% of arthritic patients used alternative therapies such as those based on herbal medicines.[37] Both adults and children use them.[24,38] In the United States, the sale of herbal remedies totaled $1.6 billion in 1994, reaching $4.0 billion by 1998.[24] From 1999 to 2004, more than $34 billion was spent on CAM treatments, with part of that going to herbal medicines.[39] In a U.S. study, 136 (70% response rate) customers who had bought dietary supplements in one of two health food stores reported that they had used 805 supplements—84.3% were taken for disease prevention and wellness, and 15.7% were taken to treat perceived health problems. Garlic, ginseng, and *Ginkgo biloba* were the most commonly named herbal products.[24] Klepser and colleagues[40] reported that the incidence of use of herbal remedies among 794 persons studied in Iowa was 41.6%. Most of the users were white women and had been educated beyond the high school level.[40] Patients with cardiovascular disease in Canada also were studied for their use of herbal products.[41] About 17% were found to use such products.[41] Products most commonly used were garlic, cayenne pepper, and ginseng.[41]

A recent study reported the use of herbal supplements by adult dental patients in a U.S. dental school.[42] During a 1-month period, 12.6% of 1119 dental patients reported the use of one or more of 21 herbal products. A majority of these patients were middle-aged educated white women. Twenty-four percent of the patients used an herbal product as a single agent, and 76% used herbal products in combination with prescription or over-the-counter (OTC) medicines, or with both types of medicines. The five most frequently used herbal medicines were green tea, garlic, echinacea, ginkgo biloba, and ginseng.

EFFICACY OF HERBAL MEDICINES

Many herbal remedies have been used for hundreds of years.[43,44] However, traditional use is not in itself a good indication of efficacy. The "gold standard" for testing efficacy is the randomized controlled trial (RCT).[43] This standard should apply as much to herbal medicines as to conventional medicines. Numerous RCTs of herbal medical products have been conducted. However, many of these studies differ in how they were conducted and in their findings.[43] Ernst and Pitler[43] suggest that the best way to evaluate RCTs undertaken to assess the efficacy of a specific herbal medicine is to do a systematic review or metaanalysis of all RCTs for that product.

HERBAL MEDICINES WITH PROVEN EFFICACY

Several herbal remedies have been repeatedly tested in placebo-controlled RCTs.[43] Systematic reviews of these studies have shown that some herbal medicines are effective for particular conditions.[43] For example, *ginkgo biloba* has been shown to be effective for the symptomatic treatment of dementia and intermittent claudication.[45,46] Echinacea and zinc lozenges were found to be beneficial for the treatment of the common cold.[29] Table E-1 lists the more commonly used herbal medicines that have proved effective for the condition(s) listed.

HERBAL MEDICINES WITH DOUBTFUL OR NO EFFICACY

Asian ginseng, one of the most popular herbal medicines in the United States, showed no convincing evidence for efficacy as a general tonic or as a means of enhancing mental and physical performance.[47] A review of studies regarding the use of valerian as a hypnotic agent was inconclusive because of flaws in study design.[48] No evidence was found in a systematic review of RCTs that evening primrose was effective in treating women with

TABLE E-1 Claims for Herbal Actions Supported by Clinical Trials

Herb	Claimed Action	Effectiveness Supported by Clinical Trials
Kava	Used to treat anxiety	Clinical trials have shown that it reduces anxiety to a significantly greater extent than placebo.
Artichoke	Used to lower lipid levels in blood	Only one randomized clinical study shows it to moderately lower elevated total cholesterol levels when given orally for several weeks.
Feverfew	Used for women's ailments and inflammatory diseases; more recently suggested as agent for treatment of headache and migraine	Three studies showed greater effect than placebo in alleviating symptoms of headache or migraine.
Garlic	Used for blood pressure reduction and lowering of blood lipid levels	Data show a small but statistically significant reduction in systolic and diastolic blood pressure. No data support the claims for lipid-lowering properties of garlic.
Ginger	Used to treat nausea and vomiting	Several studies support antiemetic uses for ginger. Used to treat or prevent nausea or vomiting.
Echinacea	Used to treat the common cold	Moderate effectiveness in 5 or 6 clinical trials
Ginkgo biloba	Used to treat cerebral insufficiency and to prevent loss of cognitive function and tinnitus	Studies have shown it to be effective in the treatment of cerebral insufficiency when given for 4 to 6 weeks. Data show that regular oral intake of *ginkgo biloba* slows the loss of cognitive function in patients with dementia.
Hawthorn	Used to treat heart failure	In various studies, shown to be effective for the early signs of congestive heart failure.
Horse chestnut	Used to treat venous congestion	Studies have shown it to be effective in reducing signs and symptoms of chronic venous insufficiency.
Saw palmetto	Used in Europe for symptoms of prostate enlargement	Clinical trials support its use for symptoms of benign prostatic hyperplasia.
St. John's wort	Used to treat depression	Studies show that it is effective for treating mild to moderate depression. The question of its effectiveness for severe depression remains unanswered.

TABLE E-2 Claims for Herbal Actions Unsupported by Clinical Trials

Herb	Claimed Action	Effectiveness Supported by Clinical Trials
Aloe vera	Used as an adjunctive oral treatment for diabetes and skin conditions such as herpes and psoriasis	At the present time, compelling data support none of the claims made for aloe vera.
Evening primrose	Used for the treatment of premenstrual syndrome	Current evidence suggests uncertain value when it is used to treat this syndrome.
Ginseng	Used to treat type 2 diabetes and herpes simplex infections. Also has been used to enhance physical and psychomotor performance, as well as cognitive function	None of the 16 double-blind, randomized clinical trials supports any effective action on physical performance, psychomotor performance, and cognitive function, nor in type 2 diabetes and herpes simplex infections.
Guar gum	Used to treat obesity and overweight	Clinical trials have not supported this use.
Mistletoe	Has been suggested for the treatment of cancer	Current studies do not support these claims.
Peppermint	Used to treat irritable bowel syndrome	Studies show that it alleviates the symptoms of irritable bowel syndrome. However, many of these trials were flawed.
Valerian	Used to promote sleep	Randomized clinical studies are needed to evaluate effectiveness. Studies to date have been flawed.

premenstrual syndrome.[49] Garlic was not found to be effective as a cholesterol-lowering agent.[50] A review of herbal products used to treat asthma found little to no effectiveness.[25] Table E-2 lists some of the more common herbal medicines that were found not to be effective for the conditions listed.

ADVERSE EFFECTS AND ADVERSE REACTIONS

Increased recent use of herbal remedies seems to have resulted from the public's view that natural products are harmless or at least have fewer adverse effects than those attributable to regular drugs.[51] The assumption that phytomedicines (herbal medicines) have only beneficial effects has proved to be incorrect.[18,19,51]

Toxicity may be associated with the use of herbal remedies. These reactions may be due to accidental or deliberate contamination of the product. For example, lead, mercury, cadmium, pesticides, microorganisms, and fumigants have been found to contaminate some herbal products.[51] Substitution of animal substances such as enzymes, hormones, or organ extracts and synthetic drugs has accounted for some of the toxic reactions to herbal products.[51] Adulteration caused by the accidental or deliberate substitution of the original plant material by other plant species also has been reported to be a source of toxic reactions to herbal products.[51]

Other adverse reactions to herbal products are intrinsic or plant-associated.[51] In some cases, the manufacturer has ignored the known toxicity of a plant or constituent in the herbal product.[51] In other cases, the product contains plants for which no or insufficient data are available regarding safety. If a highly concentrated or a specifically processed extract is used, toxic reactions may occur. If a plant contains constituents known to affect the bioavailability and/or pharmacokinetics of other drugs, serious drug interactions may occur.[51]

TABLE E-3 Selected Herbal Medicines with Potentially Serious Adverse Effects

Product	Effect
Aristolochia	Nephrotoxicity Carcinogenicity
Chaparral	Cholestatic hepatitis
Comfrey	Acute and chronic hepatitis
Digitalis leaf	Arrhythmia
Ephedra	Hypertension Stroke Myocardial infarction
Germander	Acute and chronic hepatitis
Kava	Hepatitis
Khat	Tachycardia Psychosis
Kombucha	Hepatotoxicity Lactic acidosis
Mistletoe	Anaphylaxis
Skullcap	Seizures Acute and chronic hepatitis
St. John's wort	Photosensitivity Possible hypertension with tyramine-containing foods

Long-term users, consumers of large quantities of phytomedicines, and people who use many different medicinal products may be prone to adverse effects. Pregnant or nursing women, babies, elderly persons, and patients who are sick and undernourished also are at higher risk for adverse effects.[51,52] Some of the more common adverse effects associated with herbal remedies include bleeding with *ginkgo biloba*; upset stomach, tiredness, dizziness, confusion, dry mouth, and photosensitivity with St. John's wort; high blood pressure, arrhythmia, nervousness, headache, heart attack, or stroke with ephedra; and feeling sleepy, rash, and motor dysfunction of skeletal muscles with kava.[53] Table E-3

TABLE E-4 Selected Natural Medicines that Potentiate or Interfere with Approved Drugs

Natural Medicine	Approved Drug
Ephedra	Theophylline (P) Antihypertensives (I) Corticosteroids (I)
Evening primrose	Anticoagulants (P) Antiplatelet agents (P) Low-molecular-weight heparins (P) Anticonvulsants (I)
Garlic	Aspirin (P) Clopidogrel (P) Ticlopidine (P)
Ginkgo leaf extract	Anticoagulants (P) Antiplatelet agents (P) Anticonvulsants (I)
Glucosamine	Antidiabetic drugs (I)
Panax ginseng	Anticoagulants (P) Diabetic agents (possible P) Nifedipine (P)
Saw palmetto	Hormone replacement therapies (P)
Soy	Estrogenic drugs (P)
St. John's wort	Antidepressants (P) HIV protease inhibitors (I) Cyclosporine (I)
Valerian	Sedatives (P)
Yohimbe	Antihypertensives (I)

HIV, Human immunodeficiency virus; *I,* Interferes; *P,* Potentiates.

lists some of the serious adverse reactions that can occur when natural products are used.

MEDICAL PROBLEMS

Some medical problems can make the taking of herbal medicines unsafe. Patients with high blood pressure, thyroid disease, psychiatric disorders, Parkinson's disease, enlarged prostate gland, diabetes mellitus, heart disease, epilepsy, glaucoma, blood clotting problems, or a history of stroke should check with their physician before taking any herbal remedies.[53] Persons with a history of aspirin allergy may be at risk for adverse reactions if they take a herb that contains willow bark.[54]

DRUG INTERACTIONS

Important drug interactions may occur between certain herbal products and conventional medications[18,19] (Table E-4). The drug most commonly involved with drug-herb interactions is warfarin.[55] The herb most commonly involved with such interactions is St. John's wort.[55] Markowitz and co-workers,[56] in a study undertaken to evaluate the potential of St. John's wort to alter cytochrome P-450 enzymes, found that a 14-day course of the herbal product significantly induced the activity of CYP 3A4, as measured by changes in alprazolam pharmacokinetics. These investigators concluded that long-term administration of St. John's wort may result in diminished clinical effectiveness or increased dosage requirements for all CYP 3A4 substrates, which represent about 50% of all marketed medications. By contrast, in another study, these workers found little evidence that garlic extracts would alter the disposition of coadministered medications metabolized by the CYP 3A4 pathway.[57]

Patients who take aspirin, warfarin, ticlopidine, clopidogrel, or dipyridamole should not take *ginkgo biloba,* because bleeding may occur.[53] Patients who take an antidepressant should not take St. John's wort. Patients who are taking a decongestant or a stimulant drug and people who drink caffeinated beverages should not take ephedra. Persons who are taking a benzodiazepine, a barbiturate, an antipsychotic medication, or any medicine used to treat Parkinson's disease should not take kava products.[53] It is important that patients notify their general practitioner if they are taking phytomedicines concurrently with conventional drugs—especially those with cardiac, diuretic, sedative, hypotensive, or other potentially dangerous properties.[51] Persons who are taking a prescription medicine should check with their physician before taking any herbal health product.[53]

Some patients with cancer have been found to use complementary and alternative medicine (CAM) to manage associated symptoms and in some cases as the primary treatment for their disease.[13,27,58-61] Various studies show that 30% to 60% of patients with cancer use some form of CAM in the management of symptoms and the cancer itself.[59,60] These patients are at risk for interactions between the anticancer drugs and the CAM agents they are taking. These interactions may reduce the effectiveness of conventional anticancer drugs or increase the toxicity of these drugs. An oncology database (OncoRx) is being developed to provide information regarding anticancer drugs and CAM interactions.[62]

DENTAL IMPLICATIONS

A limited number of published papers describe the use of complementary and alternative medical systems for dental problems.[63-91] Two of these papers report on the use of herbal products for the treatment of periodontal disease.[63,82]

Acupuncture may be of some benefit in dentistry. In one study, patients with radiation-induced xerostomia demonstrated increased salivary flow rates both on objective and subjective measures.[87] However, the sample size was small at 12 patients with severe xerostomia. In another study, acupuncture was found to reduce gagging in orthodontic patients.[90] A third study found that acupuncture administered before dental treatment reduced the level of anxiety in patients with severe dental anxiety.[89] A review of randomized controlled trials investigating the use of acupuncture for treatment of temporomandibular joint disorder (TMD) symptoms found moderate evidence that it was effective in alleviating symptoms.[88]

INFORMATION FOR DENTISTS

Herbal remedies have the potential to affect the safety of invasive or prolonged dental procedures.[92] Excessive bleeding may occur with some of these medications.[92] Other herbal medicines may affect the cardiovascular system, rendering the patient more susceptible to cardiac arrhythmia and other cardiovascular complications.[68] Ginseng may cause hypoglycemia.[92] Chinese patients with cancer undergoing chemotherapy who were users of Chinese herbal medicine were found to have higher scores for mucositis.[93] It is important for the dentist to include a section in the patient's medical history on taking herbal medications and OTC drugs. Because most U.S. dental schools teach very little about the use, adverse effects, toxicity, and drug interactions associated with herbal remedies, the dentist must find a way to become informed about these issues.

Important references for dentists are the *Physicians' Desk Reference for Herbal Medicines*, 4th edition (2008), and the *Physicians' Desk Reference for Nonprescription Drugs, Dietary Supplements, and Herbs*, 2nd edition (2008), both published by Physicians' Desk Reference. Dentists should use only treatment procedures that have been established as effective and involving minimal risk. Because clinical trials have shown some alternative and complementary medicine treatments to be effective and safe, those treatments may be incorporated into conventional medicine and dentistry.[94] The dentist may find that a medically compromised patient is taking an herbal remedy that is potentially harmful. This should be discussed with the patient, who should then be referred to the primary care physician for evaluation and treatment.

REFERENCES

1. Little JW: Complementary and alternative medicine: impact on dentistry, *Oral Surg Oral Med Oral Path Oral Radiol Endod* 98:137-146, 2004.
2. Straus SE: Complementary and alternative medicine. In Goldman L, Ausiello D, editors: *Cecil textbook of medicine*, ed 22, Philadelphia, 2004, Saunders, pp 170-174.
3. Micozzi MS: Characteristics of complementary and integrative medicine. In Micozzi MS, editor: *Fundamentals of complementary and integrative medicine*, ed 3, St. Louis, 2006, Elsevier, pp 3-8.
4. Ergil KV: Chinese medicine. In Micozzi MS, editor: *Fundamentals of complementary and integrative medicine*, ed 3, St. Louis, 2006, Elsevier, pp 375-417.
5. Sodhi V: Ayurveda: the science of life and mother of the healing arts. In Pizzorno JEJ, Murray MT, editors: *Textbook of natural medicine*, St. Louis, 2006, Churchill Livingstone, pp 317-327.
6. Zysk KG, Tetlow G: Traditional ayurveda. In Micozzi MS, editor: *Fundamentals of complementary and integrative medicine*, ed 3, St. Louis, 2006, Elsevier, pp 494-507.
7. Voss RW, et al: Native American healing. In Micozzi MS, editor: *Fundamentals of complementary and integrative medicine*, ed 3, St. Louis, 2006, Elsevier, pp 536-550.
8. Murray MT, Pizzorno JEJ. Nutritional Medicine. In Pizzorno JEJ, Murray MT, editors: *Textbook of natural medicine*, St. Louis, 2006, Churchill Livingstone, pp. 461-475.
9. Martinez RM: Manipulation. In Pizzorno JEJ, Murray MT, editors: *Textbook of natural medicine*, St. Louis, 2006, Churchill Livingstone, pp 417-431.
10. Nolting MH: Acupuncture. In Pizzorno JEJ, Murray MT, editors: *Textbook of natural medicine*, St. Louis, Churchill Livingstone, 2006, pp 309-317.
11. Wells RE, et al: Complementary and alternative medicine use among US adults with common neurological conditions, *J Neurol* 257:1822-1831, 2010.
12. Su D, Li L: Trends in the use of complementary and alternative medicine in the United States: 2002-2007, *J Health Care Poor Underserved* 22:296-310, 2011.
13. Bell RM: A review of complementary and alternative medicine practices among cancer survivors, *Clin J Oncol Nurs* 14:365-370, 2010.
14. Adams P, et al: Humor. In Micozzi MS, editor: *Fundamentals of complementary and integrative medicine*, ed 3, St. Louis, Elsevier, 2006, pp 351-371.
15. Barnes J: Consumer and pharmacist perspectives. In Ernst E, editor: *Herbal medicine: a concise overview for professionals*, Oxford, 2000, Butterworth & Heinemann, pp 19-33.
16. Carlston M: Homeopathy. In Micozzi MS, editor: *Fundamentals of complementary and integrative medicine*, ed 3, St. Louis, 2006, Elsevier, pp 95-110.
17. Hoffman CJ: Aromatherapy. In Micozzi MS, editor: *Fundamentals of complementary and integrative medicine*, ed 3, St. Louis, 2006, Elsevier, pp 207-220.
18. Micozzi MS, Meserole L: Herbal medicine. In Micozzi MS, editor: *Fundamentals of complementary and integrative medicine*, ed 3, St. Louis, 2006, Elsevier, pp 164-180.
19. Sierpina V, Gerik S: Common herbs for integrative care. In Micozzi MS, editor: *Fundamentals of complementary and integrative medicine*, ed 3, St. Louis, 2006, Elsevier, pp 181-206.
20. Ernst E: Homeopathy: what does the "best" evidence tell us? *Med J Aust* 192:458-460, 2010.
21. Eldin S, Dunford A: *Herbal medicine in primary care*, Oxford, 1999, Butterworth & Heinemann.
22. Lange A: Homeopathy. In Pizzorno JEJ, Murray MT, editors: *Textbook of natural medicine*, St. Louis, 2006, Churchill Livingstone, pp 387-401.
23. Murray MT, Pizzorno JEJ: Botanical medicine—a modern perspective. In Pizzorno JEJ, Murray MT, editors: *Textbook of natural medicine*, St. Louis, 2006, Churchill Livingstone, pp 327-339.
24. Eisenberg DM, et al: Trends in alternative medicine use in the United States, *JAMA* 280:1569-1575, 1998.
25. Clark CE, et al: Herbal interventions for chronic asthma in adults and children: a systematic review and meta-analysis, *Prim Care Respir J* 19:307-314, 2010.
26. Cohen PA, Ernst E: Safety of herbal supplements: a guide for cardiologists, *Cardiovasc Ther* 28:246-253, 2010.
27. Olaku O, White JD: Herbal therapy use by cancer patients: a literature review on case reports, *Eur J Cancer* 47:508-514, 2011.
28. Tabet N, Khan R, Idle H: Vitamin and herbal extracts use in patients diagnosed with dementia: What do health professionals know and think? *Aging Ment Health* 15:267-271, 2011.

29. Nahas R, Balla A: Complementary and alternative medicine for prevention and treatment of the common cold, *Can Fam Physician* 57:31-36, 2011.
30. Gyorik SA, Brutsche MH: Complementary and alternative medicine for bronchial asthma: is there new evidence? *Curr Opin Pulm Med* 10:37-43, 2004.
31. Rathbone J, et al: Chinese herbal medicine for schizophrenia, *Cochrane Database Syst Rev* 4:CD003444, 2005.
32. Sun A, et al: The Chinese herbal medicine Tien-Hsien liquid inhibits cell growth and induces apoptosis in a wide variety of human cancer cells, *J Altern Complement Med* 11:245-256, 2005.
33. Treasure J: Herbal medicine and cancer: an introductory overview, *Semin Oncol Nurs* 21:177-183, 2005.
34. Wen MC, et al: Efficacy and tolerability of anti-asthma herbal medicine intervention in adult patients with moderate-severe allergic asthma, *J Allergy Clin Immunol* 116:517-524, 2005.
35. Zhang ZJ, et al: Adjunctive herbal medicine with carbamazepine for bipolar disorders: a double-blind, randomized, placebo-controlled study, *J Psychiatr Res* 41:360-369, 2007.
36. Zick SM, Blume A, Aaronson KD: The prevalence and pattern of complementary and alternative supplement use in individuals with chronic heart failure, *J Card Fail* 11:586-589, 2005.
37. Ernst E: Herbal medicine in the treatment of rheumatic diseases, *Rheum Dis Clin North Am* 37:95-102, 2010.
38. Zuzak TJ, et al: Medicinal systems of complementary and alternative medicine: a cross-sectional survey at a pediatric emergency department, *J Altern Complement Med* 16:473-479, 2010.
39. Herman PM, Craig BM, Caspi O: Is complementary and alternative medicine (CAM) cost-effective? A systematic review, *BMC Complement Altern Med* 5:11, 2005.
40. Klepser TB, et al: Assessment of patients' perceptions and beliefs regarding herbal therapies. *Pharmacotherapy* 20:83-87, 2000.
41. Pharand C, et al: Use of OTC and herbal products in patients with cardiovascular disease, *Ann Pharmacother* 37:899-904, 2003.
42. Abebe W, Herman W, Konzelman J: Herbal supplement use among adult dental patients in a USA dental school clinic: prevalence, patient demographics and clinical implications, *Oral Surg Oral Med Oral Path Oral Radiol Endod* 111:320-325, 2011.
43. Ernst E, Pittler MH: Herbal medicine, *Med Clin North Am* 86:149-161, 2002.
44. Micozzi MS: Translation from conventional medicine. In Micozzi MS, editor: *Fundamentals of complementary and integrative medicine*, ed 3, St. Louis, 2006, Elsevier, pp 9-17.
45. Ernst E, Pittler MH: *Ginkgo biloba* for dementia: a systematic review of double-blind placebo-controlled trials, *Clin Drug Invest* 17:301-308, 1999.
46. Pittler MH, Ernst E: *Ginkgo biloba* extract for the treatment of intermittent claudication: a meta-analysis of randomized trials, *Am J Med* 108:226-281, 2000.
47. Vogler BK, Pittler MH, Ernst E: The efficacy of ginseng: a systematic review of randomised clinical trials, *Eur J Clin Pharmacol* 55:567-575, 1999.
48. Ernst E: The efficacy of herbal medicine—an overview, *Fundam Clin Pharmacol* 19:405-409, 2005.
49. Buderiri D, Li Won Po D, Dornan JC: Is evening primrose oil of value in the treatment of premenstrual syndrome? *Controlled Clin Trials* 17:60-68, 1996.
50. Stevinson C, Pittler MH, Ernst E: Garlic for treating hypercholesterolemia, *Ann Intern Med* 133:420-429, 2000.
51. Halkes SBA: Safety issues in phytotherapy. In Ernst E, editor: *Herbal medicine: a concise overview for professionals*, Oxford, 2000, Butterworth & Heinemann, pp 82-100.
52. Conover EA: Herbal agents and over-the-counter medications in pregnancy. *Best Pract Res Clin Endocrinol Metab* 17:237-251, 2003.
53. MD Consult: Complementary and alternative medicine, Elsevier, available at http://home.mdconsult.com/clinicaltours, accessed July, 2004, 2003.
54. Boullata JI, McDonnell PJ, Oliva CD: Anaphylactic reaction to a dietary supplement containing willow bark, *Ann Pharmacother* 37:832-835, 2003.
55. Brazier NC, Levine MA: Drug-herb interaction among commonly used conventional medicines: a compendium for health care professionals, *Am J Ther* 10:163-169, 2003.
56. Markowitz JS, et al: Effect of St John's wort on drug metabolism by induction of cytochrome P450 3A4 enzyme, *JAMA* 290:1500-1504, 2003.
57. Markowitz JS, et al: Effects of garlic (*Allium sativum* L.) supplementation on cytochrome P450 2D6 and 3A4 activity in healthy volunteers, *Clin Pharmacol Ther* 74:170-177, 2003.
58. Bishop FL, Yardley L, Lewith GT: Why consumers maintain complementary and alternative medicine use: a qualitative study, *J Altern Complement Med* 16:175-182, 2010.
59. Hietala M, et al: Natural remedy use in a prospective cohort of breast cancer patients in southern Sweden, *Acta Oncol* 50:134-143, 2011.
60. Rausch SM, et al: Health behaviors among cancer survivors receiving screening mammography, *Am J Clin Oncol* Feb 2, 2011. [Epub ahead of print.]
61. Bishop FL, et al: Complementary medicine use by men with prostate cancer: a systematic review of prevalence studies, *Prostate Cancer Prostatic Dis* 14:1-13, 2011.
62. Yap KY, et al: An onco-informatics database for anticancer drug interactions with complementary and alternative medicines used in cancer treatment and supportive care: an overview of the OncoRx project, *Support Care Cancer* 18:883-891, 2010.
63. Amrutesh S: Dentistry and ayurveda, *Indian J Dent Res* 14:1-5, 2003.
64. Barolet R: Acupuncture in dentistry, *J Am Dent Assoc* 97:166-168, 1978.
65. Dougherty K, Touger-Decker R, O'Sullivan MJ: Personal and professional beliefs and practices regarding herbal medicine among the full time faculty of the Newark-based schools of the University of Medicine and Dentistry of New Jersey, *Integr Med* 2:57-64, 2000.
66. Ferraris S: Alternative dentistry, *Br Dent J* 173:156-157, 1992.
67. Goldstein BH: Unconventional dentistry: part V, professional issues, concerns and uses, *J Can Dent Assoc* 66:608-610, 2000.
68. Goldstein BH: Unconventional dentistry: part III, legal and regulatory issues, *J Can Dent Assoc* 66:503-506, 2000.
69. Goldstein BH: Unconventional dentistry: part II, practitioners and patients, *J Can Dent Assoc* 66:381-383, 2000.
70. Goldstein BH: Unconventional dentistry: part I, introduction, *J Can Dent Assoc* 66:323-326, 2000.
71. Goldstein BH, Epstein JB: Unconventional dentistry: part IV, unconventional dental practices and products, *J Can Dent Assoc* 66:564-568, 2000.
72. Johnson NW: Complementary medicine in dentistry, *Oral Dis* 4:69, 1998.
73. McComb D: Unconventional dentistry, *J Can Dent Assoc* 67:190, 2001.
74. Mulrooney R: Unconventional dentistry, *J Can Dent Assoc* 67:10-11, 2001.
75. Oepen I: A critical evaluation of unconventional diagnostic and therapeutic methods in dentistry, *Fortschr Kieferorthop* 53:239-246, 1992.

76. Penzer V, Matsumoto K: Neuroanatomical and neurophysiological basis for use of acupuncture in dentistry, *J Mass Dent Soc* 36:83-84, 1987.
77. Pistorius A, et al: Efficacy of subgingival irrigation using herbal extracts on gingival inflammation, *J Periodontol* 74:616-622, 2003.
78. Romano JAJ: Acupuncture and dentistry, *J Bergen Cty Dent Soc* 44:7-9, 1978.
79. Rosted P: Introduction to acupuncture in dentistry, *Br Dent J* 189:136-140, 2000.
80. Rosted P: Use of acupuncture in dentistry, *Aust Dent J* 43:437, 1998.
81. Rosted P: The use of acupuncture in dentistry: a review of the scientific validity of published papers, *Oral Dis* 4:100-104, 1998.
82. Sastravaha G, et al: Adjunctive periodontal treatment with *Centella asiatica* and *Punica granatum* extracts: a preliminary study, *J Int Acad Periodontol* 5:106-115, 2003.
83. Thayer T: Acupuncture in dentistry, *SAAD Dig* 18:3-8, 2001.
84. Tobey HS: What dentists need to know about CADM: complementary and alternative dentistry and medicine, *J N J Dent Assoc* 67:21-24, 1996.
85. Vachiramon A, Wang WC, Vachiramon T: The use of acupuncture in implant dentistry, *Implant Dent* 13:58-64, 2004.
86. Wilcox CE: The practical uses of acupuncture in dentistry, *CDS Rev* 75:25-27, 1982.
87. Braga FP, et al: The effect of acupuncture on salivary flow rates in patients with radiation-induced xerostomia, *Minerva Stomatol* 57:343-348, 2008.
88. Cho SH, Whang WW: Acupuncture for temporomandibular disorders: a systematic review, *J Orofac Pain* 24:152-162, 2010.
89. Rosted P, et al: Acupuncture in the management of anxiety related to dental treatment: a case series, *Acupunct Med* 28:3-5, 2010.
90. Sari E, Sari T: The role of acupuncture in the treatment of orthodontic patients with a gagging reflex: a pilot study, *Br Dent J* 208:E19, 2010.
91. Shaw D: Unethical aspects of homeopathic dentistry, *Br Dent J* 209:493-496, 2011.
92. Ang-Lee MK, Moss J, Yuan CS: Herbal medicines and perioperative care, *JAMA* 286:208-216, 2001.
93. Chan CW, et al: Oral complications in Chinese cancer patients undergoing chemotherapy, *Support Care Cancer* 11:48-55, 2003.
94. Miller FG, et al: Ethical issues concerning research in complementary and alternative medicine, *JAMA* 291:599-604, 2004.

INDEX

Page numbers followed by "f" indicate figures, "t" indicate tables, and "b" indicate boxes.